Procedural Dermatology

EDITORS

MARC R. AVRAM, MD
Clinical Professor of Dermatology
Weill Cornell Medical School
New York, New York
Private Practice
New York, New York

MATHEW M. AVRAM, MD, JD
Director, MGH Dermatology Laser & Cosmetic Center, Massachusetts General Hospital
Faculty Director for Dermatology Laser and Cosmetic Training, Harvard Medical School
Assistant Professor of Dermatology, Harvard Medical School Affiliate Faculty, Wellman Center for Photomedicine
Boston, Massachusetts

DÉSIRÉE RATNER, MD
Director of Comprehensive Skin Cancer Program
Continuum Cancer Centers of New York (CCCNY)
Director, Dermatologic Surgery, Department of Dermatology
Mount Sinai Beth Israel Medical Center and St. Luke's and Roosevelt Hospitals
New York, New York

Mc Graw Hill Education

New York Chicago San Francisco Athens London Madrid Mexico City
New Delhi San Juan Singapore Sydney Toronto

Procedural Dermatology

1 2 3 4 5 6 7 8 9 9 CTP/CTP 18 17 16 15 14

ISBN 978-0-07-179506-7
MHID 0-07-179506-5

This book was set in Warnock Pro by Aptara, Inc.
The editors were Anne M. Sydor and Christie Naglieri.
The production supervisor was Catherine Saggese.
Project Management was provided by Amit Kashyap at Aptara, Inc.
China Translation & Printing Services, Inc. was printer and binder.

This book is printed on acid-free paper.

Library of Congress Cataloging-in-Publication Data

Procedural dermatology / edited by Marc R. Avram, Mathew Avram, Desiree Ratner.
p. ; cm.
Includes bibliographical references.
ISBN 978-0-07-179506-7 (hardcover : alk. paper) – ISBN 0-07-179506-5 (hardcover : alk. paper)
I. Avram, Marc R., editor. II. Avram, Mathew M., editor. III. Ratner, Desiree, editor.
[DNLM: 1. Dermatologic Surgical Procedures–methods. 2. Cosmetic Techniques. 3. Esthetics. WR 670]
RL71
616.5–dc23

2014016140

Marc R. Avram, MD

I would like to dedicate this book to my loving parents Morrell and Maria Avram. They have always given me and my family unconditional support and love. Thank you!

To my wife Robin for all of her love and being my best friend. To my sons Robert and Jacob, thank you for always bringing joy, love, and wonder to my life. I am very proud of you both.

Mathew M. Avram, MD, JD

I would like to dedicate this textbook to my parents, Morrell and Maria Avram, who have provided me with their love and support my entire life. To my beautiful wife, Alison. Thank you for your love, understanding and support. To my wonderful children Rachel, Alexander and Noah. Thank you for inspiring me with your love, joy and accomplishments.

Désirée Ratner, MD

To my parents, Marion and Paul Ratner, for always being there, to my children, Xanthe and Evan Thomas, for their love and support, and to Paul Heller, for his kindness, love, and understanding.

CONTENTS

CONTRIBUTORS

Sumaira Z. Aasi, MD
Dermatologic Surgery
Stanford Department of Dermatology
Redwood City, California

Chris G. Adigun, MD
Clinical Instructor of Dermatology
Ronald O. Perelman Department of Dermatology
New York University School of Medicine
New York, New York

John G. Albertini, MD
Vice President and Laboratory Director
The Skin Surgery Center
Winston Salem, North Carolina

Salman Alsaad, MD
Division of Mohs Surgery and Procedural Dermatology
Scripps Clinic Torrey Pines
La Jolla, California

Snehal Amin, MD
Surgical Director
Manhattan Dermatology and Cosmetic Surgery
Clinical Assistant Professor of Dermatology
Weill Cornell Medical College
Attending, Department of Dermatology
New York Presbyterian Hospital
New York, New York

Christopher J. Arpey, MD
Mayo Clinic, Department of Dermatology
Rochester, Minnesota

Mathew M. Avram, MD, JD
Director, MGH Dermatology Laser and Cosmetic Center, Massachusetts General Hospital
Faculty Director for Dermatology Laser and Cosmetic Training, Harvard Medical School
Assistant Professor of Dermatology, Harvard Medical School Affiliate Faculty, Wellman Center for Photomedicine
Boston, Massachusetts

Marc R. Avram, MD
Clinical Professor of Dermatology
Weill Cornell Medical School
New York, New York
Private Practice
New York, New York

Karen L. Beasley, MD
Clinical Assistant Professor of Dermatology
University of Maryland School of Medicine
The Maryland Laser Skin and Vein Institute
Baltimore, Maryland

Paul X. Benedetto, MD
Procedural Dermatology Fellow, Department of Dermatology
Dermatology and Plastic Surgery Institute
Cleveland Clinic Foundation
Cleveland, Ohio

Jeremy Bordeaux, MD, MPH
Assistant Professor, Director of Dermatologic Surgery
Department of Dermatology
University Hospitals
Case Medical Center
Case Western Reserve University
Cleveland, Ohio

Liza Braun, BA
Department of Dermatology and Cutaneous Surgery
University of Miami Miller School of Medicine
Miami, Florida

Jerry D. Brewer, MD
Division of Dermatologic Surgery
Department of Dermatology
Mayo Clinic College of Medicine
Rochester, Minnesota

Neil Brody, MD, PhD
Department of Dermatology
State University of New York Downstate Medical Center
Brooklyn, New York

Kimberly J. Butterwick, MD
Private Practice
San Diego, California

Erik S. Cabral, MD
Bennett Surgical Center
Santa Monica, California

Valerie D. Callender, MD
Callender Dermatology and Cosmetic Center
Glenn Dale, Maryland

John A. Carucci, MD, PhD
Associate Professor; Chief, Mohs Micrographic and Dermatologic Surgery
Director, Procedural Dermatology Fellowship Training Program
Director of Dermatologic Surgery, Ronald O. Perelman Department of Dermatology
New York University School of Medicine
New York, New York

Anna Chacon, MD
Post-Doctoral Clinical Research Fellow
Sylvester Comprehensive Cancer Center
Mohs/Laser Unit
Miami, Florida

Yoon-Soo Cindy Bae, MD
Department of Dermatology
Boston University Medical Center
Boston, Massachusetts

Joel L. Cohen, MD
AboutSkin Dermatology and DermSurgery
Englewood, Colorado

Karen L. Connolly, MD
Henry Ford Hospital Department of Dermatology
Detroit, Michigan

Nicholas B. Countryman, MD, MBA
The Laser and Skin Surgery Center of Indiana
St. Vincent Carmel Hospital, Carmel, Indiana
Volunteer Assistant Professor of Clinical Dermatology
Indiana University School of Medicine
Indianapolis, Indiana

Milène K. Crispin, MD
Dermatologic Surgery
Stanford Department of Dermatology
Redwood City, California

Clara Curiel-Lewandrowski, MD
Associate Professor, University of Arizona
Director, Pigmented Lesion and Cutaneous Oncology Clinic
Arizona Cancer Center and Section of Dermatology
Tucson, Arizona

Daniel A. Davis, MD
Departments of Dermatology and Pathology
University of Arkansas for Medical Science
Little Rock, Arkansas

Zoe Diana Draelos, MD
Consulting Professor
Department of Dermatology
Duke University School of Medicine
Durham, North Carolina

Jason Emer, MD
University of California at San Francisco
Dermatologic Surgery and Laser Center
San Francisco, California

Rachel Epstein, DO
Loma Linda University
Department of Dermatology
Loma Linda, California

Tarek M. Fakhouri, MD
Surgical Dermatology Group
Birmingham, Alabama

Richard E. Fitzpatrick, MD
Private Practice, Cosmetic Laser Dermatology
Volunteer Clinical Professor
University of California San Diego
San Diego, California

Katlein Franca, MD, MSc
Post-Doctoral Research Associate
Sylvester Comprehensive Cancer Center
Mohs/Laser Unit
Miami, Florida

Daniel P. Friedmann, MD
Private Practice
Westlake Dermatology Clinical Research Center
Austin, Texas

Nima M. Gharavi, MD, PhD
Department of Medicine, Division of Dermatology
University of California
Los Angeles, California

Charles H. Greenbaum, MD
Emeritus Clinical Professor of Dermatology
Thomas Jefferson University School of Medicine
Philadelphia, Pennsylvania

Joshua M. Greenbaum
Vanderbilt University
Nashville, Tennessee

Steven S. Greenbaum, MD
Director of Skin and Laser Surgery Center of Pennsylvania
Clinical Professor of Dermatology Drexel University School of Medicine
Clinical Associate Professor of Head and Neck Surgery Thomas Jefferson
University School of Medicine
Philadelphia, Pennsylvania

Hugh T. Greenway, MD
Division of Mohs Surgery and Procedural Dermatology
Scripps Clinic Torrey Pines
La Jolla, California

Michael H. Gold, MD
Medical Director
Gold Skin Care Center
Advanced Aesthetics Medical Spa
Tennessee Clinical Research Center
The Laser and Rejuvenation Center
Clinical Assistant Professor
Vanderbilt University School of Medicine, Department of Dermatology
Vanderbilt University School of Nursing
Nashville, Tennessee
Visiting Professor of Dermatology
Huashan Hospital, Fudan University
Shanghai, China
Hospital of China Medical University
Shenyang, China
Visiting Professor of Plastic Surgery
First People's Hospital of Foshan
Guangzhou, China

David J. Goldberg, MD
Skin Laser and Surgery Specialists
Department of Dermatology
Mount Sinai School of Medicine
New York, New York

Mitchel P. Goldman, MD
Private Practice, Cosmetic Laser Dermatology
Volunteer Clinical Professor
University of California
San Diego, California

Merete Haedersdal, MD, PhD
Bispebjerg University Hospital
Department of Dermatology
Copenhagen, Denmark

C. William Hanke, MD, MPH, FACP
The Laser and Skin Surgery Center of Indiana, St. Vincent Hospital
Carmel, Indiana
Visiting Professor of Dermatology
University of Iowa-Carver College of Medicine
Iowa City, Iowa
Clinical Professor of Otolaryngology-Head and Neck Surgery
Indiana University School of Medicine
Indianapolis, Indiana

Christopher B. Harmon, MD
Surgical Dermatology Group
Birmingham, Alabama

Jill Henley, BA
Midwestern University
College of Osteopathic Medicine
Scottsdale, Arizona

Jenny C. Hu, MD, MPH
Division of Dermatology
David Geffen School of Medicine University of California
Los Angeles, California

Andrea M. Hui, MD
Department of Dermatology
State University of New York Downstate Medical Center
Brooklyn, New York

Mussarrat Hussain, MD, MS
Manhattan Dermatology and Cosmetic Surgery
New York, New York

Omar A. Ibrahimi, MD, PhD
Director, Connecticut Skin Institute
Stamford, Connecticut
Visiting Assistant Professor of Dermatology
Massachusetts General Hospital
Harvard Medical School
Boston, Massachusetts

H. Ray Jalian, MD
Clinical Instructor
Division of Dermatology
University of California, Los Angeles
Visiting Scientist
Wellman Center for Photomedicine
Massachusetts General Hospital
Santa Monica, California

Nathaniel Jellinek, MD
Clinical Assistant Professor of Dermatology
Brown University Department of Dermatology
East Greenwich, Rhode Island

Sasha Jenkins, MD, MPH
Emory Department of Dermatology
Atlanta, Georgia

Hillary Johnson-Jahangir, MD, PhD
Assistant Professor
Director of Dermatologic Surgery
Weill Cornell Medical College
Department of Dermatology
New York, New York

Elizabeth K. Jones, BS
Jefferson Medical College
Philadelphia, Pennsylvania

Aaron K. Joseph, MD
Skin and Laser Surgery Associates
Pasadena, Texas

Kristen M. Kelly, MD
Department of Dermatology
Beckman Laser Institute and Medical Clinic
University of California
Irvine, California

Suzanne L. Kilmer, MD
Founding Director
Laser and Skin Surgery Center of Northern California
Clinical Associate Professor of dermatology
University of California
Sacramento, California

Caroline C. Kim, MD
Assistant Professor, Department of Dermatology, Harvard Medical School
Director, Pigmented Lesion Clinic
Associate Director, Cutaneous Oncology Program, Department of Dermatology
Beth Israel Deaconess Medical Center
Boston, Massachusetts

Jenny Kim, MD, PhD
Division of Dermatology
David Geffen School of Medicine University of California
Los Angeles, California

Robert S. Kirsner, MD, PhD
Department of Dermatology and Cutaneous Surgery
University of Miami Miller School of Medicine
Miami, Florida

Nils Krueger, PhD
Chief Operating Officer
Rosenpark Research
Wilhelminenstrasse
Darmstadt, Germany

Gary P. Lask, MD
Department of Medicine, Division of Dermatology
University of California
Los Angeles, California

Jennifer Ledon, BSc
Clinical Research Fellow
Sylvester Comprehensive Cancer Center
Mohs/Laser Unit
Miami, Florida

Erica H. Lee, MD
Assistant Attending Physician
Memorial Sloan-Kettering Cancer Center
Instructor, Weill Medical College of Cornell University
New York, New York

Henry Hin Lee Chan, MBBS, MD, PhD, FRCP, FHKCP, FHKAM
Honorary Clinical Professor
Division of Dermatology, Department of Medicine
Li Ka Shing Faculty of Medicine
The University of Hong Kong
Hong Kong, China
Visiting Scientist, Wellman Center for Photomedicine
Massachusetts General Hospital
Harvard Medical School
Boston, Massachusetts

Catherine Lee Tran, MD
Procedural Dermatology Fellow
Cutaneous Surgery and Oncology Unit
Department of Dermatology, Johns Hopkins Medical Center
Baltimore, Maryland

Wilfred A. Lumbang, MD
Assistant Professor of Medicine (Dermatology)
Division of Dermatology
Department of Medicine
Vanderbilt University Medical Center
Nashville, Tennessee

Ian A. Maher, MD
Assistant Professor, Department of Dermatology
Virginia Commonwealth University
Richmond, Virginia

Mary E. Maloney, MD
Division of Dermatology
University of Massachusetts Medical School
Worcester, Massachusetts

Margaret Mann, MD
Assistant Professor, Department of Dermatology
Director of Aesthetic Dermatology
University Hospitals
Case Medical Center
Case Western Reserve University
Cleveland, Ohio

Jo Martin, MD
Johns Hopkins Department of Dermatology
Baltimore, Maryland

Peter L. Mattei, MD
Johns Hopkins Department of Dermatology
Baltimore, Maryland

Riley McLean, MD
Division of Dermatology
University of Massachusetts Medical School
Worcester, Massachusetts

Bichchau M. Nguyen, MD
Procedural Dermatology Fellow
Brigham and Women's Faulkner Hospital
Jamaica Plain, Massachusetts

Christopher J. Miller, MD
Hospital of the University of Pennsylvania
Perelman Center for Advanced Medicine
Division of Dermatologic Surgery and Cutaneous Oncology
Philadelphia, Pennsylvania

Lee M. Miller, MD
Division of Mohs Surgery and Procedural Dermatology
Scripps Clinic Torrey Pines
La Jolla, California

Kira Minkis, MD, PhD
Assistant Professor, Director of Mohs and Dermatologic Surgery
Weill Cornell Medical College Department of Dermatology
New York, New York

Vineet Mishra, MD
Division of Mohs Surgery and Procedural Dermatology
Scripps Clinic Torrey Pines
La Jolla, California

Summer D. Moon, BS
Fourth Year Medical Student
Lake Erie College of Osteopathic Medicine
Saint Petersburg, Florida

Kishwer S. Nehal, MD
Associate Attending Physician
Memorial Sloan-Kettering Cancer Center
Associate Professor of Dermatology
Weill Medical College of Cornell University
New York, New York

Andrew A. Nelson, MD
Assistant Clinical Professor of Dermatology
Tufts University School of Medicine
Boston, Massachusetts
Nelson Dermatology
Saint Petersburg, Florida

Tanya Nino, MD
Loma Linda University
Department of Dermatology
Loma Linda, California

Katherine A. Nolan, BA
Mount Sinai School of Medicine
New York, New York

Keyvan Nouri, MD
Professor of Dermatology, Ophthalmology and Otolaryngology
Louis C. Skinner, Jr. M.D. Endowed Chair in Dermatology
University of Miami
Miami, Florida

Arisa E. Ortiz, MD
Assistant Clinical Professor
University of California
San Diego, California

David M. Ozog, MD
Henry Ford Hospital Department of Dermatology
Detroit, Michigan

June J. Park, BS
University of Illinois College of Medicine
Chicago, Illinois

Zena Pinnella, MD
Baylor College of Medicine
Fourth-Year Medical Student
Houston, Texas

Claire Marie Reyes-Habito, MD
Los Banos Doctors Hospital and Medical Center
Laguna, Philippines

Kerri Robbins, MD
Baylor College of Medicine
Dermatology Resident
Houston, Texas

Nicole E. Rogers, MD
Assistant Clinical Professor Dermatology
Tulane University School of Medicine
Private Practice
Metairie, Louisiana

Anthony Rossi, MD
Procedural Dermatology Fellow
Memorial-Sloan Kettering Cancer Center
Weill Medical College of Cornell University
New York, New York

James D. Russell, MD
Resident, Department of Dermatology
Virginia Commonwealth University
Richmond, Virginia

Robyn Sackeyfio, MD
Plastic Surgery Resident
New York Presbyterian Hospital
New York, New York

Neil S. Sadick, MD
Clinical Professor
Weill Cornell Medical College
Cornell University
New York, New York

Jessica Savas, BSc
Clinical Research Fellow
Sylvester Comprehensive Cancer Center
Mohs/Laser Unit
Miami, Florida

Meghan Scharf, MD
Dermatology Resident
Division of Dermatology
Department of Medicine
Vanderbilt University Medical Center
Nashville, Tennessee

Chrysalyne D. Schmults, MD, MSCE
Assistant Professor of Dermatology, Harvard Medical School
Director, Brigham and Women's Mohs and Dermatologic Surgery Center
Director, Dana Farber High-Risk Skin Cancer Clinic
Jamaica Plain, Massachusetts

Roberta Sengelmann, MD
Associate Clinical Professor
Irvine Department of Dermatology University of California
(President and Owner) Santa Barbara Skin Institute
Santa Barbara, California

Kathryn Serowka, MD
Department of Dermatology
University of California
Irvine, California

Thuzar Shin, MD
Resident Department of Dermatology
University Hospitals
Case Medical Center
Case Western Reserve University
Cleveland, Ohio

Daniel M. Siegel, MD
Department of Dermatology
State University of New York Downstate Medical Center
Brooklyn, New York

Robert Silich, MD
Assistant Clinical Professor of Surgery
New York Presbyterian Hospital
New York, New York

Meena Singh, MD
Private Practice
Kansas City, Missouri

Andrea Smith, MD
Loma Linda University
Department of Dermatology
Loma Linda, California

Maren Cotes, MD
Emory Department of Dermatology
Atlanta, Georgia

James M. Spencer, MD, MS
Professor of Clinical Dermatology
Mount Sinai School of Medicine, New York
Carillon Outpatient Center
Saint Petersburg, Florida

Henry M. Spinelli, MD
Clinical Professor of Surgery
Clinical Professor of Neurological Surgery
New York Presbyterian Hospital
New York, New York

Thomas Stasko, MD
Professor and Chair of Dermatology
University of Oklahoma Medical Center
Oklahoma City, Oklahoma

Joseph F. Sobanko, MD
Hospital of the University of Pennsylvania
Perelman Center for Advanced Medicine
Division of Dermatologic Surgery and Cutaneous Oncology
Philadelphia, Pennsylvania

Seaver L. Soon, MD
Division of Dermatology and Dermatologic Surgery
Scripps Clinic
La Jolla, California

Susan C. Taylor, MD
Society Hill Dermatology
Philadelphia, Pennsylvania

Katrine Togsverd-Bo, MD, PhD
Bispebjerg University Hospital
Department of Dermatology
Copenhagen, Denmark

Abel Torres, MD
Loma Linda University
Department of Dermatology
Loma Linda, California

Mark M. Tran, MD
Dermatopathology Fellow
Stanford Dermatopathology Service
Department of Pathology Stanford University Medical Center
Stanford, California

Joshua W. Trufant, MD
Dermatology Resident, Ronald O. Perelman Department of Dermatology
New York University School of Medicine
New York, New York

Hensin Tsao, MD, PhD
Massachusetts General Hospital
Department of Dermatology and Wellman Center for Photomedicine
Boston, Massachusetts

Allison T. Vidimos, MD, RPh
Chairman, Department of Dermatology
Vice-Chairman, Dermatology and Plastic Surgery Institute
Cleveland Clinic Foundation
Cleveland, Ohio

Heidi A. Waldorf, MD
Associate Clinical Professor of Dermatology
Icahn School of Medicine
Director of Laser and Cosmetic Dermatology
Mount Sinai Medical Center
New York, New York
Mount SinaiWaldorf Dermatology and Laser Associates, PC
Nanuet, New York

Timothy S. Wang, MD
Associate Professor of Dermatology
Director, Cutaneous Surgery and Oncology Unit
Department of Dermatology
Johns Hopkins Medical Center
Baltimore, Maryland

Molly Wanner, MD
Harvard Medical School and Department of Dermatology
Massachusetts General Hospital
Boston, Massachusetts

Robert A. Weiss, MD
Clinical Associate Professor of Dermatology
University of Maryland School of Medicine
Director, The Maryland Laser Skin and Vein Institute
Baltimore, Maryland

Michael M. Wolz, BMBCh, JD
Mayo Clinic, Department of Dermatology
Rochester, Minnesota

Samantha Yee Nam Shek, MBBS, DipClinDerm
Honorary Research Associate
Division of Dermatology, Department of Medicine
Li Ka Shing Faculty of Medicine
The University of Hong Kong
Hong Kong, China

Cherie M. Young, MD
Callender Dermatology and Cosmetic Center
Glenn Dale, Maryland

Fiona Zwald, MD, MRCP
Emory Department of Dermatology
Emory Transplant Dermatology Clinic
Mohs Micrographic surgery
Atlanta, Georgia

PREFACE

Dermatologic surgery is a discipline that has evolved dramatically from the mid-20th century to the present day. Dermabrasion, chemical peels, hair transplantation, Mohs chemosurgery, and excisional surgery were performed principally by a select group of NYU dermatologists in the 1950s, while cutaneous laser surgery was first performed at the University of Cincinnati in the 1960s. Over the years, the number of dermatologists performing these procedures increased significantly. Our knowledge of basic science has also advanced, as has our clinical expertise in wound healing and postoperative care. Dermatologic surgeons have become experts in Mohs micrographic surgery and defect reconstruction, while our cosmetic armamentarium has grown to include botulinum toxins, a variety of soft tissue fillers, sclerotherapy, ambulatory phlebectomy, nonablative and ablative lasers, fractional resurfacing, lasers for the treatment of tattoos, pigmented and vascular lesions, and liposuction. Standards of training, patient safety, informed consent, anesthesia and analgesia, preoperative evaluation, and office accreditation are now recognized to be of vital importance, and have become disciplines of their own. Now, decades after a small group of dermatologists founded the American Society for Dermatologic Surgery in 1970, surgical training has become a fundamental and required part of all dermatology residencies, while postgraduate fellowship training in procedural dermatology is an ACGME accredited subspecialty.

Developing knowledge and expertise in any field requires starting with the basics, and building upon them. To that end, we have organized this text into the following sections: surgical principles, surgical skills, skin tumors, aesthetic and laser procedures, and aesthetic problems. We have endeavored to develop a consistent format for each chapter, with high-quality photographic images and graphics to enhance the presentation of each topic. The reader may choose to progress sequentially through the book, or to focus individually on the topics of interest to them.

Our goal in developing this textbook was to compile the current, state of the art information concerning all aspects of procedural dermatology. The authors of this text are without exception leaders in their fields with a passion for teaching, and we feel fortunate to have enlisted them to assist us in this endeavor. Our hope is that this book will become a resource for all practitioners of dermatologic surgery, from the novice to the seasoned surgeon looking to refine his or her skills in a particular area. We hope you enjoy reading this book as much as we have enjoyed putting it together.

Marc R. Avram, MD
Mathew M. Avram, MD, JD
Désirée Ratner, MD
2014

ACKNOWLEDGMENTS

We extend our heartfelt thanks to the staff at McGraw Hill, most notably Christine Barcellona, Christie Naglieri, and Anne Sydor, for making this book possible and helping us see it through to completion.

SECTION 1

Surgical Principles

CHAPTER 1

Superficial Head and Neck Anatomy

Hugh T. Greenway, Vineet Mishra, Lee M. Miller, & Salman Alsaad

INTRODUCTION

Mastering surgical anatomy is crucial for the dermatologic surgeon, not only to obtain the best cosmetic outcome but also to avoid complications related to injury of underlying anatomic structures. Since a significant number of dermatologic surgeries are performed on the head and neck, the dermatologic surgeon ought to have full knowledge of the facial nerve and its branches, blood supply, sensory nerves, underlying musculature, and specialized structures such as the parotid duct. With a full understanding of the superficial anatomy of this complex region, the physician will have the confidence to perform a wide range of superficial surgical procedures while keeping possible risks and complications in mind.

NOSE

The external nose is shaped like a pear or pyramid with several key divisions: dorsum, tip, ala, and lateral sidewalls. The dorsum of the nose extends from the tip, the lowermost aspect of the nose, to the nasal root. In contrast to the dorsum of the nose where the skin is quite mobile, the skin overlying the tip of the nose is adherent to the underlying fibrous tissue and cartilage. The nasal bridge is the portion of the nose overlying the nasal bones. The lateral sides of the nose encompass the area from the nasal dorsum to the cheeks. The nasofacial sulcus, or margin of the nose, is the transition from the lateral aspects of the nose to the cheeks.[1]

The ala, a distinct cosmetic subunit, is demarcated from the lateral sidewalls of the nose by the alar crease and separated from the lip by the nasolabial crease. The root of the nose is the region of attachment of the nose to the glabella. The nares are the openings into the anterior nasal vestibules. They are divided by the nasal septum medially and bounded by the nasal alae laterally. The columella is the freely movable portion of the nasal septum (Fig. 1-1).[2]

The skeleton of the nose includes both bone and cartilage. The two nasal bones lie adjacent to the maxilla laterally and the frontal bone superiorly. There are also five major cartilages of the nose which provide the remainder of the nasal framework: two lateral cartilages, two greater alar cartilages, and the single septal cartilage. In the midline, the septal cartilage joins each of the lateral cartilages. The lateral aspect of the lateral cartilage articulates with the frontal process of the maxilla whereas the superior aspect of the lateral nasal cartilage articulates with the inferior aspect of the nasal bone. The greater alar cartilages are C-shaped. Each of the medial crura joins at the midline with the septal cartilage to form the nasal septum. The lateral crura articulate with the inferior aspects of the lateral nasal cartilages.[1]

There are several muscles associated with the nose: the nasalis, the depressor septi, the levator labii superioris alaeque nasi, and the procerus muscles. The transverse

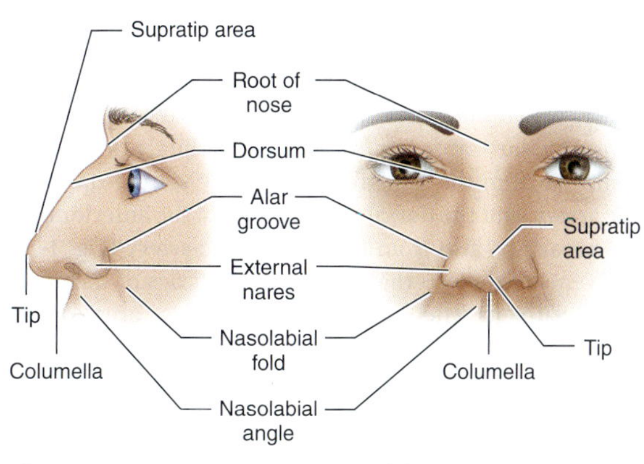

Figure 1-1 Cutaneous anatomy of the nose.

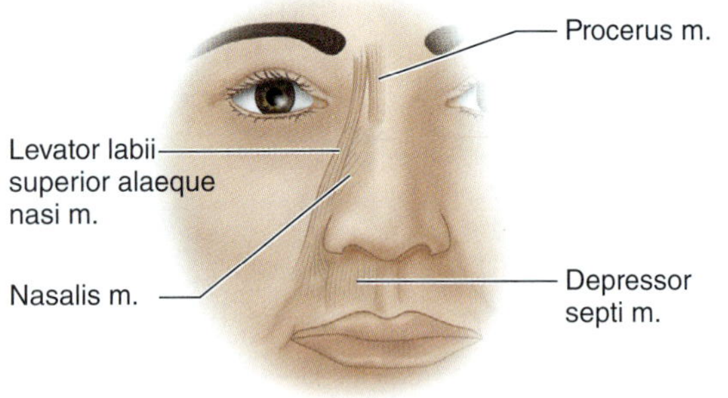

Figure 1-2 Musculature of the nose.

portion of the nasalis muscle originates from the body of the maxilla on each side and inserts into the aponeurosis that overlies the bridge of the nose. A small portion of the nasalis, the alar component, inserts into the lateral crus of the alar cartilage. Contraction of the transverse portion of the nasalis muscle compresses the nares; meanwhile, activation of the alar portion causes dilation of the nares. Innervation of the nasalis muscle occurs via the buccal branch of the facial nerve. The depressor septi muscle functions to narrow the nares. It originates from the incisive fossa of the maxilla and inserts into the columella and nasal septum. The buccal branches of the facial nerve also innervate this muscle.[3] The levator labii superioris alaeque nasi muscle originates from the frontal process of the maxilla and courses inferiorly with a portion of the muscle inserting into the ala before the main body inserts into the skin of the upper lip. The alar portion dilates the nares and is innervated by the buccal branches of the facial nerve. The procerus muscle arises from the nasal bones and inserts into the skin overlying the glabella. Contraction of this muscle leads to downward pulling of the skin while creating horizontal folds over the bridge of the nose. Unlike the other nasal muscles, the procerus is innervated by the temporal branch of the facial nerve (Fig. 1-2).[1]

Sensory innervation to the nose is provided by the terminal branches of the ophthalmic and maxillary divisions of the trigeminal nerve. The supra- and infratrochlear branches innervate the nasal root, bridge, and upper sidewall. The dorsal external nasal branch of the anterior ethmoidal nerve innervates the lower dorsum and nasal tip. The infraorbital nerve provides sensation to the lateral sidewall and ala whereas the depressor septi branch is responsible for the columella.[4]

The vasculature supply to the nose is quite robust. The arterial supply to the external nose primarily arises from the lateral nasal and septal branches of the superior labial artery, which emanates from the facial artery. There are also secondary branches from the infraorbital artery, nasal branches from the infratrochlear artery via the ophthalmic artery, and the dorsal nasal branch of the anterior ethmoidal artery, also from the ophthalmic artery (Fig. 1-3). The veins of the external nose are tributaries of the anterior facial vein. The nose lies in the "danger area" of the face given the open communication between the anterior facial vein and ophthalmic veins, which drain into the cavernous sinus.[1] The lymphatic drainage of the nose flows into the buccal nodes of the facial lymphatic chain and then subsequently into the submandibular nodes.[4]

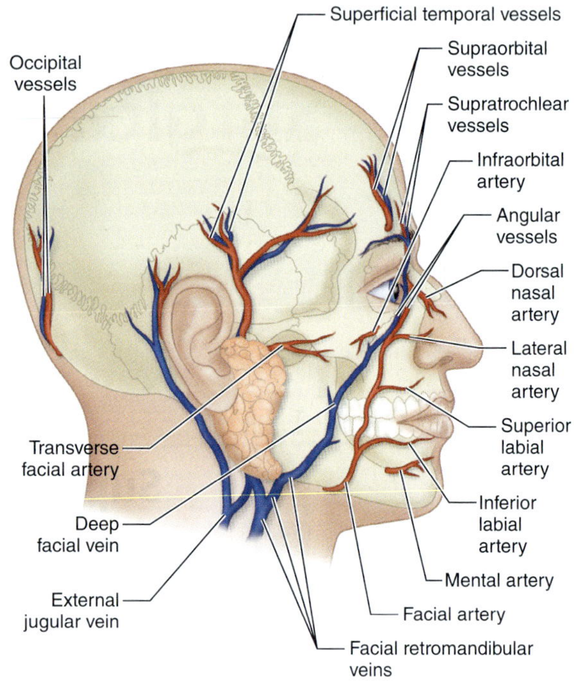

Figure 1-3 Vasculature of the face.

PERIORAL REGION

The labial area of the face is demarcated by the mental region inferiorly, the nose superiorly, and the buccal areas of the cheeks laterally. The lips are two structures defining the entrance to the mouth. The upper and lower lips are joined laterally at the labial commissures. The upper lip is separated from the cheek by the melolabial crease, which extends from the ala of the nose inferiorly and obliquely, and is divided into two halves by the philtrum. The philtrum is a depression in the central upper lip bounded by the two prominences (philtral ridges) laterally, the vermilion border of the upper lip inferiorly, and the nasal septum superiorly. The crossing of the muscle insertions within the superficial portion of the orbicularis oris muscle is hypothesized to lead to the formation of the philtrum.[2] Each lip also has a vermilion border, a region of transition from normal skin to modified epithelium without hair, sweat glands, and sebaceous glands. The junction of the vermilion border with the philtrum is known as "Cupid's bow."[1]

The oral musculature arises from different regions on the face. For purposes of simplification, these can be divided into four major groups: the muscles of the lower lip (depressors), the muscles of the upper lip (elevators), the buccinator, and the orbicularis oris. The muscles of the lower lip are comprised of the depressor anguli oris, the depressor labii inferioris, and the mentalis. The depressor anguli oris depresses the corners of the mouth. It arises from the anterolateral aspect of the body of the mandible and inserts into the skin and mucosa at the labial commissure (Fig. 1-4). Similarly, the depressor labii inferioris originates from the mandible deep to the depressor anguli oris muscle and inserts into the skin and mucosa of the lower lip, thereby depressing the lips. The mentalis originates

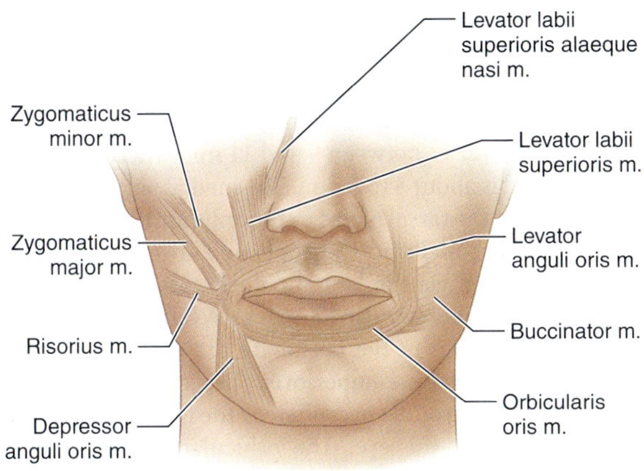

Figure 1-4 Musculature of the perioral area and medial cheek.

from the body of the mandible medial to the depressor labii inferioris and inserts into the skin overlying the tip of the chin. Upon contraction, it leads to protrusion of the lower lip and dimpling of the skin. These muscles are innervated by the marginal mandibular branch of the facial nerve with secondary innervation from the buccal branches of the facial nerve.[5]

The muscles of the upper lip consist of the risorius, zygomaticus major and minor, levator labii superioris, levator labii superioris alaeque nasi, and levator anguli oris muscles (Fig. 1-5). The risorius arises from the parotid fascia and inserts into the skin and mucosa at the corner of the mouth. This leads to pulling of the labial commissure laterally. The zygomaticus major muscle arises from the posterolateral aspect of the zygomatic bone; it inserts into the skin and mucosa of the lateral upper lip and elevates the labial commissure. The zygomaticus minor muscle arises medial to the zygomaticus major and inserts into the skin and mucosa of the upper lip, thus elevating the upper lip. The levator labii superioris originates from the maxilla just above the infraorbital foramen and inserts into the skin and mucosa of the medial upper lip, thereby elevating the upper lip. The levator labii superioris alaeque nasi arises from the medial origin from the orbit, gives off fibers to the nasal ala, and proceeds inferiorly to insert into the skin and mucosa of the medial aspect of the upper lip. This muscle not only elevates the upper lip but also dilates the

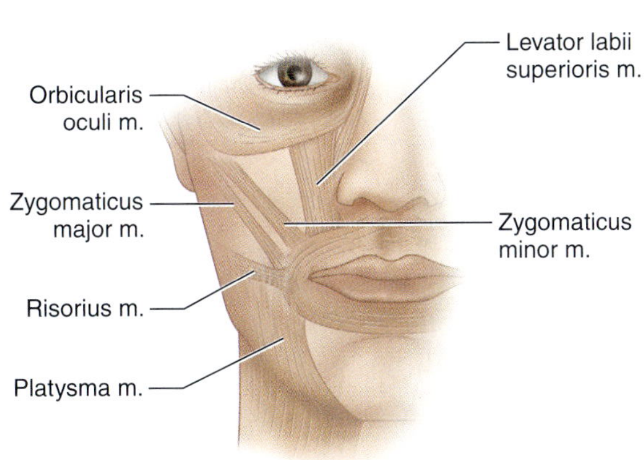

Figure 1-5 Superficial musculature of the perioral area.

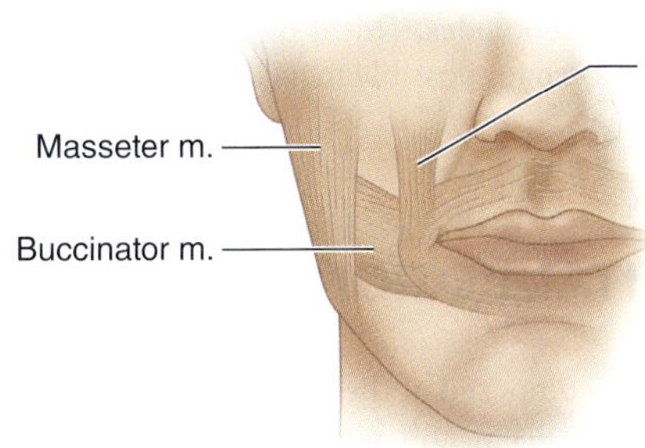

Figure 1-6 Deeper musculature of the perioral area.

nares. The levator anguli oris originates from the maxilla below the infraorbital foramen and inserts into the skin and mucosa at the labial commissure, thus elevating the corners of the mouth. These muscles are innervated by the buccal branches of the facial nerve with secondary innervation from the zygomatic branches of the facial nerve.[2]

The buccinator, also known as the cheek bulk muscle, is the key muscle of the cheek (Fig. 1-6). It originates from the posterolateral aspect of the maxilla, the medial aspect of the mandible near the last molar, and the pterygomandibular raphe. Its insertion is into the skin and mucosa of the labial commissure as well as the upper and lower lips. It serves to press the lips and cheeks against the teeth. Its innervation is from the buccal branches of the facial nerve. Of note, this is the only muscle of facial expression that receives its innervation from the superficial aspect of the facial nerve.[5]

Finally, the orbicularis oris consists of concentrically arranged fibers providing a sphincteric function, which allows for pursing and protrusion of the lips. It is mostly innervated by the buccal branches of the facial nerve.[2]

The sensory supply to the lips is provided by the branches of the trigeminal nerve. The maxillary division of the trigeminal nerve gives off the infraorbital branch, which innervates the upper lip, lower eyelid, infraorbital cheek, parts of the buccal cheek, malar cheek, and lateral aspect of the nose. The mandibular division of the trigeminal nerve branches into the mental nerve, which provides sensation to the lower lip. To identify these nerves, one may visualize an imaginary vertical line dropping inferiorly from the supraorbital notch. The infraorbital foramen and nerve are found approximately 5 mm below the inferior margin of the orbit. The mental foramen and nerve are intersected by this imaginary line and are located midway along the height of the body of the mandible.[5]

The vascular supply to the lips arises from the facial artery via the inferior and superior labial arteries. These tortuous vessels meander through the muscle fibers and anastomose across the midline; therefore, if needed, the facial artery may be ligated at its point of entry into the face without fear of ischemia to the ipsilateral face. The venous drainage from the lips occurs through the superior and inferior labial veins, which eventually join the anterior facial vein. The lymphatic drainage from the lips is multifaceted. The central and ipsilateral regions of the upper lip drain into the ipsilateral submandibular nodes. The lateral regions of the lower lip flow into the ipsilateral submandibular nodes; however, the central portion of the lower lip flows into both ipsilateral and contralateral submandibular and submental nodes. This is of great importance when there is concern for possible metastasis of tumors in this location.[1]

PERIORBITAL REGION

The orbital rim is composed of the following bones: frontal, zygomatic, maxillary, and lacrimal. Key landmarks include the supraorbital margin, supraorbital notch, and infraorbital margin. The supraorbital notch, from which the supraorbital nerve exits, is found 2 cm from the midline. The lateral orbital tubercle, also known as Whitnall's tubercle, is a small bony prominence located 10 mm below the zygomaticofrontal suture and 4 mm behind the anterolateral orbital rim. This is the site of attachment for the lateral palpebral ligament. In the area of the medial orbital rim is the anterior lacrimal crest, to which the medial palpebral ligament is attached. The lacrimal sac is located posterior to the medial palpebral ligament.[3]

The eyelids form a protective covering for the underlying globe. The upper eyelid is larger than the lower eyelid and provides the bulk of protection to the underlying eyeball. The skin of the eyelids is quite thin and continuous with the conjunctiva at the free margins. The palpebral fissure is the space between the open eyelids. The commissure or canthus is the site where the upper and lower eyelids join. The medial canthus is separated from the surface of the eyeball by the lacrimal caruncle, which appears as an erythematous structure. The space occupied by the lacrimal caruncle is the lacrimal lake. The plica semilunaris is the portion of the folded conjunctiva lateral to the lacrimal caruncle. Along the free margins of the medial eyelids are small elevations at the base of the eyelashes known as lacrimal papillae. Each papilla encircles a punctum, which marks the opening to the lacrimal canalicular system through which the fluid drains into the lacrimal sac. From there, the nasolacrimal duct, which typically runs for approximately 18 mm, empties its contents into the inferior meatus of the nose. The lacrimal gland, located behind the orbital margin of the zygomatic process of the frontal bone, consists of a larger orbital portion and a smaller palpebral portion and provides lubrication for the eye (Fig. 1-7).[4]

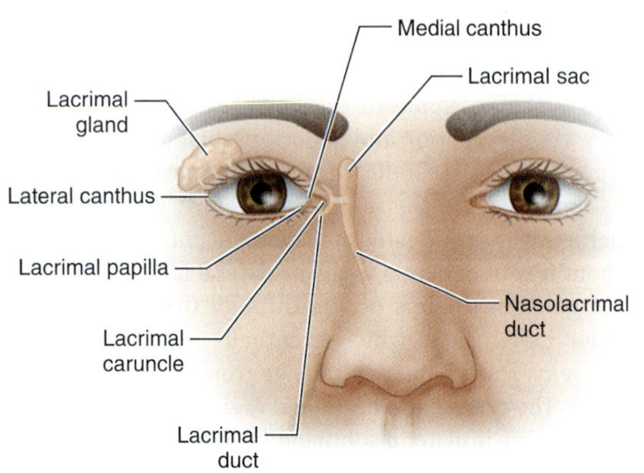

Figure 1-7 Anatomy of the lacrimal system.

The conjunctiva covers the globe and lines the inner surface of the eyelids to form the conjunctival sac. The tarsal plates of the upper and lower lids give form and shape to the eyelids. On average, the height of the tarsal plate in the upper lid varies between 9 and 11 mm whereas that of the lower lid is about 4 to 5 mm. The medial palpebral ligament secures the tarsal plates to the anterior lacrimal crest at the medial orbital rim. The upper and lower tarsal plates are also secured via the lateral palpebral ligament to the lateral orbital tubercle, also known as Whitnall's tubercle.[3]

The key muscles of the eyelid are the orbicularis oculi and levator palpebrae superioris. The orbicularis oculi allows for closure of the eye whereas the levator palpebrae superioris opens the eye. The orbicularis oculi muscle fibers encircle the eyelids, forehead, temple, and cheeks. This muscle functions as a sphincter and can be divided into palpebral and orbital portions, whose primary and secondary innervation are provided by the zygomatic and temporal branch of the facial nerve, respectively. Upon contraction, the muscle allows for protection of the globe and even spreading of tears across the surface of the eye. Damage to the muscle or its innervation may lead to ectropion of the lower eyelid. The second eyelid muscle of note is the levator palpebrae superioris muscle, which is innervated by the third cranial nerve (the oculomotor nerve).[5] This muscle originates from the orbital apex and then fans out, molding itself around the globe before inserting onto the anterior surface of the tarsus. It also has fibers above the superior border of the tarsus between the orbicularis oculi and the skin, which forms the supratarsal eyelid crease.

The orbital septum is a fibrous sheath lying beneath the orbicularis oculi muscle. This structure marks the anterior border of the orbit and encases the orbital fat. The orbital septum originates from the bony margins of the orbit and lies anterior to the tarsal plates. The septum is thinnest at its medial aspect (Fig. 1-8). There are two fat pads posterior to the orbital septum in the upper eyelid and three fat

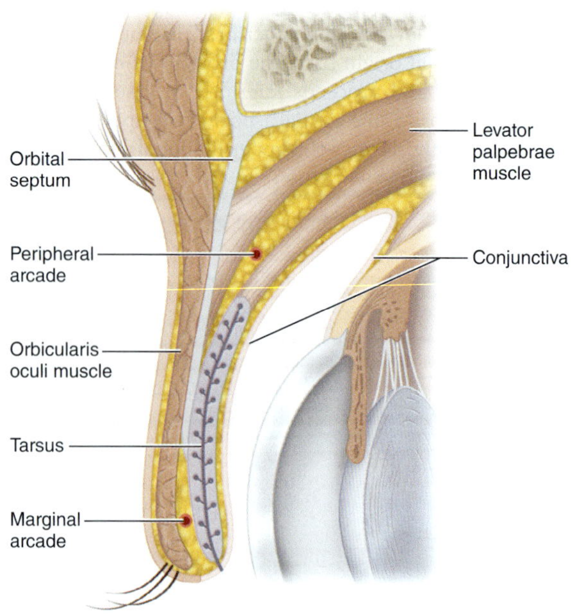

Figure 1-8 Sagittal view of the upper eyelid.

pads posterior to the orbital septum in the lower eyelid. In addition, in the upper eyelid, posterosuperior to the orbital septum, is the lacrimal gland.[1]

The nerve supply to the eyelids consists of both motor and sensory components. The zygomatic and temporal branches of the facial nerve supply motor innervation to the orbicularis oculi. The oculomotor nerve innervates the levator palpebrae superioris. Sensory innervation is provided by the ophthalmic division of the trigeminal nerve. The ophthalmic division of the trigeminal nerve gives rise to the supraorbital, supratrochlear, and lacrimal nerves, which provide sensation to the upper eyelid. The lower eyelid is innervated by the infraorbital nerve, which arises from the maxillary division of the trigeminal nerve. Of note, visual acuity should be documented prior to any surgical procedure in the periorbital region. After surgery, if the eye needs to be patched, extra care should be exercised to ensure that it is patched in the closed position to avoid corneal abrasions and injury to other structures of the eye.[4]

The vascular supply to the eyelids is derived from the rich arterial supply from both the internal and external carotid arteries. The ophthalmic artery arises from the internal carotid artery and gives rise to the supraorbital, supratrochlear, medial palpebral, dorsal nasal, and lacrimal arteries. The medial palpebral arteries include both superior and inferior components that dive through the orbital septum medially and then traverse laterally over the eyelid. Of note, the superior palpebral artery supplies both the peripheral and marginal arcades. The peripheral arcade is located in the upper body of the tarsus whereas the marginal arcade is found in the lower portion of the tarsus just superior to the eyelashes in the pretarsal space. Meanwhile, the external carotid artery gives off the maxillary and superficial temporal arteries. The maxillary artery gives rise to the infraorbital artery, which exits the infraorbital foramen and supplies the lower eyelid. The superficial temporal artery branches into the transverse facial artery, the zygomatico-orbital artery, and the frontal artery. These supply the lateral orbit and forehead. There are two key sites for anastomosis: first in the lateral eyelid, between the superficial temporal artery and the lateral distribution of the infraorbital artery, and second in the medial eyelid, between the inferior medial palpebral artery and the infraorbital artery.[1]

The venous network of the eyelid is also quite extensive, and parallels the arterial system. The veins drain into the ophthalmic venous system, the superficial temporal vein, or the angular vein. Of note, the ophthalmic venous system flows into the dural venous sinus. The lymphatic drainage of the periorbital area is divided into lateral and medial components. The lateral aspects of the upper and lower eyelids drain into the preauricular nodal basin whereas the medial aspects drain to the central facial and submandibular nodes.[3]

SCALP

The scalp consists of the skin and multiple layers of soft tissue overlying bone. The calvarium, which is composed of the frontal, occipital, and two paired parietal bones, serves as the foundation for the scalp. The scalp bones are separated by the coronal, sagittal, lambdoid, and squamosal sutures. The soft tissues above it include five distinct layers which are easily remembered using the following mnemonic:

Skin
Connective tissue (subcutaneous tissue)
Aponeurosis (galea aponeurotica)
Loose areolar connective tissue
Periosteum

On the scalp, the skin extends from the supraorbital ridges of the frontal bone posteriorly to the superior nuchal lines of the occipital bone. The lateral portions cover the parietal bones and temporalis muscle. The forehead may be considered a subsection of the scalp extending from the supraorbital ridges to the highest wrinkle overlying the frontal bone. The flat portion of the forehead is due to the underlying squamous portion of the frontal bone. Posteriorly, the inion is a protuberance which may be palpated at the midline of the occipital bone. Extending laterally from the inion are two ridges forming the superior nuchal lines (Fig. 1-9).[1]

The bones of the calvarium consist of an inner table and an outer table of cortical bone separated by a spongy diploe layer of trabecular bone. These bones receive their blood supply from both the interior and exterior surfaces. On occasion, the dermatologic surgeon may need to sample the outer table to evaluate for invasion of tumor, or may remove portions of the outer table to stimulate the formation of granulation tissue. Care must be taken to avoid penetrating the inner table if sampling is done with the osteotome and mallet. The surgeon should also avoid using an osteotome across suture lines of the calvarium or on a site which has been irradiated previously.[5]

Under the skin of the scalp lies the connective tissue layer (subcutaneous tissue), which contains most of the vascular and nerve supply for the scalp. The scalp vasculature consists of many anastomosing branches which originate from both the internal and external carotid

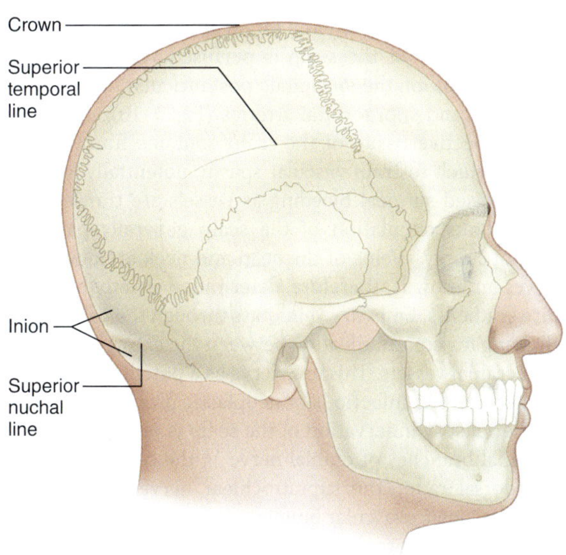

Figure 1-9 Landmarks of the scalp.

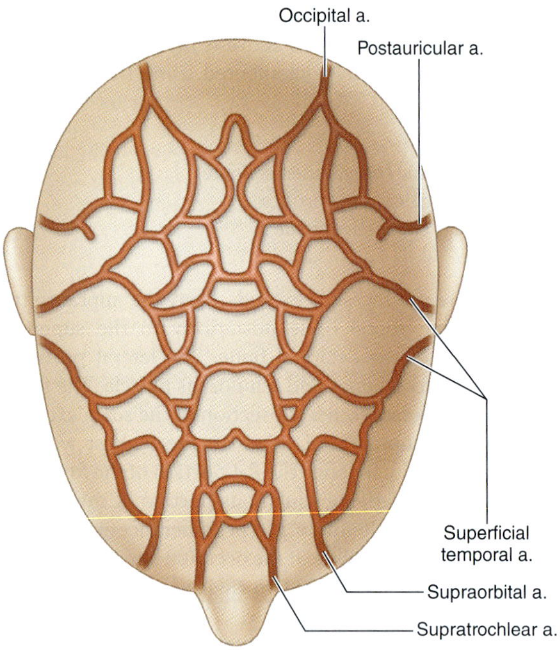

Figure 1-10 Vasculature of the scalp.

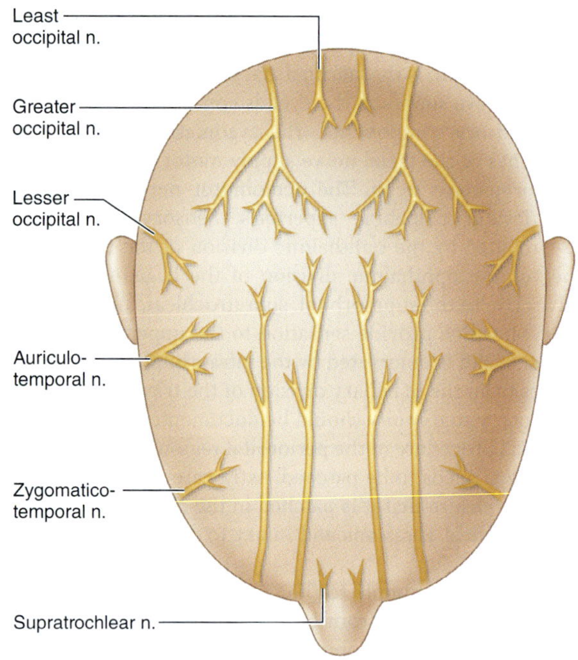

Figure 1-11 Sensory innervation of the scalp.

arteries. The occipital artery and posterior auricular artery are branches from the external carotid which supply the occipital and retroauricular scalp. The external carotid artery eventually branches into the superficial temporal artery, which is palpable at the superior pole of the parotid gland, supplying the temporal scalp. The internal carotid artery, via the ophthalmic artery, divides into the supraorbital, supratrochlear, and lacrimal arterial branches. After traversing the orbit, the supraorbital artery exits the supraorbital foramen as part of a neurovascular bundle approximately 2 to 2.5 cm lateral to the nasion along the superior orbital margin.[4] This foramen is palpable as the supraorbital notch. The supratrochlear artery also traverses the orbit and wraps around the supraorbital rim approximately 1 cm medial to the supraorbital notch to supply the medial forehead. The supraorbital and supratrochlear arteries supply the forehead and anterior scalp. The remainder of the scalp is perfused via anastomosing branches of the occipital, postauricular, superficial temporal, and supraorbital arteries (Fig. 1-10).[2] Of note, the connective tissue of the scalp contains fibrous retinacula which restrain vascular spasm, potentially leading to increased surgical bleeding as vessels are transected.[1] The venous circulation of the scalp generally parallels arterial supply.[6] Veins of the head and neck are devoid of valves and flow is, therefore, determined strictly by pressure gradients. Emissary veins pass through the calvarium, allowing for communication between the extracranial and intracranial vessels. This may serve as a potential route for spread of either infectious or neoplastic processes.

The sensory innervation of the scalp is provided by the terminal branches of cranial nerve V, the cervical plexus, and dorsal rami. The supratrochlear nerve parallels the artery as a neurovascular bundle and innervates the medial forehead. The supraorbital nerve passes through the supraorbital foramen/notch and innervates the lateral forehead. These two nerves course superiorly across the frontal bone and posteriorly along the top of the scalp to innervate the crown.[1] The auriculotemporal nerve originates from the mandibular division of the fifth cranial nerve. It courses posterior to the ramus of the mandible and follows the course of the superficial temporal artery. It supplies sensation for most of the temporal and parietal scalp as well as the anterolateral auricle and anterior half of the external auditory canal.[6] The lesser occipital nerve originates from the cervical plexus and follows the posterior edge of the sternocleidomastoid muscle to supply the skin over the mastoid and lateral occipital region of the scalp. The greater occipital nerve is the dorsal ramus of the second cervical spinal nerve. It penetrates the trapezius muscle to provide sensation to the occipital and parietal regions of the scalp extending anteriorly as far as the vertex (Fig. 1-11).[1]

Deep to the subcutaneous connective tissue of the scalp lies the galea aponeurotica which, along with the occipital and frontalis muscles, forms the most important fasciomuscular unit of the scalp. The small muscular belly of the occipital muscle originates from the posterior mastoid process and the posterior nuchal line of the occipital bone. It inserts into the galea aponeurotica and serves to pull the entire scalp posteriorly. The frontalis muscle originates from the galea aponeurosis and inserts into the skin of the forehead and eyebrows, contiguous with the superficial muscular aponeurotic system (SMAS) consists of fibrous and muscle tissues ensheathing and connecting facial muscles which allow coordinated facial expressions. The occipitalis muscle is innervated by the posterior auricular branch of the facial nerve whereas the frontalis receives its innervation from the temporal branch of the facial nerve. If the temporal branch of the facial nerve is damaged, this may result in drooping of the eyebrow or ptosis of the upper eyelid. If paralysis of the temporalis muscle occurs, the surgeon may try to correct the damage by doing a brow lift, a coronal lift, a blepharoplasty, or a combination of these procedures. The galea is a thick fibrous layer and as such serves as a barrier against tumor spread.[6] It may also impede tissue movement when considering reconstructive approaches. Galeal resection or relaxing incisions may be necessary to allow adequate motion of flaps in order to optimize reconstruction of scalp defects.

A layer of relatively avascular loose areolar connective tissue lies below the occipitofrontalis muscle and the fibrous galea aponeurotica. The loose and avascular nature of this tissue creates an ideal plane for undermining the overlying skin, connective tissue, and galea, allowing for increased tissue mobility. This area is also sometimes referred to as the "danger zone," due to its potential for accumulation of large volumes of blood or other fluids and the possibility of infection spreading intracranially via emissary veins.[1]

The lymphatic drainage of the scalp closely follows the vascular supply. The occipital scalp drains into scattered occipital nodes along the superior nuchal lines. The postauricular nodes located around the mastoid process receive drainage from the occipital, parietal, and temporal scalp. The forehead and temporal regions drain into the preauricular or superficial parotid nodes.[4,5]

EAR

In general, the ear may be divided into three portions: the inner ear, the middle ear, and the external ear. The external ear consists of the auricle and external auditory meatus, which terminates at the tympanic membrane. The auricle is composed of irregularly shaped elastic cartilage and adipose tissue suspended below in the form of the lobule. This cartilaginous support is lined with perichondrium and draped with skin. The skin of the anterior auricular surface is tightly adherent to the underlying structure as compared to the posterior surface which is rather loose. There are several anatomic landmarks which prove useful when describing the location of lesions on the ear, including the helix, scaphoid fossa, antihelix, triangular fossa, crus of the helix, crura of the antihelix, concha (conchal bowl), tragus, antitragus, incisure (intertragal notch), and lobule (Fig. 1-12). The entire auricle is fixed to the cranium by auricular ligaments.[1]

The external auditory meatus consists of cartilage and bone lined with skin, which terminates at the tympanic membrane. The anterior and inferior lateral third of the meatus is composed of cartilage, whereas the posterior and superior portions of the lateral third and the entire medial two-thirds are composed of temporal bone. The cartilaginous portion of the lateral third of the meatus is frequently perforated by fissures called the fissures of Santorini. It is important to note that the superior pole of the parotid gland lies immediately anterior and inferior to these fissures, which may, therefore, represent a potential direct route for tumor invasion of the parotid from the external meatus.[4]

The musculature of the ear consists of the anterior, superior, and posterior auricular muscles. They arise from the scalp and insert into the skin and auricle in areas named according to their location. They are innervated by posterior and temporal branches of the facial nerve, but are of minimal clinical significance if their function is lost.[2,5]

The vascular supply of the ear originates from the external carotid artery. The lateral surface receives its supply from the auricular branches of the superficial temporal artery, whereas the medial surface receives its supply from the posterior auricular and occipital arteries. Its venous drainage parallels the arterial supply and its lymphatic drainage flows to the preauricular, postauricular, and superficial cervical nodes.[1] The sensory innervation of the ear includes the auriculotemporal nerve, which originates from the mandibular branch of cranial nerve V. It innervates the anterosuperior quadrant of the anteriomedial half of the auricle, the anterior half of the external auditory meatus, the tympanic membrane, a small portion of the superior auricle on the posterosuperior surface, and most of the temporal scalp.[2,5,6] Cranial nerves VII, IX, and X supply the concha, the posterior half of the external auditory meatus, and a small patch of skin on the posterior auricle. The remainder of the auricle is innervated by the greater auricular nerve and the lesser occipital nerve, which originate from the cervical plexus. The greater auricular nerve appears at the posterior edge of the junction of the middle and upper thirds of the sternocleidomastoid muscle. It ascends across the sternocleidomastoid directly toward the inferior auricle to supply the anterolateral surface of the auricle, as well as most of its posteromedial surface. The lesser occipital nerve parallels the posterior edge of the sternocleidomastoid to supply a small portion of the posteromedial auricle and the skin overlying the mastoid.[1]

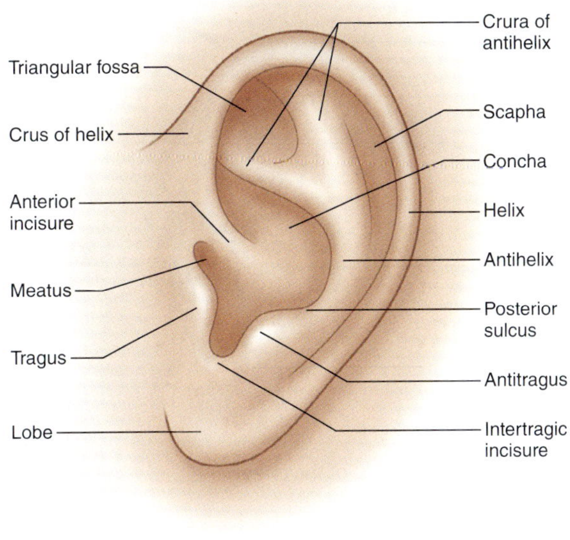

Figure 1-12 Cutaneous anatomy of the ear.

CHEEK

The cheek is a loosely defined area which extends anteriorly from the tragus of the ear to the oral commissure, and from the inferior orbital margin and the zygomatic arch inferiorly to the mandible. The nasolabial fold extends inferolaterally from the alar groove and separates the cheek from the perioral region, extending downward to become the melolabial fold. The cheek can be divided into four subsections: malar, infraorbital, masseteric, and

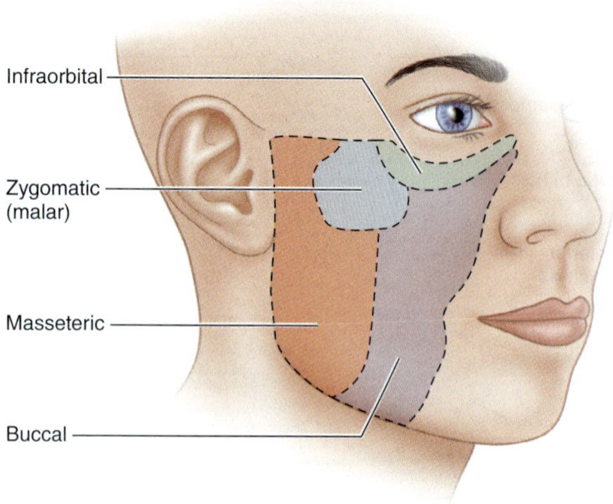

Figure 1-13 Divisions of the cheek.

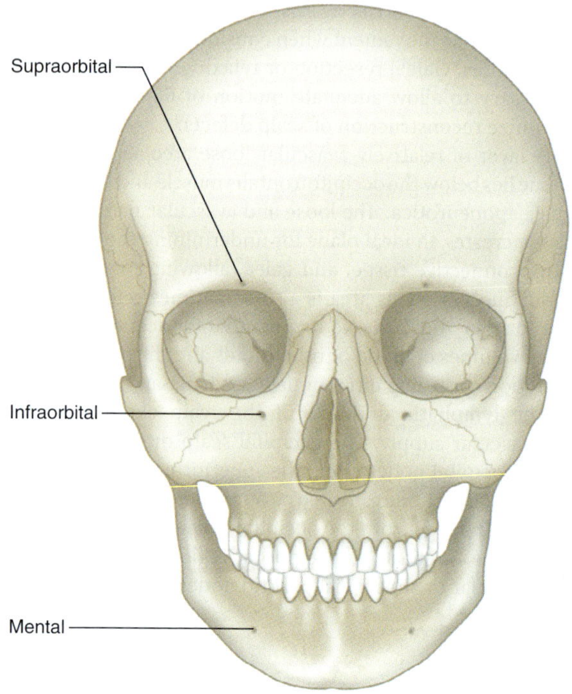

Figure 1-14 Foramina of the face.

buccal (Fig. 1-13). The malar portion of the cheek overlies the malar prominence of the zygomatic bone. The infraorbital cheek consists of the small area just below the inferior orbit. The tissue overlying the masseter muscle constitutes the masseteric cheek. The buccal cheek is the largest area and extends from the anterior edge of the masseter muscle to the oral commissure and from the infraorbital area to the mandible.[3]

The underlying bony structure of the cheek includes portions of the maxilla, the zygoma, and the mandible. The temporal process of the zygoma extends posteriorly to join the zygomatic process of the temporal bone, forming the zygomatic arch, and marking the superior aspect of the cheek.[2] While the malar prominence and zygomatic arch of the zygomatic bone contribute to the overall shape of the cheek, the maxilla is the predominant bony support of the cheek and lower face. Deep to the skin of the cheek lies the subcutaneous tissue. The fat of the cheek is thickest in an area of the buccal cheek referred to as the buccal fat pad. It is positioned between the buccinator muscle and the masseter muscle. It continues deep into the face between these two muscles and then superiorly into the temporal and infratemporal fossae. This space may serve as a possible route for deep tumor extension, possibly even as far as the maxilla or maxillary sinus, from the mid cheek.[1]

While not palpable, the parotid gland is an important structure which lies directly over the masseter muscle. The posterior edge of the parotid gland begins at the posterior edge of the mandibular ramus. Its superior pole extends nearly to the zygomatic arch and its inferior margin extends to the angle of the mandible. The anterior margin of the gland extends a variable distance over the masseter. The parotid gland is encapsulated in a thin layer of fascia. The parotid duct, Stensen's duct, is palpable halfway between the zygomatic arch and the oral commissure along the anterior edge of the masseter as the teeth are clenched.[5] This duct pierces the buccinator muscle and empties onto the mucosal cheek opposite the second upper molar. Should the duct be damaged during surgery, immediate repair is indicated.[4–6] In addition to its salivary function, this gland serves to protect the facial nerve as it courses through the gland and divides into its various branches.

The sensory innervation for the cheek is derived from multiple nerves, including the infraorbital and zygomaticofacial branches from the maxillary division of cranial nerve V and the auriculotemporal and buccal nerves from the mandibular branch of cranial nerve V. The maxilla contains the infraorbital foramen, through which travels the infraorbital nerve, which supplies the infraorbital, buccal, and portions of the malar cheek, as well as the lower eyelid, lateral nose, and upper lip. If a vertical line is drawn on the face passing through the supraorbital foramen and the pupil, the infraorbital foramen would be found approximately 0.5 to 1.5 cm from the inferior margin of the orbit along that line.[1] The mental foramen is also located approximately 1 cm above the inferior margin of the mandible along this same line (Fig. 1-14). The zygomaticofacial nerve penetrates the zygoma through small foramina in the malar prominence to supply the overlying skin of the malar cheek. As mentioned previously, the auriculotemporal nerve courses superiorly just anterior to the auricle and supplies the masseteric cheek, a portion of the ear, and the temporal scalp. The buccal nerve leaves the infratemporal fossa and descends medial to the mandible into the cheek along the superficial surface of the buccinator muscle. It innervates the overlying skin and buccal mucosa. The greater auricular nerve, which originates from the cervical plexus and ascends across the surface of the sternocleidomastoid muscle, provides the sensory innervation for the lower portion of the masseteric cheek (Fig. 1-15).

The musculature of the cheek can be divided into superficial and deep components. The superficial musculature includes the zygomaticus major and minor, the orbicularis oculi, the risorius, the levator labii superioris, and the platysma. The deeper muscle group includes the

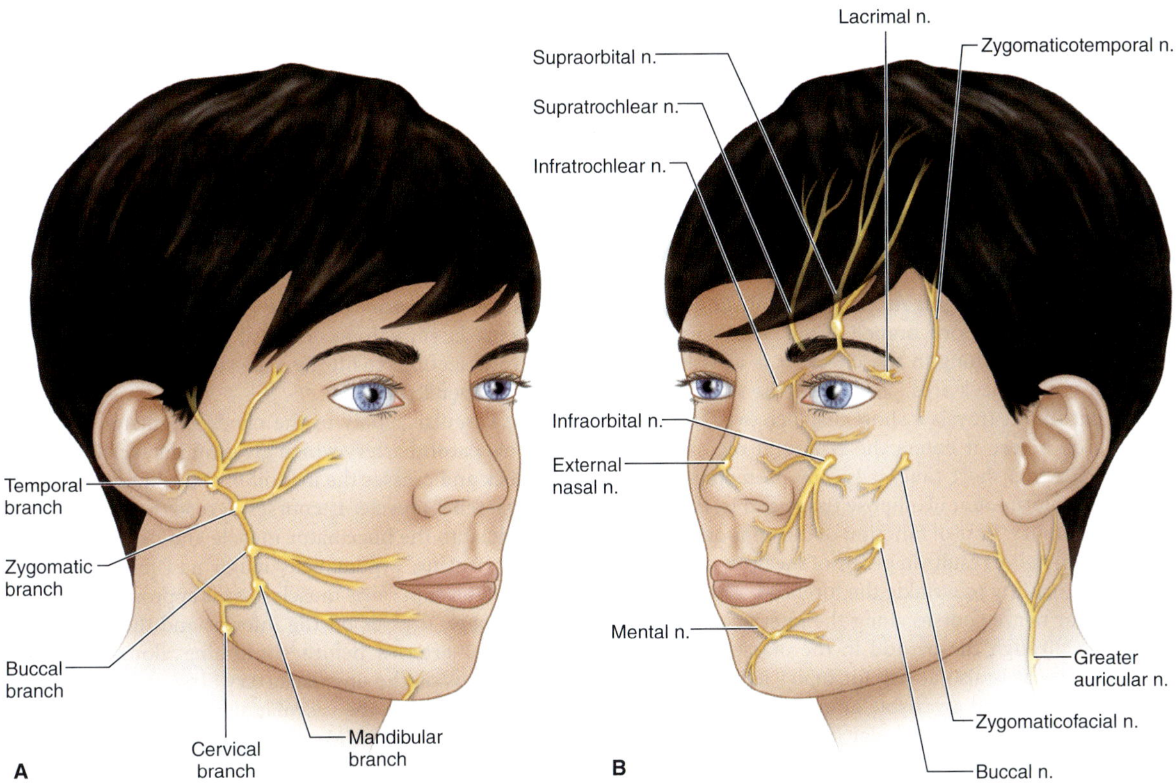

Figure 1-15 Sensory and motor nerves of the face (**A**) motor facial nerve and branches (**B**) sensory nerves.

levator anguli oris and the buccinator muscle. The zygomaticus major and minor originate from the zygoma and insert into the skin of the upper lip, serving to elevate the lip. The orbicularis oculi is a muscle which affects primarily the orbital and periorbital region, but some of its fibers extend onto the infraorbital cheek. Its circumferential course around the orbit serves to close the eye tightly. The risorius arises from the parotid fascia and inserts into the skin at the corner of the mouth, serving to pull the oral commissure laterally. The levator labii superioris originates from the maxilla just above the infraorbital foramen. It inserts into the skin of the upper lip and elevates the lip. The platysma originates from the superficial fascia of the upper thoracic region and the neck. It extends over the mandible and inserts into the skin of the oral commissures and pulls them inferiorly. The levator anguli oris arises from the maxilla below the infraorbital foramen and inserts into the corner of the mouth. It elevates the oral commissures. The buccinator muscle plays a key role in the musculature of the cheek. It originates from the pterygomandibular raphe, the posterolateral aspect of the maxilla, and the medial aspect of the mandible. It inserts into the skin and mucosa of the upper and lower lips, and this muscular wall keeps the cheek pressed against the dentition and assists in mastication.[3]

The muscles of the cheek all receive their motor innervation from the facial nerve with the exception of the platysma, which is innervated by the cervical plexus, and the masseter, which is innervated by the mandibular division of the fifth cranial nerve. The muscles of facial expression all receive their innervation from the deep surface of the muscle, except the buccinator which receives its motor innervation from its superficial surface.[6]

The facial nerve exits the stylomastoid foramen, courses inferiorly, gives off the posterior auricular nerve, and enters the posterior aspect of the parotid gland as a single nerve trunk which arborizes into five branches: temporal, zygomatic, buccal, marginal mandibular, and cervical (Figs. 1-15 and 1-16). These branches exit the parotid along its anterior edge, arborize in either one or two stages, and fan across the face. The temporal branch

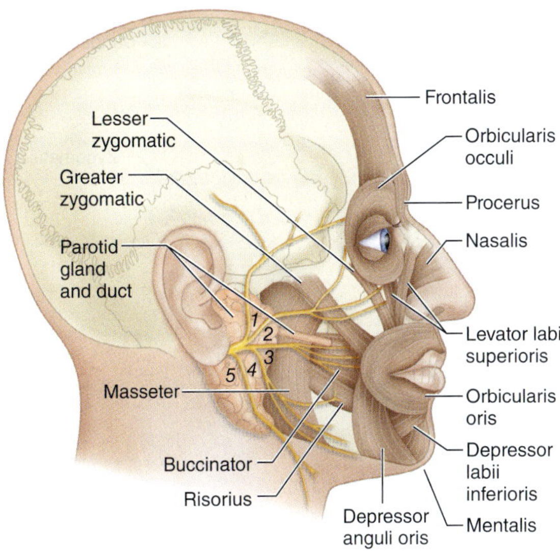

Figure 1-16 Branches of the facial nerve.

innervates the frontalis muscle. The marginal mandibular nerve innervates muscles in the perioral area and the cervical branch innervates the neck. The zygomatic and buccal branches of the facial nerve are, therefore, the only branches which provide innervation to the cheek area. The buccal branch exits the anterior edge of the parotid and parallels the course of the parotid duct. It provides innervation to the zygomaticus major and minor, levator labii superioris, risorius, levator anguli oris, and buccinator muscles. The zygomatic branch provides secondary innervation to the zygomaticus major and minor muscles. While the temporal branch of the facial nerve does not innervate anything in the cheek, it is at risk in the superior malar cheek area.[1] As it exits the superior pole of the parotid, it travels a short distance over the zygomatic arch before it enters the temporal region of the scalp.[2,4] For this short time, it is only protected by skin and a variable amount of adipose tissue and is, therefore, subject to injury. Loss of function of the temporal branch of the facial nerve results in ptosis of the brow and eyelid as well as inability to wrinkle the forehead. The marginal mandibular nerve courses along the inferior edge of the mandible through the parotid in the masseteric cheek. Once it exits, it is also at risk for injury as it too is only covered by skin and a variable amount of subcutaneous tissue. The marginal mandibular branch also remains as a trunk and fails to arborize until it nearly reaches its intended target. This means that surgical injury to this nerve may result in a more complete motor deficit.[1] It is also important to note that in the elderly, the marginal mandibular nerve may descend up to 2 cm below the margin of the mandible. Due to the risk of injury to branches of the facial nerve as they exit the parotid, a schematic "danger zone" has been devised (Fig. 1-17). To create this zone, a line is drawn parallel to and 1 cm above the zygomatic arch from the tragus to Whitnall's tubercle of the lateral margin of the orbit. A vertical line is drawn from the lateral margin of the orbit to the inferior margin of the mandible at the insertion of the masseter muscle. Finally, a line curving 2 cm below the inferior margin of the mandible, coursing posteriorly to the angle of the mandible, is drawn. Within the area delineated by these lines, the branches of the facial nerve are at risk for injury as they have not arborized extensively.[2,4–6] It may, therefore, be wise to avoid vertical incisions overlying the inferior masseter and mandible as well as deep incisions parallel to the zygomatic arch, so as to avoid injury to the marginal mandibular and temporal branches of the facial nerve. The danger zone is an area in which the surgeon may prefer to place incisions parallel to the course of the nerve regardless of the relaxed skin tension lines to minimize the chance of nerve injury. It may also be useful to use larger volumes of local anesthesia or saline for "hydrodissection" to lift the superficial tissues away from these deeper structures.

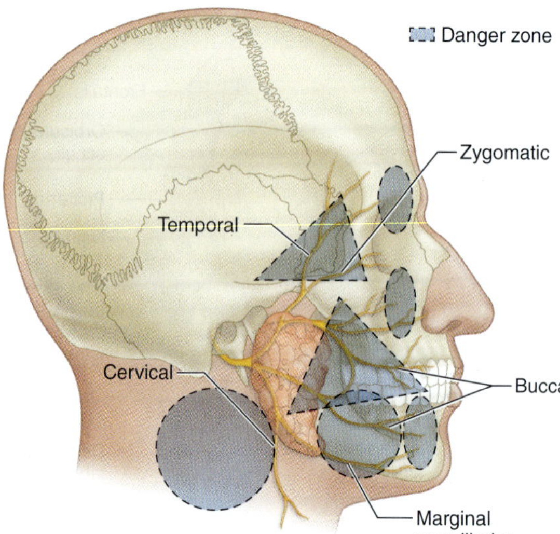

Figure 1-17 Danger zones of the face.

The vascular supply of the cheek originates from the external carotid artery which gives off the facial artery in the neck and crosses the mandible at the anterior edge of the masseter muscle. It courses across the face directly superficial to the buccinator muscle and deep to the platysma, risorius, zygomaticus major and minor, and the levator labii superioris muscles. As it approaches the oral commissure, it gives off the inferior and then the superior labial arteries before continuing along the nasofacial sulcus as the angular artery. The maxillary artery also contributes to the vascular supply of the cheek. It is another branch of the external carotid artery which ultimately branches into the infraorbital and buccal arteries. The infraorbital artery passes through the infraorbital foramen to supply the overlying area of the cheek. The buccal artery originates medial to the mandible, descends inferiorly onto the superficial aspect of the buccinator, and supplies the skin and buccal mucosa. The superficial temporal artery yields the transverse facial artery which passes through the superior pole of the parotid gland and parallels the parotid duct to supply the malar region of the cheek (Fig. 1-18). The venous circulation follows the same pattern as the arterial circulation, including the buccal, infraorbital, superficial temporal, and anterior facial veins. The anterior facial vein is the most important collecting vein for venous drainage of the face. Of note, due to the valveless nature of veins in the head and neck as well as the numerous anastomotic connections between them, it is possible for veins of the face to communicate with the cavernous sinus, most notably via the buccal or infraorbital veins.[1]

Lymphatic drainage from the cheek flows predominantly to the preauricular/parotid nodes. This nodal basin drains the masseteric cheek, the posterior half of the buccal cheek, and the lateral half of the infraorbital cheek. The facial nodes which follow the course of the facial vein drain the remainder of the anterior cheek. From there, the lymph flows into the submandibular and submental nodes (Fig. 1-19).

NECK

The neck can be divided into two triangles: anterior and posterior. The anterior triangle borders are defined by the anterior border of the sternocleidomastoid muscle, the inferior margin of the mandible, and the midline border from the tip of the chin to the jugular notch. The posterior triangle borders are composed of the sternocleidomastoid

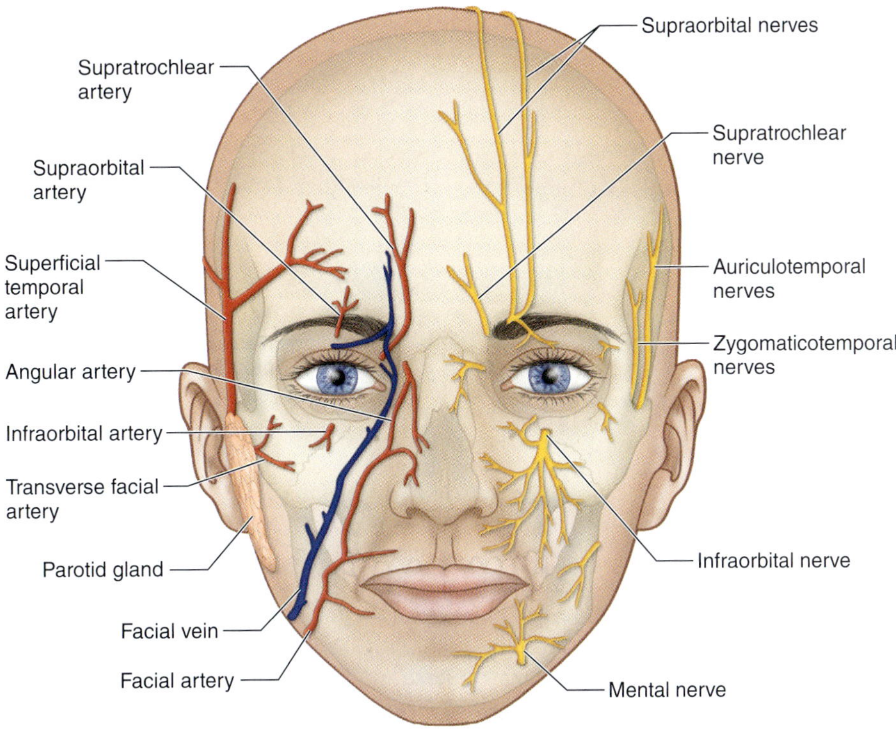

Figure 1-18 Vasculature and sensory innervation of the cheek.

muscle, the clavicle inferiorly, and the anterior edge of the trapezius muscle (Fig. 1-20).

Each triangle can be divided into smaller triangles for more precise localization of skin lesions and better understanding of neck anatomy. The anterior triangle can be subdivided into submental, submandibular, carotid, and muscular triangles. The borders of the submental triangle are the anterior belly of the digastric muscle, the hyoid bone body, and the midline of the neck. The borders of the submandibular triangle are the two bellies of the digastric muscle and the mandible. The borders of the carotid triangle are the sternocleidomastoid muscle, the posterior border of digastric muscle, and the superior belly of the omohyoid muscle. The borders of the muscular triangle are the sternocleidomastoid muscle, the superior belly of the omohyoid muscle, and the midline of the neck.[3]

The posterior triangle of the neck can also be divided into two smaller triangles: the subclavian and the occipital. The subclavian triangle's borders are composed of the clavicle, the sternocleidomastoid muscle and the inferior belly of the omohyoid muscle. The occipital triangle's borders are demarcated by the inferior belly of the omohyoid muscle, the sternocleidomastoid muscle, and the trapezius muscle.[4]

The skin of the neck exhibits various unique properties. First of, it is very delicate and thin. It also contains numerous hair follicles, sweat glands, and some sebaceous glands. The superficial cervical fascia, a thin layer of loose areolar connective tissue, allows for the skin of the neck to be pliable and mobile. Of note, the fascia is continuous with the superficial fascia of the face. The platysma, located within the anterior triangle, is the only superficial muscle in this area. It originates from the fascia of the upper chest and continues superiorly over the mandible to insert into the skin and superficial tissue of the lower face. The platysma muscle tenses the skin of the neck and depresses the mouth. The cervical branch of the facial nerve provides innervation to the platysma. Although the platysma is superficial to the sternocleidomastoid and reaches the most inferior aspect of the occipital triangle, it does not provide coverage or protection to the spinal accessory nerve in the posterior triangle. The sternocleidomastoid muscle arises from the sternum and the clavicle and passes obliquely across the neck to end at the mastoid process.[3]

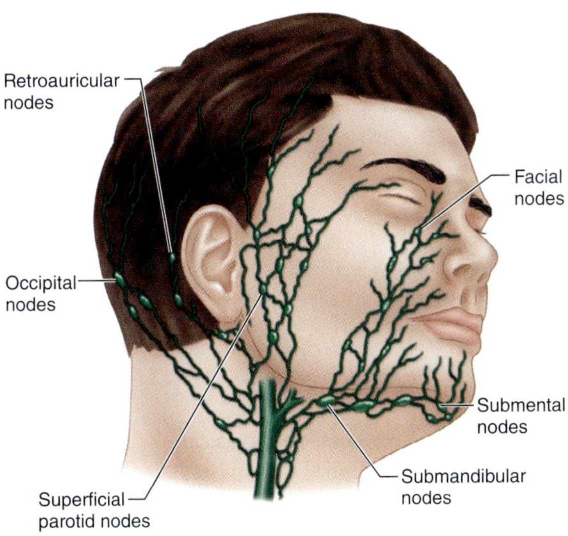

Figure 1-19 Lymphatics of the head and neck.

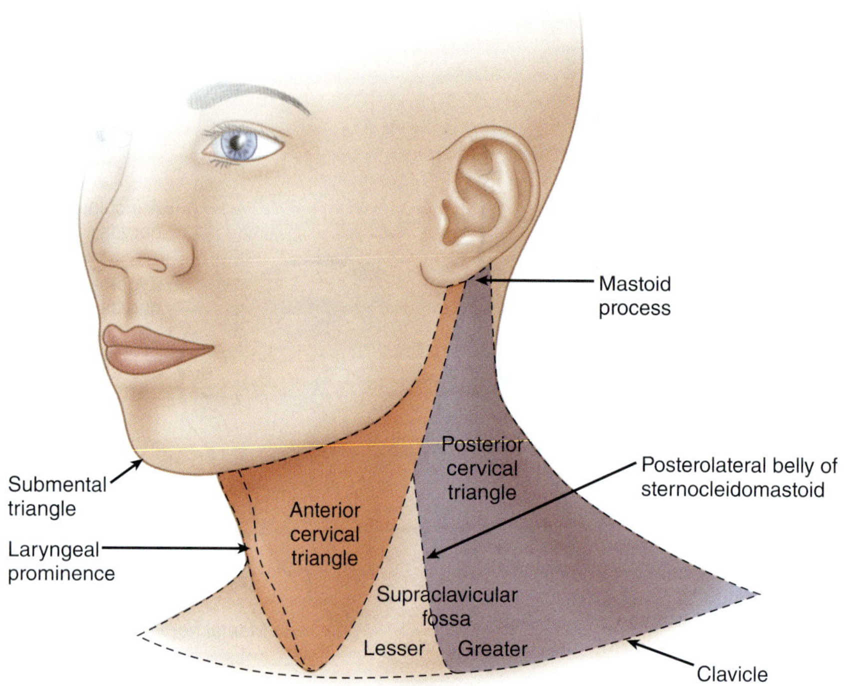

Figure 1-20 Anatomy of the neck. The neck can be further divided into the anterior and posterior cervical triangles.

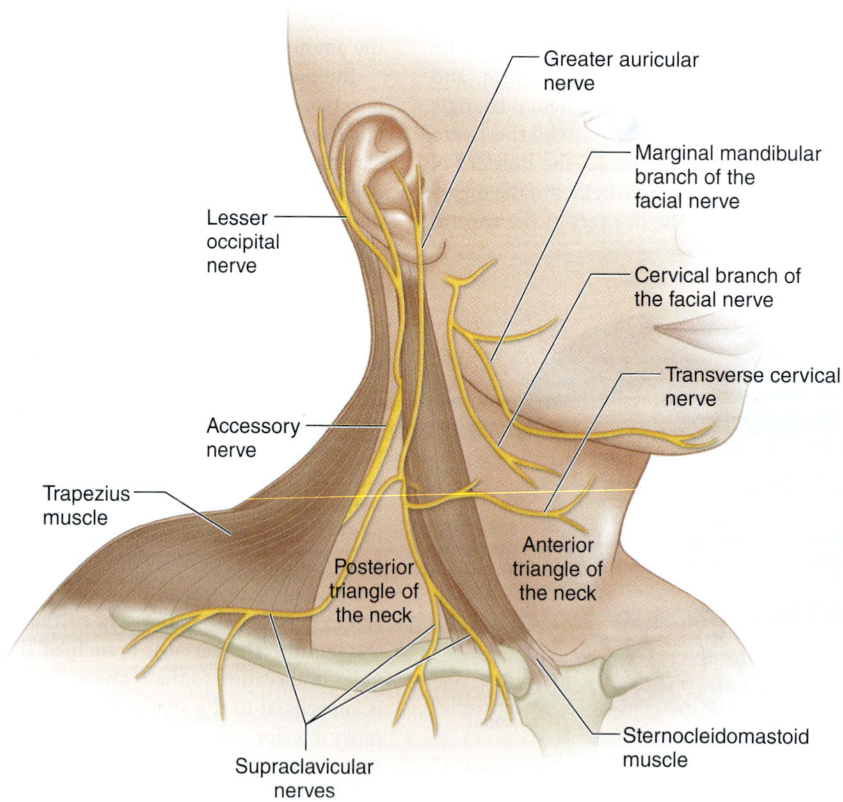

Figure 1-21 Sensory and motor supply of the neck and associated regions.

The hyoid bone is located in the anterior triangle of the neck at the second cervical vertebral level. It can be palpated just inferior to the chin within the midline of the neck. The prominence of the thyroid cartilage is also palpable just below the hyoid bone. The anterior lamina of the cricoid cartilage, along with tracheal rings and the isthmus of the thyroid gland, is located below the thyroid cartilage.[1]

The branches of the external carotid artery and the thyrocervical trunk, a branch of the subclavian artery, provide the arterial supply to the neck skin. The venous drainage of the neck occurs through the anterior superficial venous system deep to the platysma muscle. It then drains into the anterior jugular vein, which may be connected to the common facial vein via a small communicating vein. The superficial veins of the posterior cervical triangle drain into the external jugular vein.[6]

The cervical plexus provides sensory innervation to the skin of the neck. The transverse cervical nerves cross the sternocleidomastoid muscle at the midpoint horizontally to provide sensory innervation to the mid-anterior cervical triangle. A series of supraclavicular nerves pass inferior to the transverse cervical nerves to supply the skin of the anterior and posterior cervical triangles as well as the upper pectoral area. The lesser occipital nerve is found at the posterior border of the sternocleidomastoid muscle near its midpoint. It travels superiorly, paralleling the posterior border of the sternocleidomastoid muscle, to innervate the posterior ear and mastoid area. Similarly, the greater auricular nerve arises from the midpoint of the sternocleidomastoid muscle with a superior trajectory to provide sensory innervation to the lower portion of the ear.

Understanding the location of the nerves in the neck is key for every surgeon so as to avoid complications. The marginal mandibular branch of the facial nerve descends into the anterior triangle of the neck along the mandible before innervating the muscles of the lower lip. The marginal mandibular nerve is at risk during surgery in this area. The spinal accessory nerve, which supplies the sternocleidomastoid and trapezius muscles, is at risk in the posterior triangle during surgery. This is especially true as it exits from the junction of the upper and middle thirds of the sternocleidomastoid muscle to enter the posterior triangle, as it is covered only by skin and superficial fascia at this location (Fig. 1-21). Damage to the spinal accessory nerve can lead to a permanent loss of ability to elevate the shoulder on the ipsilateral side.[1]

CONCLUSION

The head and neck region contains many important anatomic structures that every dermatologic surgeon must be familiar with to provide the highest level of patient care. Preoperative anatomic knowledge and planning, along with intraoperative awareness and precision, are necessary to provide the best cosmetic result with the least possible functional disturbance. With a full understanding of this anatomically complex region, the physician will have the confidence to perform a wide range of superficial surgical procedures and the knowledge required to minimize the likelihood of complications and adverse outcomes.

REFERENCES

1. Greenway HT, Breisch EA. Anatomy of the head and neck. In: Mikhail GR, ed. *Practice of Mohs Micrographic Surgery*. Philadelphia, PA: W.B. Saunders; 1991:150–166.
2. Breisch EA, Greenway HT. Surgical anatomy. In: Moy RL, Lask GP, eds. *Principles and Techniques of Cutaneous Surgery*. New York, NY: McGraw-Hill; 1996:35–46.
3. Breisch EA, Greenway HT. *Cutaneous Surgical Anatomy of the Head and Neck*. New York, NY: Livingstone Inc.; 1991:1–133.
4. Greenway HT, Breisch EA. Superficial cutaneous anatomy. In: Robinson JK, Arndt KA, Leboit PE, Wintroub BU, eds. *Atlas of Cutaneous Surgery*. Philadelphia, PA: W.B. Saunders Co; 1996:5–19.
5. Breisch EA, Greenway HT. Fundamental anatomy for the practice of cutaneous surgery. In: Arndt KA, Leboit PE, Robinson JK, Wintroub BU, eds. *Cutaneous Medicine and Surgery*. Philadelphia, PA: W.B. Saunders Co; 1996:111–119.
6. Breisch EA, Greenway HT. Superficial anatomy of the head and neck. In: Greenway HT, Barrett TL, eds. *Preoperative and Postoperative Dermatologic Surgical Care*. New York, NY: Igaku-Shoin Medical Publishers; 1994:71–92.

CHAPTER 2

Preoperative Evaluation

Bichchau M. Nguyen & Chrysalyne D. Schmults

INTRODUCTION

Preoperative evaluation of patients undergoing cutaneous surgery serves multiple purposes: (1) it provides patients and physicians with the opportunity to discuss pertinent risks, benefits, and alternatives for the planned procedure; (2) to identify significant patient, lesion, or surgical factors that could increase the risk of complications; and (3) to plan care so as to mitigate identified risk factors.

The extent of preoperative evaluation depends in part on the type of procedure, the duration and degree of invasiveness of the procedure, and the use of topical, local, or general anesthesia. The vast majority of dermatologic surgeries are conducted under local anesthesia. A brief questionnaire addressing major risk factors for bleeding, infection, allergies, and implantable cardiac devices that may limit the use of electrocautery devices, will typically suffice for superficial procedures such as biopsies and curettage. Surgical excisions and Mohs micrographic surgery require a more thorough investigation of the patient's past medical history and lesion(s) of interest to identify and appropriately mitigate possible complications. Preoperative evaluation for elective cosmetic procedures such as laser therapies, liposuction, hair transplant, sclerotherapy, injections of fillers, and botulinum toxins varies significantly depending on the procedure and will, therefore, be covered in their corresponding specific chapters.

GENERAL OVERVIEW

A thorough preoperative evaluation provides a global overview of patient factors that can complicate the planned surgical procedure: past medical and surgical history, medications, allergies, and social history and habits (Table 2-1). Diabetes, cardiovascular heart disease, immunosuppression, blood-borne infections, bleeding disorders, and neuropsychiatric conditions are medical conditions that may influence operative planning. All prior surgeries, surgical complications and outcomes, and the presence of prosthetic joints or implantable cardiac devices should be specifically elicited from the patient.

Obtaining an accurate medication record is crucial but challenging, especially in the elderly population, whose medication lists can be extensive. It can be helpful to confirm the medication list on record with the patient and his or her caregiver, given the varying degrees of compliance and to inquire specifically about over-the-counter medications and herbal supplements as these are often underreported. Information on allergies should contain agent name and type of reaction. Patients may sometime confuse an adverse effect or vasovagal response with a true allergy. Allergic reactions can be anaphylactic (type I) or delayed hypersensitivity (type IV) reactions. Facial edema and respiratory distress are important type I reactions that should be asked about, especially with respect

TABLE 2-1
Preoperative Assessment of Surgical Patients

Past medical history	▪ Medical: cardiovascular disease, hypertension, diabetes, bleeding disorders, malignancy, immunosuppression, blood-borne infection (HIV, hepatitis C) ▪ Neuropsychiatric: claustrophobia, anxiety, panic attacks, dementia
Past surgical history	▪ Prosthetic joints, coronary artery stents, implantable cardiac devices ▪ Prior surgical complications and outcomes
Medications	▪ Prescribed medications: antiplatelet, anticoagulant, antibiotics, analgesics ▪ Over-the-counter medications (herbal supplements and vitamins)
Allergies	▪ Medications: agent and type of reaction (adverse effects vs. true allergy; delayed hypersensitivity vs. anaphylactic response) ▪ Topical preparations: cleansing antiseptics, dressings, adhesives
Social history	▪ Alcohol consumption: servings per week ▪ Smoking: pack-years ▪ Illegal drug use ▪ Social situation: caregiver, transportation, type of job, access to medical care

to antibiotic and latex allergies. Aside from medications, patients can also develop allergies (mostly allergic contact dermatitis) to antiseptic agents, topical antibiotics, and surgical dressings.

Social habits such as smoking, consumption of alcohol, and use of illicit drugs should be noted, although data on the true impact of these factors on surgical risks are mixed. Finally, difficult social situations including lack of social support, caregivers, or stable housing can make postoperative wound care challenging. Long-distance travel, lack of transportation, and limited access to local medical care may delay detection and treatment of postoperative complications. These factors should be considered in choosing appropriate surgical repairs and follow-up care.

A focused physical examination should be performed to assess the overall health status of the patient and characteristics of lesion(s) being treated. The correct procedure, diagnosis, and site should be confirmed with patients (via a mirror if needed) and/or caregivers and verified with available medical records, ideally including photographs. Use of prebiopsy photographs to identify the correct lesion is highly recommended because studies have shown that both patients and physicians are prone to identifying incorrect sites in a significant percentage of surgical cases—16% and 6%, respectively, in a prospective cohort study involving patients undergoing Mohs micrographic surgery.[1] When a lesion cannot be definitively identified using the available resources, frozen biopsy of the suspected site can be performed with continuation to surgery if biopsy is positive for malignancy, or 3 month clinical follow-up if the biopsy is negative.[2]

Once the correct lesion has been identified, the physician can proceed to assess the extent of spread, evidence of local or metastatic spread, proximity to functionally or aesthetically critical structures, feasibility of obtaining adequate surgical margins, and any potential neurologic or vascular complications. Depending on these factors, a nodal examination, imaging studies or consultation with other specialists might be warranted. The patient should be made aware of potential risks that may pertain to their procedure (such as infection, bleeding, hematoma, seroma, numbness, paralysis, asymmetry, and scarring) prior to surgery. A comprehensive discussion of these risks as well as the benefits of the proposed treatment and possible alternatives is needed in order for the patient to make a fully informed choice to proceed. Expectations regarding the anticipated extent of surgery and the length of recovery should be addressed preoperatively as well.

MEDICAL COMORBIDITIES

Patients with certain medical comorbidities deserve additional preoperative consideration due to their suspected or proven impact on the surgical risks of infection, bleeding, or wound healing. These special patient populations are discussed in more detail subsequently.

DIABETES

As of 2012, 9.3% of all children and adults in the United States were shown to have diabetes, with 25.9% of patients aged 65 years or older affected.[3] Diabetic patients have an increased risk of infection after general and cardiac surgeries. However, conflicting data exist regarding the risk of postoperative complications in diabetics undergoing dermatologic surgery. In the absence of prophylactic antibiotics, the risk of perioperative infection in these patients ranges from 1.1%[4] to 10%.[5] Some studies have found an increased risk of infections in patients with diabetes compared to those without,[6] whereas others have noted no difference between the two groups.[5] Patients with diabetes do not appear to have an increased risk of dehiscence, bleeding, or other noninfectious complications.[6] Little data exist on the effects of insulin dependence or perioperative glycemic control on the risk of dermatologic surgical complications. The variable prevalence of diabetics in study cohorts, along with different definitions of infection, inconsistent use of cultures, and the observational nature of these studies contribute to the difficulty of translating the available data into management guidelines. One may, therefore, advise patients with diabetes that they may have an increased risk of surgical site infection, but, as addressed later in this chapter, standard use of prophylactic antibiotics in this patient group is not warranted.

HYPERTENSION

The main concern in patients with uncontrolled hypertension is an increased risk of intra- and postoperative bleeding. Studies from the 1970s showed that patients with a blood pressure of 150/100 mm Hg had twice the risk of postoperative hematoma following rhytidectomy compared to normotensive counterparts.[7] More recent meta-analysis has shown that patients with blood pressures as high as 180/100 mm Hg do not have an increased risk of perioperative cardiac complications such as myocardial infarction, arrhythmia, and stroke when undergoing general anesthesia for planned surgeries.[8] Concerns exist that blood pressure lability during cutaneous surgery may be significant, raising the question of whether intraoperative monitoring is warranted for baseline hypertensive patients. However, studies have found little fluctuation in blood pressure before, during, or after cutaneous surgery in both normotensive and hypertensive patients.[9] Cutaneous surgery may be safely conducted in patients with a baseline blood pressure of 180/100 mm Hg or less. For patients with blood pressures >180/100 mm Hg, the procedure, if not urgent or emergent in nature, should be rescheduled so that further evaluation by a primary care physician or hypertension specialist may take place. A component of observed hypertension could be secondary to anxiety as well as the "white coat phenomenon" which can be effectively mitigated with use of low dose anxiolytics and nonmedical interventions such as music and maintaining a calm surgical environment. Patients should also be reminded to continue taking their prescribed antihypertensive medications on the day of surgery.

CARDIOVASCULAR DISEASE

Three main considerations in patients with cardiovascular disease undergoing dermatologic surgery are anticoagulation, implantable cardiac devices, and prophylactic antibiotics for endocarditis. These patients are often prescribed antiplatelet agents, for example, aspirin and clopidogrel, for primary and secondary prevention of coronary artery disease, or to prevent stenosis of coronary artery stents. Patients with atrial fibrillation or prosthetic valves may receive anticoagulation with warfarin to prevent clot formation, thromboembolic events, and valve failure. In general, all of these agents should be continued, since their discontinuation in patients undergoing dermatologic surgery has been associated with catastrophic thrombotic adverse events such as myocardial infarctions and stent restenosis (see Anticoagulants section under medications). Discontinuation of any prescribed anticoagulants should be discussed with and cleared by the patient's primary care physician or cardiologist. Although these agents may increase the risk of bleeding, the reported complications are often localized and not life threatening. Thus, the risks of stopping anticoagulants usually outweigh potential benefits. Rare exceptions may include patients undergoing major reconstructions such as free flaps. In such cases, decisions regarding perioperative anticoagulation can be made with input from the entire physician team. More detailed information on the specific agent and recommended management can be found in the "Anticoagulants" section. Appropriate endocarditis prophylaxis is discussed in the section on prophylactic antibiotics.

STENTS

Dual antiplatelet therapy with aspirin and typically clopidogrel is recommended for patients with recently placed bare metal or drug eluting stents as treatment for coronary arterial disease. Patients with bare metal stents should continue taking aspirin and clopidogrel for at least 1 month after stent placement, while those with drug eluting stents should be on these agents for at least 1 year after the procedure to prevent stent thrombosis.[10] Current published guidelines recommend continuation of dual antiplatelet therapy for all dermatologic procedures, including Mohs micrographic surgery with extensive reconstruction.[11–13] Elective procedures can be delayed until the patient has finished the recommended course of dual antiplatelet therapy. If medically necessary procedures in highly vascularized areas are required, one might consult the managing cardiologist to consider holding clopidogrel therapy for 1 week or ticlopidine for 2 weeks prior to the procedure.

IMPLANTABLE CARDIAC DEVICES

Implantable cardiac devices include pacemakers, defibrillators, and cardiac synchronization therapy devices. Indications for pacemakers include heart blocks, bradycardia, and atrial fibrillation. Defibrillators are indicated for primary prevention of arrhythmias in patients with heart failure, and secondary prevention for ventricular arrhythmias. Cardiac resynchronization therapy devices are designed to improve symptoms in patients with advanced heart failure through the use of ventricular synchronization. These devices contain sensing leads that connect to the patient's cardiac tissue and a pulse generator that discharges electrical signals to treat detected arrhythmias. Electromagnetic interference from electrosurgical devices can either impair the sensing capabilities of the leads or trigger inappropriate electrical discharges from the pulse generator.

The most commonly used electrosurgical device in dermatologic surgery is the hyfrecator, which generates low power, high frequency alternating current through an electrode that can either be monoterminal or biterminal. The hyfrecator itself can transmit current through the tissue through one or two prongs, that is, monopolar or bipolar, respectively. Less electrical current passes through the patient with a bipolar hyfrecator. As a result, recommendations for patients with implantable cardiac devices have included use of handheld bipolar electrocautery, short bursts of current, temporary deactivation of cardiac devices with magnets, intraoperative cardiac monitoring, and postoperative device function testing to reduce the risk of electromagnetic interference.

Recent experimental data, however, suggest that the hyfrecator is safe to use in patients with implantable cardiac devices. Weyer et al. tested the electromagnetic interference of two commonly used hyfrecators on six Medtronic devices (three pacemakers and three defibrillators) using an industry standard saline–collagen gel model that simulates human soft-tissue conduction. Tested settings include monoterminal and biterminal configurations, typical and maximum power (10 and 30 W, respectively), intermittent on/off and continuous on modes, with various distances between the hyfrecators and the cardiac devices. There was no electromagnetic interference at any of the tested settings for the defibrillators and no accidental discharge of electrical currents. Inhibition of ventricular pacing was noted at a distance of 1 cm, and of atrial pacing at 3 cm. The authors prospectively used hyfrecators for hemostasis in 40 patients with cardiac devices and noted no adverse events.[14]

Based on these data, hyfrecators may be safely used within 2 in of cardiac devices without the need for biterminal configuration, intraoperative cardiac monitoring or postoperative testing of device function. Routine dermatologic surgery utilizing only the hyfrecator for hemostasis and electrodesiccation is generally safe for all patients with pacemakers and defibrillators when the surgical site is more than 2 in away from the cardiac devices.

BLEEDING DISORDERS

The three most common congenital coagulation disorders are von Willebrand disease, factor VIII deficiency (hemophilia A), and factor IX (hemophilia B).[15] A bleeding diathesis often presents as slow but persistent oozing from multiple operative sites rather than as localized rapid bleeding. Patients with von Willebrand disease have a 10% risk of clinically significant bleeding from a decreased quantity or quality of von Willebrand factor, which provides binding sites for platelets and factor VIII. Treatment with desmopressin, 1-desamino-8-arginine vasopressin (DDAVP), or select factor VIII concentrates is typically indicated for 1 day before and 3 to 5 days after minor surgery and up to 10 days after major surgery. The patient's bleeding time should be corrected to 100% of normal for the perioperative period. For hemophilia A and B, factor VIII and factor IX concentrates, respectively, can be infused to raise factor levels to 100% of normal preoperatively and 30% to 50% postoperatively during the wound healing phase.[15] Preoperative evaluation should elicit a hemostasis history after prior surgical procedures since laboratory studies such as bleeding time, PTT, and PT cannot reliably predict intra- and postoperative bleeding. Consultation with hematology services is highly recommended for appropriate clinical and laboratory preoperative evaluation, as well as for management of transfusion products during the perioperative period. Meticulous hemostasis, minimizing undermining, and frequent postoperative follow-up are also helpful in reducing the risks of serious bleeding complications in this patient population.

BLOOD-BORNE INFECTION—HEPATITIS AND HIV

With continuing improvements in antiretroviral therapies and supportive care, patients with HIV now have a significantly longer life expectancy and are therefore more commonly encountered in the outpatient and surgical settings. Higher risks of postoperative surgical site infections in patients with HIV are often assumed but there is little available data to confirm this hypothesis. A multicenter prospective cohort study in Italy examining the incidence of surgical site infection in HIV patients undergoing a variety of inpatient surgical procedures revealed a 10% rate of infection overall and a 12.5% rate of infection following plastic/dermatologic surgical procedures. Antibiotic prophylaxis use varied widely among the surgical subspecialties, ranging from 50% of patients undergoing plastic/dermatologic surgical interventions, up to nearly 100% in patients undergoing cesarean sections or thoracic surgeries.[16] However, there were no data on infection rates in non-HIV patients or outpatient surgical procedures in this study, which precludes extrapolation of these data to outpatient dermatologic surgery. A meta-analysis of orthopedic surgery studies showed no statistically significant differences in the incidence of surgical site infection between HIV and non-HIV patients.[17] Given the paucity of data supporting an increased risk of infection in HIV patients, antibiotic prophylaxis for this patient population in the setting of routine outpatient dermatologic surgery is not currently recommended.

Aside from patient safety, one must also consider personnel safety when performing surgical procedures on patients with HIV, hepatitis B or hepatitis C infections. A survey of Mohs micrographic surgeons revealed an astonishingly high 65% rate of needlestick and other exposure injury within the past year, with 5% reporting exposure to patients with HIV or hepatitis. Strategies such as use of double gloves for surgeons, assistants, and laboratory technicians, formal training of laboratory personnel, and warning labels on surgical trays are associated with lower relative risk of exposure injuries. Warning labels on the patient's chart, though used by almost half of surveyed surgeons, did not impact the risk of injuries.[18] Universal precautions are recommended since depending on the clinical setting and patient population, the rate of undiagnosed HIV or hepatitis infection can be as high as 10%.[19]

MEDICATIONS

Polypharmacy, defined as using five or more prescription medications, is especially prevalent in the elderly population, with 29% of patients over the age of 65 taking 10 or more medications in a week.[20] Polypharmacy increases the risks of drug adverse events; one-third of these events relate to the use of insulin, digoxin, or warfarin.[21] Hemorrhagic complications account for nearly one in five adverse events. The remaining adverse effects result from electrolyte, metabolic, and gastrointestinal disturbances.[22] Efforts should be made to obtain an accurate and complete medication list from patients undergoing dermatologic surgery to ensure appropriate medication monitoring. Adjustments to certain medications to reduce the risks of bleeding, blood pressure lability, poor glycemic control, and altered mental status may be indicated. Specific questions regarding the use of anticoagulants and antiplatelet agents, corticosteroids, immunosuppressants, over the counter medications, and herbal supplements should be included in any preoperative questionnaire. Management of these classes of medications is detailed below.

Anticoagulants. Management of anticoagulants in the perioperative period has changed significantly in the past several years. In the past, withholding these agents before and after the procedure was common. Now, consensus guidelines recommend continuation of these agents in the vast majority of patients undergoing dermatologic surgeries, since the risks of catastrophic thrombotic events associated with their discontinuation far outweigh the increased risk of bleeding complications.

The list of medications that affect platelet function and the coagulation cascade continues to grow (Table 2-2). Aspirin and thienopyridines (e.g., clopidogrel, ticlopidine, and prasugrel) inhibit platelet function for the lifespan of the platelets. Heparin, low–molecular-weight heparin (e.g., enoxaparin and dalteparin), direct thrombin inhibitors (e.g., dabigatran, argatroban, and lepirudin), and warfarin all target specific components of the coagulation pathway.[23] Indications for these agents include primary and secondary prevention of cardiac and neurologic thrombotic events, pulmonary embolism, and deep vein thrombosis. The most commonly encountered agents in dermatologic surgery are aspirin, clopidogrel, and warfarin.[24]

Patients on anticoagulants are at increased risk of bleeding complications although the overall absolute risk for these events remains low and none of the reported complications have been life threatening. The risk of severe complications, defined as considerable intra- or postoperative bleeding, acute hematoma, flap or graft necrosis, and dehiscence, was 1.3% for patients taking aspirin, and 5.7% for those taking warfarin based on a meta-analysis of six published studies encompassing approximately 1400 patients.[25] Clopidogrel-containing regimens have a higher risk of severe complications (3%) than aspirin alone (0.5%).[26] A large prospective study on 1900 patients undergoing dermatologic surgeries

TABLE 2-2
Anticoagulants Encountered in Outpatient Setting

Anticoagulant	Mechanism of Action	Duration of Action	Risk of Severe Complication in Cutaneous Surgery	Monitoring
Aspirin	Irreversible inhibition of cyclooxygenase	7–10 d	0.5%–1.3%[25,26]	None
Clopidogrel[a] Ticlopidine Prasugrel	Irreversible inhibition of adenosine diphosphate	7–10 d	3%[a26]	None
Warfarin	Vitamin K antagonist, inhibition of synthesis of factors II, VII, IX, and X	2–5 d	5.7%[25]	PT, INR
LMWH—enoxaparin and dalteparin	Selective inhibition of factor Xa	24 h	N/A	aPTT
Dabigatran, argatroban[a], lepirudin[a]	Selective reversible direct thrombin inhibitor	24 h	N/A	aPTT

[a]Cook-Norris RH, JAAD, 2011—Table 3.

showed that clopidogrel increased bleeding risk by 4.7 fold, warfarin by 10 fold, and both agents by 40 fold.[24] A significantly increased risk of bleeding in patients on two or more anticoagulants compared to those on one or no anticoagulant was confirmed by Shimizu et al.[27] in a large retrospective study involving 1000 patients. No difference in infection rates attributable to use of anticoagulants was noted.

Several new anticoagulants and antiplatelet agents have entered the market in the last 5 years. Three new oral anticoagulants, designed to replace warfarin, have been approved for stroke and systemic embolism prevention in patients with atrial fibrillation: dabigatran, rivaroxaban, and apixaban. No data exist on the effects of these agents on bleeding risk during or after cutaneous surgery. However, Healey et al. compared the periprocedural bleeding rates in 4591 patients on dabigatran (110 mg or 150 mg) or warfarin undergoing at least one invasive procedure, including pacemaker/defibrillator insertion, dental procedures, diagnostic procedures, cataract removal, colonoscopy, and joint replacement. They found no statistically significant differences in bleeding rates among those taking dabigatran 110 mg po daily, 150 mg po daily or warfarin (3.8%, 5.1%, and 4.6%, respectively).[28] Similarly, rivaroxaban appears to have a statistically equivalent risk of major bleeding to warfarin, 3.6% versus 3.4%, in a multicenter randomized controlled trial (RCT) with over 14,000 patients.[29] Apixaban, the latest approved oral anticoagulant, has a slightly lower reported risk of major bleeding compared to warfarin, 2.1% versus 3.09% in an RCT study of over 18,000 patients[30] and a risk of major and clinically relevant nonmajor bleeding events comparable to that of aspirin (4.5% vs. 3.8%) in a randomized study of stroke prevention with 5599 patients.[31] On the basis of these data, management of these three new oral anticoagulants should mirror that of warfarin for cutaneous surgeries, namely, continuation of the agents if they are prescribed as monotherapy, unless patient comorbidities and extent of planned surgery warrant discussion with the prescribing physician regarding consideration of a brief interruption in therapy.

The management of new antiplatelet agents, prasugrel and ticagrelor, is similarly based on comparative data against clopidogrel. Prasugrel functions in a manner similar to that of clopidogrel but has higher potency. In animal models, prasugrel inhibition of platelet aggregation was 10 and 100 times more potent than that of clopidogrel and ticlopidine, respectively.[32] Clinically, this agent has a higher documented risk of fatal bleeding and the need for transfusion in a study of 13,608 patients undergoing percutaneous cardiac intervention for acute coronary syndrome.[33] On the other hand, ticagrelor, a reversible antiplatelet aggregation agent, has demonstrated a risk of severe bleeding equivalent to that of clopidogrel, 2.9% versus 3.2%, in an RCT study of 13,408 patients.[34] Consultation with cardiology regarding the perioperative management of these two agents is prudent, particularly in the case of patients taking prasugrel who may have a higher bleeding risk than those taking clopidogrel.

Heparin and low–molecular-weight heparin preparations, such as enoxaparin and dalteparin, are associated with higher risks of bleeding in patients undergoing cardiac and gynecological surgeries. However, because of their intramuscular and intravenous administration, these agents are relatively rarely seen in the outpatient setting where dermatologic surgeries are conducted.

Although anticoagulants increase the risks of bleeding and severe complications, discontinuation of these agents can result in catastrophic life-threatening thromboembolic events. There have been case reports of stroke, TIA, pulmonary embolism, DVT, MI, clotted prosthetic aortic valve, and retinal artery occlusion occurring shortly after discontinuation of anticoagulants for dermatologic surgery.[35–37] These events are thought to be secondary to a rebound hypercoagulable state due to more rapid depletion of antithrombotic protein C and S relative to clotting factors during the first few days of anticoagulant reinitiation.[38] Given that the risk of thromboembolic events outweighs the risk of bleeding from dermatologic surgery, prescribed monotherapy aspirin, clopidogrel, and warfarin should be continued in the perioperative period. For patients taking both aspirin and clopidogrel, or aspirin and warfarin, or clopidogrel and warfarin, elective procedures should be delayed until one or both of the agents are no longer medically indicated. For medically necessary procedures, the surgeon should discuss the situation with the prescribing physician to determine whether one of the agents can be safely discontinued. For monitoring of warfarin, older studies suggested that checking INR within 24 hours of surgery and use of a target INR goal of <3.5 could minimize the risks of intra- and postoperative bleeding.[39] However, even with an INR <3.5, patients on warfarin still have an increased risk of bleeding compared to patients not taking anticoagulants.[40] Appropriate surgical techniques should be employed to minimize intra- and postoperative bleeding in these cases.

In summary, all prescribed monotherapy anticoagulants and antiplatelets should be continued for dermatologic surgeries. Aspirin may only be discontinued if it is self-prescribed by the patient or used solely for pain relief. For patients on combination therapy with two or more agents, discussion with the managing physicians is warranted to determine whether any of those agents can be safely discontinued. Appropriate laboratory monitoring, meticulous surgical techniques, and close follow-up will minimize complications in this patient population.

In our practice, nonprescribed aspirin is discontinued 7 days before and 3 days after the procedure, and a preoperative INR is checked within 24 hours with a target of <3.0. Consultation with the managing physician is standard for patients on two or more anticoagulants to determine whether discontinuation of one or more agents is feasible to reduce the risk of bleeding.

CORTICOSTEROIDS

Chronic corticosteroid use carries two particular concerns relating to dermatologic surgery: (1) hypothalamus–pituitary axis (HPA) suppression requiring supplement stresses dose of steroids and (2) poor wound healing. HPA suppression can occur in patients receiving prednisone 20 mg po or higher dosing daily for more than 3 weeks. These patients should be continued on their normal daily prednisone dose and should receive additional corticosteroid for anticipated surgical stress, the dosing of which depends on the extent of the surgery. Superficial procedures such as skin biopsies and short procedures <1 hour in duration under local anesthesia typically do not require supplementation. For minor procedures or those that last longer than 1 hour, supplemental hydrocortisone 25 mg po once should be considered on the day of the surgery.[41] These recommendations are based on general surgery data since little data exist in the dermatologic surgery literature regarding perioperative steroid management. Chronic glucocorticoid use also interferes with multiple phases of healing, leading to delayed wound healing and an increased risk of infection.[42] Even mid- to high-strength fluorinated topical steroids can delay wound healing through impairment of reepithelialization, collagen formation, and angiogenesis.[43] Patients should be made aware of these potential complications prior to surgery so that nonessential topical steroid use may be discontinued.

RETINOIDS

Chemoprophylaxis with acitretin does not appear to increase the risks of infection, hypertrophic granulation tissue, scars, or dehiscence in organ transplant recipients undergoing Mohs or surgical excisions for nonmelanoma skin cancers.[44] Therefore, for nonelective surgeries, therefore, patients may continue taking acitretin in the perioperative period. For ablative resurfacing, the standard of care is discontinuation of isotretinoin for 6 months' preprocedure to avoid the risks of delayed healing and excessive granulation tissue based on the manufacturer's recommendations.[45] Acitretin can be withheld for 20 days prior to the procedure if concerns of similar complications exist, although none have been reported in the literature or by the manufacturer. In our practice, patients on low-dose (25 mg daily or less) acitretin for skin cancer prevention continue on this medication in the pre- and postoperative period surrounding Mohs surgery and reconstruction.

BIOLOGIC RESPONSE MODIFIERS

Biologic response modifiers or tumor necrosis factor (TNF) antagonists such as infliximab, etanercept, and adalimumab are most commonly encountered in patients with psoriasis, inflammatory bowel disease, or inflammatory arthropathies. These medications may increase the risks of opportunistic bacterial, mycobacterial, and fungal infections. However, available data have shown no significant increase in perioperative infections or dehiscence with TNF antagonists in rheumatoid arthritis and inflammatory bowel disease patients undergoing elective ankle and foot surgeries, joint replacements, and, abdominal surgeries.[46,47] Use of TNF antagonists in patients with inflammatory bowel disease actually improved healing of surgical wounds, fistulas, and mucosal ulcerations. A paucity of data exists on the perioperative risks of psoriatic patients on biologic response modifiers. Perioperative management options include continuing these agents with close postoperative follow-up, or discontinuing them 1 week before and 1 to 2 weeks after the surgery.[41,48] Consultation with the managing physician has been recommended for other immunosuppressive agents such as methotrexate, cyclosporine, tacrolimus, azathioprine, and mycophenolate mofetil since usage, dosing, and perioperative management vary depending on disease under treatment and other medical comorbidities. However, skin cancer is common in organ transplant patients who are often on such medications, and dermatologic surgical procedures are performed routinely in such patients without reports of increased complications. Thus, in our practice, no special perioperative considerations are made for patients taking these drugs (other than discussions with the treating team regarding dose reductions to boost immunity in patients who are developing multiple cancers and may, therefore, be overly immunosuppressed).

HERBAL SUPPLEMENTATION

Use of herbal supplements has increased dramatically in the United States, accounting for more than $5 billion

TABLE 2-3
Common Herbal Supplements and Effects on Operative Risk[50]

Herbal Supplement	Possible Effects on Surgical Risk
Garlic	▪ Increased bleeding due to direct antithrombotic effects and increased effects of warfarin, ASA/NSAIDs ▪ Hypotension due to increased effects of antihypertensive drugs
Ginseng	▪ Increased bleeding due to direct anticoagulant effects and increased effects of warfarin, ASA/NSAIDs ▪ Increased blood pressure and heart rate
Ginkgo	▪ Increased bleeding due to direct anticoagulant effects and increased effects of warfarin, ASA/NSAIDs ▪ Hypotension due to vasodilator effects
Ma Huang	▪ Increased bleeding due to inhibition of complement cascade
Vitamin E	▪ Increased bleeding due to inhibition of platelet function and vitamin K-dependent clotting factors
Echinacea	▪ Possible poor wound healing in chronic users

in sales every year. There are more than 20,000 herbal medicines available on the market, with echinacea, garlic, goldenseal, ginseng, ginkgo, aloe, ma huang, St John's wort, valerian, and cranberry as the top selling products. Up to 85% patients with skin diseases report using complementary and alternative medicines, most commonly vitamins and herbal supplements, yet only a fraction of these patients report their use to physicians.[49,50] The physiological effects are not fully understood for the majority of the herbal supplements. Studies on the more commonly prescribed agents have shown interference with hepatic cytochrome P450 enzymes, and interactions with many prescribed medications including anticoagulants, antihypertensives and antidepressants, and clinical effects on the cardiovascular, neurologic, and coagulation systems. These effects may result in prolonged anesthesia, bleeding, cardiovascular, and neurologic instability in the perioperative period (Table 2-3).[50,51] Given these potential complications, the American Society of Anesthesiologists recommends discontinuation of all herbal medications for 2 weeks prior to surgery under general anesthesia. Although no consensus recommendations exist regarding dermatologic surgery, advising patients to discontinue all herbal supplements 1 to 2 weeks before procedures such as excisions and Mohs micrographic surgery would be reasonable.

SOCIAL HABITS: ALCOHOL AND SMOKING

Alcohol may increase bleeding tendencies through inhibition of platelet aggregation, decreasing clotting factors, and increasing fibrinolysis and vasodilation.[52] Patients may therefore be instructed to stop or reduce alcohol intake 48 hours before and after surgery.

Smoking has not been definitively shown to increase the risk of surgical complications in patients undergoing routine dermatologic surgery. Large scale meta-analyses comparing complication rates between smokers and nonsmokers undergoing general surgery have found that smokers have an approximately four times higher risk of tissue necrosis, and a two times higher risk of surgical site infection, dehiscence, and healing delay. Former smokers have a significantly lower risk of surgical complications compared to current smokers but still higher than that of nonsmokers.[53] However, prospective 5 year data on surgical excisions of over 7000 skin lesions in 4100 patients revealed no difference in the rates of infection, bleeding, dehiscence, or flap/graft necrosis between smokers and nonsmokers. The same conclusions held when the two groups were matched for age, gender, geographic location, and outdoor occupational exposure. The total complication rate was approximately 4% for both groups.[54] Although smoking has deleterious effects on the overall health of the patient, it does not definitively increase complication rates in patients undergoing dermatologic surgery. Perioperative smoking cessation has produced mixed results in terms of reducing complications in smokers undergoing general surgery. Patients who stopped smoking 4 to 8 weeks before and 2 to 4 weeks after the surgical procedure had a reduction in surgical site infections but not in healing complications.[53]

ANTIBIOTIC PROPHYLAXIS

Prophylactic antibiotics serve two purposes: (1) to prevent local surgical site infection and (2) to reduce bacteremia resulting in endocarditis and prosthetic joint infections. Recent years have seen a shift away from routine prescription of prophylactic antibiotics, given that the risks of adverse effects from antibiotics outweigh their benefits in most cases based on available data. If a decision is made to provide antibiotic prophylaxis, it must be given within 1 hour of the procedure to ensure biologic availability at the time of incision. Topical antiseptics, surgical field preparation and maintenance, sterile equipment during wound closure, and surgical technique have a greater influence on risk of surgical site infection than the presence or absence of antibiotic prophylaxis.

TABLE 2-4

Dermatologic Procedures with High Risk of Surgical Site Infection[a]

Any procedure breaching oral mucosa
Any procedure involving infected skin or musculoskeletal tissue
High risk of local surgical site infection based on ▪ Anatomical site: lower legs, groin ▪ Reconstruction: grafts, wedge excision on the ear or lip

[a]Based on published guidelines from American Board of Dermatology and American Society of Dermatologic Surgeons.[57,58]

PROPHYLAXIS AGAINST LOCAL SURGICAL SITE INFECTION

The risk of surgical site infection in dermatologic surgery is quite low, ranging from 1% to 2% for excisions and Mohs micrographic surgery in multiple studies.[55] Medical comorbidities, smoking status, alcohol consumption, location and extent of tumor, and reconstruction techniques have been examined as potential factors influencing the risk of surgical site infection. Conflicting data on the degree of risk attributable to these factors make establishing consensus guidelines challenging. Diabetic patients and smokers do not necessarily have higher infection risks, as previously discussed. Surgeries on the lower legs or in the groin, wedge excisions of the lip and ear, and reconstruction with grafts carry a > 5% risk of infection based on prospective data from 5000 lesions in 2400 patients from a single practice in Australia.[4] However, prospective cohort data from the United States on 1000 patients undergoing Mohs micrographic surgery showed a culture proven infection rate of only 0.7% overall, and 3.1% for nose flaps.[56] Antibiotic prophylaxis to reduce local surgical site infections may be considered on an individual basis for surgeries on the lower legs and in the groin, wedge excisions, and grafts based on the overall clinical assessment of the patient and procedure (Table 2-4). Universal prophylaxis for all patients under these circumstances is not currently supported by available data.

The choice of antibiotic depends on the organisms that need to be covered, which varies with body location (Table 2-5). Most skin flora, such as *Staphylococcus* and *Streptococcus* species, can be treated adequately with cephalexin. Amoxicillin is the preferred agent for procedures that involve the oral mucosa. Patients with penicillin allergy may take levofloxacin for surgeries in the groin or on the lower extremities, and clindamycin or azithromycin for surgeries in other sites.[57] When local surgical site infection is suspected, a clinical evaluation should be performed and a culture should be obtained, followed by empiric treatment with penicillin- or cephalosporin-based antibiotics unless there is a high clinical index of suspicion for infection with methicillin-resistant *Staphylococcus aureus* (MRSA). The incidence of hospital and community acquired MRSA skin and soft-tissue infections has increased in recent years, especially in elderly, African–American, and male patients, and those with a history of hospitalization or surgeries in the previous year.[59] Rates of MRSA infection also vary between geographic locations and communities. For patients with a history of MRSA infection or colonization, clindamycin or trimethoprim-sulfamethoxazole may be used for empiric coverage for MRSA pending culture sensitivity results.[57]

PROPHYLAXIS AGAINST ENDOCARDITIS

Bacteremia from surgical procedures can lead to endocarditis in high-risk patients with specific valvular or cardiac defects. The American Heart Association narrowed its definition of patients at high risk for infective endocarditis in 2007 to include only those with prosthetic heart valves, cardiac transplantation with valvulopathy, cyanotic congenital heart defects that are unrepaired or repaired in the previous 6 months, or history of infective endocarditis (Table 2-6). Patients with mitral valve prolapse, rheumatic heart disease, bicuspid valve disease, calcified aortic stenosis, septal defects, and hypertrophic cardiomyopathy are no longer considered high risk. Furthermore, high-risk patients should only receive infective endocarditis prophylaxis when undergoing high-risk surgical procedures, namely surgeries involving the oral mucosa or clinically infected skin and musculoskeletal tissue.[60] The vast majority of dermatologic surgeries do not require infective endocarditis antibiotic prophylaxis even for high-risk patients. Immunocompetent patients undergoing excisions and Mohs micrographic surgery have a 1% to 3% risk of transient bacteremia,[61] a significantly lower risk than that from routine activities such as brushing teeth and eating.[62] Antibiotic prophylaxis has not been shown to protect patients from endocarditis resulting from these rare transient bacteremias. Moreover, antibiotics have a

TABLE 2-5

Antibiotic Prophylaxis for Prevention of Local Surgical Site Infection

Surgical Site	Antibiotic
Groin and lower legs	Cephalexin 2 g po ***If penicillin allergic:*** TMP-SMX-DS 1 tablet po ***OR*** Levofloxacin 500 mg po
Wedge excisions of ear or lip, grafts, nose flaps	Cephalexin 2 g po ***OR*** Dicloxacillin 2 g po ***If penicillin allergic:*** Clindamycin 600 mg po, ***OR*** Azithromycin or Clarithromycin 500 mg po

Source: Data from published guidelines from American Board of Dermatology, 2008.

TABLE 2-6
Conditions with High Risk of Infective Endocarditis

Prosthetic cardiac valves
History of infective endocarditis
Cardiac transplant recipients who develop valvulopathy
Cyanotic congenital heart defects that are unrepaired, repaired within last 6 mo, or with residual defects at or near prostheses

Source: Data from American Heart Association consensus guidelines, 2007.[60]

long list of potential side effects including gastrointestinal disturbance, drug interactions, cutaneous eruptions, anaphylactic reactions, and drug resistance. Adherence to the published guidelines will reduce the number of patients receiving unnecessary antibiotics without compromising overall protection against infective endocarditis.

PROPHYLAXIS AGAINST HEMATOGENOUS JOINT INFECTION

Total prosthetic joint infection may result from transient bacteremia during surgery, or more commonly from late onset bacteremia secondary to local surgical site infection.[63] The occurrence of either scenario may be reduced with preoperative antibiotic prophylaxis. The same principle guides antibiotic prophylaxis for joint infection as for infective endocarditis: prophylaxis is indicated only in high-risk patients undergoing high-risk procedures. Patients with an increased risk of prosthetic joint infection are generally those with prior joint infections, or a history of insulin-dependent diabetes, malignancy, or immunosuppression. Recognized causes of immunosuppression include inflammatory arthropathies such as systemic lupus erythematosus and rheumatoid arthritis, immunosuppressive medications, radiation, HIV infection, poor nutritional status, and hemophilia (Table 2-7). Patients at high risk of prosthetic joint infection require antibiotic prophylaxis when undergoing surgeries involving oral mucosa, infected skin and tissues, or procedures with high risk of local surgical site infections.[64] Assessment of surgical site infection risk was previously discussed in detail, but mainly takes into account anatomical sites such as legs and groin, and reconstruction with grafts. Routine antibiotic prophylaxis for all patients with prosthetic joints is not recommended for any other procedures including Mohs micrographic surgery. Patients with orthopedic pins, plates, or screws also do not require antibiotic prophylaxis.[57] At postoperative follow-up, both the surgical site and the area with joint prosthesis should be inspected for redness, pain, swelling, and warmth as signs of infection. Suspected local surgical site infection in patients with a prosthetic joint must be aggressively treated with initial empiric therapy designed to cover *S. aureus* and beta-hemolytic streptococci. The definitive antibiotic choice should ultimately be guided by sensitivity results from cultures.

TABLE 2-7
Patients at High Risk of Prosthetic Joint Infection

All patients soon after prosthetic joint surgery
History of prosthetic joint infection
Insulin-dependent diabetes
HIV infection
Malignancy
Inflammatory arthropathies (lupus, rheumatoid arthritis)
Drug or radiation-induced immunosuppression
Hemophilia
Poor nutritional status

Source: Data from American Association of Orthopedic Surgeons consensus guidelines, 2009.

CONSENSUS STATEMENT: PROPHYLACTIC ANTIBIOTICS

An advisory statement published by the Journal of the American Academy of Dermatology in 2008 recommended prophylactic antibiotics for high-risk patients with surgical sites that are infected or involving oral mucosa. Antibiotics may also be considered in patients with severe inflammatory dermatoses, grafts, flaps on the nose, wedge excisions of the ear or lip, and surgeries on the lower extremities or in the groin, to decrease the risk of surgical site infection.[57]

At our procedural dermatology and Mohs micrographic surgery center in a tertiary care academic institution, prophylactic antibiotics to prevent surgical site infection are routinely used only in patients with infected wounds (although surgery is usually delayed in such cases until infection has resolved), patients with extensive inflammatory skin diseases, or oral flaps/grafts. Saline irrigation is used prior to closure of all wounds. For prevention of infective endocarditis and hematogenous total joint infection, antibiotics are prescribed only for high-risk patients undergoing surgery involving the oral mucosa, groin, lower legs, or infected skin. Cephalexin 2 g po is the preferred antibiotic for cutaneous cases, and amoxicillin 2 g po for mucosal cases. Clindamycin 600 mg po or levofloxacin 500 mg po are alternatives for patients with penicillin allergies (Table 2-8).

Given that the guidelines for antibiotic prophylaxis for infective endocarditis and hematogenous prosthetic joint infection have undergone significant changes in recent years, patients may have come to expect antibiotic prophylaxis even when it is no longer indicated. Consultation with the patient's managing cardiologist or orthopedic surgeon to determine whether extenuating circumstances exist, as well as discussion of the treatment guidelines and patient education will help to clarify the appropriate course of action.

TABLE 2-8
Antibiotic Prophylaxis for Prevention of Infective Endocarditis or Total Prosthetic Joint Infection

Surgical Site	Antibiotic
Skin	Cephalexin 2 g po ***If penicillin allergic:*** Azithromycin or Clarithromycin 500 mg po ***OR*** Clindamycin 600 mg po
Oral mucosa	Amoxicillin 2 g po ***If penicillin allergic:*** Azithromycin or Clarithromycin 500 mg po ***OR*** Clindamycin 600 mg po

Source: Data from published guidelines from American Board of Dermatology, 2008.

CONCLUSION

This chapter has reviewed the major preoperative considerations of which surgeons should be aware prior to performing dermatologic surgical procedures, as well as current data and recommendations regarding antibiotic prophylaxis. Standardized checklists summarizing this information can be helpful in alerting physicians to their patients' medical conditions preoperatively, so that appropriate evaluation and/or action can be taken, and complications can be avoided. Physicians can use this preoperative screening to adjust care as needed in accordance with each individual patient's needs, thereby optimizing both patient safety and outcomes in the dermatologic surgical setting.

REFERENCES

1. McGinness JL, Goldstein G. The value of preoperative biopsy-site photography for identifying cutaneous lesions. *Dermatol Surg.* 2010;36(2):194–197.
2. Starling J III, Coldiron BM. Outcome of 6 years of protocol use for preventing wrong site office surgery. *J Am Acad Dermatol.* 2011;65(4):807–810.
3. National Diabetes Fact Sheet. National estimates and general information on diabetes and prediabetes in the United States, 2011. 2011. http://www.cdc.gov/diabetes/pubs/estimates14.htm. Accessed July 2014.
4. Dixon AJ, Dixon MP, Askew DA, Wilkinson D. Prospective study of wound infections in dermatologic surgery in the absence of prophylactic antibiotics. *Dermatol Surg.* 2006;32(6):819–826; discussion 826–827.
5. Heal CF, Buettner PG, Drobetz H. Risk factors for surgical site infection after dermatological surgery. *Int J Dermatol.* 2012; 51(7):796–803.
6. Dixon AJ, Dixon MP, Dixon JB. Prospective study of skin surgery in patients with and without known diabetes. *Dermatol Surg.* 2009;35(7):1035–1040.
7. Straith RE, Raju DR, Hipps CJ. The study of hematomas in 500 consecutive face lifts. *Plast Reconstr Surg.* 1977;59(5): 694–698.
8. Howell SJ, Sear JW, Foex P. Hypertension, hypertensive heart disease and perioperative cardiac risk. *Br J Anaesth.* 2004; 92(4):570–583.
9. Larson MJ, Taylor RS. Monitoring vital signs during outpatient Mohs and post-Mohs reconstructive surgery performed under local anesthesia. *Dermatol Surg.* 2004;30(5):777–783.
10. Levine GN, Bates ER, Blankenship JC, et al. 2011 ACCF/AHA/SCAI Guideline for Percutaneous Coronary Intervention: executive summary: a report of the American College of Cardiology Foundation/American Heart Association Task Force on Practice Guidelines and the Society for Cardiovascular Angiography and Interventions. *Circulation.* 2011; 124(23):2574–25609.
11. Chu MB, Turner RB, Kriegel DA. Patients with drug-eluting stents and management of their anticoagulant therapy in cutaneous surgery. *J Am Acad Dermatol.* 2011;64(3):553–558.
12. Douketis JD, Berger PB, Dunn AS, et al; American College of Chest Physicians. The perioperative management of antithrombotic therapy: American College of Chest Physicians Evidence-Based Clinical Practice Guidelines (8th Edition). *Chest.* 2008;133(6 Suppl):299S–339S.
13. Korte W, Cattaneo M, Chassot PG, et al. Peri-operative management of antiplatelet therapy in patients with coronary artery disease: joint position paper by members of the working group on Perioperative Haemostasis of the Society on Thrombosis and Haemostasis Research (GTH), the working group on Perioperative Coagulation of the Austrian Society for Anesthesiology, Resuscitation and Intensive Care (OGARI) and the Working Group Thrombosis of the European Society for Cardiology (ESC). *Thromb Haemost.* 2011;105(5):743–749.
14. Weyer C, Siegle RJ, Eng GG. Investigation of hyfrecators and their in vitro interference with implantable cardiac devices. *Dermatol Surg.* 2012;38(11):1843–1848.
15. Peterson SR, Joseph AK. Inherited bleeding disorders in dermatologic surgery. *Dermatol Surg.* 2001;27(10):885–889.
16. Drapeau CM, Pan A, Bellacosa C, et al. Surgical site infections in HIV-infected patients: results from an Italian prospective multicenter observational study. *Infection.* 2009;37(5): 455–460.
17. Kigera JW, Straetemans M, Vuhaka SK, Nagel IM, Naddumba EK, Boer K. Is there an increased risk of post-operative surgical site infection after orthopaedic surgery in HIV patients? A systematic review and meta-analysis. *PLoS One.* 2012; 7(8):e42254.
18. LoPiccolo MC, Balle MR, Kouba DJ. Safety precautions in Mohs micrographic surgery for patients with known blood-borne infections: a survey-based study. *Dermatol Surg.* 2012;38(7 Pt 1):1059–1065.
19. Seamon MJ, Ginwalla R, Kulp H, et al. HIV and hepatitis in an urban penetrating trauma population: unrecognized and untreated. *J Trauma.* 2011;71(2):306–310; discussion 311.
20. Qato DM, Alexander GC, Conti RM, Johnson M, Schumm P, Lindau ST. Use of prescription and over-the-counter medications and dietary supplements among older adults in the United States. *JAMA.* 2008;300(24):2867–2878.
21. Budnitz DS, Pollock DA, Weidenbach KN, Mendelsohn AB, Schroeder TJ, Annest JL. National surveillance of emergency department visits for outpatient adverse drug events. *JAMA.* 2006;296(15):1858–1866.
22. Gurwitz JH, Field TS, Harrold LR, et al. Incidence and preventability of adverse drug events among older persons in the ambulatory setting. *JAMA.* 2003;289(9):1107–1116.
23. Callahan S, Goldsberry A, Kim G, Yoo S. The management of antithrombotic medication in skin surgery. *Dermatol Surg.* 2012;38(9):1417–1426.
24. Bordeaux JS, Martires KJ, Goldberg D, Pattee SF, Fu P, Maloney ME. Prospective evaluation of dermatologic surgery complications including patients on multiple antiplatelet and anticoagulant medications. *J Am Acad Dermatol.* 2011; 65(3):576–583.
25. Lewis KG, Dufresne RG Jr. A meta-analysis of complications attributed to anticoagulation among patients following

cutaneous surgery. *Dermatol Surg.* 2008;34(2):160–164; discussion 164–165.
26. Cook-Norris RH, Michaels JD, Weaver AL, et al. Complications of cutaneous surgery in patients taking clopidogrel-containing anticoagulation. *J Am Acad Dermatol.* 2011; 65(3):584–591.
27. Shimizu I, Jellinek NJ, Dufresne RG, Li T, Devarajan K, Perlis C. Multiple antithrombotic agents increase the risk of postoperative hemorrhage in dermatologic surgery. *J Am Acad Dermatol.* 2008;58(5):810–816.
28. Healey JS, Eikelboom J, Douketis J, et al. Periprocedural bleeding and thromboembolic events with dabigatran compared with warfarin: results from the Randomized Evaluation of Long-Term Anticoagulation Therapy (RE-LY) randomized trial. *Circulation.* 2012;126(3):343–348.
29. Patel MR, Mahaffey KW, Garg J, et al; ROCKET AF Investigators. Rivaroxaban versus warfarin in nonvalvular atrial fibrillation. *N Engl J Med.* 2011;365(10):883–891.
30. Granger CB, Alexander JH, McMurray JJ, et al; ARISTOTLE Committees and Investigators. Apixaban versus warfarin in patients with atrial fibrillation. *N Engl J Med.* 2011;365(11):981–992.
31. Flaker GC, Eikelboom JW, Shestakovska O, et al. Bleeding during treatment with aspirin versus apixaban in patients with atrial fibrillation unsuitable for warfarin: the apixaban versus acetylsalicylic acid to prevent stroke in atrial fibrillation patients who have failed or are unsuitable for vitamin K antagonist treatment (AVERROES) trial. *Stroke.* 2012;43(12): 3291–3297.
32. Niitsu Y, Jakubowski JA, Sugidachi A, Asai F. Pharmacology of CS-747 (prasugrel, LY640315), a novel, potent antiplatelet agent with in vivo P2Y12 receptor antagonist activity. *Semin Thromb Hemost.* 2005;31(2):184–194.
33. Hochholzer W, Wiviott SD, Antman EM, et al. Predictors of bleeding and time dependence of association of bleeding with mortality: insights from the Trial to Assess Improvement in Therapeutic Outcomes by Optimizing Platelet Inhibition With Prasugrel–Thrombolysis in Myocardial Infarction 38 (TRITON-TIMI 38). *Circulation.* 2011; 123(23):2681–2689.
34. Cannon CP, Harrington RA, James S, et al. Comparison of ticagrelor with clopidogrel in patients with a planned invasive strategy for acute coronary syndromes (PLATO): a randomised double-blind study. *Lancet.* 2010;375(9711): 283–293.
35. Khalifeh MR, Redett RJ. The management of patients on anticoagulants prior to cutaneous surgery: case report of a thromboembolic complication, review of the literature, and evidence-based recommendations. *Plast Reconstr Surg.* 2006;118(5):110e–117e.
36. Kovich O, Otley CC. Thrombotic complications related to discontinuation of warfarin and aspirin therapy perioperatively for cutaneous operation. *J Am Acad Dermatol.* 2003; 48(2):233–237.
37. Alam M, Goldberg LH. Serious adverse vascular events associated with perioperative interruption of antiplatelet and anticoagulant therapy. *Dermatol Surg.* 2002;28(11):992–998; discussion 998.
38. Grip L, Blomback M, Schulman S. Hypercoagulable state and thromboembolism following warfarin withdrawal in post-myocardial-infarction patients. *Eur Heart J.* 1991;12(11): 1225–1233.
39. Ah-Weng A, Natarajan S, Velangi S, Langtry JA. Preoperative monitoring of warfarin in cutaneous surgery. *Br J Dermatol.* 2003;149(2):386–389.
40. Blasdale C, Lawrence CM. Perioperative international normalized ratio level is a poor predictor of postoperative bleeding complications in dermatological surgery patients taking warfarin. *Br J Dermatol.* 2008;158(3):522–526.
41. Hernandez C, Emer J, Robinson JK. Perioperative management of medications for psoriasis and psoriatic arthritis: a review for the dermasurgeon. *Dermatol Surg.* 2008;34(4):446–459.
42. Karukonda SR, Flynn TC, Boh EE, McBurney EI, Russo GG, Millikan LE. The effects of drugs on wound healing–part II. Specific classes of drugs and their effect on healing wounds. *Int J Dermatol.* 2000;39(5):321–333.
43. Hengge UR, Ruzicka T, Schwartz RA, Cork MJ. Adverse effects of topical glucocorticosteroids. *J Am Acad Dermatol.* 2006;54(1):1–15; quiz 16–18.
44. Tan SR, Tope WD. Effect of acitretin on wound healing in organ transplant recipients. *Dermatol Surg.* 2004;30(4 Pt 2): 667–673.
45. Abdelmalek M, Spencer J. Retinoids and wound healing. *Dermatol Surg.* 2006;32(10):1219–1230.
46. Bibbo C, Goldberg JW. Infectious and healing complications after elective orthopaedic foot and ankle surgery during tumor necrosis factor-alpha inhibition therapy. *Foot Ankle Int.* 2004;25(5):331–335.
47. Colombel JF, Loftus EV Jr, Tremaine WJ, et al. Early postoperative complications are not increased in patients with Crohn's disease treated perioperatively with infliximab or immunosuppressive therapy. *Am J Gastroenterol.* 2004;99(5):878–883.
48. Rosandich PA, Kelley JT III, Conn DL. Perioperative management of patients with rheumatoid arthritis in the era of biologic response modifiers. *Curr Opin Rheumatol.* 2004; 16(3):192–198.
49. Fuhrmann T, Smith N, Tausk F. Use of complementary and alternative medicine among adults with skin disease: updated results from a national survey. *J Am Acad Dermatol.* 2010;63(6):1000–1005.
50. Broughton G II, Crosby MA, Coleman J, Rohrich RJ. Use of herbal supplements and vitamins in plastic surgery: a practical review. *Plast Reconstr Surg.* 2007;119(3):48e–66e.
51. Ang-Lee MK, Moss J, Yuan CS. Herbal medicines and perioperative care. *JAMA.* 2001;286(2):208–216.
52. Salem RO, Laposata M. Effects of alcohol on hemostasis. *Am J Clin Pathol.* 2005;123(Suppl):S96–S105.
53. Sorensen LT. Wound healing and infection in surgery. The clinical impact of smoking and smoking cessation: a systematic review and meta-analysis. *Arch Surg.* 2012;147(4):373–383.
54. Dixon AJ, Dixon MP, Dixon JB, Del Mar CB. Prospective study of skin surgery in smokers vs. nonsmokers. *Br J Dermatol.* 2009;160(2):365–367.
55. Shurman DL, Benedetto AV. Antimicrobials in dermatologic surgery: facts and controversies. *Clin Dermatol.* 2010; 28(5):505–510.
56. Maragh SL, Brown MD. Prospective evaluation of surgical site infection rate among patients with Mohs micrographic surgery without the use of prophylactic antibiotics. *J Am Acad Dermatol.* 2008;59(2):275–278.
57. Wright TI, Baddour LM, Berbari EF, et al. Antibiotic prophylaxis in dermatologic surgery: advisory statement 2008. *J Am Acad Dermatol.* 2008;59(3):464–473.
58. Rossi AM, Mariwalla K. Prophylactic and empiric use of antibiotics in dermatologic surgery: a review of the literature and practical considerations. *Dermatol Surg.* 2012;38(12):1898–1921.
59. Awad SS, Ehabash SI, Lee L, Farrow B, Berger DH. Increasing incidence of methicillin-resistant *Staphylococcus aureus* skin and soft-tissue infections: reconsideration of empiric antimicrobial therapy. *Am J Surg.* 2007;194(5):606–610.
60. Wilson W, Taubert KA, Gewitz M, et al. Prevention of infective endocarditis: guidelines from the American Heart Association: a guideline from the American Heart Association Rheumatic Fever, Endocarditis, and Kawasaki Disease Committee, Council on Cardiovascular Disease in the Young, and the Council on Clinical Cardiology, Council on Cardiovascular Surgery and Anesthesia, and the Quality of Care and Outcomes Research Interdisciplinary Working Group. *Circulation.* 2007;116(15):1736–1754.
61. Carmichael AJ, Flanagan PG, Holt PJ, Duerden BI. The occurrence of bacteraemia with skin surgery. *Br J Dermatol.* 1996;134(1):120–122.
62. Everett ED, Hirschmann JV. Transient bacteremia and endocarditis prophylaxis. A review. *Medicine (Baltimore).* 1977; 56(1):61–77.
63. Berbari EF, Hanssen AD, Duffy MC, et al. Risk factors for prosthetic joint infection: case-control study. *Clin Infect Dis.* 1998;27(5):1247–1254.
64. American Academy of Orthopaedic Surgeons, American Dental Association. *Prevention of Orthopaedic Implant Infection in Patients Undergoing Dental Procedures Guideline.* Rosemont, IL: American Academy of Orthopaedic Surgeons; 2012.

CHAPTER 3

Informed Consent

Tanya Nino, Rachel Epstein, Andrea Smith, & Abel Torres

INTRODUCTION

A physician's duty has been succinctly described in medicine's famous oath "To Do No Harm." Although this concept may seem straightforward, defining harm can be more complex. A physician is in a unique position, possessing knowledge of the possible harm that may occur as a result of a procedure, which must then be communicated to the patient. There are many types of informed consent, which are generally based on the risk of the procedure to be performed. Traditional informed consent depends on the patient's capacity to comprehend and appreciate the nature and consequences of a decision regarding medical treatment; however, even routine situations can be complicated when they involve patients with individual needs and challenges. Our ultimate goal as physicians is to have open communication with informed and engaged patients. We will address how physicians can do their utmost to appropriately inform every patient in their practice about the risks inherent in the procedures that have been recommended for them, with emphasis on ways to improve the informed consent process.

UNDERSTANDING CONSENT: THE BASICS

Obtaining proper consent is of paramount importance in dermatologic surgery. By obtaining consent for treatment, a physician invites the patient to take part in medical decision-making. Consent can fall into the categories shown in Figure 3-1.

Implied consent is typically employed in basic office situations, where a patient's conduct can be considered to be an inferred acceptance of a proposed medical intervention. Examples include the following:

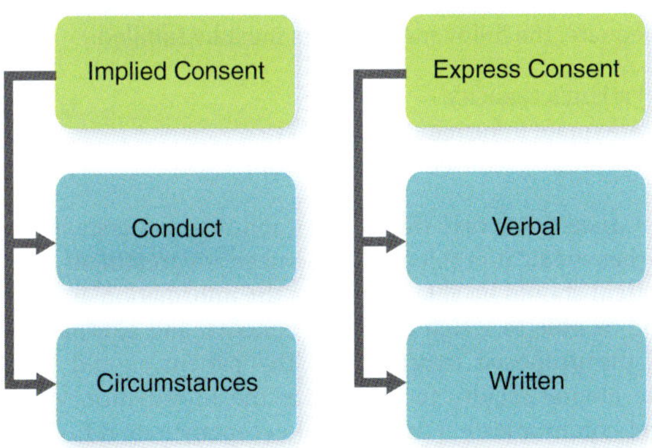

Figure 3-1 Types of consent.

- A patient does not withdraw or object when the medical assistant obtains the vital signs.
- A patient removes his or her shirt to show a skin lesion prior to the examination of the area.
- A patient applies sun block when advised to protect the skin from ultraviolet light.

In these situations, the patient's agreement is assumed by his or her conduct in response to the proposed intervention. This type of implied consent, otherwise known as simple consent, is appropriate for low-risk decisions. Accordingly, it is an accepted practice for the dermatologic surgeon to explain the low-risk intervention in simple terms and to accept the patient's implied consent.[1]

As circumstances become more complex, however, it becomes more precarious to rely on implied consent alone. This is because the burden of proof usually lies with the physician to show that the patient consented through his or her conduct.[2] Even in some low-risk situations, it may be wise to obtain express consent. Examples include the following:

- Performing a physical examination of a sensitive area.
- Low-risk procedures that are potentially painful (i.e., cryotherapy, intralesional injection).
- Prescription medications that pose some risk of an undesirable result (i.e., topical chemotherapy).

In the aforementioned examples, it is prudent at minimum to obtain verbal consent as well as verbalization of understanding from the patient.

As circumstances begin to involve a greater degree of risk to the patient, informed consent with shared decision-making comes to the forefront. Examples include the following:

- Using isotretinoin to treat severe acne in a fertile woman.[1]
- Surgical excision versus topical imiquimod for the treatment of a superficial basal-cell carcinoma on the arm.
- The option of a sentinel lymph node biopsy for a Stage II melanoma.

Often, it is best to obtain written consent from the patient. It is important to remember that informed consent is more than a patient's signature on a form; rather, it encompasses a process during which the physician can explore the patient's needs, values, and beliefs and invite patients to participate in their own healthcare decisions. During this process, physicians should discuss the nature of the medical intervention at length, including the purpose, risks, benefits, and alternatives, after which the patient should explicitly agree to or refuse the proposed intervention.[1]

DEVELOPMENT OF THE INFORMED CONSENT PRINCIPLE: LEGAL BACKGROUND

Informed consent law derives from the principles of human autonomy and self-determination.[3] These basic human rights are fundamental to medical ethics and provide a basis for informed consent and shared decision-making. In addition, the concept of informed consent derives from the intentional torts of *assault* and *battery.* Assault is a volitional act intended to cause another person to fear harmful or offensive contact.[3,4] Battery takes place when there is intentional physical contact to a person against his or her wishes, which a reasonable person would consider harmful or offensive.[3,4] In medical battery cases, the patient (plaintiff) must prove that the unauthorized contact resulted in harm.[3,4] In surgical dermatology, a physician may be subject to allegations of battery under the following circumstances[4,5]:

- The surgeon performs a procedure without a patient's consent.
- The surgeon performs a procedure that is significantly different from the one to which the patient consented.
- The surgeon surpasses the scope of the consent.

As such, obtaining proper consent and acting accordingly are of paramount importance in dermatologic surgery.

The law also recognizes the concept of negligence as a completely separate distinct cause of action from battery law. Medical negligence takes place when a breach of duty occurs that compromises the standard of care and results in unintended harm to the patient. The components required to prove medical negligence are listed in Table 3-1.

Each of these components must be present in order to prove a case of medical negligence. First, physicians have a *duty* of reasonable care to patients to avoid foreseeable risks of harm. Medical malpractice may take place when a treatment falls below the accepted standard of care (*breach of duty*), which results in injury to the patient (*causation and damages*).

Central to the theory of medical negligence is the term *standard of care*, which refers to the conduct and degree of prudence expected of a similarly situated physician in a particular (similar) circumstance. If a plaintiff (patient) brings a claim that informed consent was absent or defective, it must be shown that the defendant (physician) did not conform to the standard of care when disclosing the pertinent risks, benefits, and alternatives of a procedure.[3,4] In other words, one must determine what a reasonably prudent physician in a similar situation would have disclosed regarding the given procedure.[3,4] But what determines the standard against which a defendant may be measured? Many jurisdictions will consider the community standard to be that prevailing within a physician's local geographic area; however, with advances in communication, technology, and electronic documentation, the scope of the duty has expanded. Thus, a physician's "community" may include a national and even an international level.

In addition to determining what a reasonable physician would disclose to a patient, in most jurisdictions it is important to assess what a reasonably prudent patient would have expected in order to make a decision in a given situation, based on the information presented to that patient. Inadequate information could lead a patient to choose an option that results in an unfavorable outcome. This approach means that in most jurisdictions the dermatologic surgeon should disclose all information that a patient would consider material to his or her decision-making.[6]

What makes a risk material? The answer lies in the risk's frequency of occurrence, as well as its severity.[6] It may not be relevant to focus on risks that are remote or unlikely to arise; however, if such risks could have severe consequences, they could become pertinent to the patient.

It is important to keep in mind that damages must also be incurred in order for an action for medical negligence to be present. In other words, even if informed consent was lacking or defective, the other elements of medical negligence must be satisfied in order for a patient to recover damages. This means that the actual injury must have arisen as a result of occurrence of the nondisclosed risk.[6]

TABLE 3-1
Components of Negligence

Duty
Breach of Duty
Causation
Damages

ADEQUATE INFORMED CONSENT: ELEMENTS

Shared decision-making and respect for patient autonomy are the key concepts behind the doctrine of informed consent. The basis for having appropriate informed consent is to promote a patient's self-determination in deciding what can be done to his or her body.[5] In order for consent to be adequate, the following elements must be fulfilled:

- Patient's capacity
- Adequate information
- Freedom to consent (noncoercion)

Capacity refers to the patient's ability to understand his or her medical problem and the need for treatment. The patient should be able to process the information at hand and be able to weigh the risks, benefits, and alternatives of the proposed treatment.[5–7] The patient should have the mental faculty to rationalize the information given and communicate a meaningful acceptance or refusal of that treatment. This hinges on the requirement that the patient be without cognitive impairment. Specifically, a patient's reasoning should not be impaired by medications, substance abuse, psychiatric conditions (i.e., depression, anxiety), or external pressures (such as from family members).[5] Accordingly, patients who have been deemed incompetent secondary to dementia should have their decision-making rights transferred to an authorized surrogate, as is discussed later in this chapter.

When it comes to the actual medical consent document, certain requisites should be present to show that the patient was presented with adequate information. First, there should be an acceptable description of the proposed procedure in terms that are easily understood by the patient. The nature of the patient's illness or injury should be addressed, along with the purpose of the proposed medical intervention. The form should contain the risks and benefits of the proposed procedure with the probability of success. Documentation of alternative treatment options (including the option of no treatment) should be included with the respective advantages and disadvantages. A checklist for an informed consent document is shown in Table 3-2.[2,4–7]

In order for an informed consent to be valid, the patient's consent must be *voluntary*.[5–7] This means that the consent must be given by free will, without any undue persuasion or duress. The patient must not be coerced, meaning that there must be no threats or intimidation involved. While this may seem obvious, it may be considered coercive if one were to exaggerate the risks of harm from foregoing a given treatment, or to mislead the patient through misrepresentation of the facts.[7]

During the informed consent process, a meaningful dialogue should take place, and the physician should assess the patient's values and beliefs. Subject to HIPAA regulations, it may also be appropriate to include family members and healthcare surrogates in the decision-making process so that patients can lean on their support network.[5] Obtaining proper informed consent and ensuring patient comprehension can be an important way to avoid future litigation. Most importantly, the informed consent process is a unique opportunity to build trust between the physician and the patient.

TABLE 3-2
Checklist for the Informed Consent Document

Nature of illness or injury
Description and purpose of procedure
Common, even if not serious, risks
Uncommon but serious risks
Benefits
Probability of success
Alternative strategies
Risks of foregoing treatment
Patient's signature
Physician's signature
Witness' signature
Date of signatures

SPECIAL CIRCUMSTANCES

Central to the spirit of informed consent is the concept that a patient should be able to participate fully. Ideally, patients are able to appreciate their current condition, how the procedural intervention (or lack thereof) will affect their future, the likelihood of expected and unexpected outcomes, and alternatives to the offered treatment that they may consider;[8] however, in the field of medicine, there are circumstances in which the patient is unable to participate in this manner. These circumstances may include occasions when the patient does not have the intellectual capacity to participate, when the patient is a minor, or when the patient refuses the surgical intervention.[8] In these circumstances, much thought and consideration must be devoted to balancing the needs of the patient, respecting the patient's autonomy, and understanding the patient's beliefs and values, so as to guide the decisions that are made.[8]

PATIENTS WHO REFUSE SURGERY

When a patient refuses a recommended intervention, it can be difficult for the physician not to take personal umbrage or question the validity of the patient's decision; nevertheless, the patient should be supported and questioned in order to elicit the reasoning for the decision in a nonthreatening and professional manner.[8] Common reasons for refusal of the procedure can include a "state of indecision" where the patient feels unprepared to make a decision in an immediate time frame, a lack of understanding, consideration of alternative treatments, mistrust of the surgeon, or feelings of anxiety or depression.[8]

For example, when a patient is offered Mohs surgery for a basal-cell carcinoma of the nose, reasons for declining may include: wishing to discuss the diagnosis with family, not understanding the concept of Mohs surgery, wanting to try less invasive treatments such as topical preparations, being concerned about the surgical skills of the physician, or being concerned about the potential impact of the surgery on physical appearance.

If the physician is able to maintain a nonthreatening and supportive atmosphere, he or she may be able to address the patient's specific concerns in a way that results in a reasonable treatment solution and preserves the best interest of the patient.

In the aforementioned example, the following could be options:

- Allowing the patient to return with a family member to discuss the surgery further.
- Drawing diagrams and providing written information detailing what will be expected on the day of Mohs surgery.
- Considering a trial of topical therapy such as 5-fluorouracil or imiquimod with a date set for the lesion to be reevaluated.
- Consideration of referral to another surgical specialist for assistance in the repair of the Mohs surgical defect.
- Discussion of likely repair options so that the patient has a reasonable expectation of possible final results.

With many dermatologic conditions, the outcome of delaying surgery is not life-threatening; therefore, these may be appropriate and acceptable treatment options. However, there are a few circumstances in which delaying surgery can be life-threatening, such as when patients present with a diagnosis of invasive melanoma, Merkel cell carcinoma, or squamous cell carcinoma in high-risk areas. In these circumstances, it is imperative that patients understand the ramifications of their decision to delay or decline treatment. In addition, the physician needs to make a concerted effort to understand the underlying system of values guiding the patient's decision-making process. For certain patients, discussing how a proposed surgical intervention will or will not affect them in the context of their belief system may be essential in determining whether they will accept or decline treatment.

All patients have a value system that drives them toward the goals they have for their lives. Physicians need to make an effort to understand these values so that they can discuss how the surgical intervention does or does not affect them. While physicians usually recommend the "gold standard" for treatment, whether this is the best option for the patient must be considered within the context of the patient's individual circumstances. In declining the procedure, patients may be choosing the option that helps them achieve their values best, even if the cancer poses a significant risk to their health.

Examples where declining the offered treatment may be the most appropriate choice for the patient include the following:

- The patient has other life-threatening conditions that preclude him or her from any life-lengthening benefit from the procedure; for example, a patient who has metastatic colon cancer may reasonably decline treatment for the Merkel cell carcinoma on the scalp in favor of comfort care.
- The patient has had multiple previous treatments of the same type; for example, a patient who has had multiple resections of a melanoma with frequent recurrences thereafter may appropriately decide that he/she does not wish to have further surgeries, even if that decision ultimately results in death.
- There is an alternative treatment that may be adequate even though not first line; for example, a patient with a basal-cell carcinoma on the nose may elect for a trial of topical imiquimod rather than Mohs surgery.

If the physician is not able to determine a reasonable basis for the patient's refusal to consent, it may be reasonable to consider whether the patient has adequate cognitive understanding to decline the procedure.[8] This may prompt the physician to consider a Surrogate Consent or at least an evaluation to determine whether that might be appropriate.

SURROGATE CONSENT

As reviewed earlier, the elements of Informed Consent include Patient's Capacity, Adequate Information, and Freedom to Consent; therefore, in order for any patient to participate fully in informed consent, he or she must be free from any cognitive impairment. In most cases, this is clear, but in some cases it is difficult to determine whether or not a patient has decision-making capacity. Legally, every patient is considered competent or to have the capacity to make autonomous decisions until there is clear evidence that they do not.[9] If a patient is determined not to have the capacity, then a surrogate decision-maker should be sought.

In general, the more high-risk a surgical intervention, the more important it is for the patient to have a high level of capacity;[9] for example, when treating a patient for an actinic keratosis with liquid nitrogen, receiving confirmation from the patient that he or she has a spot that needs treatment may be sufficient. If Mohs surgery for a skin cancer of the temple is planned, however, the patient should have the capacity to understand that there is a risk of nerve damage in addition to other surgical risks in this anatomical area. It is important, therefore, that clinicians assess the patient's capacity or at least recognize signs that warrant further evaluation by someone more experienced. Before determining that a patient lacks the capacity, the physician must have given sufficient information to the patient in a way that is considered "reasonably" understandable,[9] such as the following:

- Describing things in simple terms that are easy to understand.
- Using drawings, diagrams, and other visual aids.
- Discussing the procedure at a time when the patient is most lucid.
- Assuring that there are no language barriers, using translators when necessary.

A study published by Sessums et al.[10] in the *Journal of the American Medical Association* describes four aspects of capacity. These include the following:

- Recognizing your current situation.
- Identifying the consequences of your choices.
- Identifying the important information with relation to important risks, benefits, and alternatives.
- Communicating a choice.

The most common reasons in the United States for a patient's capacity to be questioned include being elderly, mentally ill, or objecting to recommended treatment.[9] All of these groups have unique and complicated needs.

If the patient is determined to lack the capacity for medical decision-making, it is then appropriate to find a person to be the surrogate for giving consent. Often this is an individual who has been legally empowered with full authority for medical decision-making ahead of time. This is usually called Durable Power of Attorney for healthcare. The physician should first determine whether the patient has appointed such a designated person. Another legal alternative is called the Living Will, in which the patient has created a document outlining preferences regarding treatment, should the patient lose the capacity to make these medical decisions.[9] If these arrangements have not been previously made, then a person should be sought out to help make decisions in accordance with the patient's wishes, preferably someone who is intimately familiar with the patient's values. The order in which these individuals usually have priority has been documented in Table 3-3.[9]

TABLE 3-3
Priority of Surrogate Decision-Makers

1. Guardian
2. Spouse
3. Adult Children
4. Parents
5. Adult Siblings
6. Other Close Adults
7. Court-Appointed

It is important to remember that while patients may designate a surrogate to help make their medical decisions, an effort should still be made to develop a joint decision and explain and obtain consent from patients themselves to the degree that they are able.[11]

PEDIATRIC PATIENTS: CONSIDERATIONS

In most states, an individual is considered a Minor until the age of 18 years. Until this threshold is reached, in general the parents or the Legally Authorized Representative (LAR) must give consent for any treatment or procedure.[12,13]

There are some legal exceptions for emergent care and special circumstances such as religious factors where there is precedent for treatment without consent from an LAR. However, these exceptions aside, any treatment or procedure that is done on a minor usually requires informed consent from the LAR with the same requirements as for adults.[12] This does not mean, however, that there should not be an effort to gain the minor's engagement in the decision-making. In fact, every effort should be made on the part of the clinician to include the minor in decision-making appropriate to his or her level of understanding and ability to participate. As in every patient population, care should be taken to approach the consent at a level that can be reasonably understood and not cause undue concern. In the case of a child, this frequently involves employing analogies and very simple language.

For example, if a young child requires a biopsy, informed consent should be obtained from the LAR with the standard information regarding scar, bleeding, and infection. However, cooperation may be obtained from the child with terms such as "bee sting" for the injection and "owie" to describe the biopsy site. Clearly, the level of involvement of children should increase with their age and ability to participate.

Minors present a unique challenge in that they often present for evaluation and treatment without their LAR. Children are often brought in by other family members, caretakers, and noncustodial parents. Careful attention should be paid by the clinician in those circumstances, because if the LAR has not given informed consent, the physician may be held accountable legally for assault as described earlier.[12] If emergent treatment is required or the LAR is not available, then most states frequently have a predetermined hierarchy concerning who will be next in line to give informed consent. An example of this hierarchy is illustrated in Table 3-4.[12,13]

TABLE 3-4
Consent by Proxy

1. Step-parent
2. Grandparent of a Minor
3. Adult Brother/Sister
4. Adult Uncle/Aunt
5. Power of Attorney/Court Appointed

Adolescents are another unique population as they are beginning to function independently and learning to make decisions that affect their personal health. All states have recognized this by writing unique legislation for this age group. Physicians should be aware of the following special circumstances in which the minors are entitled to confidentiality and may legally give their own consent. These include minors who are married or considered emancipated and situations where their reproductive health, mental health, or substance use is concerned.[12] It is important to note that the age at which a patient is considered an adolescent may vary from state to state. Finally, adolescents may also consent to their own treatment when a parent has agreed to confidentiality between the physician and the adolescent.

There is also substantial common law supporting a practice known as the "mature minor law." If an adolescent has been living in a proven responsible manner, he or she is entitled to give his or her own consent; however, this should be carefully scrutinized on a case-by-case basis.[12]

PARTICIPATION OF SUPERVISED TRAINEES

The process of obtaining consent for procedures in which a trainee will be involved presents a unique conundrum for the medical community. It is well established that the common reasonable risks of a procedure should be reviewed with the patient as a part of informed consent. However, the common risks are based on the performance of an experienced and competent practitioner. Trainees present a possible additional risk in that they have not performed the procedure numerous times and have not yet been declared competent to practice without supervision. Nevertheless, society as a whole has been amenable to allowing trainees to learn with supervision because physicians must be trained for the future of healthcare.

The question then becomes: to what extent should patients be informed that a trainee might be involved in their procedure? Pallin et al. proposed that this question should be examined starting with how much patients want to know about the involvement of trainees. These authors performed a study interviewing patients waiting to be seen in the emergency room. The study found that most patients do not understand the hierarchy of training. Only 30% of patients were able to correctly identify the definition of a Medical Student, an Intern, and a Resident.[14] Once patients become informed, they are even less willing to have a trainee participate in their care;[14] therefore, the study demonstrates that patients want to know whether a trainee will be involved, and physicians should consider including this in their informed consent. The American Medical Association Council on Ethical and Judicial Affairs agrees and in their position statement states: "Patients should be informed of the identity and training status of individuals involved in their care, and all healthcare professionals share the responsibility for properly identifying themselves."[8]

In an Editorial regarding informing patients of surgeon-specific outcomes, Dr. Margaret Schwarze states that it is the job of the medical specialty to ensure that all surgeons perform at an acceptable standard. If this standard is upheld by the medical specialty, patients should be able to trust that every certified surgeon meets that standard. This would preclude the necessity to provide patients with a surgeon's personal "safety and complication record."[15] Dr. Schwarze, however, also clearly states that every patient has a right to know his or her options and be given a chance to "opt out" should he or she feel uncomfortable with the situation.[15] These principles should apply to procedures involving trainees as well. Trainees should not be allowed to participate in procedures during which they are not adequately trained or supervised. The burden lies with the training institutions to ensure that these standards are upheld, for patients to be assured that an acceptable standard of care will be met even when trainees are involved. Should patients be hesitant to proceed, they should be given the option of obtaining care where trainees are not involved.

IMPROVING INFORMED CONSENT

Informed consent forms the ethical foundation for the modern practices of shared decision-making and patient-centered care.[16] It should be viewed as an ongoing process of communication, education, question answering, and listening to the patient or the surrogate that proceeds through the continuum of care.[7] It has been well established that effective communication reduces the likelihood of litigation and that the level of rapport between a physician and a patient is a better predictor of the risk of litigation than the actual documented content of any particular discussion.[17,18]

Legally and ethically, physicians have an obligation to strive to establish a strong patient–physician relationship. Theoretically, improvements in health outcomes occur when patients are better informed and more engaged in treatment decisions because they select treatments that better fit their values and lifestyle.[19] It is a physician's duty to educate patients and improve informed consent. To make improvements, one must evaluate the pitfalls, anticipate complications, and use various tools to implement change.

Some practical suggestions to improve the informed consent process include: improving information retention and communication with the patient and/or surrogates, discussing all treatment options regardless of insurance coverage, using an ABCDEF mnemonic (detailed later in this section), avoiding guarantees about procedures, and documenting discussions thoroughly.[17,20]

Several studies have demonstrated that patients' information retention rates are approximately 25% to 57%.[21–25] Patients undergoing elective Mohs micrographic surgery had an overall retention rate of 26.5% only 20 minutes after being informed of 10 possible complications, with no significant differences in recall based on age, gender, source of referral, or education.[20]

Hence, methods must be developed to aid in communication and retention. One model for more effective communication is the "teach-back" approach in which the physician identifies the principal messages of the discussion and then asks the patient to paraphrase them.[18] Patients should be encouraged to actively ask questions and restate information in their own words. Some physicians even have the patients fill in the procedure and risks discussed on the informed consent form. Other improvements could include the use of technology, such as videos or photos, to demonstrate potential risks or complications. The use of technology and its role in informed consent will be addressed further in the next section.

Staying up-to-date with the medical literature as well as the risks and benefits of all treatment alternatives is imperative. The goal is to present patients with enough data to be able to understand and better stratify the risks of their treatment options. The need for laboratory and radiographic studies should also be discussed including their advantages, disadvantages, and limitations. It is also important to discuss how test results can be communicated to reduce error and liability. Physicians should make no presumptive conclusions and should also consider a patient's financial situation in the shared decision-making process. It is important to customize the discussion with patients as it relates to their occupation, restrictions on lifestyle, physical appearance, and so on. One can also provide patients with medical literature and contact information for support groups so that they can make a more educated decision.

The ABCDEF mnemonic is useful for guiding physician discussion and documentation. It is as follows: **A**lternative therapies available, **B**enefits of the therapy proposed, **C**ommon but not devastating risks, **D**evastating but not common risks, **E**xtra considerations specific to this patient, and **F**acial expressions, body language, and questions.[17]

A discussion of risks, benefits, and alternatives for any procedure, whether elective or not, is critical to informed consent. The discussion should include any associated risks of medication and anesthesia. No guarantees should be made regarding any procedure, since guarantees are nearly impossible in life and can sometimes be the impetus for legal action (breach of warranty claim) should the promised outcome not occur. It is important to remember that one can refer a patient for another opinion if a patient's expectations are out of line or if the procedure is outside one's realm of expertise. The physician should be open and honest about all qualifications and representations, and should make sure these representations are accurate, so as not to undermine the validity of the informed consent.

Finally, it is essential to document well. While documentation is of the utmost importance, there are no clear-cut laws dictating what represents adequate documentation.

With the advent of electronic medical records, patient charts have become more legible and easier to store. Physician offices must keep up-to-date with the documentation requirements from the various insurance companies, as well as with federal and state legislation.

Improving informed consent not only protects the physician but also enhances the doctor–patient relationship. Traditional informed consent methods have often proven inadequate in this day and age. As educators, physicians also have an ethical obligation to continue to optimize informed consent for all patients.

FUTURE OF INFORMED CONSENT

Reform is required in order to adapt to the ever-changing medical and social environment. This section will focus on the use of technology for advancement of informed consent. It is vital to be prudent and knowledgeable about common law, medical ethics, and statutory law. Be sure to check with the state in which you practice medicine, as some state laws regarding informed consent may vary.

The traditional process of informed consent can be inadequate, inconsistent among physicians obtaining consent, and variably comprehensible among patients with different educational levels.[26] Decision aids such as pamphlets, videos, and photographs may significantly improve retention rates, comprehension, and ultimately patients' decision-making. There are multiple benefits to utilizing decision aids during the informed consent process, which aid in improving two major pitfalls that have been identified in surgical consent: lack of time for dialogue with a patient and poor timing of the consent.[27] Decision aids offer patients the opportunity to learn about their disease or condition and their treatment options in the comfort of their home at a less stressful time. Patients can also review the information multiple times on their own or with family and friends. Furthermore, patients can have more time to think about personal preferences and values for different risks/benefits and can be more prepared to discuss options with their physician.[19] A Cochrane review conducted in 2009 concluded that shared decision-making with decision aids improves patient knowledge of the risks and benefits of treatment, the accuracy of risk perceptions, patient comfort with decisions, and participation in decision-making and lessens the number of patients remaining undecided concerning their treatment.[28]

A newer concept using portable video media for presenting informed consent has recently come into the spotlight. Several prior studies suggest that video-based patient education may lead to greater patient comprehension and satisfaction as well as a significant reduction in patient anxiety.[29–33] Dermatologists routinely obtain informed consent and provide pre- and postprocedure instructions for patients undergoing biopsies and other procedures. Armstrong et al.[26] demonstrated a statistically significant increase in knowledge and satisfaction following video education on informed consent and wound care instruction for skin biopsies, as opposed to following traditional verbal education. These decision aid modalities, however, do not necessarily replace verbal discussions between the physician and the patient. Patients should have the opportunity to ask questions regarding the indications, alternatives, and complications of any procedure they may need to undergo. Physicians can make decision aids especially effective by being culturally sensitive to their target population.

In conclusion, decision aids such as videos, photographs, diagrams, and pamphlets are effective tools that can strengthen the informed consent process. They provide highly reproducible dissemination of information with a high degree of patient satisfaction.[26] Decision aids can also potentially help patients with their retention and comprehension, which has been associated with improved clinical outcomes.[34] It is useful to document the secondary sources that are used, suggested, or given to a patient.

Another important topic to address here concerns the ethical and legal aspects of informed consent with respect to photography. The use of photography is an integral part of multiple specialties including dermatology and plastic surgery. Photographs are part of the patient's medical record and thus are covered both by federal and state privacy laws. Some states have specific requirements as to the manner in which these photographs are taken and what claims may appear as text with the photographs.[35] Prior to taking a photograph, one should obtain and record consent adequately.[36] The photography consent form should include the name of the individual, subject matter (i.e., soft-tissue augmentation, scar revision, etc.), and nature of use and distribution (i.e., patient care, lecture, manuscript for publication, brochure, etc.). Patients have the right to review photographs for accuracy and have the right to revoke their consent at any time before publication. Once the information has been committed to publication, however, it may not be possible to revoke the consent.[35] It is paramount to respect the patient's autonomy, privacy, and confidentiality by de-identifying all photographs and images. Patients should be aware that there are no current efficient controls once an image is electronically published.[37] One should respect ethical principles and use images with anonymous information to avoid future legal consequences.

CONCLUSION

The field of dermatology, like medicine in general, is constantly changing and becoming more vulnerable to medical–legal implications. Dermatologists are performing more cosmetic and surgical procedures which add to the inherent risks. Informed consent and the concept of shared decision-making should be implemented, not only to help protect against lawsuits but also to strengthen the dynamic physician–patient relationship. Patients are more likely to take legal action if they perceive their doctors to be lacking in empathy and communication skills.[38] Physicians should be cognizant of patient values and preferences and view informed consent as a shared therapeutic alliance that is ongoing.

The physician is ultimately responsible for obtaining informed consent. The consent should be individualized and can be written, verbal, and/or manifested by conduct. Decision aids can be a very useful tool for both parties involved such that physicians can provide reproducible information to their patients in more effective ways. Patients can also use these aids to improve retention and comprehension. Technology will continue to be an integral tool in evolution of the informed consent process.

Remember that informed consent varies from state to state and country to county. If you are interested in learning more about informed consent, it would be wise to contact your state medical board and/or your attorney for additional information.

REFERENCES

1. Whitney SN, McGuire AL, McCullough LB. A typology of shared decision making, informed consent, and simple consent. *Ann Intern Med.* 2003;140:54–59.
2. Torres A, et al. Medical and legal aspects of skin cancer patients. In: Rigel D, ed. *Cancer of the Skin.* 2nd ed. China: Elsevier Saunders; 2011.
3. Dobbs DB. *The Law of Torts.* St. Paul, MN: West Group; 2000.
4. Pape T. Legal and ethical considerations of informed consent. *AORN J.* 1997;65(6):1122–1127.
5. Paterick TJ, Carson GV, Allen MC, Paterick TE. Medical informed consent: general considerations for physicians. *Mayo Clin Proc.* 2008;83(3):313–319.
6. Sprung CL, Winick BJ. Informed consent in theory and practice: legal and medical perspectives on the informed consent doctrine and a proposed reconceptualization. *Crit Care Med.* 1989;17:1346–1354.
7. Bernat J, Peterson L. Patient-centered informed consent in surgical practice. *Arch Surg.* 2006;141:86–92.
8. Jones JW, McCullough LB, Richman BW. A comprehensive primer of surgical informed consent. *Surg Clin North Am.* 2007;87:903–918.
9. Venesy BA. A clinician's guide to decision making capacity and ethically sound medical decisions. *Am J Phys Med Rehabil.* 1994;73:219–226.
10. Sessums LL, Zembrzuska H, Jackson JL. Does this patient have medical decision-making capacity? *JAMA.* 2011;306(4):420–427.
11. Whitely L, Kuwahara RT, Garcia C. Dermatologic surgery in the demented patient. *Dermatol Surg.* 2003;29:241–244.
12. Berlan ED, Bravender T. Confidentiality, consent and caring for the adolescent patient. *Curr Opin Pediatr.* 2009;21:450–456.
13 McAbee GN; Committee on Medical Liability and Risk Management American Academy of Pediatrics. Consent by proxy for nonurgent pediatric care. *Pediatrics.* 2010;126:1022–1031.
14. Pallin DJ, Harris R, Johnson CI, Giraldez E. Is consent "informed" when patients receive care from medical trainees? *Acad Emerg Med.* 2008;15:1304–1308.
15. Schwarze ML. The process of informed consent: neither the time nor the place for disclosure of surgeon-specific outcomes. *Ann Surg.* 2007;245:514–515.
16. Laine C, Davidoff F. Patient-centered medicine: a professional evolution. *JAMA.* 1996;275:152–156.
17. Kaibara P. 8 ways to improve the informed consent process. *J Fam Pract.* 2010;59(7):373–375.
18. National Quality Forum. *Implementing a National Voluntary Consensus Standard for Informed Consent: A Users Guide for Healthcare Professionals.* Washington, DC: National Quality Forum; 2005:13,15,27.
19. King J, Eckman M, Moulton B. The potential of shared decision making to reduce health disparities. *J Law Med Ethics.* 2011;39(Suppl 1):30–33.
20. Fleishman M, Garcia C. Informed consent in dermatologic surgery. *Dermatol Surg.* 2003;29:952–955.
21. Godwin Y. Do they Listen? A review of information retained by patients following consent for reduction mammoplasty. *Br J Plast Surg.* 2000;53:121–125.
22. Hekkenberg RJ, Irish JC, Rotstein LE, Brown DH, Gullane PJ. Informed consent in head and neck surgery: how much do patients actually remember? *J Otolaryngol.* 1997;26:155–159.
23. Herz DA, Looman JE, Lewis SK. Informed consent: is it a myth? *Neurosurgery.* 1992;30:453–458.
24. Kriwanek S, Armbuster C, Beckerhinn P, Blauensteier W, Gschwantler M. Patients' assessment and recall of surgical information after laparoscopic cholecystectomy. *Dig Surg.* 1998;15:669–673.
25. Priluck IA, Robertson DM, Buettner H. What patients recall of the preoperative discussion after retinal detachment surgery. *Am J Opthalmol.* 1979;87:620–623.
26. Armstrong AW, Alikhan A, Cheng LS, Schupp C, Kurlinkus C, Eisen DB. Portable video media for presenting informed consent and wound care instructions for skin biopsies: a randomized controlled trial. *Br J Dermatol.* 2010;163:1014–1019.
27. Edwards WS, Yahne C, Thomas G. Orr Memorial Lecture: surgical informed consent: what it is and is not. *Am J Surg.* 1987;154:574–578.
28. O'Connor AM, Bennett CL, Stacey D, et al. Decision aids for people facing health treatment or screening decisions. *Cochrane Database Syst Rev.* 2009;(3). http://decisionaid.ohri.ca/cochsystem.html.
29. Idriss NZ, Alikhan A, Baba K, Armstrong AW. Online video-based patient education improves melanoma awareness: a randomized controlled trial. *Telemed J E Health.* 2009; 15:992–997.
30. Miller JS, Litva A, Gabby M. Motivating patients with shoulder and back pain to self-care: can a videotape of exercise support physiotherapy? *Physiotherapy.* 2009;95:29–35.
31. Hill AM, McPhail S, Hoffman T, et al. A randomized trial comparing digital video disc with written delivery of fall prevention education for the older patients in hospital. *J Am Geriatr Soc.* 2009;57:1458–1463.
32. Ong J, Miller PS, Appleby R, Allegretto R, Gawlinski A. Effect of a preoperative instructional digital video disc on patient knowledge and preparedness for engaging in postoperative care activities. *Nurs Clin North Am.* 2009;44:103–115.
33. Jlala Ha, French JL, Foxall GL, et al. Effect of preoperative multimedia information on perioperative anxiety in patients undergoing procedures under regional anesthesia, *Br J Anaesth.* 2010;104:369–374.
34. Schillinger D, Piette J, Grumback K, et al. Closing the loop: physician communication with diabetic patients who have low health literacy. *Arch Intern Med.* 2003;163:83–90.
35. Segal J, Sacopulos MJ. Photography consent and related legal issue. *Facial Plast Surg Clin North Am.* 2007; 18(2):237–244.
36. Hill K. Consent, confidentiality and record keeping for the recording and usage of medical images. *J Vis Commun Med.* 2006;29(2):76–79.
37. Mavroforou A, Antoniou G, Giannoukas AD. Ethical and legal aspects on the use of images and photographs in medical teaching and publication. *Int Angiol.* 2010;29(4):376–379.
38. Farmer ER, Gonin R, Hanna MP. Discordance in the histopathologic diagnosis of melanoma and melanocytic nevi between expert pathologists. *Human Pathol.* 1996;27:528–531.

CHAPTER 4

Anesthesia and Analgesia

Nima M. Gharavi & Gary P. Lask

INTRODUCTION

Local anesthesia is an essential part of surgical dermatology. A proper understanding of the selection and administration of anesthesia, including indications, contraindications, potential side effects, and toxicities, is necessary to maximize patient safety and comfort.

HISTORY

The biologic effects of local anesthestics were first described in the ninteenth century, when Albert Niemann, a graduate student in pharmacology in Gottingen, Germany, extracted cocaine from the leaves of the coca plant (*Erythroxylum coca*) and noted numbness after application to his tongue.[1] Niemann, however, did not consider cocaine's utility as an anesthetic during surgery. Approximately 25 years later, Sigmund Freud, then a graduate student in Vienna who had read Niemann's work, began experimenting with cocaine. In the 1880s, he published a famous paper "Uber Coca," in which he advocated this agent as a means of treating patients with morphine addiction, dyspepsia, fatigue, hysteria, and headaches, as well as a number of mental disorders.[1] In 1884, Karl Koller, a resident in ophthalmology and a colleague of Freud, introduced cocaine into the clinical arena by publishing a paper on its use in ophthalmologic surgery.[1] Although the medical establishment was slow to accept this new anesthetic and its vast potential, most practitioners eventually began to adopt the use of cocaine as an aid in preventing pain during a variety of operations. As its use for local anesthesia expanded, however, reports of potential toxicities and addictive effects also began to emerge.

In the twentieth century, a number of safer anesthetics were identified. In 1904, Alfred Einhorn synthesized procaine hydrochloride, an ester of para-aminobenzoic acid (PABA).[2] In 1905, Heinrich Braun became the first to use this new anesthetic in surgery.[1] Soon, Höechst and Company marketed procaine under the trade name Novocain. However, it was soon learned that procaine, a vasodilator, caused a profound drop in blood pressure, by allowing the anesthetic to travel widely from the site of injection. In fact, a number of deaths were reported after infiltration of procaine. Fortunately, this was overcome by combining procaine with epinephrine, initially at a ratio of 1 to 20,000, which shortly became 1 to 200,000. In 1930, tetracaine, a more potent PABA ester, was introduced. Additional side effects such as allergic reactions were noted in some patients. In 1943, Lofgren and Lundqvist synthesized lidocaine, an amide derivative of diethylaminoacetic acid.[1,2] This new anesthetic displayed superior safety and efficacy, which has since led to its widespread use in cutaneous surgery, as well as its claim as the prototype of local anesthetics. Following the introduction of lidocaine, additional amide derivatives were developed.

Currently, there are multiple local anesthetics and modes of delivery available for cutaneous surgery. A comprehensive understanding of the pharmacological properties, as well as techniques for administration of local anesthesia, is necessary in order to maximize patient safety, minimize pain and discomfort, and improve the ease with which surgical procedures are performed.

STRUCTURE AND PHYSIOLOGY

Local anesthetics have similar chemical structures. The three major components include an aromatic ring, an intermediate chain, and an amine portion. These three components and their modification determine the pharmacological properties of anesthetic agents. The aromatic ring, which is lipophilic, facilitates diffusion of the anesthetic through membranes and nerve sheaths, and correlates with both the onset of action as well as the potency of the anesthetic.[3,4] In contrast, the terminal amine portion may exist in a tertiary form (3 bonds) that is lipid soluble or as a quaternary form (4 bonds) that is positively charged and renders the molecule water soluble.[5] While the aromatic ring determines the actual degree of lipid solubility, the terminal amine portion acts as an "on–off switch" allowing the local anesthetic to exist in either a lipid-soluble or a water-soluble conformation.[5] The amine portion is also postulated to bind to the sodium channel and determine the anesthetic's duration of action.[6] Connecting these two chemical residues is an intermediate chain, which biochemically is either an amide or an ester. Disruption of the intermediate chain mediates the metabolism of anesthetics and determines the reversible nature of these drugs (Fig. 4-1).

Local anesthetics can be classified into two groups, esters or amides, as determined by the structure of the intermediate chain (Table 4-1). These two groups behave differently in several ways, namely their duration of action, metabolism, and potential for sensitization.[3,4] In general, ester anesthetics have a shorter duration of action due to rapid hydrolysis by plasma pseudocholinesterase and excretion via the kidneys.[5] The potential for toxicity as a side effect may, therefore, be higher in individuals with low levels of pseudocholinesterase. In addition, a major

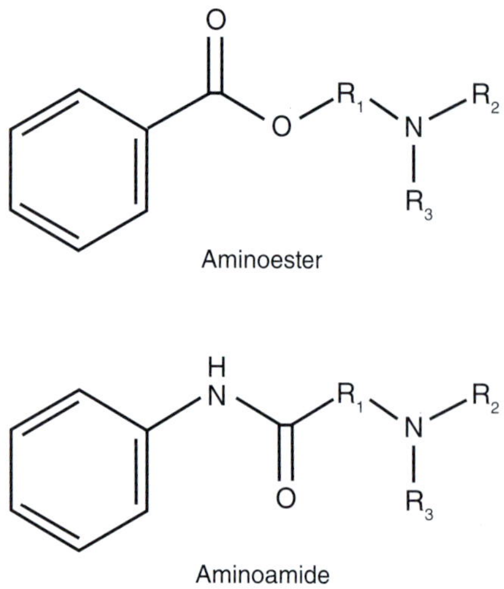

Figure 4-1 Chemical structure of amide and ester anesthetics.

metabolic byproduct of ester anesthetics (and amides to a much lesser degree) is PABA, which in turn is responsible for a higher incidence of allergic reactions.[5,7] In addition, cross-reaction may occur with other agents, including thiazide diuretics, sulfa drugs, and azo dyes.

In contrast, amide anesthetics are not readily hydrolyzed. They are metabolized in the liver by the P450 system of microsomal enzymes (namely CYP 3A4), and subsequently excreted via the kidneys.[5] Caution is warranted in individuals with compromised liver function, who may be more susceptible to potential toxicities.[8]

MECHANISM OF ACTION

Local anesthetics reversibly block nerve propagation and depolarization.[9] In a resting cell, the intracellular electric potential is negative relative to the extracellular space, mainly as a result of an ionic gradient of sodium and potassium ions. The cell membrane and the Na+/K+ adenosine triphosphatase (ATPase) pump help maintain this gradient.[10] During depolarization of a neuron, sodium channels open, allowing for entry of sodium ions across the cell membrane into the cell to generate an action potential. Local anesthetics prevent this depolarization and subsequent nerve activation by interfering with the influx of sodium ions into the cell.[9] The exact mechanism by which local anesthetics inhibit this sodium transport remains unclear, but one hypothesis is that it occurs through direct binding of the local anesthetic to a receptor in the sodium channel, which in turn undergoes conformational changes, rendering the sodium channel inactive.[10] This receptor site is thought to be located at the cytoplasmic (inner) portion of the sodium channel. Local anesthetic drugs bind more readily to sodium channels in an activated state, leading to the more rapid onset of neuronal blockade in neurons that are rapidly firing. This is referred to as state-dependent blockade.[11,12]

There are three main categories of nerve fibers: A, B, and C fibers (Table 4-2).[7] A and B fibers are myelinated, whereas C fibers are unmyelinated. A fibers have the largest diameter and the highest conduction velocities, and are divided into four subtypes: alpha, beta, gamma, and delta. A-alpha fibers conduct motor impulses, A-beta fibers conduct pressure and light touch, A-gamma fibers conduct proprioception, and A-delta fibers, which are the smallest A fibers, conduct pain and temperature. B fibers are preganglionic sympathetic fibers. C fibers are the smallest fibers, and similar to A-delta fibers, conduct pain and temperature. As a general rule, larger myelinated fibers are more difficult to block than smaller myelinated fibers. Therefore, the sensations of pain and temperature are eliminated before loss of vibration, pressure, and proprioception.[7] Clinically translated, this means that while a patient may be locally anesthetized to pain and temperature, he or she may continue to feel a pressure sensation during the surgical procedure.

TABLE 4-1
Anesthetic Classification

Class	Generic Name	Trade Name
Ester	Benzocaine	HurriCaine
	Chloroprocaine	Nesacaine
	Procaine	Novocaine
	Tetracaine	Pontocaine
Amide	Bupivicaine	Marcaine
	Dibucaine	Nupercainal
	Etidocaine	Duranest
	Levobupivacaine	Chirocaine
	Lidocaine	Xylocaine
	Mepivicaine	Carbocaine
	Prilocaine	Citanest
	Ropivacaine	Naropin

TABLE 4-2
Nerve Fibers

Type	Myelinated	Function
A fibers		
Alpha	Yes	Motor impulse
Beta	Yes	Pressure and light touch
Gamma	Yes	Proprioception
Delta	Yes	Pain and temperature
B fibers	Yes	Preganglionic sympathetic
C fibers	No	Pain and temperature

ADDITIONS TO LOCAL ANESTHETICS

In order to improve and enhance the duration, ease, and safety of local anesthetics, various substances may be admixed. It is important for the dermatologist to have a good understanding of the concentration at which these substances may be added, as well as the physiologic properties of these additives, including their impact on anesthesia.

EPINEPHRINE

Local anesthetics, with the exception of cocaine, promote relaxation of vascular smooth muscle. The resulting vasodilation can in turn lead to undesired side effects, such as increased operative site bleeding, as well as increased diffusion of the anesthetic away from the site of injection. Agents that promote vasoconstriction, such as epinephrine, may be added to local anesthetics, facilitating the ease of surgery through the following mechanisms. First, through vasoconstriction, these agents help to decrease operative bleeding. It should be noted however, that while the anesthetic may have an immediate onset of action, full vasoconstriction with epinephrine typically requires 7 to 15 minutes.[7] Second, vasoconstrictors decrease diffusion and absorption of local anesthetics, allowing the surgeon to minimize the amount of anesthetic injected and the potential for systemic toxicity. Third, by decreasing the diffusion of local anesthetics and any associated systemic toxicity, the addition of vasoconstrictors raises the maximum concentration of anesthetic that can be used during the surgical procedure. The maximum concentration of lidocaine without epinephrine, for example, is 4.5 to 5.0 mg/kg; with epinephrine, the maximum concentration is 7.0 mg/kg (Table 4-3).

Epinephrine is the most common vasoconstrictor added to local anesthetics, and is commercially available premixed with lidocaine at concentrations of 1:100,000 to 1:200,000.[13,14] Although the optimal dose of epinephrine has been debated, concentrations higher than 1:100,000 have been reported to have a higher incidence of serious adverse effects.[5] The maximum dose of epinephrine for local anesthesia injected in healthy individuals should not exceed 1 mg (100 mL of 1:100,000 solution) over approximately 8 to 10 hours (roughly equivalent to five half-lives). Careful attention must also be paid to the patient's age and any concomitant health issues which may affect the metabolism of and/or sensitivity to epinephrine.

Although epinephrine at recommended doses is a safe additive, studies on its safety during pregnancy have shown reduction of uterine blood flow in animal models.[15] Given that decreased placental perfusion can theoretically interfere with fetal organogenesis, epinephrine has been labeled as a pregnancy category C drug. Decreased uterine blood flow in the later months of pregnancy may also induce premature labor. Therefore, while not an absolute contraindication, pregnancy is considered a relative contraindication to the use of epinephrine, and nonurgent procedures requiring epinephrine should be postponed until after delivery.[16,17] It should be noted that the only absolute contraindications to epinephrine are uncontrolled hyperthyroidism and pheochromocytoma. A complete list of the relative and absolute contraindications to epinephrine is provided in Table 4-4.

TABLE 4-3
Maximum Recommended Dose of Lidocaine

Lidocaine Type	Maximal Dose (for 70 kg adult)
Plain	4.5 mg/kg or 300 mg
With epinephrine	7.0 mg/kg or 500 mg

TABLE 4-4
Contraindications to Epinephrine

Absolute Contraindications	Relative Contraindications
Uncontrolled hyperthyroidism	Pregnancy
Pheochromocytoma	Hypertension
	Coronary artery disease
	Tachycardia/Arrhythmias
	Glaucoma
	Known allergy to epinephrine

Commercially prepared lidocaine with epinephrine contains acidic preservatives to prevent the degradation of epinephrine. Such preservatives include sodium metabisulfite and citric acid.[18] Given that the resulting solution is more acidic, it tends to cause more pain on injection. However, if epinephrine is added freshly to lidocaine, the solution will be less acidic and in turn, cause less discomfort with injection.[19] Preparation of fresh lidocaine with epinephrine at a concentration of 1:100,000 and 1:200,000 can be made by adding 0.5 mL or 0.25 mL of 1:1000 epinephrine respectively to 50 mL of lidocaine. In the following section, we will describe the use of sodium bicarbonate as another means of decreasing the pain of injection of lidocaine with epinephrine.

SODIUM BICARBONATE

Lidocaine without epinephrine is slightly acidic with a pH ranging from 5.0 to 7.0. Commercially available lidocaine with epinephrine has acidic preservatives, as previously described, which lower the solution's pH to around 3.3 to 5.5, in turn leading to more pain and discomfort with injection. Sodium bicarbonate is a weak basic compound with the formula, $NaHCO_3$. When added to commercially available lidocaine with epinephrine, $NaHCO_3$ renders the solution less acidic and, therefore, less painful on infiltration.[20] Typically, an 8.4% solution of $NaHCO_3$ is used to buffer commercially available lidocaine with epinephrine and added at a ratio of 1:10 (1 part $NaHCO_3$ to 10 parts 1:100,000 epinephrine) or 1:15 (1 part $NaHCO_3$ to 15 parts 1:200,000 epinephrine). Although the resulting solution has a pH closer to physiologic range and is less painful, adjusting the pH of the solution affects other pharmacologic properties of the anesthetic as well.[21,22]

Epinephrine is less chemically stable in solutions with a neutral pH. The addition of $NaHCO_3$ to anesthetic solutions containing epinephrine decreases the epinephrine's duration of action as well as the shelf life of the mixture, and the mixture cannot, therefore, be stored for more than 24 hours.[21,22] Furthermore, addition of $NaHCO_3$ to anesthetics containing epinephrine renders the solution more neutrally charged and lipid soluble, allowing it to cross the nerve membrane more rapidly, leading to a faster onset of action.[21,22] This in turn leads to more rapid nerve blockade. Animal studies have also suggested that the addition of $NaHCO_3$ to anesthesia containing epinephrine increases the duration of action.[6]

HYALURONIDASE

Hyaluronidase is an enzyme that breaks down hyaluronic acid, one of the major natural acid mucopolysaccharides present in the extracellular matrix. It is commercially available and marketed under the trade name Vitrase. When added to local anesthetics, hyaluronidase facilitates diffusion of the local anesthetic through tissue, thereby increasing the area of anesthesia and minimizing the tissue distortion caused by any potential fluid retention.[23] It may also facilitate undermining of the subcutaneous plane by hydrodissection of tissue.[24] Clinical uses for hyaluronidase have been well documented in ophthalmologic surgery, where this enzyme has been shown to minimize the number of anesthetic injection sites, decrease the volume of anesthesia used, decrease the extent of bruising, and improve the onset of anesthesia. Although the precise dose of hyaluronidase to be used in cutaneous surgery remains unclear, most studies recommend a concentration of 7.5 IU/mL or 150 units in 20 to 30 mL of anesthetic.[24]

This enzyme does, however, have disadvantages that limit its use in cutaneous surgery. It decreases the duration of anesthesia and potentially increases the risk of toxicity due to greater diffusion and systemic absorption.[24] It also contains the preservative thimerosal, a known contact allergen. Rare allergic reactions to hyaluronidase have been documented and preoperative skin testing is, therefore, recommended.[24]

TOPICAL ANESTHESIA

Topical anesthesia may be used to alleviate pain associated with various inflammatory disorders, as well as a number of surgical, cosmetic, and laser procedures. The major barrier to the delivery of topical anesthesia is diffusion through the stratum corneum.[25] Thus, topical anesthesia is particularly effective on mucosal surfaces and areas with a relatively thin stratum corneum (Table 4-5). Novel delivery systems have been developed to allow for increased absorption and efficacy of topical anesthesia. Given the potential for systemic absorption and toxicity, careful attention must be paid to the anatomic location to which the agent is applied, the total surface area covered, and the duration of skin contact with the anesthetic.

TABLE 4-5
Topical Anesthetics

Generic Name	Trade Name	Concentration
Benzocaine	American Otic	20% (Liquid, gel, spray)
Benzocaine	HurriCaine	20%
Benzocaine/ Tetracaine	Cetacaine	14%/2%
Cocaine		2%–10%
Lidocaine	Xylocaine	2% viscous solution; 5% liquid; 5% ointment

BENZOCAINE

Benzocaine is an ester anesthetic. It is available at concentrations ranging from 5% to 20%, and in a variety of vehicles, including gels, ointments, and solutions. Benzocaine is commonly used on mucosal surfaces, and is the active ingredient in many over-the-counter anesthetic ointments, such as products for oral ulcers. The 20% gel, marketed as HurriCaine gel, can be applied with a dry gauze for 30 to 60 seconds or as a spray for less than 2 seconds to achieve anesthesia within 30 seconds.[26] Benzocaine is also commonly combined with other anesthetics, such as lidocaine and tetracaine, for more effective topical anesthesia. Since it is derived from PABA, cases of allergic contact dermatitis have been reported.[27] In addition to possible allergic reactions, benzocaine can also increase the risk of methemoglobinemia and, therefore, should be avoided in infants.[28]

LIDOCAINE

Lidocaine is an amide anesthetic which is available at concentrations ranging from 2% to 5%, and in a variety of vehicles, including gel, ointment, and solution. A 5% topical patch is also commercially available, primarily marketed to treat postherpetic neuralgia.[26] Recently, newer preparations of lidocaine, including those with higher concentrations, as well as combination anesthetics, in which it is mixed with tetracaine or with benzocaine and tetracaine, have been manufactured to provide more effective anesthesia. To facilitate penetration, newer delivery systems using microemulsion or liposomal vehicles have also been developed.

TETRACAINE

Tetracaine is a long-acting ester anesthetic. It is available as a topical cream and gel as well as a 0.5% solution. The solution is most commonly employed during ophthalmologic procedures, since one to two drops instilled into the eye provide anesthesia for up to 1 hour.[26] Tetracaine solution has also been combined with 1:2000 epinephrine and 11.8% cocaine, a mixture termed TAC, and used over the past few decades as anesthesia for repair of superficial wounds, especially in children.[28] Although this solution has limited absorption, concern regarding potential systemic toxicities of cocaine, have limited its use.[29] Furthermore, newer anesthetic mixtures, including LET (4% lidocaine, 1:2000 epinephrine, 0.5% tetracaine), BLT (20% benzocaine, 6% lidocaine, 4% tetracaine), and EMLA (eutectic mixture of lidocaine anesthesia) (2.5% lidocaine with 2.5% prilocaine) have demonstrated similar to superior efficacy compared to TAC for topical anesthesia.[30,31]

Tetracaine 4% gel (Amethocaine gel) comes in a lecithin based microemulsion vehicle. Lecithin is a mixture of phospholipids in oil; its hydrophobic properties provide enhanced penetration of tetracaine. In a recent study, Amethocaine 4% gel was demonstrated to be superior to EMLA after a 60 minute application time in a group of 29 patients prior to pulsed dye laser (PDL) treatments, as determined by visual analog and verbal rating scores.[32]

TOPICAINE

Topicaine (4% Lidocaine & 5% Lidocaine) is an amide anesthetic, found in a hydroethanolic translucent gel microemulsion vehicle. Each gram of Topicaine contains lidocaine 40 mg in a gel composed of water, ethanol (35% w/w), glycerin, jojoba oil, aloe vera oil, glyceryl monolaurate, benzyl alcohol, carbomer 940, and EDTA. The 4% preparation is applied under occlusion whereas the 5% preparation may or may not be applied under occlusion. The recommended duration of application is 30 to 60 minutes under occlusion for intact skin and 30 minutes on mucosal surfaces. One study with Topicaine noted effective anesthesia against 1064 nm Q-switched Nd:YAG laser induced pain after 30 minutes of application under occlusion.[30] The anesthetic's highest level of efficacy was achieved 30 minutes after removal of the anesthetic. In a separate study, EMLA and ELA-Max provided analgesia superior to that of topicaine at the 60 and 90 minute measurement periods.[32]

LMX

LMX (originally called ELA-Max; Ferndale, Michigan) is a topical anesthetic, which contains lidocaine encapsulated in a liposomal delivery system. A liposome is an artificially prepared vesicle composed of a phospholipid bilayer that can be used as a vehicle for administration of pharmaceutical agents. The liposomal delivery system enhances the penetration of lidocaine, and increases its duration of action by protecting it from metabolic breakdown.[32] LMX is available at concentrations of 4% and 5%, is available over the counter, and does not require a prescription. The 5% cream is labeled as an anorectal cream, and provides temporary relief for discomfort associated with anorectal disorders. LMX has a relatively fast onset of action; a 30 minute application time prior to procedures is recommended. Studies comparing LMX 5% to EMLA have shown that both are effective in reducing pain, but that LMX 5% has a longer duration of action.[33] Regarding safety, a study demonstrated that application of moderate amounts (30 to 60 g) of occluded LMX 4% in eight healthy patients had no signs of clinical or serum toxicity.[34] LMX can also be used in children but special consideration must be paid to the surface area of application. In a child weighing less than 20 kg, a single application of LMX should be limited to an area less than 100 cm^2.[32] LMX has been used without occlusion to decrease the level of pain induced during cosmetic procedures such as medium-depth chemical peels and laser hair removal.[35,36] Its use on mucosal surfaces and the conjunctiva is not recommended due to increased absorption and potential toxicity, as well as the potential for direct irritation of the cornea.[26]

EMLA

EMLA is a 5% eutectic mixture of lidocaine (2.5 mg/mL) and prilocaine (2.5 mg/mL) in an oil-in-water emulsion cream. It is also available as a patch. A eutectic mixture is one whose constituents melt at room temperature and are present in liquid phase. Broberg and colleagues[37] discovered this property serendipitously, observing that when lidocaine and prilocaine bases in crystalline form were mixed together, they became fluid at room temperature. In EMLA, the concentration of lidocaine and prilocaine achieved in the oil droplet is 80% though the overall concentration of both the active drugs is as low as 5% in the mixture. EMLA contains emulsifiers that enhance skin penetration and decrease the overall concentration and potential for systemic toxicity.[26] In addition to lidocaine and prilocaine, EMLA is composed of polyoxyethylene fatty acid esters to serve as emulsifiers, carboxypolymethylene as a thickening agent, distilled water, and no preservatives. Several studies have shown the efficacy of EMLA in alleviating pain during various dermatologic procedures, including laser surgery, chemical peels, harvesting split-thickness skin grafts (STSG), skin biopsies, curettage and electrosurgery, and application of liquid nitrogen.[26,32]

EMLA cream has to be applied under occlusion. The onset of anesthesia depends on the anatomic location and the duration of application. On the face, anesthesia can occur in less than 25 minutes for needlestick purposes.[32] On mucous membranes, given its rapid penetration, onset of anesthesia is within 5 to 15 minutes.[32] EMLA does not provide effective anesthesia on thick glabrous skin such as the palms and soles and is not recommended for procedures in these areas. The recommended application time for adequate analgesia is at least 1 hour. For painful procedures, the recommended application time is 2 hours.[32] Maximum effect is reached 2 to 3 hours after application and lasts for at least 1 to 2 hours after removal. The depth of analgesia is 3.0 mm after 60 minutes of application and 5.0 mm after 120 minutes.[26]

EMLA is contraindicated in patients with a positive history of amide hypersensitivity, liver disease, and skin diseases such as atopic dermatitis or psoriasis.[29] In the latter conditions, EMLA is contraindicated secondary to higher rates of absorption from inflamed areas. Alkaline injury to the cornea has also been reported with EMLA, and it should, therefore, not be used in this area.[38] Finally, EMLA should be used with caution in infants less than 12 months of age, in patients with glucose-6-phosphate dehydrogenase (G6PD) deficiency and those with congenital or idiopathic methemoglobinemia, given the increased risk of methemoglobenemia secondary to prilocaine. A maximum of 1 g for an hour of application is safe on intact skin of term neonates younger than 3 months (Table 4-6).[29] Central nervous system (CNS) toxicity was reported in a toddler after excessive EMLA was applied over an extensive area prior to molluscum treatment.[37]

TABLE 4-6
Recommended EMLA Use by Age and Body Weight

Age and Body Weight	Maximum Dose (g)	Maximum Area (cm^2)	Maximum Application Time (h)
1–3 mo or <5 kg	1	10	1
4–12 mo and <5–10 kg	2	20	4
1–6 yr and <10–20 kg	10	100	4
7–12 yr and >20 kg	20	200	4

For infants and children based on application to intact skin.
If a patient greater than 3 months old does not meet the minimum weight requirement, the maximum total dose of EMLA Cream should be restricted to correspond to the patient's weight.

LIDOCAINE/TETRACAINE PEEL

Lidocaine/tetracaine (LT) peel is a 1:1 eutectic mixture of 7% lidocaine and 7% tetracaine. It is delivered in a self-occlusive membrane, whereby the cream is applied to the treatment area and allowed to air dry into a flexible membrane. The thin membrane is then peeled from the skin prior to the procedure. Recommended durations for effective anesthesia are approximately 20, 30, and 60 minutes for 585 to 595 nm PDL, 30 minutes for collagen injection, cryotherapy, laser hair removal, and 1450 nm diode nonablative facial laser rejuvenation, and 60 minutes for 1064 nm Nd:YAG leg vein treatment and 1064 nm Q-switched Nd:YAG laser assisted tattoo removal.[39] One study demonstrated that when compared to a placebo peel, LT peel was more effective for local anesthesia in patients undergoing cryotherapy for facial actinic keratoses (30 minute application), collagen injections (30 minute application), PDL treatment of facial telangiectasia or port wine stains (20, 30, 60 minute applications), laser hair removal (30 minute application), nonablative facial laser resurfacing (30 minute application), 1064 nm long pulsed Nd:YAG leg vein treatment (60 minute application), and laser-assisted tattoo removal (60 minute application).[40] The LT peel also provided greater anesthesia for cutaneous carbon dioxide laser skin resurfacing of the cheek when compared to EMLA cream under occlusion after a 30 minute application time for both. Of note, serum lidocaine and tetracaine concentrations after 30, 60, and 90 minute applications to areas ranging from 50 to 200 cm^2 were below the lower limit of quantitation values.[39]

OTHER TOPICAL AGENTS

Topical anesthetics may be compounded by pharmacies for use in dermatologic procedures. Although any pharmacy may compound topical medications, most mixtures are custom prepared by specialized compounding pharmacies. Table 4-7 lists the most commonly compounded topical anesthetics. Clinical trials are not required to approve compounded topical anesthetics, as they do not fall under FDA regulation. As a result, great variability may exist among available preparations and no consensus guidelines on maximum dosages or maximum surface areas exist. Given this, and because of the narrow therapeutic window that exists with most topical anesthetics, it is essential that the clinician develop a working relationship with a reputable compounding pharmacy. Maximum doses should not exceed those established for injectable preparations. Compounded topical anesthetics should only be used under direct physician supervision.

TABLE 4-7
Compounded Topical Anesthetics

Anesthetic Preparation	Comment
Lidocaine Laser Ointment: 30% Lidocaine suspension in proprietary emulsion ointment	60 min application provides effective anesthesia for most laser procedures
23% Lidocaine: 7% Tetracaine	30–60 min application time
20% Betacaine: 8% Lidocaine: 4% Tetracaine (BLT)	30–60 min application time
7% Lidocaine: 7% Tetracaine	60 min application time
Photocaine: 6% Lidocaine: 6% Tetracaine in a lotion like vehicle	30 min application (face) Maximum treatment area = 600 cm^2 over a 2 h period
4% Tetracaine in a lecithin-gel base	30 minute application time under occlusion

CRYOANESTHESIA

Application of cold agents to the skin can reduce the level of pain associated with dermatologic procedures. This technique, using ice cubes for example, is rapid, inexpensive, and relatively convenient to minimize discomfort during needle injections.[41] Various topical freezing agents or vapocoolants can also be used for brief surgical procedures (Table 4-8). Caution should be taken to protect the eyes and avoid inhalation of vapor when using these agents. Potential risks associated with using these agents include scarring and pigment alteration. Some vapocoolants, such as

TABLE 4-8
Vapocoolants

Name	Ingredients
1) Ethyl chloride[a,b] (Gebauer Company, Cleveland, OH)	50% dichlorodifluoromethane, 50% trichloromonofluoromethane
2) Instant cold spray[a] (HL Moore, New Britain, CT)	10% isopentane, 90% butane

[a]Ozone Safe, [b]Flammable
Source: Data from Plotkin S. Clinical comparison of preinjection anesthetics. *J Am Podiatr Med Assoc.* 1998;88:73–79.

ethyl chloride, are also flammable,[42,43] while others have raised concern over potential harmful effects to the ozone.[42]

Cooling methods are particularly effective during cosmetic and laser procedures. Prior to injection of botulinum toxin and/or dermal fillers, application of icepacks may reduce pain. During laser procedures, application of cooled gels, cold glass windows, and other contact cooling devices have also been employed. Devices, such as the Zimmer air cooling device, which delivers refrigerated air onto the skin, have been used successfully during many dermatologic procedures including fractional photothermolysis and PDL. Some lasers are even equipped with dichlorodifluoromethane and tetrafluoroethane cryogen sprays that deliver transient cooling to the epidermis.[43] In addition to providing anesthesia during laser procedures, these cooling methods also protect against laser-induced epidermal thermal injury.

IONTOPHORESIS

Iontophoresis is a method of enhancing the transport of topically applied drugs using a mild electric current to increase the permeability of charged drugs through the skin. This method has been used to deliver solutions of drugs such as lidocaine into the skin without the pain of needle injections. With this system, an electrical current draws ionically charged drugs into the skin.[44,45] Iontophoresis was found to enhance the penetration of lidocaine by 20 to 60 fold when compared with topical application.[46] Lidocaine iontophoresis has been found to be 80% to 100% effective in providing anesthetic action prior to procedures such as needle injections, laser surgery, and electrosurgery, especially in the pediatric population. With lidocaine iontophoresis, the onset of action is within 10 minutes and the anesthetic effect lasts for 15 minutes.[47] The depth of anesthesia was found to be 1 to 2 cm and plasma levels of lidocaine were less than 1 μg/mL after 10 minutes of iontophoresis application.[44,46] A study comparing iontophoresis of lidocaine versus EMLA found iontophoresis more effective in achieving anesthesia.[44] However, two disadvantages to using this method are the limited depth of penetration of the anesthetic, as well as the need for additional equipment.

INFILTRATION TECHNIQUES

LOCAL INFILTRATION

The most common technique for local infiltration of anesthesia is through direct injection of anesthesia into the procedural site. Injection of anesthesia can be administered either intradermally or subcutaneously, each of which has certain advantages and disadvantages. Intradermal injection, which is more superficial than subcutaneous injection, provides a more immediate onset of anesthesia and a longer duration of action, but may be more painful and may cause more tissue distortion. The deeper subcutaneous injection may be less painful and cause less tissue distortion, but has a slower onset and duration of anesthesia. A number of techniques can be employed to improve the level of pain associated with local infiltration and optimize patient experience and comfort (Table 4-9).

TABLE 4-9
Optimizing Patient Experience

The following techniques can improve patient experience and minimize discomfort during administration of local anesthesia:

- Describe the procedure and reassure the patient.
- Provide a calm, cool and quiet environment.
- Position patient with head supported to enhance comfort.
- Minimize patient viewing of the needle.
- Use small-diameter (30 or 31 gauge) needles.
- Distract patient during administration using counterirritation of adjacent skin.
- Add sodium bicarbonate to anesthetics containing epinephrine.
- Use anesthetic solution warmed to room temperature.
- Retract and stretch skin and gently insert needle.
- Inject and infiltrate anesthetic slowly.
- Minimize the number of skin punctures.
- For repeat skin punctures, advance needle initially into areas previously anesthetized.
- Consider using topical anesthesia in children and extremely anxious patients.
- For larger areas, use nerve blocks.
- For patients with a history of bleeding or on blood thinners, use anesthetic with epinephrine and wait 7 to 15 minutes before starting surgery.
- For small children, consider conscious sedation and/or general anesthesia.

Common methods employed to improve patient comfort are providing a calm environment, having the patient recline, providing reassurance, and explaining what to expect so that the patient is not surprised when the injection occurs. Patients often describe feeling sensations of a "stick and a burn," with entry of the needle into the skin and infiltration of anesthesia. A discussion of such anticipated sensations prior to the planned procedure may help alleviate anxiety. In addition, using a small-diameter needle (i.e., 30 gauge or 31 gauge) will significantly reduce pain and discomfort as compared to larger-diameter needles. Some argue that slow injection into the skin is also associated with decreased pain and discomfort. The application of topical anesthesia, ice, or other cooling devices before the initial injection is also useful to alleviate pain, especially in children and highly anxious patients.[41] Neutralizing the pH of lidocaine with $NaHCO_3$, along with warming lidocaine to body temperature, have also been shown to help attenuate the pain of infiltration.[28] Methods of distraction, such as rubbing a distant site, or providing counterirritation by pinching or stretching the skin around the needle entry point, can also diffuse any associated pain.[17] If multiple injections are needed, initial re-entry of the needle should be into areas previously anesthetized to reduce the level of discomfort from repeat needle punctures. Finally, recently developed computer-controlled injection devices such as the Wand® or CompuDent®, as well as needle-free devices, have been developed, which control the rate of injection and limit patient discomfort. These systems have been marketed primarily for dentistry, and their use in dermatologic procedures remains to be determined.

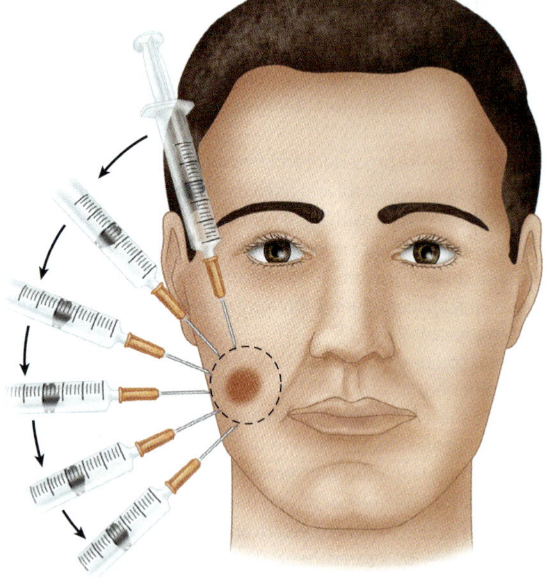

Figure 4-2 During a ring (or field) block, anesthesia is injected circumferentially around the surgical site.

TABLE 4-10
Klein Tumescent Anesthesia

Component	Final Concentration	Amount Added to 1 L Normal Saline
Lidocaine	500 mg/L	50 mL of 1% lidocaine
Epinephrine	0.5 mg/L	0.5 mL of 1:1,000,000 epinephrine
Sodium bicarbonate	10 mEq/L	10 mL of 8.5% sodium bicarbonate

Source: Data from Klein JA. Anesthetic formulation of tumescent solutions. *Dermatol Clin.* 1999;17:751–759. Reproduced with permission from Robinson JK, Hanke CW, Siegel DM, Fratlia A, eds. *Surgery of the Skin,* 2nd ed. Mosby Elsevier; 2010. Copyright Elsevier.

RING (FIELD) BLOCK

A ring block (or field block) is the injection and placement of local anesthetic circumferentially around the operative site (Fig. 4-2). It is particularly effective in surgical cases for which direct infiltration into the surgical site should be avoided, that is, excisional procedures of cysts whereby direct infiltration into the cyst may cause rupture of contents.[4] When properly performed, entry of the needle around the surgical site occurs only in areas previously anesthetized, which reduces discomfort from repeat needle punctures. The anesthetic should be injected into both the superficial and deep planes to optimize anesthesia.

TUMESCENT ANESTHESIA

Tumescent anesthesia involves the delivery of large volumes of dilute anesthesia into the subcutaneous fat until the tissue distends. It is commonly used during liposuction, appropriately named tumescent liposuction. During tumescent liposuction, the anesthetic is typically delivered through 0.5 to 1.5 mm multiport infiltration cannulas or 18 to 20 gauge blunt-tipped spinal needles. The basic tumescent solution described by Klein[48] contains 0.05% to 0.1% lidocaine with 1:1,000,000 epinephrine (Table 4-10). A special pumping device is typically used to aid infiltration of such large volumes of anesthetic. The upper dose limit of lidocaine which may be safely used with this technique is estimated at 55 mg/kg.[49] Tumescent anesthesia is a safe and effective technique for providing effective anesthesia with minimal blood loss, and without the risks of general anesthesia. Its prolonged duration of action also provides a level of postoperative analgesia.[50,51] Although its use has been best documented during liposuction, it can also be used in a number of other procedures requiring larger areas to be anesthetized, such as endovenous laser ablation, ambulatory phlebectomy and face lifts.

REGIONAL (NERVE) BLOCK

Regional blocks (or nerve blocks) involve injecting anesthesia adjacent to a sensory nerve to block the entire region served by that nerve. A detailed understanding of the anatomic distribution of the sensory nerves of the head, neck, hands, and feet, is essential to optimize effective anesthesia as well as patient comfort. These techniques are particularly effective in reducing the toxicity of anesthetic by using smaller volumes, and also decrease tissue distortion at the operative site. In cases where hemostasis is needed, local infiltration of lidocaine with epinephrine into the perioperative site may be added. Nerve blocks are particularly effective for surgical or cosmetic procedures involving the face, especially the nose and lips, as well as the digits. Additional locations in which nerve blocks are commonly employed include the ears, hands, feet, lateral thigh, and perineum.

The most common type of anesthetic used for nerve blocks is amide anesthetic. Typically, a higher concentration of the anesthetic (i.e., 2% lidocaine) is used to enhance diffusion of the anesthetic around the nerve, while using a small volume.[52] Epinephrine may be added to the anesthetic to help prolong its duration by decreasing its diffusion and absorption, and to help improve hemostasis.[53] The use of epinephrine with digital blocks is not recommended given the potential risk for vasoconstrictor-induced ischemia. That being said, some argue that this risk is only theoretical and does not occur when proper technique is used.[53,54]

In addition to recognizing the anatomic distribution of sensory nerves, a careful understanding of proper techniques for infiltration of nerve blocks is necessary to maximize patient comfort and minimize adverse effects. Proper technique involves injecting anesthesia adjacent to a nerve or within the same fascial compartment as the nerve to be anesthetized. Typically, a small, 1 inch 30 gauge, needle is used; this helps minimize pain and allows for a slow, controlled delivery of anesthesia.[54,55] After the needle is placed into the desired location, a small volume of anesthetic is injected and allowed to diffuse locally. The ensuing anesthesia allows for additional insertion of the needle without significant pain or discomfort. Careful attention must be paid not to inject the nerve itself, which can cause a neuropraxia, with resulting paresthesias; rarely, this can be permanent.[55] Furthermore, as vessels typically travel with nerves, care must also be taken to avoid intravascular injection; aspirating prior to injection may be useful in this instance. The most common potential risks associated with nerve blocks include direct nerve injury secondary to improper advancement of the needle, leading to paresis and dysesthesias, as well as vessel trauma, causing ecchymoses and potential hematomas.[52] Peripheral nerve blocks require diffusion into larger-sized nerve trunks, and as a result, these blocks have a longer onset of action than local infiltration, usually becoming effective after 5 to 10 minutes.

NERVE BLOCKS ON THE FACE

The trigeminal nerve (cranial nerve V) and branches of the cervical plexus provide the majority of the sensory innervation for the face (Table 4-11). The trigeminal nerve has three main branches: the ophthalmic (V1), maxillary (V2), and mandibular (V3) (Fig. 4-3). These nerves relay sensory innervation from the face, frontal scalp, conjunctiva, and oral cavity. Three distinct foramina serve as the bony landmarks for infiltration of trigeminal nerve blocks. In addition, the cervical plexus, a network arising from the anterior rami of the four superior cervical nerves, innervates the neck and jaw, as well as segments of the ear and occipital scalp (Fig. 4-3).[54]

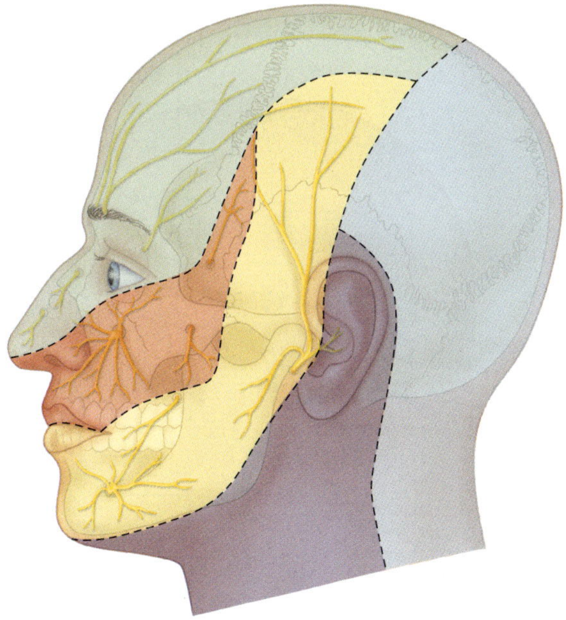

Figure 4-3 Sensory innervation to the head, showing the general distribution of the three divisions of the trigeminal nerve, as well as areas innervated by branches from the cervical plexus.

OPHTHALMIC (V1) NERVE BRANCHES

The ophthalmic (V1) nerve gives rise to the frontal nerve, which subsequently branches into the supraorbital and supratrochlear nerves (Fig. 4-4). These two nerves provide sensory innervation to the ipsilateral forehead and the frontal scalp extending to the vertex. The supraorbital nerve emerges from the supraorbital foramen or notch, which is located on the superior orbital rim in the midpupillary line.

The supratrochlear nerve is located approximately 1.2 to 1.7 cm medial to the supraorbital notch at the upper medial corner of the orbit. Blocking these nerves will provide anesthesia from the ipsilateral forehead, including the glabella, extending to the vertex of the scalp. Both nerves can be blocked through a similar approach: palpating the supraorbital notch, entering just lateral to the notch in the midpupillary line, and injecting 1 to 2 mL of anesthetic toward the midline.[56]

TABLE 4-11
Systemic Adverse Reactions

Allergic Reaction	Signs/Symptoms	Treatment
Type I (IgE-mediated)	**Mild–Moderate** Pruritus, urticaria **Severe** Wheezing, bronchospasm, angioedema, dyspnea, cyanosis, tachycardia, hypotension	**Mild–Moderate** Oral antihistamines and corticosteroids **Severe** Institute BLS protocol, alert 911, give supplemental oxygen, monitor vital signs, IM antihistamines, 0.3–0.5 mg epinephrine subcutaneously (1:1000) *Also consider:* IV access and fluids, bronchodilators, PO/IV corticosteroids
Type 4 (Delayed type)	**Allergic Contact Dermatitis** Erythema, pruritus, papulovesicular eruption within boundaries of application site	Topical corticosteroids Antihistamines

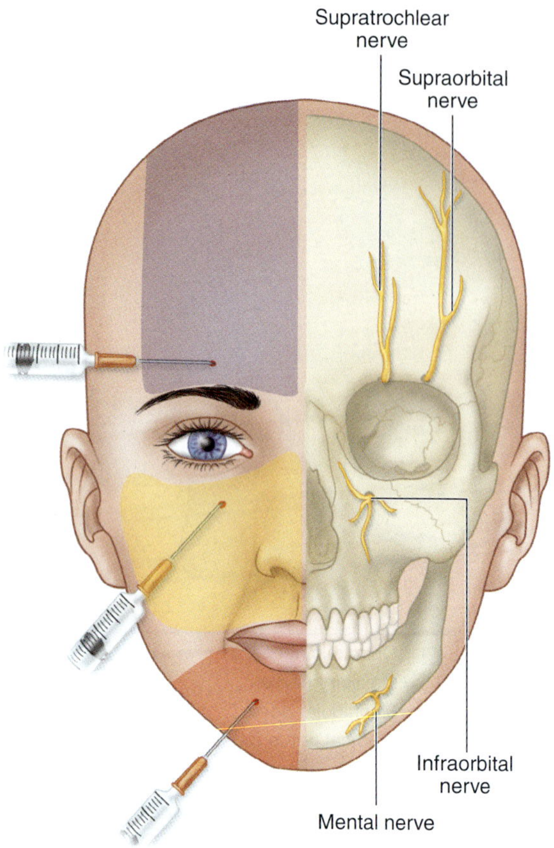

Figure 4-4 Location of supraorbital, infraorbital, and mental foramina, as well as distribution of trigeminal nerve blocks. **A.** Supraorbital and supratrochlear nerve block. **B.** Infraorbital nerve block. **C.** Mental nerve block.

Another branch of V1 is the anterior ethmoidal nerve, which gives rise to the external nasal nerve. The external nasal nerve emerges from in between the lower border of the nasal bone and the upper lateral nasal cartilage, and provides sensory innervation to the ipsilateral nasal dorsum, nasal tip, and columella. By palpating the junction between the mobile lateral cartilage and the firm nasal bones, and injecting 1 mL of anesthesia, the external nasal nerve can be effectively anesthetized.[54]

MAXILLARY (V2) NERVE BRANCHES

The maxillary (V2) nerve gives rise to the infraorbital nerve, which emerges from the infraorbital foramen or notch and provides sensory innervation to the ipsilateral lower eyelid, nasal sidewall and ala, upper lip, and medial cheek. The infraorbital notch is approximately 0.7 to 1.0 cm below the infraorbital rim and just medial to the midpupillary line (Fig. 4-4).[54] The nerve can be blocked either percutaneously or intraorally, the latter providing less pain and discomfort. The percutaneous approach is achieved by palpating the infraorbital rim, then slowly advancing the needle ~1 cm below that point, and injecting 1 to 2 mL of anesthetic. With the intraoral approach, the needle is advanced through the gingival buccal sulcus at the apex of the canine fossa for about 1 cm, at which point 1 to 2 mL of anesthetic is injected just over the periosteum (Fig. 4-5).[54] To further decrease the pain and discomfort of the intraoral approach, a topical mucosal anesthetic can be applied prior to injection.

MANDIBULAR (V3) NERVE BRANCHES

One of the branches of the mandibular (V3) nerve is the mental nerve, which provides sensory innervation to the ipsilateral chin and lower lip, including the adjacent mucosa and gingiva. The mental nerve emerges from the mental foramen, which is located midway along the height of the mandibular bone, approximately 2.5 cm lateral to midline and just medial to the midpupillary line (Fig. 4-4). With age, the mandible atrophies at the alveolar ridge and because of this, in older patients the foramen lies closer to the upper margin of the mandible.[54] Similar to the infraorbital nerve, the mental nerve can be blocked either percutaneously or intraorally. The percutaneous approach can be achieved by advancing the needle at the location of the mental foramen and injecting 1 to 2 mL of anesthetic. The intraoral approach can be achieved by advancing the needle into the inferior labial sulcus between the lower first and second premolars and injecting 1 to 2 mL of anesthetic just over the periosteum (Fig. 4-5). As previously described, the intraoral approach is less painful, especially when coupled with topical mucosal anesthetics.

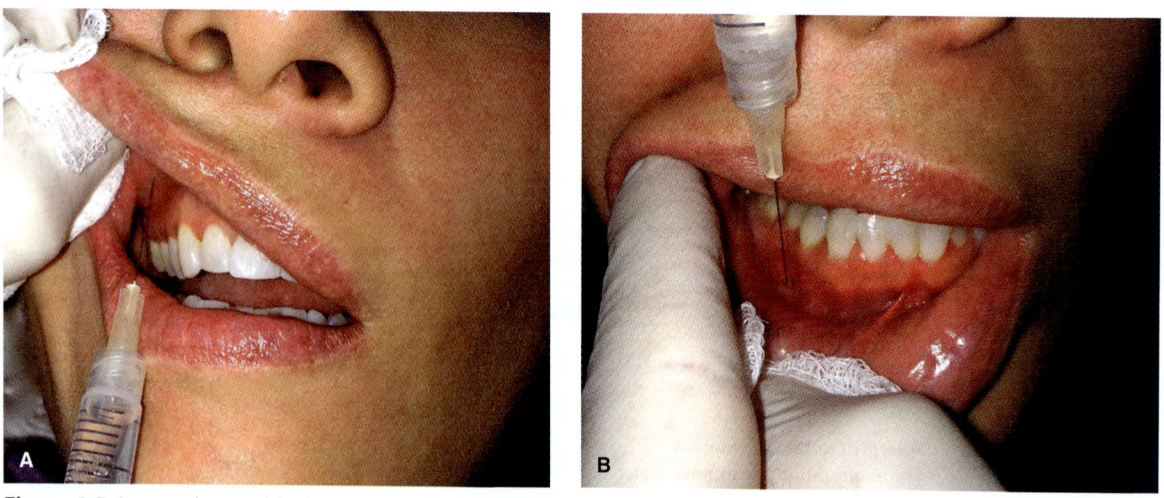

Figure 4-5 Intraoral nerve block technique for the **(A)** infraorbital and **(B)** mental nerves.

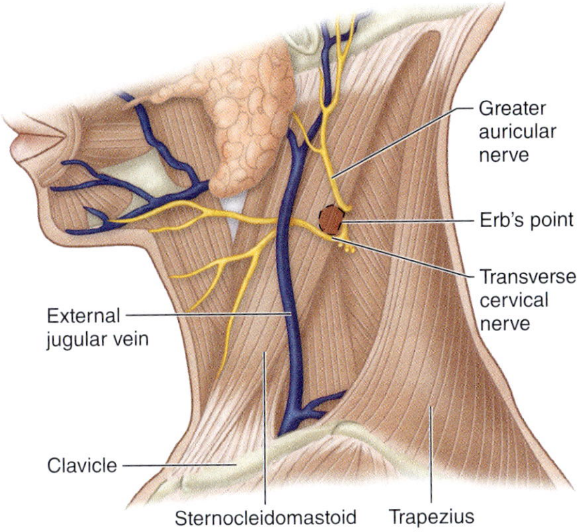

Figure 4-6 Erb's point and the posterior triangle of the neck.

Another branch of V3 is the auriculotemporal nerve, which provides sensory innervation to the ipsilateral anterior auricle, lateral temple, and temporal scalp. This nerve runs deep and posterior to the temporomandibular joint (TMJ) before emerging superficially to travel with the superficial temporal artery. The auriculotemporal nerve can, therefore, be blocked by palpating the TMJ with the jaw open and injecting 2 to 3 mL of anesthetic superior to this joint at the zygomatic arch.[54]

GREATER AURICULAR AND TRANSVERSE CERVICAL NERVES

The greater auricular and transverse cervical nerves are branches of the cervical plexus and emerge at Erb's point (Fig. 4-6), which is located in the posterior triangle of the neck, near the midpoint of the posterior border of the sternocleidomastoid muscle. The greater auricular nerve innervates the ipsilateral angle of the jaw to the submandibular area and the posterior auricle, while the transverse cervical nerve provides sensory innervation to the ipsilateral inferior central border of the mandible and the anterior neck.[56] To help accentuate the landmarks of the posterior triangle (comprised of the clavicle inferiorly, sternocleidomastoid muscle anteriorly, and trapezius posteriorly) and identify Erb's point, the patient's head can be turned 45 degrees against resistance. Injection of 2 to 3 mL of anesthetic into Erb's point will block both nerves.[54]

NERVE BLOCKS ON THE EXTREMITIES

Nerve blocks are particularly useful for surgical procedures involving the hands, feet, and digits. A thorough understanding of the anatomic locations of the sensory nerves of the extremities will help with such procedures.

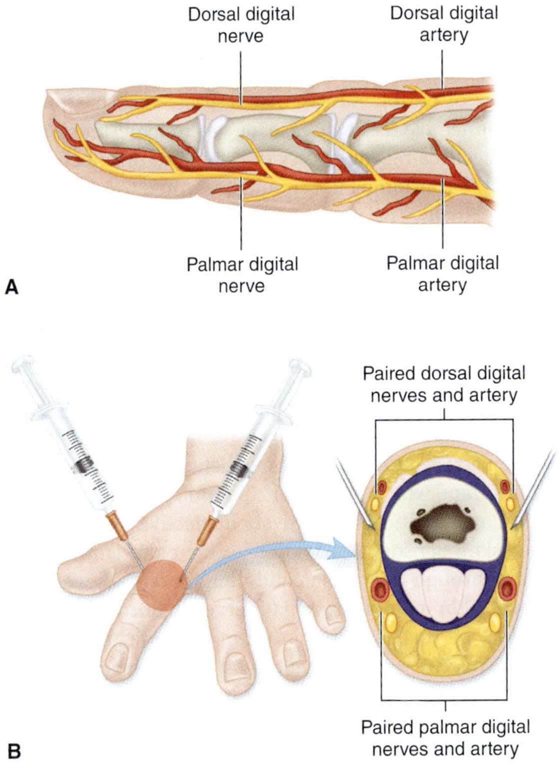

Figure 4-7 **A.** In the digit, the dorsal and palmar arteries and nerves run together. **B.** Dorsal approach for digital nerve block.

DIGITAL BLOCKS

Digital nerve blocks can be used to provide anesthesia for procedures involving the phalanges and nails. Each digit receives sensory innervation from four nerves, two dorsal and two ventral, which lie on the lateral aspects of the digit (Fig. 4-7). In order to provide anesthesia to the entire digit, anesthetic is placed around these four nerves at the base of the digit. Typically, 1% to 2% lidocaine without epinephrine is used, out of concern that epinephrine may increase the risk of vascular compromise to the digit. This potential phenomenon, however, has been refuted in several studies.[57,58] In order to achieve adequate vasoconstriction and minimize the risk of bleeding, proper use of a tourniquet can be employed.[53,59]

The most widely used approach for digital blocks is the dorsal approach, which is less painful, whereby the needle is initially advanced from the dorsal side of the digit and subsequently to the palmar/plantar side of the digit (Fig. 4-7). Using this approach, the needle is placed into the web space at the dorsolateral side of the digit and advanced slowly while injecting approximately 1 mL of anesthesia. The needle is then partially withdrawn, redirected to the ventrolateral side of the digit, and slowly advanced while injecting an additional 1 mL of anesthesia. The procedure is then repeated on the opposite side.[59]

While an extremely rare potential complication, careful consideration must be taken to avoid digital ischemia. Several factors may contribute to digital ischemia, including the use of epinephrine, excessive pressure from tourniquets, or excessive time under tourniquet application, circumferential ring blocks, and postoperative burns to anesthetized fingers.[59] As mentioned previously, use of epinephrine should be avoided, especially in patients with a history of peripheral vascular disease, vasospastic disease, connective tissue disease, or severe hypertension, or in those with a recent history of trauma to or infection of the digit.[58] Tourniquet use should be limited to 15 minutes or less. Finally, the maximum recommended volume of anesthesia for digital blocks should be 8 mL per digit, out of concern for potential vascular compromise.[7]

HAND NERVE BLOCKS

Hand (wrist) blocks can be used to provide anesthesia to select regions of the hand, especially for procedures on the palm where multiple anesthetic injections may be required, and which can be quite painful, particularly since topical anesthetics are relatively ineffective on thick glabrous skin. Sensory innervation to the palm is mediated mainly through the median and ulnar nerves, as well as a superficial branch of the radial nerve. A thorough understanding of the anatomic location of these nerves and their respective sensory regions will help with appropriate placement of nerve blocks of the hand. Potential complications associated with improper technique include intraneural and intra-arterial injections of anesthesia.

The median nerve provides sensory innervation to the first three and one-half of palmar digits, the corresponding two-thirds of the palmar surface, and a portion of the dorsal hand extending from the proximal interphalangeal joint to the tip of the fingernail on the second, third, and medial half of the fourth digit (Fig. 4-8). The median nerve is located in the midline of the volar side of the wrist between the palmaris longus tendon and the flexor carpi radialis tendon.[57] By having the patient appose the thumb and fifth digits, the palmaris longus tendon can be accentuated (Fig. 4-8). The needle can be inserted at the proximal wrist crease, and advanced medial (ulnar) to the palmaris longus tendon and under the flexor retinaculum, where 3 to 5 mL of anesthetic can be injected to provide anesthesia to most of the radial side of the palm.[57]

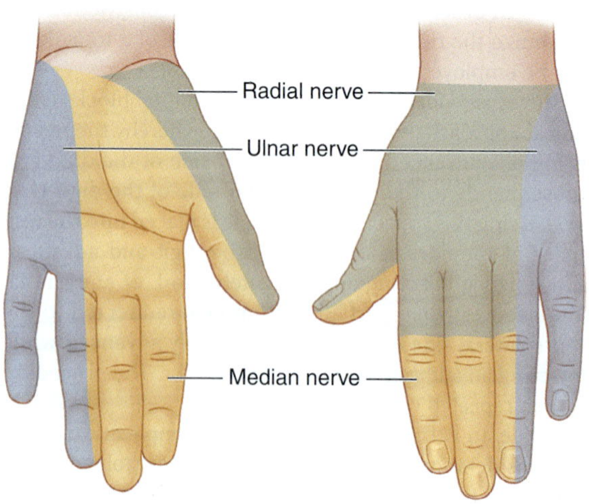

Figure 4-8 Sensory innervation of the dorsal and palmar hand and digits by the median, radial, and ulnar nerves.

The ulnar nerve provides sensory innervation to the palmar and dorsal sides of the last one and one-half digits (Fig. 4-8). This nerve runs deep to the flexor carpi ulnaris tendon and its insertion into the pisiform bone.[57] The flexor carpi ulnaris tendon can be accentuated by flexing the wrist in a slightly ulnar direction. An ulnar block can be performed by injecting 3 to 5 mL of anesthetic just lateral (radial) to flexor carpi ulnaris tendon on the proximal crease of the wrist.[57] In addition, one can also use the ulnar pulse as a landmark and inject just medial to the ulnar artery. A third technique for performing an ulnar block involves placement of the injections at the elbow, where the ulnar artery travels between the olecranon process and epicondyle of the humerus.[57]

The radial nerve provide sensory innervation to two-thirds of the dorsal hand extending from the wrist to the proximal interphalangeal joint of digits two to four and the dorsal side of the first digit. This nerve runs on the lateral border of the radius dorsal to the radial styloid process and deep to the flexor carpi radialis tendon. A radial nerve block can be performed by injecting 4 to 5 mL of anesthetic in the area lateral to the radial artery and deep to the flexor carpi radialis.[57]

FOOT NERVE BLOCKS

Sensory innervation to the foot is provided through five nerves: the posterior tibial, the superficial peroneal, the deep peroneal, the sural, and the saphenous nerves (Fig. 4-9). A thorough understanding of the anatomic location of these nerves and their respective sensory regions will help with appropriate placement of nerve blocks for the foot. The posterior tibial nerve innervates the plantar surface of the foot, except for the medial surface, which is innervated by the saphenous nerve, the lateral surface, which is innervated by the sural nerve, and a small region between the first and second toe, which is innervated by the deep peroneal nerve. On the dorsum of the foot, the superficial peroneal nerve innervates the middle dorsum, while the sural nerve and the saphenous nerves innervate the lateral and medial sides, respectively; the deep peroneal nerve innervates a small area between the first and second toes (Fig. 4-9). Nerve blocks for the foot are primarily performed around the ankle. Prior to starting any nerve blocks, the areas around the ankle should be thoroughly prepped with antiseptic solution to minimize the risk of infection.

The posterior tibial nerve can be blocked at the medial ankle. Here, the nerve runs posterior to the posterior tibial artery en route toward the plantar surface of the foot. With the patient in a supine position and the foot externally rotated, one can palpate the posterior tibial artery, then advance the needle posterior to the artery at the upper half of the medial malleolus and anterior to the calcaneal tendon, and inject 3 to 4 mL of anesthetic.[55]

The sural nerve travels on the lateral side of the ankle more superficially than the posterior tibial artery, passing between the Achilles tendon and the lateral malleolus on its way toward the lateral border of the foot. With the patient in a prone position, the needle is advanced at the posterior distal tip of the lateral malleolus between the Achilles tendon and lateral malleolus, and 3 to 4 mL of anesthetic is injected.[55,60]

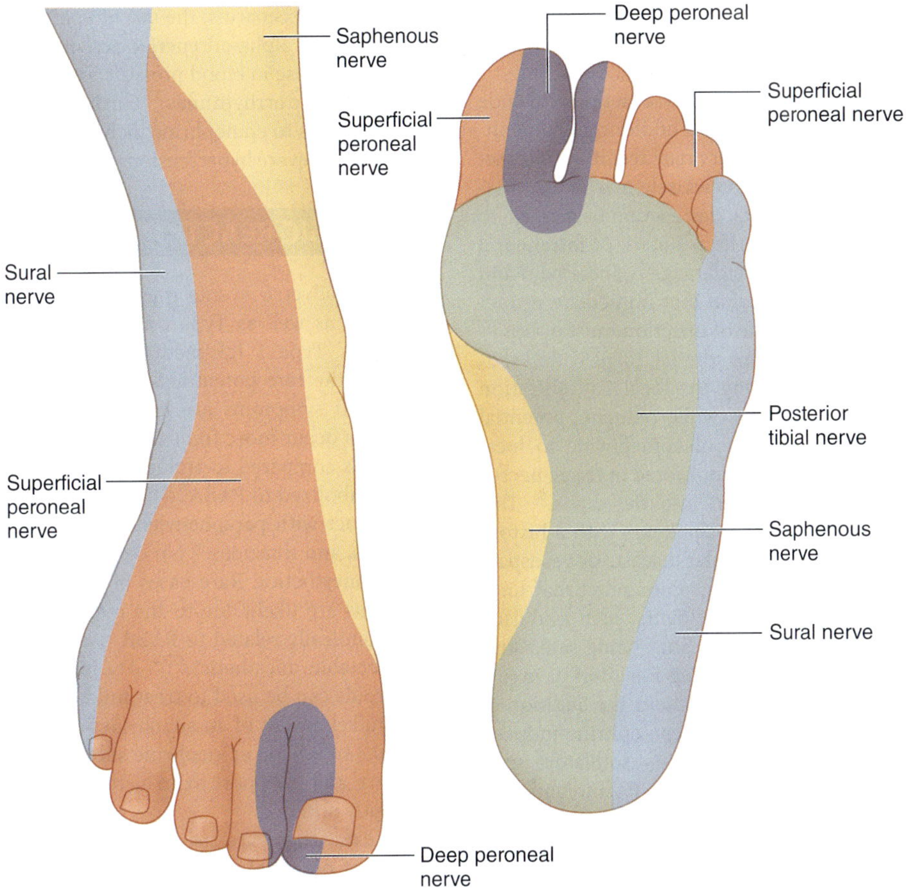

Figure 4-9 Sensory innervation of the dorsal and plantar foot and digits by the posterior tibial, saphenous, deep peroneal, superficial peroneal, and sural nerves.

The saphenous nerve travels along the medial surface of the calf and passes subcutaneously anterior to the medial malleolus and medial to the saphenous vein on the way toward the medial surface of the foot. A saphenous nerve block can be performed advancing the needle anterior to the medial malleolus and medial to the saphenous vein and injecting 3 to 4 mL of anesthetic into the subcutaneous tissue.[55]

The common peroneal nerve gives rise to both the superficial and deep peroneal nerves. The superficial peroneal nerve runs deep along the anterolateral border of the calf to the ankle, where it pierces the deep fascia to become superficial, and subsequently splits into the medial dorsal and the intermediate dorsal cutaneous nerves, which give rise to the dorsal digital nerves. To perform a superficial peroneal nerve block, a line is drawn from the distal anterior aspect of the lateral malleolus to the anterior border of the medial malleolus. The needle is then advanced into the subcutaneous tissue midway between the anterior tibial surface and the lateral malleolus, in a traverse fashion, and 3 to 6 mL of anesthetic is injected toward the medial malleolus.[55]

The deep peroneal nerve lies lateral to the extensor hallucis longus tendon and the dorsalis pedis artery. This nerve innervates only a small portion of the foot, the first web space. As such, given that this small area can be anesthetized adequately with local infiltration, deep peroneal nerve blocks are rarely performed. Nonetheless, in order to properly perform a deep peroneal nerve block, a needle can be advanced immediately lateral to the extensor hallucis longus tendon but medial to the dorsalis pedis artery, and 3 to 5 mL of anesthetic can then be injected.[55]

ADVERSE REACTIONS

Although generally safe to administer, local anesthetics can cause regional and systemic adverse reactions. Regional, or local, reactions are those that occur around the site of application or injection. Systemic reactions include allergic reactions and toxicities, as well as rare conditions, such as methemoglobinemia, which may occur in certain predisposed individuals. In the following sections, we will discuss these potential adverse reactions, including their assessment and management.

LOCAL ADVERSE REACTIONS

Local adverse reactions occur at the site of injection or topical application. Typically, with topical anesthetics, these reactions include erythema, edema, tingling or stinging, and color changes such as blanching, petechiae, purpura, and/or temporary hyperpigmentation. Local side effects are self-limiting and resolution is seen after withdrawal of the anesthetic. Topical corticosteroids may hasten recovery.

With infiltration, causes of local reactions include improper injection technique or the addition of epinephrine. With the former, nerve injury may result from direct nerve transection, pressure-induced ischemia, and/or vascular compromise secondary to destruction or damage to local vasculature.[61] Typically, the hallmark of intraneural injection and impending nerve damage is acute pain and paresthesias, which should signal that immediate retraction of the needle from the site of injection must occur.

Epinephrine is added to anesthetics to provide vasoconstriction, thereby increasing the local concentration and duration of the anesthetic, while reducing potential systemic toxicity. The addition of epinephrine to local anesthetics, however, has been implicated in tissue necrosis, particularly with infiltration into the digits.[53] This theoretical risk is even higher for patients with a history of hypertension, peripheral vascular disease, or vasospastic disease. As such, it is often recommended that local infiltration of epinephrine into the digits, such as during digital blocks, should be avoided. That being said, digital ischemia can also occur following injection of excessive volumes of anesthesia, even without the addition of epinephrine. Treatment options for epinephrine-induced digital vasospasm and ischemia include vasodilators, such as phentolamine and nitroglycerin.[58,62] Phentolamine is an alpha-adrenergic blocker that produces vasodilation, while nitroglycerin induces vasodilation through production of nitric oxide. Local injection of phentolamine (0.5 mg/mL) and topical application of nitroglycerin have been used to reverse epinephrine-induced digital vasospasm.

SYSTEMIC ADVERSE REACTIONS

True systemic adverse reactions to local anesthesia are rare.[63] When they do occur, these reactions may be subdivided into toxic reactions or hypersensitivities. Such adverse reactions must be differentiated from psychogenic attacks and epinephrine reactions. The latter typically present as vasovagal episodes, often in response to procedural anxiety felt by the patient, including fear of needles and/or fear of pain. The resulting increased parasympathetic tone manifests as lightheadedness, diaphoresis, nausea, bradycardia, hypotension, presyncope, and/or syncope.[6] The most important step in treating such reactions is to recognize their psychogenic nature and to differentiate these symptoms from those due to toxicity and/or hypersensitivity. Subsequently, to alleviate psychogenic symptoms, the patient can be reassured, placed in a calm environment, and brought into the Trendelenburg position. Some patients are more sensitive to epinephrine, and may appreciate flushing, palpitations, and anxiety, even with small doses of local anesthesia. The adrenergic effects of epinephrine may be mistaken for an allergic reaction, especially since they share many similar symptoms, including tachycardia. Measurement of blood pressure may be helpful in this situation, as blood pressure tends to drop during anaphylaxis, but will be elevated during epinephrine reactions.

Epinephrine should be used with caution in patients taking beta-blockers and tricyclic antidepressants. In these clinical scenarios, the use of epinephrine can result in unopposed alpha-adrenergic activity, which may cause a significant rise in blood pressure and heart rate, and can lead to cardiac arrhythmias.[15] Furthermore, absolute contraindications to epinephrine include uncontrolled hyperthyroidism, severe hypertension, and pheochromocytoma.

ALLERGIC REACTIONS

Systemic adverse events may be subdivided into toxic reactions as well as Type I and Type 4 hypersensitivity reactions. Type 1 IgE-mediated reactions are immediate with the rare potential for fatal anaphylactic events. Signs and symptoms are listed in Table 4-11. Allergic reactions occur more frequently with ester-derived anesthetics as compared to amide-derived anesthetics. Esters are metabolized to PABA, a common allergen, which can cross-react with paraphenylenediamine hair dyes, sulfonylureas, and thiazides.[64] No cross-reactivity occurs with amide anesthetics. Rare cases of amide-induced allergic reactions are likely due to the methylparaben preservative chemically related to PABA used in the preparation of injectable anesthetics.[63,64] Antihistamines and corticosteroids can be used to treat mild allergic reactions. In the unlikely event of an anaphylactic reaction, treatment with 0.3 to 0.5 mg epinephrine subcutaneously, basic life support, and transport to an acute care facility should be promptly initiated.

To date, there are no specific recommendations for testing of potential allergic reactions to anesthetics. The possibility of a reaction to preservatives should always be considered.[64] If a patient has a positive history of allergic reaction to PABA or methylparabens, preservative-free anesthetic may be used. If the history is unclear, intradermal skin testing with a small aliquot of preservative-free lidocaine or patch testing may be a rational approach.[65] Alternatively, in patients with suspected allergy to anesthetics, other agents may be employed for local anesthesia. Examples include diphenhydramine 1% and benzyl alcohol 0.9%, as well as intradermal tramadol and metoclopramide.[17,66,67] Studies with diphenhydramine, however, have shown that it has a smaller duration of action than lidocaine, can be potentially more sedating, and even elicits more pain.[66] In one patient, skin necrosis was reported with diphenhydramine.[67] Studies with intradermal tramadol have demonstrated effective anesthesia in comparison to prilocaine, but also a higher incidence of injection-site reactions.[68,69] Therefore, given that alternatives to local anesthetics are often subobtimal, we recommend consultation for allergy testing to rule out a true allergy to local anesthetics and to identify safe anesthetic options.

SYSTEMIC TOXICITY

Systemic toxicity may affect the CNS and cardiovascular systems. This occurs when blood levels of anesthetic rise above a certain threshold, which can occur from administering excessive amounts, inadvertent intravascular injection, rapid absorption, or abnormal drug metabolism.[63]

Rapid absorption is seen with application of topical anesthesia to the mucous membranes. Abnormal drug metabolism is seen in patients with a history of liver disease, renal disease, pseudocholinesterase deficiency, and secondary to interaction with other medications.[27,70] Among anesthetics, lidocaine toxicity is the most likely severe adverse event the clinician may encounter. Lidocaine is an amide anesthetic rapidly metabolized by the hepatic P450 system (CYP1A2 and CYP3A4) into two major metabolites, monoethylglycinexylidide (MEGX) and glycinexylidide (GX). GX is pharmacologically similar to MEGX but less potent. Lidocaine is plasma protein bound and has a half-life of 1.5 to 2 hours.[71] Liver disease raises the level of lidocaine whereas renal disease raises the level of its metabolites. Certain medications which inhibit the cytochrome P450 system, can subsequently theoretically alter the levels of lidocaine (Table 4-12). With topical anesthesia, location of application may play an important role. Due to the absence of the stratum corneum on mucosal surfaces, blood levels of topically applied lidocaine are increased because of enhanced penetration. In fact, serum lidocaine levels after application to mucosal surfaces have been demonstrated to approach those associated with parenteral administration.[71,72] The maximum doses of topical lidocaine should not, therefore, exceed the maximum doses associated with intravenous lidocaine injection.

Lidocaine has a narrow therapeutic window where the therapeutic dose approaches the toxic dose. Signs and symptoms may be subtle at first, but may progress rapidly toward cardiovascular and respiratory depression if left unrecognized (Table 4-13).[27] In fact, there have been a few reported cases of topical anesthetic-induced fatality as a result of negligent prescribing, instruction, oversight, and monitoring. The victims were all in their early twenties receiving topical anesthetics for laser treatment. Areas of gross negligence included application to excessive surface areas under occlusion for extended periods of time without direct supervision. Two cases involved application of compounded anesthetics to the bilateral legs, from the groin to ankles under occlusion for longer than 60 minutes.[34] Another case involved application to the entire back, which generally represents 18% of the total body surface area.[73] All persons applied the anesthetic themselves prior to arriving at the treatment centers. No direct physician supervision, prescription, or clear directions regarding application were provided.

Anesthetic potency directly correlates to the degree of systemic toxicity. More potent anesthetics, such as bupivacaine and etidocaine, appear to be more cardiotoxic than other anesthetics.[27] In fact, given that bupivacaine enters the sodium channel rapidly but leaves slowly, it has a greater potential to induce a serious re-entrant arrhythmia that may be refractory to defibrillation. In pregnancy, the potential cardiac toxicity of bupivacaine is even more severe, likely due to increased progesterone levels as well as impeded venous return.[6]

The most important step in the management of anesthetic toxicity is early recognition. Initial management includes stopping the delivery of the anesthetic and maintaining ventilation and oxygenation. Hypoxia and acidosis can decrease the seizure threshold and enhance the cardiotoxicity of local anesthetics.[27] Seizures can be treated and potentially prevented with diazepam, thiopental sodium, and propofol.[27] Hypotension is initially treated with administration of intravenous fluids, and if marked, may require vasopressors.[27] Bradycardia and decreased myocardial activity may require inotropic agents, such as epinephrine or ephedrine.[27] Bretylium is used to treat recalcitrant dysrhythmias. Amrinone, a phosphodiesterase inhibitor that increases cAMP in the myocardium and enhances contractility, can be used when conventional inotropes are ineffective. A detailed algorithm for treatment of anesthetic-induced cardiovascular toxicity and seizures has been recently published.[27]

TABLE 4-12
Cytochrome P450 Inhibitors

Amiodarone	Methylprednisolone
Azoles (flucon-, itracon-, ketocon-)	Metronidazole
Benzodiazapines	Nicardipine
Carbamazepine	Nifedipine
Cimetidine	Pentoxifylline
Clarithromycin	Propofol
Chloramphenicol	Propranolol
Cyclosporine	Quinidine
Danazol	SSRIs
Dexamethasone	Tetracycline
Diltiazem	Terfenadine
Erythromycin	Thyroxine
Isoniazid	Valproic acid
Methadone	Verapamil

TABLE 4-13
Lidocaine Toxicity

Serum Lidocaine Level	Signs and Symptoms
1st Stage: 1–6 μg/mL	Talkative, agitated, apprehensive, lightheaded, drowsy, disoriented, tinnitus, circumoral numbness, metallic taste
2nd Stage: 6–12 μg/mL	Nausea, vomiting, muscle twitching, tremors, blurred vision, seizures (generalized tonic/clonic)
3rd Stage: >12 μg/mL	Cardiac and respiratory depression, dysrhythmias, cardiac arrest

METHEMOGLOBINEMIA

Methemoglobin is the oxidized form of hemoglobin. In this form, iron exists in its ferric 3+ state and is unable to adequately carry oxygen. Normal physiological conditions

TABLE 4-14
Methemoglobinemia

Methemoglobin Concentration (%)	Signs and Symptoms
0–3	Normal levels
3–15	Skin discoloration (pale, blue, gray)
15–20	Cyanosis
25–50	Lightheadedness, headache, confusion, weakness, dyspnea, palpitations, chest pain
50–70	Altered mental status, delerium, death

permit the constant reduction of iron back to the ferrous 2+ state by NADH methemoglobin reductase, allowing low levels of methemoglobin to be maintained. However, when this natural process is interrupted, methemoglobin levels may rise and oxygen delivery to tissue falls. Progressively worsening signs and symptoms ensue with greater methemoglobin concentrations (Table 4-14). Prilocaine and benzocaine are two topical anesthetics which have been shown to precipitate methemoglobinemia.[74] Rare cases have also been reported with the topical use of EMLA, due to the presence of prilocaine in the preparation.[27] The onset of symptoms may be delayed for a few hours as the metabolites of the above anesthetics, rather than the anesthetics themselves, lead to the adverse reactions.

Certain patient populations are at higher risk of developing methemoglobinemia. Among them are individuals with G6PD deficiency, methemoglobin reductase deficiency, and those simultaneously taking methemoglobinemia precipitating drugs such as sulfonamides and antimalarials.[74] Infants and children are in a high-risk group because doses are often greater per kilogram of body weight, hemoglobin F is more susceptible to oxidation, and newborns have low levels of reductive enzymes. Diagnosis is best achieved through arterial blood gas and serum methemoglobin levels. Pulse oximetry generally is unreliable. Management includes removal of the offending agent, supplemental oxygen, and observation in mild cases when levels are below 30%. Intravenous methylene blue 1 to 2 mg/kg is indicated in more severe cases. Ascorbic acid 300 to 1000 mg/d IV over 3 to 4 doses is reserved for patients with G6PD deficiency in whom methylene blue is contraindicated.[74]

PRACTICAL APPLICATIONS

The majority of cutaneous surgical procedures are performed using 1% lidocaine with or without epinephrine for anesthesia. For more involved procedures, longer-acting anesthetics, such as bupivacaine, may be added and/or mixed to maximize the duration of anesthesia while minimizing risks. Commonly, local anesthetic is initially drawn from the bottle using a large 16 or 18 gauge needle (which allows for more rapid fluid suction) and the needle is subsequently switched to a smaller 30 gauge needle. Local infiltration is delivered using 30 gauge, 0.5 or 1 inch needles. Needles with a larger bore diameter are not commonly used due to increased pain and discomfort. Conversely, the 32 gauge needle is too small and flexible, limiting the ease of injection. The operative site should be outlined with appropriate markings, given that infiltration of the skin may distort lesional and anatomic borders. In patients on blood thinners and/or with a history of excess bleeding, lidocaine with epinephrine may be used and allowed to sit for 7 to 15 minutes after infiltration, to allow for adequate vasoconstriction. Finally, on infected areas, a greater volume of anesthesia may be required, given that local anesthetics are less effective in acidic environments.

For surgical procedures that require multiple injections of anesthesia, it is helpful to advance the needle into previously anesthetized sites to help minimize pain and discomfort. This is particularly useful when performing ring blocks. Ring blocks are practical for cyst excisions and/or incision and drainage of abscesses. They are also effective for procedures involving the scalp, pinna of the ear, and nose. For procedures involving large surface areas of the face, especially the nose and lips, as well as the scalp, hands, feet, and digits, nerve blocks are particularly useful. A clear prerequisite is the availability of regional nerves to be blocked. The benefits of nerve blocks include the decreased amount of anesthetic needed, fewer injection sites, and reduced tissue distortion. Disadvantages include the lag time to complete anesthesia of distal structures, as well as the lack of hemostasis that would otherwise occur with local infiltration. Nerve blocks are particularly useful for surgical excisions on the acral surfaces, digits, and the face, ablative laser resurfacing of the face, botulinum toxin injections to the palms and soles, hair transplantation, medium and deep chemical peels of the face, and for some practitioners, perioral filler injections.[54,75]

In large areas where nerve blocks are not possible (i.e., trunk and limbs), tumescent anesthesia can be employed to deliver large volumes of dilute anesthetic. With this technique, higher maximum doses of lidocaine are delivered without toxicity. While this technique is most popular for tumescent liposuction, its utility has also expanded to other procedures including laser resurfacing, face/neck lifting, ambulatory phlebectomy, and soft-tissue reconstruction.[76–78] The concentration of lidocaine and epinephrine can be varied based on anatomic location. For example, fibrous areas including the back, upper abdomen, and breasts tend to require a higher concentration of lidocaine (1000 to 1250 mg/dL), whereas less fibrous areas, such as the hips and thighs, require a lower concentration of lidocaine (500 to 700 mg/dL).

Topical anesthesia is particularly effective for surgical and cosmetic procedures. While more effective on mucosal surfaces and areas with a thinner stratum corneum, topical preparations such as EMLA and topical lidocaine, including compounded formulations, allow for effective anesthesia for superficial surgical procedures, laser procedures, filler injections, and chemical peels. Topical anesthesia is particularly helpful in performing cutaneous procedures in children, including treatment of warts and molluscum, as well decreasing the pain associated with intralesional injections, including infiltration of local anesthetic.

The techniques described above can be combined and used in cutaneous surgical procedures to achieve optimal anesthesia without the need for general anesthesia. In certain patients, low-dose benzodiazepines, such as diazepam (2 to 5 mg) and lorazepam (1 to 2 mg), may be used to minimize anxiety and allow for a more pleasant surgical experience for the patient. Finally, in some circumstances, local anesthesia may not suffice, and options may include conscious sedation and/or general anesthesia. In general, each patient must be assessed on a case-by-case basis.

CONCLUSION

Local anesthesia is an essential part of cutaneous surgery. A detailed and comprehensive understanding of the indications and contraindications of local anesthetics, their pharmacologic properties, potential adverse effects, and proper techniques for administration, will maximize patient safety and comfort. The use of topical application, local infiltration, field blocks, nerve blocks, tumescent techniques, alone or in combination, has enhanced the field of local anesthesia without the risks of general anesthesia. As the field of surgical dermatology expands, the emergence of novel agents and delivery systems will likely follow, providing the practitioner with an arsenal of tools with which to adequately and efficiently deliver local anesthesia.

REFERENCES

1. Ring ME. The history of local anesthesia. *J Calif Dent Assoc.* 2007;35:275–282.
2. Calatayud J, González A. History of the development and evolution of local anesthesia since the coca leaf. *Anesthesiology.* 2003;98:1503–1508.
3. Covino BG. Local anesthesia. 1. *N Engl J Med.* 1972;286:975–983.
4. Covino BG. Local anesthesia. 2. *N Engl J Med.* 1972;286:1035–1042.
5. Becker DE, Reed KL. Essentials of local anesthetic pharmacology. *Anesth Prog.* 2006;53:98–108; quiz 9–10.
6. Tetzlaff JE. The pharmacology of local anesthetics. *Anesthesiol Clin North America.* 2000;18:217–233, v.
7. Grekin RC, Auletta MJ. Local anesthesia in dermatologic surgery. *J Am Acad Dermatol.* 1988;19:599–614.
8. Selden R, Sasahara AA. Central nervous system toxicity induced by lidocaine. Report of a case in a patient with liver disease. *JAMA.* 1967;202:908–909.
9. Covino BG. Pharmacology of local anaesthetic agents. *Br J Anaesth.* 1986;58:701–716.
10. Fink BR. The long and the short of conduction block. *Anesth Analg.* 1989;68:553–555.
11. Butterworth JF IV, Strichartz GR. Molecular mechanisms of local anesthesia: a review. *Anesthesiology.* 1990;72:711–734.
12. Ragsdale DS, McPhee JC, Scheuer T, Catterall WA. Molecular determinants of state-dependent block of Na+ channels by local anesthetics. *Science.* 1994;265:1724–1728.
13. Fante RG, Elner VM. The use of epinephrine in infiltrative local anesthesia for eyelid reconstruction. *Plast Reconstr Surg.* 1998;102:917.
14. Siegel RJ, Vistnes LM, Iverson RE. Effective hemostasis with less epinephrine. An experimental and clinical study. *Plast Reconstr Surg.* 1973;51:129–133.
15. Lawrence C. Drug management in skin surgery. *Drugs.* 1996;52:805–817.
16. Richards KA, Stasko T. Dermatologic surgery and the pregnant patient. *Dermatol Surg.* 2002;28:248–256.
17. Auletta MJ. Local anesthesia for dermatologic surgery. *Semin Dermatol.* 1994;13:35–42.
18. Moore DC, Bridenbaugh LD, Thompson GE, Balfour RI, Horton WG. Factors determining dosages of amide-type local anesthetic drugs. *Anesthesiology.* 1977;47:263–268.
19. Howe NR, Williams JM. Pain of injection and duration of anesthesia for intradermal infiltration of lidocaine, bupivacaine, and etidocaine. *J Dermatol Surg Oncol.* 1994;20:459–464.
20. McKay W, Morris R, Mushlin P. Sodium bicarbonate attenuates pain on skin infiltration with lidocaine, with or without epinephrine. *Anesth Analg.* 1987;66:572–574.
21. Stewart JH, Chinn SE, Cole GW, Klein JA. Neutralized lidocaine with epinephrine for local anesthesia–II. *J Dermatol Surg Oncol.* 1990;16:842–845.
22. Stewart JH, Cole GW, Klein JA. Neutralized lidocaine with epinephrine for local anesthesia. *J Dermatol Surg Oncol.* 1989;15:1081–1083.
23. Lewis-Smith PA. Adjunctive use of hyaluronidase in local anaesthesia. *Br J Plast Surg.* 1986;39:554–558.
24. Clark LE, Mellette JR Jr. The use of hyaluronidase as an adjunct to surgical procedures. *J Dermatol Surg Oncol.* 1994;20:842–844.
25. Adriani J, Dalili H. Penetration of local anesthetics through epithelial barriers. *Anesth Analg.* 1971;50:834–841.
26. Huang W, Vidimos A. Topical anesthetics in dermatology. *J Am Acad Dermatol.* 2000;43:286–298.
27. Naguib M, Magboul MM, Samarkandi AH, Attia M. Adverse effects and drug interactions associated with local and regional anaesthesia. *Drug Saf.* 1998;18:221–250.
28. Chen BK, Eichenfield LF. Pediatric anesthesia in dermatologic surgery: when hand-holding is not enough. *Dermatol Surg.* 2001;27:1010–1018.
29. Rincon E, Baker RL, Iglesias AJ, Duarte AM. CNS toxicity after topical application of EMLA cream on a toddler with molluscum contagiosum. *Pediatr Emerg Care.* 2000;16:252–254.
30. Friedman PM, Fogelman JP, Nouri K, Levine VJ, Ashinoff R. Comparative study of the efficacy of four topical anesthetics. *Dermatol Surg.* 1999;25:950–954.
31. Zempsky WT, Karasic RB. EMLA versus TAC for topical anesthesia of extremity wounds in children. *Ann Emerg Med.* 1997;30:163–166.
32. Friedman PM, Mafong EA, Friedman ES, Geronemus RG. Topical anesthetics update: EMLA and beyond. *Dermatol Surg.* 2001;27:1019–1026.
33. Bucalo BD, Mirikitani EJ, Moy RL. Comparison of skin anesthetic effect of liposomal lidocaine, nonliposomal lidocaine, and EMLA using 30-minute application time. *Dermatol Surg.* 1998;24:537–541.
34. Nestor MS. Safety of occluded 4% liposomal lidocaine cream. *J Drugs Dermatol.* 2006;5:618–620.
35. Altman DA, Gildenberg SR. High-energy pulsed light source hair removal device used to evaluate the onset of action of a new topical anesthetic. *Dermatol Surg.* 1999;25:816–818.
36. Koppel RA, Coleman KM, Coleman WP. The efficacy of EMLA versus ELA-Max for pain relief in medium-depth chemical peeling: a clinical and histopathologic evaluation. *Dermatol Surg.* 2000;26:61–64.
37. Juhlin L, Evers H, Broberg F. A lidocaine-prilocaine cream for superficial skin surgery and painful lesions. *Acta Derm Venereol.* 1980;60:544–546.
38. Eaglstein NF. Chemical injury to the eye from EMLA cream during erbium laser resurfacing. *Dermatol Surg.* 1999;25:590–591.
39. Bryan HA, Alster TS. The S-Caine peel: a novel topical anesthetic for cutaneous laser surgery. *Dermatol Surg.* 2002;28:999–1003; discussion.
40. McCafferty DF, Woolfson AD, Handley J, Allen G. Effect of percutaneous local anaesthetics on pain reduction during pulse dye laser treatment of portwine stains. *Br J Anaesth.* 1997;78:286–289.
41. Kuwahara RT, Skinner RB. Emla versus ice as a topical anesthetic. *Dermatol Surg.* 2001;27:495–496.
42. Plotkin S. Clinical comparison of preinjection anesthetics. *J Am Podiatr Med Assoc.* 1998;88:73–79.
43. White JM, Siegfried E, Boulden M, Padda G. Possible hazards of cryogen use with pulsed dye laser. A case report and summary. *Dermatol Surg.* 1999;25:250–252; discussion 2–3.

44. DeCou JM, Abrams RS, Hammond JH, Lowder LR, Gauderer MW. Iontophoresis: a needle-free, electrical system of local anesthesia delivery for pediatric surgical office procedures. *J Pediatr Surg.* 1999;34:946–949.
45. Greenbaum SS, Bernstein EF. Comparison of iontophoresis of lidocaine with a eutectic mixture of lidocaine and prilocaine (EMLA) for topically administered local anesthesia. *J Dermatol Surg Oncol.* 1994;20:579–583.
46. Gangarosa LP Sr, Ozawa A, Ohkido M, Shimomura Y, Hill JM. Iontophoresis for enhancing penetration of dermatologic and antiviral drugs. *J Dermatol.* 1995;22:865–875.
47. Lener EV, Bucalo BD, Kist DA, Moy RL. Topical anesthetic agents in dermatologic surgery. A review. *Dermatol Surg.* 1997;23:673–683.
48. Klein JA. Anesthetic formulation of tumescent solutions. *Dermatol Clin.* 1999;17:751–759, v–vi.
49. Ostad A, Kageyama N, Moy RL. Tumescent anesthesia with a lidocaine dose of 55 mg/kg is safe for liposuction. *Dermatol Surg.* 1996;22:921–927.
50. Klein JA. The tumescent technique. Anesthesia and modified liposuction technique. *Dermatol Clin.* 1990;8:425–437.
51. Lillis PJ. Liposuction surgery under local anesthesia: limited blood loss and minimal lidocaine absorption. *J Dermatol Surg Oncol.* 1988;14:1145–1148.
52. Hawkins JM, Moore PA. Local anesthesia: advances in agents and techniques. *Dent Clin North Am.* 2002;46:719–732, ix.
53. Denkler K. A comprehensive review of epinephrine in the finger: to do or not to do. *Plast Reconstr Surg.* 2001;108:114–124.
54. Eaton JS, Grekin RC. Regional anesthesia of the face. *Dermatol Surg.* 2001;27:1006–1009.
55. Cohen SJ, Roenigk RK. Nerve blocks for cutaneous surgery on the foot. *J Dermatol Surg Oncol.* 1991;17:527–534.
56. Randle HW, Salassa JR, Roenigk RK. Know your anatomy. Local anesthesia for cutaneous lesions of the head and neck–practical applications of peripheral nerve blocks. *J Dermatol Surg Oncol.* 1992;18:231–235.
57. Earle AS, Blanchard JM. Regional anesthesia in the upper extremity. *Clin Plast Surg.* 1985;12:97–114.
58. Wilhelmi BJ, Blackwell SJ, Miller JH, et al. Do not use epinephrine in digital blocks: myth or truth? *Plast Reconstr Surg.* 2001;107:393–397.
59. O'Donnell J, Wilson K, Leonard PA. An avoidable complication of digital nerve block. *Emerg Med J.* 2001;18:316.
60. Sarrafian SK, Ibrahim IN, Breihan JH. Ankle-foot peripheral nerve block for mid and forefoot surgery. *Foot Ankle.* 1983;4:86–90.
61. Ben-David B. Complications of peripheral blockade. *Anesthesiol Clin North America.* 2002;20:695–707.
62. Heard CM, LaJohn S, Fletcher JE. An accidental ringblock of the great toe? *Paediatr Anaesth.* 2001;11:123.
63. Faccenda KA, Finucane BT. Complications of regional anaesthesia Incidence and prevention. *Drug Saf.* 2001;24: 413–442.
64. McCaughey W. Adverse effects of local anaesthetics. *Drug Saf.* 1992;7:178–189.
65. Mackley CL, Marks JG Jr, Anderson BE. Delayed-type hypersensitivity to lidocaine. *Arch Dermatol.* 2003;139:343–346.
66. Bartfield JM, Jandreau SW, Raccio-Robak N. Randomized trial of diphenhydramine versus benzyl alcohol with epinephrine as an alternative to lidocaine local anesthesia. *Ann Emerg Med.* 1998;32:650–654.
67. Dire DJ, Hogan DE. Double-blinded comparison of diphenhydramine versus lidocaine as a local anesthetic. *Ann Emerg Med.* 1993;22:1419–1422.
68. Altunkaya H, Ozer Y, Kargi E, Babuccu O. Comparison of local anaesthetic effects of tramadol with prilocaine for minor surgical procedures. *Br J Anaesth.* 2003;90:320–322.
69. Pang WW, Mok MS, Chang DP, Yang TF, Lin CH, Huang MH. Intradermal injection of tramadol has local anesthetic effect: a comparison with lidocaine. *Acta Anaesthesiol Sin.* 1998;36:133–136.
70. Klein JA, Kassarjdian N. Lidocaine toxicity with tumescent liposuction. A case report of probable drug interactions. *Dermatol Surg.* 1997;23:1169–1174.
71. Oni G, Brown S, Burrus C, et al. Effect of 4% topical lidocaine applied to the face on the serum levels of lidocaine and its metabolite, monoethylglycinexylidide. *Aesthet Surg J.* 2010;30:853–858.
72. Oni G, Brown S, Kenkel J. Comparison of five commonly-available, lidocaine-containing topical anesthetics and their effect on serum levels of lidocaine and its metabolite monoethylglycinexylidide (MEGX). *Aesthet Surg J.* 2012;32: 495–503.
73. Berkman S, MacGregor J, Alster T. Adverse effects of topical anesthetics for dermatologic procedures. *Expert Opin Drug Saf.* 2012;11:415–423.
74. Coleman MD, Coleman NA. Drug-induced methaemoglobinaemia. Treatment issues. *Drug Saf.* 1996;14:394–405.
75. de Almeida AR, Kadunc BV, de Oliveira EM. Improving botulinum toxin therapy for palmar hyperhidrosis: wrist block and technical considerations. *Dermatol Surg.* 2001;27:34–36.
76. Keel D, Goldman MP. Tumescent anesthesia in ambulatory phlebectomy: addition of epinephrine. *Dermatol Surg.* 1999;25:371–372.
77. Hanke CW. The tumescent facial block: tumescent local anesthesia and nerve block anesthesia for full-face laser resurfacing. *Dermatol Surg.* 2001;27:1003–1005.
78. Coleman WP III, Klein JA. Use of the tumescent technique for scalp surgery, dermabrasion, and soft tissue reconstruction. *J Dermatol Surg Oncol.* 1992;18:130–135.

CHAPTER 5

Aseptic Technique

Jill Henley & Jerry D. Brewer

INTRODUCTION

Surgical site infections (SSI) represent a leading cause of morbidity following inpatient surgical procedures, and constitute up to one-third of all nosocomial infections.[1,2] Fortunately, there is a much lower risk of infection following dermatologic procedures than there is with more invasive surgical procedures. Dermatologists perform over 3.9 million procedures each year and are estimated to have an infection rate of only 3.5%.[3–9] Although the risk of infection is low, SSI can lead to increased morbidity, expense, and distress for the patient during the postoperative period.[10]

Historically, surgical procedures were associated with high rates of infection and sepsis, as well as patient mortality. It was not until 1865 that Joseph Lister significantly improved patient outcomes after his experimentation with various antiseptic techniques.[11] Lister required the patient's wounds to be cleansed with carbolic acid prior to surgery.[11] He also required the surgical staff to scrub their hands with the acid prior to procedures and to soak instruments and towels in carbolic acid before using them in surgery.[11,12] As a result, surgeries that had once been associated with a 50% mortality rate due to infection showed vast improvements in patient survival.[11,12] In the years that followed, other scientists and researchers continued to improve upon Lister's techniques, which ultimately led to the strict standards of antisepsis in place today.

This chapter discusses the current recommendations for sterile technique with specific application to dermatologic procedures. It is important to recognize that the bacterial load on the patient's skin strongly correlates with the risk of SSI; therefore, proper preoperative precautions and aseptic technique are imperative to decrease the patient's bacterial load and the subsequent risk of infection.[13–15] This chapter will also provide information regarding the antiseptic agents available today, proper preoperative preparation of the patient and surgical staff, and proper outpatient sterilization and storage of surgical instruments.

DEFINITION OF SURGICAL SITE INFECTION

The Centers for Disease Control (CDC) have formally defined what constitutes an SSI to help ensure prompt recognition by healthcare professionals. As dermatologic procedures are mostly confined to the superficial tissues, the definition of a superficial SSI is provided here. A superficial SSI is defined as an infection confined to the epidermis, dermis, or subcutaneous tissues occurring within 30 days of the surgical procedure in the presence of at least one other sign of infection: purulent drainage from the incision site, aseptic isolation of microbes, the diagnosis of a SSI made by an attending physician, or other signs of infection such as erythema, edema, tenderness, or warmth at the incision site (Table 5-1) (Fig. 5-1).[16,17]

In addition, certain factors endogenous to the patient can increase the risk of infection. Advanced age, obesity, immunosuppression, diabetes mellitus, malignancy, chronic obstructive pulmonary disease (COPD), infectious diseases, malnutrition, chronic alcohol or tobacco use, or a bleeding diathesis all lead to a greater risk of postoperative infection.[3,15,17] Although these chronic conditions can be well managed, it can be difficult to fully eliminate these risk factors prior to cutaneous procedures. Knowledge of these conditions beforehand, along with a thorough preoperative evaluation, can allow the physician to take additional precautions before the procedure, such as placing the patient on an appropriate antibiotic.

Factors that are considered exogenous to the patient also contribute to the development of infection. Exogenous factors are largely modifiable and correlate with the quantity of microbes transferred to the patient during the procedure from patient care personnel, surgical equipment, and the surrounding environment.[17,18] The risks associated with exogenous factors can be minimized by proper antiseptic preparation of the surgical staff and proper sterilization of the surgical instruments. The length of the surgical procedure also positively correlates with the development of SSI. For every hour of surgery performed, the risk of infection is doubled.[19]

TABLE 5-1
CDC Definition of a SSI

CDC Definition of a Superficial Surgical Site Infection
The development of an infection within 30 d of the surgical procedure that is confined to the skin and subcutaneous tissues, plus one additional sign or symptom: 1. Purulent drainage from the incision site 2. Isolation of organisms from the incision site 3. At least one of the following: pain or tenderness, localized swelling, redness, or heat 4. Diagnosis of a SSI by the surgeon or attending physician[15–18]

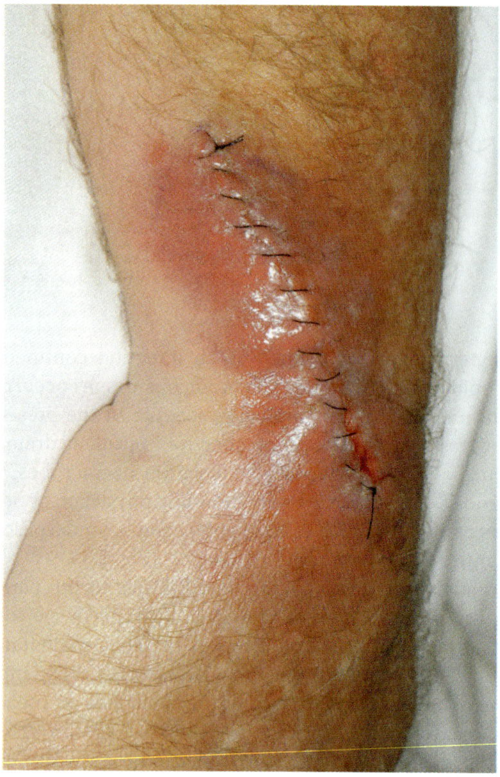

Figure 5-1 An example of a surgical site infection.

In order to estimate the patient's risk of SSI postoperatively, a set of guidelines categorizing wounds into four different classes were created (see Table 5-2). Most dermatologic procedures are performed on clean, class I wounds, with a less than 5% risk of postoperative infection. As the wounds themselves are not infected, it is often the microbial flora of the surrounding skin that poses the greatest risk of infection.[20,21]

SKIN RESIDENT AND TRANSIENT FLORA

One of the skin's major functions is to provide a protective barrier against the external environment and its microorganisms. It is estimated that over 10^{14} bacteria colonize the human body, inhabiting specific anatomic locations which depend upon the pH, temperature, oxygen, water, and nutrient availability for the bacteria.[24] Most microbial flora are considered commensal organisms that reside in the superficial layers of the skin and hair follicles, and can be further categorized into resident or transient flora.[24,25]

Resident flora is comprised of multiple, stable microorganisms that live and multiply on the skin.[26] It is largely composed of gram-positive bacteria such as *Staphylococcus epidermidis,* which comprises up to 90% of the population of aerobic bacteria.[24] The number of people colonized with *Staphylococcus aureus* is increasing, with an estimated colonization rate of 30% to 50%.[27] As a result, the number of people colonized with community-acquired strains of MRSA has also increased.[17,27] It is important to recognize that *S. aureus* remains the most common pathogen isolated from SSI (followed by *S. epidermidis, Enterococcus, and Escherichia coli*) with as few as 3×10^{14} staphylococci required for pus formation.[17,28] Because *S. aureus* is the most common pathogen isolated from SSI, it is important to place the patient on an antibiotic that has excellent coverage for *S. aureus* if a wound becomes infected postoperatively.

Transient flora consists of the microbes temporarily transferred to the skin from direct contact with a person, object, or the surrounding environment. Gram-negative bacteria and *Streptococcus* species are considered to be transient because they cannot survive on the skin for a long time.[24,29] Patients who have been hospitalized recently or who have diabetes mellitus are also more likely to be transiently colonized with gram-negative bacteria.[20,30] Since transient flora causes the majority of SSI, it is,

TABLE 5-2
Wound Classification and Estimated Infection Risk

Class	Type	Description	Examples	Infection Risk
Class I	Clean	Noncontaminated wounds created using sterile technique[17,20,22,23]	Most dermatologic procedures	<5%[20,22]
Class II	Clean-Contaminated	Wounds that are located in contaminated areas such as the oral mucosa, respiratory tract, axilla, and perineum; or in which minor breaks in sterile technique occurred during the procedure[17,20,22,23]	Procedures located on the oral or genitalia mucosa	10%[20,22]
Class III	Contaminated	Wounds that are contaminated secondary to trauma or are acutely inflamed; or in which major breaks in sterile technique occurred during the procedure[17,20,22,23]	Procedures on inflamed tissue	20%–30%[20,22]
Class IV	Infected	Wounds that are grossly purulent or necrotic[17,20,22,23]	Infected cysts or abscesses	30%–40%[20,22]

TABLE 5-3 Microbial Flora of the Skin	
Gram-Positive Bacteria	
S. epidermidis	Comprises up to 90% of the aerobic skin flora[24,25,29,31]
S. aureus	Estimated to colonize 30%–50% of healthy people[17,29] Most commonly colonizes the intertriginous areas, nares, perineum, axilla, and toe webs[27,29,31] The rate of MRSA[a] colonization is increasing with a rising proportion of community-acquired strains[32]
Micrococci	Less common than staphylococci[29,31] There are at least 8 different species of *Micrococcus* that are present on the skin with *Micrococcus luteus* being the most common[24,29]
P. acnes	Most commonly colonizes areas rich in sebaceous glands and reaches its peak around puberty[24,29,31]
Streptococcus	*Alpha*-hemolytic *Streptococcus* most commonly colonizes the oropharynx[24,25,29] *Beta*-hemolytic *Streptococcus* does not commonly colonize the skin due to the high lipid content of the skin, which inhibits growth of the species[24,29]
Gram-Negative Bacteria	
Acinetobacter, E. coli, Proteus, Klebsiella, Enterobacter, P. aeruginosa	Do not commonly comprise the resident microbial flora and are more likely to be found transiently on the skin. Most commonly found in areas of high moisture, such as the axilla, toe web spaces, and intertriginous areas.[24,25,29,31] Patients that have undergone long-term hospitalization, hospital workers, and patients with diabetes mellitus are at an increased risk for gram negative colonization.[29,33] *Acinetobacter* is estimated to colonize up to 25% of people.[25,29,31] *Pseudomonas* frequently colonizes the external ear[34]
Fungi	
Pityrosporum	Requires lipids for growth and most commonly colonizes areas rich in sebaceous glands[25,31]
Candida albicans	Can be found on the mucous membranes[25,29,31] More common in immunosuppressed and diabetic patients[29,31]

[a]Methicillin-resistant *Staphylococcus aureus.*

therefore, important to reduce the number of microorganisms that are temporarily transferred to the patient's skin by using antiseptic preparations and proper sterile technique (Table 5-3).[15]

Patients undergoing more extensive dermatologic procedures are at an increased risk of infection and should be placed on a prophylactic antibiotic before the procedure. This helps to decrease the overall bacterial load on the patient's skin at the time of surgery.[15,35] More information regarding the types of patients who could benefit from prophylactic antibiotics will be found in the chapter entitled, *Antibiotic Prophylaxis.*

PREPARATION OF THE PATIENT

Preoperative preparation is an essential element in prevention of SSI. The amount of preparation required depends on the invasiveness of the procedure. Ideally, a thorough preoperative evaluation should be conducted for dermatologic procedures that are scheduled in advance; specific infectious precautions, such as prophylactic antibiotics or preoperative bathing, can then be recommended for patients at an increased risk of infection.[20] Depending on the extent of the procedure, the patient's street clothes may need to be removed and replaced with a freshly laundered hospital gown. Other precautions, such as hair removal and antiseptic skin preparation, can be addressed on the day of the procedure.

PREOPERATIVE BATHING

Currently, there are no recommendations regarding bathing prior to dermatologic procedures; however, preoperative bathing may be beneficial for patients undergoing extensive procedures who are more likely to be at an increased risk of infection. It is thought that bathing the day before surgery with an antiseptic or bar soap helps to decrease the overall bacterial load. A 2012 Cochrane review found that patients who washed themselves using 4% chlorhexidine gluconate or regular bar soap prior to surgical operations had lower rates of infection than those who did not bathe preoperatively.[30] More research with specific application to dermatologic procedures needs to be conducted however, so that more formal recommendations can be made.

HAIR REMOVAL

Procedures located in hair bearing areas may require hair removal prior to surgery. Excess hair can interfere with suturing of the incision site, application of adhesive dressings, and the visibility of the operative field.[36,37] Hair has been speculated to increase the rate of SSI, although a 2011 Cochrane review failed to find evidence to support this claim.[38] Clipping the hair is preferable to shaving because shaving traumatizes the skin, leading to enhanced bacterial proliferation and an increased risk of infection.[3,19,21,26,38] Clipping the hair is quick, atraumatic, and leaves the hair about 1 mm in length.[38] Depilatory creams can also be used for hair removal in areas that are difficult to clip or shave, but must be applied the day before surgery to be effective, and are thought to carry the same risk of infection as shaving.[31,38]

ANTISEPTIC SKIN PREPARATION

Reducing the bacterial load on the skin prior to dermatologic procedures can significantly decrease the patient's risk for developing a SSI. Use of effective antiseptic agents as well as irrigation of the area with normal saline can help to diminish some of the bacterial load.[25,39] Numerous antiseptic agents are available for dermatologic procedures (Table 5-4). The optimal antiseptic agent would remove most of the resident and transient flora quickly and remain active for the entire procedure.[40] Two of the most commonly used antiseptics are chlorhexidine gluconate and povidone–iodine. Although larger studies have failed to show a significant difference between the two agents, smaller studies have shown chlorhexidine gluconate to be superior.[41] Chlorhexidine may be even more effective when combined with isopropyl alcohol. In 2010, a study conducted by Darouiche et al.[42] found 2% chlorhexidine gluconate in combination with isopropyl alcohol (70%) to be more effective than povidone–iodine (10%) in preventing SSI following clean-contaminated surgical procedures.

ANTISEPTICS

Chlorhexidine is one of the most effective and popular antiseptic agents used today. Its activity is concentration dependent.[44] At higher concentrations, it is bactericidal with a quick onset of action and a broad spectrum of antimicrobial

TABLE 5-4
Antiseptic Agents

Antiseptic Agent	Mechanism	Onset of Activity	Residual Activity	Antimicrobial Activity	Comments
Chlorhexidine (Chloraprep) (Hibiclens)	Biguanide that binds to the stratum corneum of the skin.[43] Bactericidal at high concentrations[44]	Rapid onset of activity.[21,45] Do not need to wait until dry[44]	Yes (up to 48 h)[27,46]	Gram-positives Gram-negatives Fungi Viruses[45,47]	Can be more expensive than other products[44] Is not inactivated by blood or other protein-rich substances[45] Many preparations contain isopropyl alcohol, which can increase the flammability of the product[48] Should not be used near the eyes or ears because of the risk of ototoxicity and irritation to the cornea and conjunctiva of the eye[26,44,49–54]
Iodophors (Betadine) (Povidone–iodine)	Bound to water-soluble carriers such as povidone; iodine is bactericidal[55]	Requires 3–5 min to dry to reach full activity[21,55,56]	Little residual activity.[43,55] Povidone prolongs the bactericidal activity of iodine[44]	Gram-positives Gram-negatives Fungi Viruses[27,55]	Inactivated by blood and other protein-rich substances.[30,55] Does not effectively kill spores.[27,55] Iodine can be irritating and lead to temporary staining of the skin [55] Can rarely lead to systemic toxicity if large amounts are applied on the mucosal surfaces, especially in infants[21,26,44,50]
Alcohol (Isopropyl alcohol) (Ethyl alcohol)	Denatures bacterial cell wall proteins.[47,57] Activity is concentration dependent[47]	Quickest onset of action of all the antiseptics	No residual activity once evaporated[55,58]	Gram-positives Gram-negatives Fungi Less viral coverage[57,58]	Can be flammable when exposed to heat[48] Little activity against spore-producing bacteria[59] Cannot remove organic material or surface dirt from the skin[60]
Phenolic compounds (Hexachlorophene) (Triclosan) (Chloroxylenol)	Bacteriostatic; Forms a film over the skin[59,61]	Slow onset of action[58,59]	Yes (Up to 6 h)[58]	Gram-positives Less gram-negative coverage (especially *P. aeruginosa*) Less fungal coverage Less viral coverage[58,59,61]	Hexachlorophene is absorbed from the skin and at high concentrations which can be toxic, particularly in neonates[58,62] Hexachlorophene can become contaminated by gram negative bacteria[61,62]; not commonly used today[63]

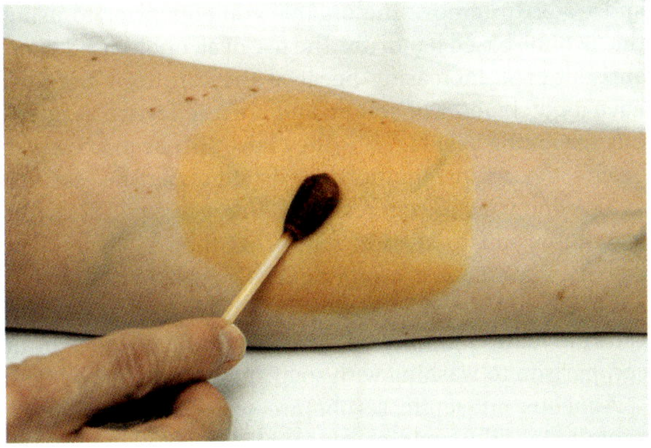

Figure 5-2 Povidone–iodine antiseptic application.

activity.[47] In addition, it binds to the stratum corneum of the skin, which prolongs the duration of activity.[3,64] Chlorhexidine does not become inactivated when it is wiped away from the skin or when it comes into contact with bodily fluids.[3] It should not be used near the eyes or the inner ear because the detergent can be irritating to these structures.[26,49–52] Rarely, serious complications such as deafness and blindness have occurred.[4,49–51,53,65]

Historically, iodine has been used as an antiseptic agent since the early 1900s. Iodine bound to water-soluble iodophors, such as povidone, is currently used, because its direct application is too irritating to the skin.[55] Moreover, the iodophor prolongs the duration of iodine's antiseptic activity on the skin.[55,59] Iodine is bactericidal with a broad antimicrobial range, but requires several minutes to dry to reach full activity.[41,56] Other disadvantages of iodine are that it can stain the skin temporarily, and that it can also be inactivated by bodily fluids, including blood.[3,4,64] In addition, the product loses its antimicrobial activity when it is wiped from the skin.[1] Iodine containing products should not be used in patients who have an iodine or shellfish allergy (Fig. 5-2).[4]

Alcohol is a commonly used antiseptic for minor dermatologic procedures. It is the most rapidly acting of the antiseptic agents, but has no residual activity once it evaporates from the skin.[4,17,55,58] Alcohol has broad antimicrobial activity but does not effectively kill spores.[17,59] Isopropyl alcohol is generally recommended over ethyl alcohol because it causes less skin irritation and has greater antimicrobial activity.[26,55,58] In general, alcohols have been found to be more effective when used in conjunction with other antiseptic agents such as chlorhexidine.[26,42] It is important to keep in mind that alcohol can become flammable in the presence of heat, such as with electrocoagulation.[48]

Phenol-derivatives such as hexachlorophene are slow-acting bacteriostatic agents that have excellent gram-positive coverage but lack adequate gram-negative coverage, especially against *Pseudomonas aeruginosa*.[59] Hexachlorophene has a very slow onset of action, requiring multiple days of application in order to be as effective as the other antiseptic agents, but has a longer duration of activity (up to 6 hours).[58] It has been found to be toxic when applied to large body surface areas and bottles of hexachlorophene are also prone to bacterial contamination.[61,62] As a result, this agent is not commonly used today.[59]

Before application of any antiseptic, it is important to remove any dirt or organic material from the skin with soap and water.[17] The antiseptic should be applied to the area in concentric circles, beginning from the operative site with extension outward to the surrounding skin.[17] Applying the antiseptic to the surrounding skin is important both to decrease the bacterial load and to prevent the surrounding bacteria from migrating to the incision site.[4] This action will also decrease the likelihood of surgical instrument contamination if the instrument comes in contact with the surrounding skin during the procedure.[4] In addition, the concentric motion used when applying the antiseptic creates friction on the surface of the skin, allowing for deeper penetration.[64] Antiseptic agents are available in disposable, one-time-use packages or in multi-use bottles. Disposable, one-time-use packages are effective, user friendly, and have a lower risk of bacterial contamination than multi-use bottles.[66]

Another technique currently being implemented by general surgeons to decrease the risk of infection is the application of a cyanoacrylate microbial sealant to the skin before clean surgical operations.[67] The sealant can be applied with a sterile applicator after antiseptically prepping the skin. Use of a sealant may be beneficial for extensive dermatologic procedures as an additional way to prevent normal flora from migrating into the operative area; however, studies have failed to find any significant differences on the incidence of SSI after preparation of the skin with a cyanoacrylate sealant.[67]

PREOPERATIVE MARKING PENS

Skin lesions are commonly outlined with a marking pen prior to dermatologic procedures both to verify the location and to accurately identify the borders of the lesion.[68] Nonetheless, preoperative marking pens have been associated with bacterial cross-contamination between patients.[69,70] Old or dried out marking pens (greater than 3 months) have been found to harbor bacteria and should not be used on patients.[69,71] Instead, an ethanol-based ink permanent marking pen or a gentian violet marking pen should be used.[71] There should also be a 2 to 10 minute interval between uses to prevent cross-contamination.[69,70,72,73] The ethanol-based ink in permanent marking pens is bactericidal and can decrease the risk of infection.[69,72,73] Gentian violet marking pens have broad antimicrobial coverage as well but do not effectively kill *Mycobacterium* species.[71] As a result, bottled solutions of gentian violet need to undergo periodic autoclaving, because they are prone to contamination with *Mycobacterium chelonae*.[74] Furthermore, the use of disposable marking pens is encouraged in patients who are immunosuppressed or who have known colonization with a multidrug resistant organism.[68–70]

DRAPING

Sterile drapes are placed around the incision site prior to dermatologic procedures to prevent the surrounding bacteria on the skin from entering the incision site as well as from coming into contact with the instruments and gloves of the surgical staff. Unfortunately, studies have failed to find a reduction in the rate of infection with the use of plastic adhesive drapes during surgical procedures, and have actually found patients to be at a slightly increased risk of infection with their use.[2] This is thought to be due to increased moisture being trapped beneath the drapes, creating an environment that enhances bacterial proliferation.[75] As a result, the drapes should be chemically pretreated to be moisture resistant. The drapes can be cloth, plastic, or paper and can be prepackaged within disposable surgical kits. Cloth drapes are not commonly used in the outpatient setting, but they should be composed of at least a 270 thread count pima cotton to provide a more effective moisture barrier.[26,76] Most of the drapes used for dermatologic procedures are disposable paper drapes. These drapes should be laminated prior to surgery to provide an adequate moisture barrier.[76] In addition, some plastic drapes come with an adhesive on the margins of the drape, to better hold the drape in place.[26]

PREPARATION OF THE SURGEON

Preparation of the staff is one of the most important ways to prevent SSI. It has been postulated that the highest rate of bacterial transfer occurs due to physical contact with the surgical staff during the procedure.[13] In order to diminish the quantity of bacteria transferred from the staff to the patient, it is important to decrease the bacterial load of the staff with preoperative hand washing and proper sterile attire. Recent studies have found that by incorporating specific infection-control practices in dermatologic surgery, such as wearing surgical caps with the hair tied back in a ponytail or bun, jewelry restrictions (only a smooth wedding band allowed), use of chlorhexidine–alcohol handrub preoperatively, and sterile gloves, the rate of SSI can be decreased from 2.5% to 0.9%.[5] Although these practices may be effective in infection prevention, they may not be cost effective. Another study with similar infection rates minimized costs by only using sterile gloves and cloth drapes for more extensive, reconstructive procedures and nonsterile gloves for the rest.[77]

WASHING HANDS

During dermatologic procedures, gloves of the surgical staff can become perforated or torn, thereby exposing the underlying skin; it is, therefore, important to thoroughly rid the skin of potential pathogens prior to procedures. Washing hands with soap and water removes most of the transient flora of the skin, but fails to inhibit the growth of the resident flora. On the other hand, antiseptic hand preparations remove all of the transient flora in addition to inhibiting the growth of the resident flora.[78]

There are three types of antiseptic hand preparations available: alcohol-based handrubs, aqueous hand scrubs, and alcohol-based handrubs containing active ingredients such as chlorhexidine gluconate or povidone–iodine.[59] Alcohol-based hand antiseptics can contain ethanol, isopropanol, or n-propanol and require rubbing of the hands until the solution has fully evaporated.[59] If the hands are visibly soiled, they should be thoroughly washed with soap and water to remove the organic contents prior to using the alcohol-based handrub. The use of alcohol-based hand antiseptics is increasing because they are user friendly, have a quick onset of action, and are as effective as aqueous scrubbing agents.[59,78,79] They have also been shown to be effective against multidrug resistant organisms, such as MRSA and vancomycin resistant *Enterococcus* (VRE), but it is important to keep in mind that they lack sufficient activity against *Clostridium difficile*.[80] An additional benefit of alcohol-based handrubs is that they are less likely to cause irritant contact dermatitis or drying of the skin in comparison to washing with soap and water.[78]

Aqueous antiseptic scrubs are water-based solutions containing chlorhexidine gluconate or povidone–iodine which require the hands and arms to be wet prior to scrubbing with a sponge or brush.[59] Chlorhexidine based aqueous scrubs are slightly more effective than povidone–iodine based aqueous scrubs in decreasing the number of colony forming units on the skin.[59]

Alcohol-based handrubs that contain chlorhexidine gluconate or povidone–iodine are extremely effective because the added ingredients prolong the duration of antiseptic activity of the alcohol in addition to broadening the antimicrobial coverage.[59] A 2008 study requiring dermatologic surgical staff to use an alcohol-based, chlorhexidine gluconate handrub found a significant decrease in the number of postoperative SSI.[5,6]

In addition to hand antisepsis, there has been a recent debate over the potential consequences of the presence of finger nail polish and jewelry during preoperative antiseptic preparation. It has been proposed that finger rings decrease the effectiveness of antiseptic handrubs by acting as a reservoir for bacteria, although there has been insufficient evidence to support this statement.[78,81] There is also the concern that rings can tear surgical gloves more readily, thereby increasing the risk of skin exposure during the procedure.[59,81] It is also thought that nail polish might harbor excess bacteria and increase the risk of SSI, but there is insufficient evidence to support this claim.[81] On the other hand, artificial nails have been found to harbor bacteria and fungi, increasing the patient's exposure to microorganisms during the procedure.[17] As a result, artificial nails are generally not recommended during extensive surgical procedures.

STERILE ATTIRE

The surgical attire worn for dermatologic procedures varies with each institution, although it often corresponds to the invasiveness of the procedure. A recent survey of dermatologic surgeons found that they are more likely to wear additional surgical garments such as surgical caps and masks for more invasive procedures like ablative resurfacing, liposuction, blepharoplasties, and Mohs micrographic surgery, in comparison to minor procedures such as shave or punch biopsies.[82]

GLOVES

Wearing gloves during surgical procedures not only provides protection for the patient against potential pathogens, but also protects the surgical staff from being exposed to bodily fluids. Since the beginning of their use in the early 1900s, sterile gloves have largely reduced the number of SSI.[83] They have been the standard of care during invasive surgical procedures for many years, although recent studies with specific application to dermatologic procedures have found nonsterile gloves to be equally effective in the prevention of SSI.[84,85] There have been similar findings in studies conducted by specialists in other fields.[86] It is important to keep in mind that the results of these studies did not pertain to longer, more invasive dermatologic procedures such as reconstruction after Mohs surgery. Wearing an additional set of gloves, which is known as double gloving, does not reduce the rate of SSI;[87] however, double gloving does decrease the risk of glove perforation.[87]

MASKS

Surgical face masks were originally designed to decrease the expulsion of microorganisms from the mouth and nasopharynx of the surgical staff during surgery to reduce the rate of infections.[88] Unfortunately, studies have failed to find evidence to support a reduction in the rate of infections with their use.[88] This may be a consequence of the mask being worn inappropriately, such as being tied too loosely around the back of the neck. This allows bacteria from the mouth and nasopharynx to flow out from the sides of the mask.[88,89] More importantly, it is hypothesized that the bacteria shed from the skin of surgical staff during the procedure has an even greater impact on the rate of infection than the bacteria shed from the respiratory tract.[88–90] The risk of infection is increased with each person that enters the operating room,[89] which is why protective clothing may be more beneficial for infection prevention than face masks.

Masks carry the additional benefit of providing protection for the surgical staff from the patient's bodily fluids during the procedure.[91] Some of the disposable face masks have a protective shield that protects the eyes from splashes during the procedure. The Occupational Safety and Health Administration (OSHA) regulations require all surgical staff to wear protective eyewear in addition to face masks during all procedures at heightened risk for exposure to bodily fluids (Fig. 5-3).[17]

HAIR COVERS

Hair covers are an essential part of the surgeon's attire for inpatient surgical procedures, although there is no evidence to support a reduction in the risk of SSI with their use.[89] Hair has been found to harbor *Staphylococcus* and *Streptococcus* species, and if shed while in contact with the patient's incision site, could potentially increase the patient's risk of infection;[92] thus, hair coverings may be beneficial in dermatologic procedures as they should be helpful in preventing bacteria on the scalp and hair from being shed during the procedure.

SCRUBS AND GOWNS

As previously mentioned, protective clothing worn by the surgical staff may be the most beneficial method of infection prevention by protecting the patient from being exposed to bacteria shed from their skin.[89] Surgical scrubs are recommended for dermatologic surgeries. They should be freshly laundered, as scrubs worn for longer periods of time tend to harbor more bacteria.[93] If the scrubs are visibly soiled with blood or other fluids, OSHA regulations require the scrubs to be exchanged for a freshly laundered pair.[17]

Sterile surgical gowns can be worn over scrubs to prevent the bacteria on the skin and clothing of the surgical staff from directly contacting the patient and from becoming airborne.[32] Most surgical gowns worn today are composed of nonwoven materials and are disposable, one-time-use gowns.[32] Reusable gowns are associated with a greater risk of infection;[94] however, more research needs to be conducted regarding the rates of infection with sterile versus nonsterile surgical gowns in outpatient dermatologic surgery.

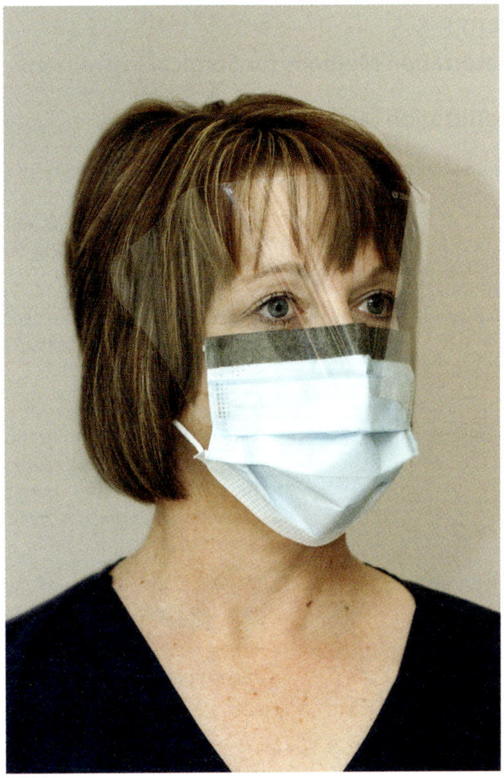

Figure 5-3 Protective face mask.

STERILIZATION AND PACKAGING OF INSTRUMENTS

As most dermatologic procedures are performed in an outpatient setting, there is great variability as to how surgical instruments are managed. Some offices may utilize disposable surgical instruments for dermatologic procedures, whereas other offices may employ their own method of instrument sterilization. Dermatologic offices see a high volume of patients daily and need to have a large amount of supplies available; therefore, the ideal method of sterilization would be quick, effective, and able to sterilize large amounts of materials at one time.

TABLE 5-5
Sterilization Methods for Surgical Instruments

Sterilization Method	Description	Comments
Steam autoclave	Produces 100% humidity at a temperature of 121°C; Effectively sterilizes instruments within 15 min at a stable, high pressure of 2 atmospheres[96]; Must allow 5–10 min for the instruments to dry[76]	Very effective. Can be used for glass beakers, cloth and paper towels, gauze, and plastic devices.[97] Must have a control, such as a biologic indicator, in place to monitor effectiveness.[17,96] The high steam can dull sharp edges of instruments[76]
Dry heat	Higher temperatures are used for a longer period of time due to lack of moisture[76]	Very effective for heat-resistant materials, that is, instruments and glassware, but cloth, paper, and plastic cannot be sterilized with this method.[82] Cost-effective and does not dull instruments[99]
Cold sterilization	Due to incomplete sterilization, it is considered a disinfectant method; glutaraldehyde is the most commonly used agent but takes 10 h to take effect and must be buffered to a pH of 8.5 to become sporicidal[76]	Not commonly used in practice due to incomplete sterilization; not effective against bacterial spores or virus particles.[82,97] Inactivated by organic materials; Buffered solutions only last up to 4 wk[76]
Chemiclave	Version of the steam autoclave; A chemical solution keeps the humidity to less than 15%[76]	Lower moisture decreases the risk for instrument dulling; Less time required for drying[76]
Gas sterilization	Ethylene oxide sterilizes the instrument over many hours at a low temperature[96]	Effective for instruments that are heat- and moisture-sensitive.[96] Ethylene oxide is toxic and a carcinogen.[97] Area must be isolated from the general work area. Not commonly used[76]

Source: Data from Sebben JE. Survey of sterile technique used by dermatologic surgeons. *J Am Acad Dermatol*. 1988;18:1107–1113.

Before instruments can be disinfected or sterilized, organic debris such as blood, dirt, or bodily fluids must be removed.[95,96] This can be accomplished by cleaning the instruments with water and a detergent manually or by a mechanical unit such as an ultrasonic cleaner, washer–disinfector, or a washer–sterilizer.[96] The advantages of an ultrasonic cleaner over manual cleaning are that the instruments are cleaned faster (within 5 minutes) and that the staff are not at risk for injury from handling the sharp instruments.[76] Instruments should be cleaned immediately following surgery to prevent drying of the organic material on the surface of the instrument.[76] All instruments should be thoroughly inspected after cleaning and, if their hinges need lubrication, instrument milk should be applied.[76] Oils should not be used for lubrication because they cause the instruments to become stiff after autoclaving.[76]

Sterilization destroys all microbes and spores and can be accomplished by various methods (Table 5-5). Most offices that sterilize surgical instruments use steam autoclaving as their preferred technique.[97] Steam autoclaving is generally very quick and effective. In a survey conducted among 614 dermatologic surgeons, 67% reported using steam autoclaving as their desired method of instrument sterilization.[82] On the other hand, more and more offices are using disposable one-time-use surgical kits. The disposable instruments can be slightly more expensive, but are user friendly and reliable. If the surgical equipment or packaging appears discolored or damp, there is a risk of bacterial contamination and the package should be replaced with another sterile surgical kit.[98]

SURGICAL INSTRUMENT PACKAGING AND STORAGE

Instruments can be packaged with cloth or paper, or placed in a plastic self-seal sterilization pack (Fig. 5-4).[76] For self-seal sterilization packs, one side of the package is transparent and the other side is paper, which can be sealed with a special autoclave tape or heat sealer.[76] Instruments should be autoclaved in the open position (e.g., hemostats) so that all areas of the instrument are sterilized. Additionally, rubber or gauze can be placed over the sharp edges of the instruments to prevent dulling.[76] On

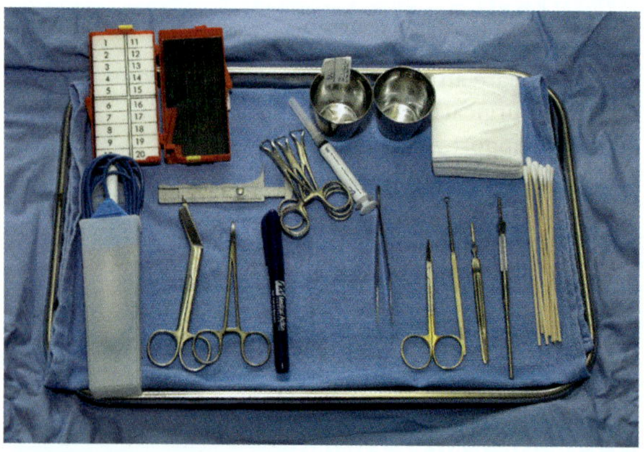

Figure 5-4 Surgical instrument tray setup with a sterile drape.

the other hand, instruments can be placed openly in the autoclave and then stored in a disinfectant holding solution upon removal, such as glutaraldehyde or peracetic acid. It is important to keep in mind that disinfectants do not adequately kill spores, which increases the risk of bacterial contamination and shortens the shelf life.[76,96] As a result, this technique is not commonly used.

The time allotted for storage depends on the material in which the instruments are packed and the moisture content of the storage environment. The sterilized instruments should be stored in a closed cabinet with adequate bug and dust control; the date and time of sterilization should be externally visible on each individual pack.[100] There should also be an external indicator, indicating that the instrument pack has been adequately sterilized.[76] The more impermeable the packaging is to moisture, the longer the instruments can be safely stored. This is why instruments that are placed in sealed packages have a longer shelf life.[100] The self-seal sterilization packs can be stored for up to 1 year.[76] Instruments wrapped in two layers of 140 thread-count muslin can be stored for approximately 7 weeks, but the storage time can be increased up to 9 months when the packs are sealed in a polyethylene bag.[100] Instruments wrapped in a single layer of crepe paper can be safely stored for approximately 8 weeks.[100] Multi-use surgical instruments that require packaging in between uses are more likely to become contaminated. It is important to thoroughly inspect the package before use, because a puncture as small as 1.1 mm has been shown to cause bacterial contamination of the instruments.[101]

PREPARATION OF THE SURGICAL SUITE

The ideal surgical suite would have a ventilation system in place that maintains a positive pressure in the room, preventing less clean air from flowing in the direction of cleaner air.[17] Some hospital operating rooms use laminar airflow systems that pass through a high-efficiency particulate air (HEPA) filter.[17] In addition, OSHA requires all equipment and environmental surfaces contaminated with blood or other bodily fluids to be disinfected in between procedures and at the end of each day with an Environmental Protection Agency (EPA) approved disinfectant.[17]

It is also important to prepare the surgical suite prior to dermatologic procedures. Primarily, this includes setting up a table or mayo stand with a sterile drape and then placing the sterile surgical instruments over the drape (Fig. 5-5). Anticipating which instruments may be needed prior to the operation may also be helpful in maintaining sterile technique during the procedure. Particularly if the patient is suspected to have a bleeding diathesis, it is important to set up the electrocautery equipment beforehand. This includes application of a disposable, sterile tip and a sterile sleeve or surgical glove around the handle of the electrosurgical unit so the surgeon can maintain sterile technique while grasping the equipment during the procedure.[26]

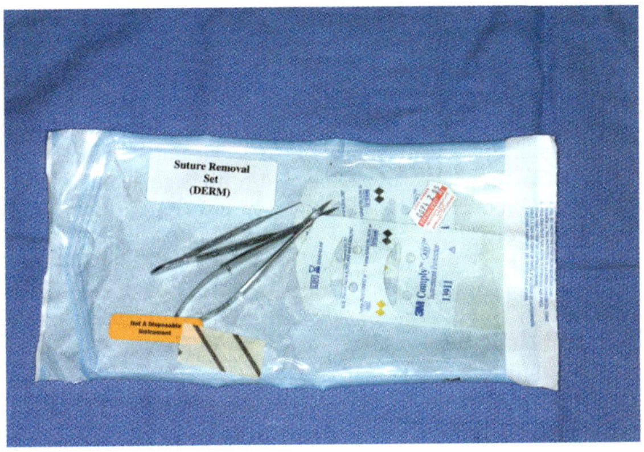

Figure 5-5 Self-seal sterilization packs for surgical instruments.

POSTOPERATIVE WOUND DRESSINGS

After the procedure, white petrolatum can be applied to the wound before the sterile dressing is placed. There is no significant difference in the rate of infection with the application of white petrolatum in comparison to topical antibiotic ointments.[102,103] White petrolatum may also be beneficial over topical antimicrobial agents because antimicrobials are more likely to cause an allergic contact dermatitis.[104] A sterile postoperative wound dressing should remain in place for at least 24 to 48 hours.[17] If a wound is left to heal by secondary intention, it should be packed with sterile gauze and then covered with a sterile dressing.[17] It is important to follow up with the patient to ensure that their wound is healing appropriately and to have them return to the office as soon as possible if they exhibit any signs of infection.

CONCLUSION

In summary, the risk of SSI following dermatologic procedures is quite low. Specific factors place certain patients at greater risk of infection over others, but it is the overall bacterial load of the patient that has the greatest impact on the rate of SSI. This can be minimized with adequate antiseptic preparation of the patient and surgical staff and proper sterilization of the surgical equipment. If the patient begin to experience signs and symptoms suggestive of infection during the postoperative period, he or she should return to the office for further evaluation and management to avoid more serious sequelae.

REFERENCES

1. Towfigh S, Cheadle WG, Lowry SF, Malangoni MA, Wilson SE. Significant reduction in incidence of wound contamination by skin flora through use of microbial sealant. *Arch Surg*. 2008;143:885–891; discussion 91.
2. Webster J, Alghamdi AA. Use of plastic adhesive drapes during surgery for preventing surgical site infection. *Cochrane Database Syst Rev*. 2007;(4):CD006353.

3. Hurst EA, Grekin RC, Yu SS, Neuhaus IM. Infectious complications and antibiotic use in dermatologic surgery. *Semin Cutan Med Surg.* 2007;26(1):47–53.
4. Wood LD, Warner NM, Billingsley EM. Infectious complications of dermatologic procedures. *Dermatol Ther.* 2011;24:558–570.
5. Martin JE, Speyer LA, Schmults CD. Heightened infection-control practices are associated with significantly lower infection rates in office-based Mohs surgery. *Dermatol Surg.* 2010;36:1529–1536.
6. Cook JL, Perone JB. A prospective evaluation of the incidence of complications associated with Mohs micrographic surgery. *Arch Dermatol.* 2003;139:143–152.
7. Maragh SL, Brown MD. Prospective evaluation of surgical site infection rate among patients with Mohs micrographic surgery without the use of prophylactic antibiotics. *J Am Acad Dermatol.* 2008;59:275–278.
8. Bordeaux JS, Martires KJ, Goldberg D, Pattee SF, Fu P, Maloney ME. Prospective evaluation of dermatologic surgery complications including patients on multiple antiplatelet and anticoagulant medications. *J Am Acad Dermatol.* 2011; 65:576–583.
9. Rogers HD, Desciak EB, Marcus RP, Wang S, MacKay-Wiggan J, Eliezri YD. Prospective study of wound infections in Mohs micrographic surgery using clean surgical technique in the absence of prophylactic antibiotics. *J Am Acad Dermatol.* 2010;63:842–851.
10. Sebben JE. Sterile technique and the prevention of wound infection in office surgery–part I. *J Dermatol Surg Oncol.* 1988;14:1364–1371.
11. Pitt D, Aubin JM. Joseph Lister: father of modern surgery. *Can J Surg.* 2012;55:E8–E9.
12. Hurwitz B, Dupree M. Why celebrate Joseph Lister? *Lancet.* 2012;379:e39–e40.
13. Ibrahimi OA, Sharon V, Eisen DB. Surgical-site infections and routes of bacterial transfer: which ones are most plausible? *Dermatol Surg.* 2011;37:1709–1720.
14. Pomerantz RG, Lee DA, Siegel DM. Risk assessment in surgical patients: balancing iatrogenic risks and benefits. *Clin Dermatol.* 2011;29:669–677.
15. Saleh K, Sonesson A, Persson B, Riesbeck K, Schmidtchen A. A descriptive study of bacterial load of full-thickness surgical wounds in dermatologic surgery. *Dermatol Surg.* 2011;37:1014–1022.
16. Horan TC, Gaynes RP, Martone WJ, Jarvis WR, Emori TG. CDC definitions of nosocomial surgical site infections, 1992: a modification of CDC definitions of surgical wound infections. *Infect Control Hosp Epidemiol.* 1992;13:606–608.
17. Mangram AJ, Horan TC, Pearson ML, Silver LC, Jarvis WR. Guideline for prevention of surgical site infection, 1999. Centers for Disease Control and Prevention (CDC) Hospital Infection Control Practices Advisory Committee. *Am J Infect Control.* 1999;27:97–132; quiz 33–34; discussion 96.
18. Horan TC, Andrus M, Dudeck MA. CDC/NHSN surveillance definition of health care-associated infection and criteria for specific types of infections in the acute care setting. *Am J Infect Control.* 2008;36:309–332.
19. Cruse PJ, Foord R. The epidemiology of wound infection. A 10-year prospective study of 62939 wounds. *Surg Clin North Am.* 1980;60:27–40.
20. Nestor MS. Perioperative use of antibiotics: preventing and treating perioperative infections. *J Drugs Dermatol.* 2005; 4:s34–s36.
21. Haas A, Grekin R. *Atlas of Cutaneous Surgery.* Philadelphia, PA: WB Saunders; 1996.
22. Haas S. The use of a surgical patch coated with human coagulation factors in surgical routine: a multicenter post-authorization surveillance. *Clin Appl Thromb Hemost.* 2006;12:445–450.
23. Culver DH, Horan TC, Gaynes RP, et al. Surgical wound infection rates by wound class, operative procedure, and patient risk index. National Nosocomial Infections Surveillance System. *Am J Med.* 1991;91:152S–157S.
24. Davis CP. Normal flora. In: Baron S, ed. *Medical Microbiology.* 4th ed. Galveston, TX: University of Texas Medical Branch at Galveston; 1996.
25. Gould D. Skin flora: implications for nursing. *Nurs Stand.* 2012;26:48–56; quiz 58.
26. Sebben JE. Sterile technique and the prevention of wound infection in office surgery–part II. *J Dermatol Surg Oncol.* 1989;15:38–48.
27. Coia JE, Duckworth GJ, Edwards DI, et al. Guidelines for the control and prevention of meticillin-resistant *Staphylococcus aureus* (MRSA) in healthcare facilities. *J Hosp Infect.* 2006;63(Suppl 1):S1–S44.
28. Nichols RL. Preventing surgical site infections: a surgeon's perspective. *Emerg Infect Dis.* 2001;7:220–224.
29. Roth RR, James WD. Microbiology of the skin: resident flora, ecology, infection. *J Am Acad Dermatol.* 1989;20:367–390.
30. Webster J, Osborne S. Preoperative bathing or showering with skin antiseptics to prevent surgical site infection. *Cochrane Database Syst Rev.* 2012;9:CD004985.
31. Thur de Koos P, McComas B. Shaving versus skin depilatory cream for preoperative skin preparation. A prospective study of wound infection rates. *Am J Surg.* 1983;145: 377–378.
32. Eisen DB. Surgeon's garb and infection control: what's the evidence? *J Am Acad Dermatol.* 2011;64:960.e1–960.e20.
33. Curie K, Speller DC, Simpson RA, Stephens M, Cooke DI. A hospital epidemic caused by gentamicin-resistant *Klebsiella aerogenes. J Hyg (Lond).* 1978;80:115–123.
34. Bagger-Sjöbäck D, Mendel L, Nord CE. The role of prophylactic antibiotics in middle ear surgery. A study on phenoxymethylpenicillin prophylaxis. *Am J Otol.* 1987; 8:519–523.
35. Rosengren H, Dixon A. Antibacterial prophylaxis in dermatologic surgery: an evidence-based review. *Am J Clin Dermatol.* 2010;11:35–44.
36. Miller JJ, Weber PC, Patel S, Ramey J. Intracranial surgery: to shave or not to shave? *Otol Neurotol.* 2001;22:908–911.
37. Kumar K, Thomas J, Chan C. Cosmesis in neurosurgery: is the bald head necessary to avoid postoperative infection? *Ann Acad Med Singapore.* 2002;31:150–154.
38. Tanner J, Norrie P, Melen K. Preoperative hair removal to reduce surgical site infection. *Cochrane Database Syst Rev.* 2011;(11):CD004122.
39. Becerro de Bengoa Vallejo R, Losa Iglesias ME, Alou Cervera L, Sevillano Fernández D, Prieto Prieto J. Efficacy of preoperative and intraoperative skin and nail surgical preparation of the foot in reducing bacterial load. *Dermatol Surg.* 2010;36:1258–1265.
40. Dzubow LM, Halpern AC, Leyden JJ, Grossman D, McGinley KJ. Comparison of preoperative skin preparations for the face. *J Am Acad Dermatol.* 1988;19:737–741.
41. Noorani A, Rabey N, Walsh SR, Davies RJ. Systematic review and meta-analysis of preoperative antisepsis with chlorhexidine versus povidone-iodine in clean-contaminated surgery. *Br J Surg.* 2010;97:1614–1620.
42. Darouiche RO, Wall MJ, Itani KM, et al. Chlorhexidine-alcohol versus povidone-iodine for surgical-site antisepsis. *N Engl J Med.* 2010;362:18–26.
43. Larson EL. APIC guideline for handwashing and hand antisepsis in health care settings. *Am J Infect Control.* 1995; 23:251–269.
44. Lee I, Agarwal RK, Lee BY, Fishman NO, Umscheid CA. Systematic review and cost analysis comparing use of chlorhexidine with use of iodine for preoperative skin antisepsis to prevent surgical site infection. *Infect Control Hosp Epidemiol.* 2010;31:1219–1229.
45. Nichols RL. Current strategies for prevention of surgical site infections. *Curr Infect Dis Rep.* 2004;6:426–434.
46. Hibbard JS. Analyses comparing the antimicrobial activity and safety of current antiseptic agents: a review. *J Infus Nurs.* 2005;28:194–207.
47. Edwards PS, Lipp A, Holmes A. Preoperative skin antiseptics for preventing surgical wound infections after clean surgery. *Cochrane Database Syst Rev.* 2004:(3):CD003949.
48. Arefiev K, Warycha M, Whiting D, Alam M. Flammability of topical preparations and surgical dressings in cutaneous and laser surgery: a controlled simulation study. *J Am Acad Dermatol.* 2012;67:700–705.

49. Bicknell PG. Sensorineural deafness following myringoplasty operations. *J Laryngol Otol*. 1971;85:957–961.
50. Mac Rae SM, Brown B, Edelhauser HF. The corneal toxicity of presurgical skin antiseptics. *Am J Ophthalmol*. 1984; 97:221–232.
51. Igarashi Y, Suzuki J. Cochlear ototoxicity of chlorhexidine gluconate in cats. *Arch Otorhinolaryngol*. 1985;242: 167–176.
52. Hamill MB, Osato MS, Wilhelmus KR. Experimental evaluation of chlorhexidine gluconate for ocular antisepsis. *Antimicrob Agents Chemother*. 1984;26:793–796.
53. Dormans JA, van Logten MJ. The effects of ophthalmic preservatives on corneal epithelium of the rabbit: a scanning electron microscopical study. *Toxicol Appl Pharmacol*. 1982;62:251–261.
54. Perez R, Freeman S, Sohmer H, Sichel JY. Vestibular and cochlear ototoxicity of topical antiseptics assessed by evoked potentials. *Laryngoscope*. 2000;110:1522–1527.
55. Durani P, Leaper D. Povidone-iodine: use in hand disinfection, skin preparation and antiseptic irrigation. *Int Wound J*. 2008;5:376–387.
56. Lenhardt HF, Lachapelle NC. Povidone-Iodine as a topical antiseptic. *Va Med Mon (1918)*. 1961;88:454–457.
57. Webster J, Bell-Syer SE, Foxlee R. Skin preparation with alcohol versus alcohol followed by any antiseptic for preventing bacteraemia or contamination of blood for transfusion. *Cochrane Database Syst Rev*. 2009;(3):CD007948.
58. Chlorhexidine and other antiseptics. *Med Lett Drugs Ther*. 1976;18:85–86.
59. Tanner J, Swarbrook S, Stuart J. Surgical hand antisepsis to reduce surgical site infection. *Cochrane Database Syst Rev*. 2008;(1):CD004288.
60. Hobson DW, Woller W, Anderson L, Guthery E. Development and evaluation of a new alcohol-based surgical hand scrub formulation with persistent antimicrobial characteristics and brushless application. *Am J Infect Control*. 1998; 26: 507–512.
61. Crowder VH, Welsh JS, Bornside GH, Cohn I Jr. Bacteriological comparison of hexachlorophene and polyvinylpyrrolidone-iodine surgical scrub soaps. *Am Surg*. 1967; 33: 906–911.
62. Kimbrough RD. Review of the toxicity of hexachlorophene, including its neurotoxicity. *J Clin Pharmacol*. 1973;13:439–444.
63. Ehrenkranz NJ. Bland soap handwash or hand antisepsis? The pressing need for clarity. *Infect Control Hosp Epidemiol*. 1992;13:299–301.
64. Tanner J. Methods of skin antisepsis for preventing SSIs. *Nurs Times*. 2012;108:20, 22.
65. Morgan JP, Haug RH, Kosman JW. Antimicrobial skin preparations for the maxillofacial region. *J Oral Maxillofac Surg*. 1996;54:89–94.
66. Woodhead K, Taylor EW, Bannister G, Chesworth T, Hoffman P, Humphreys H. Behaviours and rituals in the operating theatre. A report from the Hospital Infection Society Working Party on Infection Control in Operating Theatres. *J Hosp Infect*. 2002;51:241–255.
67. Lipp A, Phillips C, Harris P, Dowie I. Cyanoacrylate microbial sealants for skin preparation prior to surgery. *Cochrane Database Syst Rev*. 2010;(10):CD008062.
68. Cronen G, Ringus V, Sigle G, Ryu J. Sterility of surgical site marking. *J Bone Joint Surg Am*. 2005;87:2193–2195.
69. Tadiparthi S, Shokrollahi K, Juma A, Croall J. Using marker pens on patients: a potential source of cross infection with MRSA. *Ann R Coll Surg Engl*. 2007;89:661–664.
70. Ballal MS, Shah N, Ballal M, O'Donoghue M, Pegg DJ. The risk of cross-infection when marking surgical patients prior to surgery - review of two types of marking pens. *Ann R Coll Surg Engl*. 2007;89:226–228.
71. Russell PG, McKinnell TH. Cross infection risk in surgical marking pens. *J Plast Reconstr Aesthet Surg*. 2007;60:572–573.
72. Cao LY, Taylor JS, Vidimos A. Patient safety in dermatology: a review of the literature. *Dermatol Online J*. 2010;16:3.
73. Thomas RJ, Goodbourne C, Goldie B. The transmission of MRSA via orthopaedic marking pens–fact or fiction. *Ann R Coll Surg Engl*. 2004;86:51–52.
74. Chen TM, Castaneda M, Wanitphakdeedecha R, Nguyen TH, Tarrand JJ, Soares MK. Precautions with gentian violet: skin marking made sterile, effective, and economical. *Am J Infect Control*. 2009;37:244–246.
75. Chiu KY, Lau SK, Fung B, Ng KH, Chow SP. Plastic adhesive drapes and wound infection after hip fracture surgery. *Aust N Z J Surg*. 1993;63:798–801.
76. Sebben JE. Sterilization and care of surgical instruments and supplies. *J Am Acad Dermatol*. 1984;11:381–392.
77. Lilly E, Schmults CD. A comparison of high- and low-cost infection-control practices in dermatologic surgery. *Arch Dermatol*. 2012;148:859–861.
78. Messina MJ, Brodell LA, Brodell RT, Mostow EN. Hand hygiene in the dermatologist's office: to wash or to rub? *J Am Acad Dermatol*. 2008;59:1043–1049.
79. Parienti JJ, Thibon P, Heller R, et al. Hand-rubbing with an aqueous alcoholic solution vs traditional surgical hand-scrubbing and 30-day surgical site infection rates: a randomized equivalence study. *JAMA*. 2002;288:722–727.
80. Gordin FM, Schultz ME, Huber RA, Gill JA. Reduction in nosocomial transmission of drug-resistant bacteria after introduction of an alcohol-based handrub. *Infect Control Hosp Epidemiol*. 2005;26:650–653.
81. Arrowsmith VA, Taylor R. Removal of nail polish and finger rings to prevent surgical infection. *Cochrane Database Syst Rev*. 2012;5:CD003325.
82. Sebben JE. Survey of sterile technique used by dermatologic surgeons. *J Am Acad Dermatol*. 1988;18:1107–1113.
83. Ritter MA, French ML, Eitzen H. Evaluation of microbial contamination of surgical gloves during actual use. *Clin Orthop Relat Res*. 1976;(117):303–306.
84. Xia Y, Cho S, Greenway HT, Zelac DE, Kelley B. Infection rates of wound repairs during Mohs micrographic surgery using sterile versus nonsterile gloves: a prospective randomized pilot study. *Dermatol Surg*. 2011;37:651–656.
85. Rhinehart MB, Murphy MM, Farley MF, Albertini JG. Sterile versus nonsterile gloves during Mohs micrographic surgery: infection rate is not affected. *Dermatol Surg*. 2006;32:170–176.
86. Chiu WK, Cheung LK, Chan HC, Chow LK. A comparison of post-operative complications following wisdom tooth surgery performed with sterile or clean gloves. *Int J Oral Maxillofac Surg*. 2006;35:174–179.
87. Tanner J, Parkinson H. Double gloving to reduce surgical cross-infection. *Cochrane Database Syst Rev*. 2006; (3): CD003087.
88. Lipp A, Edwards P. Disposable surgical face masks for preventing surgical wound infection in clean surgery. *Cochrane Database Syst Rev*. 2002;(1):CD002929.
89. Ritter MA, Eitzen HE, Hart JB, French ML. The surgeon's garb. *Clin Orthop Relat Res*. 1980;(153):204–209.
90. Ritter MA, Eitzen H, French ML, Hart JB. The operating room environment as affected by people and the surgical face mask. *Clin Orthop Relat Res*. 1975;(111):147–150.
91. Weber A, Willeke K, Marchioni R, et al. Aerosol penetration and leakage characteristics of masks used in the health care industry. *Am J Infect Control*. 1993;21:167–173.
92. Dineen P, Drusin L. Epidemics of postoperative wound infections associated with hair carriers. *Lancet*. 1973;2: 1157–1159.
93. Krueger CA, Murray CK, Mende K, Guymon CH, Gerlinger TL. The bacterial contamination of surgical scrubs. *Am J Orthop (Belle Mead NJ)*. 2012;41:E69–E73.
94. Moylan JA, Kennedy BV. The importance of gown and drape barriers in the prevention of wound infection. *Surg Gynecol Obstet*. 1980;151:465–470.
95. Harrison SK, Evans WJ, LeBlanc DA, Bush LW. Cleaning and decontaminating medical instruments. *J Healthc Mater Manage*. 1990;8:36–42.
96. Goss LK. Staying up to date on disinfection and sterilization techniques: brush up on AORN's recommendations for perioperative practice. *Plast Surg Nurs*. 2012;32: 112–116.
97. Geisse JK. The dermatologic surgical suite. *Semin Dermatol*. 1994;13:2–9.

98. Dancer SJ, Stewart M, Coulombe C, Gregori A, Virdi M. Surgical site infections linked to contaminated surgical instruments. *J Hosp Infect.* 2012;81:231–238.
99. Pollack SV. Rapid instrument sterilization. *J Dermatol Surg Oncol.* 1990;16:438–439.
100. Mallison GF, Standard PG. Safe storage times for sterile packs. *Hospitals.* 1974;48:77–78, 80.
101. Waked WR, Simpson AK, Miller CP, Magit DP, Grauer JN. Sterilization wrap inspections do not adequately evaluate instrument sterility. *Clin Orthop Relat Res.* 2007;462:207–211.
102. Smack DP, Harrington AC, Dunn C, et al. Infection and allergy incidence in ambulatory surgery patients using white petrolatum vs bacitracin ointment. A randomized controlled trial. *JAMA.* 1996;276:972–977.
103. Dixon AJ, Dixon MP, Dixon JB. Randomized clinical trial of the effect of applying ointment to surgical wounds before occlusive dressing. *Br J Surg.* 2006;93:937–943.
104. Sheth VM, Weitzul S. Postoperative topical antimicrobial use. *Dermatitis.* 2008;19:181–189.

CHAPTER 6

Digital Imaging in Dermatologic Surgery

Andrea M. Hui, Neil Brody, & Daniel M. Siegel

INTRODUCTION

Dermatology has always been a visual field, dependent on visible changes on the skin for correct diagnosis and monitoring of therapy. Before the invention of photography, dermatological disease was painstakingly catalogued with drawings, paintings, and moulages. Photography, especially digital photography, has transformed the way dermatology is practiced by capturing a patient's dermatological complaint as it is presented and integrating these images into patient care.

As far back as the 1860s, silvered copper plate daguerreotypes and early photographs were found in specialized dermatological publications such as Alexander John Balmanno Squire's Atlas of the Diseases of the Skin.[1] It was therefore natural for dermatology to continually adopt new technologies and techniques in photography and printing as they became available. This allowed for dermatology to flourish as a specialty in which a patient's disease process could be visually documented in detail along with its histology. The development of the 35 mm Kodachrome (Eastman Kodak Company, Rochester, NY) became the gold standard of clinical dermatologic photography.[2] However, film photography was limiting due to its cost and processing time. Despite these limitations, it endured for over a century.

Digital photography is a relatively recent advance in the capture and storage of visual information. As digital photographic technology has advanced and increased in accessibility and cost-effectiveness, dermatologists have been at the forefront of its utilization in patient care. Digital photography has quickly become the standard method for photographic documentation for both clinical applications and publication purposes.[3] In addition to replacing film photography in dermatological study and practice, digital photography also offers many advantages. Some of these are straightforward, such as a switch from a film medium with a limited existence under routine storage to a reproducible, immortal digital medium. For example, the archival and quick retrieval of digital images is made significantly simpler and more cost-effective than retrieval of film images as they can be stored and searched on a computer. Beyond these types of advantages, however, are entirely new options that are made possible by digital photography.

With many dermatologic diseases, it is important to know whether a particular lesion is new or recurrent. To accomplish this goal, multiple photographs can be compared over time by documenting the patient's initial presentation and then obtaining serial photographs over time or at definitive endpoints. In addition, in a process termed *image registration*, multiple images of the same subject area are aligned and overlaid in a manner that allows one to compare changes over a period of time using both visual and computational methods[4] in a manner far simpler than could be accomplished with film. Photography provides a uniquely visual medical record that cannot be obtained by descriptive documentation alone.

There have also been advances in computerized assessment of pigmented lesions and early identification of melanoma. By performing analysis on large numbers of digital photographs of melanoma, software systems are able to "learn" the visual characteristics of both malignant and nonmalignant lesions. After doing so, these systems can then rapidly and consistently identify melanomas, even when the lesion is atypical, thereby potentially avoiding unnecessary biopsies.

DIGITAL PHOTOGRAPHY FUNDAMENTALS

Conceptually, a digital camera is similar to a film camera. Light from the scene to be photographed enters the camera, passes through a lens and potentially some mirrors, and is eventually "captured." The fundamental difference is that instead of film, the light lands on a charge-coupled device (CCD). It is this device that converts the light into digital information that is interpreted by the camera to produce a digital image. The CCD transforms the light into voltage, which then becomes converted into binary data that is stored on the camera's memory card. The CCD is of critical importance in a digital camera because the CCD's "resolution," or the density of the digital pixels in the CCD, greatly affects the quality of the image.[3] Digital photography has now achieved such high resolution that it rivals the quality of film photography with the added advantages of ease of use and efficiency.

Digital photograph resolution requires enough pixels to create an image in which the individual pixels produce the desired details on viewing. As a baseline comparison, a typical 35 mm Kodachrome 25 slide (in which the photosensitive elements of the 24 × 36 mm image are silver grains as compared with pixels) has about the equivalent resolution of a 20 megapixel (MP) image.[5] CCD resolution varies greatly by camera make and model. Studies have shown that a minimum resolution of 768 × 512 is sufficient for in-office dermatological use.[6] With this minimum resolution in mind, a trade-off must be made between higher-resolution images (which because of their higher pixel density, require more computer memory to store) and lower-resolution images (which require less computer memory). A CCD with a resolution comparable to that of film would require 33.6 MB of storage before compression. From a practical perspective, any image of greater than a single MP will suffice for clinical use.

SELECTING A CAMERA

Like film cameras, digital cameras come in both "single lens reflex" (SLR) and point-and-shoot (PAS) varieties. SLR cameras are generally more flexible, often offering an external flash and interchangeable lenses. The result of this flexibility is generally higher image quality, but SLR cameras are consequently bulkier and costlier than PAS cameras.

PAS digital cameras are an excellent choice for inexperienced photographers because they are easy to use. These cameras are less expensive because they utilize a fixed lens and built-in flash, and are subsequently much smaller and lighter in weight than SLR cameras. Photographers will often set PAS cameras on "automatic," which allows the camera to make all the choices regarding exposure, white balance, color balance, focus, and flash. As the name implies, "pointing and shooting" is exactly how these types of digital cameras may be used, and end results are often quite acceptable and useful in a clinical setting. One should be aware that automatic mode does not always provide optimal results because variables such as ambient lighting or patient position may affect image consistency especially when serial photographs are desired. For the vast majority of office photography, the latest generation of PAS cameras is an excellent choice.

SLR cameras have interchangeable lenses and flashes. The lenses may be focused manually to allow for precise capture of the object. The photographer may control all aspects of image capture, including exposure, white and color balance, and flash synchronization. The SLR camera body tends to be much larger than a PAS body, which allows for a bigger CCD and thus higher resolution images, sometimes as high as that of film photography. An SLR system is the best choice to obtain publication-quality photographs. However, due to the cumulative cost of the SLR body, lens, flash, and other accessories, the SLR system may be an order of magnitude more costly than a PAS camera.

One should select a digital camera system based on clinical requirements and cost. For example, if one plans to take photographs solely for clinical use, a PAS may be more than sufficient. If the clinician plans on publishing photographs or cost is not a large factor, an SLR system may be more appropriate. Also, if image quality and consistency is paramount, an SLR system is the best choice as it allows the photographer to precisely control all aspects of image capture. For aesthetic procedures, high-quality cameras and self-contained systems such as the VISIA Complexion Analysis or OMNIA Imaging systems[7] allow precise, reproducible capture from the same perspective, which can be a highly desirable feature in the current medicolegal climate.

There are many excellent online resources that one may utilize to learn and compare digital camera systems (Table 6-1).

TABLE 6-1
Digital Camera Online Resources

General Information and Reviews	
http://www.dpreview.com/	
http://www.digitalcamerareview.com/	
http://reviews.cnet.com/digital-cameras/	
http://www.pcmag.com/reviews/digital-cameras	
http://www.steves-digicams.com	
Manufacturer Websites	
Canon	http://www.usa.canon.com/cusa/consumer/products/cameras
Fujifilm	http://www.fujifilm.com/products/digital_cameras/
Hasselblad	http://www.hasselbladusa.com/
Kodak	http://store.kodak.com/cameras
Leica	http://us.leica-camera.com
Nikon	http://www.nikonusa.com
Olympus	http://www.olympusamerica.com/cpg_section/index.asp
Panasonic	http://shop.panasonic.com/shop/cameras-and-camcorders
Pentax	http://www.pentaximaging.com/
Ricoh	http://www.ricoh.com/r_dc/
Sony	http://www.sony.com/cameras

SELECTING HARDWARE

COMPUTER

Although professional digital artists and others in similar professions require very powerful computers for their day-to-day work, the requirements of a dermatological practice looking to store and annotate digital imagery are not as stringent.

The first choice to be made is the platform. As of 2012, the two most popular platforms are Microsoft Windows and Apple OS X.[8] In previous years, the ability of these platforms to share data was somewhat limited, so the best choice was usually whichever platform was already in use in a practice/organization. This is less of a concern with more recent systems and therefore the choice is primarily based upon personal preference, unless local information technology (IT) policies dictate otherwise.

After a platform is chosen, the decision between a desktop and a laptop can be made. If portability is not required, the best decision is likely a desktop machine, which for a given price always provides more processing power/storage when contrasted with an equivalently priced laptop. In either case, the next important attribute is the amount of hard drive space. The larger the drive, the more images can be stored.

TABLE 6-2
Data Storage Devices

External hard drive	These are hard drives (often of the same kind found in laptops) that are placed into external enclosures and connected to a computer via a temporary connection (such as a USB). While connected, the hard drive can be accessed similarly to an internal hard drive but the connection is often substantially slower than connections used internally by the computer. Because these are actual hard drives, their sizes are often large, with 2 terabytes being common as of 2012. Gradually these drives with moving parts are being supplanted by solid-state drives (SSD), which are readily available in sizes up to 960 gigabytes.
USB-stick, or "thumb drive"	These are small "sticks" that plug into a computer's USB port. They are typically cheaper, and therefore slower and smaller, than most hard drives. Typical USB stick sizes are in the hundreds of megabytes to the 128 gigabyte range.
Compact flash or SD cards	These are storage cards that are often used as the primary storage mechanism for digital cameras, and typically have sizes ranging from megabytes to 128 gigabytes.
Network storage	This type of storage refers to the accessing of storage on another computer system over a network. This sort of setup might be made available by an IT department or third party storage solution. Network storage devices and systems often have large capacities but are generally slower to access than local storage. This may be ideal for dermatology practices, which utilize serial photography and total body photography.
Cloud storage	"Cloud" storage refers to the accessing storage systems over the internet in the "cloud." This is similar to network storage in concept, but because internet connections are often slower than local network connections, this type of storage can be significantly slower than local storage. However, there may be legal implications to storing patient data on a cloud, such as access audit logs, that cannot be provided by most cloud storage providers.

DATA STORAGE

While the local computer's hard drive is usually the primary storage mechanism, there are many other types of storage. A few types are listed in Table 6-2.

STORAGE REQUIREMENTS

When choosing how to store data, it is important to know how extensive that data will be. In the context of digital photography, the two main factors are the number of photos to be stored and the resolution of each photo. The higher the resolution, the more storage is required per photo. Multiplying by the number of images to be stored gives a rough estimate of the required amount of storage. Table 6-3 lists some common image storage requirements, with some other storage sizes for context.

In Table 6-4, "compression" refers to the removal of superfluous information to reduce the storage requirements for a particular set of data. There are two types of compression: lossy and lossless. Lossless compression is compression that is reversible: one can always obtain the original data from the compressed data. A common file format for lossless compression is Tagged Image File Format (TIFF). Images may be edited and resaved without losing image quality.[9] The quality of TIFF images is independent of camera manufacturer and is ideal for record-keeping and sharing as its interpretation is universal. RAW file format is the "raw" uncompressed data that comes directly from the camera's sensor. Each camera manufacturer has its own version of the RAW format.[10] As would be expected, lossless formats result in very large file sizes. Lossy compression is compression that actually "loses" information, and the original information cannot

TABLE 6-3
Storage Requirements for Digital Photography

Storage Element	
1 megapixel photo, uncompressed	2–5 MB
5 megapixel photo, uncompressed	5–15 MB
1 megapixel photo, compressed	0.5–1 MB
5 megapixel photo, compressed	2–8 MB
1 DVD-ROM (single layer)	4.7 GB
1 Blu-ray disc (single layer)	25 GB
Human DNA	~800 MB

TABLE 6-4
Methods of Digital Mapping in MMS[a]

Preoperative image only	Outline of excised tissue and margins is marked on the preoperative image only. Subsequent stages are marked on additional copies of the same image.
Prestage image	An image is obtained prior to each stage. Outline of excised tissue and margins are marked. For each subsequent stage, the defect of the prior stage is accurately depicted.
Intraoperative image	During each stage, the excision margins are marked on the patient. After examining the tissue histologically, the positive margins are marked. The map then accurately depicts the planned defect.
Postoperative image	An image of the defect is obtained after the tissue is excised. Margins are then marked.

[a]Data from Lin et al.[20]

be retrieved or rebuilt from the compressed information. In digital photography and imagery, lossy compression is used to remove visual information that does not greatly affect the appearance of the image. A popular file format utilizing lossy compression is the JPEG image. Lossy image file size is significantly smaller when compared with lossless compression images.

DIGITAL IMAGING AND COMMUNICATIONS IN MEDICINE

It is vital to maintain secure, Health Insurance Portability and Accountability Act (HIPAA) compliant image storage and transmission. Although there are specific rules and regulations regarding the protection of private health information, there are no standards for de-identifying clinical data such as digital images in dermatology.[11] On the forefront is Digital Imaging and Communications in Medicine (DICOM), the international standard for medical images and related information, which defines the necessary format and quality of medical images for clinical use.[12] DICOM was first developed in the 1980s for use in dose planning in radiation therapy and its standards were developed by the American College of Radiology and the National Electrical Manufacturers Association. In 1993, the first standard was published. DICOM quickly became implemented in almost every radiological device, allowing for a completely digital workflow to replace film.[12]

Recently, DICOM released Supplement 142, which provided guidelines on de-identification.[11,13] Although digital dermatologic imaging was not specifically mentioned, "the removal or distortion of the actual pixel data where there is possibility of visually identifying the individual in the images" is pertinent to our field and may be accomplished by using a black bar over features such as the eyes or identifying tattoos.

It is highly likely that DICOM may also be the future for digital imaging sharing in dermatology as well. More information can be found at http://dicom.nema.org/.

IMAGING SOFTWARE

Many digital cameras come with basic photography software which allows the user to adjust variables such as contrast and brightness, and make changes such as removing red eye. Some software programs also aid in sorting and archiving. However, dermatologic photography and medical records require a more efficient workflow which allows the clinician to take a photograph and rapidly integrate the image into the medical record. Most importantly, the software must be compliant with the HIPAA.

Some basic features of photography software include pan and zoom controls, side-by-side comparison, measurement and annotation, and linking to consent forms. Some software also includes "live image overlay," which is a method of superimposing the live preview from the camera with prior digital photographs of the patient or lesion in question.[14] This is particularly helpful in acquiring serial photographs used to compare changing or new lesions such as in total body photography (TBP). HIPAA-compliant software such as Canfield's Mirror Suite can allow the practitioner to quickly select "before" and "after" photos and position them side-by-side. This is especially useful in the office setting to review results with the patient during an appointment. The Mirror system may be customized with diagnosis and procedure libraries so that practitioners can easily search and organize their images.[15] Several electronic medical record systems designed specifically for dermatology such as NexTech Dermatology Software[16] or Modernizing Medicine[17] offer easy integration of digital photographs into the patient's chart, streamlining diagnosis, planning, and results. For cloud-based sharing of clinical images, point-of-care HIPAA-compliant systems such as ClickMedix work well. For sharing of nonidentifiable clinical images, online services such as Picasa, Flickr, or Photobucket are easy and often free to use.

High-end packages such as Adobe Photoshop are valuable for manipulating images, although open source software such as GIMP offers many of the same features. From an ethical perspective, image manipulation may be a useful way to show a patient possible outcomes, but it should not be used to create images that do not reflect reality.

PHOTOGRAPHIC TECHNIQUES

Excellent clinical photography depends on the consistency of the images captured. In a series of images concerning a particular patient or procedure result, all images should accurately represent the differences at each time point without variables introduced by the photography itself. A basic understanding of photographic principles such as focus, exposure, lighting, and framing is necessary to achieve a high level of image consistency.

PATIENT POSITIONING

The clinical presentation of the patient or lesion should be as clear as possible. In all photographs, it is ideal to utilize a solid-color neutral background. Neutral grey, which reflects 90% of visible light, is soothing to the eye and makes a good wall color, although lighter skin is best captured on dark backgrounds while darker skin is best captured on light backgrounds. The photographic frame should be free of distractions such as clothing, jewelry, makeup, and excess hair. Brightly colored clothing or surroundings may render a color cast upon the subject, and items or furniture in front of the light source may result in unwanted shadows. For body photography, clothing should ideally be removed or at least covered with a drape; clothing should never be visible in the photograph. Disposable gowns may be provided to the patient when taking half-body photography.

For facial photography, the patient should present with a clean face free of any makeup or excess oil. The sheen from makeup containing minerals or from natural oils may interfere with the image especially if a flash is utilized. If a patient cleans his or her face prior to being photographed, a few minutes (or more for cosmetic images, since the facial state of hydration is critical) should elapse to allow any transient erythema to dissipate. Men should trim, or ideally shave, their facial hair. Excess hair should be secured behind the face with a headband or ponytail holder. The patient should keep a relaxed, neutral expression in all photographs unless the photograph is meant to demonstrate a pathological (i.e., Bell's palsy) or therapeutic (i.e., botulinum toxin injection outcome) process.

For surgical photography, the area of interest should be carefully "framed" with drapes. The field should be free of as much excess fluid as possible to allow for clear visualization of the area. Again, all distractors such as hair and shadows should be eliminated.

COMPOSITION

Consistent scene composition helps to ensure that the quality of photographic results and serial photography are also consistent. Clinicians may utilize just a few standard distances in order to achieve this consistency; for example, a half-body shot followed by a body area shot (such as the upper arm) followed by a close-up of the lesion in question. Ideally, each distance should have similar framing, lighting, and camera settings. Using a camera's zoom function (as made popular by PAS cameras) is suboptimal because zooming does not achieve consistent magnification; in addition, digital zoom lenses cause loss of image quality due to interpolation of data as the magnification increases. To achieve consistent image results, it is best to move the camera itself than to use the zoom function, especially in serial photography. Standard anatomic positioning is a requirement for TBP. Face-on shots of the head and neck with the nasal tip at the level of the earlobe allow consistency when creating a series. Side views of the face taken at a 90 degree angle allow for further consistency. Oblique shots may be taken where necessary to highlight a particular finding.

The patient can also be moved into predetermined positions. It may be helpful to put a mark on the floor (e.g., with tape) to guide patients into standard positions. Any external lighting should also be in its usual position to provide the most uniform illumination of the patient. Close-up photos of an individual lesion or eruption may be taken with an indexed measurement scale, which is often attached to the bottom of the camera. The ruler at the end of the scale is pressed gently against the lesion and appears in the photograph. This accessory also provides a consistent distance from which the photograph may be taken and stabilizes the camera against shaking. Printed sticker rulers such as those produced by Delasco are useful both to identify patients and to provide a size reference. The sticker should be placed below the lesion and should be visible within the frame of the photograph to provide a measuring scale.

LIGHTING

It is important that lighting remain consistent when taking serial photographs. Differences in lighting may inaccurately represent changes in the skin at each time point. A camera's built-in flash is not ideal for dermatologic photography. Its head-on illumination tends to flatten contours. Oblique lighting is superior in that it can reveal textures and shapes with much more three-dimensionality. This type of lighting may be obtained by utilizing an external flash mount system, twin-light mounted system, or several external flashes in a studio setting. Ring flashes are useful for images of the anogenital area or oropharynx, as they provide even lighting, although a loss of depth perception is the price of even illumination. These lighting systems may be metered (configured) to achieve excellent three-dimensional, evenly lit subjects. PAS systems that "wash out" or overexpose on close imaging may be "fixed" by covering the flash with a diffuser made of white tissue or a piece of soda bottle roughened with sandpaper. The flash cover itself can be treated in a similar manner. All of these approaches reduce battery life as the flash may fire at a higher output setting; the latter may also affect resale value.

CAMERA SETTINGS

EXPOSURE

In an ideal world, small apertures (f/22 or f/32) combined with lighting that emulates the color temperature of daylight (5500 K) can allow both excellent depth of field and minimal blurring. To attain ideal sharpness and illumination of the subject, the aperture of the lens (the diameter of the opening) should be set as wide open as possible. The larger the aperture, the faster the shutter speed will be, which allows for the sharpest photos by minimizing potential blurring from subject movement. In addition, the larger the aperture, the thinner the depth of field (the range of distance that is acceptably sharp). A thin depth of field can be utilized to focus specifically on one lesion or even one aspect of the lesion. The camera can be set to "Aperture Priority" to allow for the best control of depth of field and image sharpness. In contrast, one can set the camera to a small aperture such as f/22 to allow a larger range of distance to be in focus. Flash (discussed later) may be used to ensure maximal sharpness and illumination of the subject.

FOCUS

Manual lens focus is best for accomplishing exact focus upon the lesion or area of attention. For the purposes of dermatologic imaging, a portrait lens with focal length of 60 to 100 mm focal length equivalent is an excellent choice. Most 60 mm lenses, for example, allow for close focus at a usual distance of 8 inches for excellent close-up photography, although a 90 to 100 mm lens is ideal for recording aesthetic procedures where foreshortening is undesirable.

Many of today's SLR and PAS systems have autofocus systems using low power reflected infrared light that achieve superb focus with less effort. In both systems, the focused area appears as a "box" within the viewfinder or camera display, which illuminates and then adjusts the lens focus when the shutter button is depressed halfway down. One should be sure that the area of interest is completely in focus before taking the photo. Equally important to proper focusing is holding the camera steady by bracing it with two hands. The elbows should be held against the body. If a viewfinder is used, the camera should be braced against the face while looking through the viewfinder.

A method for manually focusing a fixed-focal length lens such as 60 mm is called "body focusing."[14] The focus ring can be set to desired distance index points, which are found on the top of the lens. The focus ring is usually marked with distances such as 1 foot, 5 feet, infinity, and may be changed by rotating the ring. The photographer sets a desired index point and then looks through the viewfinder, moving back and forth until the subject is focused in the viewfinder, and then the photograph is taken. This simple method allows for highly reproducible photographs in a clinical setting.

WHITE BALANCE

Adjustment of white balance permits accurate rendering of color depth by ensuring that neutral colors such as white and grey are accurately represented in the same light. Generally, the auto white balance function in either SLR or PAS systems is excellent in today's cameras. One may also select a preset white balance to adjust for certain lighting conditions, such as Daylight, Flash, Fluorescent, Cloudy, or Tungsten. To assure maximal control of white balance, one may use a grey card or manually adjust the white balance within the camera, and then save the preset for use in the same lighting conditions.

RESOLUTION

Image resolution is the amount of detail which a camera can capture, measured as pixels. The more pixels an image has, the more detail may be depicted in the final image. Image resolution setting may be found on a camera as "image quality" or "image size." For dermatologic photographs, we recommend setting the camera to as high quality a resolution as possible. One must keep in mind that the higher quality the image, the larger the file size will be; this must be taken into consideration for image storage purposes.[6] One MP is adequate for the vast majority of images. For images above 5 MP only discerning imagers will see differences.

USES OF DIGITAL PHOTOGRAPHY IN DERMATOLOGIC SURGERY

Although dermatologists are less frequently the targets of malpractice litigation than practitioners of other fields, cosmetic and surgical procedures do present legal risks. With respect to Mohs surgeons, a leading cause of malpractice suits has been operating on the wrong site.[18] Digital photography allows for dermatologic surgeons to achieve precise verification of biopsy sites, anatomical landmarks, and Mohs mapping, thus protecting themselves against errors and providing a superior level of care and safety.

Prior to performing a surgery, dermatologic surgeons depend upon multiple sources to correctly identify surgical sites. These sources often include patients and their family, physician referral letters, written descriptions and diagrams on medical records, gauze dermabrasion, and biopsy-site scars. Weeks and even months may pass between the time of the biopsy and the surgery date, resulting in a well-healed, often indiscernible scar. Surgeries are sometimes cancelled due to inability to find the site, and patients are sometimes sent back to their referring physicians to verify the site. In addition, biopsy sites may be very difficult to find on immunocompromised or severely sun-damaged patients, who may have many skin cancers in one area as well as a history of multiple prior procedures.

Dermatology is unique in that biopsy site descriptions include much more than laterality. Although some may consider terms such as "medial," "temporal," or "mandibular" helpful, multiple procedures may at times have been performed in those areas or within the same cosmetic units. Errors still occur. Triangulation of biopsy sites from two points such as an anatomical landmark and a different lesion may be helpful, but triangulation is time-consuming, sometimes inaccurate (e.g., if a triangulation point such as a seborrheic keratosis changes in appearance), and open to interpretation especially if a triangulation point is a cosmetic unit such as "temple." Additionally, measurements may change after a biopsy site heals and the tissue contracts.

Photography, with consistent camera angles and focal distances, allows for the most accurate demarcation and documentation of the biopsy site, when used to supplement the information documented in the physical examination, such as size and location. In a 2009 study by McGinness et al., 271 Mohs surgical sites were identified on the day of the surgery by patient, physician, or both, and then identified using a preoperative biopsy-site photograph. The patient incorrectly identified 16.6% of surgical sites, surgeons 5.9%, and both patient and surgeon 4.4%. When preoperative biopsy-site photographs were utilized, photography reduced the site identification error rate in the sampled Mohs surgical operations to zero.[19]

BIOPSY SITE PHOTOGRAPHY

In order for biopsy-site photographs to be useful, they must be accurate. The lesion should be identified on the patient with a surgical marker prior to taking the photograph. The composition should include useful anatomic landmarks such as the lips, eyes, or nose. Ideally, two photographs should be obtained: a photograph taken from a distance to identify nearby anatomy, and a close-up or macro photograph to identify the biopsy site in detail and possibly some nearby landmarks. If there are many potential biopsy and/or surgical sites which are visible within one image, markings may be made electronically with a tablet or mouse at later appointments. When performed properly, biopsy-site photography leaves little to no ambiguity. Proper imaging using a consistent array of views of anatomical sites ensures the accuracy of images.

MOHS MICROGRAPHIC SURGERY MAPPING

Mohs micrographic surgery (MMS) is a technique that examines 100% of the margins of excised tissue histologically in order to remove skin cancers completely. MMS has been extensively utilized and studied for the treatment of nonmelanoma skin cancers (NMSC), particularly in areas where tissue conservation is vital, such as the face. Accurate mapping of excised tissue in its correct anatomical position on the patient is a fundamental aspect of MMS. Typically a hand-drawn map is utilized to diagram excised specimens and margins relative to anatomical landmarks, often with preprinted templates for specific anatomic sites. However, hand-drawn figures are limited by inaccuracies or inconsistencies and nonstandardized templates. Errors in margin status may then occur. Instant film has been utilized for margin mapping but is limited by small print size (no larger than 3 × 4 inches), film that is one-time-use only (thus increasing cost), and a glossy film surface, which makes writing difficult.

Digital photography has recently allowed for fast, accurate mapping in MMS. This method quickly produces high-quality images precisely by depicting the actual defect in relation to its anatomic location for MMS mapping. Images may be obtained preoperatively, intraoperatively, and postoperatively (Table 6-4). While the specimens are being prepared, the images may be quickly downloaded to the computer. MMS map markings may be made on printed images or on the computer using a tablet or digital imaging software. Histologic findings are precisely correlated with margins and location on the patient. Maps can then be printed out or saved to the patient's electronic medical record. This will likely be the way that the procedure will be done in the future everywhere, but for now paper is still the standard of care.

TOTAL BODY PHOTOGRAPHY

The early detection of malignant melanoma is vital, as earlier diagnosis and treatment is associated with better prognosis. The 5 year survival after treatment of melanoma less than 1 mm thick (stage IA) is 95%, compared with a survival rate of less than 45% for melanomas more than 4 mm thick.[21] Routine full-body skin checks can help detect early melanomas but are limited by lack of precise documentation and the naked eye.

Patients with a history of melanoma, multiple dysplastic nevi or a strong family history of melanoma may be followed closely with TBP, also known as whole body integumentary photography. TBP has shown to aid in the detection of early melanomas by detecting slight changes in existing lesions and recognizing clinically subtle early malignant melanoma.[22] TBP establishes a baseline from which to compare future changes in lesions and on the body as a whole. Photographs of multiple anatomical areas are obtained, usually according to a template of standardized positions.[23] Specific moles may be followed with serial dermatoscopic photography, which may also be added to the medical record. TBP may be performed in a clinic, ideally with photography studio set-up and template software. Several manufacturers also offer TBP systems, or patients may go to designated TBP centers and bring the photographs back to their dermatologist.

Comparison of serial photographs is an important step in detecting subtle changes on the patient's skin. Multiple digital photographs taken at different time points may be aligned by a technique termed *image registration*.[4] This relies on optimal standardization of patient positioning, lighting, and conditions to ensure that the only variable within the photograph is the patient's skin. Transparency image overlay software is available, which allows the physician to correctly position the patient prior to taking the photographs. Subtle clinical changes may then be easily detected by comparing changes over time using both visual and computational methods.

TBP is also helpful in preventing excess prophylactic excisions in patients with a history of dysplastic nevi and/or melanoma. In these patients, multiple unnecessary excisions can result in an increase in disfigurement, morbidity, and expense. In a study by Cohen et al.,[24] 1630 pigmented lesions were prophylactically excised from 78 patients with stage I or II melanoma; only 12 unsuspected melanomas were found, and thus 136 lesions were removed for each melanoma found. The lifetime rate at which an individual mole from a 20 year-old transforms into a melanoma by the age of 80 years is estimated to be 0.03% in men and 0.009% in women.[25] Even if all dysplastic nevi were surgically excised in a patient, new nevi would continue to occur *de novo*. TBP allows for precise, close monitoring of all existing nevi and aids in detection of new lesions, thus potentially saving patients from unnecessary excisions of pre-existing, stable nevi. Consumer applications for whole body photography exist, such as UMSkinCheck, that are excellent when used as part of a well-thought-out surveillance protocol.

OTHER DIGITAL IMAGING MODALITIES FOR USE IN DERMATOLOGIC SURGERY

IN VIVO CONFOCAL MICROSCOPY

In vivo confocal microscopy allows for digital noninvasive high-resolution high-contrast optical imaging in real time. It has been utilized to examine NMSC, melanomas, and other skin conditions.[26–28] Confocal microscopy utilizes near-infrared laser and water immersion objective lenses to examine thin sections of human skin in vivo.[29] Skin is then examined by horizontal "en face" sections of skin instead of the vertical sections found in routine histology. Section thickness is between 3 and 5 μm thick, thus providing a very high resolution. Skin may be examined to the level of the papillary and upper reticular dermis. Compared with routine histology, the skin is imaged in its native state without the need for biopsy, fixing, sectioning, and staining. All images obtained with an in vivo confocal microscopy system may be saved and reviewed at a later date.

Confocal microscopy is probably best known for its use in identification of basal cell carcinoma. Excellent correlations between confocal microscopy and standard histological examination have aided with in vivo diagnosis of basal cell carcinoma.[28] Although several more studies need to be performed to determine sensitivity and specificity, the use of in vivo confocal microscopy may at some point eliminate the need for biopsy altogether.

OPTICAL COHERENCE TOMOGRAPHY

Optical coherence tomography (OCT) is another digital, noninvasive, cross-sectional imaging modality for skin, conducted in vivo and in real time. OCT is similar to ultrasound imaging but utilizes infrared light to measure echo delays and intensity of back reflection. It provides two-dimensional vertical images with a depth of up to 1.5 mm, which allows for examination of the epidermis and upper dermis, as well as some appendages. Lateral resolution is quite high at 10 to 15 µm.[30] Many dermatologic conditions, both benign and malignant, have been characterized by OCT and correlated with histopathology.[31] Because OCT is noninvasive and reproducible, it may be useful in monitoring and evaluating the effects of treatments for inflammatory skin conditions over time. In addition it may be useful for diagnosing skin cancers and may help to avoid biopsies. OCT appears to allow for very sensitive and specific identification of basal cell carcinoma and work is ongoing to confirm this early data.

MELAFIND

MelaFind is an FDA-approved digital, noninvasive, fully automatic, computerized diagnostic system for aiding detection of early melanoma and to identify pigmented lesions that should be considered for biopsy to rule out melanoma. MelaFind utilizes visible and infrared light to illuminate the skin dermatoscopically with 10 narrow spectral bands emitted from a hand piece. The depth of analysis extends to 2.5 mm beneath the skin surface. Each band is captured by a camera within the hand piece and transmitted to the attached computer for automatic processing and analysis. The resulting images are high resolution at 1280 × 1000 pixels and may be saved in the patient's medical record. The entire process of image capturing takes a few seconds. The multispectral images are analyzed using preset algorithms, which then provides an objective assessment in under 1 minute.[32]

In a multicenter prospective trial by Monheit et al., MelaFind achieved a sensitivity of 98.4% for thin melanomas (125 of 127 melanomas) with a biopsy ratio of 10.8:1, compared with the average biopsy sensitivity of 78% in a dermatologist reader study. When borderline lesions were included (high-grade dysplastic nevi, atypical melanocytic proliferations, or hyperplasias), the sensitivity of MelaFind was 98.3%, with a biopsy ratio of 7.6:1. Its specificity was 9.5%, significantly higher than that of investigators (3.7%).[33] Dermatologists must be aware that due to low specificity, a higher number of biopsies may be recommended by the MelaFind system for many benign lesions. Thus, only lesions that are clinically suspicious for melanoma should be assessed by MelaFind.

CONCLUSION

The practice of dermatology relies on visual evaluation of the patient. Surgical and therapeutic outcomes are assessed based on visual changes occurring on the patient's skin. Digital photography has provided an efficient, valuable, and permanent way to document a patient's baseline and then monitor progress and outcomes, and also plays an important role in improving surgical accuracy. Photographs can be easily integrated into the medical record for accurate patient assessment. Digital imaging can also be utilized to detect cancerous lesions, which may otherwise be missed by the trained eye. With the basic principles discussed in this chapter, any dermatologic surgeon can consistently produce high quality digital photographs, which will help him or her achieve the highest level of care.

GLOSSARY

Aperture: the diameter of the lens opening that determines the amount of light to which the camera sensor may be exposed.[34]

CCD: a device that converts the light into digital information that is interpreted by the camera to produce a digital image.

Depth of field: distance between the closest and farthest in-focus area of a photograph. Inversely proportional to the aperture.

Resolution: the amount of detail a camera can capture, measured as pixels.

Shutter speed: length of time that the aperture of the lens is open, exposing the camera sensor to light. For example, a shutter speed of 1/250 will expose the sensor for 1/250th of a second.

White balance: adjustment that permits accurate rendition of color depth such that neutral colors such as white and grey are accurately represented in the same light.

REFERENCES

1. Squire AJB. *Atlas of the Diseases of the Skin*. London: J Churchill; 1878.
2. Siegel DM. Resolution in digital imaging: enough already? *Semin Cutan Med Surg*. 2002;21(3):209–215.
3. Ratner D, Thomas CO, Bickers D. The uses of digital photography in dermatology. *J Am Acad Dermatol*. 1999;41(5):749–756. doi:10.1016/s0190-9622(99)70012-5.
4. Joshua E L. Image registration of sequential transparent photographs to localize and detect new versus recurrent tumors in dermatologic and Mohs micrographic surgery. *Am Acad Dermatol*. 2011;64(4):786.e1–786.e2. doi:10.1016/j.jaad. 2010.08.035.
5. Langford M. *Basic Photography*. 7th ed. Burlington, MA: Oxford: Focal Press; 2000.
6. Bittorf A, Fartasch M, Schuler G, Diepgen TL. Resolution requirements for digital images in dermatology. *J Am Acad Dermatol*. 1997;37(2 Pt 1):195–198.
7. http://www.canfieldsci.com/imaging_systems/facial_systems/VISIA_Complexion_Analysis.html. Accessed July 28, 2014.
8. http://stats.wikimedia.org/archive/squid_reports/2012-09/SquidReportOperatingSystems. Accessed July 28, 2014.
9. http://partners.adobe.com/public/developer/en/tiff/TIFF6.pdf. Accessed July 28, 2014.
10. http://www.adobe.com/content/dam/Adobe/en/products/photoshop/pdfs/understanding_digitalrawcapture.pdf. Accessed July 28, 2014.
11. Freymann JB, Kirby JS, Perry JH, Clunie DA, Jaffe CC. Image data sharing for biomedical research–meeting HIPAA requirements for De-identification. *J Digit Imaging*. 2012;25(1):14–24.
12. http://medical.nema.org/. Accessed July 28, 2014.
13. http://www.dclunie.com/papers/DR_Clunie_20051202.pdf. Accessed July 28, 2014.

14. Witmer WK, Lebovitz PJ. Clinical photography in the dermatology practice. *Semin Cutan Med Surg.* 2012;31(3):191–199. doi:10.1016/j.sder.2012.06.004.
15. http://www.canfieldsci.com/imaging_systems/imaging_software/Mirror_software/Mirror_PhotoFile.html. Accessed July 28, 2014.
16. http://www.nextech.com/dermatology. Accessed July 28, 2014.
17. http://www.modmed.com/dermatology/integrate-seamlessly/. Accessed July 28, 2014.
18. Perlis CS, Campbell RM, Perlis RH, Malik M, Dufresne RG Jr. Incidence of and risk factors for medical malpractice lawsuits among Mohs surgeons. *Dermatol Surg.* 2006;32(1):79–83.
19. McGinness JL, Goldstein G. The value of preoperative biopsy-site photography for identifying cutaneous lesions. *Dermatol Surg.* 2010;36(2):194–197. doi:10.1111/j.1524-4725.2009.01426.x.
20. Lin BB, Taylor RS. Digital photography for mapping Mohs micrographic surgery sections. *Dermatol Surg.* 2001;27(4):411–414. doi:10.1046/j.1524-4725.2001.00316.x.
21. http://www.cancer.org. Accessed July 28, 2014.
22. Feit NE, Dusza SW, Marghoob AA. Melanomas detected with the aid of total cutaneous photography. *Br J Dermatol.* 2004;150(4):706–714.
23. Halpern AC, Marghoob AA, Bialoglow TW, Witmer W, Slue W. Standardized positioning of patients (poses) for whole body cutaneous photography. *J Am Acad Dermatol.* 2003;49(4):593–598.
24. Cohen MH, Cohen BJ, Shotkin JD, Morrison PT. Surgical prophylaxis of malignant melanoma. *Ann Surg.* 1991;213(4):308–314.
25. Tsao H, Bevona C, Goggins W, Quinn T. The transformation rate of moles (melanocytic nevi) into cutaneous melanoma: a population-based estimate. *Arch Dermatol.* 2003;139(3):282–288.
26. Gonzalez S, Gonzalez E, White WM, Rajadhyaksha M, Anderson RR. Allergic contact dermatitis: correlation of in vivo confocal imaging to routine histology. *J Am Acad Dermatol.* 1999;40(5 Pt 1):708–713.
27. Langley RG, Rajadhyaksha M, Dwyer PJ, Sober AJ, Flotte TJ, Anderson RR. Confocal scanning laser microscopy of benign and malignant melanocytic skin lesions in vivo. *J Am Acad Dermatol.* 2001;45(3):365–376.
28. Gonzalez S, Tannous Z. Real-time, in vivo confocal reflectance microscopy of basal cell carcinoma. *J Am Acad Dermatol.* 2002;47(6):869–874.
29. Rajadhyaksha M, Gonzalez S, Zavislan JM, Anderson RR, Webb RH. In vivo confocal scanning laser microscopy of human skin II: advances in instrumentation and comparison with histology. *J Invest Dermatol.* 1999;113(3):293–303.
30. Welzel J. Optical coherence tomography in dermatology: a review. *Skin Res Technol.* 2001;7(1):1–9.
31. Gambichler T, Jaedicke V, Terras S. Optical coherence tomography in dermatology: technical and clinical aspects. *Arch Dermatol Res.* 2011;303(7):457–473.
32. http://www.melafind.com. Accessed July 28, 2014
33. Monheit G, Cognetta AB, Ferris L, et al. The performance of MelaFind: a prospective multicenter study. *Arch Dermatol.* 2011;147(2):188–194.

CHAPTER 7

The Surgical Suite: Equipment and Accreditation

Riley McLean & Mary E. Maloney

The surgical suite sets the tone of the office for the patient and staff and helps create the first impression of any practice. The suite is more than the four walls and also includes the important surgical equipment (Fig. 7-1, Table 7-1). To create a positive atmosphere for patient care, it is crucial to consider all aspects of surgical suite design and function.

This chapter will review both practical tips for the design of the surgical space as well as the recommended standards of major accrediting organizations. In the ideal world, the surgeon would design their space from the ground up. This is usually not possible however, and retrofitting existing space is the norm. Some aspects of design are expensive, whereas others may be impossible given the structural components of an existing building. The result is almost always a compromise. This chapter covers what would ideally be included in a dermatologic suite, with the caveat that most surgeons will likely not be fortunate enough to be able to include everything. Furthermore, since products change rapidly both as a result of technological advances and because companies come, go and merge, it would be inappropriate to endorse any particular product or brand. The recommendations here will focus on features of equipment rather than specific models.

Regulations concerning many office features will be mandated by state departments of health rather than national organizations or accreditation bodies. A review of such state regulations is beyond the scope of any text. Be advised that you should obtain your state regulations early in any renovation project. Renovation may lead to the requirement to comply with new regulations, from which older space may have been exempted due to "grandfathering." Reputable contractors should have copies of the regulations and will be a valuable asset in the process of build-out or renovation of pre-existing space.

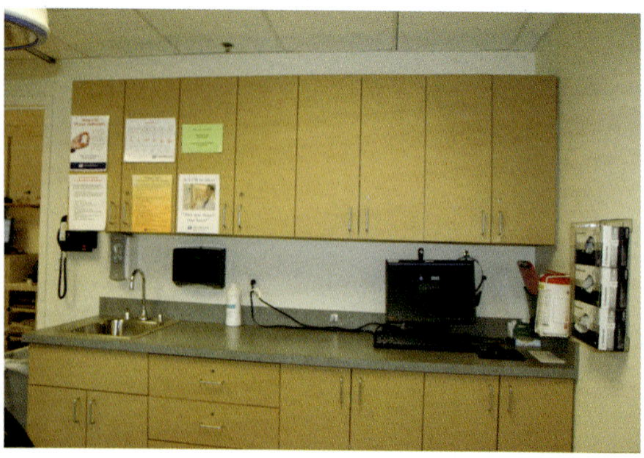

Figure 7-1 Storage and work space. Note that the counter is clear of storage items, upper cabinets have locks, and there are 18 in between the cabinet and the ceiling with nothing stored in this space.

SURGICAL SUITE

The room needs to be large enough to allow adequate movement around the surgical table. Accreditation standards require at least 3 ft around each side of the table and 150 sq ft of open floor space at a minimum. Counter space, an electrosurgical unit, a surgical tray, one or two chairs for consultation, a rolling stool, and possibly a computer station will all require a floor space footprint. The layout will take into account the shape of the room, the amount of equipment that can be wall mounted and the amount of floor equipment. Other equipment such as lasers or light banks for PDT may be stored in the surgical suites or may be rolled in for use at the appropriate time. It is important to know what functionality is needed for each room so as to plan the space accordingly. If you are going to keep lasers in each room, be sure to add that square footage to the floor plan.

Ventilation is crucial and the building must have a ventilation system. Surgical suites cannot have open windows. Although windows are important for natural light and aesthetics, they are not considered to be ventilation sources.

If at all possible, individual thermostatic control of each room should be provided. The laboratory must be kept cool to assist in maintaining cryostat temperatures. However, a cool temperature will be uncomfortable for many patients when they are immobile and in a gown, necessitating a higher room temperature.

Walls and floors must be both washable and durable. A durable neutral paint is best for walls. Because equipment frequently mars the walls, choosing a standard color will allow for retouching paint to keep the room looking fresh. Flooring is an important choice, with several factors to consider. The first is the slippery nature of flooring materials. Ceramic may be much more slippery when wet, and because many spills occur, the floor of surgical space is frequently wet. A second consideration is leg fatigue. Hard surfaces are much more difficult to stand on for long periods of time. There are several flooring surfaces available that have greater give or are "softer" and reduce fatigue. Carpet was at one time popular, but is harder to keep clean, and cannot be recommended.

Halls should be wide enough for a stretcher to turn and doors wide enough to allow stretcher access. In hospitals and hospital clinics, regulations (either Joint Commission on Accreditation of Health Care Organizations (JCAHCO) and/or state agencies) will mandate these standards,

TABLE 7-1
Surgical Suite Specifications and Equipment Parameters

	Basic Examination Room	Procedure Room	Class A Operating Facility
Corridors	Public hallways must be at least 5 ft wide without obstruction from equipment, vending machines, or drinking fountains.		
Doorways	If wheelchairs or stretchers will be regularly used, doorways should be at least 3 ft 8 in wide. If not, doorways must be at least 2 ft 10 in wide.		
Minimum size of room	80 sq ft of clear floor area. There must be at least 28 in of clear space at the foot, head, and sides of examination table.	120 sq ft of clear floor area with a minimum dimension of 10 ft. 3 ft of clear space should be at the foot, head, and sides of examination table.	150 sq ft of clear floor space with minimum dimension of 12 ft. There must be 3.5 ft of clear space at the head, foot, and sides of examination table.
Ceiling height	Minimum height of 7 ft 10 in. Rooms with ceiling-mounted equipment and lighting should be high enough to accommodate equipment.		
Ceiling material	Smooth, nonabsorptive, and able to withstand scrubbing and chemical cleaning.	Smooth, nonabsorptive, and able to withstand scrubbing and chemical cleaning.	Monolithic, scrubbable. No cracks. Penetrations in the ceiling for pipes, lighting, and other necessities should be gasketed.
Wall finishes	Washable, water resistant, able to withstand chemical cleaning and scrubbing.	Washable, water resistant, able to withstand chemical cleaning and scrubbing.	Monolithic, scrubbable, and tightly sealed.
Flooring choices	Slip resistant, low glare material. Carpet is permissible if tightly glued down. Floors should be easy to maintain, clean, and ambulate on	Slip resistant, low glare material. Carpet is permissible if tightly glued down. Floors should be easy to maintain, clean, and ambulate on	Scrubbable, monolithic, smooth. Slip resistant and easy to move wheeled equipment on.
Bathrooms	Handicapped accessible with grab bars. Doors to restrooms should open outward to ensure access in a medical emergency. For patient hand washing stations, sinks should be hands free. If a sensor activated sink is used, a backup power source is required. For sinks using single levers, blade handles should be at least 4 in in length.		
Nursing stations	Nursing station with work counter, communication system, charting space, and room for supplies.	Nursing station with work counter, communication system, charting space, and room for supplies.	Nursing station with work counter, communication system, charting space, and room for supplies. If postoperative recovery does not occur in the operating room, the recovery space should be visible from the nursing station.
Hand washing	Hand sanitizer as well as hand washing stations should be available in numbers great enough to satisfy the facility's Infection Control Risk Assessment requirements. Sinks must be 144 in^2 in area at a minimum, well fitted with sealed basins, and the distance from the point of faucet discharge to the bottom of the sink must be at least 10 in. Splash should be minimized by offsetting the sink drain from below the sink waterspout. Nothing can be stored below the sink space. Sinks in examination rooms should be hands-free. If sinks are sensor operated, they must have an alternate energy source in the event of a power outage. Nonautomatic sinks must have single levers or wrist blades at least 6 in in length. Each sink should be accompanied by a liquid or foam soap as well as a hands-free drying device such as an automatic hand dryer or paper towel dispenser.		Scrub facilities must be hands-free and operated by knee, foot, or sensor control. Sensor controlled sinks must have power supply backup. The scrub facility may be located outside of the operating suite and can service two adjacent rooms. The design of the surgical sinks should minimize splash and regulate water pressure and temperature. Proper antiseptic scrub washes should be provided.

(continued)

TABLE 7-1 (*Continued*)
Surgical Suite Specifications and Equipment Parameters

	Basic Examination Room	Procedure Room	Class A Operating Facility
Sterilization facilities	The facility must have a system for equipment sterilization and designated space for handling and storage of both clean and dirty supplies. Carts or other vehicles used for transport of supplies must be cleaned and sanitized regularly. A soiled holding area for offsite sterilization or a soiled work room for onsite sterilization should be separated from the storage space for sterile equipment. If sterilization is completed onsite, an adequate work surface, sink, and the required sterilizers and washing equipment should be provided as well as a separate clean room for assembly and terminal sterilization of equipment. Biohazard waste services and receptacles should be readily accessible in areas where soiled equipment is held or processed. The design of the storage space should demonstrate consideration for ventilation, humidity, and temperature control.		
Medical emergencies	A crash cart should be available for surgical facilities. Its storage space should include a port for charging and there should be an alternative source of power.		
Drug distribution	Medication distribution stations should be locked and in the event that controlled substances are available on site, the refrigerator that they are stored in should be double locked. The drug distribution station should also have a work counter and sink available.		
Patient safety and security	Patients' privacy should be maintained throughout their visit. Examination rooms should have closable doors, recovery areas should have curtain enclosures, and hallways leading to patient care rooms should have restricted access. Patient medical records of all media types should be maintained in a secure space as determined by facility layout and function. The records should be restricted through remote location or limited staff access and all efforts should be made to ensure that they are not lost or damaged.		

whereas private offices may only be regulated by the state. Exit signs and emergency lighting are safety features that will be dictated by the type of practice and/or state policy.

STORAGE

Deciding on the function of each room and storing enough supplies within the space will facilitate efficient procedure flow. Keeping sufficient supplies of commonly used materials within procedure rooms will keep staff in the room instead of running for supplies elsewhere in the office. Keeping inventory low while maintaining adequately stocked rooms can be a delicate balance to achieve.

There are many storage limit regulations that the surgeon should be aware of when designing a surgical suite. For example, the JCAHO requires 18 in of empty space between the ceiling and the highest storage unit. In clinical spaces, nothing can be stored underneath the sink, even if a cabinet is present. To ensure that staff does not unwittingly violate this regulation, a solid front can be installed, rather than a door which should not be used.

Choosing the type of cabinets is a decision for the surgeon to make. Cabinets come in all styles, materials (such as wood or laminate) and prices. Some physicians like glass doors on some or all of the cabinets, which allows for easy location of materials, and which can be useful to determine when rooms require restocking. However, with glass door cabinets, any "mess" can easily be seen by patients and their families, necessitating organization.

Similarly, counters are available in many styles, colors, and finishes. The surface should be nonporous and easily cleanable. Countertops adjacent to hand washing stations should be made of porcelain, stainless steel, a solid surface material, or laminate with an impervious seal to ensure adherence to JCAHO regulations (Fig. 7-2).[1]

Locks must be kept on any cabinets in which medications or sharps are stored. These can be a keyed lock or a key pad combination lock. The latter frees staff from needing a key.

HAND CLEANSING

SINK

Hand cleansing is the cornerstone of infection control and should include a surgical scrub at the beginning of each surgical session. As accreditation requirements include a sink in each room with a minimum clearance from spout to sink basin of 10 in, designing a deep sink to minimize "splash" adds little expense. These can be fitted with foot pedals which limit bacterial re-exposure, in contrast to hand faucets. If applying for JCAHO accreditation, the use of foot, knee, or sensor controlled sinks is a necessity.

Another alternative is designed scrub sinks which come as multiple or single stations. These are much larger and deeper than standard sinks, but also have a larger footprint, which can take up valuable space.

HAND SANITIZER

Foam hand sanitizer dispensers should be both outside and inside the room, allowing all health care personnel to apply foam both when entering and leaving the room. It is best to have a standard location for mounting these units so that each room provides the same time efficient motion for hand cleansing. Accreditation standards require the use of hand sanitizers in addition to sinks but do not address the location of the units.[1]

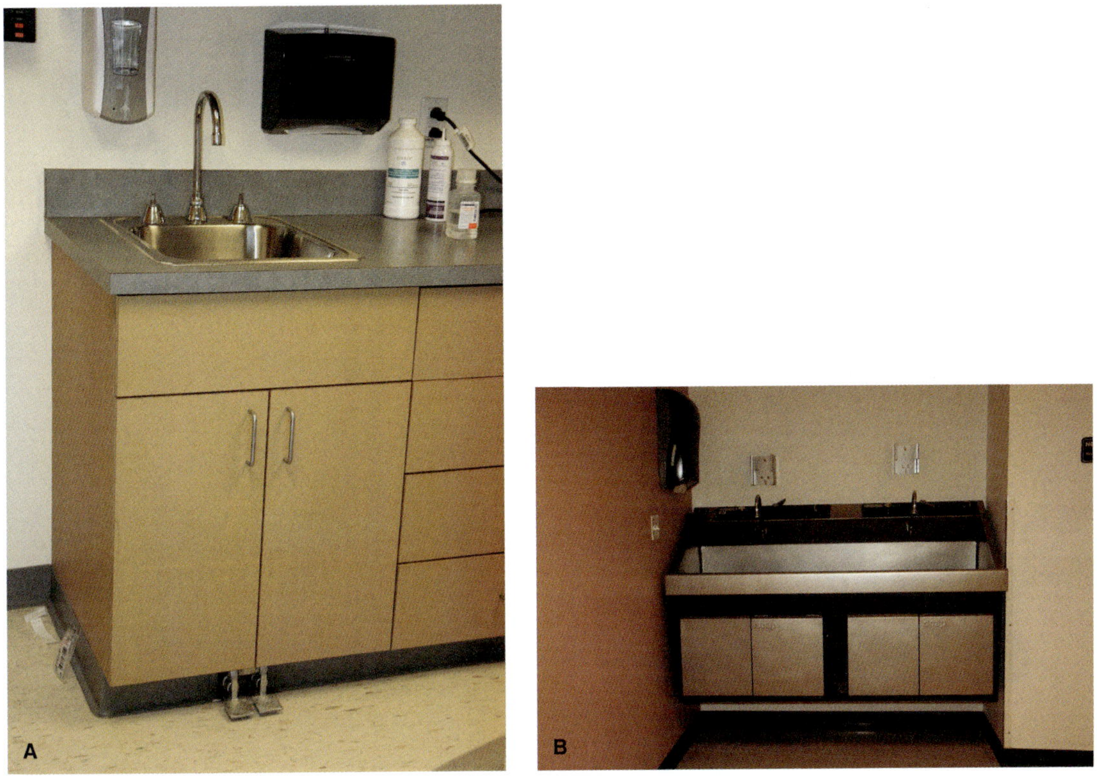

Figure 7-2 **A.** Sink with foot pedals to activate water. **B.** Large, traditional scrub sinks.

WASTE

There should be a covered trash receptacle in every room,[1,2] as well as one rolling trash receptacle, usually known as a kick bucket. The kick bucket should be emptied between patients so that there is no bloody or soiled gauze remaining in the room at the start of the next case (Fig. 7-3). In addition, the rolling kick bucket can easily be moved to a position that optimizes use and prevents bloody waste from soiling the floor. Best practice would dictate that the covered trash receptacle should be operated by a foot lift top, but this is not mandated by any regulations at this time. Red liner bags, indicating contaminated waste, need to be used in any receptacles used for disposal of blood saturated gauze or tissue.

Each room must also have a sharps container. There are several options for maintaining these, the most common one being to have a contract with a pickup and disposal company. The size of the bin and the time interval of collection can be set to match the volume of sharps waste produced in the office. In smaller communities, there may be an option to receive and return bins through a package delivery service.

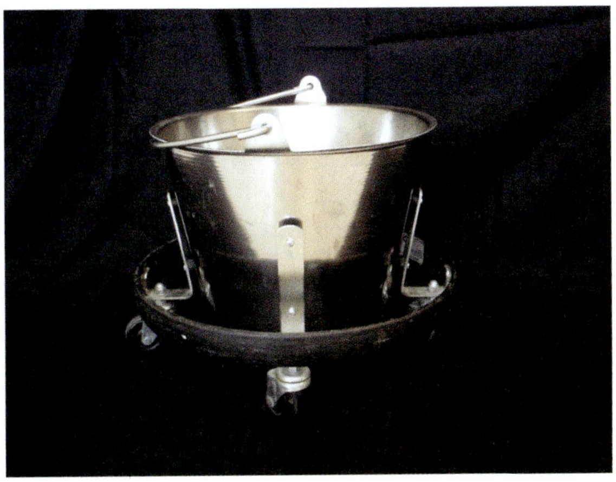

Figure 7-3 "Kick bucket" waste receptacle is on wheels.

WALL-MOUNTED ITEMS

Wall mounting reduces clutter on counters, leaves more open floor space, and minimizes trailing cords. Items that may be wall mounted include otoscopes, ophthalmoscopes, hyfrecators, blood pressure cuffs, oxygen, suction, racks for forms and anything else that has wall mount capability. Any items requiring wall mounting should be appropriately sized. Electrical cords pose a hazard for patients and staff alike and may lead to falls if not hard wired or if they do not have a dedicated outlet (Fig. 7-4).

EQUIPMENT

Suction and oxygen are not required by JCAHO in procedural rooms if sedation is not being used, although they may be helpful if the building has already been configured to provide one or both of them. Centrally sourced oxygen

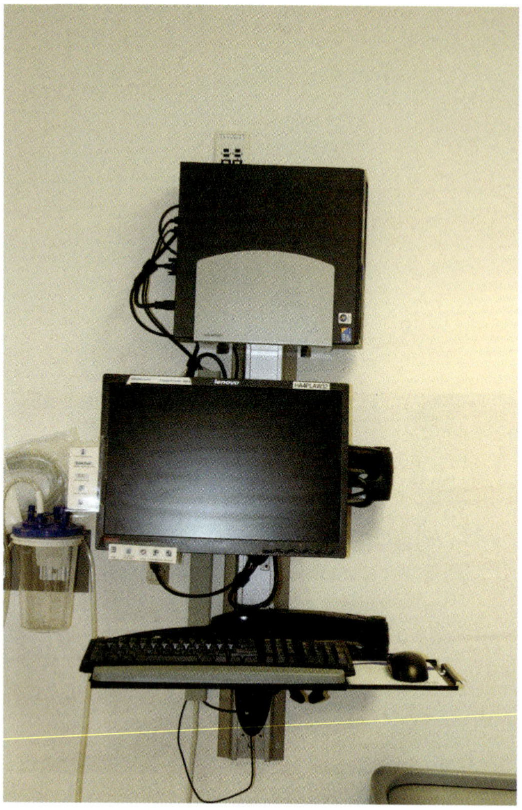

Figure 7-4 This is a wall computer mount with keyboard and monitor at eye level and the hard drive wall mounted above.

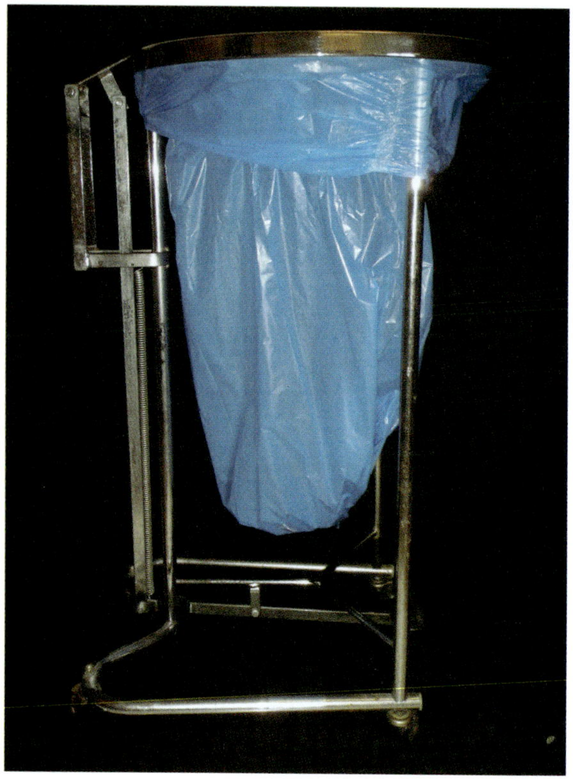

Figure 7-5 Rolling soiled linen bin. This can be stored inside or outside of the room.

is particularly useful for the patient requiring constant supplementary oxygen or who has a vasovagal episode. If unavailable from a central source, bottled oxygen kept in a central, easily accessible location will usually be acceptable in these situations.

The need for suction in the surgical suite is both provider and case dependent. Some surgeons like to use suction during their procedures, whereas others do not. Suction can be very helpful when used in surgery on rapidly bleeding wounds, but is not essential. If wall suction is available, this alleviates the need to have an additional piece of rolling equipment, lessening the potential for clutter in the office. Excellent rolling suction units are also available.

Although not required, having a phone extension in each room can be useful, especially if interpreter services are provided for patients via the telephone. Having a phone in the room can also be useful for any calls that need to be made while the patient is still in the office, such as visiting nurse follow-up, transportation, or even 911 calls (Figs. 7-5 and 7-6).

SUPPLIES

It is important to evaluate each item needed in the examination room, to find the least intrusive storage area, and to investigate options for wall rather than counter storage. Additional items that may be wall mounted include computers, chart racks, magazine racks, examination and

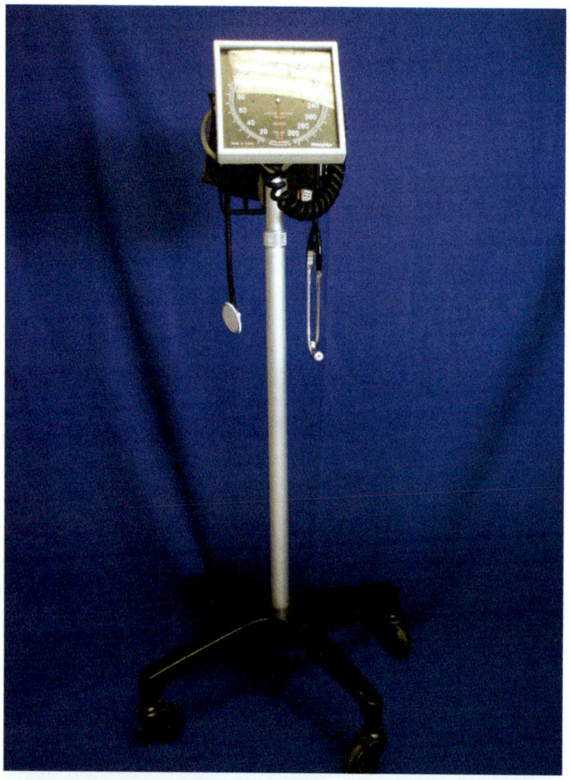

Figure 7-6 Rolling blood pressure cuff. Can be rolled out of the room to preserve floor space.

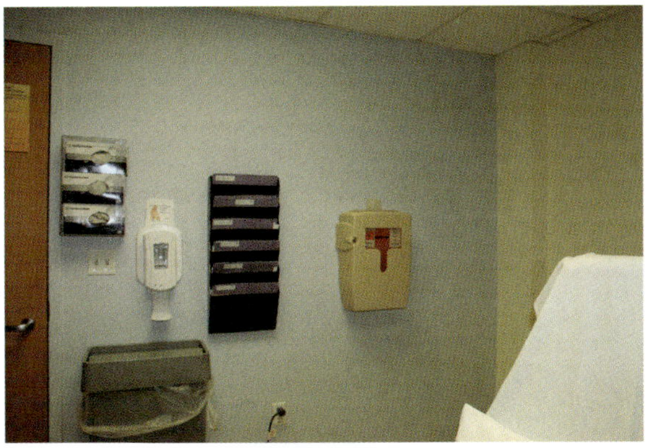

Figure 7-7 Wall mounting of all possible equipment preserves floor space. This shows mounted examination gloves, hand cleanser, forms and consents, and sharps disposal.

surgical gloves, hand cleanser dispensers, and even suture storage units. There are countless wall storage devices that can be purchased from office supply houses and medical suppliers (Fig. 7-7).

SURGICAL TABLES

Surgical tables or chairs are key equipment and care should be taken in selecting them. Patients need to rest comfortably; tables or chairs must be wide enough to fit full-figured individuals and have enough padding to be comfortable for longer procedures. They must allow the surgeon easy access to the surgical site. In dermatologic surgery this means being configured to allow the head and neck to be easily reached. Tables and chairs should be tested to ensure that they can be elevated high enough for a tall surgeon to work comfortably and that they can descend low enough for a short surgeon to work comfortably, or to allow any surgeon to sit while working. Not all tables are able to do this. Using "step ups" or stools is reasonable, but should be needed only if two people of unequal heights are working together, and should not be thought of as an alternative to a table that cannot go high enough or low enough to be functional in the operating room.

In addition to having a sufficient range of height, tables must also have mechanical head-up, tilt, and foot-up options. These features allow endless positioning possibilities for both

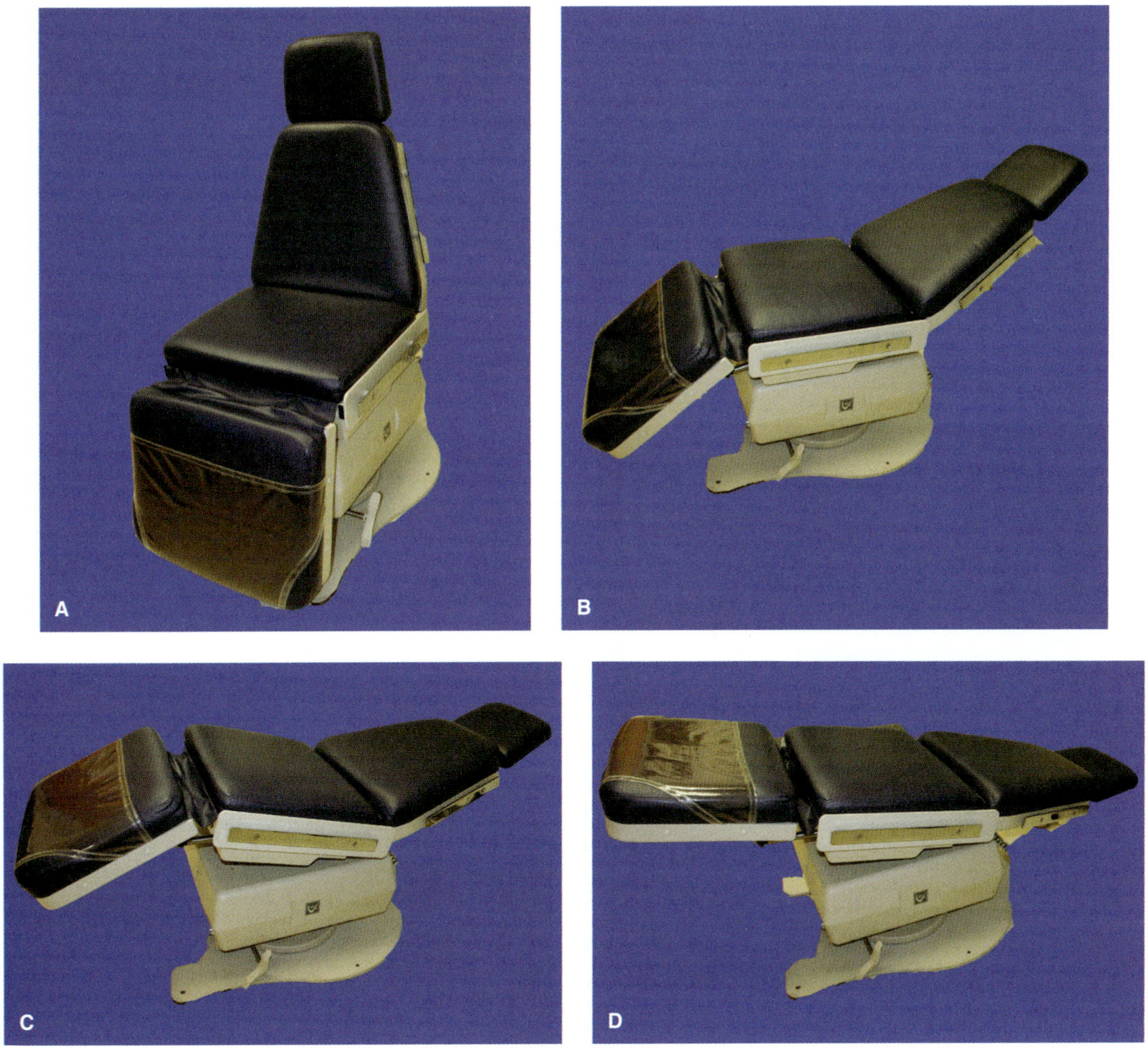

Figure 7-8 A–D. Examination table demonstrating multiple positions. **D** shows the important Trendelenburg position.

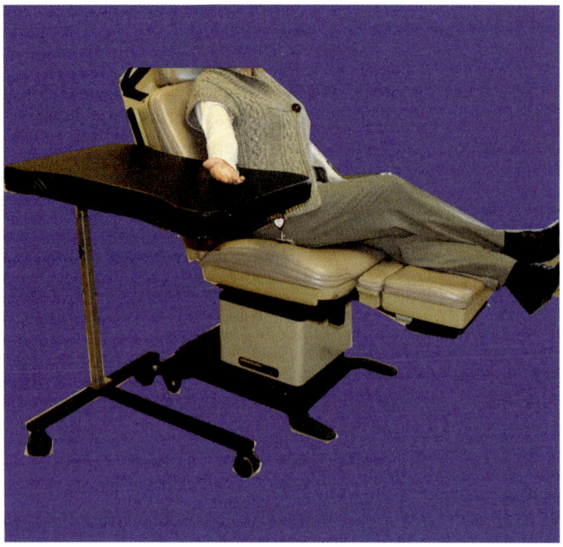

Figure 7-9 Rolling padded arm table. This can be stored in other locations and brought in the room only when needed.

patient and surgeon comfort. Although some tables come with a fixed foot position, surgery should not be performed in a setting in which the Trendelenburg position (tilt down) cannot be achieved. Tables come with foot pedals, hand controls, and the ability to preprogram certain positions. Preprogramming the Trendelenburg position may be very useful in an emergency. Because patients come in all shapes and sizes, a preprogrammed "favorite" position is only a starting point to get the patient and surgeon comfortable. Having pillows available to pad or prop up older or disabled individuals may make a substantial difference in achieving patient comfort.

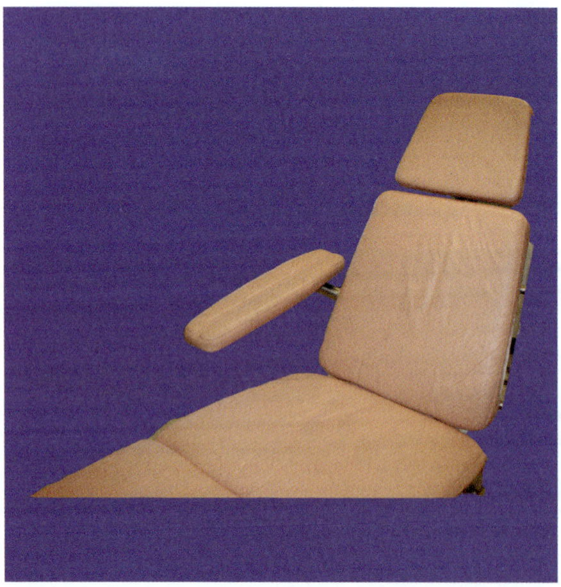

Figure 7-10 Attachable arm board. Note that it is much narrower than the arm table in Figure 7-9 but requires no floor space.

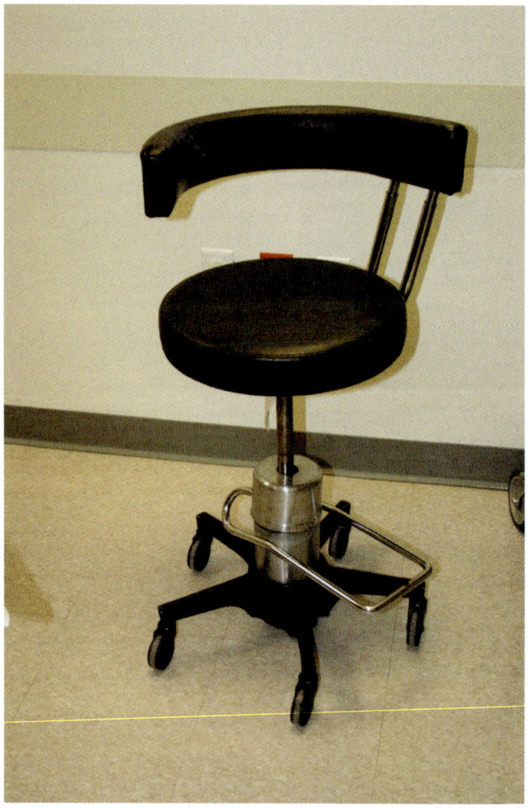

Figure 7-11 Surgeon's stool.

Some additional supplies may be necessary to provide easy access to the surgical site. An attachable arm rest or a free standing arm table should be available to allow correct positioning of the upper extremity during surgery. For surgical sites on the posterior head, neck, or back, some surgeons have a face pillow, or "donut" pillow to allow the patient to lie in a face down position with some comfort. Others simply position the patient so that the site is as accessible as possible for the surgery to be performed (Figs. 7-8 to 7-10).

Rolling stools allow the physician to sit while operating, which some practitioners find useful and others strongly dislike. The use of stools does allow surgeons of unequal heights to work at approximately the same level in relative comfort. Keep in mind, however, that stools do take up a great deal of floor space (Figs. 7-11 and 7-12).

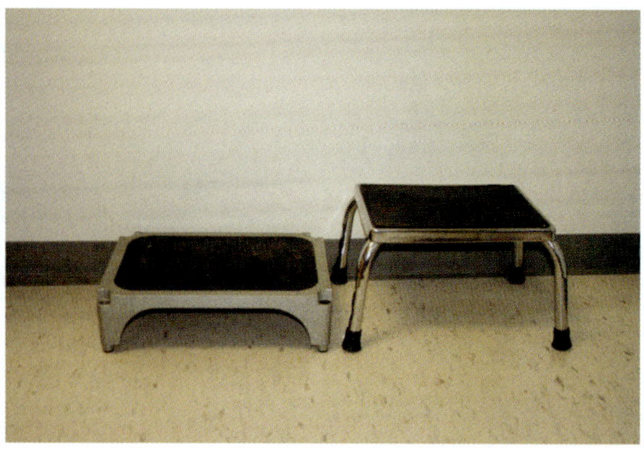

Figure 7-12 "Step ups" come in various heights.

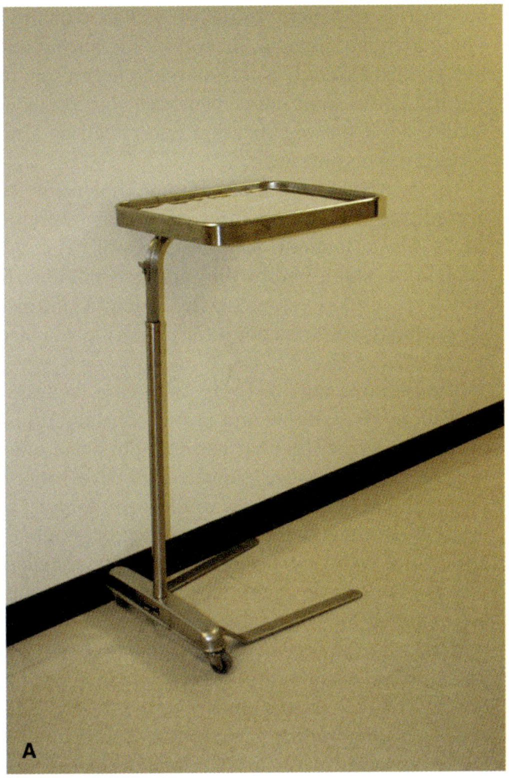

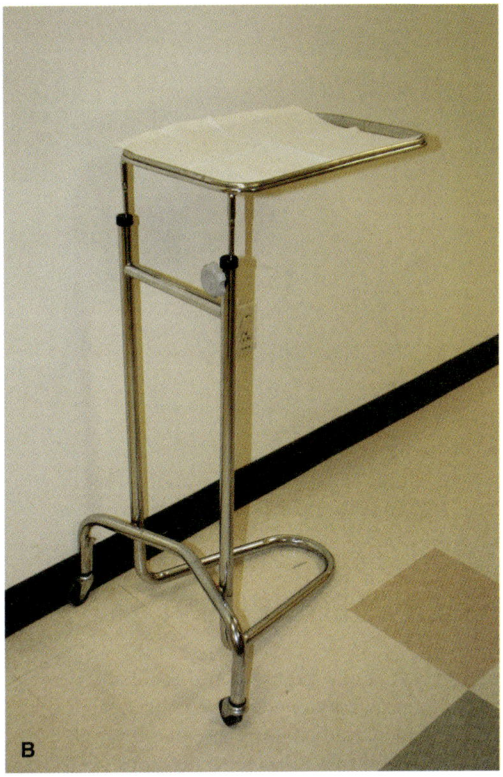

Figure 7-13 **A, B.** Mayo stand.

MAYO STANDS

Instrument stands are needed to position the instruments in an accessible place and must be mobile as surgical positioning may change. When selecting a stand, it is important to consider that some models with four wheels may be too mobile while others with two wheels are not quite as easy to move but are more stable when in position. The stand should be sturdy, as the lighter weight stands tend not to hold up to heavy use (Fig. 7-13).

LIGHTS

Surgical lights are one of the most important items in the operating suite. Adequate bright light is crucial, as is the ability to focus on deep, open wounds. Although there are many relatively inexpensive single or double light units that do not use reflective technology, these units tend to be underpowered and their arms tend to "drift" without regular maintenance and repair. Larger, reflective lights with more robust articulating arms offer greater range in positioning and better "holding" of the light source, but come with a larger price tag. These larger lights also need greater ceiling height to accommodate the articulating arms. Ceiling heights should be built to accommodate the larger lights, even if smaller lights are installed initially with the plan to upgrade at a later date, as refitting can be expensive or impossible (Figs. 7-14 and 7-15).

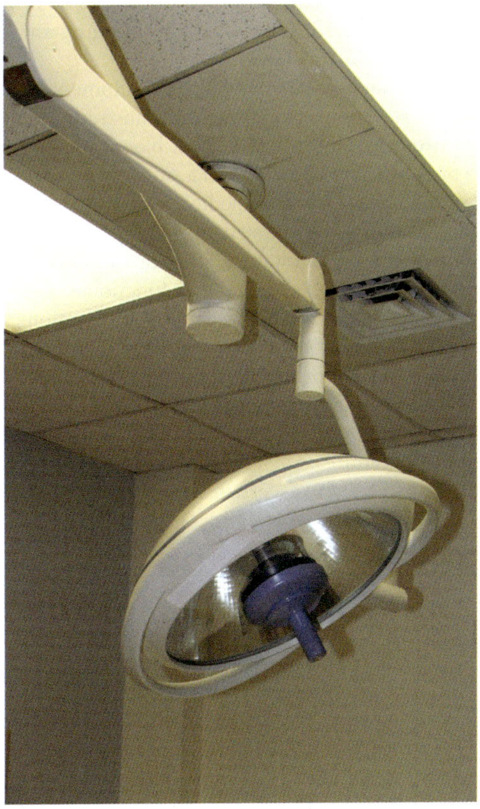

Figure 7-14 Reflective OR light with articulating arms.

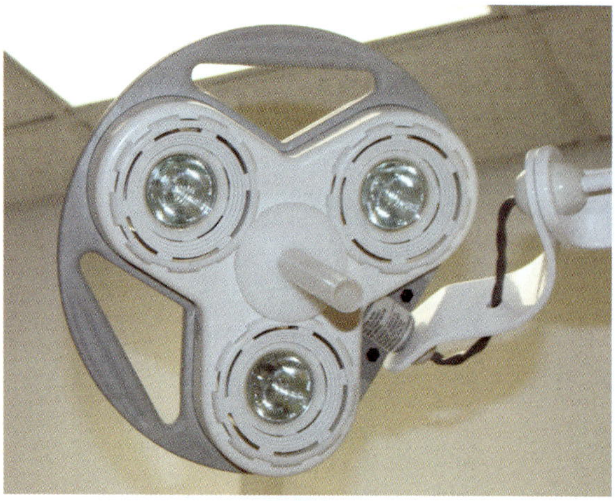

Figure 7-15 Light with three-light configuration. This tends to be hotter, with less robust articulating arms.

EMERGENCY EQUIPMENT

There are no regulatory requirements about the types of emergency equipment that need to be available in the surgical suite. There should be both an emergency plan and sufficient equipment to support a patient until emergency support arrives.

All staff should have basic life support training, and a log should be kept to be certain that all certificates are current. Surgeons and mid-level providers should consider advanced cardiac life support training. An office plan should be developed so that each staff member has a role in the event of an emergency, such as calling 911, bringing oxygen and placing it on the patient, bringing any other equipment, or starting CPR.

The minimal level of emergency equipment includes oxygen, nasal cannulas for oxygen administration, an automated external defibrillator (AED), blood pressure cuffs, and a back board to allow CPR. If a surgeon or staff is qualified, a full crash cart with medications, cardiac monitor, oxygen saturation monitor, defibrillator, and intubation equipment can be maintained. This cart requires regular maintenance to keep equipment functional, including battery checks and replacing expired medications. This cart review should be documented in a log and the log reviewed regularly for quality assurance.

Monitoring equipment includes cardiac and oxygen saturation monitoring devices. These may be important for some procedures. Each office should evaluate the procedures performed to ascertain the equipment necessary.

ACCREDITATION PROCESS

Although not currently required of dermatologic surgical facilities, accreditation by one of the major health care accreditation groups serves several purposes. First, the process of applying for accreditation serves as a reflective experience, through which the organization can identify weaknesses and seek to improve them. Secondly, the process can improve the medical team's morale and pride, and fosters the ability to deliver a higher quality of care. There are also financial incentives for having an accredited facility. Not only is this marketable as a sign of quality of care, but in some cases insurance companies will pay a facility fee if the organization is certified by a nationally recognized organization.[3*]

The JCAHO is most commonly known for its role in accrediting hospital facilities but it has developed standards for outpatient facilities as well. The outpatient guidelines established by the Facility Guidelines Institute, which are used as a standard by the Joint Commission, are an excellent reference point for preparing your facility for a JCAHO survey.

The requirements for outpatient care facilities include architectural, material, and layout considerations. As "an outpatient facility that has within it physician office(s) and space(s) for the performance of invasive procedures," a dermatologic surgical suite would need to meet the standards of an office-based surgical facility. While the operating suite is the subject of this chapter, some additional details about basic examination rooms and office layout are included for your consideration, as the surgical suite seldom exists independent of an office practice. In addition to basic examination rooms, which are self-explanatory, JCAHO has requirements for both procedure rooms and operating rooms. Under the American College of Surgeons Surgical Facility Classes, dermatologic surgical suites qualify for Class A operating facility status based on their use for minor surgeries prepared under topical and local anesthesia.

The process of accreditation begins with the selection of the accrediting agency, of which there are three well-known national groups—the JCAHO, the Accreditation Association for Ambulatory Health Care (AAAHC), and the American Association for Accreditation of Ambulatory Surgical Facilities (AAAASF). Accreditation for dermatologic surgical facilities is most commonly obtained through JCAHO or the AAAHC. Some of their standards are presented in the charts below (Table 7-2). Should the surgeon choose to have their surgical suite accredited, the handbooks for accreditation will be valuable during preparation for the site survey.

The process of accreditation is both rigorous and informative and the choice of organization should be based on what works best for each individual office. While the AAAHC requires that many procedures and protocols be provided in written format, this process enables the practitioner to tailor the way to handle issues to fit his or her practice.[2] On the other hand, the JCAHO regulations ensure that the layout and flow of the office meets standards that should lead to better patient care and quality improvement. Finally, this decision may be made for the surgeon. For example, the surgeon who is a part of a large health care organization that has pursued accreditation through one of these organizations may be expected to follow suit. We, however, strongly recommend considering both sets of standards while designing your office. The combination of well-thought-out space and safety considerations coupled with introspective protocol design should increase patient safety, satisfaction, and in turn make the surgeon's job more enjoyable.

TABLE 7-2

Standards from the Joint Commission on Accreditation of Health Care Organizations (JCAHO), the Accreditation Association for Ambulatory Health Care (AAAHC) and the American Association for Accreditation of Ambulatory Surgical Facilities (AAAASF)

Standard 1: Rights of patients	A practice must treat patients with dignity and respect through its communication with patients and with other providers, its proper use of patients' medical records, and whether the organization realistically presents the tasks it is capable of to the public.
Standard 2: Governance	There should be a selected governing body within the organization that determines the policies and procedures that are required for appropriate functioning of the organization. This governing body must initiate plans for financial health, risk management, quality improvement efforts, and proper credentialing of employees.
Standard 3: Administration	The administration of the organization seeks to enforce the policies and procedures established by the governing body, to maintain finances, to hire and manage employees, and to ensure patient and provider safety through infection and injury control plans.
Standard 4: Quality of care provided	Quality of care is assessed based on use of evidence-based medicine, judicious testing and referrals to specialists, good communication with patients and other providers, and whether the organization has an internal, ongoing assessment of their quality of care.
Standard 5: Quality management and improvement	Providers and administrators should participate in an ongoing quality performance assessment using peer review, self-reflection, and external performance measures as barometers. Quality improvement projects should document both the issue at hand and the performance goal.
Standard 6: Clinical records and health information	All aspects of patient care including office encounters, lab results, telephone encounters, and information from outside providers should be documented in a uniform way in a medical records system that is secure and confidential. In addition to inspecting individual patient charts, the AAAHC surveyor will also assess the policy for access, use, storage, discard, and release of medical records.
Standard 7: Infection prevention and control and safety	The organization should promote patient and employee safety through enforced protocols on infection prevention, disaster preparedness, and medical error reporting.
Standard 8: Facilities and environment	The facilities and layout used by the organization are appropriate for the tasks at hand and meet all state and local codes. Cleanliness, good lighting, and reduction of patient hazards (i.e., use of slip-resistant floors, employee awareness of disaster preparedness plans, adequate medical emergency training and equipment) will be assessed at the onsite visit.

The time to achieve accreditation will vary depending on the accrediting body. JCAHO accreditation will be issued when it inspects an institution, on its regular schedule. AAAHC requires an application with a fee. The organization sends the manual for compliance, and when ready, the applicant will ask for a site inspection. Preparation usually takes months. Inspection and certification by state boards depends directly on the state and always adds time to the process of building or renovation. The process, no matter which agency is involved, is slow and requires planning, work, and attention to detail.

REFERENCES

1. The Facility Guidelines Institute. *Guidelines for Design and Construction of Health Care Facilities*. Chicago, IL: American Society for Healthcare Engineering of the American Hospital Association; 2010.
2. Accreditation Association for Ambulatory Health Care. *Accreditation Handbook 2011 For Ambulatory Health Care*. Skokie, IL: Accreditation Association for Ambulatory Health Care Inc; 2011.
3. Sterling JB, Hanke CW. Office accreditation in dermatology. *Semin Cutan Med Surg*. 2005;24(3):128–132.

CHAPTER 8

Surgical Instruments

Zena Pinnella, Kerri Robbins, & Aaron K. Joseph

INTRODUCTION

Dermatologic surgery encompasses a wide range of procedures necessitating an even larger variety of surgical tools. Use of the best instruments and proper maintenance of all surgical supplies can help the surgeon achieve optimal results while capitalizing on their investment. Consistently organized surgical trays help minimize the risk of accidental injuries and maximize efficiency in the procedure room.

INSTRUMENTS

Instruments used for dermatologic surgery are typically small, easy to maneuver, and allow for delicate handling of tissues. The most commonly used tools include curettes, scalpels, scissors, skin hooks, hemostats, needle holders, and forceps. All these tools are available in a variety of qualities and costs, and it is in the surgeon's best interest to select the most economical tools that will aid in delivering the desired results. In general, higher quality instruments are more durable, easier to use, and longer lasting, and are usually covered by a warranty that ranges from 1 to 5 years. Modern instruments are most commonly made from surgical stainless steel with carbon alloy, chromium, nickel, and tungsten carbide.

CURETTES

Curettes are used for tumor removal, to better define tumor margins prior to excision, and for tumor debulking prior to Mohs micrographic surgery. They are available in disposable or nondisposable forms, or as a single-use curette blade that may be used on a scalpel handle. Ideally, a curette will remove more friable tumor-infiltrated tissue while leaving behind normal skin. Curette heads are either round or oval and vary in size from 1 to 9 mm (Fig. 8-1). A surgeon can normally purchase approximately 50 disposable curettes for the price of a single nondisposable curette. The disposable curettes have lightweight plastic handles, whereas the reusable curettes are made of stainless steel. A reusable curette may seem more cost-efficient, but it is important to remember that these instruments need to be sharpened periodically to prevent dulling of the sharp scraping edge. A dull curette may result in unnecessary damage to tissue.[1]

SCALPEL HANDLES

Scalpel handles may be flat or round, thin or thick, textured or smooth. The most commonly used handles in dermatologic surgery include the Bard–Parker #3 and Beaver handles. The Bard–Parker #3 handle may be flat or round and is available with an etched ruler. This inexpensive scalpel holds a variety of scalpel blades, including the most popularly used #10, #11, and #15 blades. The smaller, mini-Beaver handle is available in a hexagonal or round shape (Fig. 8-2). This handle is used for more delicate work around the eye or ear. It is not as versatile as the Bard–Parker #3 handle because it must be used with certain blades, such as the #64 and #67 Beaver blades, Beaver mini-blade, and the 60 degree lamellar blade. These blades

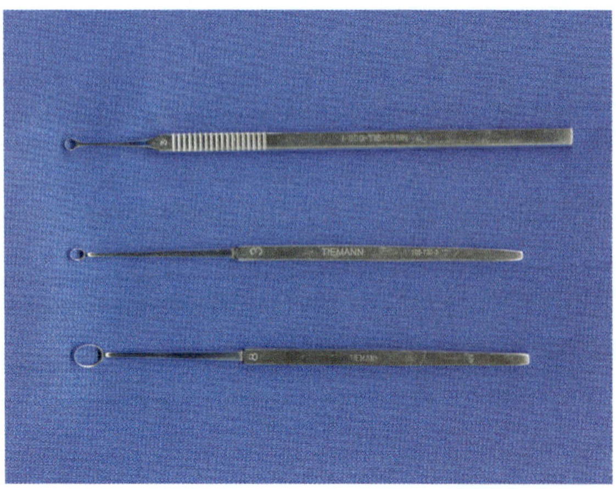

Figure 8-1 Curettes in three different sizes with round and square handles.

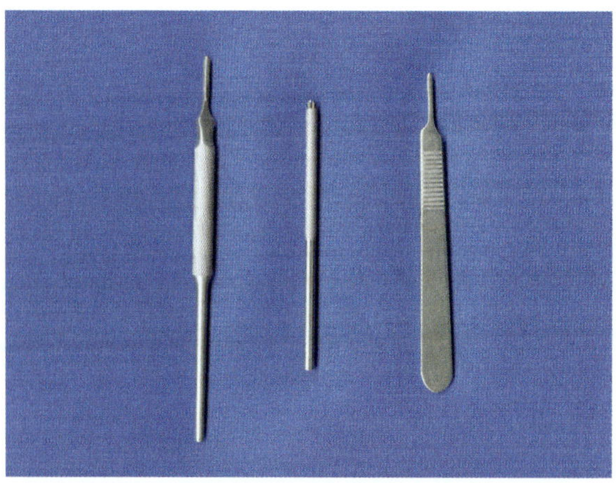

Figure 8-2 Scalpel handles: round handle; Beaver; Bard–Parker, flat (left to right).

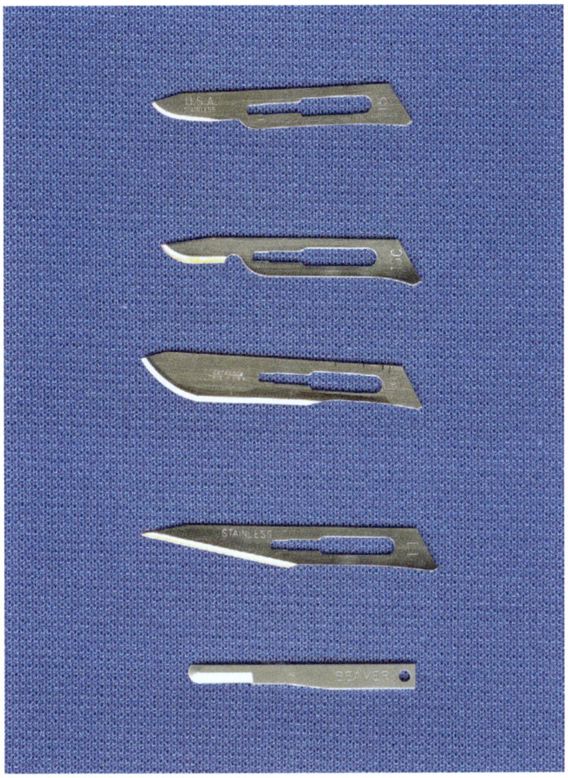

Figure 8-3 Scalpel blades: 15, 15c, 10, 11, 64 Beaver (top to bottom).

are fitted into a collet, which tightens around the blade when the scalpel handle is turned. The Siegel scalpel is favored by some surgeons when performing Mohs micrographic surgery. Its round, knurled handle allows for easy positioning when excising circular or ovoid specimens.[2]

SCALPEL BLADES

The most popular blade used in excisional surgery is the #15 blade, which has a sharp convex belly. The #15c blade is a smaller variant of the traditional #15 blade, which allows for better control when working in small confined areas. The #10 blade is a larger, wider, and more convex version of the #15 blade. It is used for excisions of thick skin such as on the back. The #11 blade is tapered to a sharp point and is thus used for incision and drainage, removal of milia, and precise cutting of flaps. The #67 Beaver blade is small with a convex belly and sharp tip. Similar to the #15c blade, the #67 blade is best for delicate work in small areas. The #64 Beaver blade has a rounded tip, which allows for easier maneuvering in arched structures such as the pinna (Fig. 8-3). Scalpel blades are available in stainless steel or carbon steel. Carbon steel is sharper; however, it is also more expensive and dulls more quickly than stainless steel blades.[1] Blades may also be coated with Teflon to decrease drag through tissue.[3]

BIOPSY BLADES

The #15 scalpel blade may also be used to perform shave biopsies. An economical alternative, which allows greater

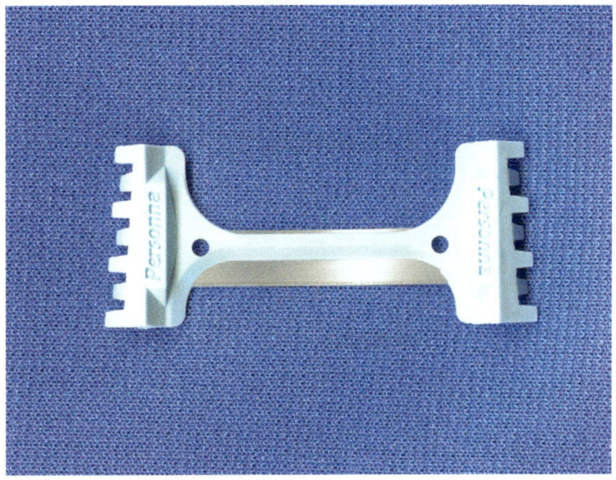

Figure 8-4 Dermablade.

precision, is the disposable razor blade. However, these blades must be separated and sterilized by office staff and can pose a sharps hazard. The unsafe use of any sharp surface is strongly discouraged by the Occupational Safety and Health Administration (OSHA).[4] A similar, more convenient (but more expensive) alternative is the prepackaged Dermablade (Fig. 8-4), which also offers a plastic holder that helps to reduce the risk of accidental injury.

SCISSORS

A wide variety of surgical scissors is available to suit the dermatologic surgeon's needs. Scissors are available in both right-handed and left-handed versions and may be short or long with either sharp or blunt-tips. Long-handled scissors are reserved for cases in which the surgeon performs extensive undermining or needs to work in deep tissue planes. Short-handled scissors are used for finer procedures on the head and neck. Scissors with blunt-tips are ideal for undermining tissue, whereas sharp-tipped scissors are used for sharp dissection. Scissor blades vary from straight to curved and serrated to smooth (Fig. 8-5). Straight blades are used for trimming skin and cutting sutures, whereas curved blades are typically used for blunt dissection. Serrated blades are particularly useful for immobilizing skin with little subcutaneous tissue when cutting. Stainless steel scissors are the most popular and least expensive. They may also have tungsten carbide inserts that strengthen the blade but increase the cost. It is important to use these instruments properly to avoid misalignment and prevent dulling of the tips.

The Gradle scissor is small, curved, and tapered to a fine point, which allows for precise cutting during skin tag removal and delicate dissection in certain areas, such as on the face. Similar to the Gradle scissor, the Westcott and Castroviejo scissors have a very fine, sharp tip that is useful for handling delicate periorbital tissue (Fig. 8-6). Unlike the Gradle scissor, these scissors are spring-loaded. The iris scissor has a short handle, sharp tip, and extremely sharp cutting edges, making it ideal for dissecting and cutting through tissue on the face and neck. The blade may be either curved or straight. This scissor is available with smooth blades, or one smooth paired with one serrated blade. The long-handled Metzenbaum scissor may have

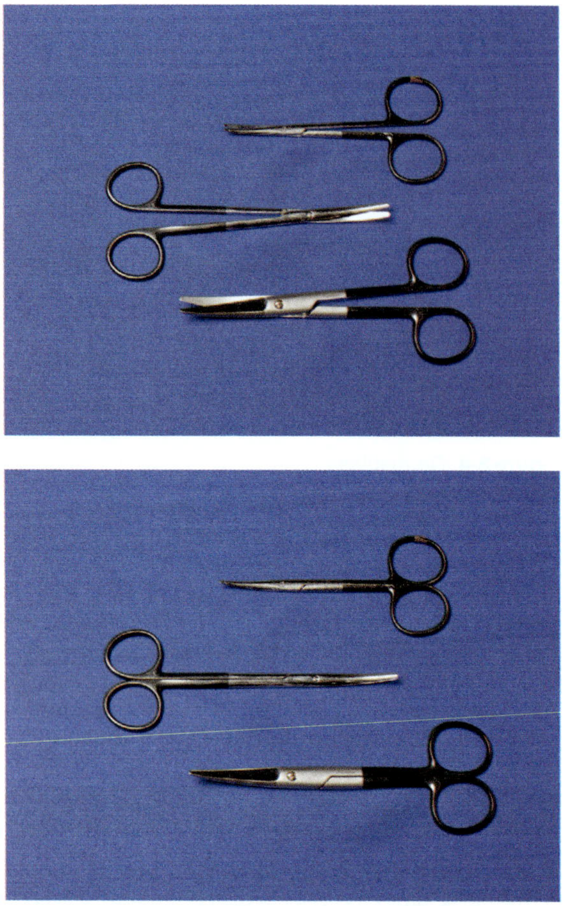

Figure 8-5 Large scissors: curved short-handled scissors, Metzenbaum, Mayo (top to bottom).

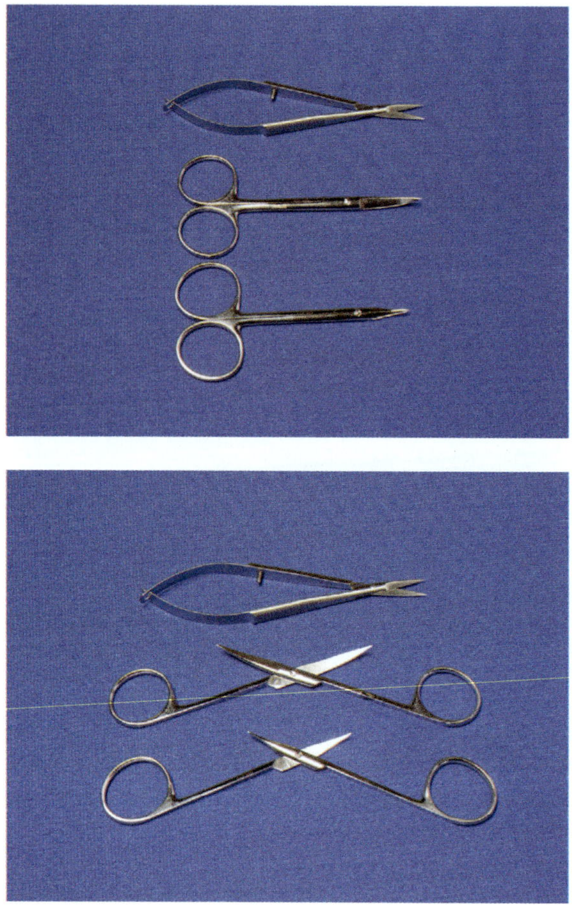

Figure 8-6 Small scissors: Castroviejo, Iris, Gradle (top to bottom).

a curved or straight blade with a sharp or blunt-tip. It is available in several sizes and is thus widely used for sharp or blunt dissection in areas that require a reach. The Mayo scissors' handle and blade are roughly equal in length; this instrument is used for blunt dissection. The S-curved LaGrange scissor is long-handled and used for undermining dome-shaped lesions, removing punch biopsy specimens, and harvesting hair transplant donor grafts. Most of these tissue scissors are available in the supercut variety, meaning that one of the blades has a fine serrated edge and that the other is sharp.

In addition to tissue scissors, dermatologic surgeons also require suture-removal scissors. While the fine, sharp Gradle, Westcott, and Iris scissors should never be used to cut sutures, other tissue scissors like the Mayo may be used for this purpose, although it is important to note that tissue scissors will dull much more rapidly when also used to cut suture. The Northbent or O'Brien scissors are specially designed scissors for suture removal. The Northbent scissor has a curved lower blade with a hook that easily catches the suture loop (Fig. 8-7). The O'Brien scissor has a short-angled blade that cuts suture at its tip, preventing unwanted nicks in the skin.

Finally, the dermatologic surgeon should be familiar with bandage-cutting scissors. The widely used Lister scissors have large, blunt-tips with gently curved blades making them ideal for cutting dressings.

SKIN HOOKS

The dermatologic surgeon may use skin hooks to manipulate tissue with minimal trauma. Skin hooks are available in single- or multiple-pronged models. The single-pronged and double-pronged hooks are used to elevate flaps, undermine very delicate skin, and stabilize

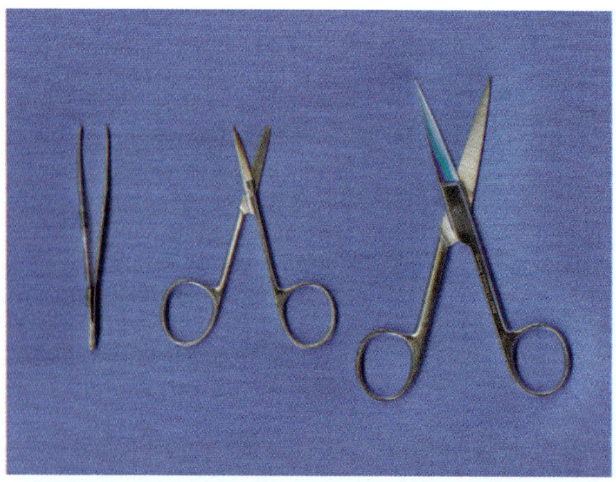

Figure 8-7 Suture removal and cutting: forceps, hooked suture removal, operative suture-cutting scissors (left to right).

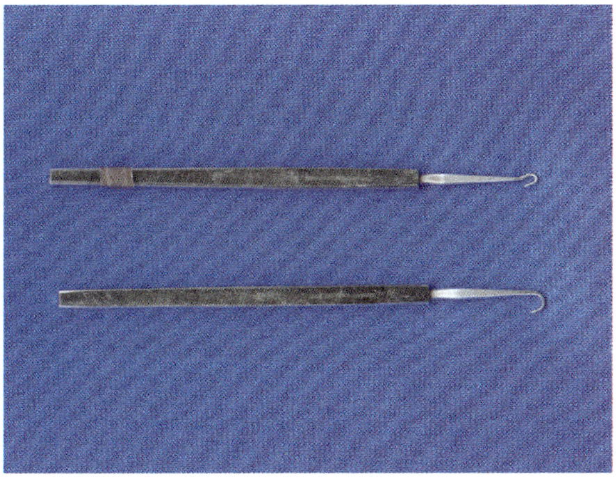

Figure 8-8 Single-pronged skin hooks: curved and shepherd's curved (top to bottom).

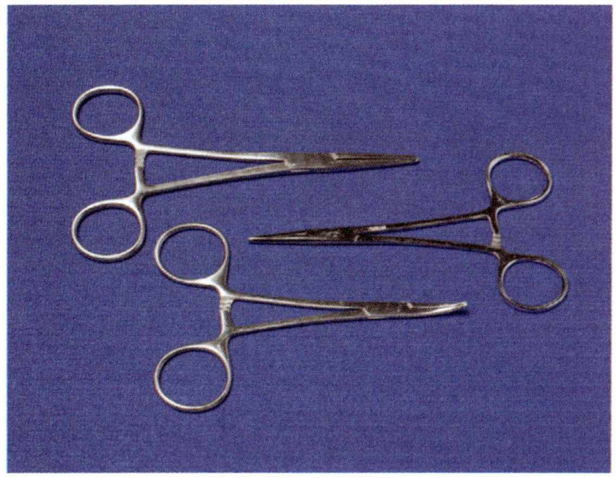

Figure 8-10 Hemostats: large straight, delicate straight, delicate curved (left to right).

tissue during dissection and prior to suturing (Fig. 8-8). The double-pronged hooks offer greater stability and thus lead to decreased risk of injury to the surgeon (Fig. 8-9). The multiple-pronged hooks are used for handling larger flaps. Skin hooks may also be used to maintain tension on the wound when placing buried or running sutures. Skin hooks vary in their degree of sharpness, curvature, and length.

HEMOSTATS

Hemostats are used to clamp bleeding vessels prior to ligation or electrocoagulation. Hemostats are available in a variety of types depending on the surgeon's preference and need. These include regular and delicate, as well as curved and straight versions (Fig. 8-10). The authors feel that the delicate versions tend to be more efficient at grasping smaller vessels. The Jacobson hemostat is ideal for dermatologic surgery because it can easily grasp small vessels with its fine tip. The Halsted Mosquito hemostat is also popular in cutaneous surgery. Hemostats should not be used as needle holders. They do not grip the needle effectively and in turn, the hard surface of the needle will damage the clamping surface of the hemostat.

NEEDLE HOLDERS

A wide variety of needle holders, available in right-handed or left-handed versions, are available to the dermatologic surgeon. To avoid damaging the instrument and associated needle, the surgeon generally pairs small needle holders with small needles and large needle holders with large needles. This is also important to prevent the needle from slipping out of the needle holder's grasp. The jaws of needle holders may be either smooth or serrated.

The Baumgartner and Mayo–Hegar needle holders are strong with serrated jaws and are used for skin surgery on the back. The Crile–Wood needle holder is long with a gently tapered, blunt-tip designed to hold larger needles (4-0 and larger), and is primarily used for skin surgery on the trunk, extremities, and scalp. Needle holders used for more delicate procedures should be small and have smooth jaws to prevent damage to the finer needles and suture (Fig. 8-11). The Neuro-smooth needle holder has a narrower tip, which is more appropriate for fine suture material (5-0 and smaller). The Webster and Halsey needle holders have narrow, smooth or finely serrated jaws that are ideal for the fine suture work that is performed in

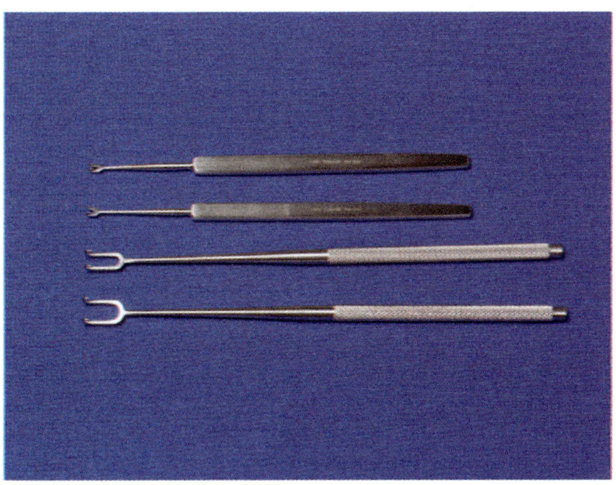

Figure 8-9 Double-pronged skin hooks: multiple sizes (close up).

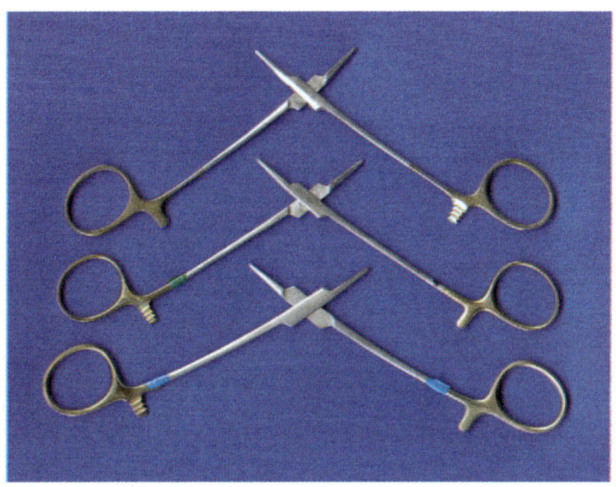

Figure 8-11 Needle holders: small left-handed, small right-handed, large right-handed (top to bottom).

cutaneous facial surgery. The Castroviejo needle holder has a detachable spring handle and self-locking device and is designed for very delicate work in the periorbital region.

Needle holders must be durable and withstand distortion from constant metal-to-metal contact. High-end needle holders, which can be identified by gold handles, have alloy inserts of tungsten carbide on the jaw surfaces to provide additional protection. However, these inserts may wear away with time, making it even more important to use the appropriately sized needle for the instrument being used.

FORCEPS

In dermatologic surgery, forceps should be lightweight and easy to manage to allow for precise manipulation of tissue and suture needles. The tips may be smooth, toothed, or serrated. Smooth forceps inflict minimal damage to tissue, but tissue is more prone to slip from its grasp. Although serrated tips allow for firm grasp of tissue, they can cause crush injury to delicate areas, resulting in suboptimal wound healing. Toothed forceps reduce crush injury and still allow for firm grasp of tissue. The tips of forceps vary from delicate (<0.6 mm), to regular (1–1.5 mm), to heavy (>1.6 mm).

Many dermatologic surgeons prefer the larger Adson forceps for grasping the thick tissue of the proximal extremities and trunk. Adson forceps have wide handles for easy grasping and their tapered tips are available in both serrated and toothed models. The Adson forceps without teeth, also called platform Adsons, may be used to grasp surgical needles for safe transfer to the needle holder during suturing. The Brown–Adson forceps are similar to the Adson forceps except that they have eight or nine teeth on each side of the forceps jaw, which allows for enhanced tissue grasping, but produces a greater risk of crush injury (Fig. 8-12). Graefe forceps have wide jaws with a row of six or eight teeth and are useful for grasping cartilage.

For more delicate work on areas with thinner skin (such as the eyelids, hands, and glans penis) the smaller, fine-tipped Bishop–Harmon forceps are popular (Fig. 8-13). They have three holes on each side of the handle, which make them even more lightweight, and they are available with or without teeth. Jewelers' forceps are small with a fine, sharp tip, which is useful for suture removal and grasping small vessels.

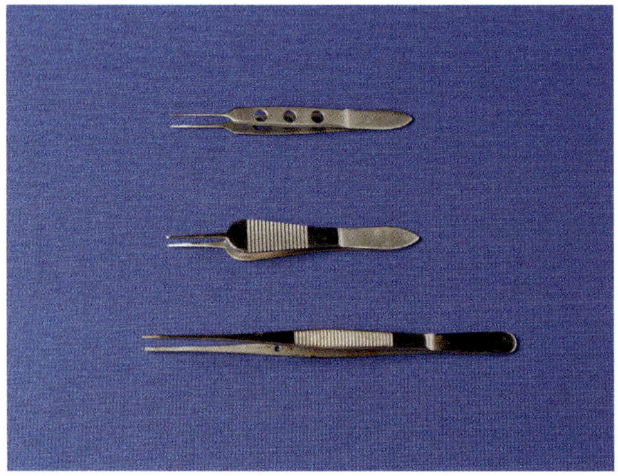

Figure 8-13 Delicate forceps: Bishop–Harmon, ophthalmic, small toothed (top to bottom).

MISCELLANEOUS INSTRUMENTS

Additional instruments used in dermatologic surgery include eye shields, chalazion clamps, Allis clamps, towel clamps, periosteal elevators, bone chisels, nail splitters, and nail elevators. Eye shields protect the eye during certain procedures that are in close proximity to the globe, such as laser, cautery, or eyelid surgery. These are available in metal or plastic varieties, but caution must be taken when using plastic eye shields as CO_2 or erbium lasers can burn through the plastic. In general, plastic shields should be used for radiofrequency treatments and metal eye shields for laser resurfacing.[5] Eye shields come with either a small handle attached or a small suction cup for easy removal.

Chalazion clamps are used to isolate eyelid, lip (mucosal), and cheek tumors. One end of the clamp has a flattened solid

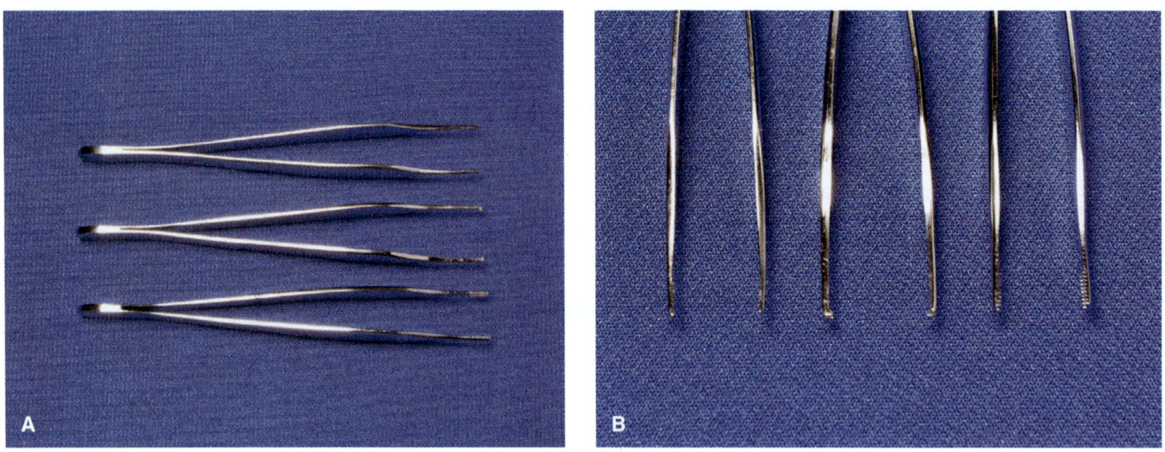

Figure 8-12 **A.** Forceps: Adson without teeth, Brown–Adson, Adson with teeth (top to bottom). **B.** Close up: Adson without teeth, with teeth, Brown–Adson (left to right).

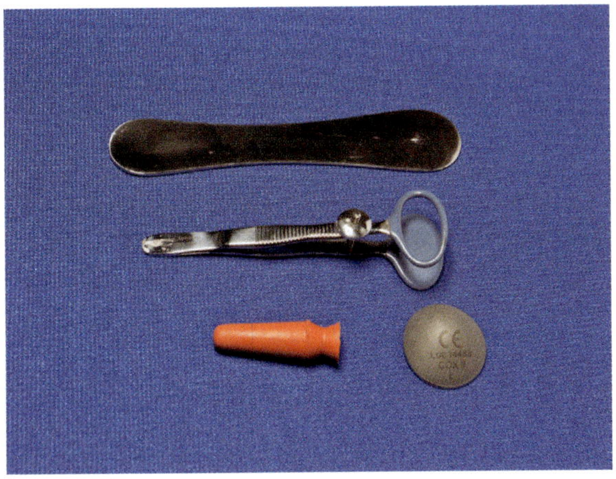

Figure 8-14 Ocular instruments: chalazion clamp, metal eye shield and suction cup, eyelid retractor (top to bottom).

plate available in several shapes, and the other end is open (Fig. 8-14). This design allows the clamps to hold delicate tissue without causing damage. Allis clamps have sharp teeth that are used to grasp tissue. As their sharp teeth can damage tissue, Allis clamps are mostly used to grasp stiff, fibrous tissue or tissue that is to be removed. They are available in a variety of sizes, the smallest with 4 × 5 teeth and the largest with 9 × 10 teeth. Towel clamps have curved ends that lock in place to anchor surgical towels and drapes within the sterile field.

Periosteal elevators are used to lift periosteum from bone and to lift full-thickness skin flaps. Periosteal elevators generally combine two different ends: a large, flat blade for retraction and a smaller, curved tip for reflection and retraction of tissue. They are commonly used with bone chisels to obtain samples of bone or periosteum that need evaluation for tumor invasion. For nail surgery, nail splitters have sharp tapered tips used to cut the nail plate. Nail elevators separate the nail from the soft tissue below without damaging the nail bed.

THE SURGICAL TRAY

A properly organized surgical tray is imperative for maximizing the efficiency and safety of a given procedure (Fig. 8-15). A sterile drape should cover the stainless steel surgical tray and stand. The Mayo surgical stand comes in two-wheeled and four-wheeled versions; both can be adjusted to the surgeon's preferred height. Surgical instruments should be placed on top of the removable surgical tray in a manner that reduces needlestick injuries. The instruments should not overlap, and gauze should not cover any sharp instruments.

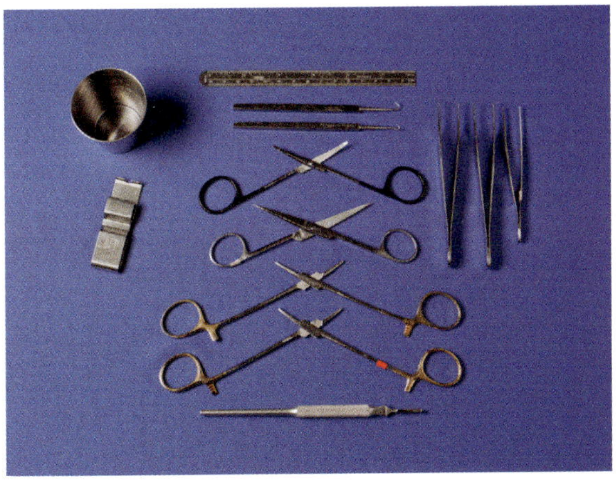

Figure 8-15 Surgical excision and repair tray: space is left between instruments for easy identification and safety.

Every excision tray should contain a marking system (commonly a marking pen or liquid gentian violet with a toothpick or wooden cotton-tipped applicator), ruler, forceps, scissors, scalpel handle, and a curette if needed for tumor debulking. Once the tray is opened, sterile gauze, scalpel blades, cotton-tipped applicators, and Telfa pads to transport surgical specimens to the laboratory should be added if desired. If a repair tray is needed, it should contain a needle holder, suture-cutting and undermining scissors, skin hooks, and a cup with sterile saline to store any skin grafts. Once the repair tray is opened, scalpel blades, sterile gauze, cotton-tipped applicators, and suture materials should be added.

INSTRUMENT MAINTENANCE

Proper sterilization and handling of surgical instruments are necessary to optimize the performance and durability of the tools. Soon after use, surgical tools should be submerged in a solution of warm water and instrument detergent. Any remaining residue may be gently removed with a plastic brush or ultrasonic cleaner.[6] Afterwards, the instruments should be rinsed with water and then completely dried before sterilization to avoid rusting or staining with water spots.[7] Before sterilization, the sharp instruments should be inspected for nicks, and tissue-grasping tools should have aligned tips. Periodic instrument sharpening and restoration are needed to optimize the ability and extend the life of surgical tools.

There are several methods of sterilization commonly utilized. Steam sterilization with an autoclave is the easiest and most commonly used method in the office setting. This autoclave uses high pressure (2 atm pressure) and high temperature (121°C) for 20 to 30 minutes to sterilize instruments. This method of sterilization is nontoxic to the patient and staff and allows prepackaging of instrument trays, which is time-efficient. However, the disadvantage to this method is that the humidity from distilled water may dull sharp instruments. The chemical autoclave uses a mixture of alcohol and formaldehyde, which decreases the humidity and causes less dulling of sharp instruments than the steam autoclave. Another method of sterilization uses dry heat to kill microorganisms. Although this method is cheap and does not dull sharp instruments, the tools cannot be placed in paper or plastic packages. As this presents a problem for preparing and storing instruments for later use, this method is usually reserved for sterilizing a particular instrument for immediate use. Gas sterilization, which has excellent microbicidal activity, is mostly used in hospitals as it is expensive, time-consuming, and uses toxic ethylene oxide gas. Cold sterilization is inexpensive, but it is not recommended as a sole method of sterilization as it is unreliable in clearing bacterial spores and the hepatitis B virus.

INJURY PREVENTION

Every surgeon, scrub nurse, and resident should take the necessary precautions to avoid inflicting injury upon themselves or others around them. Surgical personnel risk percutaneous injury and subsequent infection with blood-borne pathogens. Conversely, percutaneous injury to the surgeon may place the patient at risk of disease transfer. The major pathogens of concern are HIV, hepatitis B virus, and hepatitis C virus.

The first precaution that the surgeon and assistant should take is wearing properly fitted gloves. Loose gloves may catch on sharp instruments as well as obscure the view of the surgical field.[8] Secondly, the surgical tray should be neatly and properly set up with all instruments clearly visible and pointing away from the surgeon's hand. During the procedure, the surgeon should work away from their hand or the assistant's hand. Only one hand should be present in a surgical field when a sharp instrument is present and the instrument should not be moving. When stabilizing or manipulating tissue, the surgeon or assistant should use an instrument instead of their hands to avoid unnecessary exposure in the surgical field.[9] It is also important to use scalpel handles or needle holders when handling scalpel blades or needles, respectively. Needles should not be recapped. When removing a blade from the scalpel, a scalpel blade remover should always be used. There are various blade removal devices, including single blade removers and reusable blade removers that deposit freed blades into an attached puncture proof container (Fig. 8-16). Needle holders should never be used to remove a blade as this is an unsafe practice and will also damage the needle holder. Ideally, surgical personnel should have a "safe zone" for instrument passing, such as a tray, to avoid hand-to-hand passing of sharp instruments.

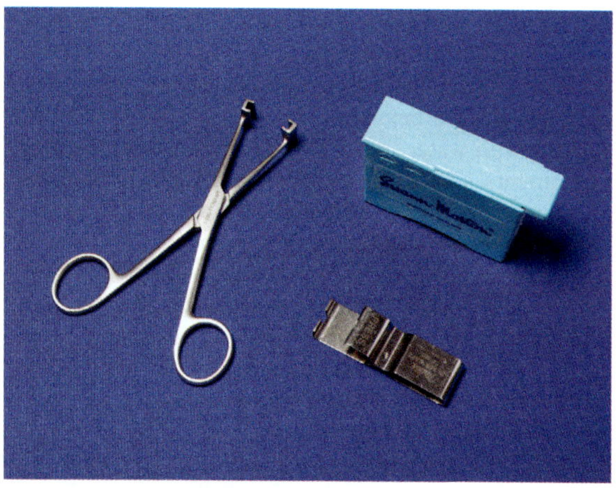

Figure 8-16 Blade removal instruments.

CONCLUSION

The dermatologic surgeon must have knowledge of the best surgical instruments and appropriate wound closure materials to effectively deliver the most precise outcome. It is important to properly handle and sterilize surgical tools to increase their longevity and maximize their utility. Appropriate scheduling and surgical tray organization will greatly enhance the speed, safety, and flow in the surgical suite.

REFERENCES

1. Neuberg M. Instrumentation in dermatologic surgery. *Semin Dermatol.* 1994;13(1):10–19.
2. Peterson SR, Goldberg LH. The rounded Siegel scalpel handle: a better instrument for curved incisions. *J Drugs Dermatol.* 2003;2(6):617–618.
3. Weber LA. The surgical tray. *Dermatol Clin.* 1998;16(1):17–24.
4. Occupational Safety and Health Administration. *Protecting Yourself When Handling Contaminated Sharps.* Washington, DC; 2011. http://www.osha.gov/OshDoc/data_Bloodborne-Facts/bbfact02.pdf. Accessed August 21, 2012.
5. Ries WR, Clymer MA, Reinisch L. Laser safety features of eye shields. *Laser Surg Med.* 1996;18(3):309–315.
6. Geisse JK. The dermatologic surgical suite. *Semin Dermatol.* 1994;13(1):2–9.
7. Sebben JE. Sterilization and care of surgical instruments and supplies. *J Am Acad Dermatol.* 1984;11(3):381–392.
8. Trizna Z, Wagner RF. Preventing self-inflicted injuries to the dermatologic surgeon. *J Am Acad Dermatol.* 2001;44(3):520–522.
9. Nori S, Greene MA, Schrager HM, Falanga V. Infectious occupational exposures in dermatology– A review of risks and prevention measures. I. For all dermatologists. *J Am Acad Dermatol.* 2005;53(6):1010–1019.

CHAPTER 9 Preoperative and Postoperative Antibiotics

Michael M. Wolz & Christopher J. Arpey

INTRODUCTION

A discussion of antibiotic use in procedural dermatology should begin with the principles of when not to use antibiotic agents, as the majority of cutaneous procedures do not require their use. The dermatologic surgeon, like any medical practitioner, should be guided by the fundamental rule *primum non nocere*—first do no harm. Medications, including topical antibiotics, have side effects. They also have costs, both to the patient and to health care systems, whether direct financial ones or indirect ones, such as from the emergence of multidrug-resistant microorganisms.

Evidence-based medicine teaches us that the use of routine antimicrobial prophylaxis, which was once common practice in dermatologic surgery, is no longer indicated. This principle applies both to topical and systemic antibiotic agents. The incidence of wound infection in cutaneous surgery is very low. Rates of surgical site infection in clean wounds typically range between 1% and 3%.[1–4] In Mohs surgery, rates fall below 3% (Table 9-1).

The risk of iatrogenic bacteremia following dermatologic surgery on clean skin has been found to be smaller than the risk of random bacteremia in healthy individuals leading a normal lifestyle.[4] For example, the risk of bacteremia following teeth brushing has been estimated to be between 20% and 40%, compared to <2% for surgery on clean, nonmucous membrane skin.[6]

Certain anatomic sites, such as the lips, ears, and groin, are susceptible to a higher risk of bacteremia.[7] Similarly, any breach in mucous membranes leads to higher risk of surgical site infection.[8] Thus, procedures on certain anatomic sites may warrant prophylactic antibiotic coverage (Fig. 9-1). Postoperatively, all wound infections require antibiotic treatment, and those that are frankly purulent or fluctuant require drainage and occasionally packing as well. This assumes, however, that one can distinguish natural wound healing from wound infections. For example, nonpurulent erythema may be the result of irritation from sutures rather than bacterial colonization. In such cases, simple removal of the sutures will alleviate the patient's symptoms and promote healing. Clinical signs which help to differentiate between these possibilities include minimal warmth, tenderness, and induration, absence of fever, and inability to express purulent material for wounds reacting to suture as opposed to infection (Fig. 9-2). Clinical experience with the normal healing process is particularly important during postoperative days 3 to 10 when low-grade cellulitis may be more difficult to distinguish from a suture reaction. Sutures have varying tissue reactivity, and familiarity with suture properties is important when assessing postsurgical wounds. Specific procedures, such as skin grafts and larger flaps, have higher associated infection risks and so may favor the use of prophylactic antibiotics.[7] Prophylaxis has been traditionally assumed necessary for certain patient populations, such as those at risk for endocarditis or prosthetic joint infection. However, even in these instances, evidence-based medicine teaches us that the uniform use of antibiotics is more likely to do harm than good.

TABLE 9-1
Comparative Incidence of Infection in Dermatologic Procedures[5]

Complication Rates	
Excisions	1.9%–2.3%
Mohs surgery	0.7%–2.3%
CO_2 resurfacing	1.1%–7.6%

IMPORTANCE OF SURGICAL PREPARATION

Avoidance of unnecessary antimicrobials requires a thorough preoperative evaluation, including clinical assessment of skin condition, a detailed medical history, information on current medications and over-the-counter supplements, drug allergies, previous surgeries, the presence of foreign

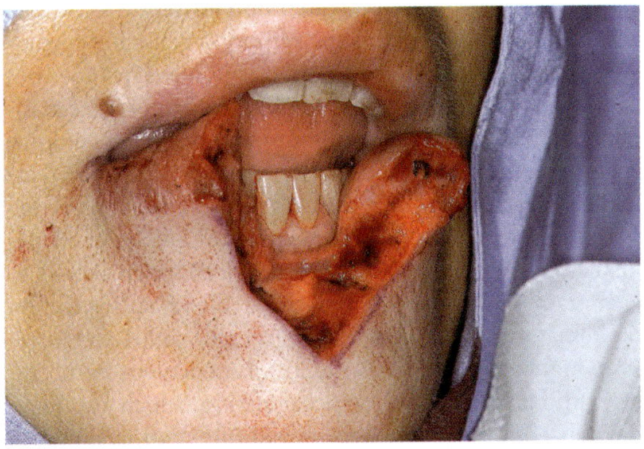

Figure 9-1 Full-thickness mucosal defect after wedge excision for squamous cell carcinoma. The anatomic site and type of procedure necessitate prophylactic antibiotic therapy with a broad-spectrum antibiotic given the presence of mouth flora.

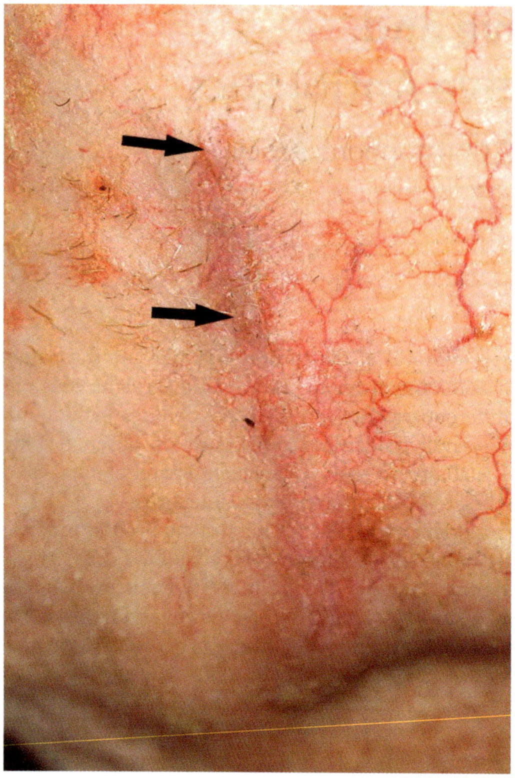

Figure 9-2 Left cheek primary repair site 6 weeks after surgery. Suture granulomas (arrows) are easily confused with late postoperative infection. The patient has minimal tenderness, no drainage, and no other clinical signs of overt infection.

objects, such as pacemakers, defibrillators or prosthetics, a history of wound infections or postsurgical endocarditis, and valvular heart disease or congenital malformations. Prior to excisional or Mohs surgery, the surgeon should also be aware of anatomic variations, tumor biology, properties of the various local anesthetic agents, instrumentation and suturing techniques. Local anesthetics frequently used in dermatologic surgery, such as lidocaine and bupivacaine, have been found to have bacteriostatic and fungistatic properties.[9] Avoidance of unnecessary antimicrobials also presupposes meticulous attention to aseptic technique and hemostasis. Dermatologic surgery is generally considered to be clean rather than sterile. This, however, does not exonerate the surgeon or the surgical team but rather mandates heightened vigilance. Improper surgical technique, such as leaving large dermal and subcutaneous defects while approximating only the epidermal edges, can predispose to fluid collection and infection. Similarly, improper instrument handling can convert a clean surgical field to a contaminated one. Subepidermal blood accumulation or hematoma formation can serve as a nidus for infection, highlighting the importance of meticulous hemostasis without excessive electrocoagulation, which can leave devitalized tissue. Although second intention healing can be useful under certain circumstances, closing a wound by first intention promotes hemostasis, reduces dead space, and decreases the risk of infection. Furthermore, while wounds that require granulation seldom become infected in normal hosts, the distinction between colonization and

TABLE 9-2
Wound Classification[10]

Classification	Location and Cutaneous Findings	Surgical Complications
I: Clean	Noninflamed skin; no contamination	None; sterile technique
II: Clean-Contaminated	Oral or respiratory mucosa, axillary or perineal skin	Minor breaks in sterile technique
III: Contaminated	Inflamed skin; trauma-induced wounds	Major breaks in sterile technique
IV: Infected	Necrotic tissue; presence of foreign material	Visible contamination

Source: Adapted with permission from Maragh SL, Otley CC, Roenigk RK et al. Antibiotic prophylaxis in dermatologic surgery: updated guidelines. *Dermatol Surg*. 2005;31(1):84.

overt infection in such cases is important to ensure that patients do not self-medicate inappropriately or seek care outside the dermatologic surgical setting because of a lack of education about the healing process. Proper wound dressings and adequate postoperative care are important tools in the effort to reduce postprocedural complications.

CLASSIFICATION OF WOUNDS

Wounds in dermatologic surgery, most of which are clean, can be classified according to surgical technique, anatomic site, and preoperative condition of the wound (Table 9-2). This classification is based on the CDC guidelines for prevention of surgical wound infections and has been found to be a strong predictor of subsequent infection.[4]

All other things being equal, class I wounds do not require antibacterial prophylaxis. For class II wounds, antibacterial prophylaxis is indicated only for immunocompromised patients, such as transplant recipients or those receiving chemotherapy.[10] This traditionally has not included HIV-infected patients unless the surgery involves the perineum.[11] Regardless of wound classification, immunocompromised patients, including HIV-infected patients, require close follow-up, because altered function of the immune system can lead to delayed or atypical presentations of wound infections. Cultures should be obtained at the first sign of infection. Appropriate, broad-spectrum antimicrobial coverage should be instituted and later tailored according to the culture results. Class III and IV wounds always require antibiotic coverage, which is aimed not only at reducing the risk of postsurgical complications but also at treating the active infection.

ANATOMIC CONSIDERATIONS

In a large prospective study, several anatomic sites were found to have significantly higher rates of postoperative infections.[1] These sites included all procedures below

TABLE 9-3 **Anatomic Sites and Procedures at Increased Risk of Infection**[7]	
Sites and Procedures at Increased Risk of Infection	
Anatomic location	Lower leg; groin Lips or ears (wedge excision)
Type of procedure	Flaps (especially nose) Skin grafts

the knee, wedge excisions of the lip or ear, and lesions in the groin (Table 9-3). In addition, skin grafts on any site and skin flaps on the nose have been associated with a higher than average risk of infection. Suboptimal circulation to these sites may contribute to their increased risk of postoperative infection. Increased density of sebaceous glands, increased humidity at mucosal or intertriginous surfaces and increased wound tension may also favor bacterial colonization and subsequent infection. Accordingly, antibiotic prophylaxis has been suggested for procedures involving certain anatomic sites or specific procedures, as summarized in Table 9-3, and as illustrated in Figure 9-3.

A prospective study of Mohs surgery revealed that 62.5% of post-Mohs wound infections occurred on the nose, although the overall infection rate on the nose was still only 0.5%.[12] On the other hand, with the inclusion of skin flaps on the nose, the infection rate rose to 3.1%. Here, too, suboptimal circulation at the surgical site likely contributed to the increased risk of infection, as well as prolonged surgical times and tissue manipulation close to the nostrils. By extension, additional anatomic locations and procedures may be considered for preoperative antibiotic prophylaxis on a case-by-case basis. For example, surgery on distal extremities, particularly on those with poor vascular supply, may warrant preoperative prophylaxis.

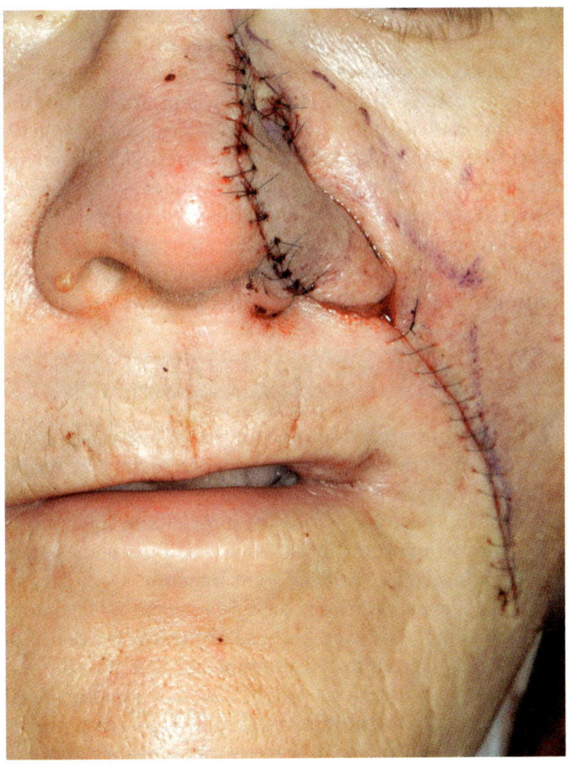

Figure 9-3 Interpolation flap and Burow's graft for a large Mohs defect involving the nasal sidewall and ala. The complexity of the repair, anatomic site and duration of the procedure warrant strong consideration for prophylactic oral antibiotics.

Anatomic sites with significant hair growth also warrant special consideration. A Cochrane Review on preoperative hair removal found that clipping or depilatory creams are associated with a reduced, statistically significant, incidence of postoperative wound infections as compared to shaving.[13] Rates of infection with shaving were statistically equivalent to the rates of infection without hair removal, which may be explained by the fact that small foci of microtrauma can allow bacteria access to the skin surrounding the surgical wound. The Cochrane Review included many nondermatologic surgeries. However, one may safely conclude that hair clipping should be the preferred method of hair removal in dermatologic procedures, if not to decrease the risk of infection, then at least to allow better visualization of the surgical field.

PATIENT FACTORS

Numerous patient and environmental factors contribute to the risk of developing postoperative wound infections. The condition of the skin surrounding the surgical site is a crucial factor. Absent other indications, procedures on noninflamed, noninfected, surgically scrubbed skin do not require prophylactic antibiotics.[14–16] However, antibiotics are necessary, both therapeutically and to prevent further spread of infection, on overtly infected skin. It is best to delay elective procedures on overtly infected skin, although avoidance may not be possible in the setting of aggressive cancers, friable tumors, or some high-risk hosts. Although the standard for cutaneous procedures is not to use antibiotic prophylaxis, patient comorbidities may mandate antibiotic use. For example, diabetes mellitus and chronic renal insufficiency are known to impair host immunological defenses. Well-controlled diabetes does not warrant antimicrobial prophylaxis, but poor glucose control is an independent risk factor for infection and should be considered in the individual patient assessment.[17] Nicotine has also traditionally been thought of as an independent risk factor for the development of wound infections, particularly after major visceral surgery.[18] However, an observational study limited to dermatologic surgical procedures disputes the presence of an increased risk of infection in smokers.[19] In any event, the microangiopathy associated with diabetes and smoking does increase the risk of necrosis, which is of particular importance in reconstructive surgery. Smokers may, therefore, be advised to stop smoking, at least perioperatively. If they are unable to cease, a reduction is helpful in the weeks prior to and after surgery. Similar to diabetes, malnutrition and obesity are independent risk factors for the development of postoperative wound infections.[18,20,21] These patient-dependent factors illustrate the importance of a thorough preoperative evaluation (Table 9-4 a and b).

TABLE 9-4

Risk Factors in the Development of Surgical Site Infections[10]

Patient Risk Factors	Common Disease Associations
Nutritional	Malnutrition, obesity
Immune defects	Inherited immune disorders; hematological malignancies; HIV/AIDS; chronic renal or liver disease; diabetes mellitus; advancing age, corticosteroid or other immunosuppressant medications (including transplant patients); concurrent infection
Wound site	Infected or colonized
Other	Excessive alcohol or tobacco use Recent hospitalization
Surgery-Related Risk Factors	
Total operative time	
Improper or nonsterile technique	
Flaps or skin grafts	
Hair shaving	

TABLE 9-5

Cardiac Conditions with the Highest Risk of Adverse Outcome[23]

Conditions for which Antibiotic Prophylaxis is Recommended	
Past medical history	Previous infectious endocarditis; transplant recipients with valvulopathy
Structural heart defects	Prosthetic valve or prosthetic material used in cardiac repair
Congenital heart defects (CHD)	Unrepaired cyanotic heart disease (e.g., shunts); repaired CHD during 6 months after procedure

INFECTIOUS ENDOCARDITIS AND NONVALVULAR CARDIOVASCULAR DEVICE-RELATED INFECTIONS

According to the American Heart Association (AHA), high-risk cardiac conditions generally warrant antibiotic prophylaxis.[22,23] The AHA provides guidelines which detail those conditions which should be classified as high risk. However, the fundamental principles of dermatologic surgery and wound classification remain the same. Surgical sites exhibiting actively infected skin require both therapeutic and prophylactic antibiotics. Similarly, high-risk surgical sites and procedures breaching mucous membranes require antibiotic prophylaxis regardless of the patient's cardiac status. It is also important to note that the majority of infectious endocarditis cases are not attributable to invasive procedures.[24,25] Moreover, approximately half of the reported cases of infectious endocarditis occurred in individuals without a detectable cardiac abnormality.

Infectious endocarditis and nonvalvular cardiovascular device-related infections are typically the result of bacteremia. The AHA categorizes risk factors for endocarditis into high, moderate, and negligible categories.[23] Generally, high-risk indications include the presence of prosthetic heart valves or substantial cardiac valvular and flow dysfunction. Other high-risk indications include a history of endocarditis and congenital heart disease (Table 9-5). Transplant patients require antibiotic prophylaxis if they have a history of valvulopathy.

The absence of hemodynamically significant flow abnormalities generally leads to a lower-risk classification. Compared to guidelines published prior to 2007, the current AHA recommendations include significantly fewer patients in the high-risk category. However, in other countries, such as the United Kingdom, expert panels have advised against any prophylaxis for infectious endocarditis.[26] From a socioeconomic perspective, this may appear reasonable, partly because prophylaxis is not 100% effective and partly because the number of treated cases needed to prevent a single case of infectious endocarditis is very large.[5]

Selection of an appropriate antibiotic is of paramount importance in preventing infectious endocarditis. Approximately one-third of infectious endocarditis cases are caused by pathogens not appropriately covered by the administered prophylaxis.[27] For keratinized skin, the predominant organisms are streptococci and staphylococci, specifically *Staphylococcus aureus* and β-hemolytic streptococci, but multiple other pathogens have been reported. Assessing individual patient risk factors is therefore important in selection of the appropriate agent.[28,29] For example, for procedures on oral mucosal surfaces, the antimicrobial agent must cover *Streptococcus viridans*.

PROSTHETIC JOINT INFECTIONS

Skin infections are a common source of late-onset artificial joint infection.[30–32] Patients with a history of recent joint replacement are also at higher risk for artificial joint infection.[33] Thus, prevention of surgical site infection is particularly important in patients with prosthetic joints. As in endocarditis, artificial joint infection secondary to dermatologic procedures is thought to occur by hematogenous seeding. However, because of the low incidence of bacteremia on noninfected, nonmucosal sites after dermatologic surgery, antibiotic prophylaxis to prevent artificial joint infection is not necessary except in high-risk patients.

High-risk patients include those with a history of previous prosthetic joint infection, patients undergoing a total joint replacement within the previous 2 years and patients with certain comorbidities, including insulin-dependent (type I) diabetes, malignancy, immunosuppression, HIV, malnourishment, and hemophilia (Table 9-6).

TABLE 9-6 Patients at High Risk of Developing Joint Infections[7]	
Conditions for which Antibiotic Prophylaxis is Recommended	
Joint specific	Prosthetic joint replacement during 2 years after the procedure; Previous prosthetic joint infection; Inflammatory arthropathies (e.g., rheumatoid arthritis)
Past medical history	Immunosuppression; insulin-dependent diabetes; HIV/AIDS; malignancy; malnourishment; hemophilia

Concerning procedures on the oral mucosa, both the American Dental Association (ADA) and the American Academy of Orthopedic Surgeons (AAOS) provide guidance.[34] The ADA–AAOS guidelines recommend antibiotic prophylaxis for all procedures in which mucosal bleeding is anticipated. This can be thought of as equivalent to procedures likely to breach mucous membranes and is therefore in keeping with the principles of dermatologic surgery which have already been discussed.

CONSIDERATION OF PROCEDURAL TECHNIQUE

More complex surgical techniques carry higher rates of postoperative wound infection than simple excisions.[1,35,36] As grafts and flaps are associated with significantly higher than average infection rates, simple reconstruction should be performed whenever possible. Hemorrhagic complications are an independent risk factor for development of postoperative wound infection, which emphasizes the importance of excellent hemostatic control.[3,35] Similarly, excessive wound tension can lead to tissue necrosis and create a nidus for infection. Excessive tissue injury, such as that due to crush injury from tissue forceps, may influence postoperative complication rates. Generally, the larger the surgical defect, the greater the risk of postoperative complications. Therefore, procedures should be performed with a view to minimizing tissue injury and avoiding high-tension closures. An adequate blood supply to the surgical site is also essential for wound healing.

Mohs micrographic surgery incorporates traditional and innovative surgical techniques but differs from most standard dermatologic procedures in that wounds are left open while surgical specimens are examined histopathologically. Patients are typically bandaged and then leave the operating room to await the results of their microscopic analysis. Sterility is therefore reduced and wound exposure time is generally thought to be a risk factor for infection. According to some authors, the infection rate doubles with each hour of surgery.[37] Nevertheless, studies examining the risk of surgical site infection involving Mohs surgery consistently reveal that the overall infection rate remains very low.[12] Thus, antibiotic prophylaxis is not generally indicated. However, due to the heterogeneity of Mohs procedures and the varying lengths of such procedures, individual assessment of risk factors and case-by-case analysis are of particular importance.

Procedural dermatology includes not only traditional surgical techniques but also numerous nonsurgical procedures. Generally, routine small-sample biopsies, such as punch and shave procedures not involving mucous membranes, typically do not require antibiotic prophylaxis.[24] Similarly, noninvasive procedures, such as nonablative laser techniques and percutaneous intravascular procedures, generally do not require prophylaxis. On the other hand, any procedure that causes more widespread destruction of the epidermis and dermis can lead to bacterial invasion and, therefore, requires consideration of antimicrobial prophylaxis. This includes laser resurfacing and other cosmetic procedures.[38]

POSTOPERATIVE INDICATIONS

Regardless of the procedure performed, the anatomic site or the patient's risk factors, postoperative complications may require the use of antibiotics. However, the threshold for antimicrobial use may be lower for certain patient populations, such as the immunocompromised, and for certain anatomic sites and procedures, such as skin grafts and flaps, for which the risk of necrosis is higher. Although the diagnosis of a postoperative wound infection may be straightforward, it is also subject to considerable inter- and intraobserver variability, which suggests that experience and a familiarity with normal variations can be helpful. The 1992 CDC definitions of nosocomial infections give some guidance[39]:

1. Purulent discharge from the incisional wound
2. Organism isolated on culture of aseptically obtained fluid or tissue
3. One or more of the following: pain, tenderness, local swelling, redness, heat
4. The surgeon deliberately reopens the wound (unless culture of the incision is negative)
5. The treating physician diagnoses a nosocomial infection

Diagnosis of a nosocomial infection is made when at least one of the above factors is present and the infection occurs within 30 days of surgery. Diagnosing an overt surgical site infection warrants aggressive and tailored therapy to prevent bacteremia and further complications. Obtaining cultures and sensitivities is crucial in directing therapy and minimizing complications.

PATHOGENS

Knowledge of anatomy and microbiology is necessary to select the antibiotic agent with the spectrum of coverage most suitable for the specific situation and procedure. Most surgical site infections are caused by resident flora.[40] This highlights the importance of adequate antiseptic preparation of the surgical site. For example, chlorhexidine has been found to significantly reduce coagulase-negative staphylococci at the end of surgery.[41] The choice of antiseptic depends on the anatomic site, type of procedure and resident microflora. Blood can neutralize certain antiseptics, and the duration of action differs markedly between the available agents.

Endogenous cutaneous flora include *S. aureus*, coagulase-negative staphylococci, *Streptococcus pyogenes*, enterococci, and *Escherichia coli*.[28] Nonbacterial organisms, such as *Candida*, can also cause infection and postoperative complications.[29] *S. viridans* and peptostreptococci are the primary pathogens arising from mucosal surfaces.[10] However, the single most important organism responsible for surgical site infection is *S. aureus*, which colonizes both mucosa and adjacent surfaces, including the nasal mucosa and perineum, and is found in particularly high concentrations in diseased skin. An epidemiological concern arises from the increasing incidence of methicillin-resistant *S. aureus* (MRSA), both community-acquired (CA-MRSA) and health care-associated (HC-MRSA).[42] HC-MRSA may be community-onset and includes invasive and noninvasive MRSA diagnosed within 12 months following a surgical procedure, hospitalization, dialysis, or residence in a long-term care facility. Invasive HC-MRSA can cause sepsis and infect cerebrospinal fluid, pleural fluid, pericardial fluid, bone, and viscera. It carries a 20% mortality rate.[7] Risk factors for invasive HC-MRSA also include age greater than 65 years, African American heritage and male gender. Because of the central role of *S. aureus* in surgical site infection, as well as the difficulties involved in treating MRSA, screening and preoperative decontamination protocols for MRSA colonization have been suggested.[43,44] However, the utility of such protocols depends on the local prevalence of MRSA, surgical technique, and procedural facilities.[45] Thus, awareness, risk factor evaluation, and case-by-case analysis remain critical.

Individual patient groups are at increased risk of infection due not only to altered immunity but also to increased microbial colonization and altered composition of resident and transient microflora. For example, colonization with disease-causing strains of *S. aureus* is more prevalent in individuals with atopic dermatitis and may be an important aggravating factor for dermatitis.[46] Similarly, diabetic patients are more prone to staphylococcal and candidal skin infections as a result of altered immunity and deranged homeostasis. Generally, patients with innate or acquired immunodeficiencies warrant special consideration, as do patients at increased risk of severe complications from surgical site infections. Although the mechanism of seeding is similar, the microorganisms responsible for infectious endocarditis and prosthetic joint infection are different. The majority of infectious endocarditis is caused by low-virulence streptococci, while artificial joint infections are typically caused by *S. aureus* and *S. epidermidis*.[47] Patient comorbidities, immune status, and associated susceptibility to specific pathogens are therefore critical in preoperative evaluation and selection of antimicrobial agents with adequate coverage.

CHOICE OF ANTIBIOTICS

Clinical context is usually the determining factor in the choice of prophylactic and therapeutic antibiotics. The anatomic site, condition of the skin, patient comorbidities and history of infection, and the type of procedure and local epidemiological data all need to be evaluated. Other considerations include the patient's history of allergies, the risk of adverse effects, expense and the emergence of multidrug-resistant microorganisms. Local knowledge of antimicrobial susceptibilities in communities and institutions is also important, particularly for MRSA infections. For purposes of daily practice, three considerations determine the choice of prophylactic antibiotics: first, the status of the wound and the condition of the surgical site; second, the anatomic site; third, whether the patient's comorbidities warrant antimicrobial prophylaxis. The choice of therapeutic antibiotics in postsurgical wound infections should be guided similarly but, in addition, cultures and sensitivities should be obtained. At minimum, this typically requires a wound swab. In some circumstances, a tissue culture may be required.

ROUTE OF ADMINISTRATION

Antibiotics can be administered topically or systemically. Use of perioperative topical antibiotics has been standard practice for many dermatologists in the past.[48] However, topical antibiotics are not indicated after clean dermatologic procedures.[49] Randomized studies have shown that the application of white petrolatum leads to statistically equivalent rates of infection compared to application of topical antibiotics, such as bacitracin.[50–52] The argument against use of topical antibiotics in standard dermatologic procedures is underscored by the risk of contact dermatitis and anaphylaxis.[53–58] In addition, white petrolatum is typically much less expensive for the dermatologist and the patient. Topical antibiotics may play a role in management of class III or IV wounds, whether preoperatively for contaminated sites or postoperatively to prevent surgical site infections. However, overtly infected wounds that are manipulated through surgical procedures should be treated aggressively with systemic antimicrobials.

Topical antimicrobial effects can also be achieved by special wound dressings. Silver sulfadiazine has been a mainstay for burn patients, as it has activity against gram-positive and gram-negative bacteria as well as yeast.[59,60] A prospective, randomized controlled study of routine infrainguinal revascularization incisions found that silver dressings reduced the risk of postsurgical complications compared to conventional dressings.[61] Although there is some evidence for the use of silver dressings in acute and chronic wounds, the data are not conclusive.[62] Silver dressings also carry the risks of argyria, contact dermatitis, anaphylaxis, and bone marrow toxicity, although this risk is probably lower than previously thought.[63] Honey-impregnated dressings are another potential tool for the topical prevention and treatment of wound infections. Honey has been found to be effective against MRSA, although one study failed to show a positive effect on chronic venous ulcers.[64–66] More studies are needed to investigate its use as a prophylactic agent.

The AHA and ADA–AAOS guidelines recommend systemic antimicrobials as prophylactic agents to prevent infectious endocarditis and prosthetic joint infection. Analogously, systemic rather than topical agents should be used to prevent other postoperative complications arising from surgical site infection. Systemic agents protect the bloodstream and prevent the dissemination of pathogens. Selection of an agent depends on patient-specific factors as well as the agent's spectrum of activity (Table 9-7).

TABLE 9-7
Common Systemic Antibiotics Used in Dermatologic Surgery[67]

Activity Spectrum of Selected Antibiotic Agents Against Commonly Encountered Microorganisms

	***Staphylococcus aureus* (MSSA)**	***Staphylococcus aureus* (MRSA)**	***Streptococcus pyogenes***	***Streptococcus viridans***	***Escherichia coli* (non-ESBL)**	**Peptostreptococci**	***Pseudomonas* species**
Penicillin	>80% resistance	Poor	Good	Good	Poor	Good	Poor
Amoxicillin	>80% resistance	Poor	Good	Good	Moderate	Moderate	Poor
Dicloxacillin	>80% resistance	Poor	Good	Moderate	Poor	Poor	Poor
Erythromycin	Moderate	Moderate	Moderate	Moderate	Poor	Moderate	Poor
Azithromycin	Moderate	Moderate	Moderate	Moderate	Poor	Moderate	Poor
Doxycycline	Moderate	Moderate	Moderate	Moderate	Moderate	Moderate	Poor
Minocycline	Moderate	Moderate	Moderate	Moderate	Inadequate data	Moderate	Poor
Cephalexin Cefazolin	Good	Poor	Moderate	Moderate	Moderate	Good	Poor
Ciprofloxacin	Poor to Moderate	Poor to Moderate	Poor to Moderate	Inadequate data	Good	No data	Good
Levofloxacin	Moderate	Moderate	Moderate	Good	Good	Moderate	Good

TIMING OF ADMINISTRATION

Antibiotics can be administered pre-, intra-, and postoperatively. Because most severe complications of surgical site infections, including infectious endocarditis and prosthetic joint infections, are caused by bacteremia, antibiotics should generally be delivered systemically. Ideally, the antibiotic should be in the bloodstream when the operation begins to prevent systemic bacterial dissemination and to ensure that the antibiotic is present in the wound coagulum at the time of surgery.[68,69] Thus, prophylactic antibiotics should be administered preoperatively within a time frame that ensures their presence in the bloodstream at the time of incision and repair. The AHA recommends 30 to 60 minutes preoperative dosing, whereas the ADA–AAOS recommends 60 minutes preoperative dosing. Intraoperative administration of topical antibiotics is probably not beneficial for standard dermatologic procedures[2,14,70] but may be indicated for procedures with delayed closures, particularly Mohs surgery.[71,72] Analogously, the need for a repeat dose of intra- or postoperative systemic antibiotics administered for prophylaxis depends on the length of the procedure, the preoperative indication, and the half-life of the antimicrobial agent.

ANATOMIC SITE

Generally, antibiotics given to prevent infections from cutaneous procedures need to target staphylococci and streptococci. Procedures performed on intertriginous, moist or macerated areas also need to target gram-negative organisms. However, staphylococci remain the most common cause of surgical site infections even in such areas. Streptococcal and coliform bacteria need to be considered in the perioral area, ear, perineum, and below the waist in diabetic patients. Systemic agents commonly used for prophylaxis on nonmucosal surfaces include cephalexin and dicloxacillin.[37] Both agents are active against gram-positive organisms and also cover common gram-negative pathogens.[73] These agents can also be used as more prolonged therapy for overt infection. To target *S. viridans* and peptostreptococci on oral mucosal surfaces, the AHA guidelines recommend the use of amoxicillin.[23] For perineal skin, a penicillinase-resistant agent, such as amoxicillin-clavulanate, should be used. Alternatives for penicillin-allergic patients include clindamycin and macrolide antibiotics, such as erythromycin and azithromycin.[7] Some fluoroquinolones, such as ciprofloxacin, have better activity against pseudomonal species and, may, thus, be indicated for procedures on the ear. For openly infected wounds or postsurgical infections, therapy should always be tailored to the cultures and sensitivities (Fig. 9-4). Dosage varies according to the individual antibiotic and the patient's comorbidities and allergies. Standardized guidelines tailored to specific anatomic sites exist but actual antibiotic use depends on patient characteristics and local epidemiological data (Table 9-8).

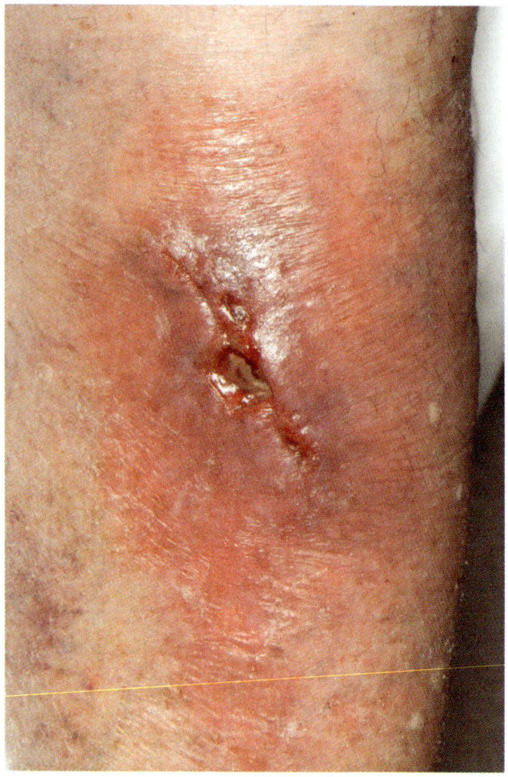

Figure 9-4 Right lower extremity wound 10 days after excision of a squamous cell carcinoma in a 76 year-old woman with leg edema and atrophic skin. Note the central partial dehiscence and asymmetric adjacent erythema due to cellulitis. Cultures revealed a polymicrobial infection with staphylococci, *Proteus*, and *Morganella* species.

TABLE 9-8
Suggested Recommendations for Antibiotic Usage in Common Clinical Settings[7]

Location	1st Line Oral Agents	Pencillin Allergy	Unable to Take PO Medications	Unable to Take PO and Pencillin Allergy
Lips or ears (wedge excision)	Cephalexin; dicloxacillin	Clindamycin; azithromycin	Cefazolin; ceftriaxone	Clindamycin
Grafts, nose flaps	Cephalexin; dicloxacillin	Clindamycin; azithromycin	Cefazolin; ceftriaxone	Clindamycin
Groin and lower leg	Cephalexin; TMP-SMX; levofloxacin	TMP-SMX; levofloxacin	Clindamycin; gentamycin	Clindamycin; gentamycin

TMP-SMX; trimethoprim-sulfamethoxazole, double-strength.

OTHER CONSIDERATIONS

Surgical site infections generally originate at the time of the procedure, but typically become clinically evident only several days later. This is one reason why antibiotic prophylaxis, if indicated, should be administered such that the antibiotic is present at the surgical site and in the bloodstream at the time of the first incision. Suture reactions and contact dermatitis from topical antibiotics or wound dressings can mimic infection. Experience should guide the clinician in making an assessment. However, if there is any concern for infection, wound cultures should be sent. While awaiting the culture results, the risks and benefits of initiating antibiotic therapy can be weighed according to the individual presentation and the patient's comorbidities and risk factors.

In addition to bacteria, fungi, and viruses may prove to be complicating factors in dermatologic procedures and wound healing. Patients with a known history of herpes simplex or zoster may require antiviral prophylaxis. Patients undergoing resurfacing procedures are at particularly high risk of viral reactivation. Thus, some authors advocate standard antiviral prophylaxis for certain cosmetic or ablative laser procedures.[38,74] Similarly, patients with a history of mucocutaneous candidiasis undergoing procedures on mucosal or intertriginous surfaces may require addition of an antifungal agent, either topically or systemically. More studies, including randomized controlled trials, are needed to investigate the utility and efficacy of antiviral and antifungal prophylaxis in dermatologic procedures.

CONCLUSION

Adhering to the generally accepted standard of care in dermatologic procedures includes knowing and applying the principles of when to use and not use antibiotic agents. This, in turn, involves familiarity with the infection risks associated with specific procedures and anatomic sites, classification of wounds, individual patient risk factors, proper surgical preparation, likely pathogens, and proper selection of antimicrobial agents. Proper procedural care does not start with the procedure itself but rather with a systematic preoperative patient evaluation and does not end with the last suture or wound dressing, but rather with a thorough postprocedural follow-up. Thus, assessing the pre- and postoperative needs for antibiotics is an integral part of patient care.

REFERENCES

1. Dixon AJ, Dixon MP, Askew DA, Wilkinson D. Prospective study of wound infections in dermatologic surgery in the absence of prophylactic antibiotics. *Dermatol Surg.* 2006;32(6):819–826.
2. Futoryan T, Grande D. Postoperative wound infection rates in dermatologic surgery. *Dermatol Surg.* 1995;21(6):509–514.
3. Rogues AM, Lasheras A, Amici JM, Guillot P, Beylot C, Taïeb A. Infection control practices and infectious complications in dermatological surgery. *J Hosp Infect.* 2007;65(3):258–263.
4. Rosengren H, Dixon A. Antibacterial prophylaxis in dermatologic surgery: an evidence-based review. *Am J Clin Derm.* 2010;11(1):35–44.
5. Shurman DL, Benedetto AV. Antimicrobials in dermatologic surgery: facts and controversies. *Clin Dermatol.* 2010;28(5):505–510.
6. Pallasch TJ, Slots J. Antibiotic prophylaxis and the medically compromised patient. *Periodontol 2000.* 1996;10:107–138.
7. Wright TI, Baddour LM, Berbari EF, Roenigk RK, Phillips PK, Jacobs MA. Antibiotic prophylaxis in dermatologic surgery: advisory statement 2008. *J Am Acad Dermatol.* 2008;59(3):464–473.
8. Wood LD, Warner NM, Billingsley EM. Infectious complications of dermatologic procedures. *Dermatol Ther.* 2011;24(6):558–570.
9. Kretschmer L, Zimmermann O, Stein A, Sebastian G; Commission for Quality Assurance of the German Dermatology Society and the Professional Association of Surgical and Oncological Dermatology. [Perioperative antibiotic therapy in dermatology. Guidelines of the Commission for Quality Assurance of the German Dermatology Society and the Professional Association of Surgical and Oncological Dermatology]. *Hautarzt.* 2001;52(7):609–614.
10. Maragh SL, Otley CC, Roenigk RK, Phillips PK; Division of Dermatologic Surgery, Mayo Clinic, Rochester, MN. Antibiotic prophylaxis in dermatologic surgery: updated guidelines. *Dermatol Surg.* 2005;31(1):83–91.
11. Nichols RL. Surgical antibiotic prophylaxis. *Med Clin North Am.* 1995;79(3):509–522.
12. Maragh SL, Brown MD. Prospective evaluation of surgical site infection rate among patients with Mohs micrographic surgery without the use of prophylactic antibiotics. *J Am Acad Dermatol.* 2008;59(2):275–278.
13. Tanner J, Woodings D, Moncaster K. Preoperative hair removal to reduce surgical site infection. *Cochrane Database Syst Rev.* 2006;19(3):CD004122.
14. Bencini PL, Galimberti M, Signorini M, Crosti C. Antibiotic prophylaxis of wound infections in skin surgery. *Arch Dermatol.* 1991;127(9):1357–1360.
15. Haas AF, Grekin RC. Antibiotic prophylaxis in dermatologic surgery. *J Am Acad Dermatol.* 1995;32(2 Pt 1):155–176.
16. Rabb DC, Lesher JL Jr. Antibiotic prophylaxis in cutaneous surgery. *Dermatol Surg.* 1995;21(6):550–554.
17. Dixon AJ, Dixon MP, Dixon JB. Prospective study of skin surgery in patients with and without known diabetes. *Dermatol Surg.* 2009;35(7):1035–1040.
18. Olsen MA, Lock-Buckley P, Hopkins D, Polish LB, Sundt TM, Fraser VJ. The risk factors for deep and superficial chest surgical-site infections after coronary artery bypass graft surgery are different. *J Thorac Cardiovasc Surg.* 2002;124(1):136–145.
19. Dixon AJ, Dixon MP, Dixon JB, Del Mar CB. Prospective study of skin surgery in smokers vs. nonsmokers. *Br J Dermatol.* 2009;160(2):365–367.
20. Bumpous JM, Johnson JT. The infected wound and its management. *Otolaryngol Clin North Am.* 1995;28(5):987–1001.
21. Malone DL, Genuit T, Tracy JK, Gannon C, Napolitano LM. Surgical site infections: reanalysis of risk factors. *J Surg Res.* 2002;103(1):89–95.
22. Baddour LM, Bettmann MA, Bolger AF, et al. Nonvalvular cardiovascular device-related infections. *Circulation.* 2003;108(16):2015–2031.
23. Wilson W, Taubert KA, Gewitz M, et al. Prevention of infective endocarditis: guidelines from the American Heart Association: a guideline from the American Heart Association Rheumatic Fever, Endocarditis, and Kawasaki Disease Committee, Council on Cardiovascular Disease in the Young, and the Council on Clinical Cardiology, Council on Cardiovascular Surgery and Anesthesia, and the Quality of Care and Outcomes Research Interdisciplinary Working Group. *Circulation.* 2007;116(15):1736–1754.
24. Dajani AS, Taubert KA, Wilson W, et al. Prevention of bacterial endocarditis. Recommendations by the American Heart Association. *JAMA.* 1997;277(22):1794–1801.

25. Durack DT. Prevention of infective endocarditis. *N Engl J Med.* 1995;332(1):38–44.
26. Richey R, Wray D, Stokes T, Guideline Development Group. Prophylaxis against infective endocarditis: summary of NICE guidance. *BMJ.* 2008;336(7647):770–771.
27. Durack DT, Kaplan EL, Bisno AL. Apparent failures of endocarditis prophylaxis. Analysis of 52 cases submitted to a national registry. *JAMA.* 1983;250(17):2318–2322.
28. National Nosocomial Infections Surveillance (NNIS) report, data summary from October 1986–April 1997, issued May 1997. A report from the NNIS System. *Am J Infect Control.* 1997;25(6):477–487.
29. National Nosocomial Infections Surveillance (NNIS) System Report, data summary from January 1992 to June 2002, issued August 2002. *Am J Infect Control.* 2002;30(8): 458–475.
30. Ainscow DA, Denham RA. The risk of haematogenous infection in total joint replacements. *J Bone Joint Surg Br.* 1984; 66(4):580–582.
31. Berbari EF, Hanssen AD, Duffy MC, et al. Risk factors for prosthetic joint infection: case-control study. *Clin Infect Dis.* 1998;27(5):1247–1254.
32. Maderazo EG, Judson S, Pasternak H. Late infections of total joint prostheses. A review and recommendations for prevention. *Clin Orthop Relat Res.* 1988;(229):131–142.
33. Advisory statement. Antibiotic prophylaxis for dental patients with total joint replacements. American Dental Association; American Academy of Orthopaedic Surgeons. *J Am Dent Assoc.* 1997;128(7):1004–1008.
34. American Dental Association; American Academy of Orthopedic Surgeons. Antibiotic prophylaxis for dental patients with total joint replacements. *J Am Dent Assoc.* 2003; 134(7): 895–899.
35. Amici JM, Rogues AM, Lasheras A, et al. A prospective study of the incidence of complications associated with dermatological surgery. *Br J Dermatol.* 2005;153(5):967–971.
36. Sylaidis P, Wood S, Murray DS. Postoperative infection following clean facial surgery. *Ann Plast Surg.* 1997;39(4): 342–346.
37. Nestor MS. Perioperative use of antibiotics: preventing and treating perioperative infections. *J Drugs Dermatol.* 2005;4(6 suppl):S34–S36.
38. Nestor MS. Prophylaxis for and treatment of uncomplicated skin and skin structure infections in laser and cosmetic surgery. *J Drugs Dermatol.* 2005;4(6 suppl):S20–S25.
39. Horan TC, Gaynes RP, Martone WJ, Jarvis WR, Emori TG. CDC definitions of nosocomial surgical site infections, 1992: a modification of CDC definitions of surgical wound infections. *Infect Control Hosp Epidemiol.* 1992;13(10): 606–608.
40. Hirschmann JV. Antimicrobial prophylaxis in dermatology. *Semin Cutan Med Surg.* 2000;19(1):2–9.
41. Veiga DF, Damasceno CA, Veiga-Filho J, et al. Povidone iodine versus chlorhexidine in skin antisepsis before elective plastic surgery procedures: a randomized controlled trial. *Plast Reconstr Surg.* 2008;122(5):170e–171e.
42. Awad SS, Elhabash SI, Lee L, Farrow B, Berger DH. Increasing incidence of methicillin-resistant Staphylococcus aureus skin and soft-tissue infections: reconsideration of empiric antimicrobial therapy. *Am J Surg.* 2007;194(5):606–610.
43. Cordova KB, Grenier N, Chang KH, Dufresne R Jr. Preoperative methicillin-resistant Staphylococcus aureus screening in Mohs surgery appears to decrease postoperative infections. *Dermatol Surg.* 2010;36(10):1537–1540.
44. van Rijen M, Bonten M, Wenzel R, Kluytmans J. Mupirocin ointment for preventing Staphylococcus aureus infections in nasal carriers. *Cochrane Database Syst Rev.* 2008; (4):CD006216.
45. Dzubow L. Apples, oranges, and methicillin-resistant Staphylococcus aureus. *Dermatol Surg.* 2010;36(10):1541–1543.
46. Kim DW, Park JY, Park KD, et al. Are there predominant strains and toxins of Staphylococcus aureus in atopic dermatitis patients? Genotypic characterization and toxin determination of S. aureus isolated in adolescent and adult patients with atopic dermatitis. *J Dermatol.* 2009;36(2): 75–81.
47. McGowan DA. Dentistry and endocarditis. *Br Dent J.* 1990; 169(3–4):69.
48. Lapolla WJ, Levender MM, Davis SA, Yentzer BA, Williford PM, Feldman SR. Topical antibiotic trends from 1993 to 2007: use of topical antibiotics for non-evidence-based indications. *Dermatol Surg.* 2011;37(10):1427–1433.
49. Levender MM, Davis SA, Kwatra SG, Williford PM, Feldman SR. Use of topical antibiotics as prophylaxis in clean dermatologic procedures. *J Am Acad Dermatol.* 2012;66(3): 445–451.
50. Campbell RM, Perlis CS, Fisher E, Gloster HM Jr. Gentamicin ointment versus petrolatum for management of auricular wounds. *Dermatol Surg.* 2005;31(6):664–669.
51. Dixon AJ, Dixon MP, Dixon JB. Randomized clinical trial of the effect of applying ointment to surgical wounds before occlusive dressing. *Br J Surg.* 2006;93(8):937–943.
52. Smack DP, Harrington AC, Dunn C, Howard RS, Szkutnik AJ, Krivda SJ. Infection and allergy incidence in ambulatory surgery patients using white petrolatum vs bacitracin ointment. A randomized controlled trial. *JAMA.* 1996;276(12): 972–977.
53. Dyck ED, Vadas P. Anaphylaxis to topical bacitracin. *Allergy.* 1997;52(8):870–871.
54. Eedy DJ, McMillan JC, Bingham EA. Anaphylactic reactions to topical antibiotic combinations. *Postgrad Med J.* 1990; 66(780):858–859.
55. Gette MT, Marks JG Jr, Maloney ME. Frequency of postoperative allergic contact dermatitis to topical antibiotics. *Arch Dermatol.* 1992;128(3):365–367.
56. Knowles SR, Shear NH. Anaphylaxis from bacitracin and polymyxin B (Polysporin) ointment. *Int J Dermatol.* 1995; 34(8):572–573.
57. Marks JG, Belsito DV, DeLeo VA, et al. North American Contact Dermatitis Group patch test results for the detection of delayed-type hypersensitivity to topical allergens. *J Am Acad Dermatol.* 1998;38(6 Pt 1):911–918.
58. Zappi EG, Brancaccio RR. Allergic contact dermatitis from mupirocin ointment. *J Am Acad Dermatol.* 1997;36(2 Pt 1): 266.
59. Hoffmann S. Silver sulfadiazine: an antibacterial agent for topical use in burns. A review of the literature. *Scand J Plast Reconstr Surg.* 1984;18(1):119–126.
60. Pruitt BA Jr, McManus AT, Kim SH, Goodwin CW. Burn wound infections: current status. *World J Surg.* 1998;22 (2): 135–145.
61. Childress BB, Berceli SA, Nelson PR, Lee WA, Ozaki CK. Impact of an absorbent silver-eluting dressing system on lower extremity revascularization wound complications. *Ann Vasc Surg.* 2007;21(5):598–602.
62. Collier M. Silver dressings: more evidence is needed to support their widespread clinical use. *J Wound Care.* 2009;18(2): 77–78.
63. Messingham MJ, Arpey CJ. Update on the use of antibiotics in cutaneous surgery. *Dermatol Surg.* 2005;31(8 Pt 2): 1068–1078.
64. Blaser G, Santos K, Bode U, Vetter H, Simon A. Effect of medical honey on wounds colonised or infected with MRSA. *J Wound Care.* 2007;16(8):325–328.
65. Jull A, Walker N, Parag V, Molan P, Rodgers A. Honey as Adjuvant Leg Ulcer Therapy trial collaborators. Randomized clinical trial of honey-impregnated dressings for venous leg ulcers. *Br J Surg.* 2008;95(2):175–182.
66. Visavadia BG, Honeysett J, Danford M. Manuka honey dressing: an effective treatment for chronic wound infections. *Br J Oral Maxillofac Surg.* 2008;46(8):696–697.
67. Wilson JW, Estes LL. *Mayo Clinic Antimicrobial Therapy Quick Guide.* New York, NY: Mayo Clinic Scientific Press/ Oxford University Press; 2012.
68. Burke JP. Maximizing appropriate antibiotic prophylaxis for surgical patients: an update from LDS Hospital, Salt Lake City. *Clin Infect Dis.* 2001;33(suppl 2):S78–S83.

69. Classen DC, Evans RS, Pestotnik SL, Horn SD, Menlove RL, Burke JP. The timing of prophylactic administration of antibiotics and the risk of surgical-wound infection. *N Engl J Med.* 1992;326(5):281–286.
70. Cruse PJ, Foord R. A five-year prospective study of 23,649 surgical wounds. *Arch Surg.* 1973;107(2):206–210.
71. Griego RD, Zitelli JA. Intra-incisional prophylactic antibiotics for dermatologic surgery. *Arch Dermatol.* 1998;134(6): 688–692.
72. Huether MJ, Griego RD, Brodland DG, Zitelli JA. Clindamycin for intraincisional antibiotic prophylaxis in dermatologic surgery. *Arch Dermatol.* 2002;138(9):1145–1148.
73. Gilbert DN, Moellering RC, Sande MA. *The Sanford Guide to Antimicrobial Therapy.* Hyde Park, VT: Antimicrobial Therapy, Inc; 2003.
74. Beeson WH, Rachel JD. Valacyclovir prophylaxis for herpes simplex virus infection or infection recurrence following laser skin resurfacing. *Dermatol Surg.* 2002;28(4):331–336.

CHAPTER 10

Wound Healing

Katherine A. Nolan, Liza Braun, & Robert S. Kirsner

INTRODUCTION

A classic definition of wound healing is that it is a dynamic process, involving multiple types of cells, cytokines, and chemical mediators that work together in a complex interaction. Although knowledge of wound healing is important in all medical fields, it is particularly significant to dermatologists as they create and care for more wounds than all other specialties.[1] The basic science of wound healing can be divided into five phases: hemostasis, inflammation, proliferation, tissue remodeling, and finally resolution (Fig. 10-1).[2] However, these phases do not always occur sequentially but are rather highly integrated and often overlap. We will describe these phases of wound healing and also discuss several important factors that impair wound healing.

WOUND MECHANISMS

ACUTE AND CHRONIC WOUNDS

Wounds can be classified as either acute or chronic on the basis of the length of the time it takes to complete epithelialization, one of the elements of the proliferative phase of the healing process. Although the exact time distinction used in classification can be arbitrary and may be affected by a number of factors such as the shape, location, and cause of the wound, chronic wounds are generally associated with physiological impairments that slow or prevent healing, such as advanced age or underlying disorders.

WOUND DEPTH

The depth of a wound has a significant impact on how wounds heal, the healing process and its clinical management. For example, if the injury is limited to the epidermis, the epidermis can relatively easily regenerate itself, without scarring. This, similar to limited injury in the liver, is one of the few instances in which regeneration, as opposed to repair, occurs after injury. However, with deeper wounds, involving part or all of the dermis and deeper layers, regeneration does not occur, but rather a repair process is initiated that usually results in scarring. Interestingly, regeneration can sometimes occur in specific situations even when the dermis is involved. One example of this is in early (first two trimesters) fetal skin wounds. Although not entirely understood, this is likely due to a reduced inflammatory response and the presence of higher concentrations of glycosaminoglycans and type III collagen and decreased levels of transforming growth factor b1 (TGF-b1), seen in fetal dermis. Overall, these factors are likely important in mediating regeneration rather than repair.[3]

Wound classification is based on the depth of involvement. Superficial wounds involve only the epidermis and

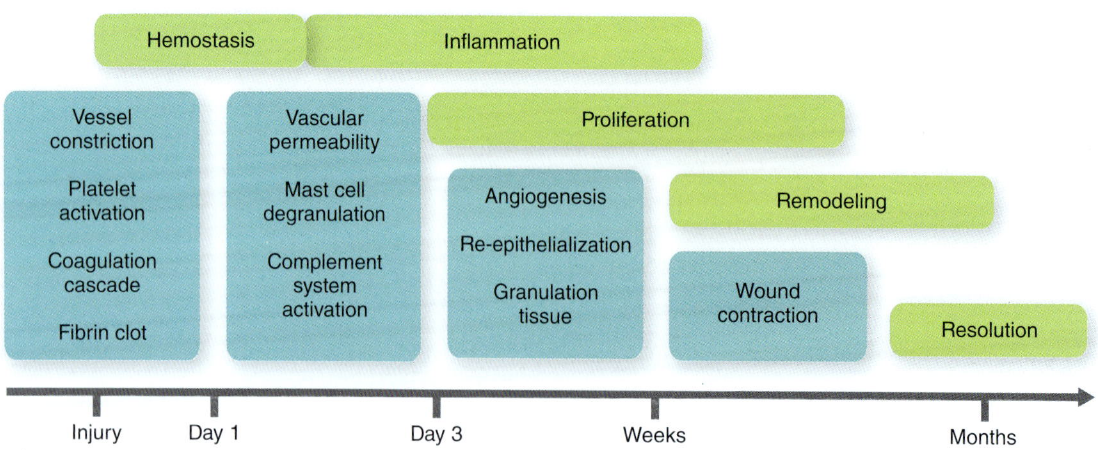

Figure 10-1 Phases of wound healing. Upon injury, the initial hemostatic response involves platelets as the primary responders. This is followed by inflammation which increases vascular permeability, allowing access for neutrophil and macrophage-derived factors. Proliferation of endothelial cells and keratinocytes promotes re-epithelialization. Ultimately progression to remodeling and resolution of the wound occurs.

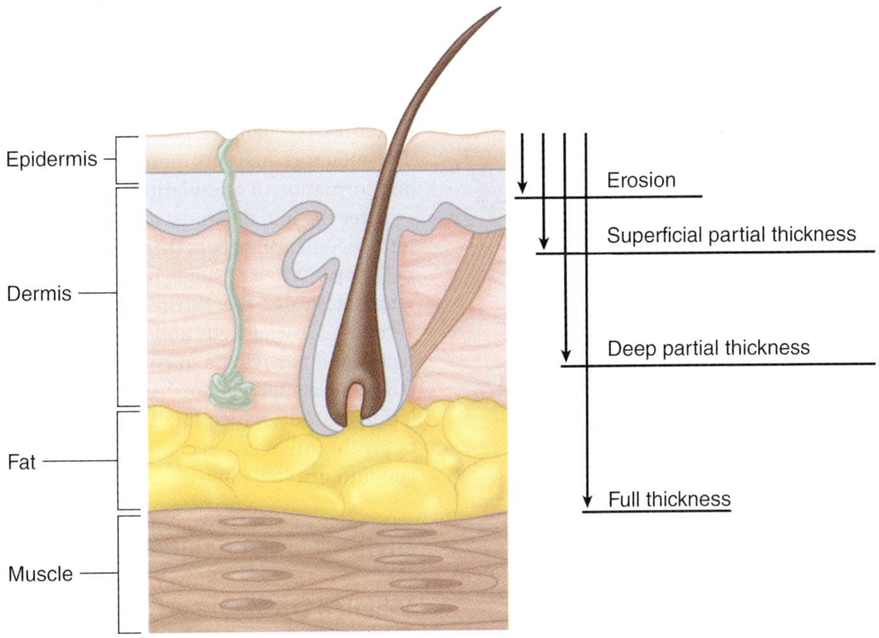

Figure 10-2 Clinical classification of wound depth. Superficial and intermediate partial-thickness wounds involve epidermis and upper dermis while deep- and full-thickness wounds involve deeper dermal layers. Partial-thickness wounds will leave remnants of dermal appendages while full-thickness wounds will not. (Redrawn with permission from Sowa MG, Leonardi L, Payette JR, Cross KM, Gomez M, Fish JS. Classification of burn injuries using near-infrared spectroscopy. *J Biomed Opt.* 2006;11(5):054002–054002–6.)

upper dermis. If only the epidermis is lost, this is termed an erosion. The term partial-thickness wound refers to tissue destruction that extends into but not completely through the dermis. This is in contrast to full-thickness wounds, which extend through the dermis to involve the subcutaneous tissue (Fig. 10-2).

These classifications are important in that partial thickness and full-thickness wounds epithelialize by different mechanisms. As the deep dermis is not affected in partial-thickness wounds, the adnexal structures that are present in the dermis are preserved. These structures act as a reservoir of keratinocytes and help repopulate the epithelial cells of the epidermis. Keratinocytes from these structures and from the edge of the wound migrate across the surface of the wound to form the new epidermis. In contrast, when the deep dermis is affected in full-thickness wounds, the adnexal structures are destroyed, and keratinocytes epithelialize the wound only from its edges. Moreover, the adnexal structures do not regenerate and are replaced with scar tissue. Full-thickness wounds often heal by contraction, while there is minimal contraction in partial-thickness wounds. Contraction involves movement of pre-existing tissue centripetally and the wound area is decreased. This may result in cosmetically disfiguring contractures.[1]

TYPES OF HEALING

Wounds heal by one of three general mechanisms. The most common mechanisms are healing by primary intention and secondary intention healing. Primary intention healing refers to the surgical closure of a wound by approximating the edges. In contrast, secondary intention healing occurs when an acute wound is left to heal on its own. A third type of wound healing, tertiary intention, is sometimes described. This refers either to delayed primary closure of a wound that is purposely left open and or when a primarily closed wound dehisces and is left to heal on its own. An example of healing by tertiary intention would be a patient who returns 3 to 4 days after an initial wound occurs, at which time debridement and wound cleansing are performed. This can be useful in the management of certain contaminated crush wounds or mammalian bites (Fig. 10-3).

PHASES OF WOUND HEALING

HEMOSTASIS

Immediately after the skin is injured, small vessels constrict in the wound area, which causes the injured small vessels to be compressed. This adhesiveness within the endothelial lining leads to vessel occlusion, a process which aids in hemostasis. Platelets are activated at the site of blood vessel injury by thrombin, as well as exposed extracellular matrix, and aggregate in the severed vessels. Platelets help initiate the clotting cascade and release many mediators from their granules including adenosine diphosphate (ADP), thromboxane A2, serotonin, fibronectin, von Willebrand factor, and fibrinogen.[1] Fibrinogen is subsequently converted by thrombin to fibrin which is deposited in the platelet plug and forms the core of the fibrin clot. This matrix stabilizes the wound and acts as a provisional scaffold for wound healing.

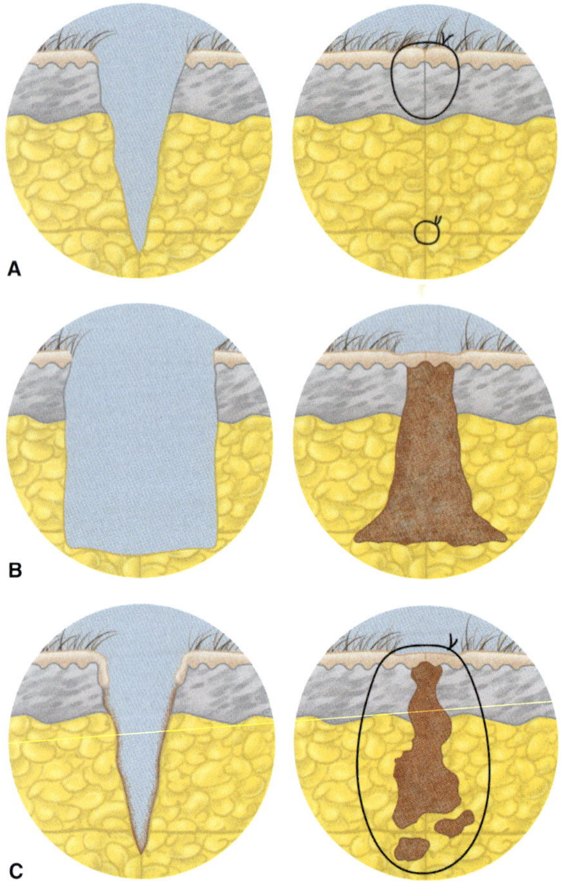

Figure 10-3 Clinical classification of primary, secondary, and tertiary wound healing. **A.** Primary intention healing involves surgical closure and apposition of wound edges. **B.** Secondary intention healing allows wound bed to fill with granulation tissue. **C.** Tertiary intention is delayed primary closure of a wound. Reproduced with permission from Timby BK. *Fundamental Nursing Skills and Concepts,* 9th ed. Philadelphia: Lippincott Williams & Wilkins;2009.

Platelets are not only essential to hemostasis, but they also contribute to re-epithelialization, fibroplasia, and angiogenesis. Platelets promote tissue regeneration through the release of growth factors like TGF-α, TGF-β, and PDGF that are part of the wound repair process.[1] These factors help promote cell migration, proliferation, and formation of granulation tissue.

After the initial hemostatic response mediated by platelets, coagulation occurs through the intrinsic and extrinsic pathways. When tissue is injured, it releases tissue factor, which activates the extrinsic coagulation pathway. Activated endothelial cells and monocytes also express tissue factor and participate in coagulation. Platelet aggregation triggers Hageman factor XII to initiate the intrinsic coagulation cascade, which finally results in the transformation of prothrombin into thrombin. This then converts fibrinogen into insoluble fibrin.

INFLAMMATION

MEDIATORS OF ACUTE INFLAMMATION.

There are several key mediators of acute inflammation (Table 10-1). Arachidonic acid (AA) metabolites are released from the phospholipid cell membrane by phospholipase A_2 and then acted upon by cyclooxygenase or 5-lipoxygenase. Cyclooxygenase then produces prostaglandins like PGI_2, PGD_2, and PGE_2, which mediate vasodilation and increased vascular permeability. PGE_2 is also an important mediator of pain and fever. 5-lipoxygenase produces leukotrienes including LTB_4, which attracts and activates neutrophils, and LTC_4, LTD_4, and LTE_4 (also known as the slow reacting substances of anaphylaxis), which in turn mediate increased vascular permeability and vasoconstriction.

In addition, mast cells have an important role in inflammation. These cells are widely distributed throughout connective tissue and can be activated by tissue trauma (as well as other mechanisms like the cross-linking of IgE in allergic reactions). Mast cells release preformed histamine granules, which mediate an immediate inflammatory response that causes vasodilation of arterioles and increases vascular permeability. They are also involved in

TABLE 10-1
Inflammatory Markers Involved in Wound Healing

Class of Mediators	Eicosanoids	Mast Cells	Complement	Neutrophils	Macrophages
Examples	Prostaglandins PGE_2, PGD_2, LTE_2 Leukotrienes LTC_4, LTD_4, LTE_4	Histamine	C1, C3a, C3b, C5a	TNF-α, IL-1, IL-4, IL-8	Fibronectin FGF, PDGF, VEGF
Functions	Prostaglandins, increased vascular permeability; leukotrienes, vasoconstriction, increased vascular permeability, neutrophil recruitment	Vasodilation, increased vascular permeability	Phagocytosis, lysis, and agglutination of microorganisms	Phagocytosis, oxidative burst	Phagocytosis, fibroblast recruitment, angiogenic

maintenance of the inflammatory response through the production of AA components like leukotrienes. Toll-like receptors (TLRs) are another important mediator of acute inflammation, especially in infection. TLRs are present on cells of the innate immune system, including macrophages and dendritic cells. TLRs are activated by pathogen-associated molecular patterns (PAMPs) that are commonly shared by microbes. For example, CD14 is a TLR on macrophages that recognizes lipopolysaccharide (a PAMP) on the outer membrane of gram-negative bacteria. The activation of TLRs results in the upregulation of NF-κB, a nuclear transcription factor that activates immune response genes leading to production of multiple immune mediators. TLRs are also present on cells involved in adaptive immunity, such as lymphocytes, and therefore play an important role in mediating chronic inflammation.

The complement system is an essential group of mediators in the acute inflammatory response. Complement describes a system of 11 proinflammatory serum proteins that circulate as inactive precursors. They are activated by three separate pathways: the classical pathway in which C1 binds IgG or IgM that is bound to antigen, the alternative pathway where microbial products directly activate complement, and the mannose-binding lectin (MBL) pathway in which MBL binds to mannose on microorganisms to activate complement. All of these pathways result in a cascade of sequential reactions, which produce multiple end products (C3a, C5a, C3b, etc.) that help destroy and prevent damage by the invading organism or toxin. In regard to wound healing, some of these end products, such as C3b, activate phagocytosis, and C5 to C9 (membrane attack complex), enhance lysis and agglutination of invading organisms. Other products like C3a and C5a (also known as anaphylatoxins) activate mast cells and basophils to release histamine.

Hageman factor or factor XII is a vital mediator of acute inflammation. It is an inactive proinflammatory protein produced in the liver and then activated upon exposure to subendothelial or tissue collagen. Hageman factor in turn helps activate the coagulation and fibrinolytic systems, complement, and the kinin system. Kinin cleaves high–molecular-weight kininogen to bradykinin, which mediates vasodilation and increased vascular permeability as well as pain.

CARDINAL SIGNS OF INFLAMMATION. There are five cardinal signs that characterize acute inflammation: rubor, calor, tumor, dolor, and loss of function. Although some of these signs may also be present in chronic inflammation, they are often absent. Rubor refers to the redness seen in acute inflammation and is often associated with calor or warmth. These signs are due to vasodilation resulting in increased blood flow. The key mediators of this process are prostaglandins, histamine, and bradykinin, which induce relaxation of arteriolar smooth muscle. The third cardinal sign, tumor, refers to the swelling seen in inflammation when fluid from postcapillary venules leaks into the interstitial space. Histamine causes endothelial cell contraction and tissue damage resulting in endothelial cell disruption and leakage. Dolor or pain is another cardinal sign of inflammation and is due to bradykinin and PGE_2 sensitization of sensory nerve endings. The final cardinal sign is *functio laesa* or "loss of function" of the inflamed area, which is a consequence of the other cardinal signs.

NEUTROPHIL ARRIVAL AND FUNCTION. Neutrophils are the first white blood cells to arrive at the site of injury. Their arrival and function can be divided into seven steps. First, in a step termed margination, vasodilation slows the blood flow in postcapillary venules and neutrophils marginate from the center of the flow to the periphery. Within 1 hour of the onset of inflammation, the endothelial margin of the venules is covered with neutrophils. Next, rolling of neutrophils occurs. This involves the upregulation of selectins on endothelial cells. Specifically, P-selectin is released from Weibel–Palade bodies, which is mediated by histamine, while E-selectin is induced by tumor necrosis factor (TNF) and IL-1. Selectins then bind to sialyl-Lewis X on leukocytes and promote the rolling of leukocytes along the vessel wall. Next, cellular adhesion molecules (ICAM and VCAM) are upregulated on the endothelium by TNF and IL-1. Also, integrins are upregulated on leukocytes by C5a and LTB_4. This interaction between the adhesion molecules and integrins results in the adhesion of leukocytes to the vessel wall. Of note, an autosomal recessive defect of integrins results in leukocyte adhesion deficiency, which is characterized by recurrent bacterial infections that lack pus formation due to impaired adhesion of neutrophils. After adhesion, leukocytes transmigrate across the endothelium of postcapillary venules and move toward chemical attractants like the bacterial products IL-8, C5a, and LTB_4. After this chemotaxis, phagocytosis occurs. This involves the consumption of pathogens or necrotic tissue and is enhanced by opsonins such as IgG and C3b. Pseudopods extend from leukocytes to form phagosomes, which are internalized and merge with lysosomes forming phagolysosomes. An example of a defect in phagolysosome formation and protein trafficking is Chediak–Higashi syndrome. This syndrome is characterized by an increased risk of pyogenic infections, neutropenia, failed bacteriolysis, and albinism because the defect in protein trafficking prevents melanin from being passed to other cells. After necrotic tissue and pathogens have been consumed by phagocytosis, they are destroyed by an O_2-dependent mechanism. O_2 is converted to O_2 radicals by NADPH oxidase, which is then converted to H_2O_2 by superoxide dismutase. Finally H_2O_2 is converted by myeloperoxidase to HOCl, which generates the oxidative burst in phagolysosomes that destroys phagocytosed material. Several diseases result from defects in these steps. First, a defect in NADPH oxidase results in chronic granulomatous disease, which leads to recurrent infections with catalase-positive organisms like *Staphylococcus aureus* and *Pseudomonas cepacia*. A deficiency of myeloperoxidase results in defective conversion of H_2O_2 to HOCl and puts patients with this deficiency at a higher risk for *Candida* infections. Finally, neutrophils undergo apoptosis and disappear within 24 hours after resolution of the inflammatory stimulus.

MACROPHAGES. In wounds, macrophages predominate after neutrophils and peak 2 to 3 days after inflammation begins. Macrophages are often considered the most important regulatory cells in the inflammatory reaction during wound healing. Macrophages are derived from monocytes in blood and arrive to the wound site by a mechanism similar to that described for neutrophils: margination, rolling, adhesion, and transmigration. Monocytes are recruited to the wound site by chemoattractants such as monocyte chemoattractant protein-1 (MCP-1)[4] and macrophage inflammatory protein-1 (MIP-1).[5] Extracellular matrix degradation products such as fibronectin fragments, collagen fragments, and thrombin are also specific chemoattractants for monocytes.[6] Similar to neutrophils, they utilize phagocytosis, but macrophages destroy phagocytosed material using enzymes in an O_2-independent process. After phagocytosis, macrophages digest and kill pathogenic organisms, destroy any remaining neutrophils, and scavenge tissue debris. These important processes help induce angiogenesis and the formation of granulation tissue essential to the structural stabilization of the wound. Macrophages also release chemotactic factors such as fibronectin, which attract fibroblasts to the wound site. These chemotactic factors also help to localize inflammation and improve adhesion of fibroblasts to fibrin in the transition between the inflammatory and proliferative phases of wound repair. Macrophages increase collagen deposition because their presence directly correlates with the deposition of collagen in the wound.[7] When macrophages are absent, significantly fewer fibroblasts migrate to the wound site, and those that do are immature. Moreover, the angiogenic capacity of macrophages has been demonstrated by inducing neovascularization in the cornea using macrophage-derived growth factor in a rat model. New blood vessel growth seems to follow a gradient of angiogenic factor produced by hypoxic macrophages, because macrophages do not produce this angiogenic factor when either fully oxygenated or anoxic. Macrophages also are an important source in the production of growth factors, and synthesize and secrete fibroblast growth factor (FGF), PDGF, vascular endothelial growth factor (VEGF), TGF-a, and TGF-b.[8] These cytokines have an important role in cell migration and proliferation as well as matrix production. Overall, macrophages play an important role in the transition from inflammation to repair.

CHRONIC INFLAMMATION. Generally the acute inflammatory response lasts approximately 2 weeks. However, as discussed previously, inflammation that persists for a long period of time (months or years) is called chronic inflammation. The presence of necrotic tissue, foreign material that cannot be phagocytosed and pathogens are all associated with chronic inflammation. Granulocytes leave the wound site through lysis and migration after the acute inflammatory phase; however, should they or other inflammatory cells persist, chronic inflammation ensues and is characterized by mononuclear cells, specifically lymphocytes, macrophages, and monocytes. In particular, macrophages that have phagocytosed foreign material remain at the wound site if they are unable to solubilize the ingested material. These macrophages then attract fibroblasts, which produce increased quantities of collagen and can slowly induce formation of a granuloma. Granulomatous inflammation is characterized by the presence of epithelioid histiocytes (macrophages with abundant pink cytoplasm) that usually surround giant cells, and a rim of lymphocytes. Granulomas are generally divided into two subtypes: caseating and noncaseating. Noncaseating granulomas lack central necrosis. Common etiologies in the formation of this type of granuloma include reactions to foreign material, sarcoidosis, catscratch disease, beryllium exposure, and Crohn's disease. In contrast, caseating granulomas exhibit central necrosis and are characteristic of tuberculosis and fungal infections. There are three important steps in granuloma formation. First, macrophages process and present antigen via MHC class II to CD4+ helper T cells. Next, this interaction leads macrophages to secrete IL-12, which induces CD4+ helper T cells to differentiate into the TH1 subtype. Finally, TH1 cells secrete IFN-γ, which converts macrophages to epithelioid histiocytes and giant cells.

As inflammation begins to resolve, inflammatory factors are broken down and fewer are secreted. The presence of macrophages has been shown to delay wound contraction and therefore macrophages may need to leave the wound site before later stages of healing occur.[9]

PROLIFERATIVE PHASE

Approximately 2 to 3 days after the initial wound was made, fibroblasts start to enter the wound site, thereby initiating the proliferative phase of healing, even if the inflammatory phase has not yet ended. The proliferative phase is generally characterized by granulation tissue formation and epithelial migration over the provisional matrix within the wound, or re-epithelialization (Fig. 10-4).

ANGIOGENESIS. Angiogenesis or neovascularization is an essential step in wound healing as it allows oxygen and nutrients to reach fibroblasts and epithelial cells. It is, therefore, required for other stages of wound healing, such epidermal and fibroblast migration, to occur. The ruby red color of healing tissue signifies the occurrence of angiogenesis and the presence of capillaries. Macrophages and other cells release cytokines that stimulate angiogenesis during wound healing. Other factors that stimulate angiogenesis include low oxygen tension, lactic acid, and biogenic amines.[10]

Normally, the dermal vasculature remains inactive, but in response to injury, endothelial cells begin the process of angiogenesis. They activate other endothelial cells, undergo cell proliferation, form a tubule structure, sprout into the wound clot, reconstruct and stabilize the basement membrane, and finally remodel the tissue. Endothelial cells located at the tips of capillaries migrate to the wound and extend cytoplasmic pseudopodia. Migration into the perivascular space also occurs and collagenase is secreted.[11] As proliferation of endothelial cells has been hypothesized to be the result of cell migration, it is believed that heparin, fibronectin, and other factors that stimulate migration also lead to endothelial proliferation.

RE-EPITHELIALIZATION. Re-epithelialization is the process through which the epidermis is restored after an injury to the skin. Re-epithelialization generally refers to basal cell proliferation and epithelial migration occurring in the fibrin bridgework inside a clot.[12] In a clean surgical wound epithelial cells generally migrate downward deep in the dermis.[13] Generally, re-epithelialization is comprised of several processes including the migration of epidermal keratinocytes from wound edges, the proliferation of keratinocytes, differentiation of the epithelium into stratified epidermis, restoration of an intact basement membrane zone,

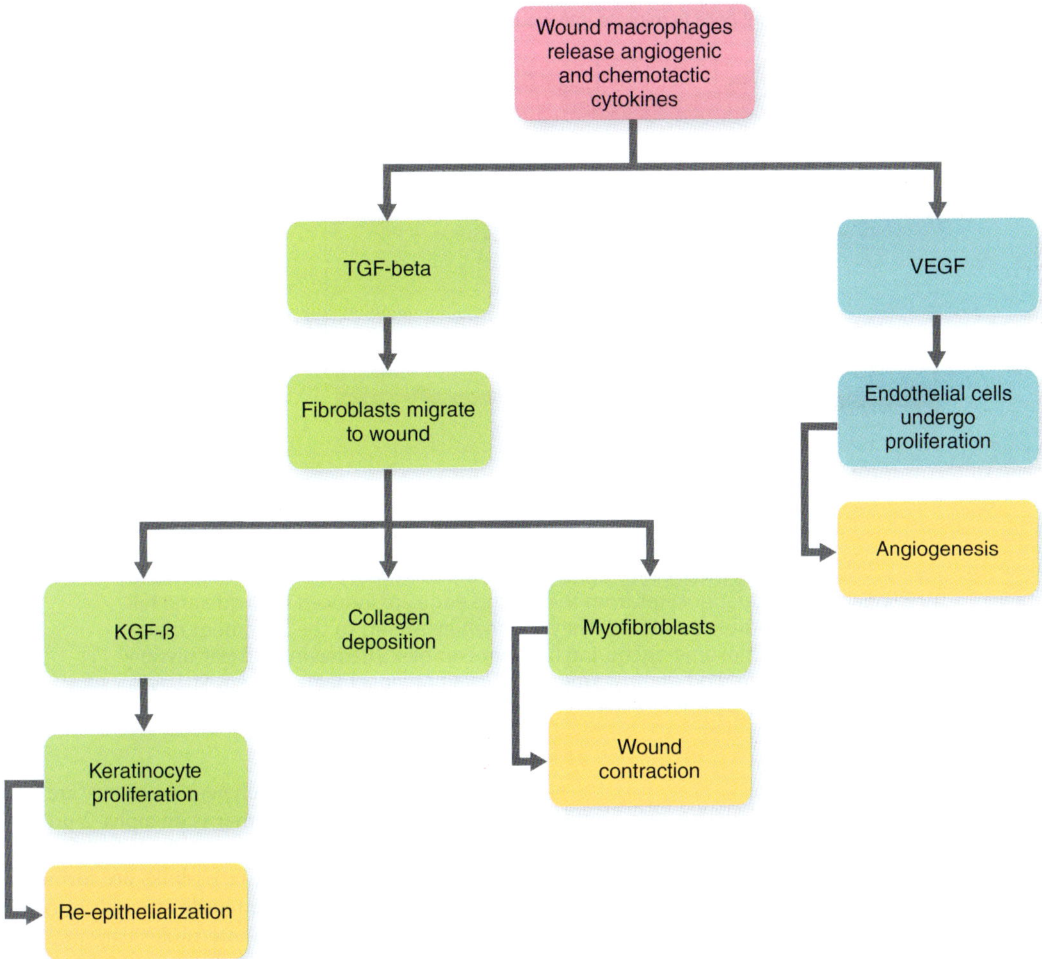

Figure 10-4 Proliferative phase in wound healing.

and the repopulation of specialized cells that direct sensory function (Merkel cells), pigmentation (melanocytes), and immune functions (Langerhans cells).[1]

Keratinocyte migration occurs early on in wound re-epithelialization, and epidermal keratinocytes initially respond to injury by migrating from the free edges of the wound within 24 hours. At approximately 12 hours postinjury, the epidermal cells become elongated and flattened, lose their cell–cell and cell–matrix attachments, develop pseudopod-like projections named lamellipodia, retract their intracellular tonofilaments, and form actin filaments at the edge of the cell cytoplasm.[1]

Although the mechanisms of re-epithelialization are still not completely understood, the "leapfrog" theory is one of the most accepted models. This theory describes the migration of epidermal cells two or three cell lengths from their initial position and the sliding or rolling of these cells over epidermal cells already in the wound.[1] The migrating cells then become fixed, and other epidermal cells migrate over these cells. As the epidermal layer progressively advances, the epithelial defect closes (Fig. 10-5).[1]

Re-epithelialization also involves increased proliferation of the keratinocytes located behind the migrating cells, in order to have an adequate supply of cells to cover the wound. When this migration stops, the keratinocytes reattach to the underlying substratum, reconstitute the basement membrane, and then recommence terminal differentiation to produce a stratified epidermis.[1]

The next important step in the re-establishment of skin integrity is the formation of an intact basement membrane zone. The basement membrane zone forms an adhesion structure and its upper portion allows attachment of basal keratinocytes through the formation of a hemidesmosome-anchoring filament complex. The lower part of the zone helps to stabilize the attachment of the underling dermis through anchoring fibrils.[1] The basement membrane zone returns to normal only 7 to 9 days after the reformation of the epidermis.[1]

FIBROPLASIA. This stage consists of the proliferation of fibroblasts, the accumulation of ground substance and collagen production. Fibroblasts are derived from mesenchymal cells and are present at the site of the wound in the first 24 hours, although they are most prevalent by the 10th day.[14]

Fibroblasts attach to the fibrin matrix of the clot at the wound site and produce mucopolysaccharides and glycoproteins, which comprise the ground substance.

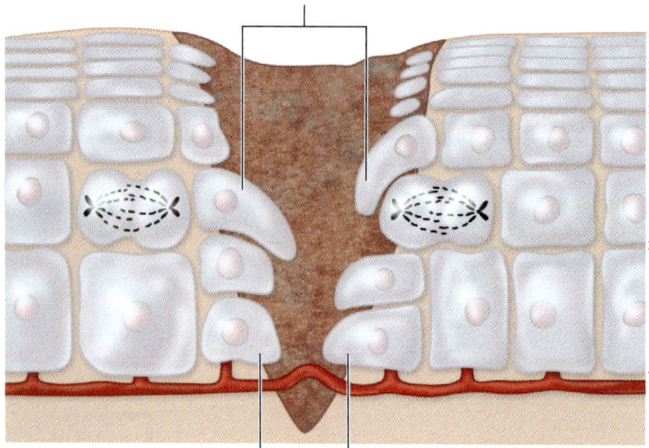

Figure 10-5 Leapfrog theory of re-epithelialization. This theory presumes that two to three cell layers of keratinocytes from the wound edge are induced to divide and fall into the bottom of the wound bed. They are then anchored to the basement membrane by a hemidesmosome-anchoring filament complex. (Redrawn with permission from Bryant RA. *Acute and Chronic Wounds: Nursing Management,* 2nd ed. St Louis, MO: Mosby; 2000. Copyright Elsevier.).

Fibroblasts also produce contractile cells called myofibroblasts. These cells are present by the fifth day after injury and are involved in pulling the edges of the wound together.

Fibroblasts are also critical to wound healing due to their role in synthesizing collagen. Collagen fibers make up approximately 80% of dry weight of the dermis and provide strength, structure, and stiffness to dermal tissue.[15] Generally, type I collagen accounts for approximately 80% of collagen found in the dermis of adults, whereas type III collagen constitutes 10% of collagen. However, during early wound healing, type III collagen is the predominant collagen synthesized.

By the second day after injury, collagen production begins. Collagen is first secreted in a form that is not strong and is analogous to an amorphous gel. Maximum production of collagen does not begin until the fifth day and then continues for a minimum of 6 weeks.[16] Fibroblasts also produce glycosaminoglycans, which together with collagen are the major components of the extracellular matrix.

MATURATION. The final phase of wound healing, maturation, includes collagen cross-linking, collagen remodeling, wound contraction, and repigmentation. Tropocollagen comprises a triple helix formed by three protein chains. Two of the polypeptide chains are identical alpha-1 proteins and the other is an alpha-2 protein. The tropocollagen molecules are initially united by hydrogen bonding but then covalent cross-links are formed, creating collagenous fibrils. The tensile strength of collagen is thought to be due to these intermolecular cross-links.[1] It has been shown that the tensile strength of the wound is directly proportional to the amount of collagen present.[17] At 6 weeks after the initial injury, approximately 80% of the original strength of the tissue has been regained. However, the morphology and diameter of the collagen fibrils do not regain their appearance in normal skin until 180 days after the initial injury.[18]

IMPAIRED WOUND HEALING AND RISK FACTORS

Various factors can lead to impaired wound healing. In general these factors can be divided into local factors that directly influence the wound itself and systemic factors that influence the overall health of the person and therefore affect their ability to heal (Table 10-2).[19]

TABLE 10-2
Local and Systemic Factors Affecting Wound Healing

Local	Hypoxia	Infection	Trauma	Edema	Ischemia	Foreign Body	
Systemic	Diabetes	Aging	Venous Insufficiency	Smoking	Hypoproteinemia	Immunosuppresion	Medications (i.e., Steroids, NSAIDs)

LOCAL FACTORS THAT IMPAIR WOUND HEALING

OXYGEN. Oxygen is an essential component for wound healing due to its central role in energy production as well as its function in the superoxide production that kills pathogens. It is vital in preventing wounds from infection, increasing keratinocyte differentiation, inducing angiogenesis, migration and re-epithelialization, promoting wound contraction, and enhancing collagen synthesis and fibroblast proliferation.[20]

In the early wound, the microenvironment is often hypoxic due to high oxygen consumption by metabolically active cells and vascular disruption. Also, some systemic conditions like diabetes can impair vascular flow, which exacerbates the hypoxia in the wound site and interferes with wound healing. Chronic wounds have been found to be significantly more hypoxic than control tissue. Studies have shown that the tissue oxygen concentration in chronic wounds when measured transcutaneously is between 5 and 20 mm Hg, whereas control tissues have oxygen concentrations of 30 to 50 mm Hg.[12]

Although chronic hypoxia delays wound healing, temporary hypoxia after injury can actually stimulate repair.[13] As discussed previously, temporary hypoxia in acute wounds can induce growth factor and cytokine production in macrophages, fibroblasts, and other cells.[13] These cytokines include TGF-β, PDGF, VEGF, endothelin-1, and TNF-α.

In normal wound healing, reactive oxygen species like H_2O_2 and superoxide can act as cellular messengers and stimulate essential wound healing processes such as angiogenesis, cell motility, and the action of cytokines. Overall, proper oxygen levels play a vital role in promoting and sustaining healthy wound healing. When oxygenation of the wound is reduced, healing is compromised and chronic wounds can result. A therapeutic option that addresses the problem of tissue hypoxia is hyperbaric oxygen therapy.[13] Although the availability of this treatment is limited, it can improve healing in hypoxic wounds.[19]

INFECTION. The disruption of the skin barrier through injury allows pathogens access to underlying tissues. Wounds can be classified by increasing levels of infection: contamination, colonization, and local infection, to invasive infection.[19] Wound contamination is defined as nonreplicating organisms present at the wound site, whereas colonization refers to replicating organisms on the wound in the absence of tissue damage. Local infection, also known as critical colonization, refers to microorganism replication in the wound and the beginning of a local tissue response. Invasive or spreading infection refers to the presence of replicating organisms within a wound and subsequent host injury.[21]

When pathogens remain in the wound site, inflammation becomes prolonged. Bacteria and endotoxins prolong the elevation of proinflammatory cytokines like IL-1 and TNF-α, which extends the inflammatory phase.[19] This leads to an increased level of matrix metalloproteases, proteases which can degrade the extracellular matrix. Conversely, there is a decreased level of natural protease inhibitors.[19] This shift in the balance of proteases can lead to the rapid degradation of the growth factors that appear in chronic wounds.[21] Also, bacteria in infected wounds form biofilms or aggregated bacteria embedded in a self-secreted extracellular polysaccharide matrix[21] and are particularly resistant to antibiotic treatment.

Common bacteria in wounds are *S. aureus*, *Pseudomonas aeruginosa*, and β-hemolytic streptococci. Biofilms containing *P. aeruginosa* are particularly prevalent among chronic ulcers and the protective microenvironment found in biofilms shields these bacteria from phagocytosis. It has been postulated that this may be an important mechanism in the resistance of chronic wounds to antibiotic treatment.

SYSTEMIC FACTORS THAT IMPAIR WOUND HEALING

DIABETES MELLITUS. Diabetes mellitus is a major problem worldwide with an estimated 346 million people suffering from this disease as of 2012.[22] Although diabetes affects many organ systems, its detrimental effects in wound healing can create some of its most devastating sequelae. This population is also particularly susceptible to the development of chronic nonhealing diabetic foot ulcers due to sensory neuropathy, which makes the patient less aware of when injury occurs. These foot ulcers occur in 15% of all people with diabetes[19] and are associated with significant morbidity, preceding 84% of diabetes-related lower-leg amputations.[23]

Several complex mechanisms underlie the pathophysiology of diabetic foot ulcers and other chronic wounds in diabetics. Diabetic foot ulcers are always associated with hypoxia, which as discussed previously, is detrimental to wound healing. Diabetes is often associated with severe peripheral artery disease with atherosclerosis affecting more distal arteries like the popliteal and tibial arteries. This peripheral artery disease in combination with diabetic neuropathy predisposes to higher rates of nonhealing ulcers and limb loss in diabetic patients.[24] Moreover, via a separate mechanism, the formation of advanced glycation end products or AGEs that are associated with hyperglycemia in diabetes are associated with impaired wound healing in diabetic mice.[25] Finally, diabetic wounds are associated with various elements of immune compromise like defects in leukocyte chemotaxis, phagocytosis, and bactericidal capacity, defective T-cell immunity and dysfunctions of fibroblasts and epidermal cells. This dysregulation is responsible for impaired bacterial clearance in individuals with diabetes as well as delayed and impaired wound repair.[26,27]

AGING. Advanced age is another systemic factor that has a detrimental effect on wound healing. With advanced age, the supply of cutaneous nerves and blood vessels decreases. Also, there is a general thinning of tissue in both the dermis and basement membrane. Finally, there is a loss of collagen as well as decreased ability to produce more collagen. Overall, these physiologic changes associated with aging result in slower and impaired wound healing in elderly individuals.[28,29]

VENOUS INSUFFICIENCY.

Chronic venous insufficiency plays a major role in impaired wound healing, and venous leg ulcers account for 40% of wounds on the lower extremities.[23] The pathogenesis of venous insufficiency involves incompetent venous valves, venous obstruction, and inadequate muscle pump function. Some risk factors for the development of chronic venous disease include a family history of venous disease, advanced age, prolonged standing, obesity, smoking, sedentary lifestyle, and high estrogen states.[30–39] These changes lead to congestion and pooling of blood in superficial veins causing venous hypertension. If sustained, this venous hypertension is associated with venous hypertensive microangiopathy. Also, these changes result in a pericapillary fibrin cuff. The combination of high venous pressure and abnormal capillaries results in vessels that are abnormally permeable and leads to the accumulation of water, large proteins, and red blood cells in the interstitial space.[40,41] These macromolecules are thought to trap matrix material and growth factors, making them unavailable for tissue repair. Moreover, the formation of the perivascular fibrin cuff decreases delivery of oxygen and nutrients. This contributes to skin hypoxia and cell death causing venous ulcers.[42]

SMOKING.

Smoking is associated with impaired wound healing and adverse outcomes following surgery. Mechanisms for this impairment include vasoconstriction which induces ischemia in the wound area, impaired bacteriocidal mechanisms, altered collagen metabolism, and a reduced inflammatory healing response.[43]

A review of four randomized trials evaluating the effect of preoperative smoking cessation on postoperative wound healing found that smoking cessation significantly reduced the incidence of surgical site infection (odds ratio 0.40, 95% CI 0.20–0.83).[44] Other studies have shown that active smoking is associated with postoperative complications and particularly increases the risk of such complication in people with other risk factors for impaired healing, such as diabetes.[45]

MEDICATIONS.

Several major categories of medication have significant adverse effects on wound healing. The three major classes of drugs we will discuss are chemotherapeutics, nonsteroidal anti-inflammatory drugs (NSAIDs) and glucocorticoids.

Most chemotherapeutic drugs inhibit rapid cell division, angiogenesis, and cellular metabolism, all critical elements of wound healing. Many of these medications inhibit DNA, RNA, and protein synthesis and therefore cause decreased fibroplasia and neovascularization of wounds.[46,47] Also, some chemotherapeutic agents' detrimental effects on wound healing may be due to their effect on VEGF, an important factor in angiogenesis in the early stages of wound healing.[48]

NSAIDs, like ibuprofen, are widely used in the treatment of pain and inflammation. Although there is little data to support the idea that short-term usage of NSAIDs interferes with wound healing, some studies have shown that long-term usage of NSAIDs can negatively impact wound healing. Systemic use of ibuprofen has been shown to have an antiproliferative effect on wound healing in animal models, and results in weakened breaking strength, decreased numbers of fibroblasts, delayed epithelialization, reduced wound contraction,[49–51] and impaired angiogenesis.[52]

Systemic glucocorticoids, also commonly used in the treatment of inflammatory conditions, are widely known to inhibit wound repair through their suppressive effects on cellular wound responses, including collagen synthesis and fibroblast proliferation.[19] Steroids also cause wounds to heal with reduced wound contraction and incomplete granulation tissue.[47] In addition to these effects on repair, systemic corticosteroids also predispose to wound infection, which as discussed previously, is detrimental to the healing process.[19]

Interestingly, topical steroids actually seem to be beneficial to wound healing. Low-dose topical corticosteroids have been shown to suppress hypergranulation, reduce exudate, and accelerate wound healing.[19] However, caution should be used with these agents as there is potentially an increased risk of infection with long-term use.[53]

CONCLUSION

Wound healing is critical to understanding dermatology and optimizing results of dermatologic surgery. In addition to understanding the normal repair process, appreciating the differences between acute and chronic wounds and having insight into factors that hasten and delay healing are of great importance. Opportunities to enhance clinical outcomes exist through improved healing.

REFERENCES

1. Li J, Chen J, Kirsner R. Pathophysiology of acute wound healing. *Clin Dermatol.* 2007;25:9–18.
2. Gosain A, DiPietro LA. Aging and wound healing. *World J Surg.* 2004;28:321–326.
3. Scheid A, Wenger RH, Schaffer L, et al. Physiologically low oxygen concentrations in fetal skin regulate hypoxia-inducible factor 1 and transforming growth factor-beta3. *FASEB Jl.* 2002;16:411–413.
4. Kunkel SL, Standiford T, Kasahara K, Strieter RM. Stimulus specific induction of monocyte chemotactic protein-1 (MCP-1) gene expression. *Adv Exp Med Biol.* 1991;305:65–71.
5. Sherry B, Tekamp-Olson P, Gallegos C, et al. Resolution of the two components of macrophage inflammatory protein 1, and cloning and characterization of one of those components, macrophage inflammatory protein 1 beta. *J Exp Med.* 1988;168:2251–2259.
6. Postlethwaite AE, Kang AH. Collagen-and collagen peptide-induced chemotaxis of human blood monocytes. *J Exp Med.* 1976;143:1299–1307.
7. Lewis JS, Lee JA, Underwood JC, Harris AL, Lewis CE. Macrophage responses to hypoxia: relevance to disease mechanisms. *J Leukoc Biol.* 1999;66:889–900.
8. Falanga V. Growth factors and wound healing. *J Dermatol Surg Oncol.* 1993;19:711–714.
9. Newton PM, Watson JA, Wolowacz RG, Wood EJ. Macrophages restrain contraction of an in vitro wound healing model. *Inflammation.* 2004;28:207–214.
10. Remensnyder JP, Majno G. Oxygen gradients in healing wounds. *Am J Pathol.* 1968;52:301–323.
11. Sethi KK, Yannas IV, Mudera V, Eastwood M, McFarland C, Brown RA. Evidence for sequential utilization of fibronectin, vitronectin, and collagen during fibroblast-mediated collagen contraction. *Wound Repair Regen.* 2002;10:397–408.
12. Tandara AA, Mustoe TA. Oxygen in wound healing–more than a nutrient. *World J Surg.* 2004;28:294–300.

13. Rodriguez PG, Felix FN, Woodley DT, Shim EK. The role of oxygen in wound healing: a review of the literature. *Dermatol Surg*. 2008;34:1159–1169.
14. Doillon CJ, Dunn MG, Bender E, Silver FH. Collagen fiber formation in repair tissue: development of strength and toughness. *Coll Relat Res*. 1985;5:481–492.
15. Booth BA, Polak KL, Uitto J. Collagen biosynthesis by human skin fibroblasts. I. Optimization of the culture conditions for synthesis of type I and type III procollagens. *Biochim Biophys Acta*. 1980;607:145–160.
16. Howes EL, Harvey SC. The strength of the healing wound in relation to the holding strength of the catgut suture. *N Engl J Med*. 1929;200:1285–1291.
17. Dodson MK, Magann EF, Meeks GR. A randomized comparison of secondary closure and secondary intention in patients with superficial wound dehiscence. *Obstet Gynecol*. 1992;80:321–324.
18. Walters MD, Dombroski RA, Davidson SA, Mandel PC, Gibbs RS. Reclosure of disrupted abdominal incisions. *Obstet Gynecol*. 1990;76:597–602.
19. Guo S, Dipietro LA. Factors affecting wound healing. *J Dent Res*. 2010;89:219–229.
20. Bishop A. Role of oxygen in wound healing. *J Wound Care*. 2008;17:399–402.
21. Edwards R, Harding KG. Bacteria and wound healing. *Curr Opin Infect Dis*. 2004;17:91–96.
22. Ginter E, Simko V. Type 2 diabetes mellitus, pandemic in 21st century. *Adv Exp Med Biol*. 2012;771:42–50.
23. Brem H, Tomic-Canic M. Cellular and molecular basis of wound healing in diabetes. *J Clin Invest*. 2007;117:1219–1222.
24. Santilli JD, Santilli SM. Chronic critical limb ischemia: diagnosis, treatment and prognosis. *Am Fam Physician*. 1999;59:1899–1908.
25. Huijberts MS, Schaper NC, Schalkwijk CG. Advanced glycation end products and diabetic foot disease. *Diabetes Metab Res Rev*. 2008;24(suppl 1):S19–S24.
26. Loots MA, Lamme EN, Zeegelaar J, Mekkes JR, Bos JD, Middelkoop E. Differences in cellular infiltrate and extracellular matrix of chronic diabetic and venous ulcers versus acute wounds. *J Invest Dermatol*. 1998;111:850–857.
27. Gary Sibbald R, Woo KY. The biology of chronic foot ulcers in persons with diabetes. *Diabetes Metab Res Rev*. 2008;24:25–30.
28. Mendelsohn FA, Divino CM, Reis ED, Kerstein MD. Wound care after radiation therapy. *Adv Skin Wound Care*. 2002;15:216–224.
29. Bowering CK. Diabetic foot ulcers. Pathophysiology, assessment, and therapy. *Can Fam Physician*. 2001;47:1007–1016.
30. Brand FN, Dannenberg AL, Abbott RD, Kannel WB. The epidemiology of varicose veins: the Framingham Study. *Am J Prev Med*. 1988;4:96–101.
31. Callam MJ. Epidemiology of varicose veins. *Br J Surg*. 1994;81:167–173.
32. Chiesa R, Marone EM, Limoni C, Volonte M, Petrini O. Chronic venous disorders: correlation between visible signs, symptoms, and presence of functional disease. *J Vasc Surg*. 2007;46:322–330.
33. Scott TE, LaMorte WW, Gorin DR, Menzoian JO. Risk factors for chronic venous insufficiency: a dual case-control study. *J Vasc Surg*. 1995;22:622–628.
34. Fowkes FG, Lee AJ, Evans CJ, Allan PL, Bradbury AW, Ruckley CV. Lifestyle risk factors for lower limb venous reflux in the general population: Edinburgh Vein Study. *Int J Epidemiol*. 2001;30:846–852.
35. Sadick NS. Predisposing factors of varicose and telangiectatic leg veins. *J Dermatol Surg Oncol*. 1992;18:883–886.
36. Iannuzzi A, Panico S, Ciardullo AV, et al. Varicose veins of the lower limbs and venous capacitance in postmenopausal women: relationship with obesity. *J Vasc Surg*. 2002;36:965–968.
37. Evans CJ, Fowkes FG, Hajivassiliou CA, Harper DR, Ruckley CV. Epidemiology of varicose veins. A review. *Int Angiol*. 1994;13:263–270.
38. Browse NL. The etiology of venous ulceration. *World J Surg*. 1986;10:938–943.
39. Browse NL, Burnand KG. The cause of venous ulceration. *Lancet*. 1982;2:243–245.
40. Franzeck UK, Haselbach P, Speiser D, Bollinger A. Microangiopathy of cutaneous blood and lymphatic capillaries in chronic venous insufficiency (CVI). *Yale J Biol Med*. 1993;66:37–46.
41. Leach RD, Browse NL. Effect of venous hypertension on canine hind limb lymph. *Br J Surg*. 1985;72:275–278.
42. Falanga V, Eaglstein WH. The "trap" hypothesis of venous ulceration. *Lancet*. 1993;341:1006–1008.
43. Turan A, Mascha EJ, Roberman D, et al. Smoking and perioperative outcomes. *Anesthesiology*. 2011;114:837–846.
44. Sorensen LT. Wound healing and infection in surgery. The clinical impact of smoking and smoking cessation: a systematic review and meta-analysis. *Arch Surg*. 2012;147:373–383.
45. Wukich DK, McMillen RL, Lowery NJ, Frykberg RG. Surgical site infections after foot and ankle surgery: a comparison of patients with and without diabetes. *Diabetes Care*. 2011;34:2211–2213.
46. Waldron DR, Zimmerman-Pope N. Superficial skin wounds. In: Slatter D, ed. *Textbook of Small Animal Surgery*. Philadelphia, PA: Saunders; 2002:259–274.
47. Franz MG, Steed DL, Robson MC. Optimizing healing of the acute wound by minimizing complications. *Curr Probl Surg*. 2007;44:691–763.
48. Erinjeri JP, Fong AJ, Kemeny NE, Brown KT, Getrajdman GI, Solomon SB. Timing of administration of bevacizumab chemotherapy affects wound healing after chest wall port placement. *Cancer*. 2011;117:1296–1301.
49. Dong YL, Fleming RY, Yan TZ, Herndon DN, Waymack JP. Effect of ibuprofen on the inflammatory response to surgical wounds. *J Trauma*. 1993;35:340–343.
50. Dvivedi S, Tiwari SM, Sharma A. Effect of ibuprofen and diclofenac sodium on experimental would healing. *Indian J Exp Biol*. 1997;35:1243–1245.
51. Krischak GD, Augat P, Claes L, Kinzl L, Beck A. The effects of non-steroidal anti-inflammatory drug application on incisional wound healing in rats. *J Wound Care*. 2007;16:76–78.
52. Jones MK, Wang H, Peskar BM, et al. Inhibition of angiogenesis by nonsteroidal anti-inflammatory drugs: insight into mechanisms and implications for cancer growth and ulcer healing. *Nat Med*. 1999;5:1418–1423.
53. Hofman D, Moore K, Cooper R, Eagle M, Cooper S. Use of topical corticosteroids on chronic leg ulcers. *J Wound Care*. 2007;16:227–230.

CHAPTER 11

Dressings and Postoperative Care

Daniel A. Davis

THE PURPOSE OF WOUND CARE

Mother Nature has been able to repair damaged integuments for at least half a billion years. Scars and scabs are evident in the fossil record since the beginning of terrestrial life.[1] So why has there been an explosion of interest in wound care since the last World War? Quite simply, because of faster and better healing. Smugly one-upping Mother Nature, modern dressings are an entire paradigm shift from the standard approach taken since time immemorial.

As there are hundreds of dressings, bandages, and wound-care products available, the purpose of this chapter is not to catalog the daily changing varieties, but rather to provide a compendium of wound-care classes in order to understand their advantages and disadvantages.[2] These products include specialty items marketed for leg ulcers, decubitus ulcers, burns, and stoma care, which may have crossover potential for postsurgical skin care, especially for granulating surgical defects.[3]

In the United States particularly, nomenclature may be confusing. A dressing is generally something placed directly on a wound, whereas a bandage supports that dressing, while being external to it and the wound. The purpose of all wound coverings, including scabs or crusts, is to provide a barrier between the internal and external world. Presuming that there is no infection, many consider the most important function of this barrier to be wound hydration or at least antidehydration. However, an ideal covering will also protect and support the wound, provide hemostasis and analgesia, absorb exudate, debride slough, regrow what is missing, will be easily applied and removed, and be inexpensive.[4] Exudate absorption is a close second in importance to wound hydration. Dressings absorb exudate by capillarity, which is defined as the sum of the hydrophilic surface forces that cause liquid to move along the surface of a solid, like watercolor paint between the hairs of a paintbrush. Wound debridement is also important. There are four types of debridement: autolytic, mechanical, chemical, and surgical. The latter two are exogenous and, although part of wound care, are generally not a part of wound dressings. Autolytic debridement occurs naturally when a dressing hydrates a wound, and it is yet another reason why moist healing is so important. Wounds are mechanically debrided when dry adherent dressings are removed, taking bits of crust with them.

CHARACTERIZATION OF WOUNDS

Wounds may be described as acute or chronic, full thickness or partial thickness, endogenous, such as vascular wounds, or exogenous, which may be infectious, surgical, or traumatic wounds. There is also a surgical classification of wounds. Class I are clean wounds or a clean surgical site sparsely colonized with bacteria; Class II are clean-contaminated wounds or a clean surgical site heavily colonized with bacteria, such as the groin. Class III wounds are contaminated, either due to unclean technique or colonization with bacteria before surgery, such as from trauma. Class IV wounds are infected. As the class number increases, complications increase and outcomes worsen.

Wounds may also be classified into four stages of healing: hemostatic, inflammatory, proliferative, and remodeling.[5] Although healing is a continuum, each one of these stages is a macroscopic benchmark indicating a change in the wound microenvironment.[6] Hemostasis begins immediately after wounding and is usually measured in minutes. The inflammatory stage also begins immediately as neutrophils are recruited to digest the wound margins. This stage lasts less than a week, at which point the proliferative phase is recognized. As the neutrophils diminish, macrophages enter the wound and master dermal cells begin the process of rebuilding the skin from the dermis up. Rebuilding human skin during this proliferative phase takes months and is considered to last from the first week to the third month. Finally, as proliferation subsides, the wound contracts and remodels into a mature structure with vasculature that will permanently sustain it. Most wound healing is complete by 6 months, but final maturation can take up to a year.

DRESSINGS

There are more than a handful of dressing classifications (Table 11-1). None are all-inclusive; there is always some composite bandage that does not neatly fit the scheme.

TABLE 11-1
Schemes to Classify Dressings

Primary versus secondary
Adhesive versus nonadhesive
Occlusive versus nonocclusive
Traditional versus modern
Natural versus synthetic
Nonbiologic versus biologic versus biosynthetic
Gas or liquid permeable versus impermeable

They are not exclusive either, and it is often helpful to use several commonly used classifications together. Any modern bandage will be self-crafted or prefabricated in layers.[7] From internal to external, the six typical parts include the wound base, and the hydrating, absorbing, wound adhering, contouring, and border adhering layers.

GAUZE. The word "gauze" probably derives from a place name in the Middle East, and this type of dressing has been used for millennia. Gauze can be used as a primary or secondary dressing, can hydrate or desiccate, be cotton or synthetic, or can be used as a bandage. However, because of tradition and its low cost, by far the most common gauze is spun cotton thread woven into cloth.

Nearly all modern cotton is grown from a single species of long staple "King cotton" that, unless treated, has only modest absorption of 10% of its weight. Cotton wool, or linters, is the unspun, absorptive, curly fiber that surrounds the cotton seed and was developed as a dressing by the pioneers of aseptic surgery. By dry weight the cotton boll is 90% cellulose, an insoluble, fibrous plant polymer of repeating D-sucrose units. The 0.5% dry-weight waxes that coat the fibers substantially diminish capillarity. Waxes and off-white coloring are typically removed by bleach and heat, independent of the sterilization process. Because cotton is a biologic material, it is biodegradable and cotton dressings must be frequently changed. Unless it is coated, cotton is adherent and will mechanically debride the wound when removed. Cotton is gas and liquid permeable.

Polyester and polyamide gauzes have the same advantages over cotton gauze as synthetic clothing. These synthetic gauzes are more durable, produce less lint, and are not biodegradable, but are typically less absorptive than medical grade cotton.

Impregnated gauze has two components: gauze and its coating. The coating makes it nonadherent and limits mechanical debridement, but capillarity suffers. Impregnated gauze remains both gas and liquid permeable, and is typically made of cotton muslin, polyester, or acetate. The wide variety of coatings include saline, Ringer's solution, petrolatum or proprietary ointments, bismuth tribromophenate, iodine, silver, zinc oxide, ferric oxide, oat glucan, and scarlet red (o-tolylzo-o-tolyazo-beta-napthol) (Table 11-2). Polyesterized gauze is a cotton- or rayon-based composite dressing that is commonly used to conform a crafted, layered bandage for a well-debrided wound that makes little exudate.

ALGINATES. Alginates are manufactured from braided or matted brown seaweed polysaccharide salts. These lightweight products can absorb 20 times their dry weight of exudate to form a wound-shaped gel.[8] In its unaltered form, sodium alginate is widely used in culinary arts as a taste-free thickener. However, it is the calcium salt of alginate that is used for wound dressings, and neither its taste nor its smell are pleasant. Alginates have an inherent musty odor that turns rapidly noxious with bacterial overgrowth. Theseare gas and liquid permeable and can facilitate autolytic debridement, but are so absorptive that they can overdry a nonexudative wound.[9] Most alginate products require a secondary dressing or bandage.

HYDROCOLLOID. Hydrocolloid dressings are unique in several ways.[10] Composed of gelatin or cellulose, they are typically composite dressings, the primary purpose of which is hydration. For this reason, they are good for autolytic debridement, but they are only moderately absorptive. Although chemically similar to the collagen dressings below, the collagen that eventually becomes gelatin comes from multiple organ systems and multiple species (bovine and porcine), and is hydrolyzed into an amino acid gel. Hydrocolloids are one of the few dressing materials that are both gas and liquid impermeable. Persistent occlusion with a hydrocolloid dressing can limit oxygenation and impede healing. An added adhesive makes hydrocolloid dressings adherent to the wound and its border, but as exudate is absorbed the adhesive will release from the wound. Frequent dressing removal can deepithelialize the wound periphery. Like most occlusive, adhesive dressings, hydrocolloid dressings are often promoted as a bacterial barrier.

HYDROGELS. Hydrogels are even better autolytic dressings than hydrocolloids. Hydrogel dressings are produced as nonadhesive, water or glycerin gel sheets or gel-impregnated gauze sheets. They are gas permeable, liquid impermeable, and somewhat absorptive.[11] Specific to this large product line, hydrogels are purported to have analgesic or soothing properties. Glycerin attracts water hygroscopically rather than through capillarity. Capillarity absorption does not alter the absorbing solid molecules, but glycerin expands into a lubricating gel when hydrated by wound exudate.

FOAM. Foam dressings are like mattresses, composed of flexible and firm, but low-density, polyurethane, a synthetic isocyanate that combines the best properties of plastic and rubber.[12] These products are highly varied and absorbent open-cell sheets. Like hydrogels, they are gas permeable and liquid impermeable, but they are also hugely absorbent and thermally insulating. Many foam products have an adhesive that can strip the surrounding epithelium. The fluid-logged dressing can exacerbate maceration of the skin surrounding the wound. Because they can be used as compression bandages, they have the ideal qualities for postliposuction care.

SOLID FILMS. Polyurethane can be manufactured in a highly varied spectrum from low to high density depending on which isocyanate and hydroxyl groups are polymerized. High-density polyurethane can be rigid, as in furniture varnish, or flexible, as in plastic kitchen wrap, but as a class polyurethanes tend to be clear, thin, and tenacious. Polyurethane film dressings are self-adhesive, gas permeable, and liquid impermeable like their low-density foam counterparts, but they are specifically nonabsorbent because they are bubble-free.[13] For this reason their use is limited to nonexudative wounds, although some fluid can be drained by puncturing the dressing material. The translucence of high-density polyurethane films allows the wound to be visualized through a thin, flexible, durable dressing, which may last for more than a week. Films can be the most difficult dressings to remove because their thinness makes them challenging to grasp and their impermeability makes adhesive removers less effective.

TABLE 11-2
Wound Dressings

Product	Components	Examples	Manufacturers
Impregnated gauze	Water Saline Petrolatum Paraffin Bismuth tribromophenate Scarlet red Oat glucan Ringer's solution Iodine Silver Zinc oxide/ferric oxide	Jelonet Xeroform Scarlet red BCG matrix TenderWet Inadine Acticoat	Smith & Nephew Kendall Health Medapex AM Scientifics ltd. Medline Industries Systagenix Smith & Nephew
Polyesterized gauze	Polyester/fabric composite	Telfa	Kendall Health
Alginate	Braided or matted brown seaweed polysaccharide	CarraGinate, CarraSorb CarboFlex, Kaltostat Curasorb Maxsorb Melgisorb AlgiSite Tegagen	Carrington Lab ConvaTec Kendall Health Medline Industries Mölyncke Health Smith & Nephew 3M
Hyaluroic acid	Hyaluronic acid	Hyalofill Regenecare HA	Convatec MPM Medical
Hydrocolloid	Occlusive moderately absorptive dressings made of gelatin or cellulose	Hydrocol Primacol Comfeel plus Combiderm, DuoDERM, Signaflex Ultec Exuderm Replicare	Bertek Dumex Coloplast Co ConvaTec Kendall Health Medline Industries Smith & Nephew
Hydrogel	Water or glycerin gel sheet maximizing moist healing	CarraDress, CarraSmart, CarraSorb, CarraSyn Vigilon Aquasite Aquaflo, Curafil, Curagel DermaGel Hypergel, NormIgel FlexiGel	Carrington Labs CR Bard Inc Dumex Kendall Health Medline Industries Mölyncke Health Smith & Nephew
Foam	Highly absorbent open-cell sheets	Flexzan CarraSmart Foam Lyofoam Curafoam, Hydrasorb, Optifoam Mepilex, Mitraflex Allevyn Reston	Bertek Carrington Labs ConvaTec Kendall Health Medline Industries Mölyncke Health Smith & Nephew 3M
Collagen (also see biologic dressings)	Absorbent, insoluble protein that promotes collagen organization	Collagen-Medifil, Collagen-SkinTemp Fibracol Plus	BioCore Medical Tech Ethicon
Composite	Complex, multi-layered barrier with an adherent border	Band-Aid Viasorb Stratasorb Alldress Repel	Johnson & Johnson Kendall Health Medline Industries Mölyncke Health MPM Medical
Wound base contacts	Polyamide net that protects wound base	Mepitel Conformant, Profore N-Terface Tegapore	Mölyncke Health Smith & Nephew Winfield Labs 3M
Films	Translucent, adherent polyurethane membrane	Clearsite Bioclusive Blisterfilm, Polyskin Mefilm, Mepore OpSite, UniFlex Tegaderm	Conmed Johnson & Johnson Kendall Health Mölyncke Health Smith & Nephew 3M

LIQUID FILMS. Like solid polyurethane films, liquid films are gas permeable, but liquid impermeable. They are applied with an alcohol vehicle that evaporates leaving the film adherent as a residue. The film is most commonly composed of acrylate, a vinyl polymer common to instant glues, but also can be made of nitrocellulose lacquer.[14] The lacquer grade is less flammable than classic guncotton nitrocellulose.

COLLAGEN. Familiar as a cosmeceutical, bovine type I collagen also has a place in wound healing regimens. This insoluble protein is surprisingly absorbent and provides moist healing and autolytic debridement once saturated. It is manufactured in many forms that fill and conform to the wound bed, but requires an additional dressing to hold it in place. When exogenous collagen is placed in a wound, it stimulates host collagenesis and collagen organization.[15] As with injectable collagen and biologic dressings, bovine collagen allergy is possible, but in this instance is easily treated by removing the temporary dressing from the wound bed.

HYALURONIC ACID. Hyaluronic acid (HA) is the most common glycosaminoglycan in the human body. However, the average human body may have only 15g HA total, much of which is continuously regenerated. Humans have three hyaluronidases that daily degrade roughly a third of that 15 g.[16] More than just dermal slime, HA organizes cutaneous hydration and cellular traffic via its primary receptor, CD44. Dermal HA acts a promoter of early inflammation, facilitates inflammatory cell migration into granulation tissue, and, as a major component of the basal keratinocyte extracellular matrix, facilitates reepithelialization.[17] HA dressings can be thought of as the animal equivalent of alginate dressings as the two polysaccharides are similar; both are absorbent, biodegradable, gas and liquid permeable products that form a wound-shaped gel when hydrated.

WOUND BASE. Wound base dressings are synthetic, made from perforated polyamide, and protect the base while transferring wound exudate to secondary dressings.

COMPOSITE. Composite dressings are not a dressing type, but are rather several types or layers of dressing materials prefabricated into a single product. Like the motherboard in your computer, a bundled unit may be less expensive than purchasing each component separately, but the convenience is not itself inexpensive and there is no choice among the individual components. The most common composite dressing is the omnipresent adhesive strip, created by Band-Aid®. Although moist healing was not championed by science until the 1960s, the Band-Aid® strip was invented in 1921, machine made by 1924, sold in sterilized form by 1938, and converted to plastic and vinyl bandages in the 1950s.[18] At their best composite dressings and bandages can encourage widely available autolytic debridement. However, wound-edge maceration and adhesive contact dermatitis are not uncommon.

BIOLOGIC DRESSINGS/SKIN SUBSTITUTES

Wound dressings are designed to facilitate healing. Biologic dressings facilitate healing, but can also facilitate wound closure by incorporating some form of skin from the dressing into the wound (Table 11-3).[19] When intended as simply a covering, biologic dressings are used as briefly as other dressings, usually for a matter of days before being changed. As a skin substitute, however, the components of a biologic dressing may remain in place for as long as a year or may be permanent.[20] For convenience, biologic dressings are usually grouped by the type of skin layers they cover or replace, including epidermis, dermis, or both. The tissue source is also considered, whether xenogeneic, allogeneic, autogenic, or synthetic. The specific composition of each layer is then described. Finally, consideration is given to how the tissues are handled, and whether they are cultured or simply processed by cleaning, filtering, or radiating. Many of the products contain bovine or porcine xenogeneic components that exclude their use in sensitive patients.

EPIDERMAL. There are three types of epidermal biologic dressings. In less than a month Epicel (Genzyme Tissue Repair Corporation) can co-culture nearly 2 m^2 of mixed murine xenogeneic and autogenic epidermal cell sheets from two 6 cm excision donor sites.[21] Vancomycin, amikacin, or murine protein sensitivity exclude its use. It is generally used for extensive burns when few autogenic donor sites are available, and is considered an expensive skin substitute. Laserskin (Fidia Advanced Biopolymers), also known as Vivoderm (ER Squibb and Sons), seeds 10 day old cultured autogenic epidermal cells on laser-perforated HA sheets for immediate engraftment. It is generally used for lower-leg ulcers.[22] Suprathel (Institute of Textile and Process Engineering; Burn Department of Marienhospital) is a synthetic epidermal equivalent comprised of lactide, methylcarbonate, and caprolactone.[23] It is a thin elastic mesh, best considered as a permanent hydrating dressing and best used for its analgesic properties which are superior to those of hydrogels.

DERMAL. There are as many allogeneic dermal skin substitutes as all other biologic dressings combined. There are also two xenogeneic products. Oasis (Healthpoint) is an acellular porcine xenograft that retains its collagen scaffolding, extracellular matrix proteins, and growth factors.[24] It is marketed for lower-extremity ulcerations and is widely used as a dermal replacement. Permacol (Tissue Science Laboratories) is processed from porcine skin similar to Alloderm® (Lifecell) and has similar indications.[25]

Alloderm® is an acellular cadaveric dermal replacement widely used as a tissue filler under flaps and grafted burns.[26] GraftJacket (Wright Medical Technologies), Neoform (Mentor Corporation), and DermaMatrix (Synthes) are similar allogeneic cadaveric dermal replacements that are rendered acellular by varying proprietary techniques. Three additional allogeneic dermal substitutes do not remove fibroblasts before implantation. It is unclear how long the fibroblasts remain viable in the host, but their presence has

TABLE 11-3

Biologic Dressings

Type	Name	Composition	Source	Manufacturer
Epidermal	Epicel	Epidermal sheet	Auto	Genzyme Tissue Repair Corp, Cambridge, MA
	Laserskin	Epidermis on HA sheet	Cx auto	Fidia Advanced Biopolymers, Abano Terme, Italy
	Suprathel	Thin elastic mesh	Syn	Institute of Textile and Process Engineering, Denkendorf, Germany
Dermal	Oasis	Acellular dermal xenograft	Xeno/p	Healthpoint, Fort Worth, TX
	Permacol	Acellular dermal xenograft	Xeno/p	Tissue Science Laboratories, Andover, MA
	Alloderm®	Acellular dermal allograft	Allo	Lifecell, Branchburg, NJ
	GraftJacket			Wright Medical Technologies, Inc., Arlington, TN
	Neoform			Mentor Corporation, Santa Barbara, CA
	DermaMatrix			Synthes, Inc., West Chester, PA
	ICX-SKN	Cellular dermal allograft	Allo	Intercytex, Ltd., Manchester, UK
	Dermagraft	Cellular dermal and synthetic allograft	Cx allo	Advanced BioHealing, Inc., La Jolla, CA
	TransCyte	Cellular dermal xeno- and allograft on nylon matrix	Xeno/p Cx allo	Advanced BioHealing, Inc., La Jolla, CA
Composite	Biobrane	Porcine dermis on nylon matrix with silicone sheet	Xeno/p Syn	UDL Laboratories, Inc., Rockford, IL
	Integra	Bovine dermis with temporary silastic covering	Xeno/b Syn Auto	Integra Life Sciences Corp, Plainsboro, NJ
	Apligraf	Bovine and allogeneic dermis with allogeneic epidermis	Xeno/b Cx allo	Organogenesis, Inc, Canton, MA
	OrCel	Porcine and allogeneic dermis with allogeneic epidermis	Xeno/p Cx allo	Ortec International, Inc., New York, NY
Autograft	CSS		Cx auto	University of Cincinnati, Cincinnati, OH
	FTSG		Auto	
	STSG		Auto	
	Epidermis		Auto	
Xenograft	Porcine		Xeno/p	Brennan Medical, St. Paul, MN

Allo, allogeneic; Auto, autograft; b, bovine; CSS, cultured skin substitute; Cx, cultured; p, porcine; syn, synthetic; xeno, xenogeneic.

been confirmed at least 6 months after transfer. ICX-skin (Intercytex) includes an allogenic collagen layer that retains its fibroblasts.[27] Dermagraft (Advanced Healing) seeds neonatal fibroblasts onto a polyglactin scaffold.[28] Transcyte (Advanced Healing) manufactures a composite xeno- and allogeneic dermal replacement in which a nylon mesh scaffold is first covered with porcine collagen and later seeded with neonatal fibroblasts.[29]

COMPOSITE. Composite biologic dressings are highly complex products that replace both the dermis and epidermis. Biobrane (UDL Laboratories) is similar to Transcyte, in which porcine fibroblasts are seeded on bilaminar polyamide mesh. The mesh is then covered with a thin silicone sheet, which temporarily simulates the epidermis until marginal reepithelialization incrementally sheds it.[30] Integra (Integra Life Sciences Corp) utilizes bovine collagen and glycosaminoglycan as a dermal analogue and silastic covering as a temporary epidermal analogue. The xenogeneic matrix becomes remodeled and a vascularized autogenic dermis is formed within 1 to 2 months, at which time the silastic covering may be removed and the neodermis autografted with split-thickness skin.[31] Apligraf (Organogenesis) composite skin substitute uses bovine xenogeneic collagen and allogeneic neonatal fibroblasts as a dermal replacement and covers them with a cornified epidermis of allogeneic epidermal keratinocytes.[32] It is most frequently used for chronic lower-extremity ulcerations. OrCel (Ortec International) is a similar bilaminar product, in which neonatal fibroblasts and keratinocytes are cultured on opposite sides of a porcine collagen sponge. Although not as widely used as the well-known Apligraf, OrCel has gained a treatment niche for skin diseases such as epidermolysis bullosa.[33]

SKIN GRAFTS

Until recently, humans have historically grafted skin, whether autologous or otherwise, with poor success. Xenogeneic grafts are immunologically rejected and function only as temporary dressings. Pig-skin xenografts are still available in North America; frog skin had a small regional market in the past. Popularized use of small human allografts in the 1860s led to the published success of autografts by the end of the nineteenth century.[34,35] The end of the twentieth century saw the development of cultured bilayers of autogeneic keratinocytes and fibroblasts at the University of Cincinnati, paving the way for volume skin replacement from a small donor site (Table 11-3).

HEMOSTATIC DRESSINGS

Hemostasis is the first phase in wound healing. Hemostatic agents have multiplied in recent years and may share features with the dressings discussed previously. However, their primary purpose is to provide hemostasis in an acute wound.

STYPTICS. Chemical hemostats are topical astringents that denature proteins, plugging the orifices of the transected postcapillary venules and staunching bleeding from nicks. Common examples are silver nitrate, aluminum sulfate, aluminum chloride, and ferric sulfate. Silver nitrate and aluminum sulfate (alum) are used as solids. They are mildly hemostatic, antiseptic topicals commonly used both in medical practice and as domestic styptic pencils. Somewhat more effective than the solid styptics, aluminum chloride and ferric sulfate are liquid suspensions applied with a cotton-tip swab. Erroneously called ferric subsulfate, ferric sulfate, or Monsel's solution, may leave an iron tattoo, due to ferrugination.[36,37]

PHYSICAL HEMOSTATS. Two physical hemostatic agents are available. Bone wax is a paraffin/beeswax mixture that physically occludes small vessels in bone; its persistence in a healing wound may promote infection and granulation tissue. Its use has diminished in favor of alkylene oxide, a carbon and oxygen, hydrophilic, and water soluble polymer that does not have the disadvantages of paraffin although it has similar texture and workability.[38]

BIODEGRADABLE HEMOSTATIC AGENTS. As in chronic wound dressings, cellulose, gelatin and collagen can provide hemostasis to acute wounds and they are biodegradable. As in chronic wound dressings, cellulose, gelatin and collagen can provide hemostasis to acute wounds and they are biodegradable.[39] Oxidized cellulose has been used as a hemostatic agent since World War II. In its modern form, it looks and can be handled like cotton dressing, does not adhere to instruments, and may completely degrade in situ within months. Oxidation lowers the pH of the product and initiates clot formation, but limits its use with other hemostatic agents. Gelatin used as an absorbable hemostatic agent is whipped into a foam, baked, and then processed as a film, sponge, or powder. Gelatin swells more than other biodegradable agents, providing a physical matrix for clot formation, and can also be sutured into place. Since it is neutral in pH, it can be used with other neutral hemostatic agents. Bovine collagen I is taken from cowhide and processed into either a powder or compressed cotton-like sheets. Collagen initiates clotting by platelet activation. Patients, therefore, need to have normal platelet function for collagen bandages to provide hemostasis. In general, absorptive dressings can also staunch minor venous or capillary bleeding. In fact, many alginates were originally marketed for this indication.

BIOLOGIC SEALANTS. Thrombin, fibrin, and platelet solutions can be potent hemostatic sealants although they are not dressings.[40] Fibrin gauze is also available and will be discussed with the dressings later. Bovine, human, and recombinant thrombin is available. Because of known or potential problems including immunologic host response and venous thrombosis, use has trended toward recombinant thrombin. Thrombin is dispensed as a powder in a vial and is reconstituted with a few milliliters of sterile diluent which can then be directly dripped onto the wound with a syringe or used with an absorbent neutral pH gelatin sponge. A normal clotting cascade is required for success. There are more numerous options for fibrin sealants, which have been available in Europe for 40 years and in the United States for 20 years. All of the four fibrin sealants presently on the US market involve a double plunger syringe that mixes thrombin and fibrinogen from various sources. Tisseel (Baxter), Evicel (Ethicon), and Crosseal (Ethicon) should be reserved for venous oozing whereas Floseal (Baxter) may be superior for arteriolar bleeding because of its particular tamponade effect. There is one platelet glue available in the United States. Application of platelet gel is even more complicated than most fibrin glues, requiring the patient's centrifuged blood to provide half of the product. The platelets are thought to provide a superior clot and increased growth factors during repair.

SYNTHETIC SEALANTS. Three nonbiologic glues are available.[41] Cyanoacrylate should not be used directly on vessels because of embolization risk, but is appropriate for postcapillary venule bleeding at wound edges. Polyethylene glycols (PEG) comprise a family of large polymer molecules which are widely used in every aspect of the medical, pharmacologic, and food industries. They work rapidly, are convenient to use, and serve as moderate hemostatic agents, but since PEG swells to many times its size over several days, it should not be used where vascular compression is a concern. Like biologic glues, PEG sealant is dripped onto wounds from a dual plunger syringe. Glutaraldehyde is a simple symmetric carbon and oxygen compound most frequently used as a cytotoxic agent. When covalently bound to albumin, it provides a scaffold for clots to form, but its cytotoxicity unfortunately persists and the adjacent cells are killed. For this reason, glutaraldehyde cross-linked albumin is best reserved for adult cardiac surgery.

HEMOSTATIC DRESSINGS. Fibrin, chitin, and zeolite have been added to gauze bandages, which, in conjunction with compression, can stop catastrophic bleeding. Fibrin is available as a glue or as a dressing in which lyophilized fibrinogen and thrombin coat cotton gauze. This coating increases shelf life and eliminates premixing, but the product can be prohibitively expensive and the gauze is brittle. At the present time its use should probably be restricted to the battlefield, for which purpose the Red Cross initially created it. Chitin (acetyl glucosamine) is a long chain polymer derived from glucose, making it structurally similar to cellulose. It is found in arthropod exoskeletons, where it functions like the keratin protein found in mammals and birds. Exoskeletons of shrimp and crab can be deacetylated to yield chitosan (glucosamine), a superior hemostatic agent. Chitosan achieves hemostasis by adher-

TABLE 11-4
Hemostatic Agents

Type	Substance	Name	Manufacturer
Styptics	Silver nitrate Aluminum sulfate Aluminum chloride Ferric sulfate		Various
Physical hemostats	Paraffin/beeswax Alkylene oxide	Bone wax Ostene	Ethicon Ceremed
Biodegradable hemostats	Cellulose Gelatin Collagen	Surgicel, Surgifoam Gelfoam, Gelfilm Avitene Helistat Instat	Ethicon Pfizer Davol Integra Ethicon
Biologic glues	Thrombin glue	Thrombin JMI Evithrom Recothrom	Monarch Ethicon Zymogenetics
	Fibrin glue	Tisseel, Floseal Evicel, Crosseal	Baxter Ethicon
	Platelet glue	Vitagel	Orthovita
Synthetic sealants	Cyanoacrylate PEG Glutaraldehyde	Dermabond Coseal Bioglue	Ethicon Baxter Cryolife
Hemostatic dressings	Fibrin Chitin Chitosan Zeolite	DFSD RDH HemCon QuikClot	American Red Cross Marine Polymer HemCon Medical Z-Medica

DFSD, Dry Fibrin Sealant Dressings; PEG, Polyethylene glycol; RDH, Rapid Deployment Hemostat.

ing to the wound and mechanically occluding blood vessels.[42] Zeolite is a regularly microporous aluminosilicate mineral commercially used as an adsorbent and molecular sieve.[43] As a powder, it is useful only for low-pressure wound packing. When enclosed in cotton mesh, it is more successful in staunching arterial bleeding. Blood and zeolite yield a profoundly exothermic reaction that can cause burns. For this reason, newer zeolite dressings are partially prehydrated, lessening heat production to not much more than body temperature (Table 11-4).

BANDAGES

There is no specific feature that distinguishes a bandage from a dressing. Dressings may be layered or have adhesive, and secondary dressings may be used to secure the primary dressing to the wound. However, in classical terms a bandage is external to an underlying dressing and secures the dressing in place (Table 11-5). Most bandages are wraps and tapes.

TABLE 11-5
Roles of a Bandage

- Keep the dressing clean
- Hold a wound dressing in place
- Restrict movement of the wound edges
- Improve the peripheral wound environment
- Reduce swelling and hemorrhage
- Provide support for an injured limb
- Provide pain relief

TAPE. Tape is a common way to externally fix a dressing and provide a compact, durable bandage. Most tapes have one-sided, pre-applied adhesive that was historically latex-based and is now mostly acrylate-based. A large number of tapes are available allowing the clinician to choose the appropriate level of adhesion, strength, translucence, and permeability (Table 11-6). Hair, oil, dirt, blood, and other moisture can impede the performance of tape. Additional skin adhesives may improve the performance of both dressings and bandages, but they are most commonly used with tape.

SKIN ADHESIVE. Skin adhesives can help skin stick to tape, other skin, or medicated dressing materials. Synthetic acrylates in various forms are used for most dressings and bandages with prefabricated adhesives and are used to attach skin to skin, thereby filling the role of sutures. Horticultural adhesives are volatile liquids that, when applied and dried, can augment tape's adherence to skin.

Many common liquid adhesives are derived from plant sources with geographic niches. Mastic, gum Arabic, and benzoin tincture are some examples.[44] Mastic is a pine-scented resin of a *Pistachia* tree grown on the Greek island of Chios; and gum Arabic is a resin from an *Acacia* tree

TABLE 11-6
Common Types of Tape

Type	Features	Example	Mfr
Paper	Light adhesive, permeability	Micropore Steri-strip	3M 3M
Plastic	Translucent, tends toward occlusive	Blenderm Transpore	3M 3M
Cloth silk	Woven; durable, moldable, has variable stretch along both axes (warp and woof)	Hypafix Medipore Durapore	S&N 3M 3M
Elastic	Elasticity	Elastoplast	BAG
Silicone	Light adhesive, translucent	Kindremoal	3M
Foam	Thermal and physical buffer	Microfoam	3M
Casting	Strong, profound molding	Scotchcast	3M

Mfr, manufacturer; 3M, 3M, Minneapolis, MN; S&N, Smith & Nephew, London, UK; BAG, Beiersdorf AG, Hamburg, Germany.

that grows in the Sahel, a strip of land that extends through the Sahara from the Atlantic Ocean to the Red Sea. Compound tincture of benzoin is a vanilla-scented resin from a *Styrax* tree that grows in Thailand and Indonesia. There is no chemical benzoin in tincture of benzoin, which is though to be an adulteration of the personal name Benjamin. Mastisol (Ferndale Laboratories Inc.) contains both *Pistachia* and *Styrax* resins.[45]

Nitric acid and wood pulp yield nitrocellulose/pyroxylin, that, when dissolved in ether, makes collodion, a word that means glutinous in Greek. Nitrocellulose and ether are both combustible, but collodion is not combustible when dried on skin.[46] Rather, it is flexible and sticky, a good adhesive for bandages, and now only occasionally used in liquid dressings.

Most tapes, adhesive dressings, and transdermal patches adhere to skin with the synthetic vinyl resins methacrylate and epoxy diacrylate.[47] Like lidocaine, cyanoacrylate adhesive (CA) was discovered during World War II, but was not marketed until the postwar boom. There are several CA adhesives available that vary by the length of their carbon backbone. Typical supermarket-brand glues are methyl- or ethyl-cyanoacrylate, and are used to seal hand dermatitis fissures and to provide a protective membrane for superficial wounds in athletes and string musicians. These glues are brittle and last for 1 to 2 days. Butyl-cyanoacrylate has been used as a surgical skin adhesive in Europe and as a veterinary adhesive in the United States since the 1970s. However, it was not until 1998 that octyl-cyanoacrylate was approved for human use in the United States.[48] Butyl-CA may be stronger, but octyl-CA is more flexible. Cyanoacrylate functions by polymerizing in the presence of hydroxyl molecules found in water. Blood rapidly sets CA, but otherwise its set time is on the order of minutes. Cotton bandages adhere immediately to CA and the two should not be used together during medical application. There is a wide body of dissenting literature regarding traditional suturing versus CA glue as a suture-replacing wound closure. The popular consensus seems to be that octyl-CA is faster, suturing is stronger, and that the expense and cosmesis of the two can be equivalent depending on individual usage, the product applicator, and the amount of product applied.[49]

ADHESIVE REMOVER. Plant resins and cyanoacrylate can both be slowly removed with most oils, such as mineral oil or petrolatum. Proprietary removers generally contain hydrocarbons, including heavy naphtha, which is a roughly 10 carbon, petroleum-based alkane, and mineral spirits, which are not petroleum-based and have a longer carbon backbone. These solvents are recognized by their viscosity, smell, and orange color. Acetone, in the form of nail polish remover, is widely used to remove adhesives from skin, but its medical use is discouraged because of its toxicity.

WRAP. Gauze wraps have been in existence since prehistoric times. As mentioned previously, they are a widely available product for inexpensively securing a bandage to a dressing. They offer minimal support and compression and can mechanically debride exposed wounds; they can also be absorbent, whether moistened or medicated. Unna boot is an eponymous medicated wrap created by Paul Unna. It is a zinc and ferric oxide-impregnated gauze wrap largely used for lower-extremity ulcerations. Tube bandages, generically known as stockinette, may be gauze, net, mesh, polyester, or cotton. Stockinettes apply moderate continuous pressure across the length of the bandage and are meant for durable, lightweight dressing immobilization. Self-adhering bandages are crinkled, stretchable wraps that self-cohere. Some tape may be required for a completely coherent bandage, but the tape secures the dressing to itself so that no adhesive touches the skin. As an aside, tape should always be used to secure wraps since pins can destroy wrap, dressings, and bandages, and puncture skin. Proper wrapping tension is required with all bandages, but self-cohering bandages will not accommodate further stretch if applied too tightly. One advantage of self-coherent bandages is the ability to easily reuse or reposition them once they have been placed. Elastic bandages are generally divided into short-stretch and long-stretch categories. The classic long-stretch elastic bandage is the ACE (3M), an acronym for all-cotton elastic. ACE wraps have reached their centennial; they can stretch many times their length, but tend to bunch with time. Short-stretch or lymphedema wraps are preferred for edematous or dependent wounds as they provide greater and more even compression. Compression hose may also be used to fix a dressing in place. Compression will be discussed later.

BOLSTER. A surgical bolster is a bandage that supports a graft after its placement on its new vascular bed. Although some authors have admonished against their use, bolsters are still more often used than not. The noun bolster means pillow and the verb means to support. The classic graft bolster is some form of impregnated gauze fluff tied in place with nonabsorbable sutures radiating from the wound edge. Published bolster and bolster-equivalents have also been crafted of aquaplast, polyurethane sponge, cotton wadding, cyanoacrylate glue, mepitel, allevyn, jelonet, and vacuum dressings.[50]

BANDAGING TECHNIQUES. An entire subculture, closely associated with the military, developed around bandage application. The Esmarch triangular (cravat) bandage famously has 32 different applications, some of which have been adopted by the Boy Scouts of America for their uniform and first aid practices. Roller bandages are variants of tube bandages and are used to immobilize extremities. Tailed and tube bandages have traditional applications for common injuries. As a rule, bandages should be wrapped from distal to proximal with gradually diminishing tension.

Tourniquets developed from gauze bandages, when a strip of cloth was turned until it restricted catastrophic blood flow. Although less frequently used today and seeming to have no cutaneous application, medical variants of tourniquets can be useful in restricting procedural bleeding of the distal extremity. Temporary sequential tourniquets are used for intravenous regional anesthesia (IVRA), also known as the Bier block. IVRA provides an anesthetized, exsanguinated limb for brief procedures such as botulinum toxin injection for hyperhidrosis, nail surgery, and micrographic surgery.[51]

COMPRESSION. Compression is a key feature of bandages in general, but several special situations require compression bandages. Negative-pressure wound therapy (NPWT), or vacuum assisted wound closure, utilizes a nonadherent foam base covered by an occlusive film dressing to form a seal. A single drainage tube is connected to a vacuum that evacuates both liquid in the form of wound exudate and gas. Used mostly for chronic wounds on the lower extremity, NWPT may also be used as a bolster substitute to quickly secure a large graft in place. The negative pressure is continuous, but suction may be applied either continuously or intermittently.[52]

Compression improves healing of lower-extremity wounds and can relieve vascular discomfort.[53] There are three types of compression garments for the lower leg, a pneumatic compression garment, sequential compression stockings, and anti-embolism stockings. Over-the-counter compression hose are generally known as anti-embolism stockings and provide less than 20 mm Hg compression which is unlikely to exacerbate undiagnosed vascular disease. Four classes of prescription hose are available in roughly 10 mm Hg increments for gradually worsening venous disease. Pressure is not equally exerted along the stocking. It is greatest at the ankle and diminishes toward the knee, which is why these hose are often called sequential or gradient compression stockings. It is imperative that compression does not impair arterial flow. Distal pulses should be evaluated and the ankle brachial index (ABI) should be determined. The ABI is calculated from the blood pressure (leg divided by arm) with a Doppler flow detector and sphygmomanometer at the pressure when the pulse resumes after occlusion. An ABI of 1.0 is normal, and less than 0.8 is indicative of arterial disease, a contraindication to lower-extremity compression.[54] Pneumatic compression units are complex, restrictive garments that milk recalcitrant edema from distal to proximal with sequential pressure waves. They are used primarily for chronic lymphedema of the extremity. Compression garments are a therapeutic necessity after liposuction and specialized product lines have developed around their use.

TOPICAL ENZYMES

Three topical enzymes are available to debride necrotic wounds. The collagenase Santyl (Smith & Nephew) is an ointment that can remove thick, collagenous, dermal debris without harming the remaining fragile granulation tissue.[55] It is most frequently used for burns. Papain, known as papaya proteinase I, is a cysteine proteinase derived from the South American papaya. Accuzyme (Healthpoint) and Panafil (Healthpoint) contain papain and its activator urea to enzymatically debride necrotic wounds without damaging viable tissue. In November 2008, the FDA recommended their discontinuation, citing unregulated use which had resulted in blindness and tachycardia. However, a Web search performed in July 2012 returned over 400 cumulative hits, with many seemingly active sales sites, suggesting that the product is still readily available and its side effects should, therefore, be more widely publicized. Finally, trypsin in a castor oil vehicle is made by several companies. Trypsin is a vertebrate serine protease that digests proteins by cleaving lysine or arginine.[56]

GROWTH FACTORS

Healthy, healing wounds produce an exudate that stimulates the surrounding cell lines to proliferate. Chronic wound exudate inhibits growth.[57] There are a surprising number of identifiable factors in exudate.[58] The factors that are thought to be most important are listed in Table 11-7. In general these factors encourage angiogenesis and differentiation of cellular lines such as fibroblasts, keratinocytes, and lymphocytes.[59] Advances in molecular biology have not only allowed the identities of those growth factors to be determined, but have also allowed their production. Application of growth factors both individually and together has been shown to improve healing.

Although each factor has been investigated in turn, only three products are currently marketed for human administration.[60] First, platelet derived growth factor (PDGF) has three isomers. The BB subunit, becaplermin, has been developed and marketed as Regranex (Healthpoint) since 2002. Its use has been restricted to chronic lower-extremity wounds and it works best to promote angiogenesis on a clean vascularized base. In patients with previous known malignancy, death from metastasis is five times greater if more than two tubes (>30 g) are used, prompting the FDA to issue a black box warning in June 2009. Platelet rich plasma is a technique that produces a five times concentrated platelet product for direct autodeposition on a debrided chronic wound. It is thought that the alpha granules in the platelets provide concentrated PDGF as well as other growth factors.[61] Finally, epidermal growth factor (EGF) may improve chronic leg wound repair.[62,63] EGF is also used in anti-aging cosmetics.

TABLE 11-7
Growth Factors Known to Affect Cutaneous Healing

Growth Factor Families	Produced By	Act On	Known Primary Functions
Epidermal			
EGF	Platelets	Endothelial cells Fibroblast	Mediates angiogenesis, mesenchymal/epidermal mitogen
TGF-α	Keratinocytes Platelets	Keratinocytes	
Fibroblast			
FGF	Macrophages Fibroblasts	Endothelial cells Fibroblasts	Mesenchymal mitogen
KGF	Fibroblasts	Epithelial	Epidermal mitogen
Granulocyte			
GCSF	Endothelial cells Macrophages	WBC	Angiogenesis, hematopoietic mitogen
IL-6	T lymphocytes Macrophages	B Lymphocytes	Proinflammatory, hematopoietic mitogen
Insulin-like			
IGF	Fibroblasts Macrophages Platelets	Endothelial cells Fibroblasts	Epithelial migration, mesenchymal mitogen
Interleukin 8			
IL-8	Endothelial cells Epithelial cells Macrophages	WBC	Inflammatory chemotaxis
Platelet-derived			
PDGF	Endothelial cells Fibroblasts	Fibroblasts WBC	Mesenchymal, hematopoietic migration
VEGF	Keratinocytes Macrophages	Endothelial cells	Angiogenesis
Transforming			
TGF-β	Fibroblasts Keratinocytes Lymphocytes Macrophages Platelets	Endothelial cells Fibroblasts Keratinocytes Macrophages	Inhibits proliferation of most cell types; prominent mesenchymal regulator; angiogenesis

EGF, FGF, IGF, KGF, PDGF, TGF, VEGF, epidermal, fibroblast, insulin-like, keratinocyte, platelet derived, transforming, vascular endothelial growth factors respectively; IL, Interleukin; GCSF, granulocyte colony stimulating factor.

HYPERBARIC OXYGEN THERAPY

Hyperbaric oxygen therapy (HBOT) provides an oxygen pressure greater than that of atmospheric pressure and also provides an increased respiratory oxygen concentration, which may be helpful in treating a variety of disorders. Average sea level atmospheric pressure is roughly 1 bar (14.5 psi) and decreases with elevation. Professional medical HBOT chambers can be pressurized to 6 bar, but utilization requires proximity to a regional medical center. Prescription home medical or portable units can be pressurized to 0.5 bar above local atmospheric pressure which may not be great enough for many indications. Oxygen concentration is generally increased to as much as 100% with an oxygen helmet or mask with intermittent air breaks during which 21% oxygen (air) is breathed. Professional treatment sessions, called dives, are pressurized cycles lasting 60 to 90 minutes. In the United States, the expense can vary widely, but hospital-based sessions cost $1000 to $2000. More than 50 sessions are typically prescribed.[64] When approved by Medicare, collections maximized at $50,000 are allowed. Proponents of HBOT for lower-leg ulcerations, specifically diabetic foot and leg ulcerations, state that its use is statistically associated with fewer patient procedures, fewer amputations, and greater wound healing.[65]

POSTPROCEDURAL WOUND CARE

HISTORY. By the mid-nineteenth century, scientific bias was firmly settled on escherization, the fathers of antisepsis believing that less purulence in an undressed wound meant fewer infections. After World War II, lesser-known studies reported that occlusion improved healing

TABLE 11-8
Topical Antiseptics[75]

	Spectrum	Use	Disadvantages
Liquids			
Isopropyl/ethyl alcohol	Broad	Site prep	Drying, flammable
Povidone	G+	Site prep	Efficacy removed by washing, blood, cytotoxic (at high concentrations)
Chlorhexidine	Broad	Site prep; Persistent effect if removed	
Acetic acid	Broad		Cytotoxic (at high concentrations)
Hydrogen peroxide	Minimal	Post-op scrub; Effervescence and chemical debridement	
Sodium hypochlorite	Broad	Staphlococcal decolonization wash	Drying
Creams and ointments			
Bacitracin			Contact allergy
Neomycin	G+		Staphylococcal resistance, contact allergy
Mupirocin	Broad	Staphylococcal decolonization around nares	
Sulfadiazine	Broad	Popular for burns	Inhibits reepithelialization
Nitrafurazone	Broad		Inhibits reepithelialization
Benzoyl peroxide	Broad	Many vehicles	10% contact allergy

G+/−, Gram positive, negative; [hi], high concentration.

in human burn scars and vascular stasis ulcerations.[66–69] This culminated in the now-famous George Winter study showing that controlled porcine skin wounds healed better and faster with a hydrating dressing.[70] Two years later, dermatologists repeated this study in humans and the era of moist healing was born.[71] Moist healing increases eschar autolysis, increases local growth factors, and reduces barriers to epidermal migration while creating a voltage gradient that improves epidermal migration.

WOUND INFECTION. Anti-infectives may be used as prophylaxis or treatment, may be used before, during, or after the procedure, and may be orally ingested or topically applied. Oral antibiotics are covered elsewhere. Topical antiseptics are typically liquids or ointments (Table 11-8). For mechanical reasons, ointment use is limited to postprocedure care. Most liquids are used for site preparation, but they may also be used for postprocedure care, like hydrogen peroxide. Isopropyl alcohol and chlorhexidine are common and effective liquids for site preparation. The flammability of alcohol may limit its use for some procedures. Bleach baths and nasal mupirocin can be helpful to preoperatively limit staphylococcal colonization. Because of their limited bacterial spectrum and widespread resistance, there is no compelling evidence that antibiotic ointments are superior to vehicle for routine wound care.[72,73] Both bacitracin (2003) and neomycin (2010) have been nominated in the past as the contact allergen of the year.[74]

PROTOTYPICAL CARE FOR A POSTSURGICAL CUTANEOUS WOUND. Most of the products listed in this chapter are intended for chronic wounds. The very existence of a chronic wound implies that something is awry. However, surgical wounds are acute and most heal without expensive or complicated care. Surgical wounds heal by either primary intent, that is, by approximation of some sort, secondary intent, which is granulation, grafting, or a combination of these techniques.

Primarily approximated wounds will epithelialize in about a week depending on site, blood supply, and other factors, at which point the superficial sutures will have accomplished their goal. The purpose of postoperative approximated-wound care is to (1) remove crust and (2) prevent its reformation. For crust removal, clinicians tend to express personal preferences for water, soap and water, saline, dilute peroxide, 3% peroxide, bleach wash, or benzoyl peroxide washes. Most clinicians recommend 3% peroxide as it is inexpensive, cleans thoroughly, has some antibacterial cytotoxic effect, and has an effervescence that gratifies caregivers and patients. However, other clinicians err on the side of prudence for the same cytotoxic reasons and recommend only soap and shower water. As with chronic wounds, lubrication is the most critical step, which is easily accomplished with topical petrolatum. Dressing occlusion is generally unnecessary if lubrication is generous, but a simple composite bandage may prevent accidental removal of petrolatum, especially during sleep and under clothing.

One of the unintended successes of Mohs micrographic surgery is a detailed knowledge of normal wound granulation.[3] Retrospective analysis of decades of granulated wounds resulted in a refined understanding of the timing, results, and complications of second intent healing. Any of the chronic wound-care products can certainly be used for granulating wounds. Alginates, collagens, and foams are useful for exudative wounds; hydrocolloids and hydrogels are useful for hydrating wounds. However, the techniques used for approximated wounds are often equally effective. Occlusion with a composite dressing may lessen caregiver duties, with its convenience justifying its expense.

The use of bandages, dressings, and wound care is a creative art aided by an ever-expanding armamentarium of products. Working knowledge of both time-tested standards as well as the burgeoning advances is essential for any health professional caring for cutaneous wounds. The attentive clinician should be able to discern what is good or untoward in any class of wound and craft both a bandage and a wound-care regimen to speed healing.

REFERENCES

1. Davis P, Kenrick P. *Fossil Plants*. Washington, DC: Smithsonian Books, 2004.
2. Hess CT, ed. *Clinical Guide: Wound Care*. 5th ed. Springhouse, PA: Lippincott Williams & Wilkins; 2004.
3. Falanga V, Zitelli JA, Eaglstein WH. Wound healing. *J Am Acad Dermatol*. 1988;19(3):559–563.
4. Fonder MA, Lazarus GS, Cowan DA, Aronson-Cook B, Kohli AR, Mamelak AJ. Treating the chronic wound: a practical approach to the care of nonhealing wounds and wound care dressings. *J Am Acad Dermatol*. 2008;58(2):185–206.
5. Stadelmann WK, Digenis AG, Tobin GR. Physiology and healing dynamics of chronic cutaneous wounds. *Am J Surg*. 1998;176(2A Suppl):26S–38S.
6. Midwood KS, Williams LV, Schwarzbauer JE. Tissue repair and the dynamics of the extracellular matrix. *Int J Biochem Cell Biol*. 2004;36(6):1031–1037.
7. Jones V, Grey JE, Harding KG. ABC of wound healing: wound dressings. *BMJ*. 2006;332:777–780.
8. Remminghorst U, Rehm BHA. Microbial production of alginate: biosynthesis and applications. In: Rehm BHA, ed. *Microbial Production of Biopolymers and Polymer Precursors: Applications and Perspectives*. Norfolk, VA: Caister Academic Press; 2009.
9. Piacquadio D, Nelson DB Alginates. A "new" dressing alternative. *J Dermatol Surg Oncol*. 1992;18(11):992–995.
10. Thomas S. Hydrocolloid dressings in the management of acute wounds: a review of the literature. *Int Wound J*. 2008;5(5):602–613.
11. Dumville JC, O'Meara S, Deshpande S, Speak K. Hydrogel dressings for healing diabetic foot ulcers. *Cochrane Database Syst Rev*. 2011(9):CD009101.
12. Fletcher J. Understanding wound dressings: foam dressings. *Nurs Times*. 2005;101(24):50–51.
13. Lionelli GT., Lawrence WT. Wound dressings. *Surg Clin N Am*. 2003;83(3):617–638.
14. Robins P, Goldberg L, Moy R, et al. The effectiveness of liquid bandage as an adhesive and antimicrobial agent. *J Drugs Derm*. 2008;7(8):764–766.
15. Takeda U, Izawa M, Koeda T, Shibata U. Laboratory studies of collagen wound dressing (CAS). Part I. Experimental use on skin excisions and burns. *J Dermatol*. 1983;10(5):475–486.
16. Stern R. Hyaluronan catabolism: a new metabolic pathway. *Eur J Cell Biol*. 2004;83(7): 317–325.
17. Matou-Nasri S, Gaffney J, Kumar S, Slevin M. Oligosaccharides of hyaluronan induce angiogenesis through distinct CD44 and RHAMM-mediated signalling pathways involving Cdc2 and gamma-adducin. *Int J Oncol*. 2009;35(4):761–773.
18. www.bandaid,com. Accessed July, 2012.
19. Bello YM, Falabella AF, Eaglstein WH. Tissue-engineered skin. Current status in wound healing. *Am J Clin Dermatol*. 2001;2:305–313.
20. Supp DM, Boyce ST. Engineered skin substitutes: practices and potentials. *Clin Dermatol*. 2005; 23(4);403–412.
21. Wright KA, Nadire KB, Busto P, Tubo R, McPherson JM, Wentworth BM. Alternative delivery of keratinocytes using a polyurethane membrane and the implications for its use in the treatment of full-thickness burn injury. *Burns*. 1998;24:7–17.
22. Lobmann R, Pittasch D, Muhlen I, Lehnert H. Autologous human keratinocytes cultured on membranes composed of benzyl ester of hyaluronic acid for grafting in nonhealing diabetic foot lesions: a pilot study. *J Diabetes Complications*. 2003;17:199–204.
23. Uhlig C, Rapp M, Hartmann H, Hierlemann H, Planck H, Dittel KK. Suprathel-An innovative, resorbable skin substitute for the treatment of burn victims. *Burns*. 2007;33:221–229.
24. Hodde JP, Ernst DM, Hiles MC. An investigation of the long-term bioactivity of endogenous growth factor in OASIS Wound Matrix. *J Wound Care*. 2005;14:23–25.
25. Harper C. Permacol: clinical experience with a new biomaterial. *Hosp Med*. 2001;62:90–95.
26. Wainwright DJ. Use of an acellular allograft dermal matrix (Alloderm) in the management of full-thickness burns. *Burns*. 1995;21:243–248.
27. Boyd M, Flasza M, Johnson PA, Roberts JS, Kemp P. Integration and persistence of an investigational human living skin equivalent (ICX-SKN) in human surgical wounds. *Regen Med*. 2007;2:369–376.
28. Omar AA, Mavor AI, Jones AM, Homer-Vanniasinkam S. Treatment of venous leg ulcers with Dermagraft. *Eur J Vasc Endovasc Surg*. 2004;27:666–672.
29. Lukish JR, Eichelberger MR, Newman KD, et al. The use of a bioactive skin substitute decreases length of stay for pediatric burn patients. *J Pediatr Surg*. 2001;36:1118–1121.
30. McHugh TP, Robson MC, Heggers JP, Phillips LG, Smith DJ Jr, McCollum MC. Therapeutic efficacy of Biobrane in partial- and full-thickness thermal injury. *Surgery*. 1986;100:661–664.
31. Groos N, Guillot M, Zilliox R, Braye FM. Use of an artificial dermis (Integra) for the reconstruction of extensive burn scars in children. About 22 grafts. *Eur J Pediatr Surg*. 2005;15: 187–192.
32. Trent JF, Kirsner RS. Tissue engineered skin: apligraf, a bi-layered living skin equivalent. *Int J Clin Pract*. 1998;52: 408–413.
33. Hasegawa T, Suga Y, Mizoguchi M, et al. Clinical trial of allogeneic cultured dermal substitute for the treatment of intractable skin ulcers in 3 patients with recessive dystrophic epidermolysis bullosa. *J Am Acad Dermatol*. 2004;50:803–804.
34. Hauben DJ, Baruchin A, Mahler A. On the history of the free skin graft. *Ann Plast Surg*. 1982;9(3):242–245.
35. Smahel J. The healing of skin grafts. *Clin Plast Surg*. 1977; 4(3):409–424.
36. Goldberg HC. Monsel's solution. *J Am Acad Dermatol*. 1981; 5:613.
37. Epstein E, Maibach HI. Monsel's Solution: history, chemistry, and efficacy. *Arch Dermatol*. 1964;90:226–228.
38. Wang MY, Armstrong JK, Fisher TC. A new, pluronic-based, bone hemostatic agent that does not impair osteogenesis. *Neurosurgery*. 2001;49:962–967.
39. Schonauer C, Tessitore E, Barbagallo G, Albanese V, Moraci A. The use of local agents: bone wax, gelatin, collagen, oxidized cellulose. *Eur Spine J*. 2004;13(Suppl 1):S89–S96.
40. Palm MD, Altman JS. Topical hemostatic agents: a review. *Dermatol Surg*. 2008;34(4):431–445.
41. Achneck HE, Sileshi B, Jamiolkowski RM, Albala DM, Shapiro ML, Lawson JH. A comprehensive review of topical hemostatic agents: efficacy and recommendations for use. *Ann Surg*. 2010;251(2):217–228.
42. Bhuvanesh G, Abha A, Shalini S, Mohammad SA. Preparation of chitosan–polyethylene glycol coated cotton membranes for wound dressings: preparation and characterization. *Polymers Advan Technol*. 2008;20:58–65.
43. Auerbach SM, Carrado KA, Dutta PK, eds. *Handbook of Zeolite Science and Technology*. Boca Raton, FL: CRC Press; 2003.
44. Smolinske SC, ed. *CRC Handbook of Food, Drug, and Cosmetic Excipients*. Boca Raton, FL: CRC Press; 1992.
45. Material Safety Data Sheet. Mastisol® liquid adhesive. www.delasco.com/pcat/pdf/mastisol.pdf. Accessed July, 2012.
46. Brown GI. *The Big Bang: A History of explosives*. Charleston, SC: History Press; 2005.
47. Kanerva L, Alanko K. Allergic contact dermatitis from 2-hydroxyethyl methacrylate in an adhesive on an electrosurgical earthing plate. *Eur J Dermatol*. 1998;8(7):521–524.
48. Singer AJ, McClain SA, Katz A. A porcine epistaxis model: hemostatic effects of octylcyanoacrylate. *Otolaryngol Head Neck Surg*. 2004;130(5):553–557.
49. Bernard L, Doyle J, Friedlander SF, Eichenfield LF, Gibbs NF, Cunningham BB. A prospective comparison of octyl cyanoacrylate tissue adhesive (dermabond) and suture for the closure of excisional wounds in children and adolescents. *Arch Dermatol*. 2001;137(9):1177–1180.

50. Weinfeld AB, Kelley P, Yuksel E, et al. Circumferential negative-pressure dressing (VAC) to bolster skin grafts in the reconstruction of the penile shaft and scrotum. *Ann Plast Surg.* 2005;54(2):178–183.
51. Solomon P. Modified Bier block anesthetic technique is safe for office use for botulinum A toxin treatment of palmar and plantar hyperhidrosis. *Dermatol Online J.* 2007;13(3):6.
52. Xie X, McGregor M, Dendukuri N. The clinical effectiveness of negative pressure wound therapy: a systematic review. *J Wound Care.* 2010;19(11):490–495.
53. Kantor J, Margolis DJ. Management of leg ulcers. *Semin Cutan Med Surg.* 2003;22(3):212–221.
54. McDermott MM, Criqui MH, Liu K, et al. Lower ankle/brachial index, as calculated by averaging the dorsalis pedis and posterior tibial arterial pressures, and association with leg functioning in peripheral arterial disease. *J Vasc Surg.* 2000;32(6):1164–1171.
55. Shi L, Carson D. Collagenase Santyl ointment: a selective agent for wound debridement. *J Wound Ostomy Continence Nurs.* 2009;36(6 Suppl):S12–S16.
56. Traversa B, Sussman G. The role of growth factors, cytokines and proteases in wound management. *Prim Intention.* 2001;9(4):161–167.
57. Bucalo B, Eaglestein WH, Falanga V. Inhibition of cell proliferation by chronic wound fluid. *Wound Repair Regen.* 1993; 1:181–186.
58. Braund R, Hook S, Medlicott NJ. The role of topical growth factors in chronic wounds. *Cur Drug Deliv.* 2007;4(3):195–204.
59. Fitzpatrick RE. Endogenous growth factors as cosmeceuticals. *Dermatol Surg.* 2005;31(7 pt 2):827–831.
60. Langer A, Rogowski W. Systematic review of economic evaluations of human cell-derived wound care products for the treatment of venous leg and diabetic foot ulcers. *BMC Health Serv Res.* 2009;9:115–121.
61. Schade VL, Roukis TS. Use of platelet-rich plasma with split-thickness skin grafts in the high-risk patient. *Foot Ankle Spec.* 2008;1(3):155–159.
62. Falanga V, Eaglstein WH, Bucalo B, Katz MH, Harris B, Carson P. Topical use of human recombinant epidermal growth factor (h-EGF) in venous ulcers. *J Dermatol Surg Oncol.* 1992;18(7):604–606.
63. Brown GL, Nanney LB, Griffen J, et al. Enhancement of wound healing by topical treatment with epidermal growth factor. *N Engl J Med.* 1989;321:76–79.
64. Kranke P, Bennett M, Roeckl-Wiedmann I, Debus S. Hyperbaric oxygen therapy for chronic wounds. *Cochrane Database Syst Rev.* 2004;(2):CD004123.
65. Duzgan AP, Satir HZ, Ozozan O, Saylam B, Kulah B, Coskun F. Effect of hyperbaric oxygen therapy on healing of diabetic foot ulcers. *J Foot Ankle Surg.* 2008;47:515–519.
66. Bloom H. Cellophane dressings for second degree burns. *Lancet.* 1945;246:559–563.
67. Bull JP, Squire JR, Topley E. Experiments with occlusive dressings of a new plastic. *Lancet.* 1948; 2(6519):213–215.
68. Gilje O. On taping (adhesive tape treatment) of leg ulcers. *Acta Dermato-Venereol.* 1948;28(5):454–467.
69. Schilling RS, Roberts N, Goodman M. Clinical trial of occlusive plastic dressings. *Lancet.* 1950;1(6599):293–296.
70. Winter GD. Formation of the scab and the rate of epithelialization of superficial wounds in the skin of the young domestic pig. *Nature.* 1962;193:293–294.
71. Hinman CD, Maibach HI. Effect of air exposure and occlusion on experimental human skin wounds. *Nature.* 1963;200:377–378.
72. Naidoo J, Noble WC. Acquisition of antibiotic resistance by *Staphylococcus aureus* in skin patients. *J Clin Pathol.* 1978;31(12):1187–1192.
73. Lowbury JL, Babb JR, Brown VI, Collins BJ. Neomycin-resistant *Staphylococcus aureus* in a burns unit. *J Hyg (Lond).* 1964;62(2):221–228.
74. American Contact Dermatitis Society. http://www.contactderm.org. Accessed July, 2012.
75. CDC. Disinfection & sterilization guideline:disinfection. HICPAC www.cdc.gov/hicpac/disinfection_sterilization/6_0 disinfection.html. Accessed July, 2012.

SECTION 2

Surgical Skills

CHAPTER 12

Biopsy Techniques

Anthony M. Rossi, Erica H. Lee, & Kishwer S. Nehal

INTRODUCTION

A skin biopsy is defined as sampling of the integumentary system for histologic evaluation and is a powerful diagnostic tool for the dermatologist. Although a biopsy may seem straightforward, its utility is enhanced when the clinician understands its applications and limitations. As with all diagnostic tools, the pretest probability that a patient will have a specific disease takes into account the prevalence of the disease and the clinical findings. A histological diagnosis should then be clinically correlated with the physician's differential diagnosis. A skin biopsy is considered the gold standard for the diagnosis of skin lesions and requires that the clinician be familiar with certain key concepts.

USES AND INDICATIONS

The skin biopsy has several indications[1]:

Establishing or excluding a cutaneous diagnosis
Monitoring the evolution of a disease or treatment effects
Determining the extent of a skin tumor
Tissue sampling for culture (bacterial, fungal, or viral organisms)
Tissue for genetic or gene rearrangement evaluations (T-cell lymphomas)
Cosmetic removal of tissue

After the decision to perform a biopsy has been made, prior to obtaining consent, the type of biopsy and site selection with relevant photography should be performed. In addition, relevant medical history, anesthesia selection, and consideration of antibiotic prophylaxis should be reviewed.

SITE AND LESION SELECTION

The selection of a representative lesion takes into account the best site for diagnosis and cosmesis. When there is a single lesion, biopsy site selection is straightforward. If the disease process is more diffuse, as in exanthems, then proper site selection is important. There are anatomical locations that are more amenable to healing and less prone to scar development. In addition, there are areas that may be prone to a higher background of histological change, which could then obscure key histologic findings. Generally, it is best to avoid performing biopsies below the knee if possible because of the increased risk of infection and delayed wound healing. Sites overlying joints also have a poorer healing outcome and potential for worsened scarring. The back often heals with stretched scars and is a site in which wound care can be logistically difficult to perform.[2] If possible, biopsy of the central face should be avoided for cosmetic reasons.

Of equal importance is selection of the lesion to be biopsied. Morphological appearance and the clinician's suspicion of the pathology will guide the choice of where the biopsy should be performed. For a biopsy of a possible cancer, it is best to sample the entire growth. If this is not feasible, then the thickest portion of the tumor should be biopsied to best assess the depth of the neoplasm. For inflammatory disorders, the most recent lesion will generally be most diagnostic. This is especially true when a diagnosis of vasculitis is suspected. To improve diagnostic accuracy, it is important to avoid any necrotic, excoriated, or secondarily infected lesions. For primary vesicles or bullae, the edge of the lesion and perilesional skin should be biopsied (for direct immunofluorescence (DIF) biopsy site selection, see section on TISSUE PROCESSING). In primary ulcers or necrotic lesions, the edge of the lesion and adjacent normal skin should be sampled, as many ulcer edges may show pseudoepitheliomatous or secondary changes. In annular patches or plaques, the edge will usually demonstrate more "active" disease as compared to the center (Table 12-1).

The suspected level of pathology will also guide biopsy selection, since certain dermatologic disorders affect the

TABLE 12-1
Lesion Type and Corresponding Biopsy

Lesion Type	Recommended Type and Site of Biopsy
Suspected malignant neoplasm	Excisional biopsy or sampling of thickest portion of tumor
Inflammatory disorders	Most recent lesion
Primary vesicle or bulla	Edge of lesion plus perilesional skin
Ulcer	Edge of ulcer plus perilesional skin
Annular patches/plaques	Advancing edge
Suspected panniculitis	Incisional biopsy or double punch technique

deeper layers of the dermis (i.e., morphea), subcutaneous fat (i.e., panniculitis), or fascia (i.e., eosinophilic fasciitis). If a superficial biopsy is performed in these cases, the histological diagnosis may be missed completely. A superficial biopsy of a neoplasm can also at times yield inconclusive results, leading to a need for rebiopsy.

PREOPERATIVE EVALUATION

Although a skin biopsy is a low-risk procedure, it is still important to review the patient's medical history. A standardized checklist is recommended before proceeding. Reviewing the medical history will alert the physician to any underlying conditions that may lead to poor or delayed wound healing or impaired hemostasis (Table 12-2).

TABLE 12-2
Prebiopsy Checklist

Medications	Anticoagulants: warfarin; clopidogrel; dabigatran; dipyridamole; aspirin; nonsteroidal anti-inflammatories (NSAIDs); Homeopathic medications
Allergies	Lidocaine, epinephrine, bacitracin, latex, adhesive
Medical history	Diabetes; hepatitis; bleeding diathesis; pregnancy; tobacco use; lymph node dissection; facial herpes; keloid/hypertrophic scar
Orthopedic history	Joint replacement
Cardiac history	Endocarditis; pacemaker/defibrillator; congenital heart defect; artificial heart valves/stent; hypertension/heart disease
Immunosuppression	Solid organ transplantation; immunosuppressive medication; HIV/AIDS; chemotherapy
Other relevant history	Radiation, neutropenia, other

It is currently not recommended to stop anticoagulation, including aspirin or warfarin,[3] for a routine skin biopsy. The risks and consequences of a thrombotic event secondary to changes in anticoagulation outweigh the risk of cutaneous bleeding complications.[4] Multiple studies have analyzed the outcomes of patients undergoing skin surgery while on anticoagulant medications. Alcalay reported that no significant bleeding events occurred in 16 patients undergoing cutaneous skin surgery while on warfarin therapy compared to 77 control patients.[5] Cook-Norris et al.[6] conducted a retrospective review of patients undergoing cutaneous surgery and showed that clopidogrel-containing anticoagulation was 28 times more likely than no anticoagulation and six times more likely than aspirin monotherapy to result in severe complications after Mohs surgical procedures ($p < 0.001$ and $p = 0.022$, respectively). In a meta-analysis, Lewis et al. concluded that while low, the risk of bleeding among anticoagulated patients may be greater than that of patients not taking anticoagulants. Among patients taking aspirin or warfarin, 1.3% and 5.7%, respectively, experienced a severe postoperative complication. Patients taking warfarin had an approximately seven times greater incidence of moderate-to-severe complications compared to controls (OR, 6.69; 95% CI, 3.03–14.7, $p < 0.001$), while patients taking aspirin or NSAIDs were more than twice as likely to have a moderate-to-severe complication compared to controls (OR, 2.0; 95% CI, 0.97–4.13, $p = 0.06$).[7] Although these studies examined skin surgeries, these same principles apply to biopsies as well, since even a routine biopsy can lead to significant bleeding in anticoagulated patients. The use of herbal supplements or homeopathic medications such as garlic supplements may also increase the risk of bleeding. Strict attention should be given to proper hemostasis and postoperative wound care in the anticoagulated patient.

ANTIBIOTIC PROPHYLAXIS

The risk of infection after a skin biopsy is low. Wright et al.[8] analyzed data from four different studies and estimated the risk of bacteremia from dermatologic procedures at 1.9%. There are specific circumstances, however, in which antibiotic prophylaxis is recommended for skin surgery. It is, therefore, important to be familiar with the current guidelines for antibiotic prophylaxis for bacterial endocarditis and hematologic joint infection (see chapter 9).[9] There are also certain clinical scenarios that may increase the risk of infection, requiring appropriate preprocedure precautions to be taken. For patients with total joint replacements who are in the immediate postoperative period, we recommend consulting with the patient's orthopedic surgeon. When biopsies must be performed in areas of previous lymph node dissection or lymphedema, precautions against infection should be taken. For neutropenic patients, sterile technique is recommended. It is at the discretion of the clinician to decide whether antibiotic prophylaxis should be given (Table 12-3).

Dixon et al. evaluated 5091 lesions that were surgically removed without pre- or postprocedure antibiotics. The overall rate of surgical site infections was low, but in certain situations the rate was greater than 5%, including

TABLE 12-3
Clinical Factors Favoring Use of Antibiotic Prophylaxis

Wound location	Increased risk of infection when wounds are located in particular anatomic sites such as the lip, the ear, the perineum, the inguinal area, and below the knee[10]
Type of procedure	Biopsy invading mucosa
Skin condition	Clean versus contaminated wounds
Patient variables	Lymph node dissection; immunosuppressed patients due to HIV/AIDS, malignancy, chemotherapy, uncontrolled diabetes

procedures performed in the groin, skin grafts, wedge excisions of the lip or ear, and procedures below the knee.[10]

When the biopsy site is prepped with an antimicrobial topical preparation it is considered to be a "clean" procedure, but this is not the case if the area is already infected or contaminated, or if there is mucosal involvement. For most biopsies, there is no need for pre- or post-antibiotic prophylaxis, although prophylaxis may be considered for procedures below the knee, wedge biopsies of the lip and ear, and lesions in the groin, as well as in patients with uncontrolled diabetes, alcoholism, malnutrition, and immunosuppression.

INFORMED CONSENT

Prior to the biopsy a comprehensive discussion of the technique, rationale, risks, benefits, possible outcomes, and alternatives between the clinician and patient should be performed (see chapter 3) (Table 12-4).[11]Patients are encouraged to ask questions and restate information in their own words before proceeding.

PHOTOGRAPHY

High-resolution standardized digital images are encouraged to document lesion morphology and location. A digital image will also aid in identification of the biopsy site if additional management, such as excision or Mohs micrographic surgery, is indicated at a later time. McGinness et al. conducted a study of 271 surgical sites and asked patients undergoing Mohs surgery to indentify their lesion site without preoperative photography. In this study, the patient incorrectly identified 45 of 271 surgical sites (16.6%), and the physician incorrectly identified 16 of 271 surgical sites (5.9%). However, all surgical sites were correctly identified when preoperative biopsy-site photography was used.[12] Images should be taken to capture the biopsy site and a topographical landmark to aid in future identification. Patient images are part of the medical record and therefore subject to Health Insurance Portability and Accountability Act (HIPAA) compliance (see chapter 6).

TABLE 12-4
Informed Consent Components for Skin Biopsy

Rationale/benefits	Reason for biopsy
Technique	Type of biopsy, methods of anesthesia, hemostasis, suturing and wound dressing
Alternatives	Observation
Risks	Include any potential complications (bleeding, infection, scar, numbness, pain); inconclusive diagnosis; risk of no biopsy/delay in diagnosis

BIOPSY STEPS

For all biopsies, a standardized site preparation protocol is essential both for efficiency and patient safety. The Joint Commission on Accreditation of Healthcare Organization (JCAHO) recommends a sequential order of steps. These include: marking the site with a surgical pen, a "time out" for patient and site identification, cleansing the biopsy site with a topical antimicrobial, draping the site if necessary, and finally anesthetizing the area.

ANTIMICROBIAL PREPARATION

The use of topical antimicrobial cleansing agents prior to a skin biopsy is an important step in the prevention of surgical site infections. Ideally, the antiseptic should be quick acting, provide a sustained duration of action, have a broad antimicrobial spectrum, and be nonallergenic. The most common antimicrobial agents used for biopsies include 70% alcohol, povidone-iodine, and chlorhexidine gluconate (Table 12-5).[13–16]

Darouchie et al. compared the rate of surgical site infections using povidone-iodine versus a chlorhexidine-alcohol preoperative skin scrub during clean-contaminated surgeries. The chlorhexidine-alcohol group had a lower overall rate of surgical site infection, superficial incisional infection and deep incisional infections. There were no significant differences in adverse events.[17]

ANESTHESIA

The majority of cutaneous biopsies require the use of local injectable anesthetics, though topical anesthesia may be used in select circumstances (see chapter 4). The mainstay of anesthesia for skin biopsies is injectable 1% or 2% lidocaine (Pregnancy Category B), with or without epinephrine (1:100,000 to 1:200,000). Lidocaine is an amide anesthetic and metabolized by the hepatic microsomal enzymes. Therefore, caution should be taken in patients with severe liver dysfunction. The use of epinephrine promotes vasoconstriction, which takes approximately 15 minutes to occur. Counteracting the vasodilatory effects of the anesthetic, epinephrine aids in hemostasis, and prolongs the anesthetic effect by slowing its clearance. A concentration of 1:10,00,000 is the lowest that can achieve

TABLE 12-5
Topical Antimicrobial Preparations[14–16]

Group	Spectrum	Onset	Sustained Activity	Comments
Alcohol 60%–95%	Gram +/–; *Mycobacterium Tuberculosis*; fungi; enveloped viruses	Fastest	None	No spores; flammable
Povidone-iodine	Gram +/–	Fast	None	Sensitivity
Iodophor (betadine)	Gram +/–	Moderate	Up to 1 h; intermediate to minimal if wiped from the skin	Effective dry; skin absorption; Potential systemic toxicity with neonates or large surface area
Hexachlorophene (pHisoHex)	Gram +	Slow	Yes	Teratogen; neurotoxic
Chlorhexidine (hibiclens)	Gram +/–; *M.Tuberculosis*; fungi; enveloped viruses	Fast	Yes; *Additive effect with repeated use*	Eye irritation; ototoxic
Benzalkonium	Gram +/–	Slow	None	Nonirritating

effective vasoconstriction. Epinephrine is a beta and alpha agonist and its use is contraindicated in patients with hyperthyroidism and pheochromocytoma. It should be used with caution in patients taking beta-blockers, monoamine oxidase inhibitors, tricyclic antidepressants, and phenothiazines, as these patients may be more sensitive to its effects. Caution should also be exercised when using epinephrine in patients with severe hypertension, cardiovascular disease, or narrow angle glaucoma.[18]

The use of epinephrine in anesthesia of the digits or closed spaces (ears, penis) has been controversial for fear of necrosis secondary to vasoconstriction. However, multiple studies have refuted this concern and show epinephrine to be safe.[19] In the few cases of digital necrosis, vessel compression due to the tamponade effect of excessive anesthetic volume was cited as the cause. Epinephrine is however, contraindicated for digital anesthesia in patients with severe peripheral vascular disease. Side effects associated with epinephrine include palpitations, tachycardia, elevated blood pressure, and headache, which tend to be self-limited and more common when injection occurs in highly vascular areas such as the face and scalp.

Common adverse effects of local anesthesia include vasovagal reactions (hypotension, bradycardia, diaphoresis, syncope) and can be mitigated by reassuring the patient, placing them in supine or Trendelenburg position, and using techniques to minimize pain. True allergic reactions to local anesthetics (Type I, IgE-mediated) are rare and represent less than 1% of adverse reactions to local anesthesia. If a patient has a true allergy to both amide and ester anesthetics, other choices for local anesthesia include injections of normal saline with benzyl alcohol preservative or 1% diphenhydramine with or without epinephrine.[20]

Measures taken to minimize the pain associated with local injections include:

- Use of topical anesthesia (important in children)
- Verbal distraction
- Mechanical distraction such as pinching the site, or application of cold/ice or a vibratory stimulus
- The use of smaller needles (30 gauge)
- Quick needle insertion with slow injection
- Buffering the anesthetic to a physiologic pH with sodium bicarbonate
- Warming the anesthetic

The depth of injection is guided by the type of skin biopsy. Injection into the subcutis is less painful than a dermal injection but requires 5 to 10 minutes for the anesthetic effects to reach the skin surface. Injection in the superficial dermis to create a "wheal" is more painful but provides immediate anesthesia. This wheal effect also creates an elevated firm platform, which facilitates shave biopsies.

HEMOSTASIS

The degree of bleeding is related to the type of biopsy and the anticoagulation status of the patient. The most common types of hemostatic agents include: chemical agents, electrosurgery, and suturing. Prolonged compression can also facilitate hemostasis. Certain hemostatic agents are better suited for specific biopsy techniques and will be discussed later.

For superficial biopsies such as shaves, snips, or curettes, a chemical hemostatic agent, or styptic, should suffice. Twenty percent aluminum chloride hexahydrate in an alcohol base and ferric subsulfate are commonly used agents. Although ferric subsulfate is a more effective hemostatic agent, aluminum chloride is usually preferred as the former can pigment dermal tissue causing tattooing. Both are applied using a cotton tipped applicator and pressure to the wound bed for approximately 1 to 2 minutes.[21]

If a styptic does not suffice or a greater amount of hemostasis is needed, electrosurgery may be used. (see chapter 14). Heat or electricity is delivered to the bleeding point via a metal tip (monopolar or bipolar electrode) connected to an electrosurgical source. If the patient has an implantable cardioverter defibrillator, pacemaker, or both, the electric current may interfere with normal functioning of these devices. In patients with an implantable cardioverter defibrillator, bipolar electrosurgery or heat electrocautery should be used.[22] For patients with pacemakers, electrosurgery may be used if the power output of the device is kept to a minimum and short pulses of less than 5 seconds are utilized. In patients with either device, thermocautery, also called heat cautery, is safe.[23]

BIOPSY TECHNIQUES

There are six main biopsy techniques: snip, curette, shave, punch, incisional, and excisional biopsy. As with any surgical procedure universal precautions should be followed. For most biopsies, clean surgical technique is appropriate but for incisional and excisional biopsies, sterile technique is recommended. The set-up for the biopsy tray should be standardized so the clinician is familiar with all materials.

SNIP BIOPSY

Snip or scissor biopsies are ideal for pedunculated lesions, which can be pulled away from the base and severed. Either iris or gradle scissors are often used. Local anesthesia for this type of biopsy includes formation of a wheal or bleb. It is important that the lesion be pulled but not overly extended with the forceps as this can result in a wider or deeper defect. Pressure hemostasis is often suitable for these superficial biopsies although for larger or more vascular lesions chemical hemostasis or electrosurgery can be utilized. Healing occurs by secondary intention (Fig. 12-1).

CURETTE BIOPSY

Curette biopsies are intended for superficial epidermal lesions in which a plane of dissection exists between the neoplasm and the underlying dermis. Examples of lesions suitable for a curette biopsy include seborrheic keratoses and molluscum contagiosum. Although some use curette biopsies for certain malignant neoplasms such as basal cell carcinomas, the destructive force of the curette may shear the tissue, making it more difficult to interpret histologically. There are two main types of curettes: the Volkmann spoon type and the sharper ring curette. The surrounding skin is held taut with the nondominant hand while the dominant hand, in a smooth movement, removes the lesion. Curettes should not be used on lax skin as they often cause tearing (Fig. 12-2). If the lesion is not completely removed with the first pass the process is repeated. Hemostasis can be obtained via pressure, chemical hemostasis, or electrosurgery. Healing occurs by secondary intention. The scar may be hypopigmented, especially in patients with darker skin types, which should be discussed before the biopsy.

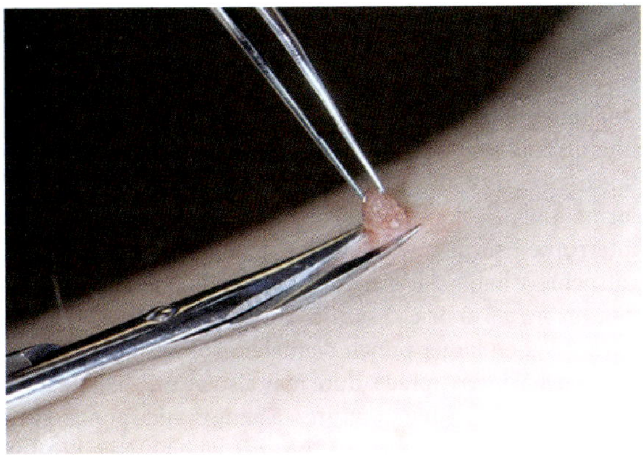

Figure 12-1 Snip biopsy (lesion is held with forceps; gradle scissor is poised at base to snip).

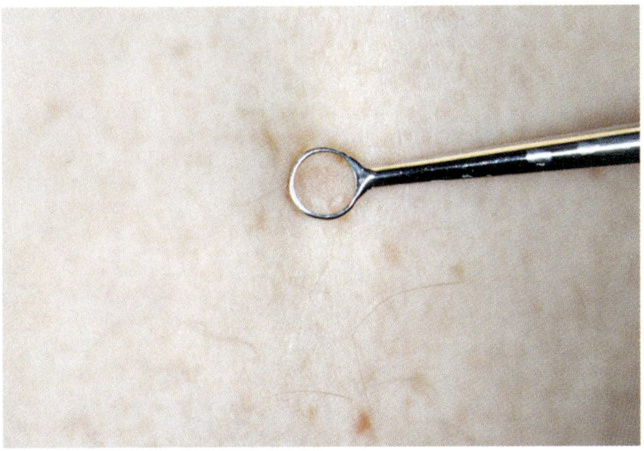

Figure 12-2 Curette (lesion is scraped using the sharp side of the curette).

SHAVE BIOPSY

The shave biopsy is a commonly performed procedure. Shave biopsies can be used to diagnose a variety of skin disorders, including neoplasms and inflammatory entities. Intradermal anesthesia with wheal formation serves to elevate the lesion while ensuring adequate anesthesia of the peripheral borders. While holding the lesion taut with the nondominant hand, forceps, or a skin hook, the dermatologist can utilize a 10 or 15 scalpel blade or a flexible concave razor blade (i.e., Dermablade®) in a parallel sawing motion (Fig. 12-3a,b). Hemostasis may be achieved with pressure, chemical hemostasis, or electrosurgery (Fig. 12-3c). Healing occurs by secondary intention. It is worth noting that as the depth of shave increases the risk of subsequent scarring increases.

There is a learning curve associated with performance of shave biopsies as the depth is guided by the operator's angulation of the blade. When greater blade angulation is utilized, the term "deep shave" or "shave excision" is used; this type of biopsy has also been referred to as a "saucerization biopsy" when it samples the epidermis along with a portion of the dermis, the whole dermis, or subcutaneous fat. Regardless of the shave biopsy technique used, the goal is to obtain a single, unfragmented, saucer-shaped biopsy specimen with consistent depth.

A saucerization biopsy is particularly useful in diagnosing lentigo maligna (malignant melanoma in situ) of the face. Lentigo maligna lesions can be quite large and a complete excisional biopsy may not be feasible. It is important, however, to obtain a sufficiently large and representative sample, as benign foci may be present within a larger

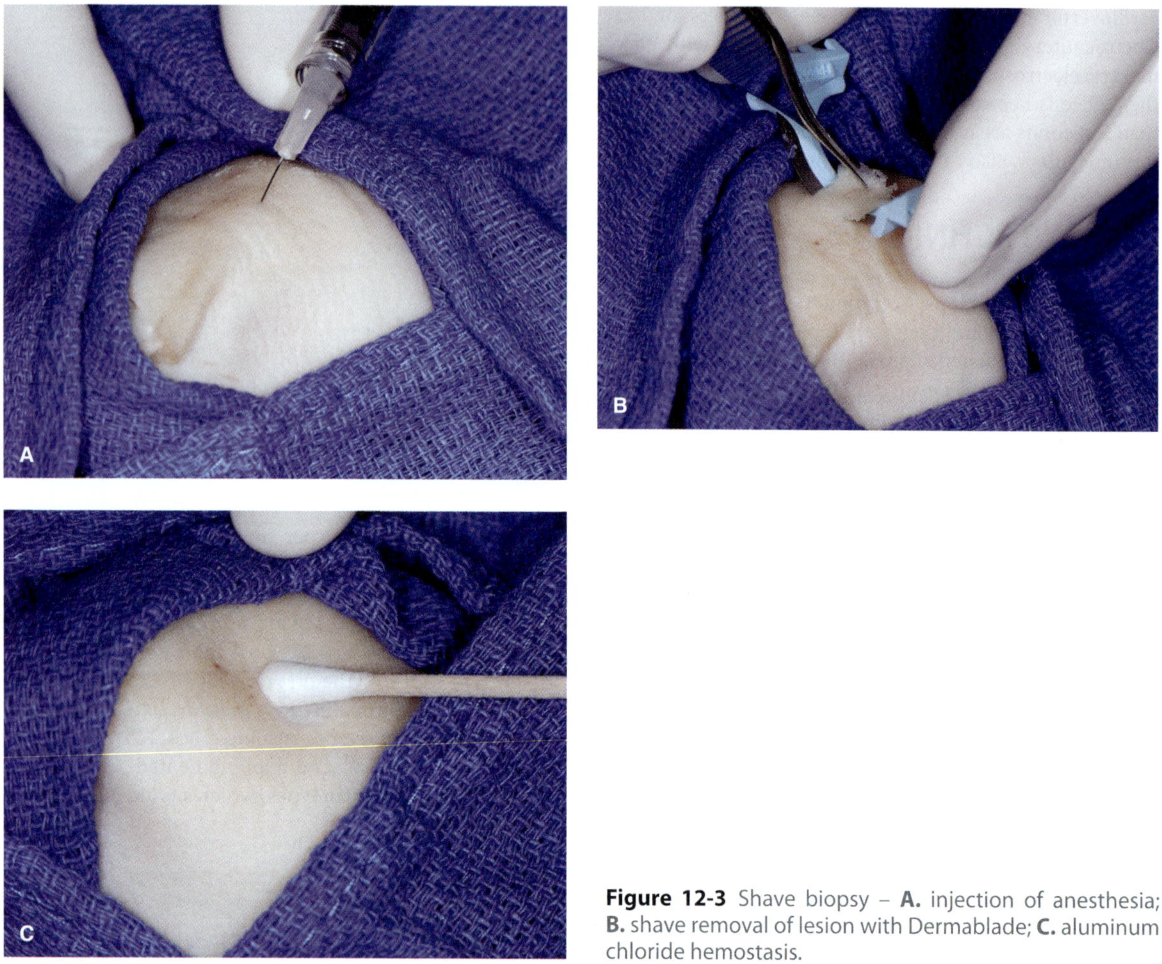

Figure 12-3 Shave biopsy – **A.** injection of anesthesia; **B.** shave removal of lesion with Dermablade; **C.** aluminum chloride hemostasis.

malignant lesion, leading to sampling error and a delay in the diagnosis of malignancy.[24] When biopsying suspected mycosis fungoides (cutaneous T-cell lymphoma), an entity that can be subtle histologically, a broad shave biopsy may be superior to a smaller biopsy. Shave biopsies can also be used for small dysplastic nevi because they allow the pathologist to visualize the epidermis at the shoulders of the lesions.[25] A superficial shave biopsy may not provide adequate depth to distinguish an invasive squamous cell carcinoma from a keratoacanthoma type squamous cell carcinoma, and it is important to obtain a sufficiently deep and wide sample when biopsying these types of lesions.

PUNCH BIOPSY

The punch biopsy is an excellent tool for sampling dermatologic processes occurring in the dermis and subcutaneous fat, including inflammatory dermatoses, neoplasms, and panniculitides. The punch instrument is a circular, hollow, metal cylinder with a cutting edge that is connected to a plastic handle. The specimen size is determined by the diameter of the cylinder (range is from 2 to 8 mm). A sample larger than 2 mm in diameter is generally recommended. However, in a study of 84 cases of 2 mm punch biopsies compared to their corresponding excisional specimens, the dermatopathologist was able to make a correct diagnosis in 79 of 84 specimens.[26] Local anesthesia of the epidermis, deep dermis, and subcutaneous fat is needed for a punch biopsy. If sutures will be used to close the defect, it is important to anesthetize the surrounding area as well.

The skin should be held taut and perpendicular to the relaxed skin tension lines of the area being sampled. The punch instrument is pushed vertically into the skin and rotated in one direction (twisting back and forth may lead to epidermal shearing). It is apparent that the subcutaneous tissue is reached when there is a loss of dermal resistance (this can be obscured in fibrosing conditions). The biopsy specimen is held gently by forceps to minimize crush artifact, and detached from the base with iris scissors (Fig. 12-4a,b). Since the skin is held at right angles to the relaxed skin tension lines, the circular defect created is transformed into an oval shape when the skin is released. This allows a linear closure with minimal dog-ear formation to be performed, which is important for optimal cosmesis. Simple interrupted sutures with slight eversion of the skin edges can achieve hemostasis and a satisfactory linear scar. On the face, using a 5-0 or 6-0 suture can avoid noticeable suture marks. When larger punch diameters are used, an absorbable dermal interrupted suture may also be utilized. In areas that are not amenable to sutures, a hemostatic sponge, such as Gelfoam®, can provide hemostasis when applied to the biopsy site and then "sealed" with a compression bandage. This material can be left in place to degrade on its own.

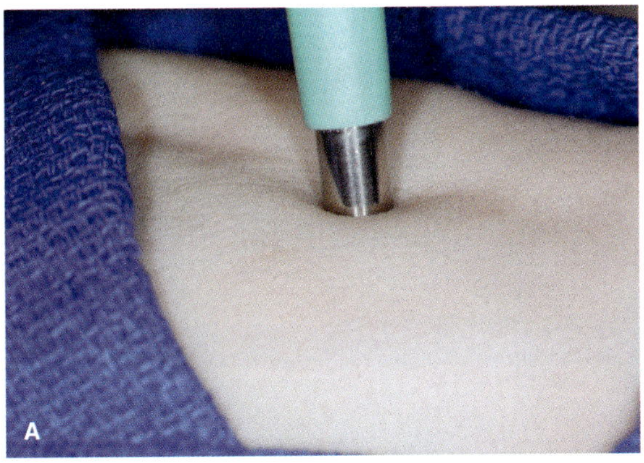

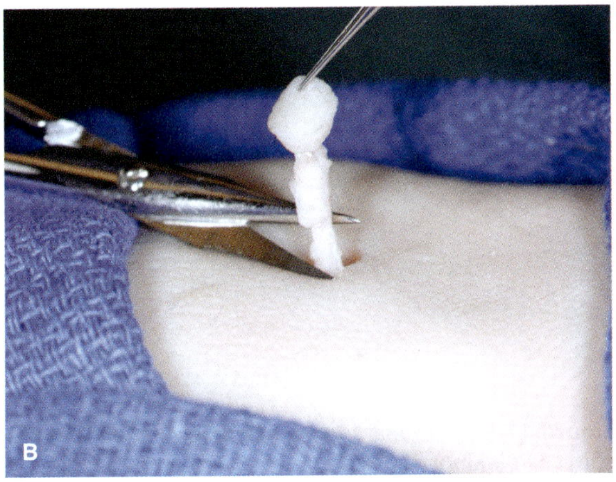

Figure 12-4 Punch biopsy – **A.** barrel rotating into skin; **B.** specimen lifted with forceps and snipped with gradle scissors.

For thicker anatomic areas or lesions in the subcutaneous fat, the "double punch" technique helps ensure adequate sampling of the dermal or subcutaneous tissue. In this technique, a larger punch instrument is used, followed by a smaller diameter punch into the defect to sample the deeper tissue. This is useful when biopsying a suspected panniculitis. Punch instruments can also be used to score around a cutaneous lesion or to incise the skin superficially in areas of thin epidermis.

For large or broad suspected malignant neoplasms a punch biopsy may not accurately define the full extent of the lesion. Russell et al. compared shave biopsies to punch biopsies for the diagnosis of basal cell carcinoma. The diagnostic accuracy rates were similar; 80.7% for punch biopsies (n = 57) and 75.9% for shave biopsies (n = 29). There was no statistically significant tendency to overdiagnose or underdiagnose any particular tumor subtype based on the type of biopsy procedure used.[27] Haws et al. reviewed 232 biopsy specimens and their corresponding wide excisions to determine the correlation between basal cell carcinoma subtypes in these specimens. Eighty-eight percent (205/232) were shave biopsies and 12% (27/232) were punch biopsies; the total specimen accuracy rate was 82%. Mixed histological subtypes were present in 54% of cases, and half contained an aggressive subtype (infiltrative, morpheaform, or micronodular). There was an 18% (42/232) discordance rate between the biopsy specimen subtypes when the growth patterns were mixed. In 40% (17/42) of these cases, an aggressive subtype was not apparent in the original biopsy.[28]

INCISIONAL BIOPSY

When the lesion in question is large or the pathology is suspected to be within the deeper dermis or subcutis, an incisional or wedge biopsy may also be utilized. The biopsy specimen may be composed exclusively of lesional tissue or may contain normal bordering skin. The skin sample is usually as wide and as deep as needed to obtain sufficient tissue. A 15 blade is routinely used and a perpendicular superficial incision is made on both sides of the area to be biopsied. The blade is incised deeply and angled toward the central axis until it reaches the appropriate depth. The biopsy tissue should be obtained in one piece to ensure precise orientation when processing. Forceps and scissors are used to grasp the specimen and detach it. Hemostasis can be obtained with electrosurgery. Deep dermal absorbable sutures and superficial nonabsorbable epidermal sutures may be used to reapproximate the skin edges.

EXCISIONAL BIOPSY

An excisional biopsy is an elliptical excision down to subcutaneous fat used to histologically evaluate a cutaneous lesion in its entirety. This technique is important when biopsying suspected malignant neoplasms, notably malignant melanoma, in which histopathologic analysis of the entire lesion is crucial for diagnosis and staging. It is important to consider the cosmesis of the resulting wound as well. Orienting the tissue along naturally occurring relaxed skin tension lines is recommended. Utilizing a 15 blade in a perpendicular orientation, an elliptical shape is incised to the subcutaneous fat or suspected lesion depth. A disc excision can also be performed instead. An advantage of a disc excision is that it allows the clinician to perform the excisional biopsy first, and then to determine the axis of closure once the tissue has been removed. With proper undermining, the defect will naturally align in the direction of least tension, or along relaxed skin tension lines. The central portion of the wound is closed with subcutaneous and epidermal sutures after which removal of redundant dog-ears can be performed (Fig. 12-5a–c). To maintain proper orientation of the specimen, a marking suture can be placed to correlate the histologic margin with the clinical orientation. When the clinical margin does not provide sufficient histological clearance, the biopsy edges will be involved with tumor and an additional excisional procedure will be indicated.

Since the degree of atypia or depth of invasion is often not uniform in malignant lesions, excisional biopsies decrease the risk of sampling error. Egnatios et al.[29] reviewed 609 melanoma biopsy specimens, of which 51% were shaves, 19% punches, and 30% excisions. Residual melanoma was seen in 240 patients (39%) after definitive wide local excision; 60% of these had undergone a shave biopsy. Ten percent (59 patients) had a tumor (T)-category upgrade after wide local excision; 64% of this group was sampled by a shave biopsy. Seven percent of patients with a T-category upgrade had negative margins initially. A

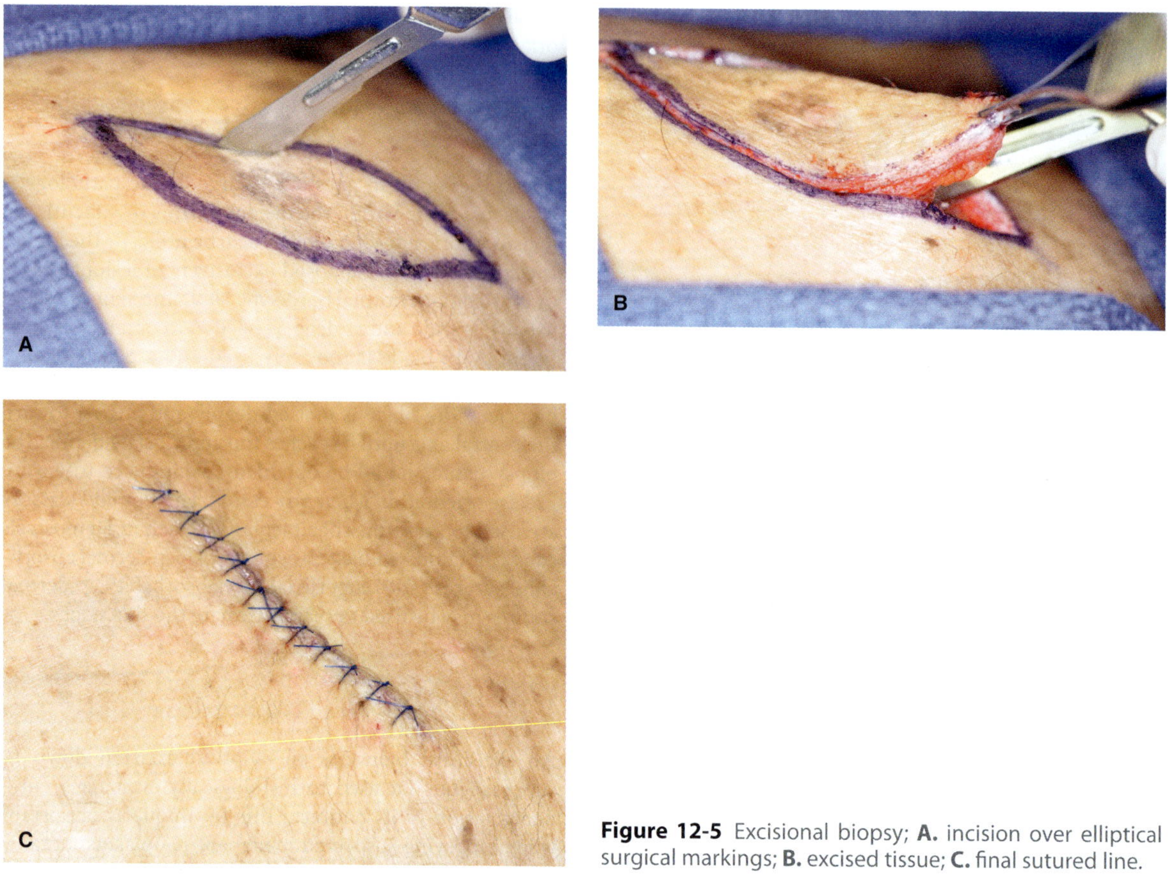

Figure 12-5 Excisional biopsy; **A.** incision over elliptical surgical markings; **B.** excised tissue; **C.** final sutured line.

positive biopsy margin and greater tumor thickness were determined to be predictors of T-category upgrade.

Johnson et al. studied the impact of incisional biopsy on melanoma microstaging. Of 1783 patients who underwent an incisional biopsy, 250 (14%) presented with a residual lesion; the mean Breslow's depth in this group was 0.66 mm compared to a mean Breslow's depth of 1.07 mm ($p = 0.001$) after complete excision. Upstaging, which was associated with a poorer prognosis because of a significant change in Breslow's depth or the presence of ulceration after completion excision, occurred in 53 of 250 patients (21%).[30] A shave biopsy significantly increased the odds of upstaging after excision of the residual lesion compared to the use of a punch biopsy. Shave biopsies increased the odds of upstaging by 2.3 compared with punch biopsies (OR = 2.3; 1.03–5.20).

Similarly, in 2010, Ng et al. compared partial and excisional biopsy techniques for accuracy of histopathological diagnosis and microstaging of cutaneous melanoma from 1995 to 2006.[31] They reported increased odds of histopathologic misdiagnosis associated with using a punch biopsy (OR, 16.6; 95% CI, 10–27) ($p < 0.001$), or shave biopsy (OR, 2.6; 95% CI, 1.2–5.7) ($p = 0.02$), compared to an excisional biopsy. Specific subgroups were associated with an increased likelihood of misdiagnosis, including acral lentiginous melanoma (OR, 5.1; 95% CI, 2–13) ($p < 0.001$), desmoplastic melanoma (OR, 3.8; 95% CI, 1.1–13.0) ($p = 0.03$), and nevoid melanoma (OR, 28.4; 95% CI, 7–115) ($p < 0.001$). The rates of microstaging inaccuracy by punch biopsy (34%) and shave biopsy (19%) were comparable to other reported rates of 16% to 43%.

There is concern that a wide excisional biopsy or a wide local excision for treatment of melanoma may preclude the use of a subsequent sentinel lymph node biopsy by disrupting lymphatic drainage. Of 1395 patients who had lymphatic mapping/sentinel lymph node biopsies for malignant melanoma, Gannon et al.[32] identified 104 patients who had wide local excision before sentinel node biopsy and compared them to patients who had had concomitant procedures. In 97/104 (93%), the surgical defects were closed primarily or with a skin graft, while seven patients (7%) had rotation flaps. Median follow-up was 51 months. In the previously excised group, 19 patients (18%) had a positive sentinel lymph node biopsy and four of these (21%) had recurrences (three distant failures and one local and distant failure). There were no lymph node recurrences in a mapped or unmapped basin in the 104 patients with a negative or positive sentinel node. The authors concluded that sentinel lymph nodes can be successfully identified and accurately reflect the regional lymph node drainage status in melanoma patients who have already had wide local excisions. However, the effectiveness of sentinel node mapping and sampling in patients who have undergone extensive reconstruction of the primary excision site remains to be defined. Leong et al. reported similarly that sentinel lymph node biopsies could be successfully performed after wide excision for truncal and extremity melanomas with no difference in relapse-free survival ($p = 0.209$) or overall survival ($p = 0.692$). They reported a single false-negative result, which occurred in a patient whose truncal excision was closed with a rotation flap.[33]

The need to assess the depth of a suspected malignancy applies to cutaneous squamous cell carcinoma as well. In 2010 the American Joint Committee on Cancer published revised staging guidelines for cutaneous squamous cell carcinoma. Based on evidence-based data, new high-risk features included: greater than 2 mm tumor thickness, Clark level greater than IV, perineural invasion, anatomic site, and degree of histological differentiation. When biopsying a suspected cutaneous squamous cell carcinoma, the physician should choose the technique that will allow the best measurement of tumor depth as this will have implications for tumor staging.

SPECIAL SITES

HEAD/NECK

It is important to exercise caution when performing biopsies in certain anatomical areas of the head and neck. The superficial temporal branch of the facial nerve lies just below the thin dermis and subcutaneous fat in the so-called "danger area." This location lies midway between the lateral eyebrow and anterior temporal hairline (the area formed by drawing a line from the tragus to the lateral eyebrow and a line from the tragus to highest forehead rhytid). The spinal accessory nerve also courses superficially in the posterior triangle at Erb's point, where the posterior edge of the sternocleidomastoid muscle meets a perpendicular line drawn midway from a line connecting the angle of the jaw and the mastoid process. Anatomical variations exist, so caution is advised in these areas.[34] The third facial danger zone is in the location of the marginal mandibular nerve that courses superficially as it exits the parotid gland at the angle of the mandible. As it crosses that angle, the nerve is only covered by skin, subcutaneous fat, and superficial muscular aponeurosis (SMAS). Most individuals have a marginal mandibular nerve that remains at or above the level of the mandible, although in about 20% of people this nerve can descend 1 to 2 cm into the neck below the angle of the mandible.

The rich vasculature of the upper and lower lip is an important consideration for biopsies in this location. The superior and inferior labial arteries are branches of the facial artery, which arises from the external carotid artery. The labial arteries are found deep to the lip mucosa but can course more superficially in older patients. The lip has a bidirectional blood source due to anastomoses and bleeding must be anticipated. A chalazion clamp may help to control bleeding while also stabilizing the tissue. This added tension can facilitate easier sampling. Another way to avoid traumatizing the biopsy sample is to use gradle scissors to sample the intended site. Sometimes a "bleb" of anesthesia may elevate the plane of the lesion facilitating easier procurement. Silk may be used as the suture material due to its soft nature and ease of handling. The mucosa of the lip heals well as long as the vermillion border has not been violated. Involvement of the vermillion border may create a more visible scar.

When performing biopsies of the ear, it is important to prevent the exposure of cartilage to minimize the risk of infection or chondritis.

SCALP

Scalp biopsies may be performed for analysis of follicular disorders. The ideal biopsy should go to the depth of the subcutis to ensure that the entire follicle is sampled. Often punch biopsies are the technique of choice. If the punch diameter is large enough the biopsy can be bisected, allowing the pathologist to cut one-half of it in transverse sections. It has been reported that noncicatricial alopecias may be better appreciated on transverse sections while scarring alopecias may be better diagnosed on longitudinal sections.[35] The plane of the biopsy should be parallel to the growing hair shafts to avoid follicle transection and resultant alopecia.

Since the scalp has a rich vascular supply, taking time for the vasoconstrictive effect of epinephrine in the local anesthetic to occur is recommended. A cross-over stitch, or cutaneous figure of eight stitch, may produce the desired hemostasis. It may be helpful to place the sutures before performing the biopsy[36] so that the suture can be tied as soon as the tissue is removed. Using rapidly dissolving sutures will circumvent the need for suture removal in an area obscured by hair growth. Gelfoam is a quick and effective hemostatic agent that can be easily placed into the punch biopsy wound as an alternative to sutures.

PALMS/SOLES

When performing biopsies on the palms, soles, digits, or toes it has been shown that local anesthesia with epinephrine is safe to use.[37] However, an excessive volume of liquid can cause tamponade of the vessels in a closed space such as the digit or toe. Addition of epinephrine actually allows for lower anesthetic volumes to be used.[38] Correct injection technique, such as aspirating to avoid vessel penetration, and proper selection of patients (absence of thrombotic or vasospastic conditions or uncontrolled hypertension) helps to minimize possible complications.

GENITAL SKIN

Genital skin, like lip mucosa, has the tendency to heal well after cutaneous biopsy if proper technique is used. The texture of the genital skin may make it difficult to obtain clean cuts with a scalpel, so using non-toothed forceps and gradle scissors may be used instead. When performing a punch biopsy, it is important not to advance the punch too deeply as it may penetrate underlying structures. Using the punch instrument to score the site to a superficial depth either on the glans penis, penile shaft, or vulva, and then using gradle scissors to snip the scored biopsy specimen will help to obtain the tissue more readily.

WOUND DRESSINGS

Postbiopsy wound care is essential for proper healing and prevention of infection. For clean biopsy wounds, petrolatum is recommended over a topical antibiotic for wound care. There are many types of dressings that can be placed, including pressure dressings for added hemostasis, or different colloid dressings for exudative wounds. For a comprehensive review, see chapter 11.

TISSUE PROCESSING

The skin biopsy is generally processed in standard 10% formalin for paraffin embedding and stained with an array of histological stains, including antibodies for immunohistochemistry. For DIF, it is important to check with the histopathology lab for their preference of media. Many labs prefer transport media such as Michel's medium or normal saline. For DIF evaluation, selection of the lesion to be biopsied is of great importance. For presumed discoid lupus, porphyria, or drug-induced pseudoporphyria, the sample is taken from exposed lesional skin, whereas for systemic lupus erythematous a biopsy from exposed normal skin is more appropriate. For cutaneous vasculitis, such as Henoch Schönlein purpura, lesional skin of less than 24 hours' duration is optimal. For suspected pemphigus or pemphigoid skin lesions the sample is taken from the edge of an intact bulla along with perilesional skin; for oral mucosal lesions a perilesional biopsy should be taken. In dermatitis herpetiformis, the optimal DIF sample would be clinically normal perilesional skin.[39]

Other diagnostic techniques that may be performed on processed tissue include polymerase chain reaction (PCR) based analysis of T-cell receptor gene rearrangement to assess clonality in cutaneous lymphomas. Cultures may also be performed on *fresh* unfixed tissue for the detection of various infectious organisms, such as bacterium, fungi, mycobacterium, and protozoa.

COMPLICATIONS

Although complications of a biopsy can include infection, bleeding, and scar, the small sample of tissue taken lessens the degree to which these occur. Hemorrhage from the biopsy site, while uncommon, usually occurs within 24 hours, and the patient should be educated regarding how to apply pressure to the area.

The infection rate seen after cutaneous biopsies is fortunately very low. Biopsies below the knee, areas affected by lymphedema, intertriginous areas or skin folds, and areas involving cartilage are more likely to develop infection. Despite the low risk of infection, many patients still use antibiotic creams or ointments, which can lead to irritant or allergic contact dermatitis and delayed wound healing. Smack et al.[40] compared the application of topical bacitracin to petrolatum after various dermatologic procedures and found no statistically significant difference in the rate of surgical site infections. The infections that did occur in the bacitracin cohort were caused by gram-negative bacilli, which were likely a result of the selective removal of gram-positive skin flora. The bacitracin group also had a higher incidence of allergic contact dermatitis. Since petrolatum has been shown to be beneficial in speeding reepithelialization and promoting the growth of natural skin flora, it may be used for wound care following routine biopsies.

Scars, whether depressed, hypertrophic, or keloidal, are potential complications of a biopsy and the patient should understand these risks. Atrophic or spreading scars can occur in areas such as the back even when the defect is closed primarily, due to the force of muscle movement. Suture marks can also be unsightly; use of rapidly dissolving sutures or the timely removal of nondissolvable sutures can lessen this risk. Persistent numbness or pain may also rarely complicate the postbiopsy course.

CONCLUSION

The skin biopsy is an essential diagnostic tool for the practicing dermatologist and dermatologic surgeon. Appropriate site and lesion selection, choosing the best biopsy method, and using proper surgical technique will all enhance the diagnostic yield with a minimum of complications. Preoperative evaluation and informed consent should be obtained and the use of standardized digital photography is recommended for comprehensive documentation. Patient expectations should be addressed to avoid any misconceptions about the procedure. While skin biopsies are generally low risk, universal precautions should always be followed and each patient should be assessed to minimize the risks due to anesthesia, infection, or poor wound healing.

With advances in cutaneous imaging such as dermoscopy and confocal microscopy, visualization of lesional architecture and cellular atypia may decrease the need for cutaneous biopsies. However, the skin biopsy will likely remain the best diagnostic tool for cutaneous lesions for many years to come.

ACKNOWLEDGMENT

We would like to thank Indira Singh for her help with the figures and illustrations.

REFERENCES

1. Dengel L, Turza K, Noland MM, Patterson JW, Slingluff CL Jr. Skin mapping with punch biopsies for defining margins in melanoma: when you don't know how far to go. *Ann Surg Oncol.* 2008;15:3028–3035.
2. Tziotzios C, Profyris C, Sterling J. Cutaneous scarring: pathophysiology, molecular mechanisms, and scar reduction therapeutics Part II. Strategies to reduce scar formation after dermatologic procedures. *J Am Acad Dermatol.* 2012;66:13–24.
3. Stables G, Lawrence CM. Management of patients taking anticoagulant, aspirin, non-steroidal anti-inflammatory and other anti-platelet drugs undergoing dermatological surgery. *Clin Exp Dermatol.* 2002;27:432–435.
4. Callahan S, Goldsberry A, Kim G, Yoo S. The management of antithrombotic medication in skin surgery. *Dermatol Surg.* 2012;38:1417–1426.
5. Alcalay J. Cutaneous surgery in patients receiving warfarin therapy. *Dermatol Surg.* 2001;27:756–758.
6. Cook-Norris RH, Michaels JD, Weaver AL, et al. Complications of cutaneous surgery in patients taking clopidogrel-containing anticoagulation. *J Am Acad Dermatol.* 2011;65:584–591.
7. Lewis KG, Dufresne RG Jr. A meta-analysis of complications attributed to anticoagulation among patients following cutaneous surgery. *Dermatol Surg.* 2008;34:160–164.
8. Wright TI, Baddour LM, Berbari EF, et al. Antibiotic prophylaxis in dermatologic surgery: advisory statement 2008. *J Am Acad Dermatol.* 2008;59:464–473.

9. National Institute for Health and Clinical Excellence. Prophylaxis against infective endocarditis: antimicrobial prophylaxis against infective endocarditis in adults and children undergoing interventional procedures. London;2008. http://www.nice.org.uk/nicemedia/pdf/CG64NICEguidance.pdf. Accessed September 23, 2013.
10. Dixon AJ, Dixon MP, Askew DA, Wilkinson D. Prospective study of wound infections in dermatologic surgery in the absence of prophylactic antibiotics. *Dermatol Surg.* 2006;32:819–826.
11. Perlis CS, Campbell RM, Perlis RH, Malik M, Dufresne RG Jr. Incidence of and risk factors for medical malpractice lawsuits among Mohs surgeons. *Dermatol Surg.* 2006;32:79–83.
12. McGinness JL, Goldstein G. The value of preoperative biopsy-site photography for identifying cutaneous lesions. *Dermatol Surg.* 2010;36:194–197.
13. Veiga DF, Damasceno CA, Veiga-Filho J, et al. Povidone iodine versus chlorhexidine in skin antisepsis before elective plastic surgery procedures: a randomized controlled trial. *Plast Reconstr Surg.* 2008;122:170e–171e.
14. Tucker KJ, Larson JL, Idris A, Curtis AB. Advanced cardiac life support: update on recent guidelines and a look at the future. *Clin Cardiol.* 1995;18:497–504.
15. Darmstadt GL, Hossain MM, Choi Y, et al. Safety and effect of chlorhexidine skin cleansing on skin flora of neonates in Bangladesh. *Pediatr Infect Dis J.* 2007;26:492–495.
16. Bibbo C, Patel DV, Gehrmann RM, Lin SS. Chlorhexidine provides superior skin decontamination in foot and ankle surgery: a prospective randomized study. *Clin Orthop Relat Res.* 2005; 438:204–208.
17. Darouiche RO, Wall MJ Jr, Itani KM, et al. Chlorhexidine-Alcohol versus povidone-iodine for surgical-site antisepsis. *N Engl J Med.* 2010;362:18–26.
18. Dzubow LM. The interaction between propranolol and epinephrine as observed in patients undergoing Mohs' surgery. *J Am Acad Dermatol.* 1986;15:71–75.
19. Wilhelmi BJ, Blackwell SJ, Miller J, Mancoll JS, Phillips LG. Epinephrine in digital blocks: revisited. *Ann Plast Surg.* 1998;41:410–414.
20. Eggleston ST, Lush LW. Understanding allergic reactions to local anesthetics. *Ann Pharmacother.* 1996;30:851–857.
21. Palm MD, Altman JS. Topical hemostatic agents: a review. *Dermatol Surg.* 2008;34:431–435.
22. Voutsalath MA, Bichakjian CK, Pelosi F, Blum D, Johnson TM, Farrehi PM. Electrosurgery and implantable electronic devices: review and implication for office-based procedures. *Dermatol Surg.* 2011;37:889–899.
23. Senthuran S, Toff WD, Vuylsteke A, Solesbury PM, Menon DK. Implanted cardiac pacemakers and defibrillators in anaesthetic practice. *Br J Anaesth.* 2002;88:627–631.
24. Stevens G, Cocherell CJ. Avoiding sampling error in the biopsy of pigmented lesions. *Arch Dermatol.* 1996;132:1380–1382.
25. Abbasi NR, Shaw HM, Rigel DS, et al. Early diagnosis of cutaneous melanoma: revisiting the ABCD criteria. *JAMA.* 2004;292:2771–2776.
26. Todd P, Garioch JJ, Humphreys S, Seywright M, Thomson J, du Vivier AW. Evaluation of the 2-mm punch biopsy in dermatological diagnosis. *Clin Exp Dermatol.* 1996;21:11–13.
27. Russell EB, Carrington PR, Smoller BR. Basal cell carcinoma: a comparison of shave biopsy versus punch biopsy techniques in subtype diagnosis. *J Am Acad Dermatol.* 1999;41: 69–71.
28. Haws AL, Rojano R, Tahan SR, Phung TL. Accuracy of biopsy sampling for subtyping basal cell carcinoma. *J Am Acad Dermatol.* 2012;66:106–111.
29. Egnatios GL, Dueck AC, Macdonald JB, et al. The impact of biopsy technique on upstaging, residual disease, and outcome in cutaneous melanoma. *Am J Surg.* 2011;202:771–777.
30. Karimipour DJ, Schwartz JL, Wang TS, et al. Microstaging accuracy after subtotal incisional biopsy of cutaneous melanoma. *J Am Acad Dermatol.* 2005;52:798–802.
31. Ng JC, Swain S, Dowling JP, Wolfe R, Simpson P, Kelly JW. The impact of partial biopsy on histopathologic diagnosis of cutaneous melanoma: experience of an Australian tertiary referral service. *Arch Dermatol.* 2010;146:234–239.
32. Gannon CJ, Rousseau DL Jr, Ross MI, et al. Accuracy of lymphatic mapping and sentinel lymph node biopsy after previous wide local excision in patients with primary melanoma. *Cancer.* 2006;107:2647–2652.
33. Leong WL, Ghazarian DM, McCready DR. Previous wide local excision of primary melanoma is not a contraindication for sentinel lymph node biopsy of the trunk and extremity. *J Surg Oncol.* 2003;82:143–146.
34. Symes A, Ellis H. Variations in the surface anatomy of the spinal accessory nerve in the posterior triangle. *Surg Radiol Anat.* 2005;27:404–408.
35. Ozcan D, Ozen O, Seckin D. Vertical vs. transverse sections of scalp biopsy specimens: a pilot study on the comparison of the diagnostic value of two techniques in alopecia. *Clin Exp Dermatol.* 2011;36:855–863.
36. McKerrow KJ, Grande DJ. Figure eight closure. *J Am Acad Dermatol.* 1991;24:146–148.
37. Firoz B, Davis N, Goldberg LH. Local anesthesia using buffered 0.5% lidocaine with 1:200000 epinephrine for tumors of the digits treated with Mohs micrographic surgery. *J Am Acad Dermatol.* 2009;61:639–643.
38. Krunic AL, Wang LC, Soltani K, Weitzul S, Taylor RS. Digital anesthesia with epinephrine: an old myth revisited. *J Am Acad Dermatol.* 2004;51:755–759.
39. Minz RW, Chhabra S, Singh S, Radotra BD, Kumar B. Direct immunofluorescence of skin biopsy: perspective of an immunopathologist. *Indian J Dermatol Venereol Leprol.* 2010;76:150–157.
40. Smack DP, Harrington AC, Dunn C, et al. Infection and allergy incidence in ambulatory surgery patients using white petrolatum vs bacitracin ointment. A randomized controlled trial. *JAMA.* 1996;276:972–977.

CHAPTER 13

Hemostasis

Wilfred A. Lumbang, Meghan Scharf, & Thomas Stasko

INTRODUCTION

Management of bleeding is fundamentally important in any surgical procedure. Historically, surgeons applied boiling oil solution and soothing balms to detoxify and cauterize wounds. It was in the sixteenth century that the French surgeon, Ambroise Paré, revolutionized the practice of surgery by introducing the use of vascular ligatures to control bleeding in amputations, sucking chest wounds and chronic ulcers.[1] The fields of medicine and surgery have undergone significant transformation since then. Dermatologic surgeons have become more cognizant of hemostasis because they now perform invasive office-based procedures, often on patients with complicated medical histories. Adequate control of bleeding during these procedures is vital to achieving optimal outcomes. The overall safety of dermatologic surgery is well established, but complications do arise and are often attributable to bleeding.

This chapter will review the principles of hemostasis as they relate to cutaneous surgery. Normal hemostasis, as well as disorders, medications, and supplements that affect hemostasis will be discussed. Various surgical approaches and relevant hemostatic agents used to control bleeding during procedures will be presented.

BIOLOGY OF NORMAL HEMOSTASIS

Understanding the principles behind hemostasis can lead to better utilization of the various tools available to achieve hemostasis during dermatologic surgery. It is also important to understand the mechanisms behind the medications that alter coagulation. The hemostatic process can be divided into four physiologic events that are intimately linked and occur in conjunction with each other – vasoconstriction, platelet plug formation, fibrin clot formation, and fibrinolysis. A schematic of normal hemostasis is shown on Figure 13-1, and is discussed in detail below.

VASOCONSTRICTION

Damage to blood vessels during surgery precipitates the process of hemostasis. Vascular constriction is the initial response to this injury and is dependent on local contraction of smooth muscle. This process is closely linked to platelet plug formation. When platelets adhere and aggregate at the site of injury, they induce factors that further potentiate vasoconstriction. Thromboxane A_2, made from arachidonic acid on platelet membranes; endothelin, released from the injured endothelium; and serotonin, released from activated platelets, are all powerful vasoconstrictors. Bradykinin and fibrinopeptides, both involved in the coagulation scheme, are also capable of contracting vascular smooth muscle.[2]

PLATELET PLUG FORMATION

There are three steps necessary for effective platelet plug formation – platelet adhesion, granule release, and platelet aggregation. Injury to the intima of a vessel wall exposes collagen fibrils in the subendothelium, leading to platelet adherence. This process requires von Willebrand factor (vWF), a subendothelial protein that cements platelet adhesion by binding to glycoprotein receptors on the platelet membrane.[3]

Platelet adhesion is followed by activation, whereby the release of storage granules is initiated. The granules contain important signaling factors, including adenosine diphosphate (ADP), calcium, serotonin, thromboxane A_2, and α-granule proteins. These mediate the recruitment of circulating platelets to the site of injury causing platelet aggregation, with ADP playing a critical role. ADP causes conformational changes in glycoprotein IIb/IIIa to allow for binding of fibrinogen, a key component in the formation of the fibrin clot. Platelets adhere to one another via the glycoprotein IIb/IIIa receptor-fibrinogen complex.[3]

As a result of platelet adhesion and aggregation, phospholipase C and A2 are activated, producing arachidonic acid. Cyclooxygenase transforms arachidonic acid to prostaglandin, which is converted to thromboxane A_2. Thromboxane A_2 is a potent vasoconstrictor and reinforces platelet aggregation by stimulating platelet activation and degranulation.[3]

The result of the release reaction is compaction of platelets into a plug. Concurrently, alterations occur in the phospholipids of the platelet membrane allowing calcium and clotting factors to bind to the platelet surface, which is important in the formation of active complexes of the coagulation pathways.[2]

FIBRIN CLOT FORMATION

Although platelet plug formation occurs within seconds of injury, the fibrin clot forms over several minutes, following

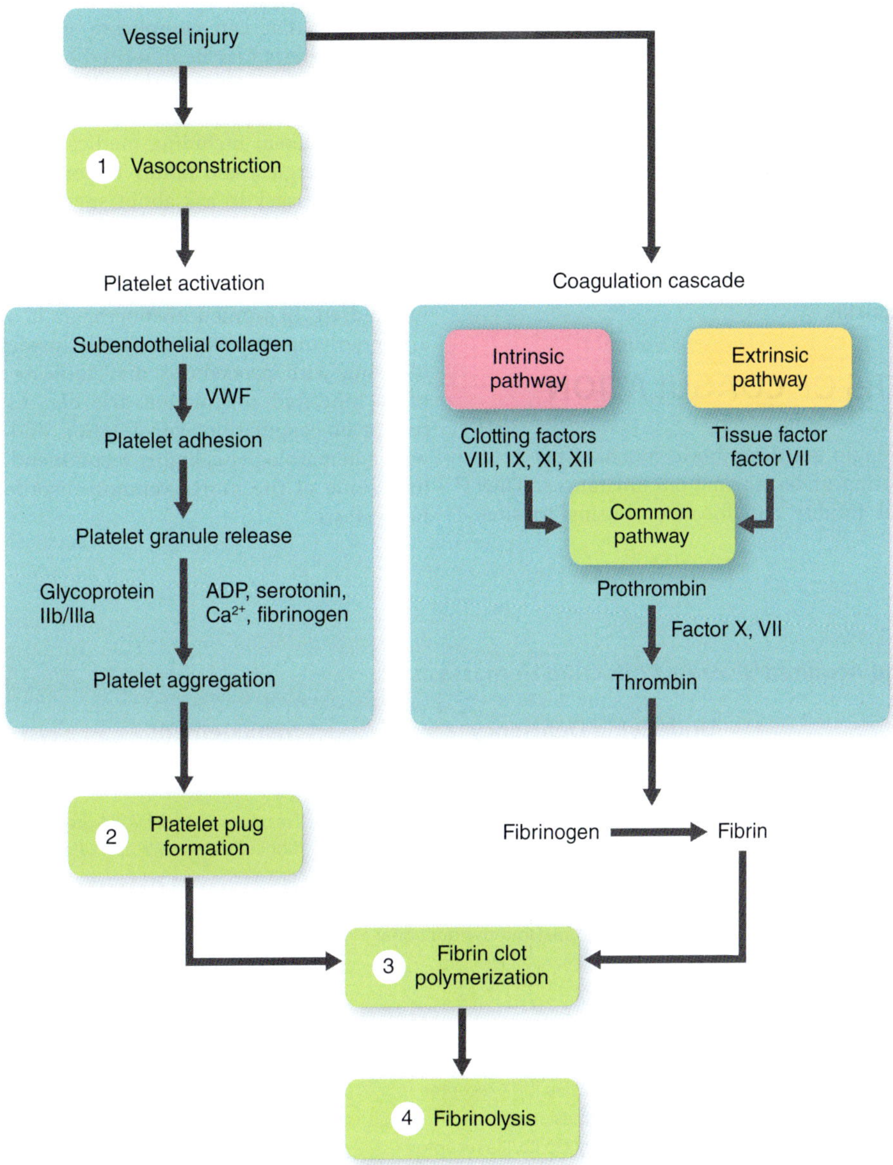

Figure 13-1 Schematic of the four interrelated physiologic processes of hemostasis. vWF, von Willebrand factor; ADP, adenosine diphosphate; Ca^{2+}, calcium)

a series of steps through what is known as the coagulation cascade. The final product is a stabilized hemostatic plug. Fibrin clot formation involves two exquisitely regulated pathways. The intrinsic pathway begins with factor XII, and through a series of enzymatic reactions, leads to activation of factors XI, IX, and VIII.[3] The intrinsic pathway components are intrinsic to the circulating plasma and do not require a surface to initiate the process. The extrinsic pathway, however, can only be initiated upon exposure of tissue factor on the injured vessel wall, and begins when tissue factor activates factor VII in the presence of calcium. Ultimately, the two converge to a common pathway with activation of factor X, which converts prothrombin to thrombin. Although thrombin has several functions, its most important role is in transforming fibrinogen to fibrin, which then polymerizes to form the fibrin clot.[3,4]

FIBRINOLYSIS

In addition to the clot formation that must occur to prevent bleeding at the time of vascular injury, two related processes exist to prevent clot propagation beyond the site of injury. First, there is feedback inhibition on the coagulation cascade, which deactivates the enzyme complexes leading to thrombin formation. Second, mechanisms of fibrinolysis allow for fibrin clot breakdown and subsequent repair of the injured vessel.[2]

During wound healing, the fibrin clot is lysed to restore blood flow. The main enzyme in this process is plasmin, which degrades the fibrin mesh. Plasmin is converted from plasminogen by several activators, including tissue plasminogen activator and urokinase plasminogen activator. Other mechanisms ensure that fibrinolysis occurs at a controlled rate and preferentially at the site of clot formation. For example, tissue plasminogen activator is more efficient when bound to fibrin, so that plasmin is formed selectively on the clot. There are also plasmin inhibitors, such as α2-antiplasmin, which ensure that clot lysis does not occur too quickly.[2]

DISORDERS OF COAGULATION

Several physiologic antithrombotic mechanisms exist to prevent clotting under normal circumstances. They preserve blood fluidity and localize clotting to sites of vascular injury. There are, however, disorders of hemostasis that can complicate surgical procedures. These disorders may be inherited or acquired. Integral to dermatologic surgery should be proper screening of patients for these disorders. A preoperative history should be taken, including medical conditions, medications, allergies, and family history. Although it may not be necessary to ask about specific disorders, simple historical questions can provide hints to underlying bleeding disorders. For example, a history of nosebleeds or excessive bleeding with tooth loss should be elicited in children. In women, menorrhagia is often a clue to an underlying condition. A family history of excessive bleeding with procedures may indicate the presence of an inherited coagulation disorder. As with all disorders of coagulation, consultation and management with a hematologist is highly recommended. Table 13-1 lists some of the more common disorders that affect hemostasis.

TABLE 13-1
Inherited and Acquired Disorders Affecting Hemostasis[3,5,6]

Conditions	Underlying Deficiency	Management
Inherited		
von Willebrand disease	Type 1 ▪ vWF and Factor VIII levels low ▪ Most common and mildest Type 2 ▪ vWF levels normal, but dysfunctional ▪ Four subtypes: 2A, 2B, 2M, 2N Type 3 ▪ vWF absent ▪ Factor VIII levels low	Desmopressin (DDAVP) preoperatively Concentrated vWF and Factor VIII infusion

Platelet disorders
▪ Bernard—Soulier
▪ Glanzmann thrombasthenia
	▪ Dysfunctional Gp Ib/IX receptor
	  ▪ Platelet adhesion defect
	▪ Dysfunctional Gp IIb/IIIa receptor
	  ▪ Platelet aggregation defect
		Consultation with hematologist recommended

Hemophilia A	Factor VIII deficiency ▪ X-linked recessive	Factor VIII replacement +/− DDAVP ▪ 50 U/kg initially, then 25 U/kg q12h
Hemophilia B (Christmas disease)	Factor IX deficiency ▪ X-linked recessive	Factor IX replacement
Hemophilia C (Rosenthal syndrome)	Factor XI deficiency ▪ Autosomal recessive, Ashkenazi Jews	Daily fresh-frozen plasma infusions
Acquired		
Uremia	Impaired platelet function	
Splenomegaly	Platelet sequestration	
Bone marrow failure	Low platelet production	Platelet infusion
Autoimmune thrombocytopenia	Idiopathic, drug-induced or secondary to viral infection; autoantibodies formed against platelets	Glucocorticoids, cessation of drug
Liver failure	Abnormal synthesis of vitamin K-dependent clotting factors ▪ Factors II, VII, IX, and X	

vWF, von Willebrand Factor; Gp, glycoprotein.

INHERITED DISORDERS OF HEMOSTASIS

PLATELET DISORDERS. Approximately 1% of the population is affected with von Willebrand disease, making it the most common congenital bleeding disorder. However, only 10% of patients experience significant bleeding.[5] As discussed above, vWF plays a key role in platelet aggregation. Patients with von Willebrand disease can either have low, dysfunctional, or absent vWF. Most commonly, patients have low levels and mild disease. Surgical prophylaxis with desmopressin or 1-desamino-8-arginine vasopressin (DDAVP) causes release of endothelial stores of vWF and is effective in 80% of patients. Twenty percent of patients with severe disease require selective factor VIII replacement, which contains high levels of vWF. Treatment is recommended for 3 to 5 days after minor surgery, and for up to 10 days following major surgery.[5]

Other rare inherited disorders of platelet function exist, including deficiencies in platelet receptors and abnormalities associated with platelet granules. Bernard–Soulier syndrome is the absence or dysfunction of the glycoprotein Ib/IX receptor. Glanzmann thrombasthenia is the absence or dysfunction of the Gp IIb/IIIa receptor. These two inherited disorders cause severe platelet dysfunction resulting in abnormal plug formation, and therapy is always needed prior to surgery.[6]

COAGULATION CASCADE DISORDERS. Disorders of the coagulation cascade pathways can be inherited or acquired. Most of the inherited disorders of coagulation involve a single component of the coagulation cascade, the most common being factor VIII deficiency or hemophilia A. This is an X-linked recessive disorder affecting one in 10,000 males. Levels of factor VIII below 5% are usually seen in patients with symptomatic disease; however, patients can present with milder disease with levels up to 25%. Severe disease is seen with levels below 1%, which often causes bleeding even without discernible trauma. Patients with hemophilia A will characteristically bleed into soft tissues, muscles, and weight-bearing joints. Postsurgical bleeding is often delayed, occurring hours to days later; large hematomas may form.[3] Treatment with plasma products enriched with factor VIII prior to surgery is key. The use of desmopressin (DDAVP) will also transiently increase the level of factor VIII by two- to threefold.[5]

Hemophilia B (Christmas disease) is an X-linked recessive disorder caused by deficiency of factor IX. It occurs in 1 in 100,000 males. Clinically hemophilia B is indistinguishable from hemophilia A. Factor IX replacement therapy is the treatment.[5] Factor XI deficiency (Rosenthal Syndrome) is inherited in an autosomal recessive fashion and is most commonly seen in Ashkenazi Jews. In contrast to factors VIII and IX, levels of factor XI do not correlate well with propensity for bleeding. Perioperative treatment with daily infusions of fresh-frozen plasma is needed.[3]

Deficiencies of factors V, VII, X, and II (prothrombin) are exceedingly rare autosomal recessive conditions. Therapy with fresh-frozen plasma is indicated for surgical procedures, although concentrated prothrombin may also be utilized.[3]

Inherited deficiencies of the intrinsic pathway involving factor XII, high–molecular-weight kininogen, and prekallikrein can result in prolonged PTT, but patients have normal hemostasis and do not require plasma replacement for surgery. Activation of the extrinsic pathway via tissue factor VIIa complex is sufficient for hemostasis in these patients.[3]

ACQUIRED DISORDERS OF HEMOSTASIS

CHRONIC DISEASES. Disorders of hemostasis can be acquired due to chronic disease or use of medications affecting critical steps in the hemostatic pathways. Patients with uremia and paraproteinemias may have excessive bleeding due to dysfunctional platelets. Patients with bone marrow failure due to malignancies can have low platelet levels. There are autoimmune conditions that can cause thrombocytopenia, which are easily treated with glucocorticoids or cessation of the offending agents. Patients with liver disease from alcoholic or nonalcoholic related causes can have coagulopathies due to abnormalities in vitamin K-dependent clotting factors (Table 13-1).

MEDICATIONS. Most acquired coagulation deficiencies are secondary or related to medications. Often patients are on medications that may affect hemostasis. A full list of medications including supplements and herbal products is important to obtain. Understanding the mechanism of action of these medications is important to properly address potential hemostasis issues prior to surgery. Medications can be subdivided into platelet inhibitors or coagulation factor inhibitors. Table 13-2 lists these medications.

Platelet inhibitors affect hemostasis by inhibiting enzymes or receptors that are critical in platelet activation, adhesion, aggregation, and ultimately plug formation. These agents are used in treating coronary artery disease, peripheral vascular disease, or strokes. Some patients use these medications as a means of preventing such conditions from occurring. The most common drug used is aspirin, an irreversible cyclooxygenase inhibitor often taken in combination with other antiplatelet agents. Thienopyridines are a class of drugs that reversibly inhibits ADP-receptor binding to decrease platelet aggregation. Clopidogrel (Plavix) is widely used and recognized. Prasugrel (Effient) is a newer drug that is more potent than clopidogrel.[7] Dipyridamole (Persantine) actually has no clinical effects on hemostasis even though it has anti-platelet activity. However, when mixed with aspirin (Aggrenox), it can impair hemostasis. This drug is used following mechanical heart valve placement and in stroke patients.

Prior to 1993, guidelines for dermatologic surgery were to stop antiplatelet agents up to 7 to 10 days prior to surgery.[8] In recent years, the paradigm has shifted to support continuing medically necessary aspirin. Although the use of these antiplatelet agents can elevate the risk of bleeding,[8–12] temporary cessation can result in life-threatening complications. Reports of thrombotic complications such as strokes, transient ischemic attacks, myocardial infarctions, and pulmonary emboli have been widely publicized.[10,13,14] As a result, it is now recommended to continue medically necessary aspirin in patients undergoing cutaneous surgery. If aspirin is used primarily for prophylaxis or pain management, discontinuation 7 to 10 days prior to surgery is recommended.

TABLE 13-2
Medications that Affect Hemostasis[7–17]

Medication	Mechanism of Action	Comments
Oral Platelet inhibitors		
Aspirin	Irreversible inhibition of COX-1 and COX-2 ▪ Decreased thromboxane A2 production ▪ Decreased platelet aggregation and degranulation	Effects last for life of platelet
Nonsteroidal anti-inflammatory drugs	Reversible inhibition of COX-1 and/or COX-2	Discontinue 2–3 d prior to surgery
Thienopyridines ▪ Ticlopidine (Ticlid) ▪ Clopidogrel (Plavix) ▪ Prasugrel (Effient)	Reversible inhibition of ADP receptor binding ▪ Decreased platelet aggregation and activation	Prasugrel more potent than clopidogrel
Dipyridamole (Persantine) Dipyridamole + Aspirin (Aggrenox)	Phosphodiesterase inhibitor, increases cAMP and blocks ADP binding ▪ Decreased platelet aggregation ▪ Vasodilation	Very little effect on hemostasis, unless mixed with aspirin
Parenteral Platelet inhibitors		
Glycoprotein IIb/IIIa inhibitors ▪ Abciximab (ReoPro) ▪ Eptifibatide (Integrilin) ▪ Tirofiban (Aggrastat)	Inhibit binding to glycoprotein IIb/IIIa ▪ Decreased platelet aggregation	Used in conjunction with aspirin and heparin; used during acute coronary syndromes
Oral Coagulation Factor Inhibitors		
Warfarin	Inhibits vitamin K epoxide reductase ▪ Decreased function of Factors II, VII, IX, and X	Monitored with INR
Dabigatran (Pradaxa)	Directly inhibits thrombin ▪ Decreased fibrin formation	No monitoring required
Rivaroxaban (Xarelto)	Factor Xa inhibitor	No monitoring required
Parenteral Coagulation Factor Inhibitors		
Heparin, Low–molecular-weight Heparin (Lovenox)	Accelerates antithrombin activity, inhibits Factor Xa	Heparin monitored with PTT Administered subcutaneously or intravenously
Fondaparinux (Arixtra)	Factor Xa inhibitors	Administered subcutaneously, no monitoring required

Trade names of drugs are in parenthesis.

Glycoprotein IIb/IIIa inhibitors are a newer class of antiplatelet agents and include abciximab (ReoPro), eptifibatide (Integrilin), and tirofiban (Aggrastat). These medications are given intravenously and are used in the setting of acute coronary syndromes. They are, therefore, more commonly encountered in the inpatient setting.

Medications can also affect hemostasis by inhibiting coagulation factors. The most widely known and used drug in this category is warfarin, which inhibits vitamin K-dependent clotting factors.[15] Warfarin activity is highly variable depending on dietary vitamin K intake, liver function, coexisting medical conditions, concurrent medications, and variations in cytochrome activity. The goal INR usually ranges from 2 to 3, unless the indication is for a mechanical heart valve (2.5–3.5). Indications for the use of warfarin include prophylaxis and treatment of venous thrombosis, thrombosis prophylaxis in patients with atrial fibrillation and mechanical heart valves, and reduction of the risk of death, recurrent myocardial infarction, and stroke in patients with recent myocardial infarctions. As with antiplatelet agents, there are studies showing elevated risk of bleeding in patients taking warfarin.[9] The previous recommendation was to stop warfarin 3 days prior to surgical procedures. However, given the recorded complications of thromboembolic events in patients who discontinue this medication, it is no longer advisable to discontinue it, provided it is within therapeutic range.[13,16] INR should be checked within 24 hours before surgery to ensure that levels are not supratherapeutic, in which case the surgery should be delayed until appropriate levels are reached.

There are newer anticoagulants that dermatologic surgeons will likely encounter in their practice. Dabigatran (Pradaxa) is an oral medication that directly binds to thrombin, and is indicated for thromboembolic prophylaxis in patients with atrial fibrillation.[17] Factor Xa inhibitors are another new group of antihemostatic drugs. Rivaroxaban (Xarelto) falls in this category and is taken orally for the prevention of deep vein thrombosis and thromboembolic complications of atrial fibrillation. As with the thienopyridines, there is no means of monitoring the level of anticoagulation on these newer drugs.[17] Their ability to increase bleeding risks during cutaneous surgery as compared to older drugs has yet to be established.

HERBAL, DIETARY, AND HOMEOPATHIC SUPPLEMENTS

Supplements come in a variety of forms, including herbs, botanicals, minerals, vitamins, and hormones. It is interesting to note that a significant number of surgical patients use supplements; 22% take herbs and 51% use vitamin supplements.[18] More and more patients turn to supplements as an alternative to conventional pharmaceuticals. Because these products are thought to be naturally occurring, they are perceived to be safe. Many supplements can have an effect on coagulation, and are therefore important to physicians who perform surgery. When obtaining a list of medications from patients, dermatologic surgeons should also ask for over-the-counter drugs and supplements so that patients can be assessed and counseled regarding their risk for bleeding.

There are various proposed mechanisms by which supplements can impair hemostatic function (Table 13-3).

TABLE 13-3
Herbal, Dietary and Homeopathic Supplements that Affect Hemostasis[18–22]

Supplements with Antiplatelet Capability	**Proposed Mechanism**	***Coumarin-containing Supplements* (Continued)**	**Proposed Mechanism**
Arnica Montana	A, B	Red clover (*Trifolium pratense*)	
Bladderwrack (*Fucus vesiculosus*)	F	Sweet clover (*Melilotus officinalis, Melilotus alba*)	
Chinese agrimony (*Agrimonia pilosa*)	A	Sweet woodruff (*Galium odoratum*)	
Danshen	A, C	***Supplements with Unknown Antiplatelet/ Anticoagulation Mechanisms***	
Dong quai (*Angelica sinensis*)	C	Anise (*Pimpinella anisum*)	Unknown/ uncertain
Evening primrose (*Oenathera biennis*)	B	Bilberry (*Vaccinium*)	
Fish oil	B	Bromelain	
Garlic	A, B, C, F	Cat's claw (*Uncaria tomentosa*)	
Ginger	B	Devil's claw (*Harpagophytum procumbens*)	
Gingko	D	Cayenne fruit (*Capsicum frutescens*)	
Ginseng	B, C, D	Celery (*Apium graveolens*)	
Glucosamine	B	Chinese peony (*Paeoniae rubra*)	
Grape seed extract	A, C, F	Chondroitin	
Green tea (*Camellia sinensis*)	B	Coleus (*Solenostemon*)	
Guarana (*Paullinia cupana*)	B	Feverfew (*Tanacetum parthenium*)	
Horse chestnut seed (*Aesculus hippocastanum*)	C	*Fritillaria cirrhosa*	
Horseradish (*Armoracia rusticana*)	B, C	*Geum japonicum*	
Horsetail rush (*Equisetum*)	C, E	Guggul (*Commiphora wightii*)	
Licorice	D	*Lonicera japonica*	
Onion (*Allium cepa*)	B	Oil of wintergreen (methyl salicylate)	
Poncitrin (*Poncirus trifoliate*)	B, E	Papain (*Carica papaya*)	
Scutellaria baicalensis	C	Red chili pepper (*Capsaicin*)	
Turmeric root (*Cucuma longa/aromatica*)	A	Reishi fruit (*Ganoderma lucidum*)	
Coumarin-containing Supplements		St. John's wort (*Hypericum perforatum*)	
Alfalfa (*Medicago sativa*)	Similar to warfarin	Saw palmetto (*Serenoa repens*)	
Fenugreek (*Trigonella foenum-graecum*)		White willow (*Salix alba*)	

A, Inhibits collagen-induced platelet aggregation; B, Inhibits thromboxane formation; C, Inhibits adenosine diphosphate; D, Inhibits platelet activating factor; E, Inhibits thrombin; F, inhibits fibrin formation.

Some can affect platelet function via inhibition of platelet aggregation, acting as inhibitors of various factors that promote platelet aggregation, while others contain coumarin or coumarin-like ingredients that behave like warfarin.

Ginkgo (*Ginkgo biloba*) is a popular supplement used to enhance memory and treat peripheral vascular disease, erectile dysfunction, macular degeneration, tinnitus, and vertigo. It inhibits platelet-activating factor, which is an important mediator of platelet aggregation.[19] Garlic (*Allium sativum*) has been shown to inhibit ADP-induced platelet aggregation and degranulation. There have been reports of spontaneous postoperative bleeding in patients taking garlic, but most problems are encountered in patients taking higher-than-recommended dosages or in patients also taking antiplatelet agents.[20]

Ginseng (*Panax ginseng*) is thought to be the most popular supplement worldwide. It is used to improve physical, mental, and sexual performance, as well as to treat and prevent cancers and improve immunity. The active components of ginseng are steroidal compounds called ginsenosides, which inhibit cyclooxygenase and thromboxane A_2 synthase in vitro.[19] However, the clinical evidence for increased bleeding with ginseng is limited to a few case reports.[20] The second best-selling herbal supplement in the United States is St. John's wort. Its antidepressant effects are attributed to hypericum which inhibits serotonin reuptake and downregulates serotonin receptors. Although St. John's wort will interfere with metabolism of warfarin, it does not directly affect coagulation.[19]

There have been several studies on the hemostatic effects of fish oil. The omega-3 fatty acids in fish oil are responsible for its antiplatelet activity. However, study results have been mixed, with some studies showing moderately increased bleeding times and reduced in vitro platelet aggregation, while others show no effect on hemostatic parameters. When combined with antiplatelet agents such as aspirin, a few studies have shown increased bleeding times.[20] Vitamin E also has antiplatelet activity, but this appears to be dose dependent. Studies have shown that low doses of vitamin E (lower than 400 IU/d) do not affect platelet activity. However, when taken at doses higher than 400 IU/d (up to 1200 IU/d), inhibition of arachidonic acid metabolism resulting in reduced platelet function has been reported.[20]

It is difficult to draw solid conclusions about the effect of supplements on hemostasis, or to determine how clinically significant these effects are. Well-controlled clinical trials are lacking, and most of the literature consists of case reports and anecdotal evidence of an increased propensity for bleeding while taking certain herbal medications. For now, one of the best and safest methods of preparing patients for surgery is to adequately screen them for supplements and homeopathic remedies. Dermatologic surgeons should familiarize themselves with the list offered in Table 13-3. It is not necessary to discontinue supplements for less invasive dermatologic procedures, such as biopsies or excisions. However, cessation of these products prior to more invasive procedures (liposuction) may be beneficial as discontinuation of supplements will cause little to no harm. Agents with antiplatelet activity should be stopped 7 to 10 days prior to surgery.

OPERATIVE MANAGEMENT OF HEMOSTASIS

PREOPERATIVE PREPARATION

A certain amount of bleeding is expected during cutaneous surgery, although bleeding can become overwhelming when it occurs in multiple areas of the surgical field. There are basic preparations prior to surgery that can make intraoperative bleeding more manageable. As cutaneous surgery patients are awake and only undergo local anesthesia, nothing could be more aggravating or anxiety-provoking than an ill-prepared physician who is about to perform surgery in a disorganized procedure suite. The room should be properly prepared for surgery, with all surgical instruments in place and the appropriate electrosurgical tool ready. There should be enough supplies on the surgical tray, including gauze or cotton-tip applicators for blotting. Some surgical offices also utilize suction to manage bleeding. Suturing materials should be easily accessible. Assistants should be properly trained, especially in simple maneuvers such as direct pressure application on the bleeding site until more permanent measures are in place. There should be ample lighting, and the patient should be properly positioned. It should be common practice that patients are in a reclining position, with gauze at the most dependent portion of the surgical field to avoid pooling of the blood. Knowledge of anatomy, specifically the vasculature of the surgical site, is vital in preparing for expected bleeding.

Dermatologists have a variety of tools to control excessive bleeding during surgery – from the most basic method of direct pressure to hemostatic agents that initiate the coagulation scheme.

VASOCONSTRICTION

Epinephrine is added to anesthetics for vasoconstriction to localize the anesthetic effects of the medication and provide hemostasis. Epinephrine can be diluted to 1:100,000 or 1:300,000 and added to the anesthetic prior to injection. Although the onset of action of anesthetics is very fast, epinephrine has a slower onset of action, and at least 15 minutes should be allowed for full vasoconstrictive effect. There has been controversy over using epinephrine in digital blocks, but recent literature suggests that in patients with no prior history of peripheral vascular disease, uncontrolled hypertension, diabetes mellitus, or vasospastic or thrombotic disease, small volumes of dilute epinephrine (1:200,000) are safe to use for digital anesthesia.[23] Epinephrine, mixed at 1:1,000,000 dilution, can provide dramatic hemostasis during liposuction in the form of tumescent anesthesia.[24]

COMPRESSION AND SUTURING TECHNIQUES

The oldest mechanical method of halting bleeding is the application of pressure. Mechanical pressure takes many forms in dermatologic surgery. Direct digital pressure or clamping of profusely bleeding vessels with a hemostat

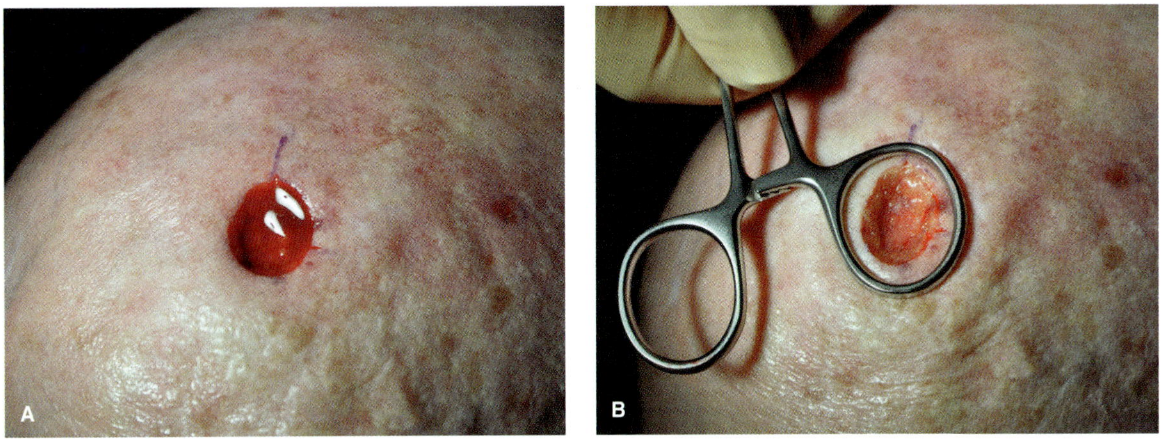

Figure 13-2 Handle of steel surgical instrument used to achieve rapid hemostasis. **A.** Bleeding surgical site in anticoagulated patient. **B.** Bleeding controlled with circumferential compression of wound using hemostat handle.

achieves temporary hemostasis until a more definitive action can be performed. Depending on the anatomic site, certain instruments can also be helpful. The chalazion clamp, used for mucosal surfaces such as the lip, provides stabilization as well as hemostasis while performing a procedure. At the nasal ala, compression from the inside of the nasal vestibule using cotton-tipped applicators helps to tamponade vessels as well as retract and immobilize the free edge of the ala. The looped handles of steel surgical instruments can provide compression during procedures, as shown in Figure 13-2. These can be particularly useful on convex areas such as the forehead or the scalp. Handles of steel instruments can be used to compress open wounds circumferentially so that the surgical field can be kept dry for cautery. This technique can be particularly useful in controlling bleeding while biopsies on the scalp are performed and in providing rapid compression of arterial bleeds.

Tourniquets are another mechanical means of achieving hemostasis. In cutaneous surgery, tourniquets are more commonly used on digits, especially during nail surgery (Fig. 13-3). Properly used, tourniquets provide compression of digital arteries and better visualization of the surgical field. There are various methods to place a digital tourniquet. A quarter-inch Penrose drain can be wrapped around the base of the proximal phalanx and clamped and drawn taut with a hemostat, or the tip of a surgical glove can be snipped and rolled proximally, exsanguinating the digit. Pneumatic tourniquets and Marmed digital tourniquets also exist for this purpose.[25] Although the exact relationship between tourniquet pressures and neurovascular injury is not clearly defined, the application of digital tourniquets should be limited to no more than 15 minutes to minimize the possibility of neurovascular damage.[26]

Suture ligation and various suturing techniques are excellent tools to control bleeding. There are situations when pressure and electrosurgery may be inadequate, especially when vessels greater than 2 mm in diameter are involved. If arteries are visualized and need to be sacrificed during surgery, ligation of the vessels in advance will prevent excessive bleeding. Vessels should be clamped with fine-tipped hemostats and absorbable sutures (such as polyglactin 910) should be used in ligating them. This technique is especially useful during extirpation of deeply infiltrating tumors on the lip, temple, and preauricular cheek. A figure-of-eight stitch or a square stitch can be used around bleeding vessels that may be difficult to visualize. For slow oozing at the wound edge, a singular or running horizontal mattress suture will provide compression and assist with hemostasis. Another useful technique is the purse string suture, which can be placed in a transcutaneous or subcuticular fashion (Fig. 13-4). Tension is applied by pulling at the ends of the suture, thus applying circumferential pressure by constricting the center of the wound. This can be particularly helpful for large defects of the scalp left to heal by second intention. Another helpful suturing technique for the highly vascularized skin of the scalp is the running-locked suture, which permits rapid closure of wounds and control of bleeding (Fig. 13-5). Although bolsters are commonly used to secure skin grafts, they can be particularly useful in providing compression and achieving hemostasis, especially in areas that are very difficult to bandage. Tie-over bolsters are useful when placed over open wounds that are allowed to heal by secondary intention, especially in patients with coagulopathies (Fig. 13-6). Bolsters can be left in place for 1 week postoperatively without the need for dressing changes.

ELECTROSURGERY

Electrosurgery is one of the most common hemostatic techniques used in dermatology. During electrosurgery, an electric current is applied to tissues. The tissue does not conduct the current efficiently, and this resistance to flow results in conversion of the electric energy to heat energy which coagulates proteins and damages tissue. The four main modalities of electrosurgery are electrodesiccation, electrofulguration, electrocoagulation, and electrosection. Both electrodesiccation and electrofulguration use monoterminal and are sufficient in thrombosing small superficial vessels.

Electrocoagulation and electrosection use biterminal devices and cause deeper ablation. Because electrocoagulation provides deeper penetration of current, it is the best modality to use for hemostasis. The bipolar electrode allows the current to pass directly between two tips of the electrode forceps. It creates less surrounding tissue damage

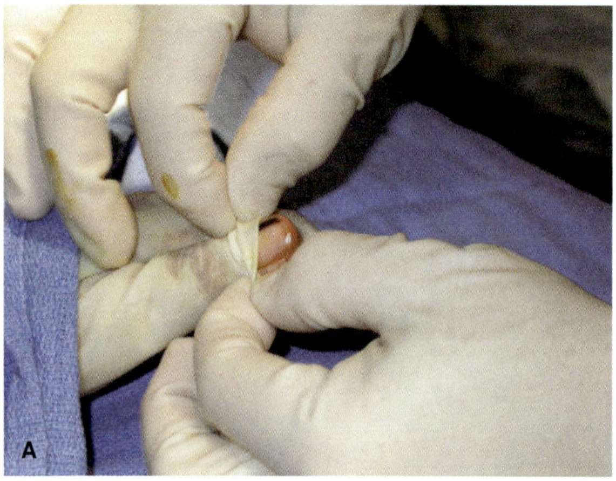

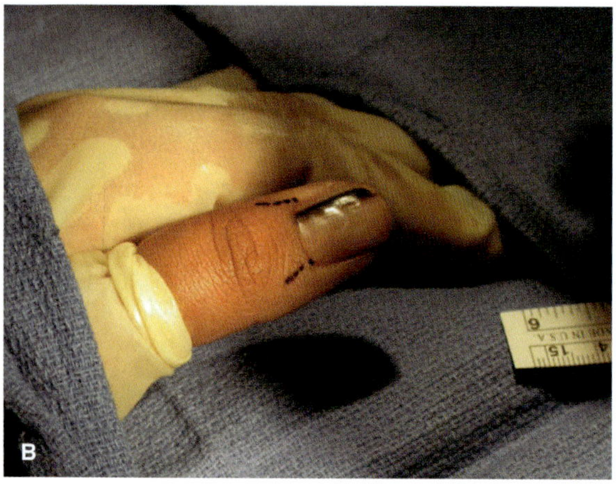

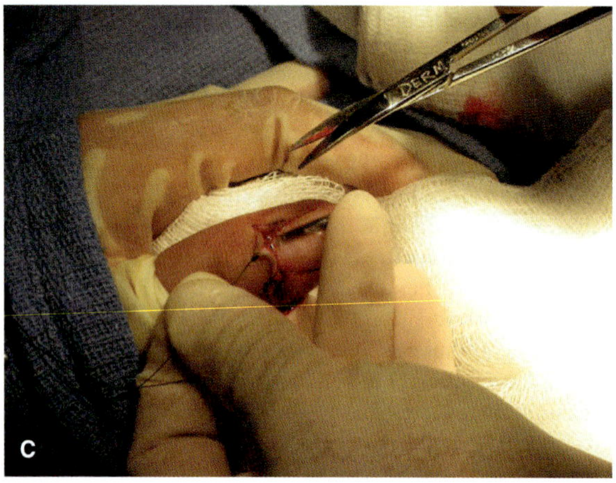

Figure 13-3 Tourniquet used during nail surgery for hemostasis. **A.** Patient dons a larger glove and the glove tip over the affected finger is cut. **B.** Compression of vasculature is achieved as the glove is rolled proximally. **C.** Note the bloodless field during the procedure.

while achieving hemostatic effects to those of the unipolar electrode.

Electrocautery does not transfer current to the tissues, but converts electric energy to thermal energy within the device, which is then passed to tissues. This technique only works to control minimal bleeding and is best when used in a dry field. Because current is not transferred to the patient, it is the safest modality to use in patients with implantable electronic devices, but electrocoagulation with the bipolar electrode is also safe.

It is important to maintain a dry surgical field, as electric current does not effectively pass through blood. It is also important to minimize the amount of excess charred tissue, as it may lead to inflammation and poor wound healing.[27]

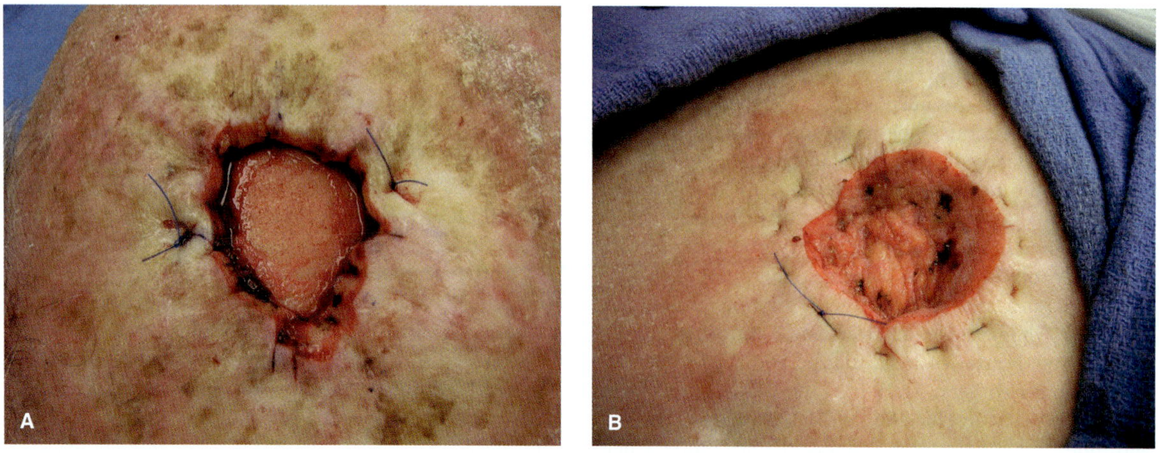

Figure 13-4 Placement of pursestring suture helps reduce the risk of bleeding. Polypropylene suture can be placed **A.** subcuticularly with an escape loop, or **B.** transcutaneously.

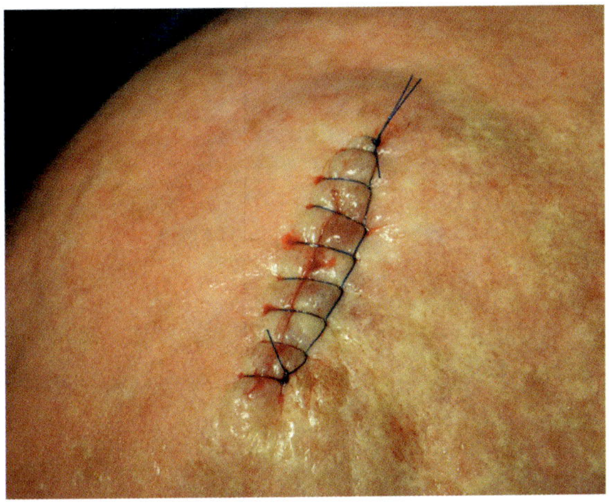

Figure 13-5 A running-locked suture on the scalp allows for rapid closure and control of bleeding.

TOPICAL HEMOSTATIC AGENTS

Topical hemostatic agents play an important role in both common and complex dermatologic procedures. These agents can be classified based on their mechanism of action and include physical or mechanical, caustic, biologic, and physiologic agents. Some agents induce protein coagulation and precipitation that results in occlusion of small cutaneous vessels, whereas others take advantage of the later stages of the coagulation cascade. Hemostatic ability, tissue reactivity, biodegradability, ease of sterilization, and cost are important considerations when choosing a topical hemostatic agent.[28]

Table 13-4 reviews topical hemostatic agents that are readily available. Some are used in dermatology on a day-to-day basis, whereas others have very limited use.

CAUSTIC AGENTS. Caustic agents are some of the most commonly used products in dermatology, especially for minor procedures. The common mechanism of action in this group is tissue necrosis, causing protein precipitation that promotes tissue coagulation and thrombus formation. These styptic agents are inexpensive and easy to handle. They are rubbed onto the wound using gauze or cotton-tipped applicators. One particular disadvantage is the risk of pigmentary alteration at the site of application. Ferric subsulfate (Monsel's solution) and silver nitrate can cause tattooing of the skin by leaving dermal deposits of iron and silver, respectively. Aluminum chloride solution (Drysol), commonly used following superficial biopsies, is less likely to leave pigment particles. Excessive application of caustic agents should be avoided as they can cause localized inflammatory reactions and impede wound healing.[28,29] An added benefit of these agents is their antimicrobial properties.[29,30]

One new caustic agent that has been recently approved by the government and has been extensively used in the battlefield is mineral zeolite (QuikClot). This agent is derived from lava rock and is made up of silicon, aluminum, sodium, and magnesium. It causes an exothermic reaction at the site of application by rapidly absorbing water, leaving behind a concentrated quantity of platelets and clotting factors that leads to rapid clotting. Older formulations have caused severe thermal burns, but the new formulation can only reach a maximum wound temperature of 105°F.[31]

Zinc chloride paste, a product of important historical value in the field of Mohs micrographic surgery, is still available as a hemostatic agent (Z squares).[32] Like other caustic agents, it is applied directly to the bleeding site, but can cause significant discomfort. Because of their antitumor properties, zinc paste compounds are touted as homeopathic agents for curing skin cancer.[33]

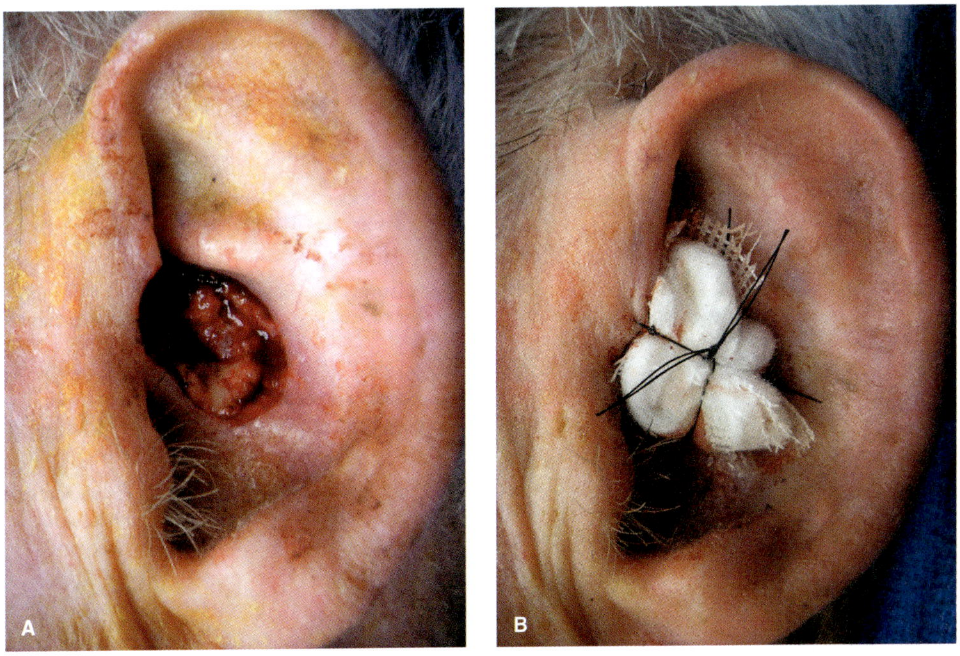

Figure 13-6 **A.** An open wound left to heal by secondary intention in conchal bowl of a patient with coagulopathy. **B.** A tie-over bolster with silk sutures serves as a compressive dressing to help control bleeding.

TABLE 13-4
Topical Hemostatic Agents[26–41]

Hemostatic Agent	Formulations	Mechanism of Action	Comment
Caustic agents			
Zinc chloride	Paste Gauze (Z-squares)	Protein coagulation leading to thrombus formation	Use limited by pain
Ferric subsulfate (Monsel's solution)	20% Solution	Protein coagulation due to low pH and oxidation by subsulfate group	Iron particles can tattoo tissues
Silver nitrate	Sticks, 10% solution	Free silver ions cause protein coagulation	Precipitated proteins leave thin eschar, small risk of tattoo
Aluminum chloride	20%–70% solution	Hydrolyzed to HCl, causing protein coagulation and vasoconstriction	
Mineral Zeolite (QuikClot)	Powder	Absorbs water molecules and causes exothermic reaction; concentrates platelets and clotting factors for rapid coagulation	Minimal risk of thermal injury
Biologic physical agents			
Gelatin (Gelfoam, Gelfilm, Surgifoam)	Foam, powder, film, sponge	Absorbs water, creates structural meshwork for platelet aggregation	May be soaked in ferric subsulfate or thrombin
Oxidized cellulose (Surgicel, Oxycel)	Mesh, gauze, sponges, and fibrillar tufts	Provides a structural meshwork for platelet aggregation	Antimicrobial properties
Poly-N-acetyl glucosamine (HemCon, ChitoSeal, SyvekPatch, Clo-Sur P.A.D.)	Film	Positive charge attracts negatively charged erythrocytes	Expensive; little use in dermatology
Microfibrillar collagen (Avitene, Helistat, Instat)	Powder, foam, film	Provides matrix for platelet adherence and activation	
Pro QR powder (Biolife)	Powder	Forms artificial scab with hydrophilic polymers and potassium salts	Over the counter
Physiologic hemostatic agents			
Epinephrine	Solution	Vasoconstrictor	Commonly administered with anesthetic
Cocaine	Solution, powder, gel	Vasoconstrictor	
Thrombin (Thrombin-JMI, FloSeal, Evithrom)	Solution, powder	Converts fibrinogen to fibrin, activates platelets and other clotting factors	Bovine and human derived; may cause disseminated intravascular coagulopathy
Fibrin sealants (Tisseel, Crosseal, Evicel)	Injectable dual syringe, spray	Thrombin and fibrinogen mixed at application site resulting in fibrin formation	
Platelet gels (SmartPReP)	Gel	Concentrated platelets and growth factors augment coagulation	Bovine, or can be individually prepared from patient's platelets
Mechanical			
Bone wax (Ostene)	Wax	Tamponades bleeding on exposed bone	Tissue reactions; inhibition of osteogenesis; limited use in dermatology
Cyanocrylates (Dermabond, Band-Aid Liquid Bandage, Tissu-Glu)	Liquid glue	Self-polymerizing causing adhesion of tissue and physical barrier to bleeding	Best used in pediatric patients and superficial wounds; some antibacterial properties

Trade names of agents are in parenthesis.

BIOLOGIC PHYSICAL AGENTS.

Biologic physical hemostatic agents mimic physiologic mediators of platelet aggregation. They vary in origin (plant, algae, bovine, human), but they work similarly by providing a matrix to which platelets adhere and promote thrombus organization. These products can be left intact on the wound, since they would be absorbed or metabolized completely within a few weeks, but they carry the risk of infection.[28] They are relatively inexpensive, readily available, pliable, and easy to handle.

Gelatin (Gelfoam) is a hygroscopic substance, absorbing many times its weight in water or liquid. It creates a moist environment to promote clotting and granulation tissue formation. It works best for diffuse small-vessel oozing and can be combined with topical agents such as ferric subsulfate or thrombin to increase efficacy.[34] Cellulose (Oxycel, Surgicel) is an oxidized plant product formulated as a mesh, gauze, sponges, or fibrillar tufts. The material is placed in the wound bed with firm pressure until the bleeding stops. It can be left in place and allowed to absorb over a few weeks,[34] with low rates of infection due to antibacterial properties of the cellulose.[28] The use of cellulose creates a low-pH environment and thus it inactivates other biologically active topical agents such as thrombin.[34]

A complex polysaccharide produced by fermenting microalgal cultures called poly-N-acetyl glucosamine (HemCon, SyvekPatch, Clo-Sur PAD, ChitoSeal) is available for small wounds and is more often used in trauma, maxillofacial, and neurosurgery because of its ability to stop significant arterial bleeding. This agent is positively charged and attracts the negatively charged erythrocytes to create a clot, and may induce vasospasm to enhance hemostasis.[31]

Microfibrillar collagen (Avitene, Instat, Helistat, Helitene, Collastat, Collatene) is composed of refined bovine collagen fibrils that provide a matrix for platelet adhesion, which results in initiation of the coagulation cascade.[35] This product is marketed as sheets, sponges, or powder and is applied to the wound bed with dry instruments and firm pressure. Despite its bovine origin, it has low immunogenicity.[32] A physical hemostatic agent that is available over-the-counter is Pro QR Powder (Biolife), which contains hydrophilic polymers and potassium salts that creates an artificial crust when applied to a bleeding wound.[28]

PHYSIOLOGIC AGENTS.

Physiologic agents can be subdivided into two subgroups – those causing vasoconstriction (epinephrine, cocaine) and those containing clotting products (thrombin, fibrin sealant, platelet gel). Epinephrine, as discussed earlier, is commonly administered with injectable anesthetics. It can be topically applied on the wound bed with gauze or dispersed with a hypodermic needle. Concentrations ranging from 1:1,000 to 1:1,000,000 are typically used.[36] Rare tachyarrhythmias have been reported to cause fatality,[37] but this is usually a result of systemic administration.

Cocaine is a potent vasoconstrictor that has been used for medicinal purposes since 1884. It has a mode of action similar to that of epinephrine, activating adrenergic receptors on blood vessels. Adverse reactions, such as tachycardia and hypertension, exist at even low dosages. More serious reactions include cardiac arrhythmias, chest pain, myocardial infarction, syncope, stroke, seizures, and death. It is available in 4% and 10% solutions, as well as in a mixture of 0.5% tetracaine, 1:2,000 epinephrine, and 11.8% cocaine gel (TAC). This product is of minimal use in dermatology. It is utilized in otolaryngology and ophthalmology when performing procedures on mucosal surfaces.[38]

Thrombin-derivative products (Thrombostat, Thrombin-JMI, FloSeal) direct the conversion of fibrinogen to fibrin. They take advantage of natural physiologic processes, thereby avoiding foreign body or inflammatory reactions. Topical thrombin may be applied to the wound bed as a solution via a saturated gauze or spray, or as a powder applied directly to the wound bed. Newer formulations require mixture at the bedside and skill on the part of the applicator. Care must be taken to avoid introducing thrombin into larger caliber vessels, as systemic exposure may lead to disseminated intravascular coagulation or death.[32] Bovine-derived thrombin should not be used in patients allergic to bovine products. The high cost of thrombin-derived products may be prohibitive for routine use, but they can be useful in patients with platelet dysfunction.[28]

Fibrin sealants (Tisseel, Crosseal) are prepared from cryoprecipitates (homologous or synthetic) and have the advantage of not promoting inflammation or tissue necrosis. Like some of the newer formulations of thrombin products, they require skill during application and are very expensive. The sealant is administered using a dual syringe compartment system. In one compartment are fibrinogen, factor XIII, fibronectin, and fibrinolysis inhibitors. The second compartment contains thrombin and calcium chloride.[39] Proper mixing of the two sets of components is important to achieve maximum effect. Onset of action is usually within 30 seconds, and the clot is reabsorbed over 5 to 10 days. Applications in dermatologic surgery include improving graft survival, particularly in difficult locations with high shearing forces and its use in patients with coagulopathies such as hemophilia and von Willebrand disease.[28]

Platelet gels (Vitagel) have been used as hemostatic agents following cosmetic procedures such as liposuction and laser resurfacing.[40,41] They are made of a concentrated bovine collagen-platelet combination, which speeds the conversion of fibrinogen to fibrin when applied to bleeding sites. They are superior to fibrin glues in that they improve overall clot strength and facilitate tissue regeneration.[40]

MECHANICAL AGENTS.

Bone wax is used to tamponade bleeding over exposed bone, and acts as a physical barrier to bleeding. It is composed of beeswax and isopropyl palmitate and may contain almond oils or salicyclic acid.[42] Although it is relatively inexpensive, the use of bone wax may lead to an increased risk of infection, foreign body granulomatous reactions, and inhibition of new tissue growth. A synthetic, water-soluble alternative to bone wax, Ostene, does not impede osteogenesis or increase risk for infection.[43]

Cyanoacrylates (Dermabond, Band-Aid Liquid Bandage) are glue polymers that create tissue adhesion, causing a physical or mechanical means of stopping bleeding. They are typically used in the emergency setting to treat superficial wounds in the pediatric population or patients with cognitive deficits.[28]

POSTOPERATIVE MANAGEMENT

Bleeding complications are inevitable, even in cutaneous surgery. Management of bleeding does not end at the completion of the procedure. Equally critical is the postoperative period, especially during the first 48 hours when bleeding is likely to occur. Dermatologic surgeons should be particularly aware of the varied presentations of bleeding complications (arterial bleeding, hematoma formation) and their potential sequelae (flap failure, tissue necrosis, dehiscence, infection).

Immediately after surgery, the patient should have an appropriate pressure dressing placed. Various forms of pressure dressings can be used. Folded absorbent gauze over a nonadherent dressing can be reinforced with adhesive tape. Dental rolls are particularly useful as a pressure dressing over small surgical sites. Close attention should be paid when dressing a site in which complex reconstruction following tumor extirpation has been performed. A bulkier dressing should be placed to provide compression and immobilization and avoid shearing forces over the site. A bolster dressing may be sutured in place over graft sites to increase take and provide compression.

Patients should receive specific written instructions, not only regarding postoperative wound care, but also reviewing the signs and symptoms of bleeding complications. They should be instructed in the use of direct pressure over bleeding or oozing sites and be provided a contact number to receive further guidance if needed. When true emergencies do occur, the physician should be easily accessible to address the complication. Persistent bleeding despite prolonged direct pressure should be investigated. The surgical site may need to be reopened and explored so that bleeding vessels can be cauterized or ligated. In patients with altered coagulation, appropriate topical hemostatic agents may need to be used. In the event of a hematoma, evacuation may be necessary to address the source and prevent necrosis or infection. It is of critical importance that an expanding hematoma near the eye or on the neck be addressed to prevent catastrophic damage to the eye or compression of the airway. Anticoagulated patients and those undergoing extensive procedures, such as extensive reconstruction following skin cancer surgery and cervicofacial liposuction, are at a much higher risk of developing bleeding complications.

CONCLUSION

Successful hemostasis in dermatologic surgery is not limited to knowing the various techniques of controlling bleeding during the intraoperative period. Patients must be properly assessed for risks of bleeding and have underlying conditions addressed prior to surgery. Patients must be closely followed and instructed regarding the proper care of the operative site during the postoperative period. Multiple hemostatic agents are now available, and more are being developed as our knowledge and understanding of the physiologic basis of hemostasis continue to evolve. These agents, however, should not serve as substitutes for meticulous surgical technique.

REFERENCES

1. Drucker CB. Ambroise Pare and the birth of the gentle art of surgery. *Yale J Biol Med.* 2008;81:199–202.
2. Gonzalez EA, Jastrow KM, Holcomb JB, et al. Hemostasis, surgical bleeding, and transfusion. In: Brunicardi FC, Andersen DK, Billiar TR, et al. eds. *Schwartz's Principles of Surgery.* 9th ed. New York, NY: McGraw-Hill; 2010.
3. Konkle B. Bleeding and thrombosis. In: Longo DL, Fauci AS, Kasper DL, et al. eds. *Harrison's Principles of Internal Medicine.* 18th ed. New York, NY: McGraw-Hill, 2012.
4. Kumar A, Kar S, Fay WP. Thrombosis, physical activity, and acute coronary syndromes. *J Appl Physiol.* 2011;111:599–605.
5. Peterson SR, Joseph AK. Inherited bleeding disorders in dermatologic surgery. *Dermatol Surg.* 2001;27:885,
6. Seligsohn U. Treatment of inherited platelet disorders. *Haemophilia.* 2012;18:161–165.
7. Lazar LD, Lincoff AM. Prasugrel for acute coronary syndromes: faster, more potent, but higher bleeding risk. *Cleve Clin J Med.* 2009;76:707–714.
8. Goldsmith SM, Leshin B, Owen J. Management of patients taking anticoagulants and platelet inhibitors prior to dermatologic surgery. *J Dermatol Surg Oncol.* 1993;19:578–581.
9. Lewis KG, Dufresne RG Jr. A meta-analysis of complications attributed to anticoagulation among patients following cutaneous surgery. *Dermatol Surg.* 2008;34:160–164.
10. Cook-Norris RH, Michaels JD, Weaver AL, et al. Complications of cutaneous surgery in patients taking clopidogrel-containing anticoagulation. *J Am Acad Dermatol.* 2011;65:584–591.
11. Holmes DR Jr, Kereiakes DJ, Kleiman NS, Moliterno DJ, Patti G, Grines CL. Combining antiplatelet and anticoagulant therapies. *J Am Coll Cardiol.* 2009;54:95–109.
12. Bunick CG, Aasi SZ. Hemorrhagic complications in dermatologic surgery. *Dermatol Ther.* 2011;24:537–550.
13. Kovich O, Otley CC. Thrombotic complications related to discontinuation of warfarin and aspirin therapy perioperatively for cutaneous operation. *J Am Acad Dermatol.* 2003;48:233–237.
14. Alam M, Goldberg LH. Serious adverse vascular events associated with perioperative interruption of antiplatelet and anticoagulant therapy. *Dermatol Surg.* 2002;28:992–998.
15. Stewart LC, Langtry JA. Clopidogrel: mechanisms of action and review of the evidence relating to use during skin surgery procedures. *Clin Exp Dermatol.* 2010;35:341–345.
16. Schanbacher CF, Bennett RG. Postoperative stroke after stopping warfarin for cutaneous surgery. *Dermatol Surg.* 2000;26:785–789.
17. Davis EM, Packard KA, Knezevich JT, Campbell JA. New and emerging anticoagulant therapy for atrial fibrillation and acute coronary syndrome. *Pharmacotherapy.* 2011;31:975–1016.
18. Tsen LC, Segal S, Pothier M, Bader AM. Alternative medicine use in presurgical patients. *Anesthesiology.* 2000;93:148–151.
19. Beckert BW, Concannon MJ, Henry SL, Smith DS, Puckett CL. The effect of herbal medicines on platelet function: an in vivo experiment and review of the literature. *Plast Reconstr Surg.* 2007;120:2044–2050.
20. Stanger MJ, Thompson LA, Young AJ, Lieberman HR. Anticoagulant activity of select dietary supplements. *Nutr Rev.* 2012;70:107–117.
21. Dinehart SM, Henry L. Dietary supplements: altered coagulation and effects on bruising. *Dermatol Surg.* 2005;31:819–826.
22. Wong WW, Gabriel A, Maxwell GP, Gupta SC. Bleeding risks of herbal, homeopathic, and dietary supplements: a hidden nightmare for plastic surgeons? *Aesthet Surg J.* 2012;32:332–346.
23. Krunic AL, Wang LC, Soltani K, Weitzul S, Taylor RS. Digital anesthesia with epinephrine: an old myth revisited. *J Am Acad Dermatol.* 2004;51:755–759.
24. Klein JA. Tumescent technique for local anesthesia improves safety in large-volume liposuction. *Plast Reconstr Surg.* 1993;92:1085–1098.
25. Harrington AC, Cheyney JM, Kinsley-Scott T, Willard RJ. A novel digital tourniquet using a sterile glove and hemostat. *Dermatol Surg.* 2004;30:1065–1067.

26. Rich P. Nail biopsy: indications and methods. *Dermatol Surg.* 2001;27:229–234.
27. Hainer BL. Fundamentals of electrosurgery. *J Am Board Fam Pract.* 1991;4:419–426.
28. Palm MD, Altman JS. Topical hemostatic agents: a review. *Dermatol Surg.* 2008;34:431–445.
29. Olmstead PM, Lund HZ, Leonard DD. Monsel's solution: a histologic nuisance. *J Am Acad Dermatol.* 1980;3:492–498.
30. Spacciapoli P, Buxton D, Rothstein D, Friden P. Antimicrobial activity of silver nitrate against periodontal pathogens. *J Periodontal Res.* 2001;36:108–113.
31. Alam HB, Burris D, DaCorta JA, Rhee P. Hemorrhage control in the battlefield: role of new hemostatic agents. *Mil Med.* 2005;170:63–69.
32. Larson PO. Topical hemostatic agents for dermatologic surgery. *J Dermatol Surg Oncol.* 1988;14:623–632.
33. Brown CW Jr, Goldstein GD, Birkby CS. Auto-Mohs.com. *Dermatol Surg.* 2001;27:975–978.
34. Sileshi B, Achneck HE, Lawson JH. Management of surgical hemostasis: topical agents. *Vascular.* 2008;16:S22–S28.
35. Alexander JM, Rabinowitz JL. Microfibrillar collagen (Avitene) as a hemostatic agent in experimental oral wounds. *J Oral Surg.* 1978;36:202–205.
36. Glasson DW. Topical adrenaline as a hemostatic agent. *Plast Reconstr Surg.* 1984;74:451–452.
37. Vaughan RW. Ventricular arrhythmias after topical vasoconstrictors. *Anesth Analg.* 1973;52:161–165.
38. Long H, Greller H, Mercurio-Zappala M, Nelson LS, Hoffman RS. Medicinal use of cocaine: a shifting paradigm over 25 years. *Laryngoscope.* 2004;114:1625–1629.
39. Martinowitz U, Schulman S. Fibrin sealant in surgery of patients with a hemorrhagic diathesis. *Thromb Haemostasis.* 1995; 74:486–492.
40. Bhanot S, Alex JC. Current applications of platelet gels in facial plastic surgery. *Facial Plast Surg.* 2002;18:27–33.
41. Farrior E, Ladner K. Platelet gels and hemostasis in facial plastic surgery. *Facial Plast Surg.* 2011;27:308–314.
42. Howard TC, Kelley RR. The effect of bone wax on the healing of experimental rat tibial lesions. *Clin Orthop Relat Res.* 1969; 63:226–232.
43. Vestergaard RF, Jensen H, Vind-Kezunovic S, Jakobsen T, Søballe K, Hasenkam JM. Bone healing after median sternotomy: a comparison of two hemostatic devices. *J Cardiothorac Surg.* 2010;5:117.

CHAPTER 14

Electrosurgery

Jo Martin & Timothy S. Wang

INTRODUCTION

Electrosurgery refers to the use of high-frequency alternating current (AC) to fulgurate, coagulate, desiccate or cut living tissue. In true electrosurgery, an electrical current is used to generate heat within the tissue itself. Electrosurgery is used widely in the field of dermatology to provide hemostasis in surgical procedures and is a fundamental component of electrodesiccation and curettage. Furthermore, it is also commonly used to destroy small benign superficial lesions such as angiofibromas, fibrous papules, acrochordons, seborrheic keratoses, verrucae, pyogenic granulomas, and molluscum contagiosum.[1] Electrosurgical devices were developed in the early twentieth century, and remain widely used today.

In contrast, electrocautery (from Greek *kauterion*, branding iron), is not a true form of electrosurgery because no electrical current enters the patient.[2,3] In electrocautery, electrical current is used to heat a conductor, which then directly heats the tissue.

HISTORY

The forerunners of electrosurgery were developed in the late nineteenth century. The Oudin coil was developed in 1899 as a transformer designed to produce high voltage arcs and discharges that could cause superficial tissue damage or destruction. In 1891, Jacques Arsène d'Arsonval, a French physician, noted that currents with frequencies higher than 10 kHz passed through human tissue without neuromuscular stimulation or tetany.[4] In 1900, a Parisian physician, Joseph Rivière, described treating an ulcer on a patient's hand using high-frequency sparks.[2] Walter de Keating-Hart and Pozzi used sparks from an Oudin coil on the skin in 1907, and introduced the term *fulguration* to describe the superficial carbonization that resulted.[5] Fulguration derives from the Latin word, *fulgur*, which means lightning.

The term *electrocoagulation* (derived from Latin *coagulare*, to curdle) was first used by Doyen in 1909 to describe coagulation of tissue from direct contact with an electrode.[6] Doyen added an indifferent electrode to the circuit to allow electricity to flow back into the electrosurgical device. The indifferent electrode prevented shocks by providing a path for the return of the current and enhanced its penetration into tissues.[5] Soon after, the term *electrodesiccation* entered the lexicon to describe the slow dehydration of tissues using an electrical current.

The largest advancements in the field were made by William Bovie, Ph.D. and Harvey Cushing, M.D. In 1920, Bovie, "an eccentric inventor with a doctorate in plant physiology," developed the first electrosurgical device that offered both cutting and coagulation.[2] Cushing, a neurosurgeon at Peter Bent Brigham Hospital in Boston, became interested in this device and started using electrosurgery in his surgical cases in 1926. When these devices were first used in the operating room, Bovie controlled the output of the electrosurgical device. Throughout the years, Bovie and Cushing made many modifications to the original electrosurgical units (ESUs), adding monopolar and bipolar electrodes with blended waveforms. Because of their influence, electrosurgical devices are still often colloquially called "Bovies."[5]

In 1937, the low-powered hyfrecator was developed by the Birtcher Corporation. It was named as a portmanteau of "high frequency eradicator," and became the first nonground return electrosurgical device. Many outpatient offices today use a nonground return electrosurgical device similar to the original hyfrecator.[7]

ELECTRICITY BACKGROUND

A comprehensive review of the physics of electricity is beyond the scope of this discussion, although an understanding of basic electrical principles is useful. Both electrocautery and electrosurgery use the flow of electrons to perform work. The flow of electrons is termed current (I) and is defined as the number of electrons that move through a conductive medium over time. A common analogy used to illustrate current is to imagine a pump pushing water through a pipe: Just as water molecules flow through the pipe, electrons flow through a conductive medium. In this analogy, current describes the number of water molecules that pass through the pipe over time. Current is measured in amperes (amps); one amp is equivalent to 6.24×10^{18} electrons passing through an electrical circuit every second.

Resistance, measured in ohms, is impedance to the flow of electrons. In the analogy above, the diameter of the pipe is analogous to the resistance (R) of an electrical circuit. Voltage is the electrical potential energy between two points and is measured in volts (joules per coulomb); it can be conceptualized as the electromotive force that drives the current through the medium. A water pump provides a pressure difference in a pipe circuit and causes water to flow; voltage is analogous to the difference in water pressure. Current, voltage, and resistance are related by the formula, voltage (V) = current (I) × resistance (R).

A difference in potential energy can be used to do work. Just as flowing water can drive a turbine, an electric current can be used to convert potential energy into kinetic energy,

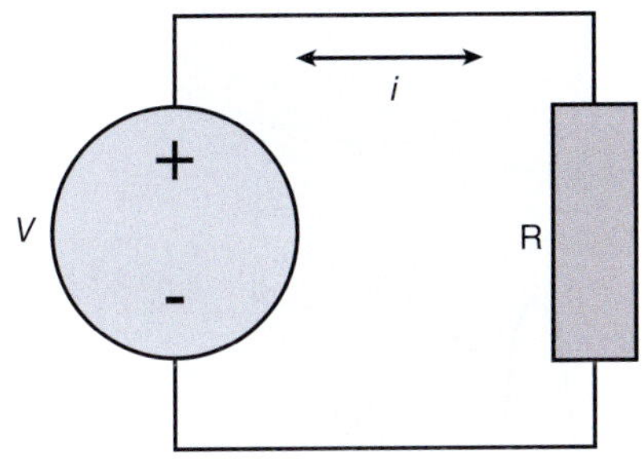

Figure 14-1 Alternating Circuit.

light, or heat. Power describes the rate at which an electrical charge is transferred or used and is measured in watts (joules per second). Power also describes the rate at which work is performed. Power, current, and voltage are related by the formula, power (P) = current (I) × voltage (V).

For current to flow, there must be potential difference between the primary electrode and the method of grounding or dispersion. In a Direct Current (DC) circuit, electrons flow in one direction only, whereas in an AC circuit, electrons flow first in one direction and then in the other direction (Fig. 14-1). When depicted graphically against time, DC voltage has constant polarity and is seen as a horizontal line. AC voltage is seen as a sine wave that alternates between positive and negative around 0 (Fig. 14-2). The frequency at which the current changes polarity is described in hertz (Hz), or cycles per second. In the United States, household wall outlets typically supply 110 to 120 V AC at 50 to 60 Hz. AC is used to supply electrical power throughout the United States because high voltages can be transmitted across great distances with minimal loss in energy.

The frequency of electrical output also affects the tissue response. For example, electrical current at 50 to 60 Hz provokes muscle contraction and tetany by causing depolarization of the neuromuscular junction. However, frequencies above 100,000 Hz do not cause muscle contraction or tetany. Electrosurgical instruments used today emit current from 100,000 to 4,000,000 Hz (0.1–4 MHz); a range that falls into the radiofrequency range.[8,9] Thus electrosurgery is sometimes referred to as radiofrequency electrosurgery.

ELECTROSURGERY

MECHANISM OF HEATING

In electrosurgery, radiofrequency current enters the patient and generates heat that is used to cut, coagulate, or desiccate. Radiofrequency electricity can heat tissue through two mechanisms: ohmic heating or dielectric heating. In ohmic heating, heat is generated by resistance to the flow of electrons. As electrons collide with atoms in the tissue, they release kinetic energy, producing heat at the site of application. Living tissue conducts electricity poorly, and ohmic heating is the mechanism utilized in electrosurgery.[8] In dielectric heating, atoms align themselves in an electromagnetic field. As the electromagnetic field oscillates at a high frequency, the molecules rotate to align with it, thereby colliding with other molecules and distributing energy in the form of heat. Dielectric heating occurs at frequencies above 500 MHz and is the mechanism by which microwave ovens operate.

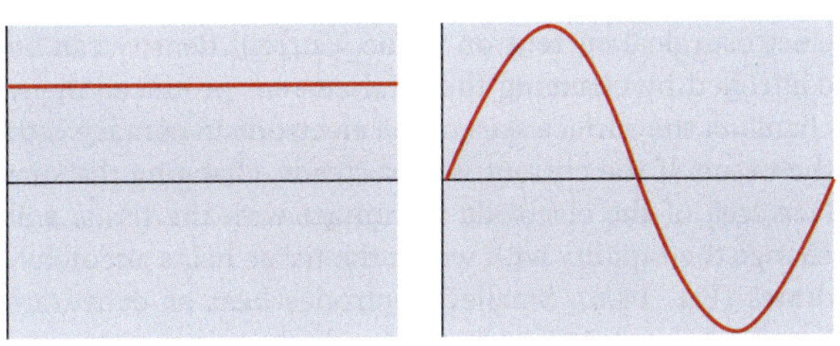

Figure 14-2 Direct and Alternating current.

ELECTROSURGICAL DEVICES

Although a variety of electrosurgical devices are available on the market today, most consist of three or four main components: a transformer to increase the current's voltage; an oscillating circuit; an electrode to transfer the current to the patient; and in some devices, an electrode return.[10]

In most ESUs, current from a standard household outlet first passes through a transformer that increases its voltage. The current then passes through an oscillating circuit that increases its frequency. The oscillating circuit may be composed of a spark gap, thermionic vacuum tube, or solid state transistor, though modern ESUs almost exclusively use transistors. Once the current's voltage and frequency are increased, it is delivered to the treatment electrode and to the patient's tissue. The active electrode delivers the current to the patient; current returns to the ESU through the passive, indifferent, or dispersive electrode. Alternately, in low-powered electrosurgical devices such as the hyfrecator, the patient's capacitance acts as a sink for the current and no return electrode is needed.

Once the electrical current enters the tissue, Ohmic heating produces heat. Below 45°C, no permanent damage to cells occurs. From 45°C to 60°C, proteins fix, solidify and become opaque, similar to cooked egg whites. This process is termed coagulation.[11] As temperature increases to 100°C, aqueous contents evaporate and the tissues "dry," a process termed desiccation. Above 100°C, the tissues begin to char and are reduced to carbon, a process aptly called carbonization.

The effect of an electrosurgical current on tissue is dependent on many factors including: the degree of heating (as described previously); the waveform and mode; the type of electrode (monopolar versus bipolar); the current density; the power setting; the shape of the electrode tip; the type of tissue; the time in contact with tissue; and the surgeon's technique.

WAVEFORM AND MODE – "CUT, COAGULATE, AND BLEND".

All ESUs emit a sinusoidal waveform of AC. These sine waves can be continuous or interrupted, which affects the tissue response. A continuous sinusoidal waveform heats the tissue rapidly, causing vaporization of water within cells and tissue cutting (Fig. 14-3). The tissue heats rapidly and relatively little heat is dispersed into the surrounding tissue.[12] Thus, cutting current vaporizes

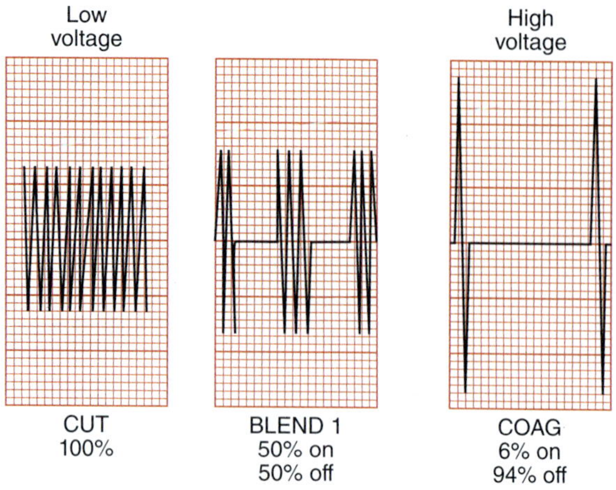

Figure 14-3 Cutting, blended, and coagulation waveforms. A purely cutting waveform is an uninterrupted sine wave. The voltage is relatively low, but current is high because it is on continuously. A blended current has progressive drops in electrical current so that the gaps between the current flow are longer. A coagulation waveform is an interrupted waveform with frequent gaps in which no current is being delivered, leading to higher voltage.

tissue without causing surrounding coagulation (Fig. 14-4). In the cutting waveform, the voltage is relatively low, but the average current is high.

In contrast, coagulation is achieved by slower tissue heating. In the coagulation setting, proteins are fixed, and tissue gradually dehydrates (Fig. 14-4). To achieve slower heating in the coagulation setting, the output waveform is either interrupted or damped, allowing heat to dissipate during the interruptions in current flow. As an analogy, imagine placing a pan over a flame and removing it: the pan heats only while over the flame, so the net effect is slower heating of the pan's contents. In coagulation modes, the unit is switched off for short periods of time, interrupting the output of continuous sine waves (Fig. 14-3). This on/off cycle is termed the duty cycle. Alternatively, the current can be damped with a diminution of voltage over time. A damped wave occurs when the wave's amplitude decreases over time due to resistance within the circuit (Fig. 14-5).[13]

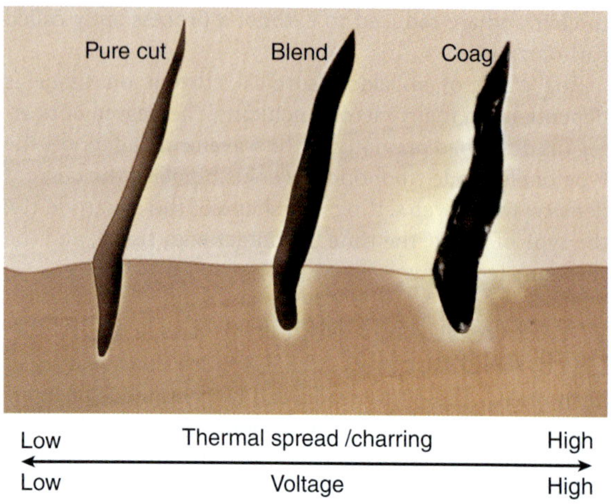

Figure 14-4 Tissue effects differ depending on electrosurgical unit setting.

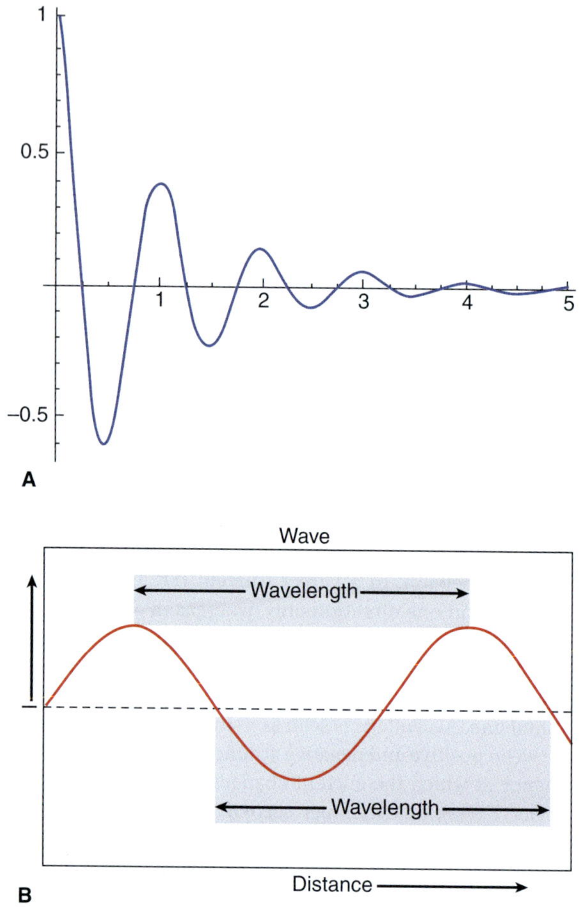

Figure 14-5 **A.** Damped sine wave. The amplitude of the sine wave decreases over time due to resistance in the system. **B.** A typical sine wave with the wavelength shown on the x axis and amplitude shown on the y axis.

"Blended" modes are used to obtain both cutting and coagulation. In "blended" modes, the unit is switched off for short periods of time, interrupting the output of continuous sine waves (Fig. 14-3). A blended mode is achieved by altering the duty cycle of the ESU output. ESUs achieve different amounts of cutting and coagulation by altering the duty cycle.[6] Different "blends" utilize preset duty cycles to provide varying combinations of cutting and coagulation. These blends are determined by ESU manufacturers.

CURRENT DENSITY

Current density significantly modulates the effect of an electrosurgical current on tissue. Current density can be controlled by changing the total current produced or by changing the surface area of the electrode in contact with the tissue. If the current is held steady, changing the surface area of the electrode in contact with the tissue will change the rapidity with which the tissue heats and dehydrates (Fig. 14-6). Smaller electrodes heat or dehydrate tissue much more quickly due to a higher current density, and thus are better for cutting. In contrast, larger electrodes are more appropriate for coagulation.

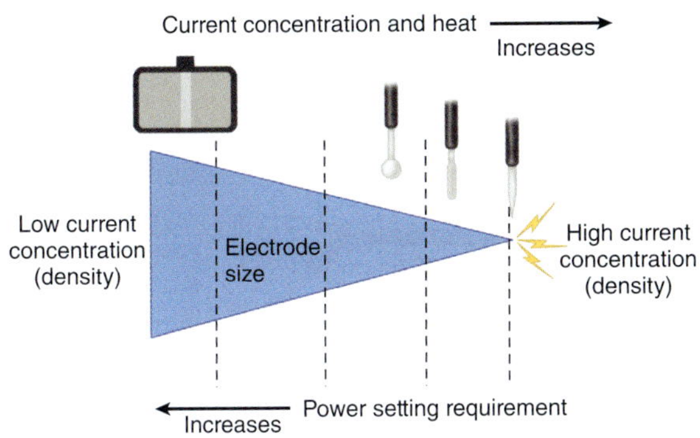

Figure 14-6 Current density depends on electrode size and power. Current density can be controlled by changing the surface area of the electrode in contact with the tissue. Large electrodes produce low current density and heat tissue more slowly. Small electrodes concentrate the current, rapidly heating the tissue.

Current density is greatest at the active electrode and dissipates as it moves from the treatment area. Monopolar, biterminal ESUs utilize return electrodes with a large surface area to lower current density as the current exits the patient and decrease the risk of a burn or shock. If the return electrode is poorly applied and only a small portion of the return electrode is in contact with the patient, current concentrates at the place of exit and can burn the patient.

MONOPOLAR VERSUS BIPOLAR

There are two types of electrodes used in electrosurgery: monopolar and bipolar (Fig. 14-7). In most monopolar applications, the surgeon manipulates the active electrode and current returns to the ESU through the return electrode (Fig. 14-8). Monopolar electrosurgery can deliver different modes of energy that result in the clinical effects of cutting, desiccating, or coagulating tissues. The monopolar electrode can either directly contact tissue or can be used in close proximity to further modulate the current's clinical effect.

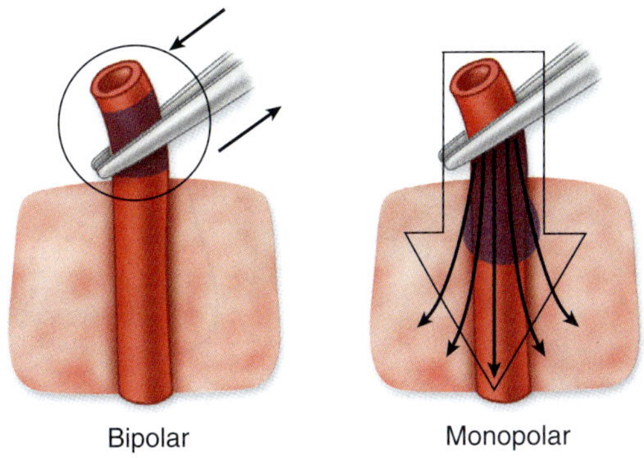

Figure 14-7 Bipolar and monopolar electrodes (the direction of current is depicted with arrows).

The hyfrecator is a specialized low power form of monopolar electrosurgery. As noted previously, in this instrument, the body's capacitance functions as a ground for electrons and current flows without the use of a return electrode. Because there is no return electrode if the patient is in contact with a grounding electrode, current will exit through the skin at the site of contact with grounding electrode. The high current density at the exit point can lead to a burn or shock. Hyfrecators are best used on conscious patients who will be able to indicate if they are inadvertently touching an object that can act as a grounding electrode.

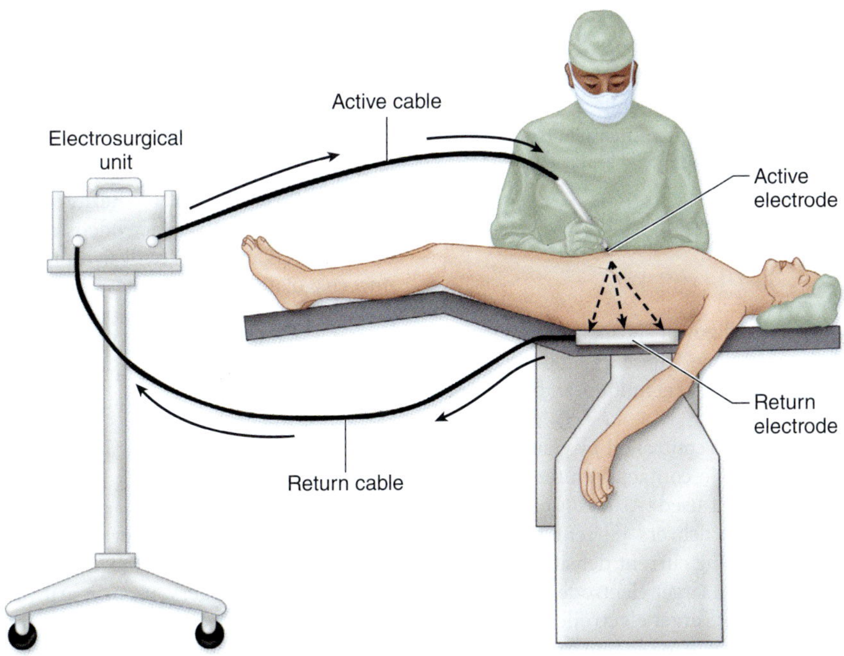

Figure 14-8 Monopolar electrosurgical unit. The current travels from the electrosurgical unit to the active electrode, through the patient and disperses through the return electrode.

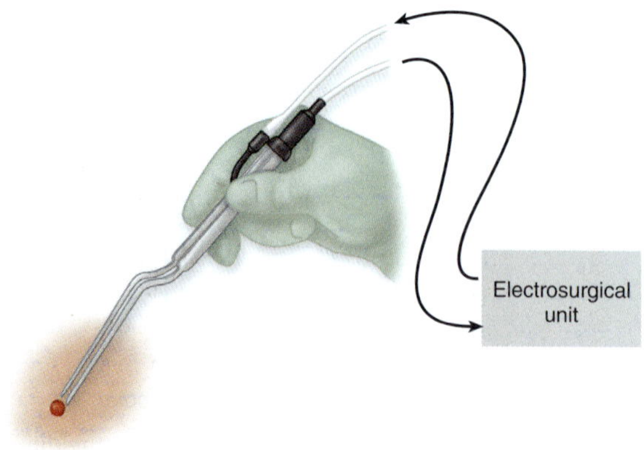

Figure 14-9 Bipolar electrosurgical unit. The current travels from the electrosurgical unit to one pole of the electrode, through the tissue, and through the other pole of the electrode.

In bipolar electrosurgery, the surgeon manipulates both the active and passive electrode in the form of electrically isolated forceps (Fig. 14-9). Current flows down the active electrode into the patient and returns via the passive electrode. Electricity only enters the tissue that is held between the electrodes. Bipolar electrosurgery is a low-power application, and is less likely to cause significant surrounding tissue damage. However, the full spectrum of electrosurgical outcomes such as cutting or fine desiccation is not possible using bipolar electrosurgery.

MONOTERMINAL VERSUS BITERMINAL

Monoterminal electrosurgery refers to an electrosurgical unit that has an active electrode without a return or dispersive electrode. In contrast, biterminal units have an active electrode and a return electrode. Monopolar units (one active electrode) can either be monoterminal or biterminal. Monopolar biterminal units consist of an active electrode and a distant return electrode. In contrast to monopolar units, bipolar units are always biterminal. Bipolar units utilize an active and return electrode in an electrically isolated pair of forceps.

OTHER FACTORS AFFECTING CLINICAL OUTCOME

In addition to waveform and power settings, other factors affect the final clinical outcome. These include the shape of the electrode, the surgeon's technique and the type of tissue.

The current density can be controlled by changing the surface area of the electrode in contact with the tissue or by changing the total current used. At a constant power setting, a smaller electrode delivers current through a smaller surface area, increasing current density and heating tissue more quickly than a larger electrode, and thus is better for cutting. In contrast, larger electrodes heat more slowly and are more appropriate for coagulation or desiccation. There are significant variations in electrosurgical electrodes to reflect the different uses (Fig. 14-10), and some are designed for very specific applications. A blade

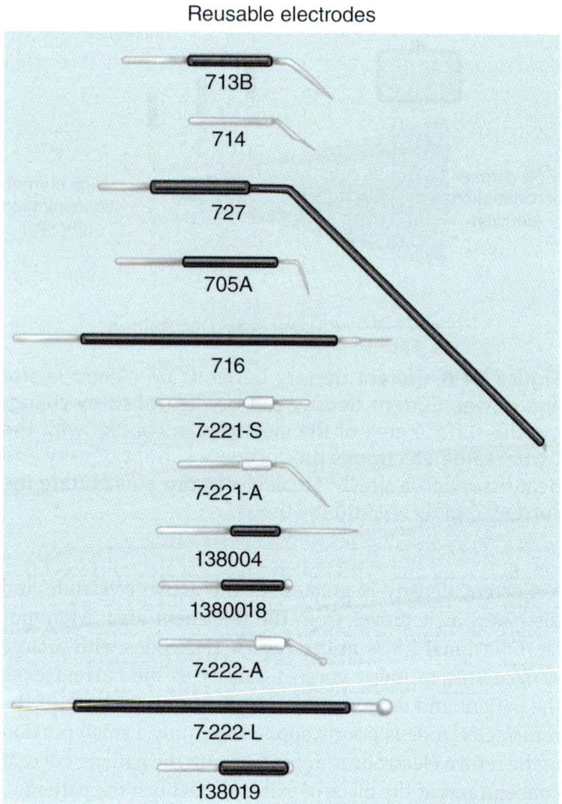

Figure 14-10 There is wide variation in electrode tip size and configuration.

or wire loop is effective at cutting tissues. A needle electrode can also be used for cutting, but is more commonly used for fine desiccation or destruction of small cutaneous lesions. A ball electrode is often used in laparoscopic surgery for blunt dissection, although the large surface area could be used successfully to provide hemostasis. Forceps that clasp tissue are often used for hemostasis, cauterizing the vessel being grasped. A variety of other electrode tips have been developed for different indications in dermatology, obstetrics and gynecology, and surgery.

Surgical technique also determines outcomes. Depending on how the active electrode is used and how far from the tissue it is applied (i.e., desiccation vs. fulguration), cutting, coagulation, or desiccation can all occur with the same power and mode settings. Tissue type affects outcomes as well. For the dermatologist, this is perhaps less important, but it should be noted that dermis, adipose tissue, muscle, and fascia vary in their response to electrical current.

TERMINOLOGY OF ELECTROSURGERY

Several terms have been developed to describe different types of electrosurgery. The differences between these forms of electrosurgery are primarily of historical importance, although electrofulguration is often differentiated from cutting, electrodesiccation, and electrocoagulation because the electrode tip is above the surgical field rather than in contact with the tissue. Furthermore, electrocautery is not a true form of electrosurgery.

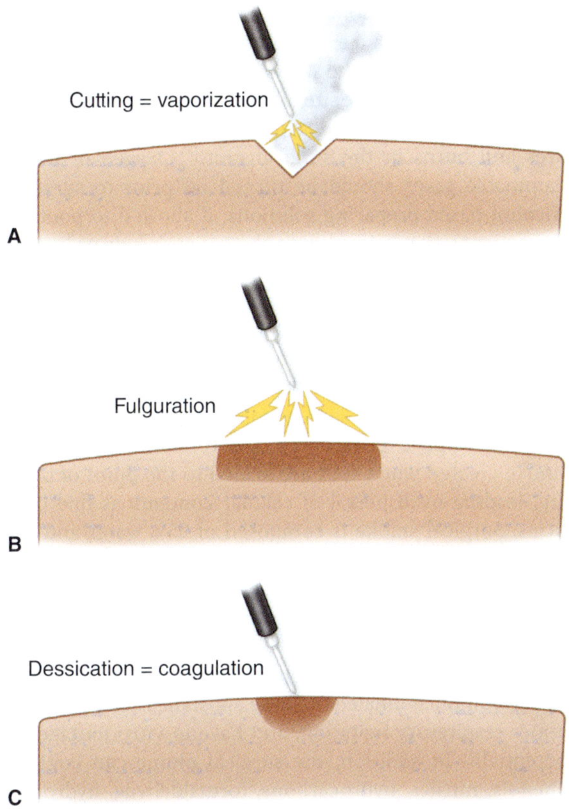

Figure 14-11 **A.** Tissue cutting using electrosurgery. Rapid heating of tissue to high temperatures leads to vaporization and the production of steam, leading to tissue cutting rather than coagulation. Cutting can either be accomplished by using high, constant current or using lower current for sufficiently long periods of time. **B.** Electrofulguration. Fulguration describes the destruction of soft tissue by an electric spark that jumps the gap from an electrode to the tissue without the electrode touching the tissue. High-voltage sparks result in rapid temperature changes in the tissue, leading to superficial coagulation and carbonization. **C.** Electrodesiccation and electrocoagulation. The electrode is placed in contact with the tissue, allowing the current to diffuse readily through the tissue. In electrodesiccation, the tissue heats slowly and gradually dehydrates. Electrocoagulation in contrast to the rapid changes in temperature caused by electrocoagulation.

ELECTROFULGURATION

Fulguration describes the destruction of soft tissue by an electric spark that jumps from an electrode to the tissue without the electrode touching the tissue (Fig. 14-11). When held close to the tissue, the current sparks in a cone-shaped distribution to the tissue. Electrofulguration utilizes a low-amperage current with high voltage. To perform electrofulguration, the current must be of sufficiently high voltage to spark across the gap between the electrode and the tissue. High-voltage sparks result in rapid temperature changes in the tissue, leading to superficial coagulation and carbonization. The carbonization often protects the underlying tissue from further damage. Electrofulguration can be used to control bleeding in small vessels up to 2 mm in diameter.[14] The surgical field must be dry or the current will simply disperse without affecting the underlying tissue. Electrofulguration is used clinically for light hemostasis of a surgical site. It can also be used to treat superficial tumors of the epidermis, such as seborrheic keratoses, verruca plana, epidermal nevi, actinic keratoses, acrochordons, or angiomas.

ELECTRODESICCATION

In 1914, William Clark described dehydration of tissue without carbonization by using very fine sparks generated from an Oudin coil. Clark used the term desiccation (from Latin *desiccare*, to dry out) to describe this action.[15] In contrast to electrofulguration, during electrodesiccation, the electrode is placed in contact with the tissue (Fig. 14-11). Classically, monoterminal units are used to achieve electrodesiccation. With the correct combination of power setting and electrode tip, the tissue heats more slowly and gradually dehydrates. Like electrofulguration, electrodesiccation is best used to treat superficial epidermal tumors. If performed correctly, electrodesiccation should result in little scarring because treatment is directed primarily at the epidermis. Lesions that can be treated well with electrodesiccation include telangiectasias, seborrheic keratoses, verruca plana, angiomas, and colloid milia.

ELECTROCOAGULATION

Electrocoagulation is the process by which proteins in the tissue are denatured. Electrocoagulation and electrodesiccation occur by a similar process, though electrodesiccation occurs through slow tissue dehydration, while electrocoagulation occurs through protein denaturation. Classically, electrocoagulation is performed with a biterminal unit. As a result, the current can penetrate more deeply into the dermis. Therefore, electrocoagulation is useful for treating dermal tumors or adnexal neoplasms. It is also very effective at providing hemostasis in the surgical field.

Both electrodesiccation and electrocoagulation can be used with curettage to treat superficial cutaneous neoplasms such as basal cell or squamous cell carcinomas. In this technique, the tumor is first treated with electrocoagulation or electrodesiccation. The electrode is moved slowly across the tumor until the tissue is charred. Following the first pass of electrodesiccation, a curette is used to remove the charred tissue and tumor. In order to ensure that the borders of the tumor are adequately treated, the curette should be applied in all directions (north–south, east–west, clockwise, and counterclockwise) around the surgical site. Tumors are typically softer than the underlying normal dermis and separate easily when treated with a curette. When this technique is used to treat keratinocyte derived skin cancers, two more passes of electrodesiccation and curettage should be applied to ensure adequate removal. Note that this technique is not appropriate for aggressive growth patterns, such as morpheaform, infiltrative, or micronodular basal cell carcinomas, or for aggressive or deep squamous cell carcinomas. Electrodesiccation and curettage works in part because of the difference in texture between tumor and normal dermis.

In lesions that are infiltrative, the borders of the tumor cannot be appreciated and there is a risk of undertreating the neoplasm.

ELECTROSECTION

A cutting current uses an undamped current to quickly heat and vaporize tissue in the treatment area. An ESU's cutting setting generates high temperatures at the electrode quickly, allowing for easy cutting through tissue while preventing significant surrounding damage. Due to the local effect of the electrode, a purely cutting current will not provide much hemostasis. However, a blended current can both cut and provide hemostasis. Hemostasis is the main benefit of using electrosection with a blended current rather than scalpel excision. Electrosection can be used to cut the skin, provide undermining, remove acrochordons, intradermal nevi, or other papillomatous or exophytic skin lesions. Dermatologic surgeons have also used electrosection to debulk large tumors or lesions such as rhinophyma or acne keloidalis nuchae.

ELECTROCAUTERY

For centuries, metal objects have been heated by fire and applied to tissue to cauterize and provide hemostasis. Today, electricity is used to heat a metal filament that is placed in direct contact with tissue, resulting in cautery and hemostasis.[16] Resistance is placed in the path of the electron flow, resulting in heat formation in a wire filament. This principle is also used to heat the wire filament of a kitchen toaster, electrical stove element, and conventional light bulbs.

In electrocautery, electrical current does not enter the patient, and thus it is safe to use in patients with pacemakers and implantable cardioverter-defibrillators (ICDs). However, electrocautery can cause damage to adjacent tissues because substantial heat is often required to obtain hemostasis. Electrocautery devices can use either DC or AC and are currently sold as disposable battery powered units (DC) or permanent units that utilize AC supplied by wall outlets. Because no current enters the patient, electrocautery is not a true form of electrosurgery.

SAFETY

Several safety concerns are associated with the use of electrosurgical devices: shock, burns, inhalation of the surgical smoke plume, and specific risks of using electrosurgery around the eye. The risk of electric shock can be minimized by ensuring that the patient is not in contact with an alternate ground. It is essential to avoid this both in "grounded" devices with a dispersive electrode and with "ungrounded" devices such as a hyfrecator. Care must also be taken to prevent close contact to other nonelectrically active wires to prevent electrical transfer to another circuit.[17]

To prevent electrosurgical burns, it is important to properly place the return or dispersive electrode. The dispersive electrode should be placed overlying muscle, which is much more conductive than adipose tissue or bone. It should also not be placed over a prosthetic device, which can also lead to a shock. Hair inhibits contact between the pad and the skin and it is recommended that all hair be shaved at the site of return electrode placement.

It is essential to take a few precautions to prevent fires and burns in the surgical unit.[18] Oxygen or other flammable gases should be turned off prior to surgery. Alcohol-based preparing solutions, if allowed to pool on the patient's skin or wick into the patient's hair or linens, can ignite during electrosurgery. Therefore, the cleanser used to prepare the skin should not be flammable or should be allowed to dry thoroughly prior to draping. Extreme care and caution should be used when performing electrosurgery around the eye. Sparks from the electrode can easily cause damage to the cornea or globe.

Electrosurgical procedures also result in a plume of smoke created when cells are heated to the point of boiling, leading to dispersal of cellular contents as fine particles. Surgical smoke is composed of 95% water and 5% particulate matter, including blood and tissue particles, chemicals, viruses, and bacteria.[19] Traditional surgical masks capture particles greater than 5 μm in diameter, but will not filter particles of smaller size. Unfortunately, most ESUs create particles of roughly 0.07 μm, which deposit in the alveoli once inhaled.[20] These substances can produce upper respiratory irritation, and have in vitro mutagenic potential.[21] In addition, the surgical plume can contain phenols, nitriles, hydrocarbons, formaldehyde, hydrogen cyanide, and a variety of trace toxic gases.[22,23] Although there has been no documented transmission of infectious disease through surgical smoke, the potential for generating infectious viral fragments, particularly following treatment of verrucae, may exist.[24–27] An effective smoke evacuation or ventilation system should be considered to prevent the inhalation of noxious smoke and vapors produced during electrosurgical operations.[28] Consideration should also be given to wearing high filtration masks during electrosurgical procedures.[29]

ELECTROSURGERY AND IMPLANTABLE DEVICES

When treating patients with implantable cardioverter-defibrillators or pacemakers (cardiovascular implantable electrical devices, or CIEDs), it is important to exercise care. Electrosurgical devices can interfere with CIEDs in several ways. Skipped beats, inhibition, reprogramming of a pacemaker, firing of an ICD, asystole, bradycardia, triggering unneeded tachyarrhythmia therapy and battery depletion have all been reported as possible complications, though the rates are quite low (0.8 cases/100 years of surgical practice).[30,31]

Monopolar electrosurgery is the most common source of electrical interference with cardiac devices in the operating room. In order to prevent adverse events, caution should be used in this setting. A position paper by the Heart Rhythm Society/American Society of Anesthesiologists recommended that a patient's cardiovascular device specialist be consulted by the procedural team prior to surgery. Factors that affect the treatment plan include the type of device, type of surgery, and whether the patient is pacemaker dependent.[32] Because of the complexity of the devices available on the market, there is no longer one standard recommendation for performing electrosurgery in patients with cardiovascular devices. In order to minimize complications, particularly given the variety of modern CIED, many centers perform electrosurgery in coordination with a pacemaker team in order to minimize complications.[33,34] In addition, the Heart Rhythm Society/American Society of Anesthesiologists recommends that all pacemakers, ICDs and cardiac resynchronization devices be interrogated within 1 month following an electrosurgical procedure using a monopolar device.[32] If electrosurgery must be performed, techniques that can be used to limit complications include the use of bipolar forceps, low power, short bursts of power (less than 5 seconds), and avoiding the area around the ICD or pacemaker.[35] Bipolar forceps are generally safer to use in patients with a CIED because the electrical current only passes through the tissue between the forceps, thus minimizing the chance that the current will interfere with the cardiovascular device. Low power and short bursts help minimize the amount of current that the patient is exposed to, thus potentially decreasing the risk to the cardiovascular device.

If the patient's cardiovascular device specialist cannot be reached prior to surgery, it should be noted that electrocautery can be safely used in these patients in all locations. Electrocautery uses heat rather than an electrical current to provide hemostasis, so it will not interfere with the CIED. Although electrocautery results in more tissue burning than electrosurgery, it does not require intraoperative monitoring and is safe to use in unstable patients.

Similar precautions are taken with patients with cochlear implants. Cochlear implants are electrical devices that are surgically implanted under the periosteum of the cranium and electrically stimulate the auditory nerve. Cochlear implants can be damaged by an electrical current in the vicinity of the device, and use of electrosurgical devices around the cochlear implant may compel surgical replacement of the implant. The British Cochlear Implant Group safety guidelines dictate that monopolar electrosurgery should not be used on the head and neck, and bipolar electrosurgery should not be used within 2 cm of the implant.[36] Monopolar electrosurgery can be safely performed below the neck in patients with implants.[37] Electrocautery can be safely performed in the head and neck region of patients with cochlear implants.

CONCLUSION

Over the past 100 years or so, electrosurgery has become a fundamental tool in the dermatologists' armamentarium. Electrosurgical tools have evolved, becoming safer and more efficient with technological advances. Furthermore, dermatologists have expanded the uses of electrosurgery beyond hemostasis and cutting to include the treatment of benign and malignant neoplasms, superficial and deep ablations, and cosmetic purposes. Due to the wide range of uses for electrosurgery, it will likely continue to play an important role in clinical care.

REFERENCES

1. Elliott JA. Electrosurgery: its use in dermatology, with a review of its development and technologic aspects. *Arch Dermatol.* 1966;94:340–350.
2. Frew JW. Performing surgery with a single electron: electrosurgery and quantum mechanics. *ANZ J Surg.* 2009;79:680–682.
3. Blankenship ML. Physical modalities. Electrosurgery, electrocautery, and electrolysis. *Int J Dermatol.* 1979;18:443–452.
4. D'Arsonval A. Action physiologque des currants alternatifs. *CR Soc Biol (Paris).* 1891;43:283.
5. Pollack SV, Carruthers A, Gerkin RC. The history of electrosurgery. *Dermatol Surg.* 2000;26:904–908.
6. Massarweh NN, Cosgriff N, Slakey DP. Electrosurgery: history, principles, and current and future uses. *J Am Coll Surg.* 2006;202:520–530.
7. Sebben JE. The status of electrosurgery in dermatologic practice. *J Am Acad Dermatol.* 1988;19:542–549.
8. Zinder DJ. Common myths about electrosurgery. *Otolaryngol Head Neck Surg.* 2000;123:450–455.
9. Friedman J. The technical aspects of electrosurgery. *Oral Surg Oral Med Oral Pathol.* 1973;36:177–187.
10. Pollack SV, Grekin RC. Electrosurgery and electroepilation. In: Roenigk RK, Roenigk HH, eds. *Roenigk & Roenigk's Dermatologic Surgery: Principles and Practice.* New York, NY: Marcel Dekker; 1996: 220–221.
11. Eggleston JL, Von Maltzahn WW. Electrosurgical devices. In: Bronzino JD, ed. *The Biomedical Engineering Handbook.* 2nd ed. Boca Raton, FL: CRC Press LLC; 2000.
12. Wright VC. Contemporary electrosurgery: physics for physicians. *J Fam Pract.* 1994;39(2):119–122.
13. Sebben JE. Electrosurgery: high-frequency modalities. *J Dermatol Surg Oncol.* 1988;14:367–371.
14. Brill AI. Electrosurgery: principles and practice to reduce risk and maximize efficacy. *Obstet Gynecol Clin North Am.* 2011;38:687–702.
15. Clark WL. The desiccation treatment of congenital and new growths of the skin and mucous membranes. *JAMA.* 1914;LXIII:925–929.
16. Gandsas A, Adrales GL. Energy sources. In: Talamini MA, ed. *Advanced Therapy in Minimally Invasive Surgery.* Hamilton, ON: BC Decker; 2006; 3.
17. Robinson TN, Barnes KS, Govekar HR, Stiegmann GV, Dunn CL, McGreevy FT. Antenna coupling – a novel mechanism of radiofrequency electrosurgery complication: practical implications. *Ann Surg.* 2012;256:213–218.
18. Spruce L, Braswell ML. Implementing AORN recommended practices for electrosurgery. *AORN J.* 1995;95:373–384.
19. Gonzalez-Bayon L, Gonzalez-Moreno S, Ortega-Perez G. Safety considerations for operating room personnel during hyperthermic intraoperative intraperitoneal chemotherapy perfusion. *Eur J Surg Oncol.* 2006;32:619–624.
20. Ulmer BC. The hazards of surgical smoke. *AORN J.* 2008; 87:721–738.
21. Barrett WL, Garber SM. Surgical smoke: a review of the literature. *Surg Endosc.* 2003;17:979–987.
22. Gatti JE, Bryant CJ, Noone RB, Murphy JC. The mutagenicity of electrocautery smoke. *Plast Reconstr Surg.* 1992;89:781–784.
23. Moot AR, Ledingham KM, Wilson PF, et al. Composition of volatile organic compounds in diathermy plume as detected by selected ion flow tube mass spectrometry. *ANZ J Surg.* 2007;77:20–23.
24. Baggish MS, Poiesz BJ, Joret D, Williamson P, Refal A. Presence of human immunodeficiency DNA in laser smoke. *Lasers Surg Med.* 1991;11:197–203.
25. Garden JM, O'Banion MK, Bakus AD, Olson C. Viral disease transmitted by laser-generated plume (aerosol). *Arch Dermatol.* 2002;138:1303–1307.
26. Gloster HM Jr, Roenigk RK. Risk of acquiring human papillomavirus from the plume produced by the carbon dioxide laser in the treatment of warts. *J Am Acad Dermatol.* 1995;32: 436–441.

27. Garden JM, O'Banion MK, Sheinitz LS, Pinski KS, Bakus AD, Reichmann ME. Papillomavirus in the vapor of carbon dioxide laser treated verrucae. *JAMA.* 1988;259:1199–1202.
28. Bigony L. Risks associated with exposure to surgical smoke plume: a review of the literature. *AORN J.* 2007;86(6):1013–1024.
29. Lewin JM, Brauer JA, Ostad A. Surgical smoke and the dermatologist. *J Am Acad Dermatol.* 2011;65:636–641.
30. El-Gamal HM, Dufresne RG, Saddler K. Electrosurgery, pacemakers and ICDs: a survey of precautions and complications experienced by cutaneous surgeons. *Dermatol Surg.* 2001;27:385.
31. Matzke TJ, Christenson LJ, Christenson SD, Atanashova N, Otley C. Pacemakers and implanatable cardiac defribillators in dermatologic surgery. *Dermatol Surg.* 2006;32:1155–1162.
32. Crossley GH, Poole JE, Rozner MA, et al. The Heart Rhythm Society (HRS)/American Society of Anesthesiologists (ASA) Expert Consensus Statement on the perioperative management of patients with implantable defibrillators, pacemakers and arrhythmia monitors: facilities and patient management this document was developed as a joint project with the American Society of Anesthesiologists (ASA), and in collaboration with the American Heart Association (AHA), and the Society of Thoracic Surgeons (STS). *Heart Rhythm.* 2011;8:1114–1154.
33. Misiri J, Kusumoto F, Goldschlager N. Electromagnetic interference and implanted cardiac devices: the medical environment (part II). *Clin Cardiol.* 2012;35:321–328.
34. Stone ME, Salter B, Fischer A. Perioperative management of patients with cardiac implantable electronic devices. *Br J Anaesth.* 2011;107:i16–i26.
35. Healey JS, Merchant R, Simpson C, et al. Canadian Cardiovascular Society/Canadian Anesthesiologists' Society/Canadian Heart Rhythm Society joint position statement on the perioperative management of patients with implanted pacemakers, defibrillators, and neurostimulating devices. *Can J Cardiol.* 28(2):141–151.
36. Frampton SJ, Ismail-Koch H, Mitchell TE. How safe is diathermy in patients with cochlear implants. *Ann R Coll Surg Engl.* 2012;94:585–587.
37. Poetker DM, Runge-Samuelson CL, Firszt JC, Wackym PA. Electrosurgery after cochlear implantation: eighth nerve electrophysiology. *Laryngoscope.* 2004;114:2252–2254.

CHAPTER 15

Cryosurgery

James M. Spencer & Summer D. Moon

INTRODUCTION

Cryosurgery is among the most powerful and efficient tools used in dermatology. This minimally invasive and cost-effective procedure is valuable for the treatment of many benign, premalignant and certain superficial malignant lesions, and is an alternative for patients who are bedridden, have blood-borne illnesses, or simply do not wish to undergo a surgical excision. As with any procedure, the risks and benefits must be properly explained. Cryosurgery has truly stood the test of time and with proper training may be used to treat a wide variety of cutaneous lesions with ease.

HISTORY

Cryosurgery is one of the oldest and most versatile procedures in dermatology. The medical use of cold dates back over 4,000 years, when ancient Egyptians used it as a local anesthetic to minimize the pain of trauma and decrease inflammation. Baron Dominique Larrey, the military surgeon of Napoleon's army, used ice and snow to pretreat injured limbs before amputation. In 1851, James Arnott of London pioneered a local analgesic using ice and saline for palliative treatment of cancerous tumors in terminally ill patients. As the first to achieve temperatures around −24°C, Arnott is often described as the father of "modern" cryosurgery.[1] In 1899, Campbell White, a New York dermatologist, became the first to successfully treat warts, nevi, keratoses, and skin cancers with a cotton-tipped applicator dipped into liquefied air. In 1907, another dermatologist, H. H. Whitehouse, engineered the first spray device delivering cryogen.[2] Soon thereafter, W. A. Pusey promoted carbon dioxide to treat acne and nevi.[3,4] Liquid nitrogen (LN) replaced carbon dioxide as the primary cryogen in 1948. During this time, LN was applied to lesions using a cotton-wool swab. In the mid-1960s with the help of Whitehouse's ideas, Setrag Zacarian and Douglas Torre made cryogen delivery more efficient. Zacarian designed the method of indirectly administrating LN by cooling copper cylinders while Torre developed a reliable LN spraying system.[5] Around the same time, Irving S. Cooper, a neurosurgeon, found a way to bring LN to a controlled temperature of −195°C, which is the temperature we use in dermatology today. In 1968, Michael Bryne developed the first commercially available handheld cryosurgical device.[6,7]

BASIC PRINCIPLES

Cryosurgery is unique because it provides a safe, effective, and economically feasible method of treating a variety of dermatological conditions. The subzero temperatures which it achieves cause cellular damage and death through heat extraction. The cellular damage itself occurs through direct injury, vascular stasis, apoptosis, and immunologic effects.

Freezing temperatures cause direct injury by creating an osmotic gradient. Crystallization outside the cells causes water to rush outward, which leads to internal dehydration, organelle damage, cell membrane and cytoskeleton changes which compromise the integrity of the cell. Additional freezing creates internal crystallization, which causes cell lysis. During the thawing process the osmotic gradient reverses as ice crystals reorganize within the cell; this leads to further destruction as water moves back into the cells, causing further swelling and cell lysis.

The initial effect of cryosurgery on blood vessels is vasoconstriction, which leads to cellular hypoxia and blood stasis. As the tissue thaws, a compensatory vasodilatation occurs, which brings in free radicals, causing peroxidation of membrane lipids.

Apoptotic cells are thought to contribute to cell death and are found at the periphery of the central necrotic area.[8,9] Apoptosis increases progressively 2 to 8 hours after the initial freezing.[9,10]

Cryosurgery's ability to generate long-term memory cells is attributed to a cytokine and delayed T-cell response induced by cryoablation.[11] The first reports of the immunologic effect of cryosurgery showed a reduction of metastatic disease after cryoablation of the primary tumor.[12,13] Murine models demonstrate inhibition of secondary and metastatic tumor growth through cryoablation of tumor tissue.[14] Further analysis has revealed that cryosurgery may enhance the uptake of tumor antigens by dendritic cells, resulting in induction of tumor-specific $CD8^+$ T cells responsible for in vivo regression of both treated and distant tumors.[15]

Necrosis occurs at the center of the treatment area where temperatures reach −40° to −50°C. The rate of freezing determines the final temperatures achieved by the target tissue. The recommended temperature and rate at which freezing temperatures are achieved differ for benign and malignant lesions. A moderate-to-rapid freeze speed with a goal of −20° to −25°C is recommended for benign lesions. A rapid freeze, with a goal of −50°C or lower, is required to treat malignant lesions.

Flash freezing with LN kills the cell whereas slow thawing prolongs the time at which the tissue remains at subzero temperatures, which increases intracellular ice formation. A single freeze–thaw cycle may be sufficient for benign lesions; repeated cycles are usually needed for malignant lesions. Using multiple freeze–thaw cycles on premalignant or malignant lesions allows the cryogen to penetrate more deeply and leads to greater cellular destruction.

The space between the lesion and the cryogen determines the final temperature of the target tissue. Air and keratin are poor thermal conductors, and it may therefore be helpful to debulk lesions with excess keratin prior to treatment. A plastic cone shield or an otoscope nasal speculum may be used between the cryogen tip and the tissue to localize therapy and prevent overspraying.

When treating benign lesions in sensitive locations, one may consider using a cotton-tipped applicator dipped in LN instead of using an open spray. This technique is usually less painful and more easily tolerated. A small amount of LN is poured into a cup or stainless steel bowl to reduce the risk of contamination, which may occur if the applicator is reintroduced into the container following treatment of warts or other infectious lesions.

EQUIPMENT

Cryosurgery requires a cryogen and a delivery unit. In dermatology, the ideal cryogen is LN, most commonly delivered in a handheld spray unit (Fig. 15-1). These units are equipped with interchangeable apertures and probe tips of various sizes (Fig. 15-2). Spray tips are available starting from 1 to 2 mm in size. Cones are available to prevent overspray and to localize tissue destruction. LN is widely accepted as the ideal cryogen because of its ease of transport, safety, low cost, ease of storage, and low temperatures.[16] Storage tanks for LN are available in capacities of 5, 10, 25, 30, 35, and 50 L (Fig. 15-3).

Cotton-tipped applicators or a metal probe dipped in LN are acceptable treatment options for benign lesions but do not achieve the temperatures necessary to treat premalignant or malignant lesions. Cotton-tipped applicators work well for patients who have lesions in sensitive areas or for those who cannot tolerate the freezing temperatures achieved by the spraying or probe techniques. Thermocoupling devices can be added to monitor the temperatures achieved by the tissue, through needles placed beneath the lesion. Thermocouples are not used frequently by dermatologists but may be helpful for the novice.

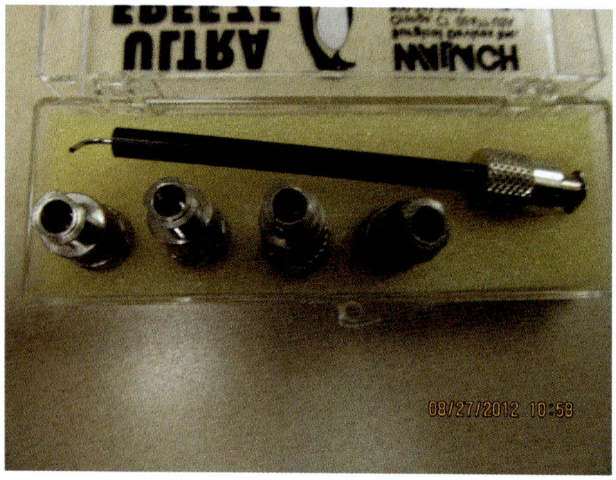

Figure 15-2 Different types of probes.

TECHNIQUES

There are five main methods used for the delivery of cryogen in dermatology: open spray, cone defined spray, chamber, probe, and intralesional.

- Open spray is the most versatile way to freeze lesions and is the preferred method of most dermatologists. Open spray delivers LN through an attachment at the spray unit's open end. Attachment tips come in a variety of diameters: A (largest), B, C, D, or E (smallest). The larger the diameter, the more cryogen delivered per unit time. Freeze time is relative to the speed of the cryogen as it is released from the gun. Larger tips (A) are reserved for larger malignancies. The most commonly used tips are B and C. The E tips come with a back vent that allows for a more precise and streamlined spray, making its use ideal for small, circumscribed, or delicate lesions. The open-spray technique is ideal for irregular lesions. If the system clogs while spraying, this is a sign that the LN is not clean and should be replaced.

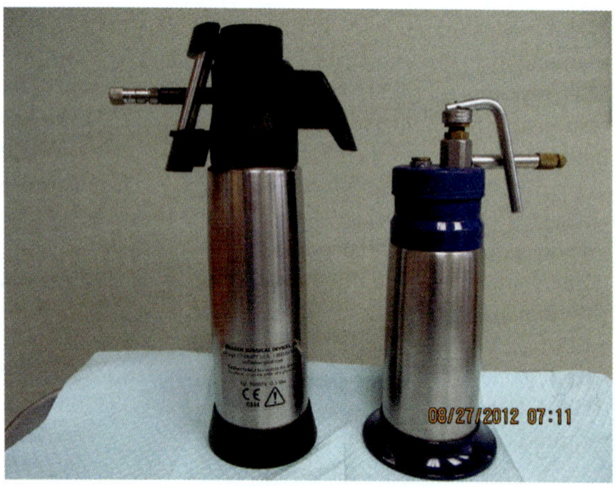

Figure 15-1 Handheld liquid nitrogen spray units.

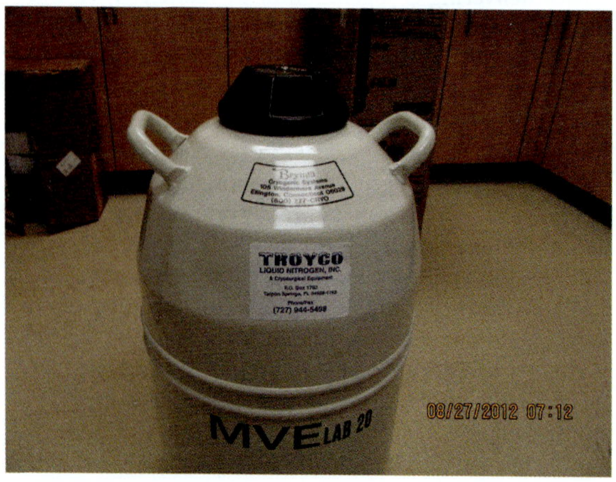

Figure 15-3 Liquid nitrogen storage container.

- Cone defined spray uses the same methods as the open spray but adds a cone between the lesion and the unit. Using this technique concentrates the spray for greater accuracy and penetration. It is essential to apply pressure to the cone in order to eliminate lateral leakage. Cones come in various sizes and materials, and should be washed in between patients to prevent contamination and the spread of infection.
- Chambers should be reserved for thick malignancies because of the technique's rapid delivery of LN. The chamber technique uses metal cylinders with a rubber base on one side, which is applied firmly to the target tissue. The opposite end allows a large amount of LN to flow into the chamber at a constant rate. Chambers are available in various sizes. For malignant lesions, it is important to select a chamber size that fits the lesion and includes the proper margins for the lesion.
- Probe techniques are reserved for contact cryosurgery. A probe is used to deliver LN from the unit via a conduit line, which maintains a closed system. Ideally, the probe should fit the shape of the lesion. It is better to use a smaller rather than a larger probe that does not fit properly; using a smaller probe avoids freezing healthy tissue.
- The intralesional technique should be reserved for deep-seated tumors. It consists of inserting one to several sterile open, closed, or double cannula probes into one side of the tumor and running the probe interstitially along the largest axis of the lesion at its deepest point until it appears on the surface at the other side.[16] LN is then sprayed into the cannula. Ice forms within the core of the lesion with minimal surface destruction in comparison to the other techniques.

A more recent technique utilizes an infrared sensor attachment placed at the probe tip to measure temperatures attained on the skin surface before and during cryosurgery.[17] This device uses a three-color–coded light system to indicate the temperature at the skin's surface. It also includes an integrated tracker, which displays the total freeze time as well as the time at which the desired temperature is reached. The duration of most treatments ranges from 5 to 10 seconds. A recent paper on the treatment of actinic keratoses (AKs) with the integrated infrared sensor achieved a 100% response rate when controlling the temperature to −5°C.[17]

When performing cryosurgery, it is essential to keep the following concepts in mind:

- The optimal freeze–thaw sequence consists of a fast freeze and slow thaw.
- One freeze–thaw cycle is usually sufficient for benign lesions.
- Premalignant or malignant lesions typically require two freeze–thaw cycles.
- Complete thawing is required when performing multiple cycles.
- Proper contact with the lesion is essential.
- Air, keratin, and cotton are poor thermal conductors.
- To direct treatment, use of a cone or nasal speculum may be considered.
- The diameter of the lesion treated is essentially equal to the depth.
- It is better to undertreat than to overtreat benign lesions.
- Do not treat a lesion that is bleeding.
- Malignant cells are more resistant to freezing than normal cells.
- Cartilage and bone are very resistant to freezing.
- Melanocytes, basal cells, and keratinocytes are very sensitive to freezing.
- Connective tissue, fibroblasts, and viruses are less sensitive to freezing.
- Healing time increases away from the face.
- Cryosurgery on the lower extremities may take months to heal.

PATIENT SELECTION AND PREOPERATIVE PREPARATION

The indications for cryosurgery are extensive but the decision to treat depends on a number of factors. Patient expectations, skin type, and overall health are important aspects to consider. Cryosurgery itself is usually well tolerated, but erythema, swelling, pain, and blistering commonly follow treatment. Depending on the location and depth of the freezing, symptoms may take up to 6 weeks for complete resolution. Patients with Fitzpatrick skin types III–VI are particularly prone to hypopigmentation. All patients should be warned of the possibility of hypo- or hyperpigmentation following treatment. Although most patients heal with minimal complications, cryosurgery should be avoided in patients with severe arteriosclerosis of the lower extremities. Treating leg lesions in patients with this condition may lead to prolonged healing times as well as the possibility of additional complications.

The portability of cryosurgery makes it particularly useful for patients in nursing homes and for those who have difficulty leaving home. Additional patient populations who may benefit from cryosurgery include high-risk surgical candidates, patients with poor wound healing, and those with allergies to local anesthesia. Cryosurgery has the benefit of being blood free, therefore making it an excellent option for managing dermatologic manifestations in patients with blood-borne diseases such as HIV or Hepatitis B and C.

CLINICAL APPLICATIONS

VIRAL VERRUCAE

Treating warts with cryosurgery can be a challenge and may require multiple attempts (Table 15-1). Some patients prefer the use of a cotton-tipped applicator, whereas others prefer the LN spray. Paring down lesions or pretreating warts with a keratolytic agent may result in higher cure rates.

ACROCHORDONS (SKIN TAGS)

Treating skin tags with LN requires a cup and forceps. The LN is poured into a cup and the forceps is allowed to soak in the LN for about 20 seconds. When the forceps are covered by frost, the stalk of the tag is grasped for approximately 10 seconds (Fig. 15-4). Tags can also be removed by scissors or electrosurgery.

TABLE 15-1
Duration of Time in Seconds to Treat Benign and Malignant Lesions with Liquid Nitrogen

Benign Lesions: Flow Rate >100°C/min	Duration (seconds)
Verruca vulgaris	10
Acrochordon	10
Molluscum contagiosum	10–20
Granuloma annulare	10–60
Prurigo nodularis	15–30
Cutaneous larva migrans	5–7
Seborrheic keratosis	5–15
Solar lentigo	3–7
Acne	5–7
Hypertrophic scars/keloids	30
Hemangiomas	10–20
Pyogenic granulomas	20–30
Vascular malformations	30
Premalignant and malignant lesion: Flow Rate >100°C/min	
Actinic keratosis	5–30
Lentigo maligna	2 × 30
Basal and squamous cell carcinoma	2 × 30
Kaposi's sarcoma	2 × 30

MOLLUSCUM CONTAGIOSUM

Molluscum contagiosum can be treated with either open or closed techniques. The lesion should be centered about 2 mm below the open-spray nozzle and the freeze allowed to spread just outside the margin of the lesion. For the probe technique, a fine-point probe the same size or slightly smaller than the lesion should be used.

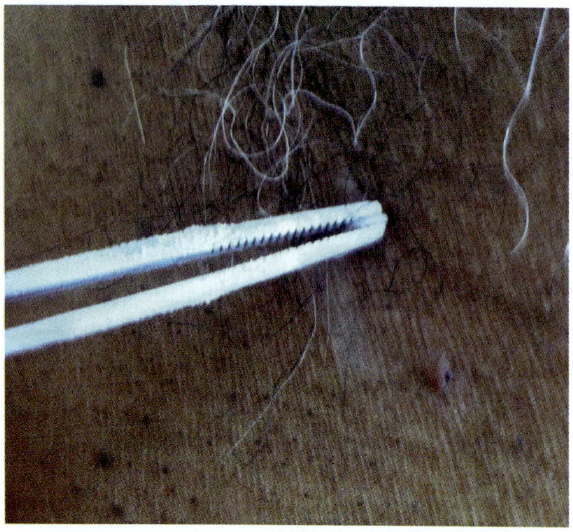

Figure 15-4 Treatment of acrochordon with forceps.

GRANULOMA ANNULARE

Cryosurgery can be used in the treatment of granuloma annulare. A prospective trial in Germany found that one freeze–thaw cycle with LN or nitrous oxide using a closed probe technique for 10 to 60 seconds produced excellent results. Resolution of the lesions occurred in 25 of the 31 patients (80.6%); only one relapse occurred during 2 years of follow-up.[18]

PRURIGO NODULARIS

Cryosurgery is one of the treatments of choice for prurigo nodularis. The open-spray technique is commonly used for 15 to 30 seconds depending on the thickness of the lesion. The use of cold tends to relieve symptoms by breaking the itch–scratch cycle.

CUTANEOUS LARVA MIGRANS

Resistant cases of cutaneous larva migrans may respond to the open-spray technique of cryogen applied at both ends of the trail. Freezing should be carried out for 5 to 7 seconds.[16]

SEBORRHEIC KERATOSES

Cryosurgery is among the fastest and most efficient way to treat seborrheic keratoses (SKs). It is essential that treatment be performed only when the diagnosis is certain since freezing a pigmented melanocytic lesion could potentially harm the patient. Most lesions are treated with the open-spray technique and commonly require only one treatment. SKs should be frozen for 5 to 15 seconds and should include a 1 to 2 mm rim around the lesion (Fig. 15-5).

SOLAR LENTIGINES

Melanocytes are particularly susceptible to cold, making cryosurgery an excellent choice for treatment of solar

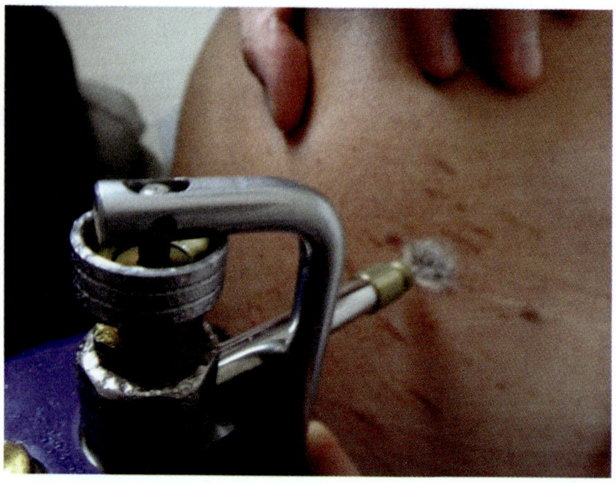

Figure 15-5 Treatment of seborrheic keratosis with hand-held liquid nitrogen spray unit.

lentigines and ephelides. It is a good idea to confirm the diagnosis by dermoscopy prior to treatment. When in doubt, it is always safer to biopsy the lesion. Once the diagnosis is confirmed, an open-spray technique directed perpendicular to the lesion for 3 to 7 seconds is usually sufficient for treatment, being certain to freeze the entire lesion.

ACNE

Cryosurgery can be particularly useful during pregnancy or as an alternative treatment for patients who do not wish to use systemic or topical treatments for pustules and/or cysts. Cold initially has an inflammatory effect and within 24 to 48 hours the pustules and cysts tend to resolve more quickly than without any treatment.[16] An open-spray technique is used, freezing the entire lesion for 5 to 7 seconds. Patients should be educated regarding the possibility of drainage after the procedure and should be instructed to apply topical antibiotics or vaseline following treatment. Spraying should never be performed on incised or draining lesions due to the risk of local crepitation or insufflation of nitrogen within the wound.

HYPERTROPHIC SCARS AND KELOIDS

Cryosurgery alone or in combination with the use of intralesional corticosteroids may treat some patients with hypertrophic scars or keloids successfully. However, there is always a risk for additional scarring. An open spray or cotton-tipped applicator dipped in nitrogen is used, and the cryogen is applied to each lesion for about 30 seconds.[19] If the lesion is large, preprocedure debulking may be considered. Multiple treatments may be necessary for thick or recurring lesions. Treatments should be spaced 1 month apart to allow for adequate healing before evaluating the patient's response to the procedure.

HEMANGIOMAS

Controversy exists regarding whether hemangiomas should be treated or left alone to resolve spontaneously. Ideally, a capillary hemangioma should be treated as soon as it appears; the decision to treat is, therefore, made immediately after diagnosis.[20] Superficial hemangiomas are treated directly using a fitted probe placed over the lesion. A single application of LN for about 10 to 20 seconds is usually sufficient, treating until the cryogen reaches 1 to 2 mm outside the lesion's border.

PYOGENIC GRANULOMAS

Pyogenic granulomas can be treated using either the probe or the open spray technique. Freezing temperatures should reach the base of the tumor for optimal treatment.

VASCULAR MALFORMATIONS

When lasers fail in the treatment of vascular malformations, cryosurgery can be a useful alternative. The ability to reduce the thickness of certain capillary lesions improves their overall appearance and makes it easier to hide them with makeup. Venous lakes can be treated with previously frozen probes applied with pressure for 4 to 5 seconds.[21] Large nodular lesions should be grasped with the probes until they are frozen down to their base.

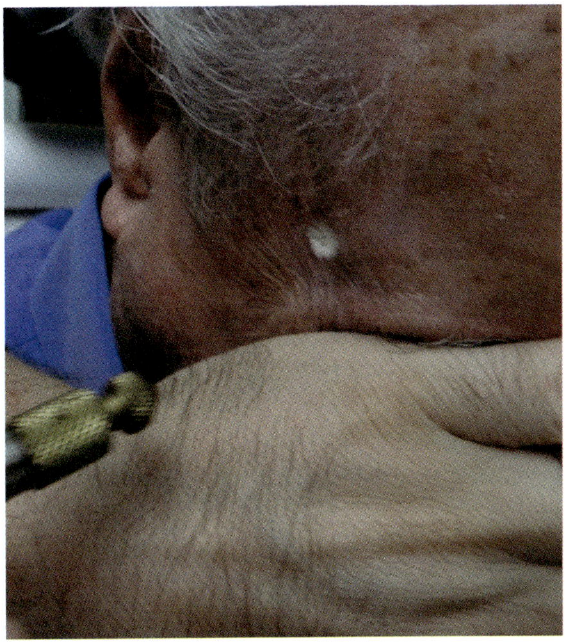

Figure 15-6 Treatment of actinic keratosis on the temporal region with handheld liquid nitrogen spray unit.

ACTINIC KERATOSES

Cryosurgery is among the most common treatments for AKs. Treatment times vary from 5 to 30 seconds depending on the amount of excess keratin on top of the lesion. Thick lesions may be debulked or pretreated with emollients. The open-spray technique is used, allowing for a 1 to 2 mm margin of freeze surrounding the lesion (Figs. 15-6 and 15-7). Treating AKs with cryosurgery is believed to be highly effective, but its actual effectiveness has been poorly documented. In 1982, Lubritz reported a single

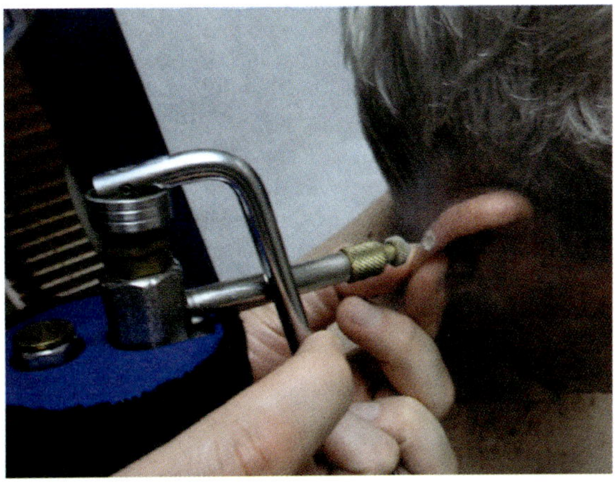

Figure 15-7 Treatment of actinic keratosis on the helix of the ear with handheld liquid nitrogen spray unit.

retrospective review of his personal experience treating 70 patients with 1018 AKs with cryosurgery. Patients were followed for 1 to 8.5 years after treatment. A 98% cure rate was reported.[22] A more recent prospective study of 89 patients with 421 AKs treated with cryosurgery at various freeze times reported only a 67.2% response rate.[23] In patients with multiple AKs, one can consider pretreatment with topical field therapy such as 5% fluorouracil or imiquimod for 2 to 4 weeks, which should lead to fewer lesions, a need for less freezing, and better cold penetration if cryotherapy is subsequently required.

LENTIGO MALIGNA

Melanocytes are sensitive to cold, and cryosurgery may therefore be considered as a treatment option for selected patients with lentigo maligna (LM) who cannot tolerate surgery. An aggressive double freeze–thaw cycle with 1 cm margins is advised.[16] Recurrence rates vary from 0% to 40% with patient follow-up ranging from 7 months to 4 years.[24–29] Biopsies are absolutely necessary following treatment, however, to confirm the absence of invasive malignancy. Cryosurgical treatment of LM has been associated with the development of amelanotic lentigo maligna melanoma (ALMM).[30] Because repigmentation can occur, close posttreatment follow-up is required.

BASAL CELL CARCINOMA AND SQUAMOUS CELL CARCINOMA

Cryosurgery is a simple and effective treatment for selected nonmelanoma skin cancers. Well-defined and superficial basal cell carcinoma (BCC) or squamous cell carcinomas (SCC) less than 2 cm in diameter are ideal candidates for this type of treatment. Treatment with open spray should consist of a double freeze–thaw cycle performed for 30 to 60 seconds depending on the thickness of the lesion. One may consider debulking thick lesions or using electrocoagulation and curettage before cryosurgery. A meta-analysis evaluating 50 patients with primary BCC followed for 5 years after LN treatment reported recurrence rates ranging from 0% to 20.4%.[31] Results from a combination treatment of curettage and cryosurgery in a 2011 prospective trial of 69 patients with 100 nonfacial tumors less than or equal to 2 cm in diameter who were followed for 1 to 5 years after treatment resulted in a 99% recurrence-free end point.[32] Tumors included in this trial consisting of superficial BCC, superficial nodular BCC with papillary dermal invasion, SCC in situ, and SCC with papillary dermal invasion. Cryosurgery in these instances should not replace surgical removal as the treatment of choice, but can be an alternative option for poor surgical candidates or patients who do not wish to undergo an invasive procedure.

KAPOSI'S SARCOMA

Cryosurgery using an open spray or probe technique is an option for patients with Kaposi's sarcoma. A double freeze–thaw cycle for open spray and a single application when using a probe usually provides adequate treatment. The freezing circle should be allowed to advance 1 to 2 mm outside the vascular lesion.

POSTOPERATIVE CARE AND EXPECTED SIDE EFFECTS

Cryosurgery is a fast, simple, and efficient tool, but there is always a risk of side effects and potential for a long recovery process. It is important to discuss the risks and to supply patients with a list of written instructions regarding postoperative care, anticipated healing time, expected symptoms, and possible complications.

Patients should be instructed to wash the wound with soap and water once or twice daily, and to dress it if the area is draining or has a bullous reaction. They can be instructed to apply topical antibiotic ointment or vaseline daily to avoid secondary infection. Healing time depends on the number of freeze–thaw cycles, the temperature achieved, and the location and depth of the lesion. It is important to keep in mind that the deeper the freeze and the poorer the circulation at the site, the longer the recovery process.

Erythema, edema, and itching and burning are expected almost immediately following treatment. Applying a topical moisturizer following cryosurgery may ease pruritus. Pain can occur and sometimes requires topical or oral analgesics. Vesicle or bulla formation may occur 1 to 5 days after treatment; these usually contain clear fluid. Occasionally the bulla may be hemorrhagic or exudative. Postoperative erythema and discomfort can last for several weeks. As melanocytes are extremely sensitive to cold, hypo- and hyperpigmentation are always risks, which may lead to a suboptimal cosmetic result. Each patient should be educated regarding these risks and benefits before treatment is performed.

COMPLICATIONS

Proper training in cryosurgery decreases the risk for complications but does not eliminate it. Bleeding is possible with deep freezing and may require electrocoagulation or, more rarely, suturing of a vessel. Lesions may become secondarily infected if they are not properly cleaned. Patients may complain of a headache following cryosurgery to the face or scalp. Nitrogen gas insufflation is rare but can occur if open-spray technique follows a biopsy of a lesion. Syncope may occur in patients who are nervous or hypersensitive to cold. Hypopigmentation and hyperpigmentation can also occur. Pigment changes may blend over time or may be a permanent complication. Hypertrophic scarring, alopecia and paresthesias are rare but have been reported as complications following cryosurgery.

RECENT ADVANCEMENTS

Cryopeeling is a newer modality currently being evaluated as another tool for dermatologists to use as field therapy. Cryopeeling uses cryosurgery in a diffuse manner on sun-damaged skin to promote skin rejuvenation and decrease the likelihood of AKs or skin cancers developing in the future. A study by Chiarello, following 373 patients with 34,604 AKs over 6.5 years concluded that the incidence of SCC was greatly reduced with cryopeeling. Conservative estimates from the literature predict that 34 SCCs should have appeared yearly in these 373 patients if these areas were left untreated. The incidence of SCC over the entire 6.5 year study was 33, with no metastases. Not all 373 patients were followed for 6.5 years.[33] More studies will therefore be required to evaluate the long-term success of cryopeeling.

PALLIATIVE TREATMENT

Palliative treatment with cryosurgery is an excellent option for patients with large or disfiguring lesions who are unable or unwilling to undergo recommended treatment. Cryosurgery can reduce bleeding, local infection, and pain, thereby allowing the patient to have a better quality of life. The open spray and chamber techniques are commonly used. Attempting to shave or debulk large lesions prior to treatment is not advised because most have an enormous network of neovascularization. Large tumors can be treated with fractional or segmental cryosurgery. Fractional cryosurgery[34] consists of reducing the extent of the area treated by beginning treatment in the center, allowing the area to heal, and then working from the inside out. Segmental cryosurgery divides lesions into quadrants, treats one area at a time, and allows for healing between treatments.[16] Both treatments are equally effective; personal comfort and experience will be the guides for treatment.

CONCLUSION

Cryosurgery is a first-line option for treating many benign and premalignant lesions. Because of its versatility and low cost, it has become one of the most frequently used techniques in dermatology. The treatment parameters and healing times vary depending on the lesion, while complications and side effects are usually minimal and well tolerated. Offering cryosurgery as a palliative treatment option for patients who do not wish to undergo surgical excision may increase their quality of life. Using cryosurgery as an adjunct to surgical or topical treatments for premalignant or malignant lesions should in theory decrease the likelihood of recurrences although to date there has been no research to prove its effectiveness. With proper training, all dermatologists should be able to use cryosurgery with ease as a treatment option for many common cutaneous lesions.

REFERENCES

1. Arnott J. *On the Treatment of Cancers by Regulated Application of an Anaesthetic Temperature.* Edinburg, UK: Churchill Livingstone; 1955.
2. Whitehouse HH. Liquid air in dermatology; its indications and limitations. *JAMA.* 1907;49:371–377.
3. White AC. Liquid air in medicine and surgery. *Med Rec.* 1899;56:109–112.
4. Pusey WA. The use of carbon dioxide snow in the treatment of nevi and other lesions of the skin. *JAMA.* 1907;49:1354–1356.
5. Torre D. Cradle of cryosurgery. *NY State J Med.* 1967;67:465–467.
6. Rubinsky B. Cryosurgery. *Ann Rev Biomed Eng.* 2000;2:157–187.
7. Kuflik EG, Gage AA, Lubritz RR, Graham GF. Millenium paper: history of dermatologic cryosurgery. *Dermatol Surg.* 2000;26:715–722.
8. Hollister WR, Mathew AJ, Baust JG, et al. Effects of freezing on cell viability and mechanisms of cell death in human prostate cancer cell line. *Mol Urol.* 1998;2:13–18.
9. Gage AA, Baust JM, Baust JG. Experimental cryosurgery investigation in vivo. *Cryobiology.* 2009;50:229–243.
10. Forest V, Peoc'h M, Campos L, Guyotat D, Vergnon JM. Effects of cryotherapy or chemotherapy on apoptosis in non-small-cell lung cancer xenografted into SCID mice. *Cryobiology.* 2005;50:29–37.
11. Adams S, O'Neil DW, Bhardwaj N. Recent advances in dendritic cell biology. *J Clin Immunol.* 2005;25(3):177–188.
12. Gage AA. Cryosurgery for oral and pharyngeal carcinoma. *Am J Surg.* 1969;118:669–672.
13. Soanes WA, Ablin RJ, Gonder MJ. Remission of metastatic lesions following cryosurgery in prostatic cancer: immunologic considerations. *J Urol.* 1970;104:154–159.
14. Joosten JJ, Muijen GN, Wobbes T, Ruers TJ. In vivo destruction of tumor tissue by cryoablation can induce inhibition of secondary tumor growth: an experimental study. *Cryobiology.* 2001;42(1):49–58.
15. Udagawa M, Kudo-Saito C, Hasegawa G, et al. Enhancement of Immunologic Tumor regression by intratumor administration of dentric cells in combination with cryoablative tumor pretreatment and bacillus calmette-guerin cell wall skeleton stimulation. *Clin Cancer Res.* 2006;12:7465–7475.
16. Pasquali P, Sebastian GJ, Zouboulis CC, et al. Cryosurgery. *Surgery of the Skin: Procedural Dermatology.* 2nd ed. Edinburgh London, New York: Mosby Elsevier;2010:153–166.
17. Goldberg LH, Kaplan B, Vergilis-Kalner I, Landau J. Liquid nitrogen: temperature control in the treatment of actinic keratosis. *Dermatol Surg.* 2010;36:1956–1961.
18. Blume-Peytavi U, Zouboulis CC, Jacobi H, Scholz A, Bisson S, Orfanos CE. Successful outcome of cryosurgery in patients with granuloma annulare. *Br J Dermatol.* 1994;130(4):494–497.
19. Zouboulis CC, Zouridaki E, Rosenberger A, Dalkowski A. Current developments and uses of cryosurgery in the treatment of keloids and hypertrophic scars. *Wound Repair Regen.* 2002;10:98–102.
20. Castro-Ron G, Pasquali P. Management of hemangiomas. Special Symposium. *Pediatr Dermatol.* 1997;14:70–71.
21. Suhonen R, Kuflik EG. Venous lakes treated by liquid nitrogen cryosurgery. *Br J Dermatol.* 1997;137:1018–1019.
22. Lubritz RR, Smolewski SA. Cryosurgery cure rate of actinic keratoses. *J Am Acad Dermatol.* 1982;7:631–632.
23. Thai KE, Fergin P, Freeman M, et al. A prospective study of the use of cryosurgery for the treatment of actinic keratoses. *Int J Dermatol.* 2004;43:687–692.
24. Kuflik EG, Gage AA. Cryosurgery for lentigo maligna. *J Am Acad Dermatol.* 1994;31:75–78.
25. Dawber RP, Wilkinson JD. Melanotic freckle of Hutchinson: treatment of macular and nodular phases with cryotherapy. *Br J Dermatol.* 1979;101:47–49.
26. Zacarin SA. Cryosurgical treatment of lentigo maligna. *Arch Dermatol.* 1982;118:89–92.
27. Bohler-Sommereggar K, Schuller-Petrovic S, Neumann R, Müller E. Cryosurgery of lentigo maligna. *Plast Reconstr Surg.* 1992;90:436–440; discussion 441–444.
28. Bohler-Sommereggar K, Schuller-Petrovic S, Knobler R, Neumann PR. Reactive lentiginous hyperpigmentation after cryosurgery for lentigo maligna. *J Am Acad Dermatol.* 1992;27:523–526.
29. Collins P, Rogers S, Goggin M, Manning W. Cryotherapy for lentigo maligna. *Clin Exp Dermatol.* 1991;16:433–435.
30. McKenna DB, Cooper EJ, Kavanagh GM, Davie RM, McLaren KM, Tidman MJ. Amelanotic malignant melanoma following cryosurgery for atypical lentigo maligna. *Clin Exp Dermatol.* 2000;25(8):600–604.

31. Thiessen MR, Neumann MH, Schouten LJ. A systemic review of treatment modalities for primary basal cell carcinomas. *Arch Dermatol.* 1999;135:1177–1183.
32. Peikert JM. Prospective trial of curettage and cryosurgery in the management of non-facial, superficial, and minimally invasive basal and squamous cell carcinoma. *Int J Dermatol.* 2011;50:1135–1138.
33. Chiarello SE. Cryopeeling (Extensive Cryosurgery) for treatment of actinic keratoses: an update and comparison. *Dermatol Surg.* 2000;26:728–732.
34. Goncalves JC. Fractional cryosurgery. A new technique for basal cell carcinomas of the eyelids and periorbital area. *Dermatol Surg.* 1997;23:475–481.

CHAPTER 16

Suture Closure Materials and Techniques

Ian A. Maher, James D. Russell, Thuzar Shin, Margaret Mann, & Jeremy Bordeaux

INTRODUCTION

Suturing is one of the foundational skills of dermatologic surgery.[1] Dermatologic surgeons must familiarize themselves with both the physical properties of suture material, as well as the available suturing techniques in order to ensure the best results for their patients.

BASIC SUTURE PROPERTIES AND TERMINOLOGY

Before he or she can select the proper suture material for a given closure, the dermatologic surgeon must understand the properties that differentiate the various suture materials, and the terminology used to describe these properties.

CONFIGURATION AND COATING

Configuration refers to whether a suture material has a single strand (monofilament), or multiple braided strands (multifilament).[2] Monofilament sutures generally exhibit less resistance when being pulled through tissue and have a lower risk of infection.[3] However, they exhibit greater memory – the suture's tendency to retain its packaged shape – and are consequently more difficult to handle than their multifilament counterparts.

Multifilament sutures, on the other hand, are more pliable and handle more easily. The braided nature of multifilament sutures creates natural crevices for bacteria, and higher rates of surgical site infection have been demonstrated relative to monofilament sutures.[4,5]

Braided sutures have more surface area than their monofilament counterparts. This increase in surface area increases resistance to being pulled through tissue and allows inflammatory cells better access to the suture material. Thus, multifilament sutures tend to be more reactive and are absorbed more quickly. In an attempt to negate the infection risk associated with multifilament sutures, antibacterial coatings have been added to multifilament sutures. Although triclosan-coated polyglactin 910 (Vicryl PLUS, Ethicon Inc., Summers, NJ) has been shown to decrease postoperative pain in the pediatric surgery population,[6] no consistent decrease in wound infection rates relative to uncoated suture has been demonstrated.[7–9]

TISSUE REACTIVITY

Although all sutures will initiate some degree of host response, the magnitude of this response can vary widely. In general, there are several guidelines which can be reliably followed. First, larger sutures will cause a larger host response, further supporting the general recommendation of using the smallest suture that is reasonable for a given defect. Second, multifilament sutures will elicit a larger inflammatory host response than monofilament due to their larger relative surface area. Third, natural materials such as silk will cause a larger response than their synthetic cousins. Finally, absorbable sutures tend to cause a larger response than nonabsorbable sutures.

DIAMETER AND USP SIZE

The size of suture is reported by the United States Pharmacopeia (USP) as the diameter of a given suture material necessary to obtain a certain tensile strength. This diameter is then reported as a number of zeroes, with fewer zeroes representing larger diameter. For example, 3-0 Prolene (Ethicon Inc., Somerville, NJ) has a larger diameter than 6-0 Prolene. However, given the fact that not all materials have the same inherent strength, it follows that not all sutures with the same USP size have the same diameter. 4-0 Ethilon (Ethicon), with its relatively high tensile strength, is significantly finer than 4-0 silk, which is an inherently weaker material. After choice of suture material, it is generally advocated to select the smallest diameter possible to achieve the necessary tensile strength.

TENSILE STRENGTH

The tensile strength of suture material can be characterized in two ways – absolute and effective. Absolute tensile strength, which is reported in pounds, is the weight an untied piece of suture can withstand without breakage. Effective tensile strength, on the other hand, is the weight that suture can withstand after it has been tied. For a given suture, effective tensile strength is approximately one-third of the absolute tensile strength. In general, synthetic suture materials have a higher tensile strength than their natural counterparts.

ABSORPTION

Absorption is the result of enzymes and other biologic substances causing a loss of integrity of suture material through a variety of mechanisms. Although sutures are classically defined as "absorbable" versus "non-absorbable," it is important to note that capacity for absorption is not synonymous with tensile strength. For example, some absorbable sutures, like poliglecaprone 25 (Monocryl: Ethicon), have a very high initial tensile strength, but are absorbed very rapidly. Synthetic polymeric sutures, such as polyglactin 910, are absorbed by hydrolysis, causing less tissue reactivity than natural protein based sutures, such as gut, which are absorbed by proteolysis.

COEFFICIENT OF FRICTION

The coefficient of friction is a measure of how easily suture passes through tissue. Materials with a low coefficient of friction, such as polypropylene, pass through tissue with ease, but generally have poor knot security. Monofilament materials will often have lower coefficients of friction than multifilament sutures. A low coefficient of friction is especially desirable in the case of subcuticular sutures that are intended for removal, as decreased resistance will minimize damage to tissue during removal. Due to improved knot security, sutures with a higher coefficient of friction are preferred in high-tension wounds.

ELASTICITY VERSUS PLASTICITY

Elasticity refers to the ability of a suture material to return to its original shape and length after stretching. This is an important characteristic to consider when performing surgery in areas prone to edema, such as the eyebrows. Plasticity, on the other hand, is the tendency of suture material to maintain its new configuration after stretching. Very plastic sutures may be loosened after the resolution of postoperative edema, and this can contribute to poor wound-edge approximation.

MEMORY

The memory of suture is the tendency to retain its original shape despite manipulation. Sutures with high memory, such as nylon, are often used for superficial wound closure given their ability to maintain approximation despite edema and intermittent physical stress. These materials are, however, more difficult to handle and have less knot security than others.

KNOT SECURITY

Knot security is defined as the force necessary to cause a knot to slip or untie. This value is directly proportional to the coefficient of friction of the suture material. Silk, with its high coefficient of friction, has excellent knot security. Conversely, a suture with low coefficient of friction like polypropylene has poor knot security, and a higher number of throws is often utilized by the surgeon using these types of suture.

THE NEEDLE

The needle is an important part of the suture apparatus. Many different needle morphologies exist, but few are regularly used in cutaneous surgery. The most commonly used needle is curved, 3/8 of a circle, with a triangular shape. These needles come in two forms: reverse cutting and conventional cutting. Reverse cutting needles, which are more commonly used, have the sharp edge on the outside of the needle, which is usually away from the wound edge. For this reason, they are less likely to tear through tissue toward the surface or wound edge during closure. Conventional cutting needles, with the sharp edge on the inside of the curve, are both weaker and more prone to tissue tearing. Needles come in a number of sizes, and the nomenclature used to describe them varies greatly based on manufacturer. Tapered needles are cylindrical with a sharp point. They exhibit greater resistance to movement through tissue and dull more quickly than cutting variants making them less suitable for cutaneous surgery.

Needle size should be selected based on the thickness of the skin being sutured. Thicker skinned areas favor the use of larger needle sizes whereas smaller needles should be used in thinner skinned areas.

WOUND CLOSURE MATERIALS

Suture materials have long been classified as either absorbable or nonabsorbable. This section will review both common and historically significant types of material in each category.

THE ABSORBABLE SUTURES

Absorbable materials are commonly used for placement of dermal sutures. In this role, they provide tensile strength for the wound early in the wound healing period. The suture is broken down by enzymatic degradation and/or hydrolysis, and no removal is required. At one time, surgical gut represented the most commonly used absorbable suture. Today, however, several newer alternatives exist that are more desirable for a number of reasons. Table 16-1 summarizes the properties of the absorbable sutures.

SURGICAL GUT. All types of surgical gut are monofilament sutures composed primarily of collagen prepared from either cow or sheep intestine. Today, it comes in three distinct types: plain, chromic, and fast-absorbing. Plain surgical gut, as the name implies, consists of untreated gut fibers. It has a holding time of approximately 7 days, and is absorbed within 10 to 14 days. Although it was once among the most popular sutures, its tissue reactivity and relatively poor tensile strength limit its utility in modern surgery. Chromic gut, which has been tanned with chromate salts to increase longevity, has a holding time of 14 days, and it is usually absorbed in 3 weeks.[10] Fast-absorbing gut is plain gut that has been heated for more rapid absorption. With absorption occurring in 5 to 7 days, it is useful as a surface suture when postoperative removal would be difficult for any reason.

TABLE 16-1
Properties of Absorbable Sutures

Material	Configuration	Ease of Handling	Knot Security	Tissue Reactivity	Initial Tensile Strength	Retention of Tensile Strength	Time to Complete Absorption
Plain surgical gut	Monofilament	Fair	Poor	High	Low	0% by 7–10 d	70 d
Chromic gut	Monofilament	Fair	Poor	Moderate	Low	0% by 21–28 d	90 d
Fast absorbing surgical gut	Monofilament	Fair	Poor	High	Low	0% by 7 d	20–40 d
Polyglycolic acid (Dexon®)	Multifilament	Good	Good	Low	Moderate	35% at 21 d	60–90 d
Polyglactin 910 (Vicryl®, Polysorb®)	Multifilament	Good	Good	Low	High	75% at 14 d, 25% at 28 d	60–70 d
Polyglactin 910 (Vicryl Rapide®)	Multifilament	Good	Good	Low	High	50% at 5 d, 0% by 14 d	40 d
Poliglecaprone 25 (Monocryl®)	Monofilament	Good	Good	Very low	Very high	60% at 7 d, 30% at 14 d	90–120 d
Glycomer 631 (Biosyn®)	Monofilament	Good	Poor	Very low	High	50% at 21 d	90–110 d
Polydioxanone (PDS II®)	Monofilament	Poor	Poor	Very low	High	60% at 14 d, 40% at 28 d[a]	180–240 d
Polytrimethylene carbonate (Maxon®)	Monofilament	Fair	Good	Low	Very high	60% at 28 d, 30% at 42 d	60–180 d

[a]For suture sizes 4-0 and smaller.

POLYGLYCOLIC ACID. Polyglycolic acid (Dexon: USSDG, Norwalk, CT) is a synthetic, multifilament suture that was first released in 1970. It is coated with Poloxamer 188, a lubricant that decreases the coefficient of friction and increases ease of handling. Dexon retains 89% of its tensile strength at day 7, 63% at day 14, and 17% at day 21.[4] With the advent of newer products such as polyglactin 910, polyglycolic acid has seen its use decline, and it is no longer widely available.

POLYGLACTIN 910, AKA POLYGLACTIC ACID. Polyglactin 910 (Vicryl: Ethicon; Polysorb: USSDG) is a multifilament, synthetic suture released soon after polyglycolic acid. As a multifilament suture, with high knot security, it is useful for the closure of high-tension wounds where knot slippage could cause loosening of the dermal sutures. It is less inflammatory than surgical gut, and retains tensile strength longer than polyglycolic acid. It was found to have 65% of its original strength at 14 days, and 40% at 3 weeks. It is then completely dissolved by 60 to 90 days via hydrolysis, which partially explains its lower immunogenicity.

Vicryl is available in both dyed and undyed forms. The dyed form is rarely used in cutaneous surgery due to risk of visible sutures within the healing wound. Vicryl Plus (Ethicon) is a product that is coated with triclosan, a topical antibiotic. Studies have demonstrated decreased postoperative pain in pediatric patients but have not consistently shown any decrease in infections with triclosan coated sutures. Vicryl Rapide (Ethicon) is a gamma-irradiated form of polyglactin 910 that loses its tensile strength within 14 days, much faster than polyglactin 910. As such, it can be used as a superficial suture that does not need future removal. A small study of facial wounds found it to be equivalent to polypropylene.[11]

POLIGLECAPRONE 25. Poliglecaprone 25 (Monocryl: Ethicon) is a synthetic monofilament with the highest initial tensile strength of all the materials in this section. That tensile strength, however, rapidly degrades. This property makes poliglecaprone most suitable for facial wounds where rapid absorption is desirable and high sustained tensions are not an issue. Poliglecaprone maintains 60% of this strength at day 7, 30% at day 14, and is absorbed within 3 to 4 weeks.[12] In a head to head study, it was shown to be less reactive than Vicryl Rapide when used for dermal sutures.[13] A small study showed no difference between superficial closures with poliglecaprone 25 and polypropylene,[14] which raises the possibility of cost-effective use of a single suture for both deep and surface closure.

GLYCOMER 631. Glycomer 631 (Biosyn: USSDG) is a monofilament, synthetic suture that is similar to poliglecaprone 25, but it dissolves more slowly. It retains 49%

of its original tensile strength at 3 weeks, and it is completely absorbed in 3 to 6 months.[15] It also has a lower coefficient of friction than poliglecaprone 25, which leads to easier handling but poorer knot security.[15]

POLYDIOXANONE. Polydioxanone (PDSII: Ethicon) is a synthetic monofilament suture renowned for prolonged tensile strength. It retains 74% of its original strength at 2 weeks, 50% at 4 weeks, and 25% at 6 weeks. It is absorbed at a slow rate over 6 months. It is most useful in high-tension areas, where long-term support for the wound is required. Use on thinner-skinned areas can cause long-standing lumps and spitting sutures due to the prolonged absorption time. Although the stiffness of polydioxanone makes it relatively difficult to handle, it has low tissue reactivity and it can be safely used in areas of high tension.

POLYTRIMETHYLENE CARBONATE. Polytrimethylene carbonate (Maxon: USSDG) is another synthetic monofilament suture that is composed of a copolymer of glycolide and trimethylene carbonate. Compared with PDS, it has an increased ease of handling. The tensile strength of polytrimethylene carbonate is measurable for 42 to 92 days.[10]

ABSORBABLE STAPLES. Insorb (Incisive Surgery, Plymouth, MN) is a synthetic absorbable suture made of a polylactic and polyglycolic acid copolymer. It maintains 40% of its initial tensile strength at 2 weeks, and has a tissue half-life of 10 weeks. Although animal studies have been promising, no human studies have shown superiority in terms of cosmetic results or infection. A study in post-tissue expander breast reduction showed no difference in scar characteristics and a finding of "increased cost efficacy."[16] However, this calculation was based on $1500 per hour operating room time, and is unlikely to be applicable to outpatient procedures.

THE NONABSORBABLE SUTURES

Table 16-2 summarizes the properties of the nonabsorbable sutures. Table 16-3 summarizes the common time to removal in various areas.

TABLE 16-3
Superficial Suture Choice by Anatomic Location

Location	Gauge	Time to Removal (days)
Face	6-0	5–7
Neck and Scalp	5-0, 6-0	7–10
Extremities	4-0, 5-0	10–14
Trunk	4-0, 5-0	10–14

SURGICAL SILK

Surgical silk is a braided, natural substance that is coated with wax or silicone to decrease coefficient of friction. It is dyed black for better visualization. Surgical silk truly excels in the areas of softness, ease of handling, and knot stability. However, as a natural product, it is highly reactive in tissue. It is this tendency to elicit reactions that limits its usefulness in cutaneous surgery. Silk is useful for closing biopsy sites in sensitive areas such as the mouth or genitals.

NYLON

Nylon, in all of its forms, represents the most commonly used suture in dermatologic surgery. It is a synthetic product, chemically inert, and it is available as both a monofilament (Ethilon: Ethicon; Monosof: USSDG; Dermalon: USSDG) and braided (Nurolon: Ethicon; Surgilon: USSDG) suture. The braided forms, which are coated with silicone, are easier to handle and have better knot security, but are more expensive and have higher tissue reactivity.

POLYPROPYLENE

Polypropylene (Prolene: Ethicon; Surgipro: USSDG) is a synthetic monofilament that is primarily known for its very low coefficient of friction. As such, it is the suture

TABLE 16-2
Properties of Nonabsorbable Sutures

Material	Configuration	Ease of Handling	Knot Security	Tissue Reactivity	Tensile Strength
Silk	Multifilament	Excellent	Excellent	High	Low
Nylon (Dermalon®, Ethilon®, Monosof®)	Monofilament	Fair	Fair	Low	High
Nylon (Nurolon®, Surgilon®)	Multifilament	Good	Good	Low	High
Polypropylene (Prolene®, Surgipro®)	Monofilament	Poor	Poor	Low	Moderate
Polyester (Dacron®, Mersilene®)	Multifilament	Good	Good	Moderate	High
Polyester, coated (Ethibond®)	Multifilament	Good	Fair	Moderate	High
Polybutester (Novafil®)	Monofilament	Fair	Fair	Low	High

of choice for running subcuticular sutures, and can be removed after wound healing with minimal tissue disruption or destruction. In addition, polypropylene's high plasticity makes it useful in areas that may experience severe swelling postoperatively. Drawbacks of polypropylene include high memory, which makes handling and knot tying more difficult, and costly.

POLYESTER

Polyester sutures (Dacron: USSDG; Ethibond: Ethicon; Mersilene: Ethicon) are braided, multifilament synthetic products with good handling and very high tensile strength. In fact, of all suture materials, polyester is second only to surgical steel in terms of strength.[17] It is available plain, or coated with polybutylate. Although the coated forms have lower coefficient of friction and hence glide more easily through tissue, they are also more prone to breakage.

POLYBUTESTER

Polybutester (Novafil: USSDG) is a synthetic, thermoplastic polymer of glycol and polybutylene terephthalates. It was designed to be stronger, less stiff, and to have a lower coefficient of friction than nylon or polypropylene. It is characterized by good handling, high elasticity, and very low tissue reactivity.

SURGICAL STAPLES

Staples have long been used for wound closure by surgeons in a number of surgical specialties. They are composed of stainless steel and offer the following benefits: extremely high tensile strength, ease and speed of placement, and low tissue reactivity. When compared with sutures, steel staples have a lower incidence of infection when closing contaminated wounds.[1] Staples are commonly used for wounds on the scalp, and they are easily removed with a hemostat or specialized extractor.

TISSUE ADHESIVES

Tissue adhesives offer the chance to close surgical wounds without puncture sites, track marks, or need for postoperative removal of sutures. They can be applied quickly and easily to nearly any area of the body. They are most often used in small wound under minimal tension. Today, there are two commonly used tissue adhesives in cutaneous surgery: 2-octylcyanoacrylate (Dermabond: Ethicon) and n-butyl-2-cyanoacrylate (Indermil: USSDG; Glu-Stitch: Glu-Stitch Inc., Delta, BC, Canada).

2-OCTYLCYANOACRYLATE

2-octylcyanoacrylate (Dermabond: Ethicon) is a long chain cyanoacrylate that has been on the market in the United States since 1998. It is applied to the skin immediately surrounding, but not within, the surgical wound. Three layers are generally used, with time in between for the previous one to dry. When compared with sutures, it was shown to be faster and equally efficacious for the closure of lacerations, with no difference in cosmetic outcome.[18]

N-BUTYL-2-CYANOACRYLATE

N-butyl-2-cyanoacrylate (Indermil: Covidien; PeriAcryl: Glu-Stitch) is another long chain cyanoacrylate that is approved for use in the United States. When compared with traditional suture, it was shown to equally effective for securing full-thickness skin grafts on the face.[19] Although this adhesive is 3 to 4 times weaker than Dermabond based on bonding strength, a head-to-head study showed no difference between the two when used on facial lacerations in pediatric patients.[20] When selecting tissue adhesives, the decision comes down to cost, availability, and physician preference.

ADHESIVE STRIPS

Steri-strips (Steristrips: 3 M) are thin adhesive strips that can be used, in certain situations, for the closure of small, superficial defects. To use, they are placed on the skin, perpendicular to the direction of the wound, to bring the edges together and generate a small amount of tension. Steri-strips have been shown to be an equivalent replacement for epidermal sutures during the repair of cheek defects after excision of malignancy.[21] Although Steri-strips are occasionally used in addition to continuous subcutaneous sutures, a large review suggests this gives no benefit.[22]

WOUND CLOSURE TECHNIQUES

DEEP SUTURES

Deep, subcuticular, or buried sutures are a key element in optimizing cosmetic results. The deep suture provides tensile strength to the wound, closes dead space, and aids in everting the wound edges. Eversion of the wound edges prevents formation of a depressed scar as the wound undergoes 3-dimensional contraction during scar maturation.[23]

SIMPLE BURIED INTERRUPTED SUTURE

The classic buried interrupted suture is an inverted simple interrupted stitch entirely contained within the dermis and with the knot buried. Although suture marks are absent, it produces minimal eversion, increasing the risk of a depressed scar (Fig. 16-1).[24]

BURIED VERTICAL MATTRESS SUTURE

In contrast to the circular shape of the buried interrupted suture, the lateral aspects of the buried vertical mattress suture traverse the dermis at a higher point than the medial aspects of the stitch, providing wound edge eversion and facilitating the creation of a fine imperceptible scar.[25] Multiple groups have demonstrated good aesthetic results with

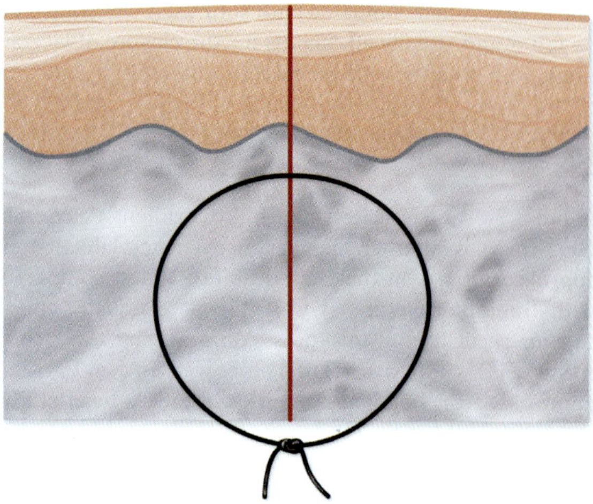

Figure 16-1 A simple buried interrupted suture.

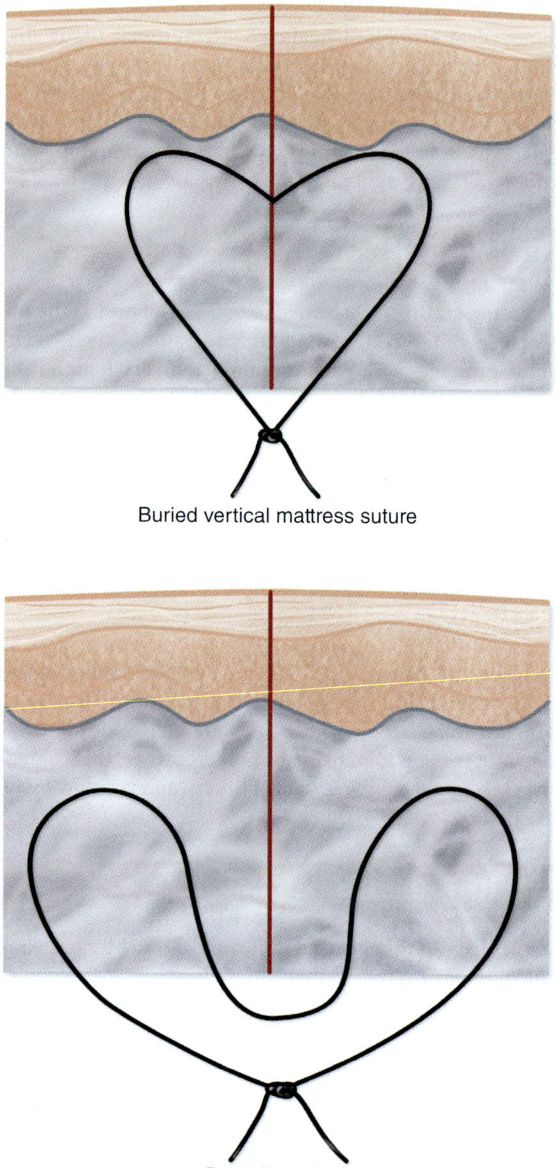

Figure 16-2 A buried vertical mattress (top), and the butterfly variant of the buried vertical mattress (bottom).

the use of buried vertical mattress sutures in the absence of epidermal sutures.[21,26]

In order to create the everting, "heart-shaped" profile of the buried vertical mattress the following steps should be taken; the needle enters the underside of the dermis in a vertical direction until upward pressure on the skin surface can be perceived. At this point forceps or a skin hook are used to turn the skin edge outward as the needle is advanced through the tissue until it exits into the wound bed at a descending angle. The needle then enters the opposite wound edge at a level equal to that of its exit and at an ascending angle. The needle is pushed out away from the wound edge and allowed to turn on its axis until it exits the dermal undersurface (Fig. 16-2).

It may be difficult to generate the heart-shaped profile of the buried vertical mattress in thin-skinned areas or when exposure is limited due to closely spaced dermal sutures. The percutaneous buried vertical mattress suture may be useful in such cases. By exiting and reentering the skin surface through the same puncture sites on either side of the wound edge, the suture material is buried within the dermis while a vertical mattress configuration is created (Fig. 16-3). When utilizing this technique it is advisable to use a low-reactivity absorbable suture such as polydioxanone or polyglecaprone to minimize the risk of transepidermal elimination.

BURIED HORIZONTAL MATTRESS SUTURE

The fully buried horizontal mattress suture consists of two horizontally oriented half loops that approach, but do not pierce, the skin surface as they travel parallel to the wound edge (Fig. 16-4).[27] The horizontal mattress provides added wound-edge eversion to the aforementioned advantages of traditional buried interrupted sutures. Superficial knot placement and a decreased ability to close dead space are weaknesses. This technique is most useful when deep sutures and eversion are required in narrow or tight spaces where it is often difficult to execute a buried vertical mattress suture.

BURIED PULLEY STITCH VARIANTS

The pulley stitch utilizes mechanical advantage to close wounds under greater tension than could be closed with other suture variants. Buried pulley stitch variants, executed with an absorbable suture, allow the tension-bearing suture to be left in vivo, thus providing added tensile strength to the wound, while eliminating the risk of suture marks associated with superficial tension bearing sutures.[28,29]

The subcutaneous inverted cross mattress stitch (SICM) is executed by throwing a vertical mattress suture. However, instead of tying that suture off, a second continuous vertical mattress pass is performed 3 to 4 mm from the first. The free ends of the suture are then tied to each other (Fig. 16-5).[29] In addition to being useful for closing wounds under high tension, the SICM is useful as the initial tension-bearing suture in thin-skinned areas such as

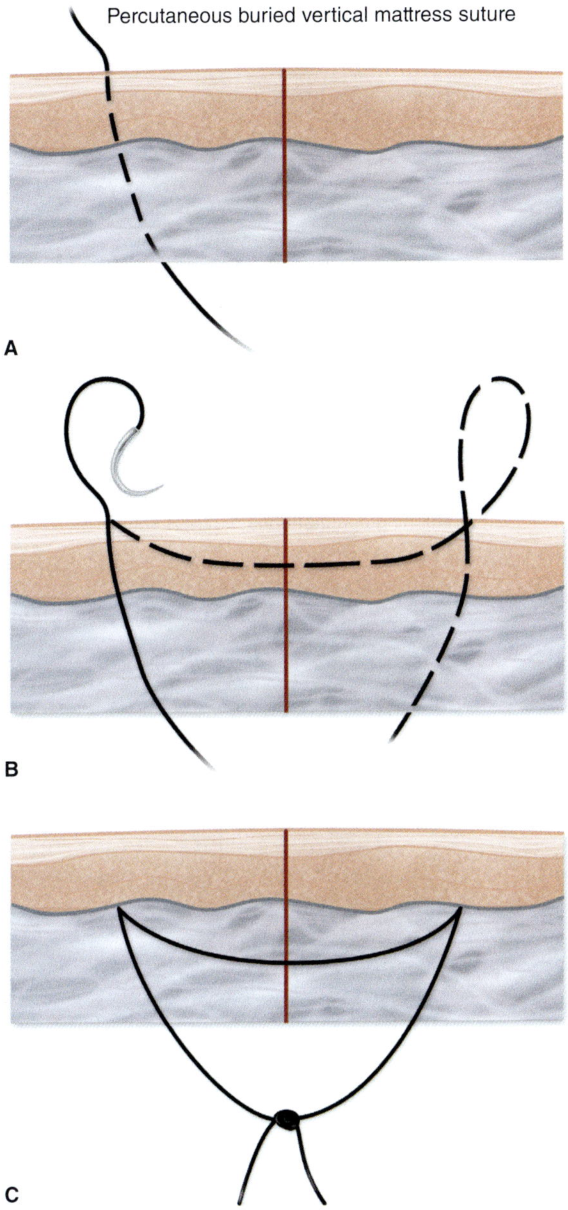

Figure 16-3 The percutaneous vertical mattress. **A.** The needle is inserted on the deep surface of the dermis and is pushed out the epidermal surface. **B.** The needle is reinserted through the same puncture hole and takes a superficial bite crossing the wound edge before exiting the skin surface on the opposite side of the wound. The needle is then reinserted into the same puncture site and pushed through the full thickness of the dermis. **C.** The final suture configuration. By entering and exiting through the same puncture sites the suture buries itself into the dermis.

atrophic, actinically damaged forearm skin. By distributing the tension across the two adjacent throws the risk of the suture tearing through thin tissue is reduced.

RUNNING SUBCUTICULAR SUTURE

Subcuticular closure is used in areas where track marks would be unacceptable and in anatomic areas with high

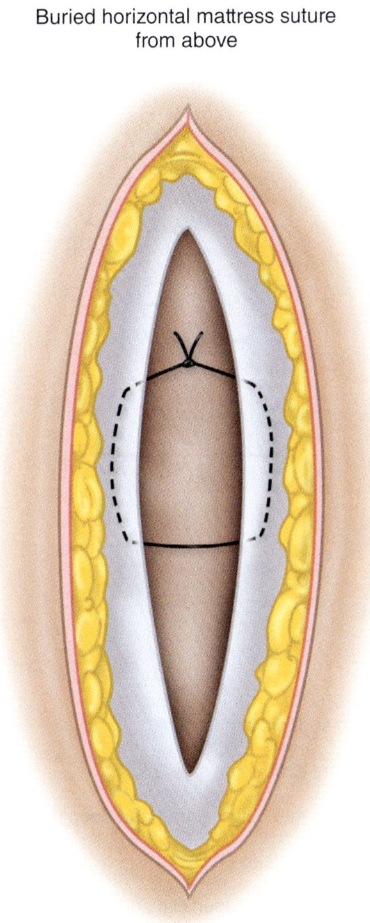

Figure 16-4 A diagram of the buried horizontal mattress suture as viewed from above.

tension.[30,31] Absorbable and nonabsorbable suture material can be used. If absorbable material is used, the suture is placed by first securing a buried dermal knot at one end of the wound before passing the needle through the apex of the wound.[30] If nonabsorbable material is selected, the tail of the suture is securely taped to the skin, or tied off with a sliding knot. The needle is then advanced by taking horizontal bites at the dermal–epidermal junction on alternate sides, with some overlap (Fig. 16-6). Once the end of the wound is reached, the suture is tied and buried if absorbable, or tied and secured to the skin if nonabsorbable. The main disadvantages of the traditional subcuticular closure are its time-consuming and technically challenging nature, decreased ability to evert wound edges, and the risk of transepidermal elimination of sutures when using an absorbable material.

Everting variants of the subcuticular closure have been reported to overcome the limited eversion provided with typical subcuticular techniques.[32] The running percutaneous vertical mattress suture technique uses the "in and out" technique of the interrupted percutaneous vertical mattress to produce eversion while burying the suture material in the dermis. The technique begins with a buried vertical mattress. The non-needle end of the suture is cut and a series of alternating deep passes paralleling the

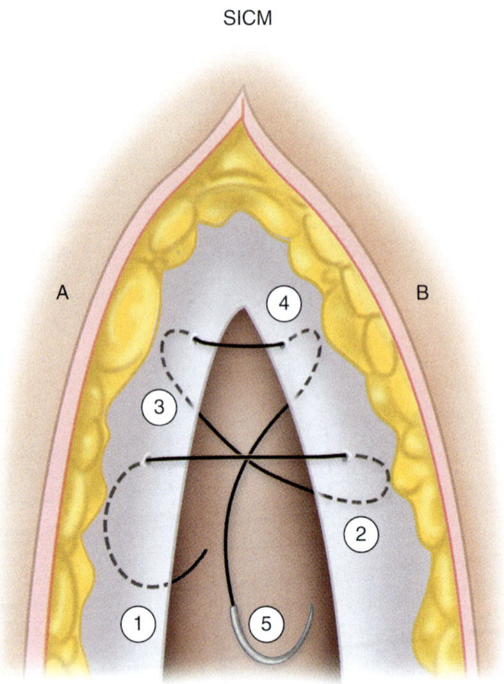

① Deep to superficial on side A

② Superficial to deep on side B

③ Advance 5 mm down wound and deep to superficial on A

④ Superficial to deep on B

⑤ Tie needle end to superficial end

Figure 16-5 A diagram of the subcutaneous inverted mattress suture. Step by step instructions are illustrated on the diagram.

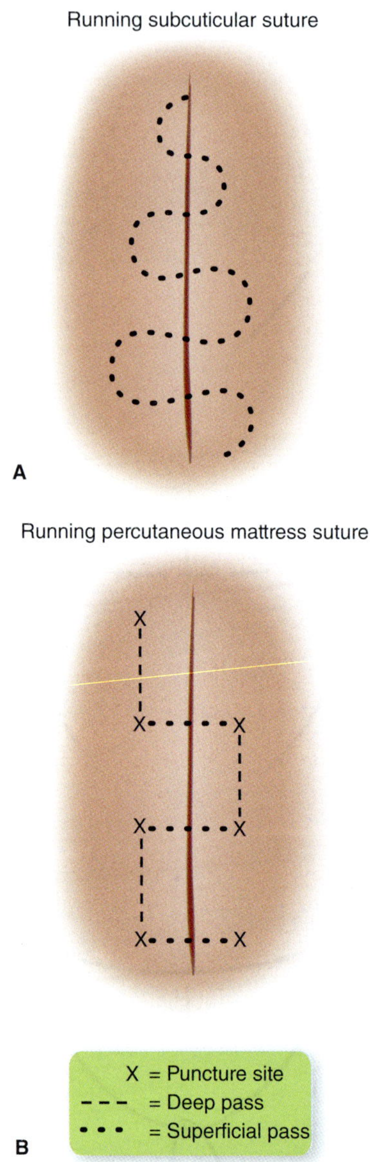

Figure 16-6 A. The typical running subcuticular closure. **B.** The running percutaneous mattress suture.

wound edge and superficial dermal passes crossing the wound edge perpendicularly continue along the length of the wound. When the end of the wound is reached, the last deep loop of suture is left long and tied off to the needle end of the suture.

SUPERFICIAL SUTURES

INTERRUPTED SUTURES

SIMPLE INTERRUPTED SUTURE. The simple interrupted stitch is the most basic suture technique in cutaneous repair (Fig. 16-7). It is performed by inserting the suture needle at an angle greater than 90 degrees approximately 5 mm from the wound edge, rotating the wrist so that the needle takes a pear-shaped path as it traverses perpendicular to the long axis of the wound and emerges from the opposite side. The epidermis is approximated and a surgeon's knot is tied. The wider base of the suture pass recruits tissue toward the center of the wound, forcing the superficial tissues upward and naturally everting the wound edges as the suture is tightened. The depth and breadth of the stitch should directly correlate with the thickness of the skin being sutured – for example, smaller bites for areas such as the thin periorbital skin. The simple interrupted can be used to correct uneven wound edges by taking a more superficial bite on the higher side and a deeper bite on the lower side.

Advantages include technical simplicity, knot security, enhanced eversion of the wound, and precise epidermal approximation. The main disadvantage is the development of track marks if sutures remain in place for an extended period of time.

HORIZONTAL MATTRESS SUTURES

The horizontal mattress suture is performed by beginning as if placing a simple stitch. Instead of securing the interrupted stitch, the needle is advanced forward approximately 5 mm down the length of the wound and a simple backstitch is

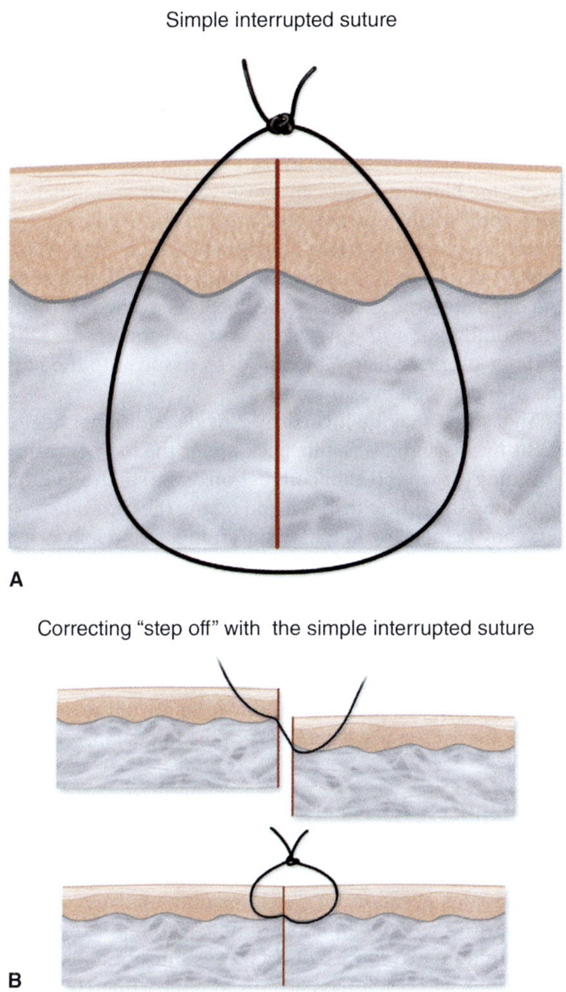

Figure 16-7 **A.** Simple interrupted suture. **B.** Illustration of step-off correction technique with the simple interrupted suture. A smaller, more superficial bite is taken on the high side.

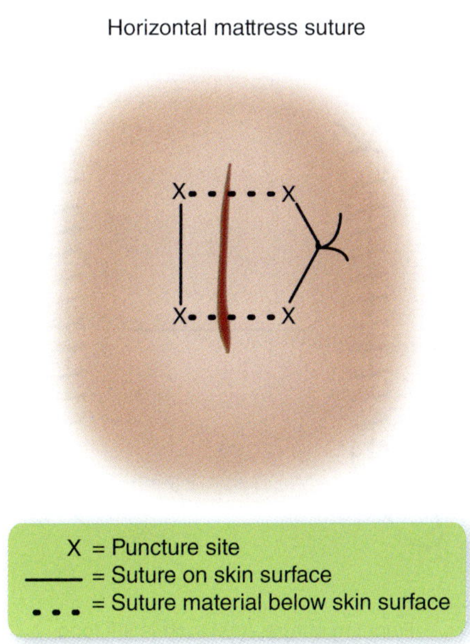

Figure 16-8 The horizontal mattress suture.

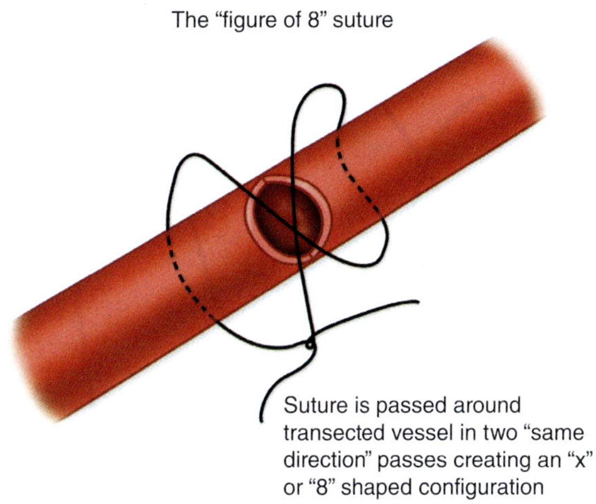

Figure 16-9 The suture is passed around a transected blood vessel with two, same direction passes. This yields an "x" or "8" shaped configuration when the suture is tied.

placed in the reverse direction. The suture is then tied with a surgeon's knot (Fig. 16-8). This technique decreases tension on, and everts, the wound edges, and it aids in hemostasis by closing dead space. However, if tied too tightly, horizontal mattress sutures may compromise the blood supply from the superficial dermal plexus resulting in epidermal necrosis. In addition, they may be difficult to remove, are more technically challenging and take more time to perform. For these reasons, the horizontal mattress stitch is often used in conjunction with other interrupted and running sutures.

The half buried horizontal mattress, or tip stitch, is a variant of the horizontal mattress that is useful for securing triangulated wound edges. By making a horizontal pass through the dermis of the triangulated flap tip, the tip stitch minimizes the risk of vascular strangulation.

FIGURE OF "8" SUTURE

The figure of "8" suture is used primarily as a hemostatic suture. Two parallel passes are performed on either side of a bleeding vessel without reversing the direction of the needle (Fig. 16-9). This suture may be performed with absorbable suture if it is placed in subcutaneous tissue, or with nonabsorbable suture if it is placed on the skin surface.

VERTICAL MATTRESS SUTURE

The far-far-near-near vertical mattress suture is performed by beginning with a wider and deeper simple interrupted stitch. Instead of tying the stitch, the needle is reversed and a second, more superficial interrupted backstitch is placed medial and superficial to the first, then secured (Fig. 16-10). The vertical mattress stitch is used to enhance wound-edge eversion at locations such as the helical rim, where a depressed scar would distort the natural contour of a free margin. As a mattress suture, it closes dead space, thereby decreasing tension and providing hemostasis. Care should be taken to avoid excessive tightening of the knot, which can strangulate the wound edges and cause necrosis. Like the horizontal mattress suture, the vertical

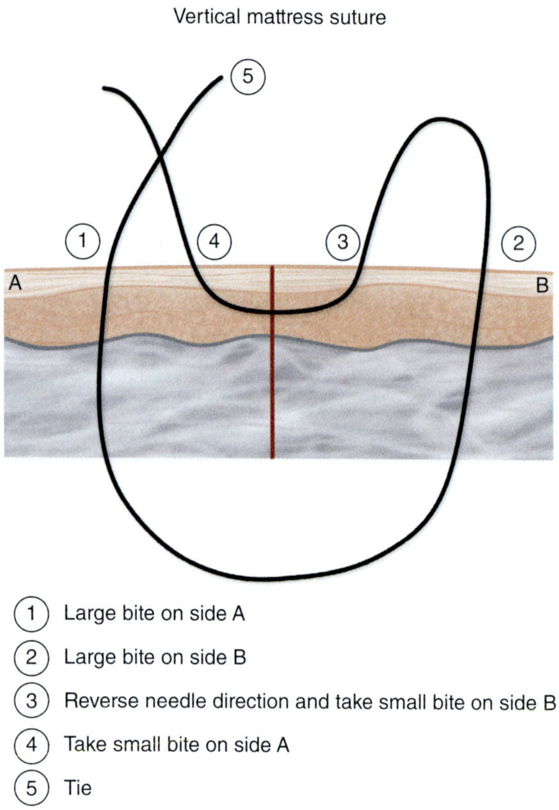

Figure 16-10 A diagram of the vertical mattress suture.

mattress is technically challenging, takes additional time to perform, and is commonly used in combination with other methods of closure.

PULLEY STITCH

The pulley stitch can be viewed as a variant of the vertical mattress. The pulley stitch is useful for relieving tension on tight wounds and may be used as a temporary suture to aid closure, or left in place. Like any superficial tension-bearing suture, the risk of suture marks are increased if this suture is left in vivo. Unlike the vertical mattress where the needle direction is reversed and the knot tied entirely on one side of the wound, in the pulley suture both passes are made in a single direction and the knot is tied across the wound.

Variants of this suture exist, but all involve multiple passes through the tissue before tying. These multiple passes allow for the creation of mechanical advantage as well as resistance to suture loosening before tying is completed.[33] Pulley sutures are useful for aiding closure in high-tension areas such as the scalp or lower extremities.

RUNNING SUPERFICIAL SUTURES

SIMPLE RUNNING SUTURE

The simple running stitch is begun as if placing a traditional simple interrupted suture at one apex of the wound. The non-needle suture tail is cut and simple stitches are placed in approximately 5 mm apart along the length of the wound (Fig. 16-10). The last loop is not tightened but left long and tied to the free end. Maintaining the fundamentals of the simple interrupted suture, such as puncturing the skin at an angle of 90 degrees or greater and taking pear-shaped bites, helps produce maximal eversion. An additional strategy to maximize eversion while minimizing tissue handling that can cause vascular strangulation is to apply slight upward pressure on the needle once it punctures the skin surface on the first wound edge. A forceps or skin hook is then used to apply inward pressure on the opposite wound edge as the needle is pushed through. The combination of upward pressure on the needle with counter-pressure helps "bunch" deep tissue onto the needle producing an everting bite.

This stitch may be locked to provide additional hemostasis by passing the needle back under the loop of suture spanning the wound after completion of the stitch and prior to pulling the suture through and taking the next bite.[34] As with any hemostatic stitch, tissue strangulation may occur if excessive tension in applied. The main advantages of the simple running are even distribution of tension, ease of placement, ability to correct uneven wound edges, and increased speed of wound closure. Disadvantages include decreased knot security and risk of epidermal necrosis if tied too tightly. In addition, the entire length of the repair is at risk for dehiscence should one of the knots fail.

RUNNING MATTRESS SUTURES

Running mattress sutures may be used to accentuate wound-edge eversion.[32,35–37] All running mattress sutures begin with the same knot as a simple running suture. The horizontal mattress variant then uses bites in alternating directions with each pass advanced approximately 5 mm down the wound edge (Fig. 16-11). The running horizontal mattress produced superior results to simple running suture in one small study (Fig. 16-12).[36] The vertical

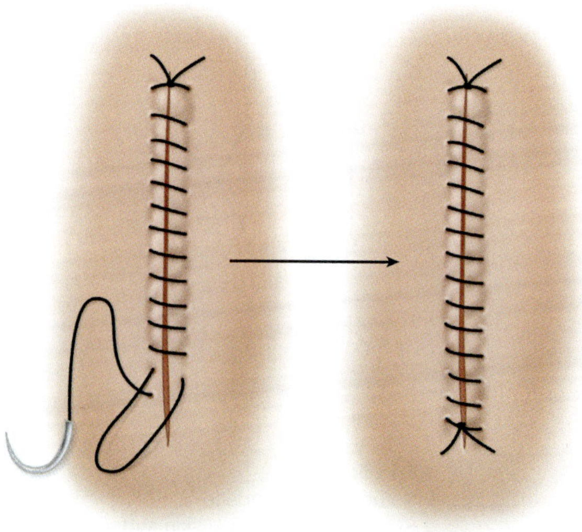

Running suture. Last loop is left long and tied to the free needle end

Figure 16-11 The simple running suture.

Horizontal running mattress suture

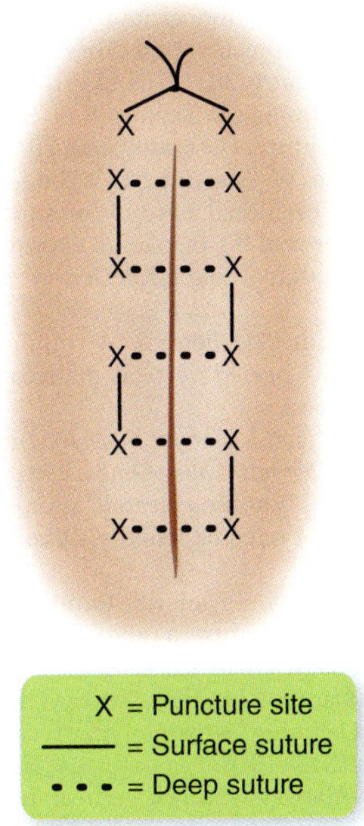

Figure 16-12 The running horizontal mattress suture.

mattress variant combines deep bites which cross the wound bed diagonally with superficial bites that cross the wound edge in the superficial plane (Fig. 16-13). As running mattress sutures are often difficult to remove, modifications with alternating simple and mattressed bites have been reported to maximize eversion while maintaining ease of suture removal.[35]

Running vertical mattress suture

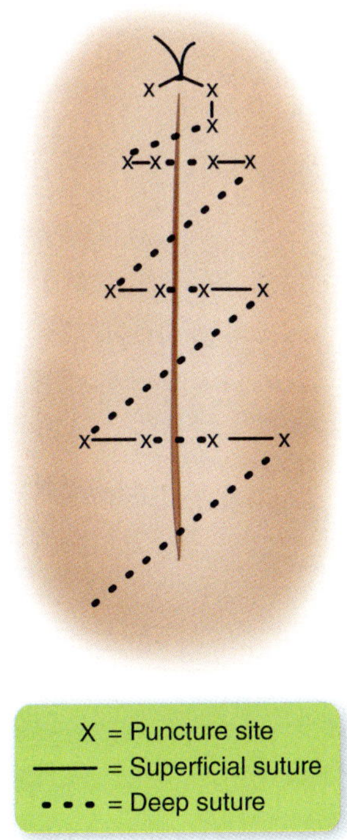

Figure 16-13 The running vertical mattress suture.

CONCLUSION

Suturing is one of the foundational skills of dermatologic surgery. A full understanding of suturing techniques and materials allows surgeons to optimize results for their patients.

REFERENCES

1. Hochberg J, Meyer K, Marion M. Suture choice and other methods of skin closure. *Surg Clin North Am.* 2009;89:627–641.
2. Bennett RG. Selection of wound closure materials. *J Am Acad Dermatol.* 1988;18:619–637.
3. Gabrielli F, Potenza C, Puddu P, Sera F, Masini C, Abeni D. Suture materials and other factors associated with tissue reactivity, infection, and wound dehiscence among plastic surgery outpatients. *Plast Reconstr Surg.* 2001;107:38–45.
4. Tajirian A, Goldberg D. A review of sutures and other skin closure materials. *J Cosmet Laser Ther.* 2010;12:296–302.
5. Bloom B, Goldberg D. Suture material in cosmetic cutaneous surgery. *J Cosmet Laser Ther.* 2007;9:41–45.
6. Ford H, Jones P, Gaines B, Reblock K, Simpkins D. Intraoperative handling and wound healing: controlled clinical trial comparing coated VICRYL plus antibacterial suture (coated polyglactin 910 suture with triclosan) with coated VICRYL suture (coated polyglactin 910 suture). *Surg Infect.* 2005;6:313–321.
7. Seim B, Tønnessen T, Woldbaek P. Triclosan-coated sutures do not reduce leg wound infections after coronary artery bypass grafting. *Interac Cardiovasc Thorac Surg.* 2012;15:411–415.
8. Chang W, Srinivasa S, Morton R, Hill A. Triclosan-impregnated sutures to decrease surgical site infections: systematic review and meta-analysis of randomized trials. *Ann Surg.* 2012;255:854–859.
9. Chen SY, Chen TM, Dai NT, Fu JP, Chang SC, Deng SC. Do antibacterial-coated sutures reduce wound infection in head and neck cancer reconstruction? *Eur J Surg Oncol.* 2011;37:300–304.
10. Sanz LE, Patterson JA, Kamath R, Willett G, Ahmed SW, Butterfield AB. Comparison of Maxon suture with Vicryl, chromic catgut, and PDS sutures in fascial closure in rats. *Obstet Gynecol.* 1988;71:418–422.
11. Parell GJ, Becker G. Comparison of absorbable with nonabsorbable sutures in closure of facial skin wounds. *Arch Facial Plast Surg.* 2003;5:488–490.
12. Bezwada RS, Jamiolkowski DD, Lee IY, et al. Monocryl suture, a new ultra-pliable absorbable monofilament suture. *Biomaterials.* 1995;16:1141–1148.
13. Niessen FB, Spauwen PH, Kon M. The role of suture material in hypertrophic scar formation: Monocryl vs. Vicryl-rapide. *Ann Plast Surg.* 1997;39:254–260.
14. Rosenzweig L, Abdelmalek M, Ho J, Hruza G. Equal cosmetic outcomes with 5-0 poliglecaprone-25 versus 6-0 polypropylene for superficial closures. *Dermatol Surg.* 2010;36:1126–1129.
15. Molea G, Schonauer F, Bifulco G, D'Angelo D. Comparative study on biocompatibility and absorption times of three absorbable monofilament suture materials (Polydioxanone, Poliglecaprone 25, Glycomer 631). *Br J Plast Surg.* 2000;53:137–141.
16. Cross K, Teo E, Wong S, et al. The absorbable dermal staple device: a faster, more cost-effective method for incisional closure. *Plast Reconstr Surg.* 2009;124:156–162.
17. Edlich R, Drake D, Rodeheaver G, et al. Syneture stainless STEEL suture. A collective review of its performance in surgical wound closure. *J Long Term Eff Med Implants.* 2006;16:101–110.
18. Sniezek PJ, Walling HW, DeBloom JR, 3rd, et al. A randomized controlled trial of high-viscosity 2-octyl cyanoacrylate tissue

adhesive versus sutures in repairing facial wounds following Mohs micrographic surgery. *Dermatol Surg.* 2007;33:966–971.
19. Craven NM, Telfer NR. An open study of tissue adhesive in full-thickness skin grafting. *J Am Acad Dermatol.* 1999;40:607–611.
20. Bernard L, Doyle J, Friedlander SF, Eichenfield LF, Gibbs NF, Cunningham BB. A prospective comparison of octyl cyanoacrylate tissue adhesive (dermabond) and suture for the closure of excisional wounds in children and adolescents. *Arch Dermatol.* 2001;137:1177–1180.
21. Plotner A, Mailler Savage E, Adams B, Gloster H. Layered closure versus buried sutures and adhesive strips for cheek defect repair after cutaneous malignancy excision. *J Am Acad Dermatol.* 2011;64:1115–1118.
22. Kolt JD. Use of adhesive surgical tape with the absorbable continuous subcuticular closure. *Anz J Surg.* 2003;73(8): 626–629.
23. Dresner H, Hilger P. Comparison of incision closures with subcuticular and percutaneous staples. *Arch Facial Plast Surg.* 2009;11:320–326.
24. Fiennes AG. Interrupted subcuticular polyglactin sutures for abdominal wounds. *Ann R Coll Surg Engl.* 1985;67:121–121.
25. Zitelli JA, Moy RL. Buried vertical mattress suture. *J Dermatol Surg Oncol.* 1989;15:17–19.
26. Singer A, Gulla J, Hein M, Marchini S, Chale S, Arora B. Single-layer versus double-layer closure of facial lacerations: a randomized controlled trial. *Plast Reconstr Surg.* 2005;116:363–368.
27. Alam M, Goldberg L. Utility of fully buried horizontal mattress sutures. *J Am Acad Dermatol.* 2004;50:73–76.
28. Giandoni MB, Grabski WJ. Surgical pearl: the dermal buried pulley suture. *J Am Acad Dermatol.* 1994;30:1012–1013.
29. Yag Howard C. Novel surgical approach to subcutaneous closure: the subcutaneous inverted cross mattress stitch (SICM Stitch). *Dermatol Surg.* 2011;37:1503–1505.
30. Genders R, Hamminga E, Kukutsch N. Securing the subcuticular running suture. *Dermatol Surg.* 2012;38:1722–1724.
31. Alam M, Posten W, Martini M, Wrone D, Rademaker A. Aesthetic and functional efficacy of subcuticular running epidermal closures of the trunk and extremity: a rater-blinded randomized control trial. *Arch Dermatol.* 2006;142:1272–1278.
32. Maher I, Bingham J, Mellette R. A running modification of the percutaneous buried vertical mattress. *Dermatol Surg.* 2012;38:1560–1562.
33. Snow SN, Dortzbach R, Moyer D. Managing common suturing problems. *J Dermatol Surg Oncol.* 1991;17:502–508.
34. Kouba D, Miller S. "Running pleated" suture technique opposes wound edges of unequal lengths. *Dermatol Surg.* 2006;32: 411–414.
35. Krunic A, Weitzul S, Taylor RS. Running combined simple and vertical mattress suture: a rapid skin-everting stitch. *Dermatol Surg.* 2005;31:1325–1329.
36. Moody B, McCarthy J, Linder J, Hruza G. Enhanced cosmetic outcome with running horizontal mattress sutures. *Dermatol Surg.* 2005;31:1313–1316.
37. Zuber T. The mattress sutures: vertical, horizontal, and corner stitch. *Am Fam Physician.* 2002;66:2231–2236.

CHAPTER 17

The Elliptical Excision and its Variations

Joseph F. Sobanko & Christopher J. Miller

INTRODUCTION

The elliptical excision is the workhorse procedure to remove cutaneous lesions. Although the term "elliptical" frequently describes the design of excisions in the dermatologic and plastic surgery literature, it inaccurately describes the surgical design in practice. As opposed to an ellipse, which has a curved shape along its entire boundary, a fusiform excision has two sides that taper to a sharp point at each end. Recognizing that most surgeons employ a "fusiform" design, this chapter will use the terms "elliptical" and "fusiform" excisions interchangeably. This chapter will focus on the design and execution of the elliptical excision and its variations. Each of the five individual steps required to successfully complete a surgical excision will be discussed in detail. The skills necessary to design and execute an elliptical excision provide the foundation to progress to more technically advanced surgical procedures, such as cutaneous flaps.

PREOPERATIVE EVALUATION AND INFORMED CONSENT

The surgeon and his or her staff should perform a thorough preoperative evaluation to ensure the patient's safety and to optimize outcomes of any cutaneous surgical procedure. Especially important items that could alter the surgeon's practice or affect outcomes include the patient's history of transmissible disease, whether the patient takes oral anticoagulants, the presence of implantable electrical devices, and concerns regarding antibiotic prophylaxis.[1] The reader is referred to other chapters in this book for comprehensive coverage of these topics.

After a thorough preoperative evaluation, the surgeon must obtain informed consent. A careful informed consent sets realistic expectations for the patient and reduces the risk of litigation from consequences that the patient had not expected. The main risks associated with an elliptical excision include scarring, bleeding, infection, and incomplete resection of the lesion. Cosmetic disfigurement and compromised function of critical anatomic structures should occur rarely with a carefully designed and executed elliptical excision. As the risks associated with an elliptical excision are relatively low, informed consent frequently focuses on ensuring that the patient has realistic expectations for the postoperative appearance and recovery. Expected immediate postoperative sequelae after the excision include mild discomfort, swelling, and bruising, which vary in severity according to the size, depth, and location of the procedure. Discomfort is most severe in the first 24 to 48 hours after surgery, swelling usually subsides by 1 week, and bruising usually subsides after 1 to 2 weeks.

Patients should have realistic expectations about the appearance of the scar. Erythema limited to the suture line often persists for 1 to 2 weeks, and eversion of the scar edges can take approximately 3 to 4 months to flatten. Changes in sensation, such as numbness, tingling, and fleeting sharp pains are common for up to several months postoperatively.[2] Patients should understand that the appearance and sensation of the scar evolve considerably over the first 3 to 6 months postoperatively. Finally, as wrong-site surgery is the most common reason for malpractice claims against dermatologic surgeons,[3] informed consent must include confirmation of the site of the excision with the patient.

INTRAOPERATIVE EVALUATION AND EXECUTION

EVALUATION OF THE LESION

Before anesthetizing the area, the surgeon must first carefully examine the lesion to be excised as well as the surrounding skin. Proper lighting is essential as the surgeon stretches the skin and palpates the lesion to detect subtle changes between normal and pathologic skin. Accurate demarcation of the clinical margins of the lesion determines the accuracy of the surgical margins of the excision. Underestimation of the clinical size of the lesion increases the risk for incomplete excision and positive pathologic margins. Overestimation of the clinical size of the lesion will result in an unnecessarily large excision that could compromise cosmetic or functional outcomes. Through visual inspection and palpation, the surgeon estimates the anatomic depth of invasion of the lesion and uses a surgical marking pen to delineate its peripheral margins. The surgeon should also meticulously inspect the surrounding skin and outline any suspicious lesions that may collide with the surgical margins or design of the excision.

After determining the clinical margins of the lesion, the surgeon must determine the surgical margin, which includes a rim of normal tissue around the periphery and deep aspects of the lesion. The size of the surgical margins will vary, depending on the clinical and/or pathologic diagnosis of the lesion as well as the intent of the excision. Narrow surgical margins are more common when the lesion is benign or when the primary intent of the excision is to obtain tissue for pathologic diagnosis. Wider surgical margins are more common when the lesion is malignant or when the primary intent of the excision is definitive removal. The surgical margins may require adjustment if there are suspicious lesions adjacent to the primary lesion.

Sound knowledge of anatomy is essential to be able to perform surgical excisions safely and efficiently. The surgeon should anticipate encountering any vital underlying anatomic structures, such as motor nerves or large caliber vessels. Preoperative marking of the expected path of these underlying structures on the skin surface optimizes intraoperative safety. Once the surgical site is adequately marked, the surgeon should again confirm with the patient that the site is correct and explain the size of the clinical and surgical margins.

STANDARD ELLIPTICAL EXCISION DESIGN

The design of the elliptical excision is the first step in optimizing the aesthetic surgical result. Optimal design respects free margins, maintains the normal contour of the skin, places the scar within cosmetic subunit junction lines, and orients incisions parallel to relaxed skin tension lines.

PRESERVING FREE MARGINS: ORIENTING THE LONG AXIS OF THE ELLIPSE PERPENDICULAR TO FREE MARGINS

To preserve the position of free margins, such as the eyelid, distal nose, lips, and helical rim, the surgeon should orient the fusiform excision with its long axis perpendicular to the free margin. This orientation will place the tension vectors of the elliptical excision parallel to the free margin, thereby avoiding distortion. The tension vectors run perpendicular to the long axis of the fusiform excision, are greatest at the central, widest portion of the fusiform design, and diminish toward each of the apices of the wound. Closing the wound requires recruitment of tissue from each side. If the fusiform excision is designed parallel to the free margin, then the tension vectors will pull the margin either up or down (Fig. 17-1). Near the lower eyelid, for example, a fusiform excision oriented parallel to the lid margin risks ectropion. By contrast, orienting the excision perpendicular to the eyelid margin preserves the position of the free margin.

PRESERVING CONTOUR: DESIGNING THE ELLIPSE WITH A SUFFICIENT LENGTH:WIDTH RATIO

Standard design of an elliptical excision has two symmetric arcs that mirror one another along a long axis and intersect to form an apex at each end.[4] The goal of this arciform design is to create a fine, straight-line scar and avoid redundant tissue cone formation after excision and suturing. Common dogma states that an ellipse with a long axis

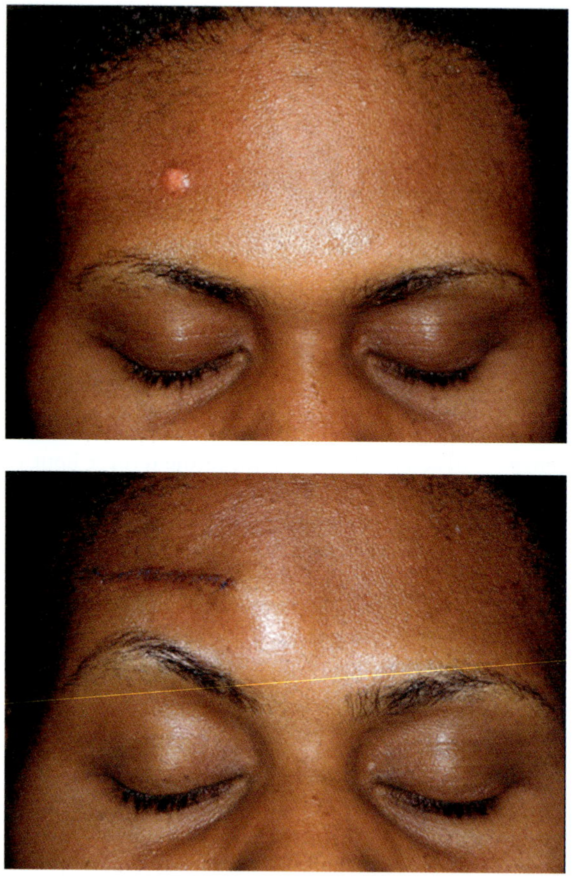

Figure 17-1 An elliptical excision that demonstrates improper orientation and has resulted in a change in a position of the free margin.

that is three times greater than its short axis will create apical angles of 30 degrees.[5] However, excisional geometry and mathematical calculations show that a design with circular arcs and a 3:1 length to width ratio actually creates apical angles closer to 70 degrees.[6] In practice, a fusiform design with 70 degree angles will result in significant tension of the wound edges and create redundant, upwardly protruding tissue at the apices of the excision.[7] Redundant tissue cones, sometimes referred to as "dog-ears," standing cones, or Burow's triangles, can compromise even the best executed closure by leaving an unaesthetic contour at the ends of a fine-line scar.

The length to width ratio and angles at the apices of the fusiform excision are the key design elements that influence contour. The most common source of contour irregularity after a fusiform excision is a standing cone, or tissue protrusion, that results from an insufficient length:width ratio (i.e., the fusiform design is too short) and excessively obtuse angles at the apices of fusiform design. Fine line contour of cutaneous surgical excisions can be maintained by lengthening the ellipse design, which subsequently creates a longer scar. In order for the arciform-designed ellipse to generate a fine line contour with apical angles of 30 degrees, a length to width ratio closer to 7:1 may be necessary.[6] A scar length that is seven times greater than the width of the excision is impractical however, given that many patients are concerned with their appearance and desire the shortest, least noticeable scar.

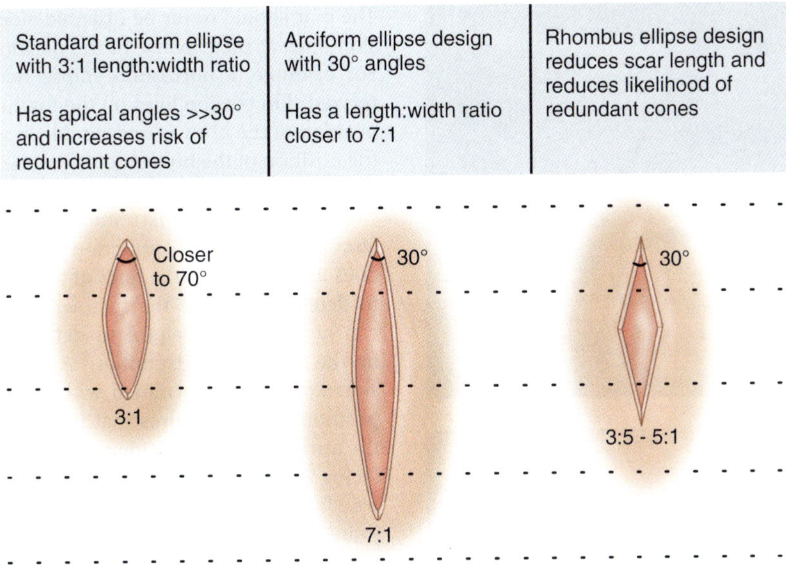

Figure 17-2 The rhombus design of the ellipse more easily creates shorter apical angles and reduces the scar length in addition to the likelihood of redundant cones.

A simple design variation to the traditional curved lines of the elliptical excision can reduce redundant cones while simultaneously minimizing the scar length. Rather than creating curved arcs around the lesion to be excised, straight-line tissue incisions that are angled in the shape of a rhombus can be made, allowing for 30 degree apical angles and generating a much shorter length to width ratio of 3 to 3.5:1.[6] Straight lines taper to the apices more rapidly than curved lines, decrease the angle at the apices, and minimize the risk of standing cones, as shown in Figure 17-2.

Tissue distensibility plays a practical role in fusiform excision design. The elasticity of skin within a given anatomic location can impact the likelihood of redundant cone formation. For example, the bound-down skin of the pretibial lower extremity or nasal tip frequently displays raised tissue cones if 30 degree apical angles are selected. The circumferential contractile forces from the surrounding skin also make these areas challenging to bring together even if a rhombus-shaped length to width ratio of 3 to 3.5:1 is chosen. By elongating the rhombus-shaped design with a length to width ratio of approximately 4:1 or 5:1 and creating apical angles closer to 15 to 20 degrees, the wound may be closed under minimal tension and with a lower risk of contour deformity.[8] Conversely, anatomic locations with elastic skin such as the dorsal hand or scrotum can be aesthetically repaired with a design that is less than 3:1 and with angles slightly greater than 30 degrees. Small residual tissue protrusions in these locations often spontaneously regress.

Most elliptical excisions are designed to have equivalent areas of skin to be removed on each side of the skin lesion, but this presumes that the laxity of skin is equivalent on both sides of the defect. This may not be the case in anatomic areas where the skin transitions between thick and thin skin or from tightly adherent to loosely bound skin. Anatomic examples of these transitions in skin quality include the temple and nasofacial sulcus. When encountering a defect to be excised in such a location, it may be advantageous to design an ellipse with triangles of unequal areas – the overall surface area of the two sides is equivalent to a traditionally designed ellipse but the larger of the two triangles is placed on the more tightly adherent skin and the looser skin has a smaller triangle of skin excised.[4] The end result remains a fine linear scar.

CAMOUFLAGING SCARS BY ORIENTING THE ELLIPSE ALONG COSMETIC SUBUNIT JUNCTION LINES

Linear scars that conform to cosmetic subunit junction lines help to camouflage scars. Orientation of the ellipse along cosmetic subunit junction lines is especially advantageous on the face, where shadows in concavities and reflections at convexities demarcate areas on the face. Common examples on the face include the shadow at the concave melolabial fold, which divides the cheek from the lip, and the convex ridge where the forehead transitions to the temple (Fig. 17-3). Orienting the elliptical excision within these cosmetic subunit junction lines makes the scar less noticeable, as the viewer expects to see a shadow or reflection in these areas.

REDUCING TENSION AND CAMOUFLAGING SCARS BY ORIENTING THE ELLIPSE PARALLEL TO RELAXED SKIN TENSION LINES

Sutured wounds that heal under minimal tension often create the least conspicuous scar lines. Minimization of scar tension may be facilitated by orienting the long axis of the ellipse parallel to the direction of a relaxed skin tension line. On the face, these lines of tension are partly the result of muscular forces under the skin being transmitted through fascial attachments. The curvilinear facial relaxed skin tension lines are perpendicular in orientation to the

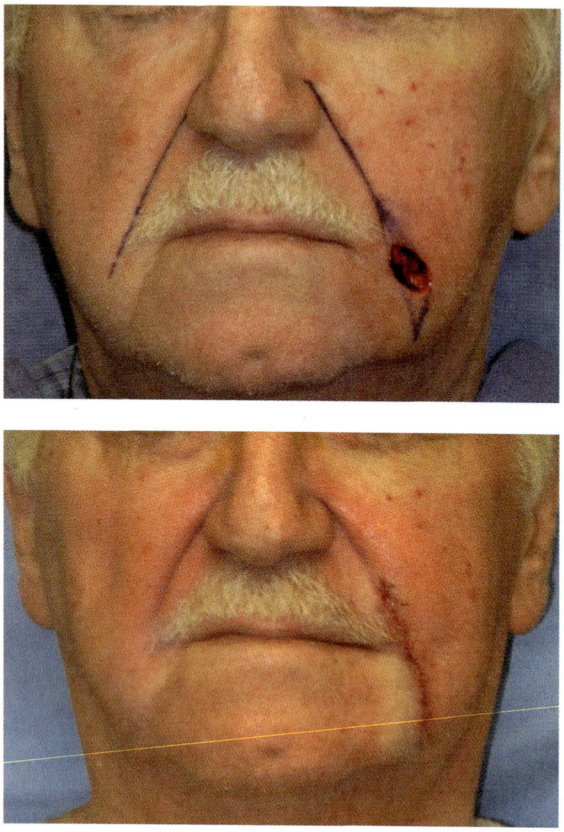

Figure 17-3 Elliptical repair along a cosmetic junction line allows for camouflaging of scars.

direction of contraction from the underlying muscles and can be accentuated by having the patient perform dynamic movements with their mouth, eyes, and forehead. A classic example on the face is to orient the long axis of the ellipse parallel to the crow's feet in the lateral canthus (Fig. 17-4).

The scar should never be oriented along relaxed skin tension lines at the expense of the position of a free margin. For example, a horizontal ellipse that conforms to the relaxed skin tension lines on the forehead but elevates the position of the brow is undesirable. It is better to preserve the position of the brow and orient the scar perpendicular to the relaxed skin tension lines.

On the trunk and extremities, the lines of tension are less apparent, since contraction of the underlying muscles does not accentuate the lines of tension. Pinching the skin to determine where the furrows and ridges are formed can be especially helpful to determine lines of tension on the trunk and extremities.[9] As a rule, the lines of tension should be determined with the patient in a neutral position, which requires that the patient be upright with the arms by his or her side and palms of the hands gently facing forward. Changes in patient position can mask the true lines of tension. A classic example in which position influences surgical design is seen in the alignment of the relaxed skin tension lines on the back. If the patient lies supine with his/her arms under his/her chin, the lines of tension on his/her back will appear to run perpendicular to the vertebral column. When he/she sits upright in the neutral position, it is obvious that the lines of tension run at an inferolateral tangent from the vertebral column. On the back, one can accentuate the lines of tension by having the patient sit at attention while bringing the scapulae together (Figs. 17-5 and 17-6).

VARIATIONS OF THE ELLIPSE

There are instances in which designing a fusiform excision that creates a straight-line scar is not ideal. Special consideration must be given to the shape of the fusiform design when the lesion to be excised is overlying a convex surface, is contained within a nonlinear relaxed skin

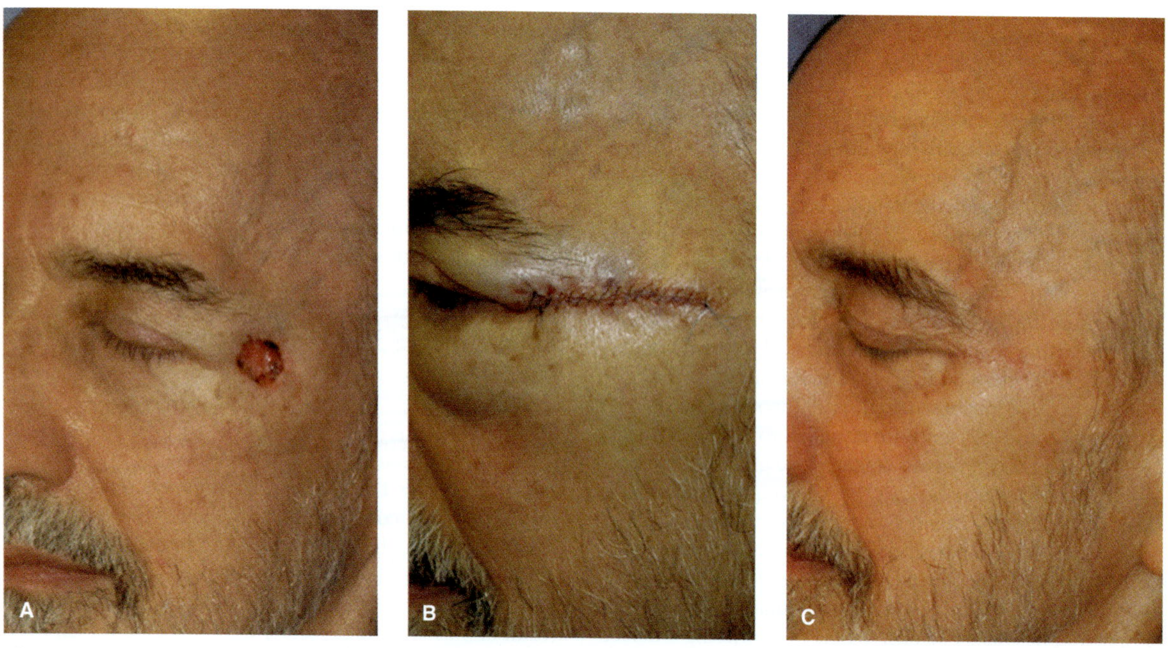

Figure 17-4 Elliptical repair within relaxed skin tension lines allows for camouflaging of scars, A. Mohs defect, B. immediate postoperative appearance, C. 6 weeks postoperatively.

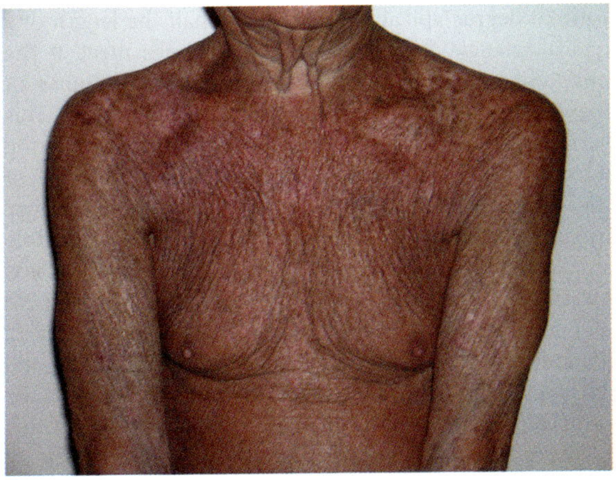

Figure 17-5 Curvilinear relaxed skin tension lines on the torso change with movement.

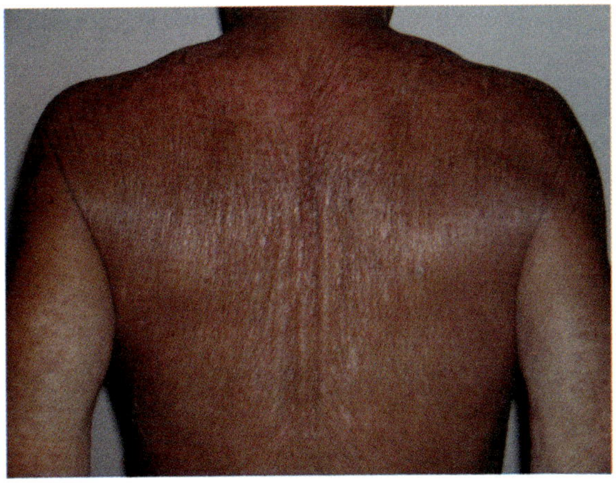

Figure 17-6 Accentuation of lines of tension on back by bringing scapulae together.

tension line, or is approaching an important anatomic structure. In these scenarios, alteration of the shape or length of the ellipse often results in enhanced cosmesis. Please see Figure 17-7 for a review of these design variations.

CRESCENT

Certain anatomic locations display relaxed skin tension lines that are curvilinear rather than simply straight lines. This is most evident on the skin of the cheek, particularly when the folds become accentuated while the patient smiles. To create a scar with a curvilinear shape that mimics the relaxed skin tension lines on the cheek, one can consider a design modification called the crescentic ellipse. Whereas the standard fusiform design has sides of equal length that join to form a linear scar, the crescentic design employs two lines of different length to create a curvilinear, arciform scar. On the cheek, the lateral or posterior limb of the crescentic design has a longer, arciform design that falls within the curvilinear relaxed skin tension lines, and the medial or anterior limb has a shorter,

Variations of ellipse

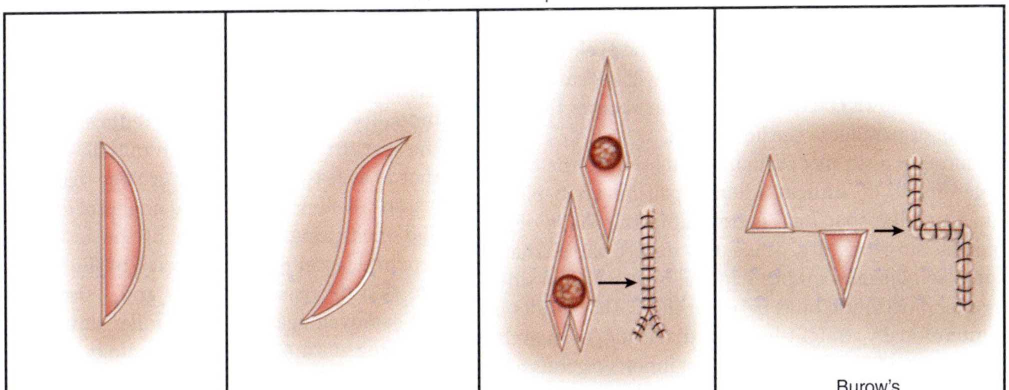

	Crescent	S-plasty	M-plasty	Burow's advancement
Design:	Straight, reverse	Lazy S	Bifurcation of fusiform design	Fusiform design with displaced triangle
Indications:	Useful in anatomic areas with curved relaxed skin tension lines (e.g. cheek)	Convex surface, (e.g. premaxillary cheek, extremities)	Shortens scar length and is useful when approaching free margins such as the eyelid	Zigzag shape allows for camouflaging of scars
Warning:	Unequal length of 2 sides requires attention to detail when suturing. Minimize redundant cones by suturing with the rule of halves.	Suture bites should be horizontal between sides. Diagonal bites between sides will create an unintentionally long, straight-line scar.	Use of 'tip stitch' allows for proper contour but risks ischemia if placed to close to distal end of skin	Orientation must ensure that tension vectors do not pull on adjacent free margins

Figure 17-7 Design variations of the ellipse that allow for enhanced cosmesis in certain situations.

straight line that runs parallel to the relaxed skin tension lines. Because these two lines are of unequal length, the resultant scar becomes curved after the two sides are sutured together. As the difference in length between the two limbs increases, the final curvature of the sutured scar increases. However, an increased discrepancy in length between the limbs will create a standing cone on the longer, curved limb, which can be minimized by distributing the excess length by suturing with the rule of halves or by excising a Burow's triangle (see section on standing cone deformities).

S-PLASTY

All scars contract up to 30% over time.[10] Although this contraction may not diminish the cosmetic nature of a scar on a planar surface, linear scars on convex and concave surfaces have the potential to become depressed or elevated, respectively. Scar inversion on convex surfaces may be avoided by lengthening the excision so that the total scar length becomes greater than the linear distance between the two ends.[11,12] Practically, this is executed by altering the straight fusiform design into a "lazy-S" shape. As the scar contracts, the "lazy-S" shape usually straightens, but the extra length gained from the modified design reduces the risk of scar inversion. Convex surfaces where this particular elliptical design variation is ideal include the premaxillary cheek, chin, and the dorsal forearms and hands. If a defect on the preseptal lower eyelid or infraorbital cheek has its long axis in a horizontal direction (i.e., parallel to the to the lid margin), the "lazy-S" design helps to redirect tension vectors to preserve the position of the free margin of the lower eyelid. By drawing superior and inferior standing cones perpendicular to the eyelid margin at each end of the defect, the surgeon will create a lazy-S shape that allows closure with tension vectors that are horizontal, or parallel to the lid margin.

The surgeon must pay particular attention to the order and placement of sutures when repairing an S-plasty design. Once the specimen is excised in the shape of an "S," novice surgeons are prone to convert the S-shape back into an ellipse by taking diagonal bites between sides rather than horizontal bites between sides. This results in an unintentionally straight-line scar that is longer than the initially designed curvilinear scar. Beginner surgeons also have a tendency to "chase" redundant tissue cones with their scalpel, creating an unnecessarily long scar. Both of these undesirable outcomes can be avoided with precise placement of the first buried suture. When aligned properly, this initial suture will create crescent-shaped defects on either side of the suture, with each crescent inverted in orientation relative to one another Thereafter, carefully placed buried sutures will convert the remaining areas into the desired S-shape.

M-PLASTY

The total length of an elliptical excision can be shortened when the scar approaches vital adjacent structures with the use of an M-plasty (Fig. 17-7).[13] One or both ends of a fusiform design are converted from a single triangle with an apical angle of 30 degrees to two adjacent triangles with 30 degree apical angles that are half the length of a typical triangle and whose adjoining limbs meet at the midpoint of the edge of the defect. The appearance of these neighboring triangles mimics the letter "M." This variation of the ellipse shortens the scar line by converting it from a straight line to a V-shape at the end. The length of the M-plasty and redundant cone can be shortened further by simply repeating the division of the "M" with multiple smaller triangles. This "nested" M-plasty allows for less excision of normal tissue and is useful for excisions on flat and concave skin surfaces.[14] Some consider the M-plasty a modified V-Y-plasty and design the shoulders of the adjacent triangles more widely in order to avoid tissue protrusions.[15] Regardless of the conceptualization of this fusiform variation, a half-buried horizontal mattress (e.g., "tip stitch") allows the sutured end to sit flat and avoid puckering. The M-plasty is a helpful modification to the fusiform closure and best used on the face when approaching vital structures such as the eyelid and lower lip or when a defect has one end that is wider than the other.

SERIAL ELLIPTICAL EXCISIONS

Complete excision of a lesion is sometimes not possible or practical because the tension on the closure would be too great to accomplish in a single stage. Congenital nevi, for example, are sometimes large enough that complete removal of the growth would result in dysfunction or disfigurement of the anatomic site. For instances in which it is impractical to excise a lesion in toto, the surgeon may take advantage of the skin's inherent tissue creep by excising the lesion via serial procedures. This method of excision allows for a lesion to be removed in stages – the number of stages being proportional to the size of the lesion relative to the specific anatomic location. This modality often significantly reduces the final length of the scar. To start, rather than initially designing an ellipse that is at least three times greater than the width of the lesion, an ellipse with apical angles of less than 30 degrees and measuring the length of the lesion is excised and repaired. After 8 to 12 weeks of healing, so the tension on the skin decreases, the scar and a similar strip of lesion are removed again with a similar design. This process is repeated until no further pathology remains on the skin (Fig. 17-8). The ultimate result is a shorter, more aesthetically elegant scar.

BUROW'S ADVANCEMENT FLAP: A VARIATION ON THE ELLIPSE

The Burow's wedge closure is often considered a cutaneous advancement flap but can also be simply conceptualized as an extension of the fusiform excision.[16] This particular elliptical variation displaces one-half of the linear scar into a more desirable location simply by modifying the typical fusiform design. Rather than to have two adjoining triangles meet in the center to form an ellipse, this design shifts one of the two triangles laterally. This tangential movement that displaces the scar produces a zigzag shape but the overall outline camouflages well when used properly in opportune locations such as the lips and eyebrow.[17]

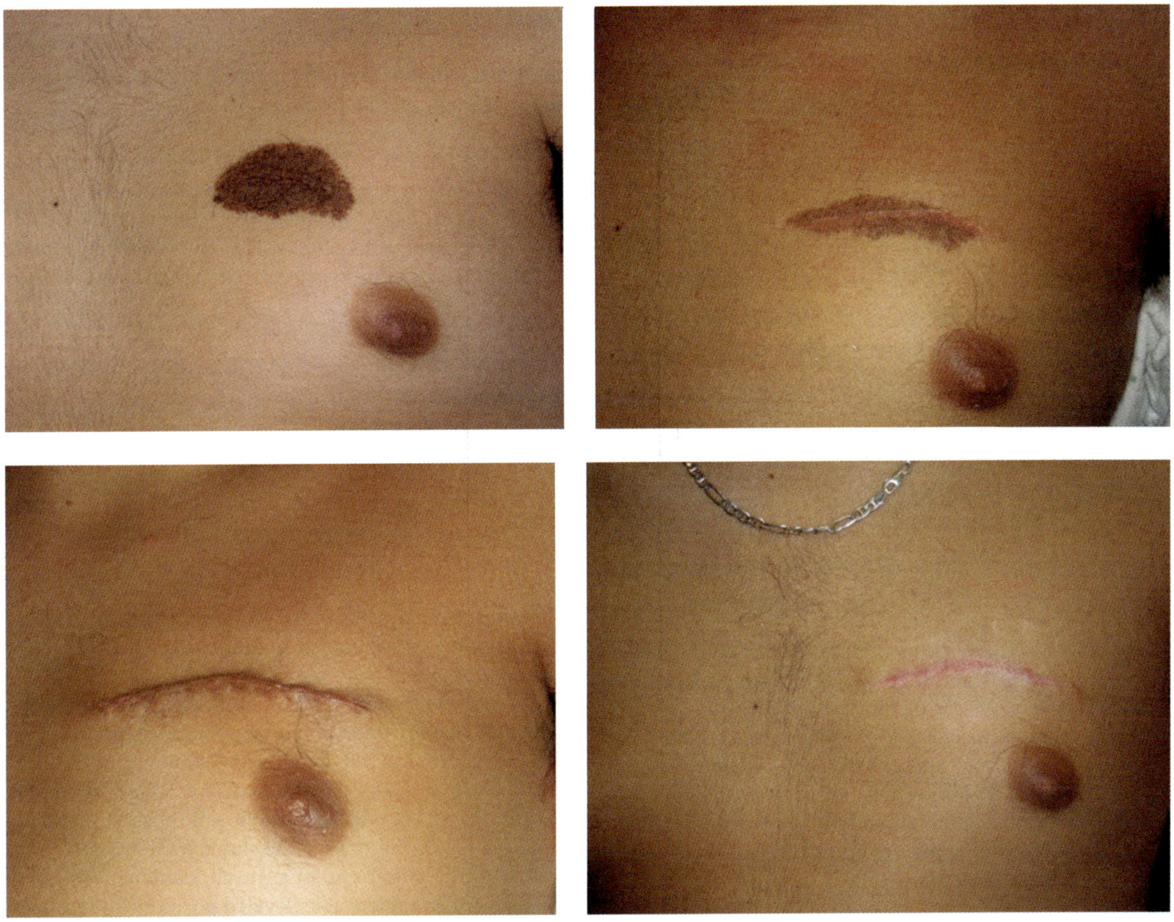

Figure 17-8 An example of serial elliptical excisions that allows for removal of a lesion with reduced scar length. An 8 week interval occurred between excisions.

ANESTHESIA

After designing the ellipse on the skin, the patient is ready for local anesthesia. Local anesthesia can distort the clinical margins of a lesion and alter tension on the skin, so it is preferable to complete the surgical design prior to anesthesia. Most elliptical excisions can be performed safely under local anesthesia in an office-based, outpatient setting. Local anesthesia often obscures the clinical margins of cutaneous lesions and should not be injected until the clinical and surgical margins have been carefully marked. One percent of lidocaine with 1:100,000 epinephrine is typically used for local anesthesia because of its favorable safety and pharmacodynamic profile. For excisions covering large surface areas, similar pain control with an even lower risk of lidocaine toxicity may obtained by using decreased concentrations of lidocaine, such as 0.5% lidocaine with 1:200,000 epinephrine, which is also commercially available.[18]

Injecting local anesthesia is the first invasive step of the procedure. Careful technique helps to minimize pain, decrease patient anxiety, and establish rapport. Anxious patients may be placed at ease by reassuring them that the procedure will not begin until complete local anesthesia has been obtained. The health professional injecting the anesthesia should make all efforts to divert the patient's attention away from the site of injection and keep the needle and the syringe away from patient's view. Holding the skin taut or pinching the skin helps to distract from the slight pain with brisk insertion of a 30 gauge needle into the subcutaneous layer. Slow delivery of anesthesia into the subcutaneous layer allows infiltration under minimal resistance. Although initial injection into the superficial dermis may provide quicker anesthesia, patients usually experience pain because the dense dermis resists the injection more than the looser fat. For larger procedures requiring excision into the subcutaneous fat, patients may feel fewer needle sticks by first infiltrating the superficial subcutaneous fat under minimal resistance, then injecting the dermis. Freshly mixed lidocaine has a higher pH (pH ~6.5) than premixed lidocaine, which improves patient comfort upon injection. Buffering the anesthetic with 1:10 ratio of 8.4% sodium bicarbonate to lidocaine raises the product pH and ultimately decreases pain with infiltration.[19] The onset of lidocaine action upon injection is almost immediate, and the duration of action is 1 to 2 hours. However, it is prudent to wait a few minutes after local infiltration has been performed to optimize the full vasoconstrictive effects of the epinephrine.[20] Clinically, vasoconstriction is evident when a ring of pallor is observed around the surgical area infiltrated with lidocaine mixed with epinephrine.

PREOPERATIVE ANTISEPSIS

After marking the clinical and surgical margins and ensuring complete anesthesia, the surgical site and the surrounding skin are scrubbed widely with an antiseptic, and sterile drapes are placed to protect the scrubbed field from contamination. The reader is referred to additional chapters on antisepsis for complete coverage of this topic. Sterile technique not only minimizes the risk for infection, but it also influences the execution of the procedure. Bulky drapes that decrease the size of the surgical field or shift while working impair operative efficiency and increase the risk of contaminating the field.

EQUIPMENT NEEDED FOR PROCEDURE

A carefully prepared surgical tray includes all the instruments and supplies necessary to complete the elliptical excision without interruption. The reader is referred to the chapter on surgical instrumentation for a comprehensive discussion. This section will briefly mention some general principles. Management of the surgical tray affects both safety and operative efficiency. A cluttered surgical tray increases the risk for exposure to sharp instruments and makes it harder to locate the desired instruments. The scalpel blade and scissors should be as sharp as possible. Dull instruments force the surgeon to use excessive pressure and increase procedure time. To avoid tissue trauma, the surgeon should use a forceps with teeth (e.g., Adson forceps). The teeth of the forceps allow manipulation of the tissue without trauma. Please see Table 17-1 for a list of the instruments and materials essential to perform an excision.

TECHNIQUE

Sound surgical design is the first step in achieving an excellent surgical outcome. After anesthetizing, cleaning and draping the field, and organizing the surgical tray, the surgeon is ready to begin the procedure. Precise surgical technique is necessary to ensure a fine, linear scar. Execution of the elliptical excision involves five successive steps: *incision, excision, undermining, hemostasis, and suturing.* Meticulous execution of each step maximizes the functional and aesthetic outcomes and results in reproducibly excellent scars. Errors in early steps will make precise execution of subsequent steps more difficult. The remainder of this chapter details the necessary steps to properly perform each of these five tasks so that successive portions may be executed with ease.

TABLE 17-1
Instruments and Materials for Surgical Excisions

Scalpel and scalpel blade
Forceps – Adson type with teeth
Needle driver
Scissors – Iris and Metzenbaum
Skin hook – single or double prong
Suture material
Sharps receptacle
Electrosurgical instrument
Gauze
Cotton-tipped applicators
Specimen container

INCISION

The goal of the initial incision is to release the skin to the desired anatomic depth and to create smooth and perpendicular wound edges without a tissue bevel. Before initiating the procedure, the surgeon should have a clear plan for the anatomic depth of the incision (Table 17-2). The desired anatomic depth will vary based on the location and intention of the procedure. In most cases, the depth of the incision will correspond to the intended anatomic plane for the subsequent steps of excision and undermining.

The incision should create wound edges that are sharply perpendicular to the skin surface, because any bevel of the dermis or fat will impede the direct apposition of the epidermal edges during suturing. Sound technique is necessary to prevent a beveled skin edge. The scalpel handle tends to fall toward the surgeon's dominant hand, similar to the eraser end of a pencil, thereby positioning the blade in an undesirable beveled position. The surgeon must compensate for this natural tendency by taking care to hold the scalpel perpendicularly to the skin surface throughout the entire pass of the incision.

Cleanly incised wound edges facilitate precise apposition of the epidermis and dermis during suturing. A sharp scalpel should incise the skin smoothly with minimal downward pressure. If the surgeon forces the scalpel with downward pressure in an attempt to reach the desired depth in one pass, or if the scalpel edge is dull, the scalpel may succumb to chatter, resulting in jagged wound edges. To avoid chatter, especially in thick or fibrotic skin, more than one pass of the scalpel may be necessary to reach the desired depth. Stabilizing the skin with the nondominant hand or the hands of a surgical assistant places tension on the skin surface and facilitates entry into the correct surgical plane. In addition, particularly in loose skin with thin dermis, creating taut skin with manual pressure assists in preventing "chatter" of the blade, which creates jagged cuts. As noted earlier, designing the fusiform excision as a rhombus rather than a true ellipse also assists in creating smooth, nonjagged strokes since a straight line is easier to incise than a curved line.

One important, yet frequently overlooked portion of incising the skin is the continuation of the incision up to and including the apical angles at the proper depth. Similar to the tendency for the blade to fall ipsilaterally, there is a tendency to incise the outer, lateral parts of the ellipse correctly but create a shallower, angled incision toward the apices. This error fails to fully release the dermis, resulting in an uneven removal of the specimen and beveled edges at the apices that can prevent proper tissue

TABLE 17-2
Ideal Surgical Planes for Excising and Undermining

Location	Preferred Anatomic Plane	Comments/Critical Structures to Consider
Trunk and extremities	Junction of subcutaneous fat and fascia. In larger individuals, it may be difficult to go all the way down to "deep" fascia.	On the trunk, proximal extremities and neck, aim for the junction between the tightly organized, compact, columnar cells adherent to the underside of the dermis and the underlying, looser, larger fat cells that invest the fascia.
Hands and feet	Junction of subcutaneous fat and dorsal superficial fascia	Take care to preserve the vessels which lie in the lamina directly beneath the dorsal superficial fascia.
Lateral face	Junction of the subcutaneous fat and SMAS	The motor nerves from the facial nerve always lie deep to the most superficial layer of SMAS[a]. Excision at the junction of the subcutaneous fat and SMAS will protect the motor nerves.
Central 1/3 of face and scalp	a. Small excisions: junction of subcutaneous fat and SMAS b. Large excisions: deep to the muscles of facial expression or SMAS	Because the branches of the facial nerve have arborized, excision deep the SMAS is less likely to cause motor deficits (e.g., excision of midline and paramedian frontalis does not leave motor deficit on the forehead).

[a]In areas where the muscles of facial expression are layered, e.g., lip depressors and elevators, the motor nerves innervate the deepest muscles from their superficial surface.

apposition when suturing. In addition, there is a tendency to take numerous passes with the scalpel toward the apices to release the tissue in this location. Single, smooth incisions are preferred at each apical angle so as to avoid jagged marks on the surface.

The scalpel blade chosen for the procedure is dictated by the anatomic location. Excisional sites with thin to moderately thick dermis, such as the cheeks, forehead, nose, lips, and distal extremities, are best incised with a #15 scalpel blade. Incision of skin with thick dermis, namely the trunk and proximal extremities, is best performed with the larger #10 blade. Finally, in thin skin with high aesthetic importance such as the eyelid, a beaver blade or #15c blade allows for smooth, sharp incisions with minimal tissue drag. With sound technique, the surgeon will accomplish a uniform release to the desired anatomic depth along the entire incision line and create clean wound edges without a bevel.

It should be noted that the epidermis and dermis have greater surface tension compared to the fat. After incising through the dermis, the epidermis and dermis immediately retract away from the incision, and the subcutaneous fat tends to lag toward the center of the wound. The lagging subcutaneous fat can impede apposition of the dermis during suturing. Most surgeons have seen fat lobules extruding through the wound after placement of a deep suture (Fig. 17-9). The lagging fat also tends to obscure visualization of the reticular dermis, which is the primary target of buried dermal sutures. Trimming the lagging fat flush with the dermis optimizes precise approximation of the dermis and allows clear visibility of the reticular dermis during placement of the buried dermal sutures. The surgeon can stabilize the lagging fat with the forceps and trim with the scissors. Excessive traction on the lagging fat should be avoided, because it frequently causes a reverse bevel (i.e., a bevel away from the wound edge), which makes it more difficult to place the deep sutures without a prominent dimple. Stabilizing the fat without tension allows the surgeon to trim flush with the dermis and create a sharply perpendicular wound edge along the full thickness of the skin flap. In many cases, trimming the lagging fat is best accomplished after undermining.

EXCISION

The excision has two purposes, either to ensure complete removal of a lesion or to restore contour by removing the standing cone or excess tissue during the reconstruction (this latter purpose is addressed at the end of this chapter). Based on the clinical examination and pathology of the preoperative biopsy, the surgeon must determine the anatomic depth of the excision. The depth of excision should maximize the likelihood of complete removal with minimal collateral damage to important anatomic structures. Deeply infiltrating tumors may require excision at a depth that causes predictable morbidity. For example, a

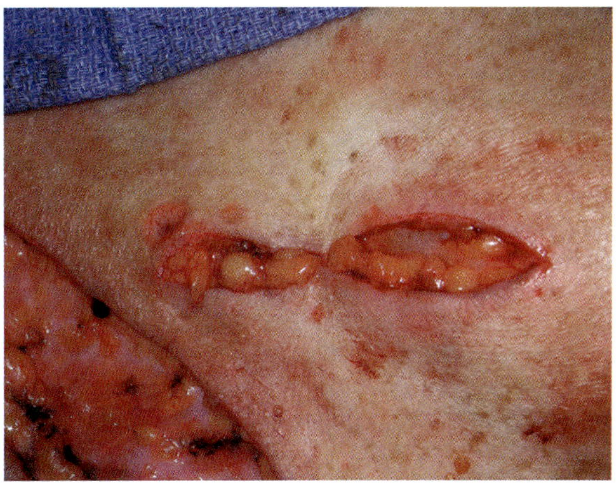

Figure 17-9 An untrimmed fat bevel impedes proper wound-edge apposition when suturing.

tumor that invades the deep fat on the temple may require excision through the superficial musculoaponeurotic system (SMAS) and may sacrifice the temporal branch of the facial nerve. By contrast, the surgeon can almost always dictate the anatomic plane when excising standing cones or excess tissue during the reconstruction.

The goal of the excision is to remove the skin in a uniform anatomic plane with minimal morbidity to the underlying structures. Ideally, the preceding incision has released the skin to the desired anatomic depth, and the excision continues a clean lift of tissue in the same surgical plane. In areas with thick subcutaneous fat, a disparity between the depths of the incision and excision may create unnecessary challenges during the closure. For example, if the incision extends to the fascia, but the tissue is excised at the level of the superficial subcutaneous fat, then the island of subcutaneous fat at the base of the wound can impede advancement of the wound edges during the closure and complicate hemostasis by obscuring blood vessels.

On the scalp, central face and temples, hands and feet, and male genitalia, the subcutaneous fat is either thin or indistinct (e.g., on the mid chin, the mentalis inserts directly into the dermis and there is not a distinct layer of fat), so the surgeon encounters the underlying muscle or fascial layer immediately after release of the dermis. On the cheeks, neck, trunk, proximal extremities, and female genitalia, there is frequently a thicker layer of subcutaneous fat. In these locations, a layer of columnar, compact, and tightly organized fat cells adheres to the underside of the dermis. A surgical plane separates these tightly organized columnar cells from a deeper layer of larger, more loosely organized fat that invests the fascia. Vigorous scrubbing with gauze can often dislodge these deeper, loosely organized, larger fat cells from the fascia. During the incision, the scalpel will find a releasing point at the junction of these two layers of fat. Using the scissors to feel the release, the surgeon can effortlessly excise the specimen at the junction of these two fat layers.

Assuming deeper excision is not necessary for oncologic reasons, the optimal planes for excision vary by location. In general, excising at the junctions of tissue planes improves operative efficiency by minimizing bleeding and by allowing effortless dissection. On the trunk and extremities, the surgeon will usually excise tissue in the plane where the subcutaneous fat meets the deep muscular fascia. In order to preserve the underlying branches of the facial nerve on the lateral face and neck, the surgeon excises at the junction of the subcutaneous fat and fascia of the SMAS. On the scalp, where there is no risk for motor deficits, and on the central face, where there is minimal risk for motor deficits from working in a deep surgical plane, the anatomic plane of excision may vary, depending on the extent of the procedure. On the midline forehead, for example, the surgeon may choose to stay above the frontalis muscle for a small excision but may excise deep to the frontalis to remove bulk and facilitate tissue advancement for a large excision.

The surgeon can use either the scissors or the scalpel for the excision. Scissors have some advantages over the scalpel, especially when the surgeon does not have intimate

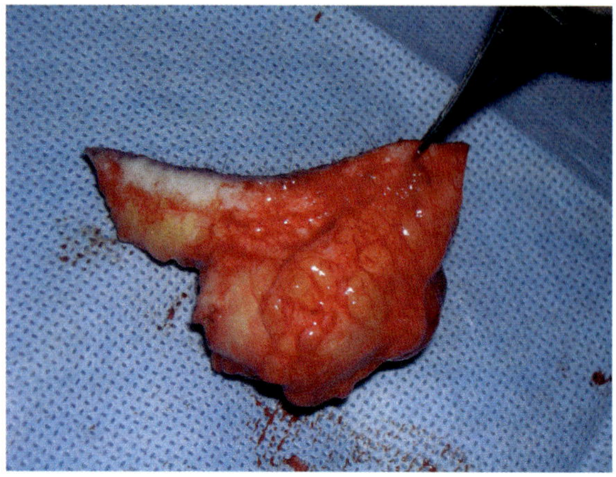

Figure 17-10 Examination of an excisional specimen demonstrates uneven removal which can translate into difficulty reapproximating the wound and/or an increased likelihood of redundant tissue cones.

knowledge of the surgical planes. Compared to the scalpel, scissors provide more tactile feedback, which helps the surgeon feel the release of tissue and maintain a uniform anatomic plane. The scissors should split the anatomic plane with ease, especially in healthy skin without fibrosis from a previous scar. Undue resistance during the excision should prompt the surgeon to reevaluate the accuracy of the anatomic plane. In contrast to scissors, the blind sharp edge of the scalpel blade more easily breaches tissue planes. Especially in areas with thick subcutaneous fat, such as the abdomen or proximal thigh, there is a tendency for the scalpel to cut progressively deeper during the excision and for the underside of the specimen to have scalloped edges (Fig. 17-10). The surgeon should aim for a clean separation of anatomic planes and an excision specimen with a uniform thickness, which reflects the accuracy of the plane of excision.

UNDERMINING

Undermining facilitates advancement of skin edges by releasing either the skin edges or flap from underlying adhesions. Undermining can also facilitate eversion of the wound edges during suturing. The surgeon must make two key decisions when undermining: (1) the ideal anatomic plane for undermining; and (2) the extent of undermining (i.e., how widely to undermine). In most cases, the anatomic plane for undermining coincides with the depth of the incision and the plane of the excision.

If the surgeon is working in an efficient surgical plane, undermining should occur with ease. Undue resistance while undermining usually signifies an inefficient anatomic plane (e.g., most commonly splitting the subcutaneous fat or attempting to split the dermis, rather than working at the junction of the fat and fascia). The ideal surgical plane varies based on the location (see Table 17-2 specifying ideal anatomic planes for excision and undermining). In some instances, undermining at a more superficial anatomic depth than the excision can minimize morbidity. For example, if excision of the SMAS is necessary for clearance of a tumor on the temple, the surgeon may decrease morbidity to the underlying temporal branches of the facial nerve by undermining the edges of the reconstruction superficial to the SMAS.

It should be noted that skin undermined too superficially (e.g., immediately subdermal) may not have adequate perfusion.[21,22] To optimize blood supply the skin is typically undermined so that a layer of tight columnar cells from the subcutaneous fat remain adherent to the underlying dermis. For example, on the central face (e.g., nose, lips, and central forehead) and scalp, undermining deep to the muscles of facial expression or galea, respectively, is desirable in most cases. By contrast, on the lateral face, temple, and posterior triangle of the neck, undermining superficial to the SMAS and investing fascia of the neck, respectively, preserves function of the underlying motor nerves.

The lateral extent of undermining varies according to the procedure. Wide undermining may be necessary when operating in areas where the dermis is firmly adherent to the fascia and muscles below, such as on the lip or chin. For most primary closures, wide undermining rarely increases mobility of the skin edges. Usually, minimal undermining (0.5–1.0 cm) suffices. In some instances, especially deep wounds and sites with thin overlying dermis such as the dorsal hands, no undermining may be necessary. Fascial plication sutures can advance tissue, decrease undermining requirements, and minimize the surface tension that is transmitted to sutures.[23] To help decide whether undermining is necessary, the surgeon can take a skin hook to place the leading edge of skin in an everted position. If underlying adhesions fix the skin in an inverted position, undermining will help.

Undermining too widely can also threaten the skin's blood supply.[22] In general, the surgeon should aim to undermine just enough to move the skin so that the edges approximate without tension. Frequent assessment of skin mobility while undermining helps to avoid unnecessarily wide undermining. Sharp undermining with scissors is much more efficient than blunt undermining. With thorough knowledge of anatomy, the surgeon can undermine sharply and with confidence. Compared to the scalpel, scissors allow sharp undermining with better tactile feedback. The scissors precisely release the skin at the desired surgical plane. After the initial releasing cut, the surgeon can efficiently undermine the remaining skin by sliding one blade of the scissors in the newly released space and use the second blade to complete the cut. Using this slide and divide technique of undermining,[24] the surgeon does not have to rediscover the preferred undermining plane with each new cut.

Countertraction with skin hooks greatly facilitates undermining. Compared to forceps, skin hooks allow forceful countertraction of the skin without epidermal trauma. The skin hook should be placed firmly at the desired depth of undermining (usually under the dermis) and immediately over the point of undermining. If the skin hook is placed too superficially, for example, in the mid dermis, the instrument tends to slip from the skin. If the skin hook is placed remotely from the point of undermining with the scissors, the forces of countertraction diminish and undermining is more difficult. Therefore, as the scissors progress to a new spot, the retracting skin hook should follow.

HEMOSTASIS

When the prior steps of incision, excision, and undermining are performed correctly, the amount of bleeding present within the surgical wound should be minimal. However, meticulous hemostasis must still be obtained prior to proceeding with suturing. Although rarely life-threatening, postoperative hematomas from cutaneous surgical excisions can significantly compromise the aesthetic outcome and are often avoidable. A detailed discussion regarding the numerous electrosurgical modalities by which bleeding vessels are treated is beyond the scope of this chapter, and readers are referred to other relevant chapters in this book for a more detailed discussion on electrosurgery. A few guiding principles may help the surgeon while attempting to stop intraoperative bleeding.

First, a thorough preoperative assessment of bleeding risk can help to avoid uncontrolled perioperative bleeding. Precise cauterization of vessels ensures optimum hemostasis and minimizes collateral tissue damage. This can be facilitated by indirect electrosurgery whereby the surgeon gently picks up the bleeding area with forceps or a delicate hemostat and an assistant touches the forceps handle with the electrosurgical device. The forceps or hemostat releases the tissue once the area has been sufficiently desiccated.

For sites that have brisk amounts of bleeding, the surgeon should firmly compress the area with gauze pads in the nondominant hand followed by a slow, rolling release of the tissue to visualize and grab the bleeding site with the forceps or hemostat. Because gravity will cause blood to move downward, hemostasis is more efficient when the surgeon begins this task at the superior pole of the wound. This will prevent pooled blood from obscuring the surgical site and allows the surgeon to find the vessels more easily.

Once the base of the wound has definitive hemostasis, the surgeon must ensure that the undermined wound edges have sufficiently stopped bleeding. The most efficient means of evaluating the undermined areas is to have an assistant "walk the edges" with skin hooks whereby the tissue is lifted, everted, and shown to the surgeon. Any culprit vessels may be stopped to ensure there will be no bleeding during and after suturing. Electrosurgery should then be applied directly with the device tip to any remaining bleeding areas that are too small for the indirect method with forceps. Hemostasis may be considered complete when the surgeon can visualize the defect without any blood pooling at the base or edges of the wound.

SUTURING

A layered wound closure allows for optimal cosmesis and the number of suture layers selected to repair a wound is dependent upon the depth and location of the wound. For full-thickness defects, a minimum of two layers allows for precise approximation of the dermal and epidermal edges, while reducing the tension on the surface of the incision via wound eversion. In this scenario, deep sutures are placed to close the dermis in a buried vertical mattress fashion followed by cuticular sutures that reapproximate the epidermis. For deeper and larger wounds, a deep layer of sutures to approximate the subcutaneous tissue may be placed prior to the buried vertical mattress sutures. This deepest layer of sutures eliminates dead space and relieves additional tension on the incision line, thus reducing the likelihood of future scar inversion. Fascial plication sutures also perform a similar function for deep excisional wounds such as on the back or cheek.[23]

DERMAL SUTURES

Deep sutures eliminate dead space, approximate the dermis and epidermis, and provide strength to the wound as the scar matures. Judicious selection of the suture and needle, a thoughtful plan for suture sequence, and positioning relative to the wound are the first steps for effective execution of the buried vertical mattress suture, the workhorse deep suture technique for cutaneous reconstruction.[25] The anatomic layers requiring suturing will vary by site, depth, and complexity of the wound, and a comprehensive discussion of these various wounds lies beyond this scope of this chapter.

The buried vertical mattress suture creates the same heart-shaped loop as a cutaneous vertical mattress suture (Fig. 17-11),[26] except that the knot lies at the bottom of the loop and there is no risk for suture marks on the epidermis. This course of the needle facilitates wound eversion and counteracts the contractile forces to prevent an inverted or depressed scar. In cross section, the buried vertical mattress suture has a heart-shaped loop with two peaks at the level of the mid dermis or deep papillary dermis and a valley at the depth of the deep reticular dermis. As the difference in depth between the peaks and valley of the suture path increases, the degree of eversion will increase.

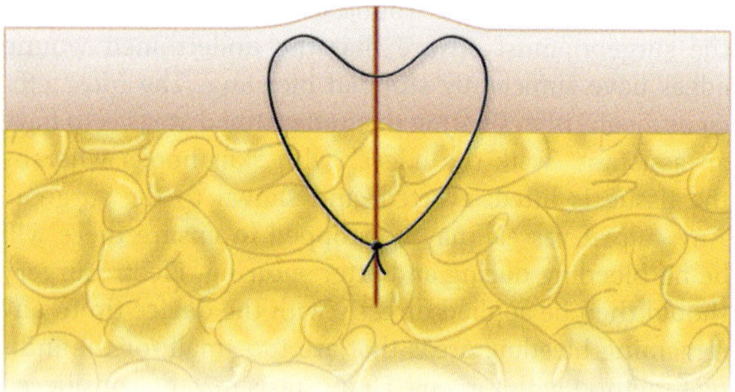

A

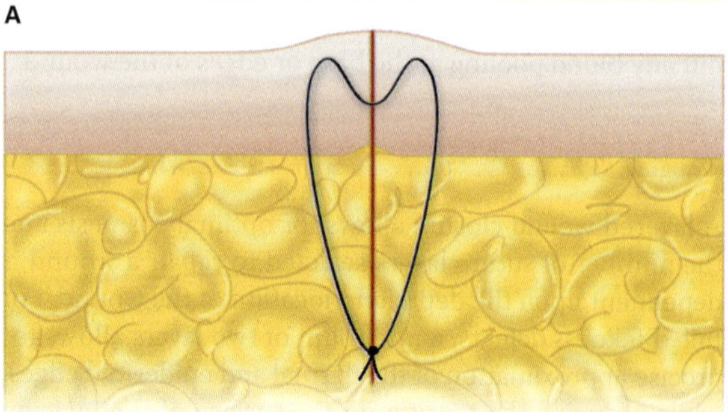

B

Figure 17-11 A. Short, broad heart-shaped loop for thick dermis. **B.** Tall narrow heart-shaped loop for thick dermis

To begin, the needle is passed starting from the undermined plane, aiming for the desired location of the peak of the heart-shaped loop. The distance of the peak of the heart-shaped loop from the incised wound edge varies depending on the thickness of the dermis. In general, thicker dermis requires a greater distance of the peak of the heart-shaped loop from the incised wound edge. Once the tip of the needle reaches the mid dermis or papillary dermis, the needle is rotated toward the incised wound edge. As the needle is rotated toward the center of the wound, the wound edge must be retracted aggressively in an everted position. This aggressive retraction ensures that the tip of the needle will reach the incised wound edge at a greater depth, usually in the reticular dermis. When the peaks lie closer to the underside of the epidermis than the valley of the heart-shaped loop, the epidermis and superficial dermis of the incised wound edge naturally snap back toward the center of the wound. The surgeon observes this natural "snap" upon release of the retracting forceps or skin hook after completing the suture bite. The "snap" of the epidermis and superficial dermis toward the center of the wound is a quality control checkpoint. If the "snap" does not occur, then there is a high likelihood of a gap between the wound edges.

The needle is then passed in the opposite side of the wound in a path that creates a mirror image of the first side. The needle enters the wound in the deep reticular dermis and must aim to create a peak of the heart-shaped loop in the more superficial dermis. Retracting the skin edge in an everted position with the skin hook or forceps naturally facilitates the proper suture path. In practice, the start of the second throw requires extension of the wrist and will feel like the tip of the needle is aiming upward. Once the tip of the needle reaches the peak, the needle is rotated toward the base of the wound and exits at the level of the undermined plane.

The thickness of the dermis determines the path of the buried vertical mattress suture. In areas with thicker dermis (e.g., the back or proximal extremities), the path of the suture must have a greater difference in height between the peaks and valley of the buried vertical mattress suture. To achieve this greater difference, the surgeon must take a wider bite (i.e., further from the wound edge) with the skin edge retracted aggressively in an everted position. In practice, a wide bite with the skin edge retracted aggressively feels like the suture needle is passing parallel to the underside of the epidermis for as long as possible. In areas with thinner dermis (e.g., eyelid and dorsal hand and forearm), the ideal difference in height between the peaks and valley of the buried vertical mattress sutures is smaller. To achieve this minimal difference, the surgeon must take a narrow bite (i.e., closer to the wound edge) with the skin edge retracted in a less aggressive vertical position. In practice, a narrow bite with a gently retracted everted edge feels like the suture needle is passing parallel to the vertical face of the incised skin edge. Another way to describe the difference in the suture path for thick versus thin dermis is to conceptualize the distance of the peaks of the heart-shaped loop from the incised wound edge. In thick dermis, the peaks of the heart-shaped loop will lie further from the incised wound edge and the path of the suture creates a broad-based, heart-shaped loop. In thin dermis, the peaks of the heart-shaped loop lie closer to the incised wound edge and the path of the suture creates a narrow, tall, heart-shaped loop (Fig. 17-11).

To achieve perfect apposition of the wound edges, the path of the buried vertical mattress suture on one side should be a mirror image of the suture path on the other side. When the paths of the buried vertical mattress suture on each side are not mirror images, the wound edges will not appose each other precisely. As a rule, the side with the bite of suture more superficial relative to the epidermis will have a wound edge that is depressed relative to the other side (see section on troubleshooting).

The suture is now ready to be tied with the knot buried at the depth of the undermined plane. An effective instrument tie is necessary to prevent an "air knot" and to ensure that the suture snugly approximates the wound edges. The surgeon may consider a "V-area" that is the empty airspace between the running end (e.g., suture point) and free end of the suture (i.e., "tail"). The needle driver does all of the work in this "V," allowing for efficient and effective knot-tying. The knot may be tied by wrapping the running end of the suture around the needle one time. The needle holder then grasps the free end of the suture and pulls it in the same direction of the previous wrapping motion and cinches the knot firmly, not forcefully, down.[27] This knot is repeated again in the same direction, while future throws are alternated in direction. If the surgeon wishes to secure the knot, which is helpful for wounds under some tension, the free end of the suture may be pulled up while the working end is relaxed after the second flat throw. Alternatively, a surgeon's knot secures the suture by performing a double wrap on the first throw of the instrument tie.[27]

The deep sutures should support the dermis along the entire wound and still allow easy manipulation of the epidermal edges. To ensure an adequate number of deep sutures, the surgeon can apply the "pull test." The pull test consists of applying lateral pressure to try to spread the wound edges from each other. Additional deep sutures may be prudent in any gap produced by the pull test. To assess proper depth of the deep suture, the surgeon can use the skin hook or forceps to retract the epidermis and superficial dermis. Resistance signifies that the suture was placed too superficially, usually as a result of using a circular, rather than heart-shaped, path of the suture.

CUTICULAR SUTURES. Even with careful technique when performing the deep sutures, the wound edges frequently benefit from an additional layer of superficial sutures for precise approximation of the epidermal edges. If the deep sutures have been placed effectively, the epidermis and dermis should not have a gap between them and the top sutures should not need to bear tension. However, minor height discrepancies after placement of the deep sutures are common. The primary purpose of the top sutures is to correct these height discrepancies.

The anatomic location of the surgical excision often dictates the manner in which "top" sutures are placed. Tension-free sites such as the head and neck lend themselves to percutaneous epidermal sutures with nonabsorbable or fast-absorbing sutures. The types of knots selected for this layer of sutures vary and include simple interrupted, running continuous, vertical mattress, and horizontal mattress.[28] Anatomic sites bearing more postoperative tension, such as the chest and back, may be best repaired with an absorbable or nonabsorbable running subcuticular suture. The nonabsorbable suture can be removed at 1 week. Because scars are inherently weaker than normal tissue, particularly early in the postoperative period, placing an absorbable running subcuticular suture at a tension-bearing site may reduce the likelihood of the scar widening or spreading.

The type and caliber of the suture, the size of the needle, and the timing of suture removal also influence execution of the top sutures. The surgeon must be aware that smaller caliber sutures have a lower risk of leaving track marks compared to thicker caliber sutures when percutaneous cuticular sutures are performed. Effective placement of buried vertical mattress sutures nearly eliminates tension on the wound edges and allows the surgeon to use lower caliber sutures. In addition, smaller suture needles (e.g., P-3) should be used to suture delicate wound edges. Larger needles increase the likelihood of tearing delicate wound edges. Finally, percutaneous epidermal sutures should be removed as early as possible to avoid track marks. In wounds with effective placement of deep sutures, the top sutures do not bear tension and can be removed within 5 to 7 days in most cases, especially on the head and neck. Leaving the sutures for a longer time offers little advantage, as the deep sutures bear the tension that keeps the wound from dehiscing.

Once the surgeon has chosen the suture materials, an important decision that must be made is selecting the frequency of the top sutures and the distance of the suture bites from the wound edge. In general, skin with a thinner dermis requires a higher frequency of sutures (i.e., sutures placed closer together) and suture bites that are closer to the wound edge. The top sutures help to accentuate the eversion, defined as upward sloping skin edges that meet perfectly at the peak without any plateau or inversion. If the bite of the suture is too far from the wound edge, it can create an eversion–inversion phenomenon.

The top sutures should be thrown with minimal tension. Excessive tension increases the risk for wound necrosis and suture marks. As a quality control measure to assess the tension on the sutures, the surgeon should be able to slide one arm of the forceps under the suture loop without difficulty. If the top sutures are thrown with tension, a gap will form at the points of entry and exit. The process of reepithelialization begins immediately to close this gap, so track marks are sure to occur, even if the top sutures are removed before 1 week.

The first step in placing accurate top sutures is to recognize which side of the wound is riding higher than the other. The high side either obscures visibility of the lower wound edge by sliding over it like a shingle on a roof or it bleeds because its superficial dermis is exposed. The high side of the wound is usually slightly more delicate and can be more challenging to manipulate. It is often more efficient to correct height discrepancies of the wound edge by biting the high side first. The general guideline to correct height discrepancies with top sutures is: "Bite high on the high side, and bite low on the low side." In other words, the needle should approach the high side with a shallow bite in the superficial dermis (i.e., close to parallel to the plane of the epidermis) that is relatively close to the wound edge. After showing the tip of the needle between the wound edges, the surgeon has control of this side of the wound. The surgeon must then depress the wound edge until it matches the height of the opposite side. The needle is then passed with a deeper and wider bite that precisely matches the wound edges.

REDUNDANT TISSUE CONES

Redundant tissue cones are commonly encountered at the end of a repair and can compromise the cosmetic outcome by creating abnormal contour at one or both ends of an elliptical excision. As wound edges are sutured together, skin becomes displaced along the central axis. This displaced skin produces raised edges that form at the distal portions of the closure due to excess tissue compression.[29] Many names have been given to these cones: dog-ears, Burow's cones, and triangles. The dermatologic surgeon must be mindful of how these cones form and of how to address them in order to obtain optimum cosmesis.

AVOIDING REDUNDANT TISSUE CONES

Three main factors affect redundant tissue cone formation. First, the apical angles directly influence the likelihood of protruding tissue cones. Conceptually, if the closure of a fusiform excision is thought of as a parallel advancement of two edges then the apical angles experience rotational forces. As this apical angle increases, particularly beyond 30 degrees, so too does the potential for creation of raised excess skin.[7,29] Second, as the length of a fusiform closure is reduced, the likelihood of redundant cones becomes higher, because there is less tissue to counteract the compression of the sutured edges. Finally, when the opposing wound edges are of different lengths, redundant cones are more likely to form if not addressed properly.

Redundant tissue cones can be avoided by many of the designs and surgical techniques noted previously in this chapter and include:

1. Creation of apical angles of 30 degrees or less with a rhombus-shaped fusiform excision
2. Ensuring that the sides of each ellipse are equal when operating on a planar surface
3. Converting the rhombus into an S-shape design on convex surfaces
4. Continuing smooth, nonbeveled incisions all the way to each apex so that excess dermal or subcutaneous tissue does not obstruct wound closure
5. Properly undermining around the entire wound, particularly beyond the apices.[7]
6. If a redundant cone is anticipated because of sides of unequal length, then the wound edges may be sutured together in a manner that progressively divides the wound into "halves" in order to equalize the length discrepancy. This technique can be enhanced even further by taking horizontal mattress bites of the longer wound edge.

CORRECTING REDUNDANT TISSUE CONES

Despite proper excision design and technical execution, the surgeon must be prepared to address redundant tissue cones that form at the edges of wound repair. Redundant tissue cones can spontaneously regress over time and the likelihood of contour improvement is proportional to the actual height of the cone as well as the length of time since surgery.[30] Although it is certainly possible to allow redundancies to "settle out," the contour deformation of the surgical site often detracts from the aesthetic result. In order to please the patient with the immediate postoperative result, these redundancies are usually best removed at the time of surgical excision.

Surgical removal of standing tissue cones can be performed in numerous ways (Fig. 17-12). The manner in which a cone is excised is influenced by the surgical site, the adjacent relaxed skin tension lines, and the location of adjacent rhytides. If a relaxed skin tension line is continuous and parallel with the sutured wound then straight elliptical excision around the tissue can be performed. In this scenario, arched incisions are made immediately around the redundancy and are extended as far distal as the conical protrusion reaches. Another method of creating a straight-line removal is to lift up the redundant cone with forceps or a hook and incise the cone directly down the center to the distal end of the raised area. Once incised, each triangle of skin can be draped over the new defect and trimmed so that a new elliptical defect can be sutured into a straight line. Attempts to remove less skin than extends to the distal raised area will result in a persistent contour deformity. Novice surgeons frequently will take less skin than is required to remove a redundant cone which results in "chasing" the contour deformity over a number of excisions, decreasing the likelihood of an elegant, aesthetic result.

There are instances in which redundant cones are removed in a curved or perpendicular fashion in order to better camouflage the scar within the relaxed skin tension lines or adjacent rhytides (Fig. 17-12). This technique is similar to the incisions necessary to surgically excise a redundant cone to create a straight-line scar. The distinguishing feature, however, is that the first incision with the scalpel occurs specifically in the direction where the new scar line is desired. Once this full-thickness incision is made through the skin to the appropriate depth, the remaining flap of skin is draped over the wound and trimmed and a new, angled defect may be sutured.

Once the surgeon becomes comfortable with excision of redundant cones, this technique may allow minimization of scars and conservation of tissue by excising lesions as a circle rather than with a fusiform ellipse design. The disadvantages of the fusiform excision design include poor compensation for the variability in regional tissue laxity that exist along redundant cone deformity sites in addition to the potential to remove excessive amounts of healthy tissue due to a predetermined design.[31] In fact, on nonwrinkled skin, optimal scar orientation can be challenging and it may be common to find that a created ellipse gapes wider and in a different direction than initially anticipated by the surgeon.[32] Circular excisions

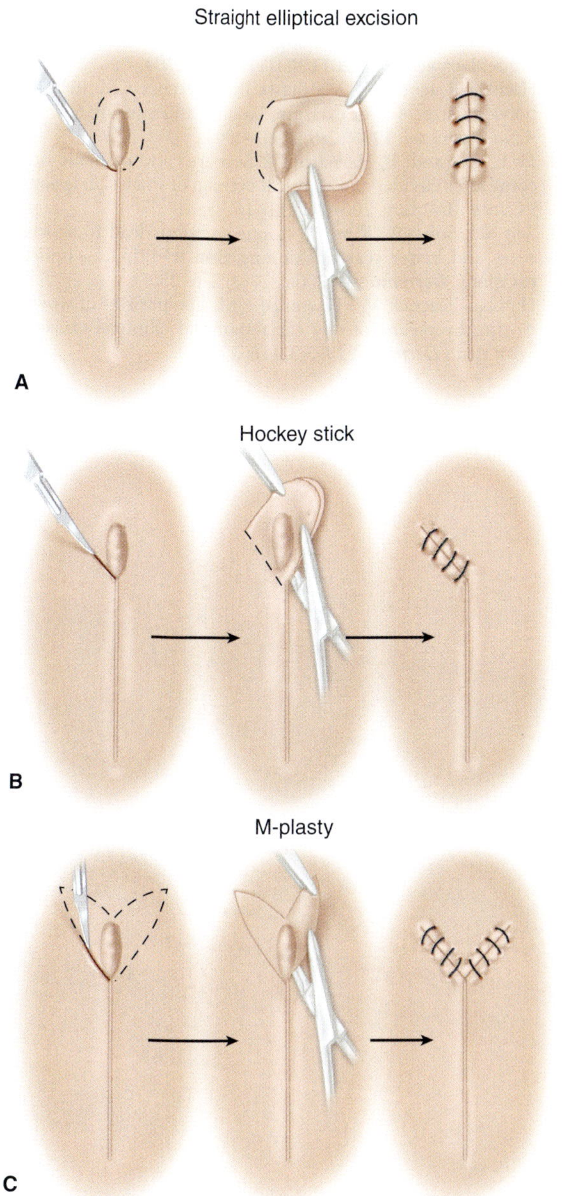

Figure 17-12 The varying methods of removing redundant tissue cones. An elliptical excision of the cone creates a continuous linear scar (**A**), while the hockey-stick (**B**), and M-plasty techniques, curve or shorten the scar, respectively. Note that in all 3 examples, the scalpel blade incises from the distal skin puckering to the base of the tissue cone, which ensures that the redundant skin is fully removed and proper scar contour is achieved.

of lesions with subsequent removal of redundant tissue cones into desired areas can reduce scar size, decrease operative time, and allows for potentially better oriented wounds.[33–35]

CONCLUSION

Proper design and execution of the elliptical excision and its variations allows for improved patient satisfaction and enhanced cosmesis. The excision may be divided into five individual steps – incision, excision, hemostasis, undermining, and suturing. Proficiency in the skills to perform these steps will allow the surgeon to begin to obtain reproducibly excellent results and progress to more technically advanced surgical procedures, such as cutaneous flaps.

REFERENCES

1. Otley CC. Perioperative evaluation and management in dermatologic surgery. *J Am Acad Dermatol.* 2006;54(1):119–127.
2. Macrae WA. Chronic pain after surgery. *Br J Anaesth.* 2001;87 (1):88–98.
3. Perlis CS, Campbell RM, Perlis RH, Malik M, Dufresne RG Jr. Incidence of and risk factors for medical malpractice lawsuits among Mohs surgeons. *Dermatol Surg.* 2006;32(1):79–83.
4. Goldberg LH, Alam M. Elliptical excisions: variations and the eccentric parallelogram. *Arch Dermatol.* 2004;140(2):176–180.
5. Dunlavey E, Leshin B. The simple excision. *Dermatol Clin.* 1998; 16(1):49–64.
6. Moody BR, McCarthy JE, Sengelmann RD. The apical angle: a mathematical analysis of the ellipse. *Dermatol Surg.* 2001; 27(1):61–63.
7. Weisberg NK, Nehal KS, Zide BM. Dog-ears: a review. *Dermatol Surg.* 2000;26(4):363–370.
8. Cook J, Zitelli JA. Primary closure for midline defects of the nose: a simple approach for reconstruction. *J Am Acad Dermatol.* 2000;43(3):508–510.
9. Borges AF. Relaxed skin tension lines (RSTL) versus other skin lines. *Plast Reconstr Surg.* 1984;73(1):144–150.
10. Robinson J, Hanke CW, Siegal DM, Fratila A. *Surgery of the Skin: Procedural Dermatology.* Philadelphia, PA: Elsevier; 2010:239–250.
11. Zitelli JA. TIPS for a better ellipse. *J Am Acad Dermatol.* 1990; 22(1):101–103.
12. Mizunuma M, Yanai A, Tsutsumi S, et al. Can dog-ear formation be decreased when an S-shaped skin resection is used instead of a spindle skin resection? A three-dimensional analysis of skin surgery techniques using the finite element method. *Plast Reconstr Surg.* 2000;106(4):845–848; discussion 9–51.
13. Salasche SJ, Roberts LC. Dog-ear correction by M-plasty. *J Dermatol Surg Oncol.* 1984;10(6):478–482.
14. Krishnan RS, Donnelly HB. The nested M-plasty for scar length shortening. *Dermatol Surg.* 2008;34(9):1236–1238.
15. Wisco OJ, Wentzell JM. When an M is a V: vector analysis calls for redesign of the M-plasty. *Dermatol Surg.* 2009;35 (8):1271–1276.
16. Gormley DE. A brief analysis of the Burow's wedge/triangle principle. *J Dermatol Surg Oncol.* 1985;11(2):121–123.
17. Oberemok S, Eliezri Y, Desciak E. Burow's wedge flap revisited. *Dermato Surg.* 2005;31(2):210–216; discussion 6.
18. Morganroth PA, Gelfand JM, Jambusaria A, Margolis DJ, Miller CJ. A randomized, double-blind comparison of the total dose of 1.0% lidocaine with 1:100,000 epinephrine versus 0.5% lidocaine with 1:200,000 epinephrine required for effective local anesthesia during Mohs micrographic surgery for skin cancers. *J Am Acad Dermatol.* 2009;60(3):444–452.
19. Stewart JH, Cole GW, Klein JA. Neutralized lidocaine with epinephrine for local anesthesia. *J Dermatol Surg Oncol.* 1989;15(10):1081–1083.
20. Sobanko JF, LJ, Swanson NA, Lee KK. Biopsy techniques. In: Rigel DS, Robinson JK, Ross MI, et al., eds. *Cancer of the Skin.* 2nd ed. Philadelphia, PA: Saunders; 2011:434–443.
21. Pearl RM, Johnson D. The vascular supply to the skin: an anatomical and physiological reappraisal–Part I. *Ann Plast Surg.* 1983;11(2):99–105.
22. Pearl RM, Johnson D. The vascular supply to the skin: an anatomical and physiological reappraisal–Part II. *Ann Plas Surg.* 1983;11(3):196–205.
23. Kantor J. The fascial plication suture: an adjunct to layered wound closure. *Arch Dermatol.* 2009;145(12):1454–1456.

24. Boyer JD, Zitelli JA, Brodland DG. Undermining in cutaneous surgery. *Dermatol Surg.* 2001;27(1):75–78.
25. Zitelli JA, Moy RL. Buried vertical mattress suture. *J Dermatol Surg Oncol.* 1989;15(1):17–19.
26. Davis JS. The on-end or vertical mattress suture. *Ann Surg.* 1933;98(5):941–951.
27. Nevarre DR. Increasing efficiency in the operative field: knot tying, instrument ties, and locking the suture. *Ann Plast Surg.* 1998;40(3):313–315.
28. Kudur MH, Pai SB, Sripathi H, Prabhu S. Sutures and suturing techniques in skin closure. *Indian J Dermatol Venereol Leprol.* 2009;75(4):425–434.
29. Dzubow LM. The dynamics of dog-ear formation and correction. *J Dermatol Surg Oncol.* 1985;11(7):722–728.
30. Lee KS, Kim NG, Jang PY, et al. Statistical analysis of surgical dog-ear regression. *Dermatol Surg.* 2008;34(8):1070–1076.
31. Lee TS, Murakami CS, Suryadevara AC. Tissue conservation using circular defect with dog-ear deformities excision technique. *Laryngoscope.* 2011;121(11):2299–2304.
32. Hudson-Peacock MJ, Matthews JN, Lawrence CM. Relation between size of skin excision, wound, and specimen. *J Am Acad Dermatol.* 1995;32(6):1010–1005.
33. Ek L, Hogstedt B, Herrstrom P. Scar area and cosmetic outcome after circular and elliptical excision of small skin lesions. *J Cutan Med Surg.* 2004;8(1):11–15.
34. Seo SH, Son SW, Kim IH. Round excisions lead to shorter scars and better scar positioning than traditional elliptical excisions. *Dermatology.* 2008;217(3):276–280.
35. Hudson-Peacock MJ, Lawrence CM. Comparison of wound closure by means of dog ear repair and elliptical excision. *J Am Acad Dermatol.* 1995;32(4):627–630.

CHAPTER 18

Random Pattern Flaps

Margaret Mann, Jeremy Bordeaux, & Roberta Sengelmann

INTRODUCTION

Random pattern flaps are an indispensable reconstruction option for closure of wounds which may not be suitable for healing by second intention or repair with a linear closure. Defects too large to close in a side-to-side fashion may be ideally suited for such flaps, which are recruited from adjacent tissue reservoirs and use tissue with a similar skin match. When second intention healing or linear closure may result in distortion of free margins, well-designed random pattern flaps can be helpful in redirecting and redistributing tension vectors and allow incision lines to be hidden along cosmetic boundaries and relaxed skin tension lines.

Random pattern flaps are so named because their blood supply is not based on a single vessel, but on the "random" albeit copious subdermal plexus. Advancement, rotation, and transposition flaps are all types of random pattern flaps, each named based on the type of movement the flap undergoes (Table 18-1). Advancement flaps slide in a straight line from the donor site to the recipient site. Rotation flaps rotate in an arc about a pivot point. Transposition flaps move from the donor site to the defect over a peninsula of uninvolved intervening skin.

GENERAL CONCEPTS

Prior to any reconstruction, the surgeon must ensure that complete tumor clearance has been obtained. The goal of a well-designed repair is to optimize functional and aesthetic outcomes. During flap design, one must identify a donor site or tissue reservoir – ideally with a color, texture, and thickness similar to that of the defect. Incision lines should be drawn along relaxed skin tension lines, and boundaries between cosmetic units should be maintained. Generous undermining is often needed for proper mobilization, but care must be taken to perform it in the proper plane (Table 18-2) and in such a way as to minimize unnecessary vascular trauma. Movement of the flap should create minimal tension and virtually imperceptible distortion of surrounding structures.

At the same time, for optimal design and survival of a random pattern flap, one must balance its blood supply with the limitations of the donor tissue. Random pattern flaps can carry a significant risk for ischemia if excessive tissue manipulation occurs or if the flap is improperly designed. Thus, careful design and surgical technique are essential to optimize flap survival. Traditional dogma dictates that a flap should have a length to width ratio no more than 4:1. Although the surviving flap length is partially dependent upon the width of its base, it is now well understood that flap ischemia is influenced to a greater extent by perfusion pressure and the tension across the wound. Ischemia occurs when the perfusion pressure drops below the critical closing pressures of the arterioles in the subdermal plexus, which can occur due to significant edema or venous congestion in the flap. Patient risk factors such as smoking and diabetes can also result in vasoconstriction. Excess tension at the flap tip or edges can constrict small arterioles, leading to the possibility of ischemia. Widening the flap recruits additional subdermal arterioles for increased collateral circulation but does not necessarily change its perfusion pressure. However, when properly designed, widening a flap can displace the defect over a larger area, which in turn, distributes the tension over a larger surface.

Minimizing tension across a flap is critical for its survival as well as a successful aesthetic and functional outcome. Poorly designed flaps can create undue secondary movement resulting in distortion of anatomic landmarks and free margins. The primary movement of a flap is its intended movement into the defect itself. Secondary movement is the movement of the adjacent skin in the opposite direction. One must anticipate the true extent of the primary and secondary movement when designing a flap. When a flap is rotated or transposed into place, pivotal restraint may limit its movement and reach or may create tension at its tip, which can lead to ischemia or free-margin distortion. Thus, one must plan in advance by oversizing the flap to compensate for pivotal restraint. With proper foresight and understanding of flap dynamics, one can maximize the likelihood of a successful outcome of any random pattern flap.

TABLE 18-1
Classification of Surgical Flaps

Movement type	Advancement Rotation Transposition Interpolation
Vascular supply	Random Arterial/Axial Musculocutaneous
Configuration	Rhombic Bilobed

TABLE 18-2
Plane of Undermining based on Location

Location	Undermining Plane	Important Structure(s)
Scalp	Subgaleal	Extensive vasculature
Forehead	Subgaleal or subcutaneous fat above frontalis fascia	Supraorbital and supratrochlear nerve
Temple/Zygomatic arch	Superficial subcutaneous fat	Temporal branch of the facial nerve
Mandible	Superficial subcutaneous fat	Marginal mandibular branch of the facial nerve
Ear	Above perichondrium	
Lip	Above orbicularis oris	Labial artery
Nose	Above perichondrium/periosteum	
Rest of face	Superficial subcutaneous fat, above the parotid duct	Parotid duct, branches of the facial nerve
Terminal hair bearing area	Subcutaneous plane	Hair papillae/bulbs
Lateral neck	Superficial subcutaneous fat	Spinal accessory nerve
Trunk/Extremities	Above muscular fascia	
Hands and feet	Subdermal	

GENERAL CONCEPTS

a. Create incisions along relaxed skin tension lines and maintain boundaries between cosmetic units.
b. Identify donor sites with potential reservoirs of tissue.
c. Avoid distortion of anatomic landmarks and free margins.
d. Maintain shape and symmetry.
e. Repair defect with skin of similar characteristics.
f. Balance blood supply and tissue restraint by
   i. understanding the effects of perfusion pressure and tension on flap ischemia.
   ii. distributing flap tension in the desired direction, over an area larger than that of the defect.
   iii. optimizing primary movement and minimizing secondary movement.
   iv. anticipating flap shortening caused by pivotal restraint.

ADVANCEMENT FLAPS

Conceptually, an advancement flap can be thought of as a variation of the linear closure, in which one or both of the redundant cones are displaced laterally. The flap slides unidirectionally in a straight line from the donor to the recipient site. The major advantage of an advancement flap compared to a linear closure is its ability to displace tissue redundancies (dog-ears) away from free margins to a more aesthetically suitable location. The advancing limb of the flap can be hidden in creases, along the hairline or between cosmetic units. Closure of the displaced dog-ears advances the flap toward the defect and distributes wound tension away from the wound.

The main drawback of these flaps is that their tension vector is unchanged from that of a direct side-to-side repair – both are oriented parallel to the primary motion of the flap. As a result, if the tension vector for a side-to-side closure is improperly designed or distorts free margins, the undesirable tension vector may not change.

Typically, the length to width ratio of an advancement flap should be no more than 3:1 on the face and 2:1 on the trunk and extremity or there will be a risk of distal ischemia, which will vary depending upon the perfusion pressure of the flap and the tension under which the wound is closed. A flap with a 4:1 ratio closed with little tension and a good perfusion pressure will survive, while a flap with 1.5:1 ratio under significant tension will be at significant risk of necrosis.

CLASSIC ADVANCEMENT FLAPS (UNILATERAL AND BILATERAL)

Advancement flaps can be designed with their redundant cones displaced either unilaterally (U-plasty) or bilaterally (H-plasty) if tissue reservoirs are available and movement from both sides of the defect is required (Fig. 18-1). The H-plasty is most often used for eyebrow defects, where scars can be hidden along the upper and lower aspects of the brow (Fig. 18-2). Similarly, one can design an advancement flap such that only a single cone is displaced unilaterally (Burow's advancement) or bilaterally (A to T or O to T) (Figs. 18-3 and 18-4). Classic advancement flaps are frequently a desirable reconstructive option because their incision lines can be well hidden along a free margin or cosmetic boundaries such as the eyebrow, hairline, and vermilion borders of the lips.

O TO L AND CRESCENTIC MODIFICATIONS

Variations on the classic advancement flap include O-to-L repair, or Burow's advancement flap, in which

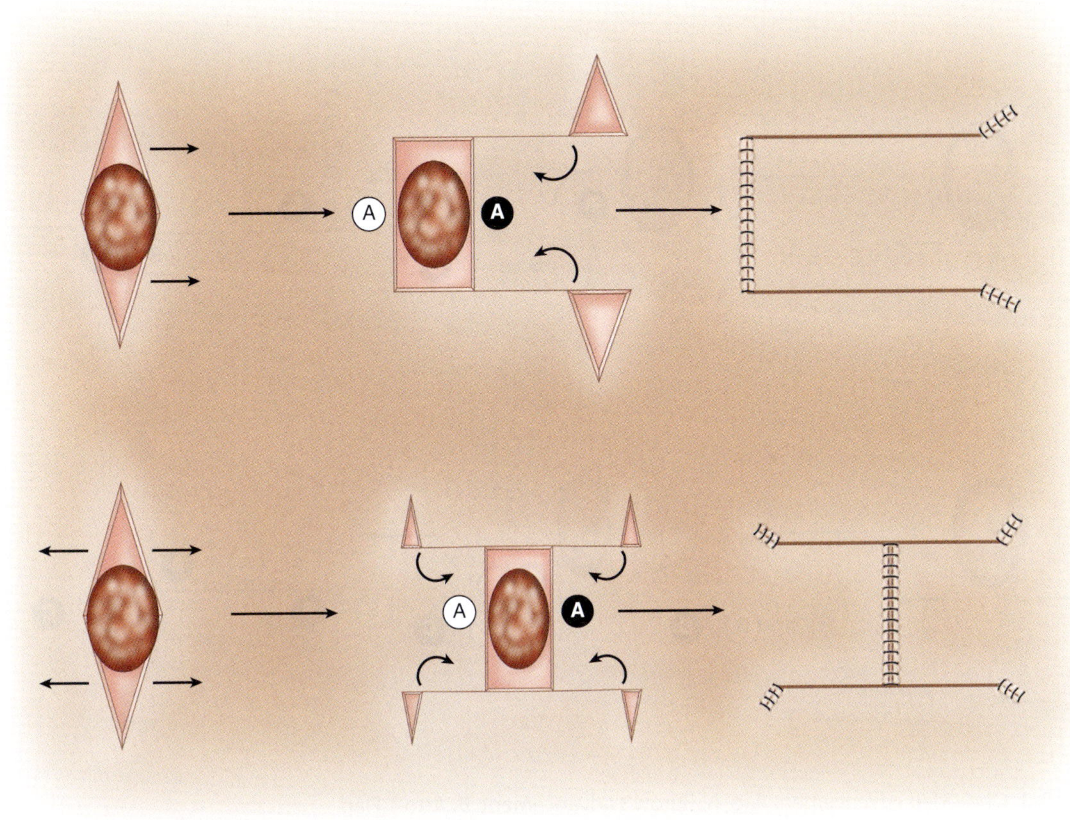

Figure 18-1 Unilateral (U-plasty) and bilateral (H-plasty) advancement flap. Redundant cones are displaced laterally.

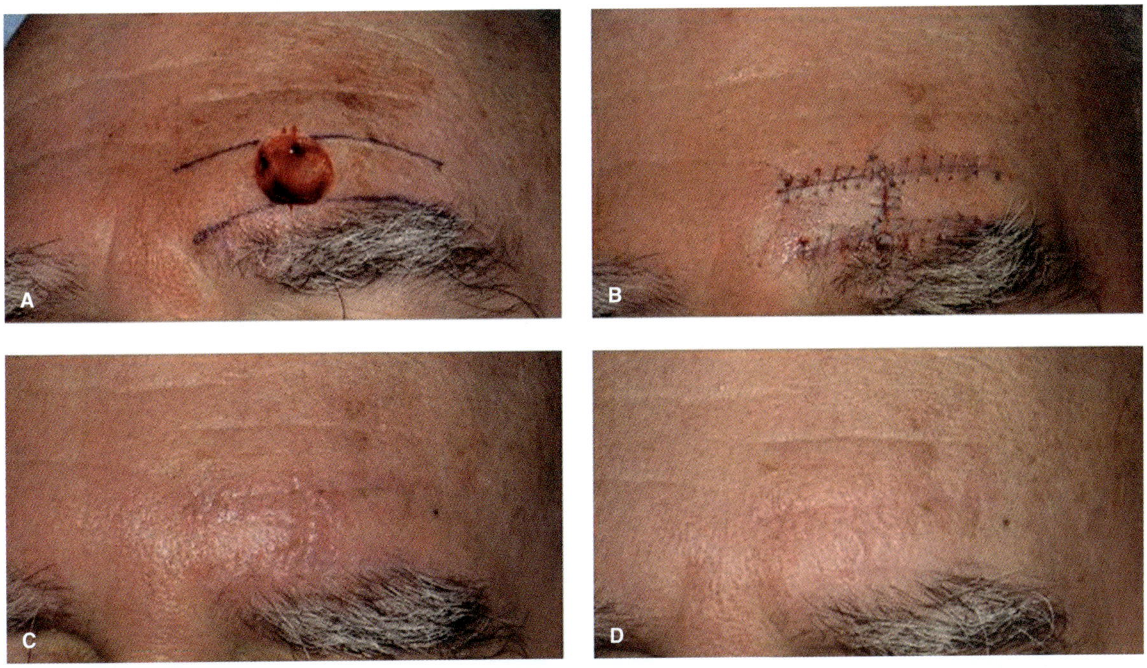

Figure 18-2 A bilateral advancement flap for a forehead defect superior to the eyebrow. **A.** Post Mohs surgery defect with design for bilateral advancement flap (H-plasty). The advancing limbs of the flap are hidden along the natural horizontal forehead rhytid and the upper aspect of the brow. **B.** Final wound closure. Note in this example, redundant tissue is evened out during closure by applying the "rule of halves," avoiding the need for standing cones. **C.** At suture removal 1 week. **D.** At follow-up in 3 months.

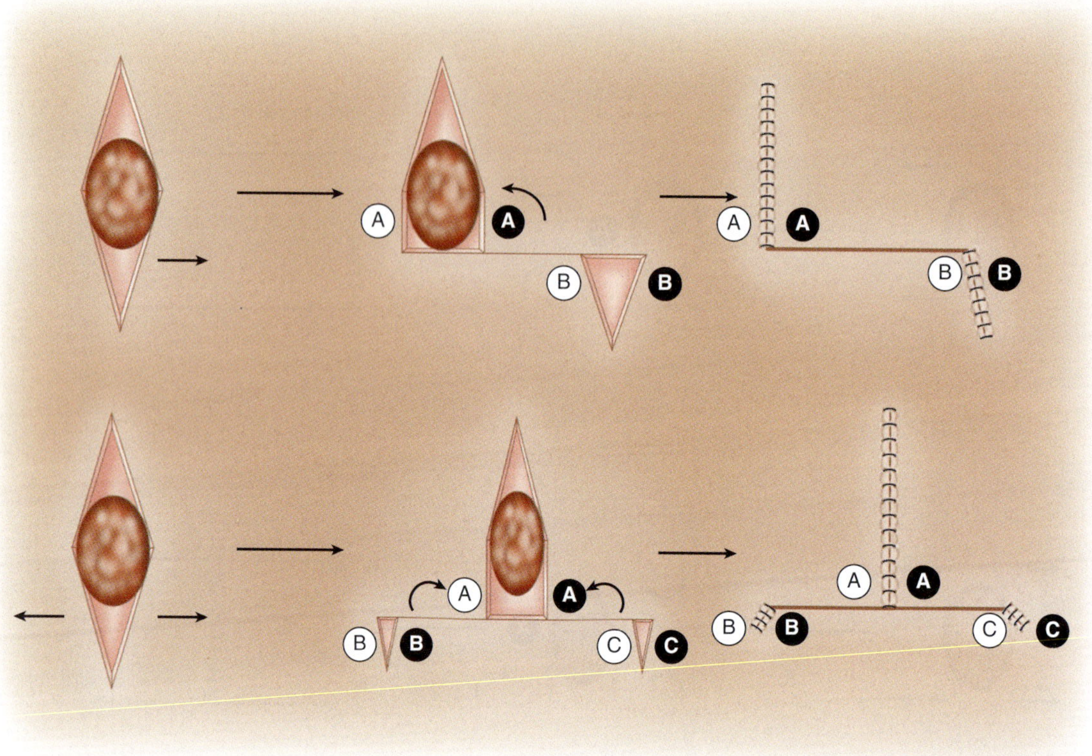

Figure 18-3 One-sided advancement flap. **A.** Burow's advancement. **B.** A-to-T Flap.

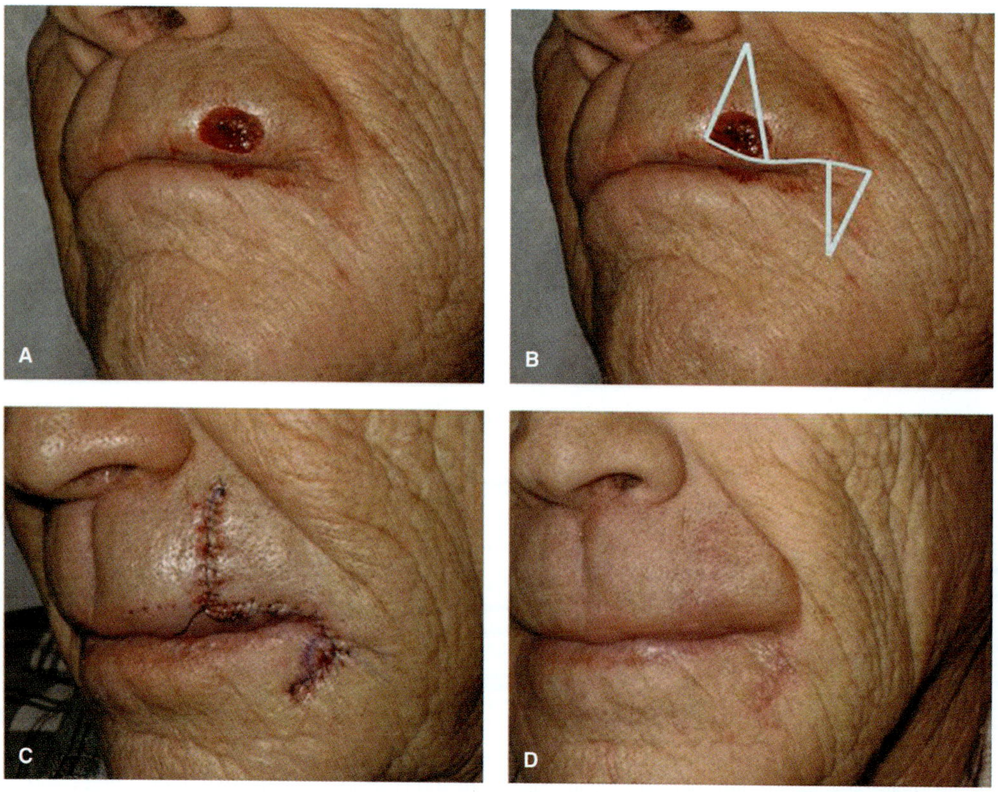

Figure 18-4 A Burow's advancement flap on the upper lip. **A.** Post Mohs surgery defect. **B.** Design for a one-sided Burow's advancement flap. Incision lines are hidden along the vertical lip line and vermillion border. **C.** Final wound closure. **D.** Suture removal at 1 week.

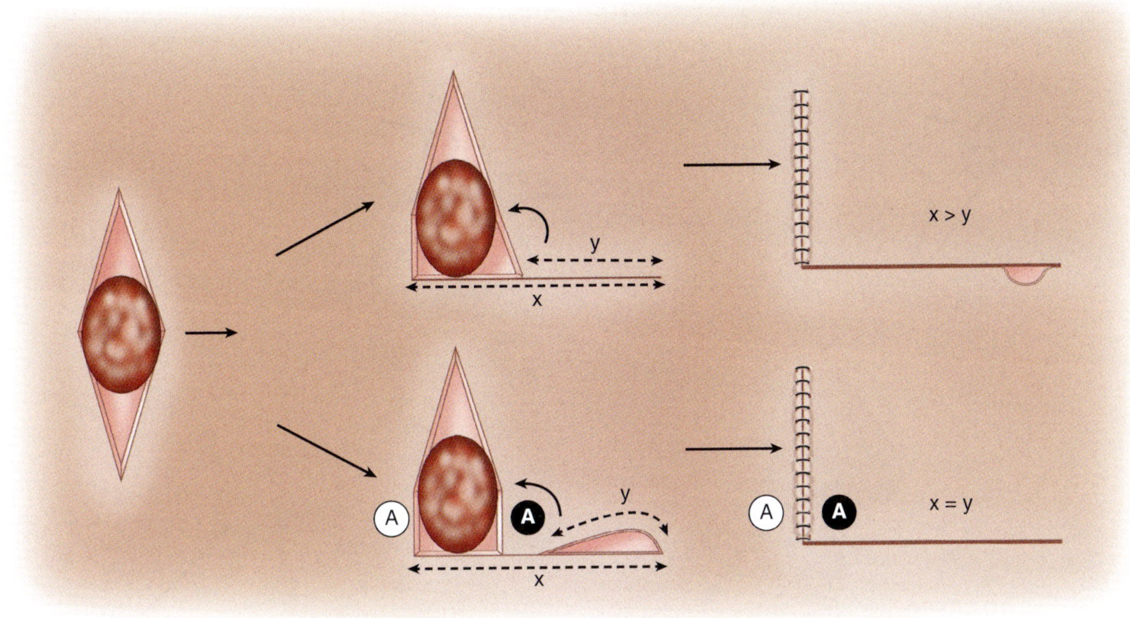

Figure 18-5 Modified crescentic advancement flap. The curvilinear design increases the effective length of the shorter horizontal limb to match the other side.

the redundant tissue is not excised as a "dog-ear" but is evened out during closure by extending the length of the flap and applying the "rule of halves." Similarly, the crescentic modification lengthens the advancing limb of the defect, making a standing cone unnecessary and avoiding the need for unsightly incisions that violate adjacent cosmetic boundaries or lines (Fig. 18-5).[1] The crescentic modification is particularly useful for upper lip, nasal sidewall, and forehead defects (Fig. 18-6).

PERIALAR CRESCENTIC ADVANCEMENT FLAP

This variation of the basic advancement flap is useful along curvilinear cosmetic units because of its curved incision lines. The classic crescentic flap is the perialar crescentic advancement flap, in which the lateral cheek is advanced into the defect with removal of a crescent shape along the ala and nasolabial fold. One disadvantage of this flap is that it can obliterate the apical or hairless triangle if the crescent is incised/resected along the alar crease and onto the nasal sill (Fig. 18-7).

EXECUTION OF THE CRESCENTIC MODIFICATION (Fig. 18-8)

1. Design a classic O-to-T or A-to-T advancement flap.
2. Lengthen the advancing limb in a curvilinear fashion, effectively creating equal lengths along both sides of the wound. The angle of the curvilinear incision should be less than 30 degrees to avoid

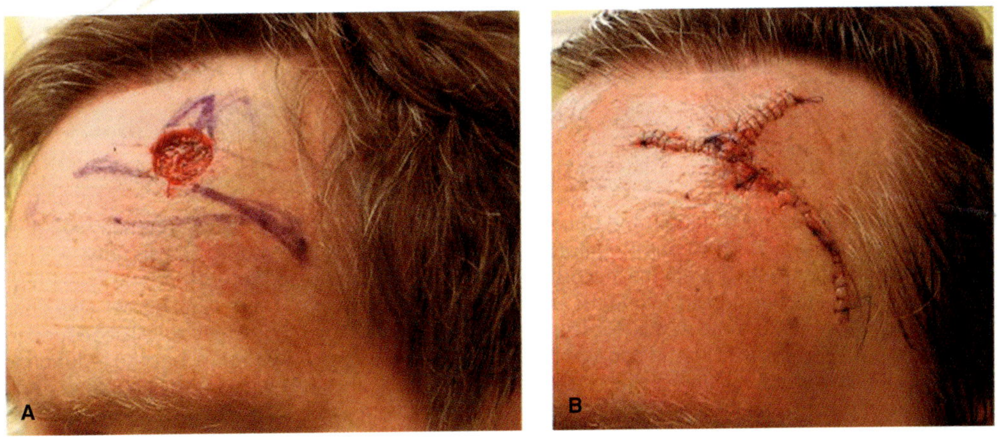

Figure 18-6 A-to-T closure with crescentic modification. **A.** Post Mohs surgery defect. Note the curvilinear design negates the need to remove standing cones. **B.** Final wound closure.

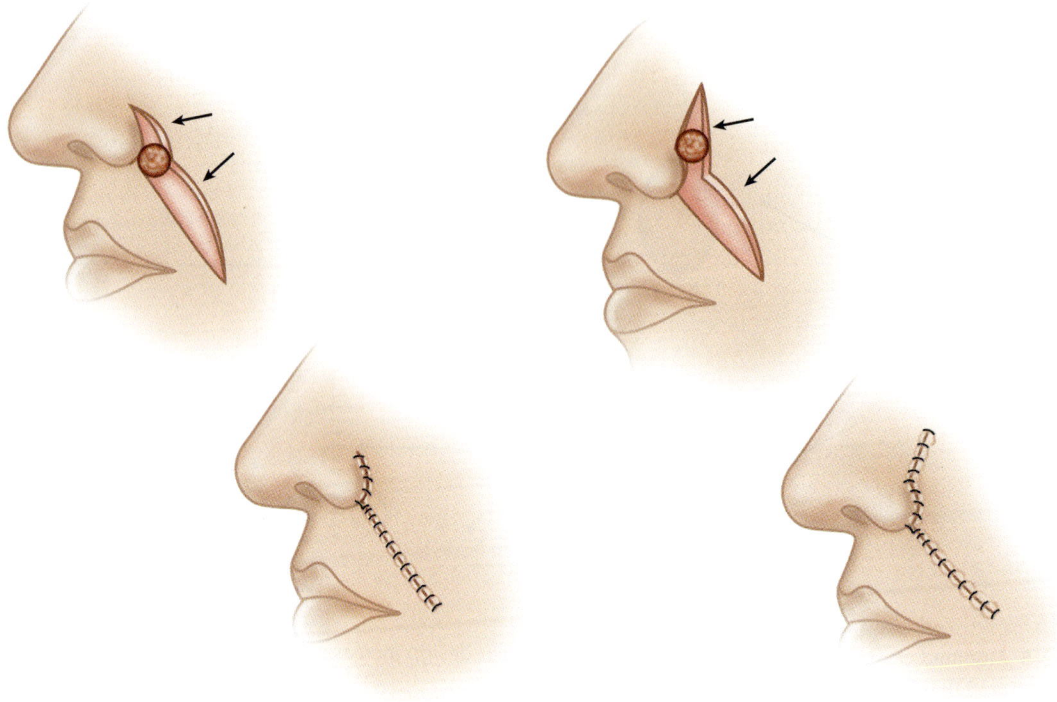

Figure 18-7 Crescentic advancement flap. The perialar design hides the incision along the alar crease and nasal sill.

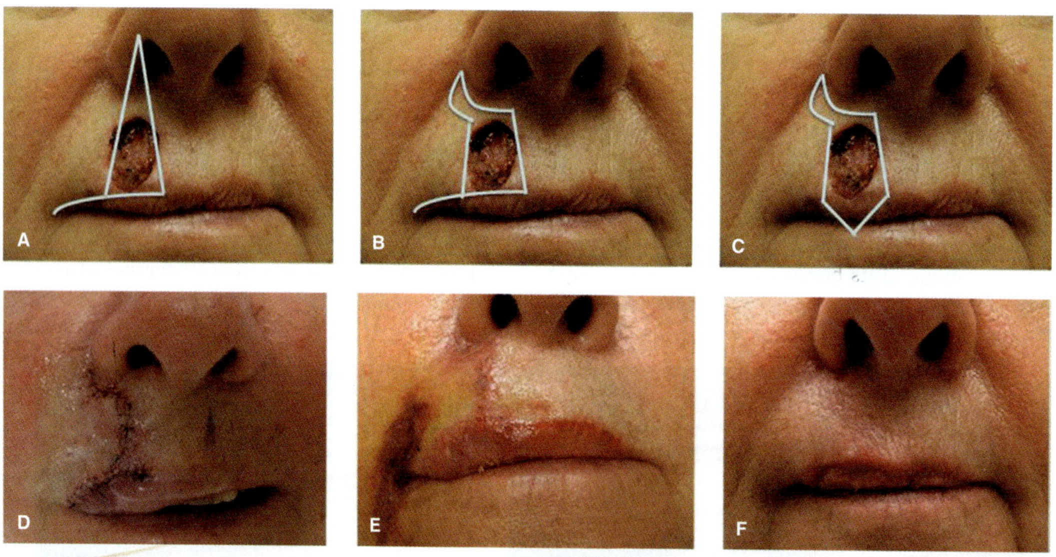

Figure 18-8 Crescentic advancement flap on the upper lip. **A.** Classically designed advancement flap would violate the cosmetic boundaries of the nose. **B.** Crescentic modification with incisions along the nasal sill and alar crease. **C.** Alternative design with removal of inferior cone through the mucosal lip. **D.** Final wound closure. **E.** Suture removal 1 week. **F.** Follow-up 3 months. Note the well-hidden incision line along the alar crease, vertical lip line, and vermillion border. One disadvantage of this advancement flap design is the potential for fullness along the mucosal lip. This is due to tissue redundancy along the mucosa when the flap is advanced in the horizontal axis. This usually improves with time but the redundancy can be removed with a small elliptical excision that can be hidden in the mucosal lip. To avoid lip fullness, rather than displacing the inferior cone horizontally along the vermillion border, one could alternatively extend the redundant cone of tissue through the uninvolved vermillion border to the mucosal lip. However, meticulous care must be taken to realign the vermillion border. In this patient, the fullness improved significantly with time and she declined any revisions. She also developed a small suture granuloma at the squared off portion of the flap that resolved with removal of the suture and intralesional kenalog.

any elevation of adjacent tissue or the necessity of removing an additional dog-ear due to secondary movement.

HELICAL ADVANCEMENT FLAP

The helical advancement flap is particularly useful for repairing helical defects involving the skin and cartilage of the mid-to-superior helix, and not occupying more than 30% of the helical circumference. The robust vascular supply to the posterior helix allows for long incisions to be made along the helical sulcus and, if necessary, through cartilage, leaving the postauricular helical skin intact with minimal risk of flap necrosis.[2] Burow's triangles can be excised from the lobule and less frequently the scapha to facilitate movement. A large postauricular standing cone is also excised. Compared to wedge repairs, the helical advancement flap preserves the natural contour of the ear and minimizes the reduction in its size. A less frequently used technique involves making a full-thickness incision along the anterior and posterior aspects of the helical sulcus. Although simpler to perform, this design has a more precarious blood supply because of the narrow pedicle of the flap. In either design, to prevent a reduction in the size of the lobule, rather than removing the Burow's triangle, a Z-plasty modification can be used.[3]

EXECUTION OF THE HELICAL ADVANCEMENT FLAP (WITH POSTAURICULAR SKIN INTACT, Fig. 18-9)

1. Extend the helical defect to the helical sulcus. Square off the margins of the wound to allow for optimal reapproximation of the helical rim and to prevent notching.
2. Incise through anterior helical skin and, if necessary, through cartilage inferiorly along the helical sulcus from the defect to the lobule. Undermine along the postauricular sulcus to maintain the broad postauricular vascular pedicle.
   a. If the defect is along the mid- or inferior portion of the helical rim, an incision can be made through and through the skin to create a thin helical pedicle.
3. To prevent helical rim notching, the epidermis along the helical rim should be hypereverted with vertical mattress sutures.
4. Redundant lobule skin
   a. Can be removed as a Burow's triangle at the lobule
   b. Modification: A Z-plasty incision can be made at the lobule to remove the redundancy without a reduction in the size of the lobule (Fig. 18-10).

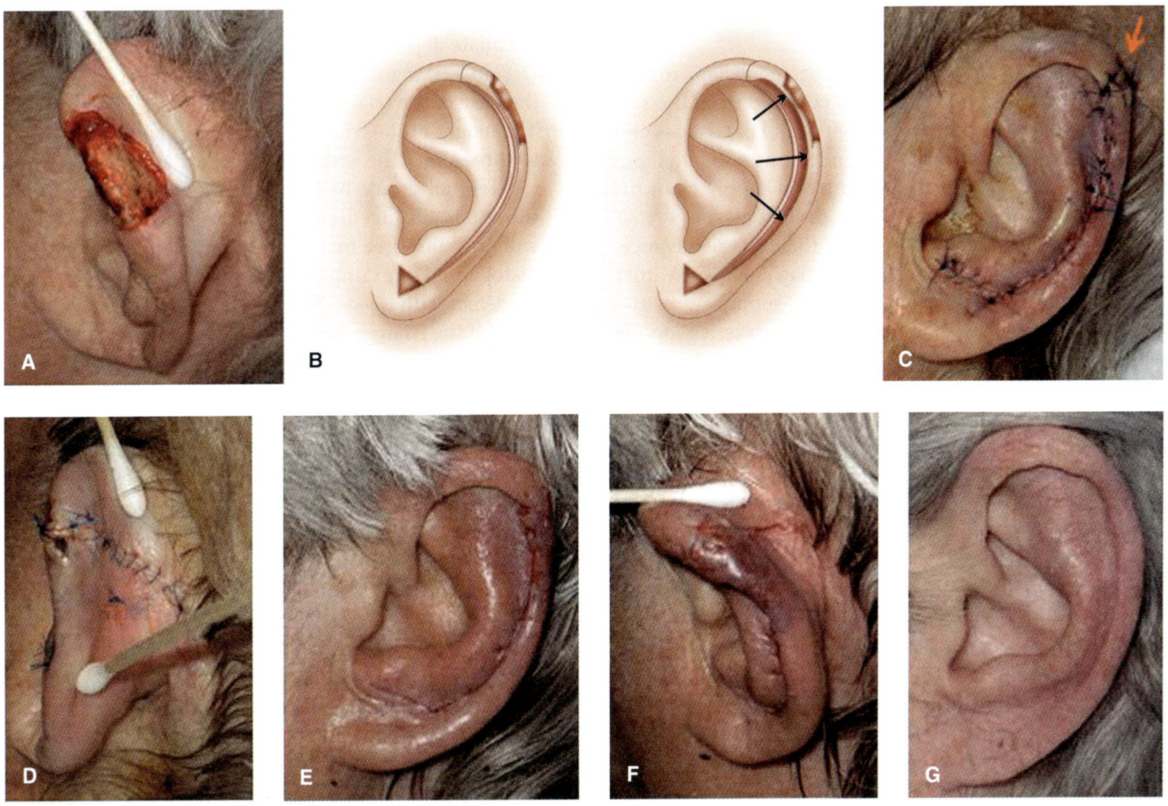

Figure 18-9 Helical advancement flap. **A.** Post Mohs defect. **B.** Design of the helical advancement flap with incision made along the helical sulcus through the dermis and cartilage, preserving the posterior cutaneous pedicle base. A Burow's triangle is excised at the lobule to facilitate movement. A large postauricular standing cone is excised. **C, D.** Final wound closure. Note the incision line hides along the helical sulcus. Vertical mattress sutures are used to close the epidermis along the helical rim to prevent notching (see arrow). **E, F.** Suture removal at 10 days. **G.** Final appearance at 3 months.

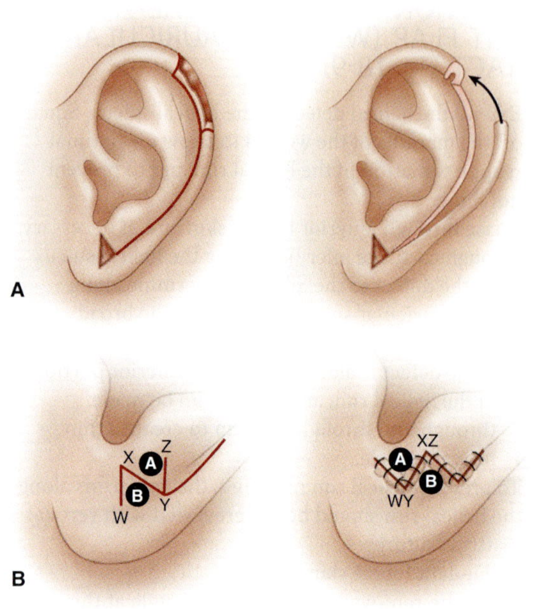

Figure 18-10 Modification to the helical advancement flap. **A.** Incision made through and through the skin. **B.** Z-plasty at the lobule to prevent reduction in the size of the lobule.

V-TO-Y FLAP (ISLAND PEDICLE FLAP, KITE FLAP)

V-to-Y flaps differ from other advancement flaps in that they have no epidermal or dermal connection to the surrounding tissue. Rather, a triangular island of tissue is created with a deep pedicle to the underlying subcutaneous fat and muscle. Due to their rich blood supply from the underlying vessels rather than the dermal plexus, V-to-Y flaps are less prone to flap necrosis than classic advancement flaps. The classic island pedicle flap denotes a V-to-Y flap harvested from a particular arterial supply.

V-to-Y flaps may be a useful reconstructive option when excessive tension prevents side-to-side closure of the defect and/or when volume restoration is required at site of tissue loss. The V-to-Y flap is also tissue-sparing and eliminates the need for standing cone resection altogether. Two-dimensionally, one of the cones in a linear closure is advanced into the surgical defect. The secondary defect is then repaired in a side-to-side fashion. The triangular geometric shape of the repair may at times become conspicuous. Because of this tendency, the V-to-Y flap is classically used for superior lip defects, as one or more limbs of the flap can be hidden in existing cosmetic junction lines, namely the lip margin and nasolabial fold. The incisions should have an angle of approximately 30 degrees between them, to avoid standing cone removal, and the height of the triangle should be roughly 2 to 3 times the width of the flap and defect. Proper design, undermining, and impeccable suture placement are of utmost importance to minimize a kite-shaped, unnatural scar.

V-to-Y flaps are ideal for repairing deep defects as they have a thick base of subcutaneous and muscular tissue. If oversized or if adjacent tissue is not undermined, this flap is prone to pin-cushioning due to wound contraction. When this occurs, it usually resolves with time, massage, and intralesional corticosteroids. To reduce the chance of trapdoor deformity, the surrounding tissue should be widely undermined to allow for the secondary motion of the skin to flatten the flap. The flap must also be carefully sized and slightly inset which occurs naturally due to the tension on the flap that occurs with advancement. Buried vertical mattress sutures can be helpful in bringing the pedicle below the level of the surrounding skin. Although undersizing the flap can minimize trap-dooring, the flap should instead be sized to fill the defect when it is located near a free margin. When the primary movement of the flap is toward the defect along the free margin, secondary movement in the opposition direction can produce anatomic distortion. Some authors advocate squaring off the defect rather than rounding off the tip of the flap, as an angulated flap may create less pin-cushioning.[4]

Flap mobility is dependent on the vertical restraint of the pedicle as well as the skin laxity. Often, the leading edge (1–3 mm) and tapered tail (distal 1/3 of flap) must be freed to remove any tethering restraints on the flap. When mobilized properly, V-to-Y flaps can traverse a much greater distance than other types of advancement flaps that are hindered by their cutaneous attachments.

EXECUTION OF V-TO-Y FLAP (Figs. 18-11 and 18-12)

1. Remove excess tissue from the wound base to ensure adequate depth to accommodate the flap
2. Design a triangular flap adjacent to the defect, with the base of the triangle being the edge of the defect. The height of the triangle should be roughly two to three times the width of the defect and flap. The tapered tail should be sufficiently long that, once the flap is advanced, closure of the secondary defect will not cause free margin or other anatomical distortion. For example, when repairing an upper lip defect with a V-to-Y flap, be sure to extend the apex of the triangle below the lateral commissure to minimize the risk of pulling the free margin of the lip upward. The angle between the two limbs should be about 30 degrees. Incise the two limbs through the epidermis and dermis to the subcutaneous plane.
   i. Modification: The tapered tail can be gently curved to rest on the adjacent cosmetic junction line.
3. Undermine widely in the surrounding subcutaneous plane. Slightly undermine the leading edge and tapered tail of the flap to allow adequate mobility.
4. Undermine the flap itself with blunt, vertical undermining to liberate it along its muscular pedicle. Elevate it and move it into the defect. Free any tethered subcutaneous restraints as needed to allow adequate movement.
   i. Modification: The flap can be rotated on its pedicle, with care, as much as 180 degrees before insetting.
5. Inset the flap with buried (vertical mattress) sutures.
6. Trim excess tissue if needed to slightly undersize the flap to minimize "pin-cushioning." Consider squaring off the defect rather than rounding the tip.

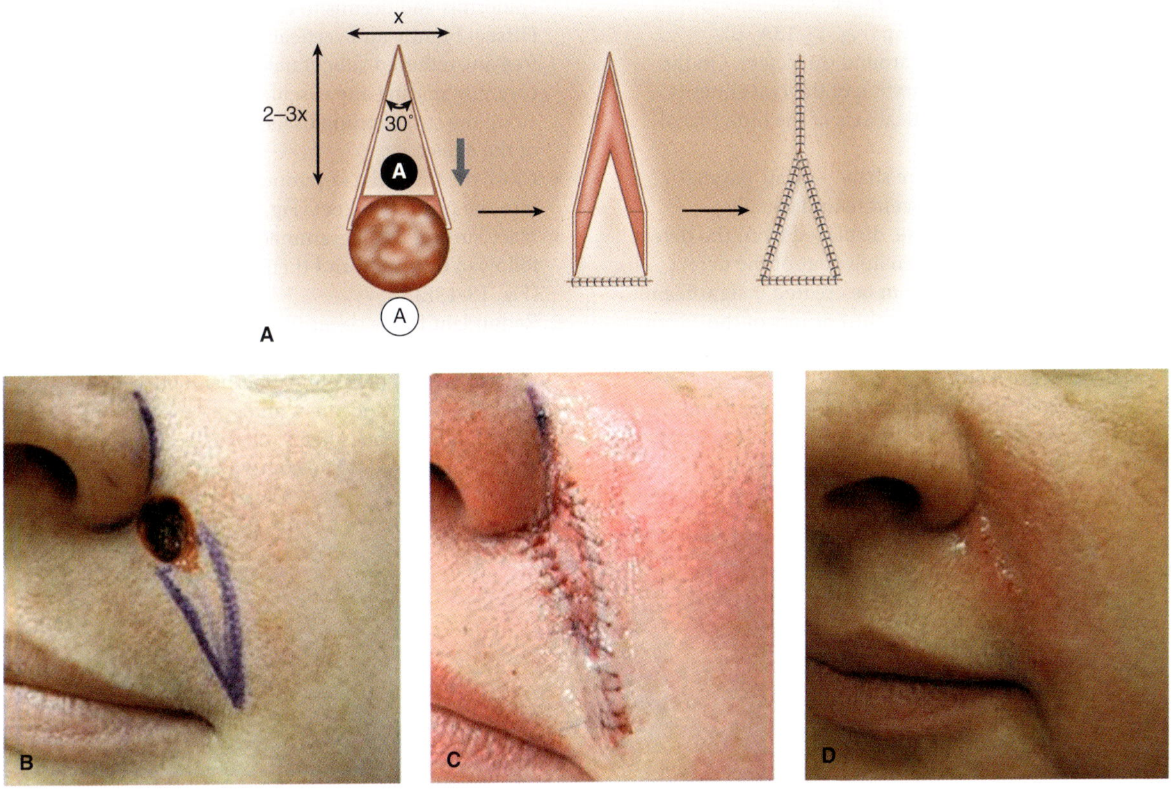

Figure 18-11 **A.** V-to-Y advancement flap.

7. Close the secondary defect and approximate the epidermal margins.

KEYSTONE FLAP

A modification to the V-to-Y flap, the Keystone fasciocutaneous flap, is designed as a curvilinear trapezoidal shape with a broader pedicle of subcutaneous fat and a minimal muscular base, making it ideal for large defect closures on the lower extremity.[5,6] Unlike primary closures that can cause undue tension to the wound and depression in the scar, the Keystone flap tends to maintain the natural convexity of the skin due to its thick pedicle base and standing tissue cone avoidance. The keystone flap is also superior to skin grafting, which tends to create atrophic and hypopigmented wounds with poorer overall survival.

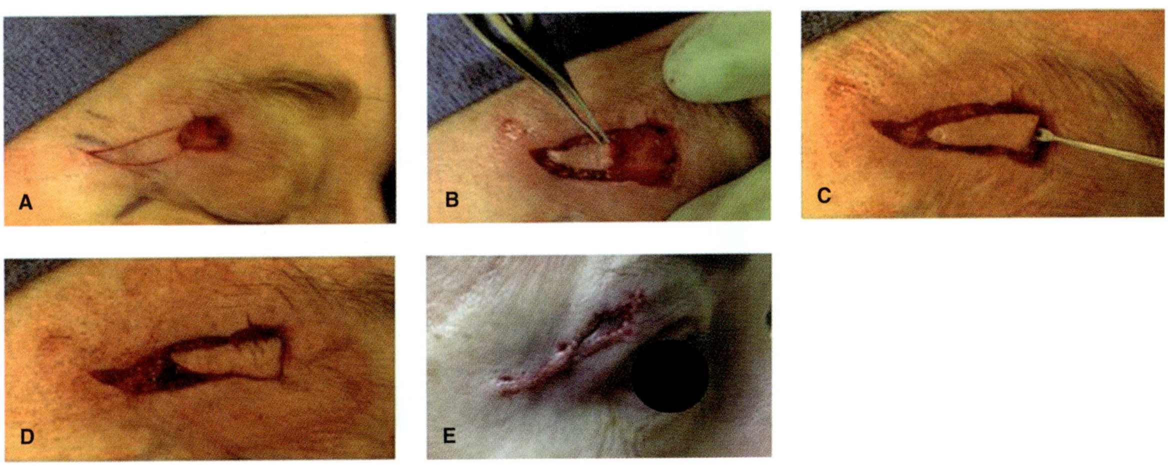

Figure 18-12 V-to-Y advancement flap. **A.** Triangular flap design with incision made through the epidermis and dermis to the subcutaneous plane. **B.** Elevate the flap by freeing any vertical restraints to liberate it along its muscular pedicle. Slightly undermine the leading edge and tapered tail to maximize movement. **C, D.** Move and inset the flap into the defect with buried sutures. **E.** Final wound closure.

EXECUTION OF KEYSTONE FLAP (Fig. 18-13)

1. To design the keystone flap (Fig. 18-13A, B)
   a. Draw a classic ellipse around the defect. On the extremities, the orientation of the two cones is usually along the vertical axis of the limb (distal and proximal)
   b. To create the keystone shape – draw parallel curvilinear lines adjacent to and usually posterior to the ellipse, displaced from the defect by a distance approximately that of the defect width. (A larger flap can be created if significant tension is anticipated). The corners of the keystone shape should be designed at an angle of 90 degrees.
2. Excise the elliptical shape around the defect and remove excess tissue from the wound base to extend the depth through the subcutis. (Fig. 18-13C)
3. Incise along the entire keystone flap through the epidermis and dermis to the subcutaneous fat. Dissect bluntly and vertically down to the fascia to free any tethered subcutaneous fibrous attachments, carefully sparing any vascular bundles. Undermine along the surrounding tissues on the opposing side of the defect.
4. Close the tip of the keystone first to advance the flap into the primary defect (Fig. 18-13D).
5. Place sutures as diagrammed to align the flap, followed by buried and then epidermal sutures (Fig. 18-13E).
6. Redundant tissue cones tend to be quite large for this flap and at the superior and inferior ends of the flap are oriented almost perpendicular to the direction of advancement and greatest tension. Excising these cones helps to transfer flap tension and ensures good tissue contours (Fig. 18-13F).

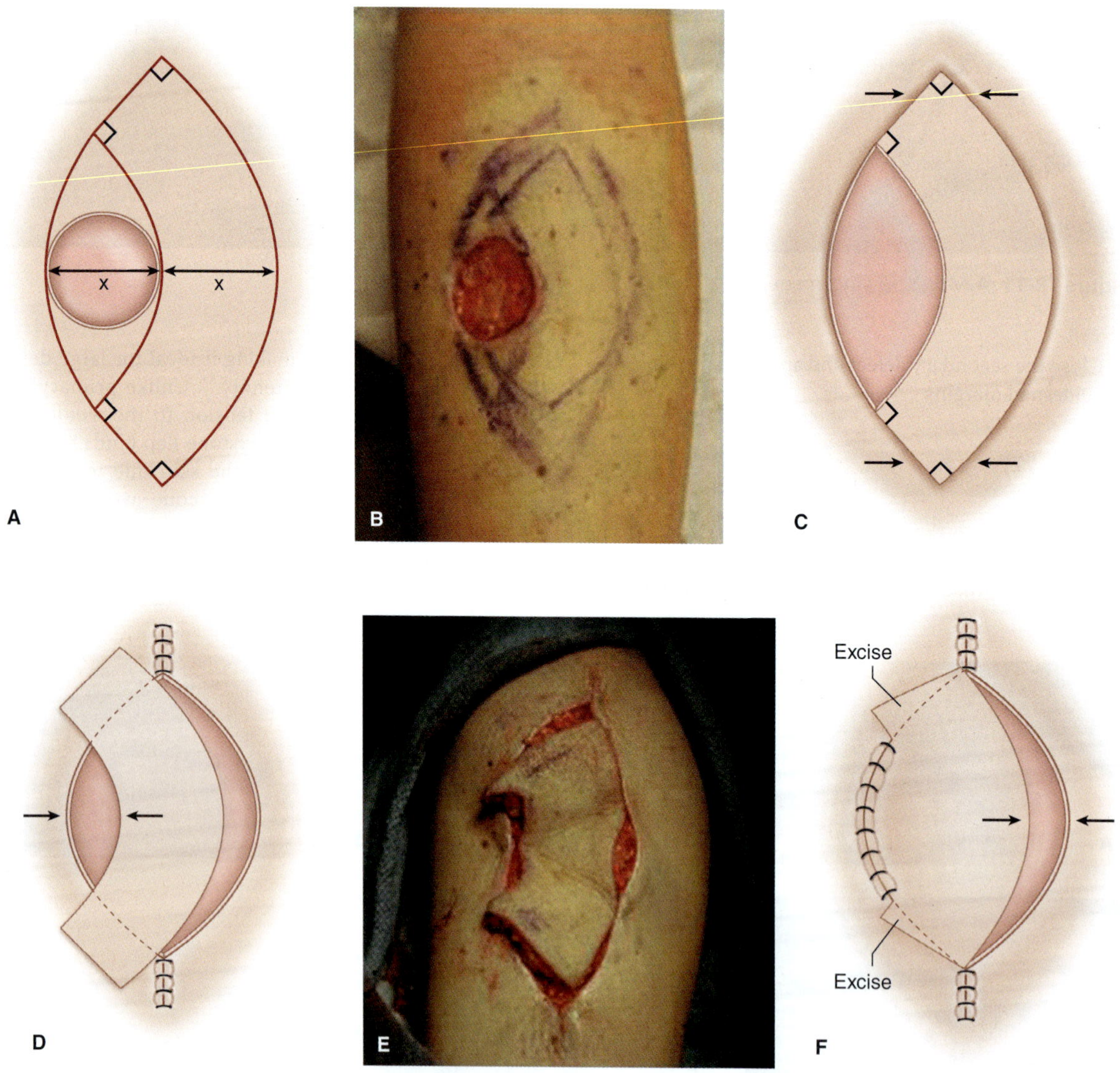

Figure 18-13 Keystone Flap. **A, B.** Keystone shape design with the width of the flap approximately that of the defect. The corner of the keystone shape should be 90 degrees. **C.** Excise the elliptical shape around the defect and incise along the keystone flap to the subcutis. Undermine along the surrounding tissue to mobilize the flap. **D, E.** Close the tip of the keystone first to advance the flap then place key sutures to align the flap. **F.** Excise redundant tissue cones at the superior and inferior ends of the flap. *(continued)*

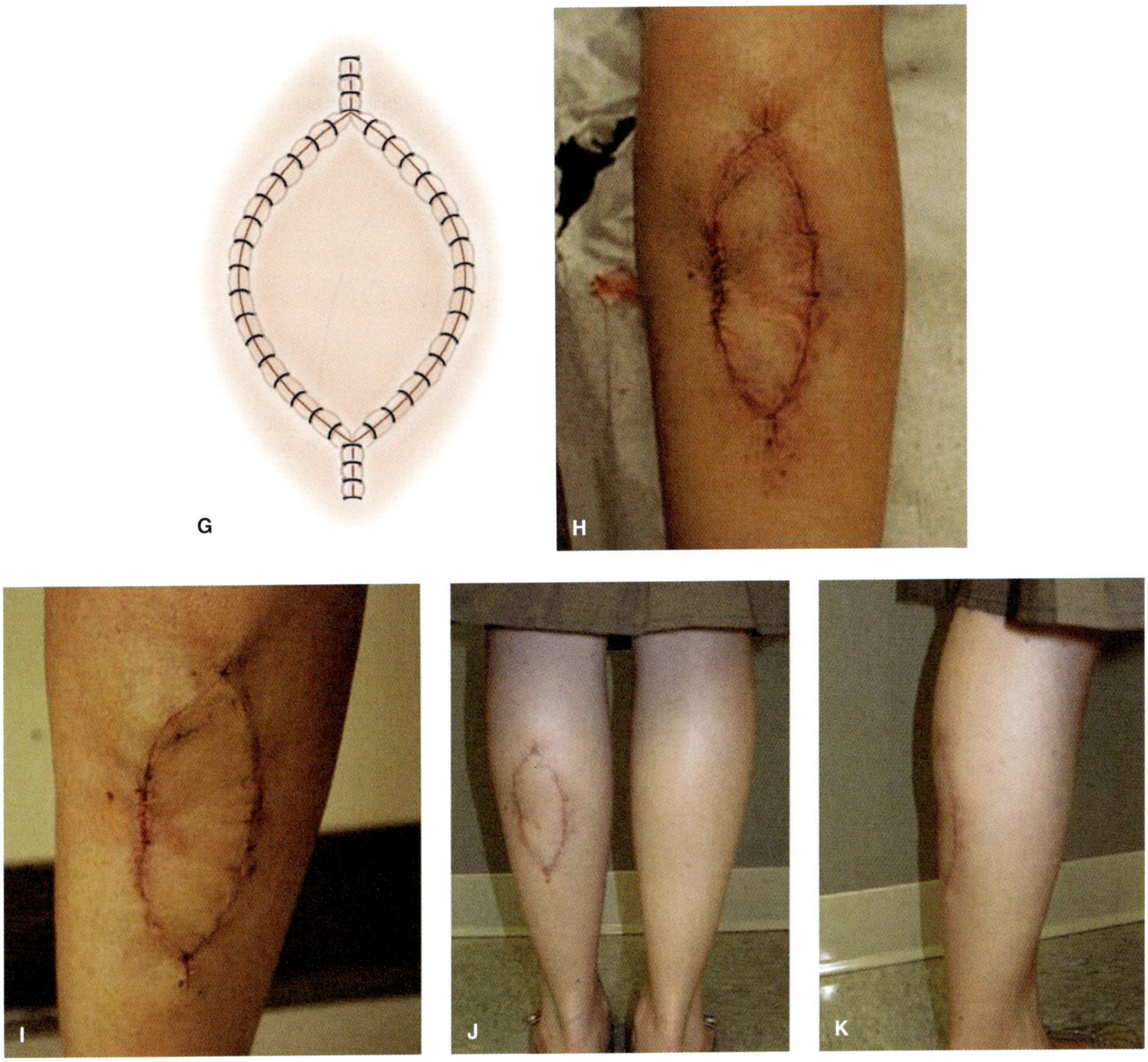

Figure 18-13 (*Continued*) **G, H.** Final wound closure. I. Suture removal at 2 weeks. **J, K.** Final appearance at 3 months. Note restoration of the natural contour of the calf.

ROTATION FLAPS

Rotation flaps rotate along an arc from the donor site to an adjacent recipient area around a pivot point. These broadly based flaps have an ample blood supply and are ideally suited for locations with an abundant surrounding tissue reservoir that may be lacking in tissue laxity. The superior viability of these flaps makes them particularly useful for repairing large defects when tissue sparing is important, such as along the lateral cheek and scalp. The curved incision lines hide well along naturally curvilinear cosmetic boundaries, relaxed skin tension lines, and the hairline.

There are several disadvantages to a rotation flap. While the tension vector is distributed along the curvilinear line of the closure, the tension vector is greatest along the flap tip. Significant tension placed at the tip may cause undesirable secondary motion, especially near a free margin. This is compounded by pivotal restraint, defined as the inherent stiffness of the tissue that limits the flap's movement at the pivot point. Several factors affect pivotal restraint: inelasticity of the skin, as in scalp skin; poorly arced rotations and broadly based flaps, especially when the incisions are not long enough to provide adequate movement; and highly arced rotations which shorten the effective length of the flap. A flap that rotates 45 degrees results in a 5% reduction in length; a 90 degrees rotation creates a 15% reduction in length (Fig. 18-14A). To minimize tip tension, the rotation arc design may need to be oversized and offset (Fig. 18-14B).[7] Undermining deeply beneath the pivot point relieves pivotal restraint and improves flap mobility, as does a backcut into the flap. Caution must be taken not to compromise the vascular supply of the flap pedicle with either of these two maneuvers.

UNILATERAL ROTATION FLAP

Several general rules are helpful in the design of a rotation flap. First, the circular defect can be converted to a triangular defect with at least a 2:1 height to width ratio.

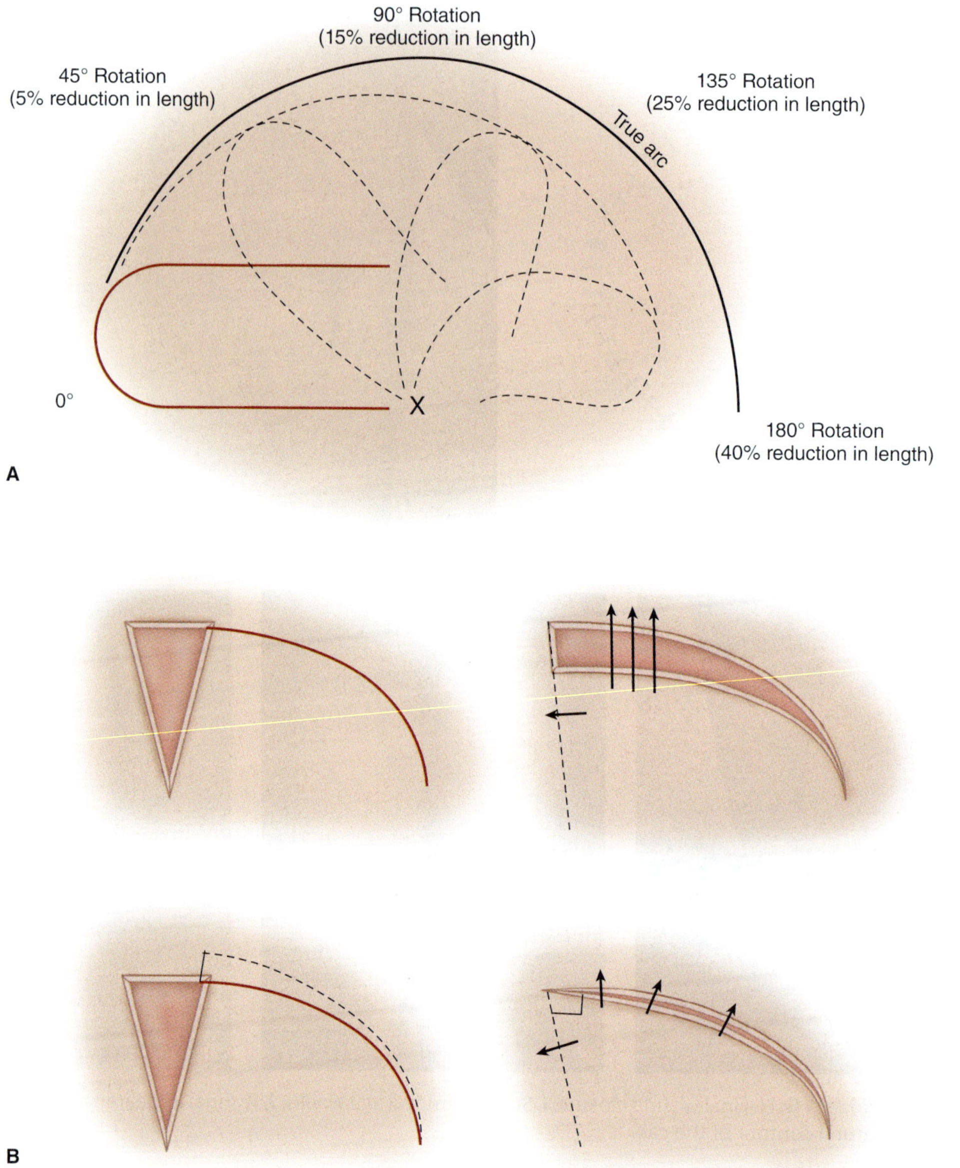

Figure 18-14 **A.** Rotation flap demonstrating pivotal restraint. Solid line denotes a true semicircular arc. Dash line demonstrates the actual path of the rotation flap as it rotates around the pivotal point "X". As the flap rotates into place, its effective length shortens. The greater the rotation, the shorter the flap length. **B.** The highest tension is along the tip of the flap. To reduce tension, a flap may need to be oversized to compensate for its predictable shortening.

This avoids the need to remove an additional standing cone at the base of the triangle. Next, the length of the flap should be designed along natural skin tension lines. A long-flap incision is usually required to maximize movement and minimize tension. The flap length is generally at least four times the height of a triangular defect on the face and at least six times the height of a defect on the scalp.

Narrow rotation flaps with a more acute arc of rotation have decreased pivotal restraint but a tendency for wider secondary defects and increased secondary tension. Wider flaps with a broader arc of rotation create more pivotal restraint but reduce the size of the secondary defect, which minimizes wound closure tension and secondary motion (Fig. 18-15).[8] Removal of the Burow's triangle is not limited to the tail of the arc; rather, it can be excised anywhere along the length of the flap that is cosmetically suitable. Redundant tissue can also be evened out by applying the "rule of halves" (Fig. 18-16).

BILATERAL ROTATION FLAPS AND O-TO-Z FLAPS

Bilateral rotation flaps are required when there is insufficient tissue reservoir and/or laxity for a unilateral flap.

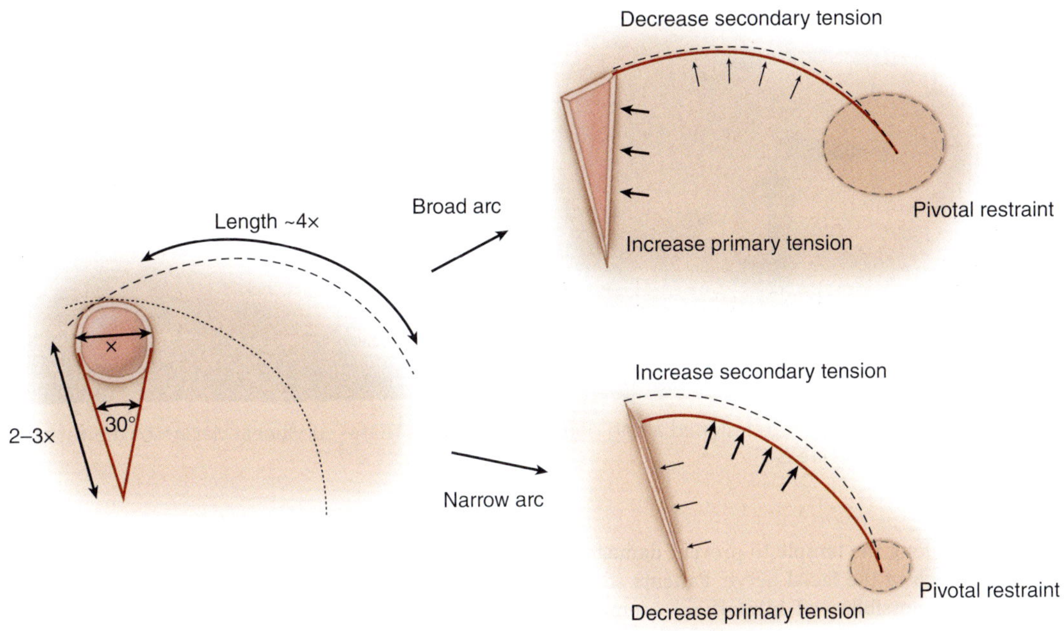

Figure 18-15 The role of rotational arc design on pivotal restraint and secondary tension. A broad arc of rotation creates a broader-based flap with increased pivotal restraint which reduces primary movement of the flap. This result in a smaller secondary defect and decreased secondary tension. On the other hand, a more acute arc of rotation creates a narrow-based flap with reduced pivotal restraint and increased primary movement, but results in a wider secondary defect and increased secondary tension.

Locations with limited skin mobility, such as the scalp, often benefit from utilizing bilateral tissue reservoirs. Bilateral rotation flaps can be designed along one rotation arc (classically along the mental crease, Fig. 18-17) or opposing arcs as in an O-to-Z rotation flap (often used on the scalp, Figs. 18-18 and 18-19).

MUSTARDE ROTATION FLAP

Described specifically for large mid-to-lateral cheek and lower eyelid defects, this laterally based rotation flap mobilizes redundant adjacent tissue along the lateral cheek and temple. To prevent ectropion, all tension at the defect site is directed horizontally. Vertical tension is prevented by creating a flap that arcs superolateral to the lateral canthus and is anchored there to support the lower lid. As the flap rotates into place, pivotal restraint shortens it. Extending the curvilinear design superior to the lateral canthus prevents the shortening of the flap that inevitably occurs due to pivotal restraint as it rotates into place (Fig. 18-20). The flap should be elevated above the orbicularis oculi muscle medially and in the superficial

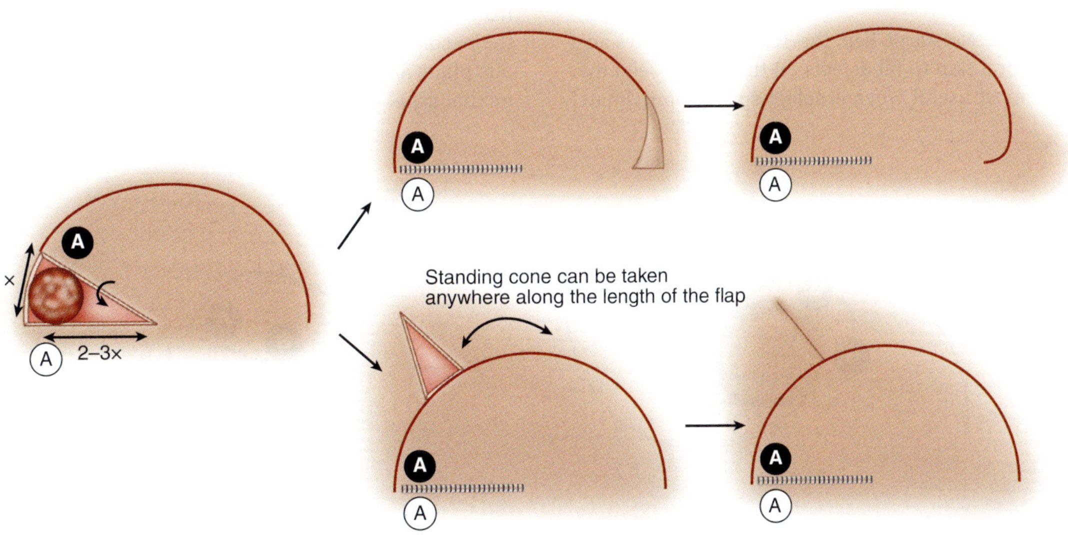

Figure 18-16 Rotation flap design. Redundancy can be removed with a backcut or standing cone anywhere along the length of the flap.

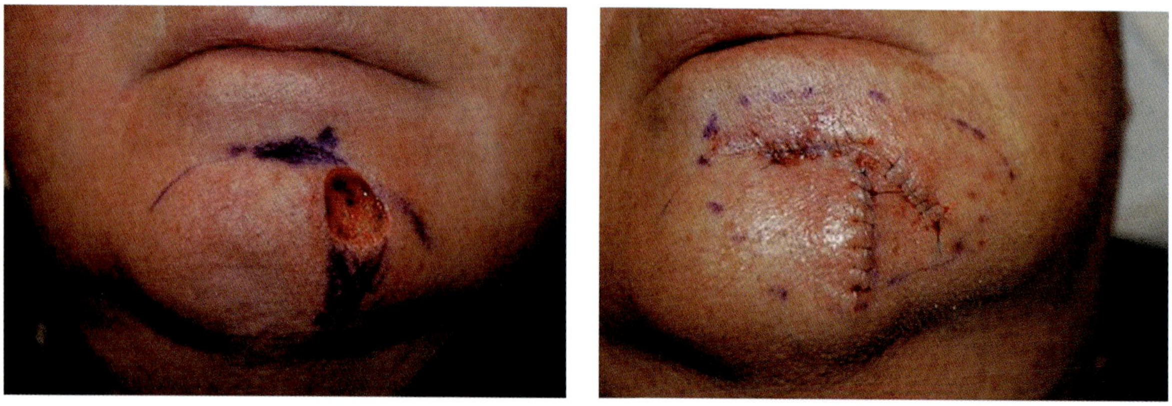

Figure 18-17 Bilateral rotation flap designed along one rotation arc. Note the curvilinear design of the rotational flap hides nicely along the mental crease.

subcutaneous fat along the temple to prevent damage to the temporal branch of the facial nerve. Patients should be warned of the possibility of infraorbital edema for several weeks due to obstruction of the laterally draining lymphatic channels.

EXECUTION OF THE MUSTARDE FLAP

1. The flap incision is made at the superior aspect of the defect laterally along the lower eyelid. Beginning at the lateral canthus, this vector extends superolaterally toward the temple. The incision then curves downward laterally just in front of the hairline and ear.
2. The flap is elevated just above the orbicularis oculi muscle medially and in the subcutaneous and supra-SMAS zone everywhere else.
3. If a large cheek and temple rotation flap is required, a periosteal suspension suture placed along the lateral orbital rim may be useful to prevent ectropion.

TENZEL SEMICIRCULAR ROTATION FLAP

Similar to the Mustarde flap, the Tenzel flap rotates adjacent temporal skin to fill defects on the lower eyelid margin. It is most useful when a defect spans approximately 50% of the lower lid. A semicircular flap is designed at the lateral canthus curving superolaterally to the temple (Fig. 18-21). To prevent ectropion, the flap should be designed with generous vertical height to support the lower lid. A flattened flap will likely pull the lid downward. A lateral canthotomy and a lower cantholysis are usually required to slide the lateral portion of the lid medially and to maximize the movement of the flap. The canthotomy is performed by creating a slightly superiorly directed horizontal incision along the lateral canthal tendon down to its periosteal insertion at Whitnall's tubercle. The inferior cantholysis is then achieved by severing the lower crus of the tendon. Finally, it is important to anchor the flap along the periosteum of the lateral orbital rim to recreate the lateral canthus.

MEDIALLY BASED ROTATION FLAPS

Inferomedially based flaps recruit tissue from the lower cheek and nasolabial fold and are helpful for repairing smaller defects along the medial lower lid and nasal sidewall. The arc of rotation is drawn inferior to the defect along the nasal sidewall and inferior cheek, starting from the inferomedial aspect of the defect and ending in the nasolabial fold. Once undermined in the subcutaneous plane and elevated, the flap is "hung" at the superomedial aspect of the defect, often suspended from nasal

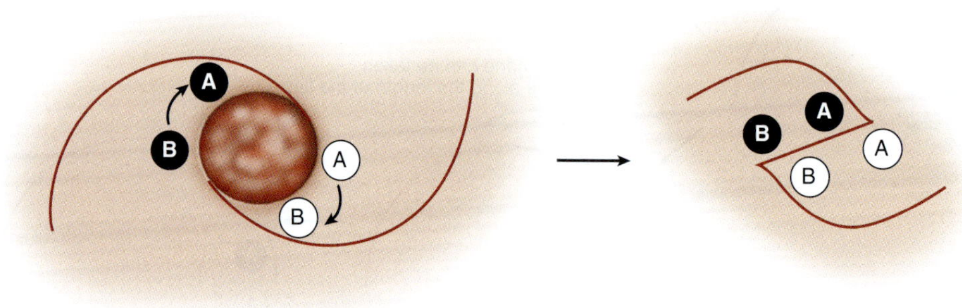

Figure 18-18 Bilateral rotation flap (O-to-Z plasty) designed on opposing rotation arcs.

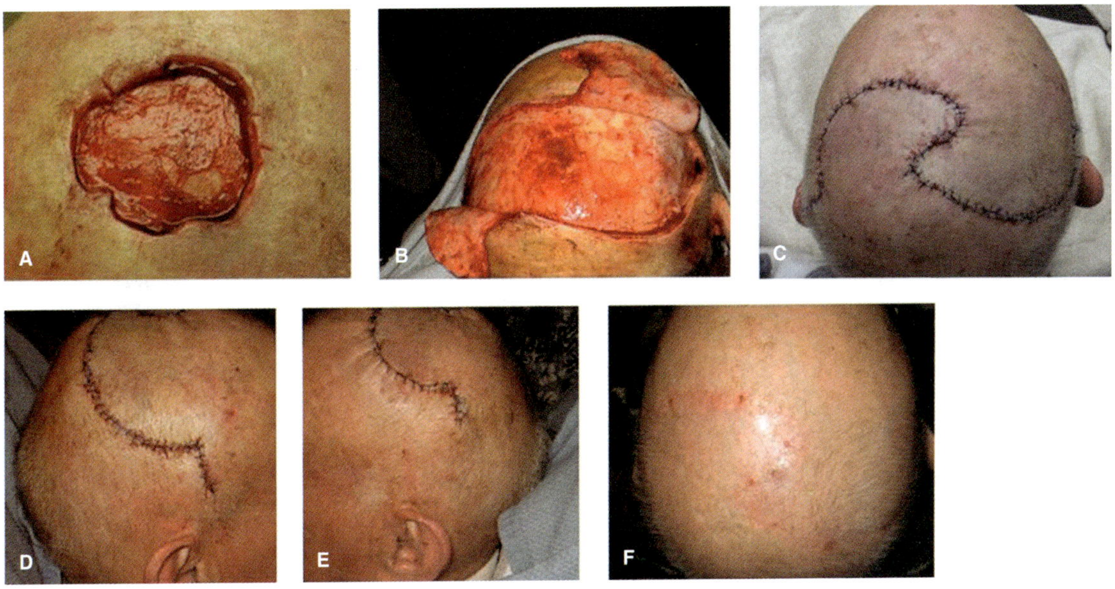

Figure 18-19 Bilateral rotation flap (O-to-Z plasty) for a large defect on the scalp. **A.** Post Mohs defect. **B.** The inelasticity of the scalp skin necessitates a large broadly based rotation flap design. Significant undermining is required to mobilize the flap. **C, D, E.** Final wound closure. **F.** Final appearance at 3 month follow-up.

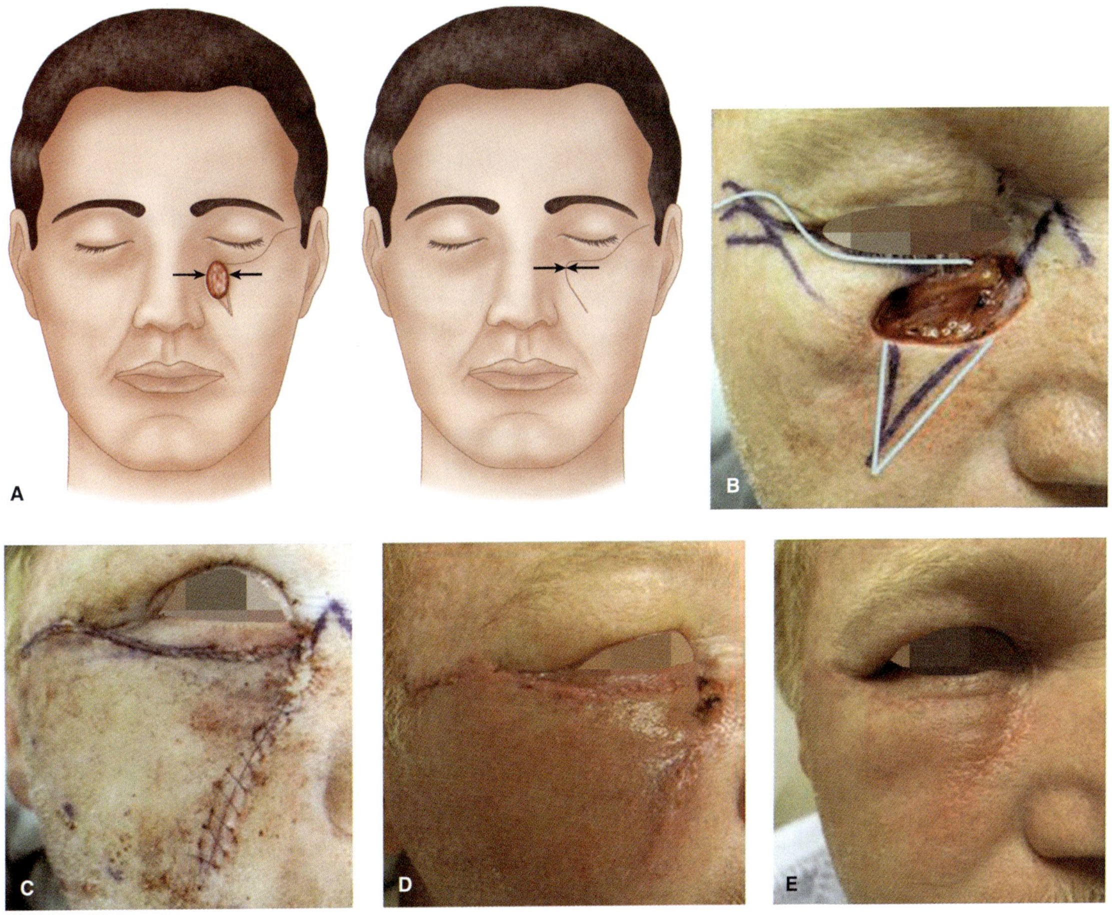

Figure 18-20 **A.** Laterally based cheek rotation flap (Mustarde flap). The primary movement is directed horizontally. A curvilinear design superior to the lateral canthus supports the lower lid. **B.** Post Mohs defect. **C.** Final wound closure. A small skin graft was placed medially to reduce tension to the flap. **D.** Suture removal at 1 week. **E.** Final appearance at 1 month with minimal residual infraorbital edema. There is minor webbing to the medial canthus which resolved with time and massage. Occasionally a Z-plasty may be required to correct more extensive medial canthal webbing.

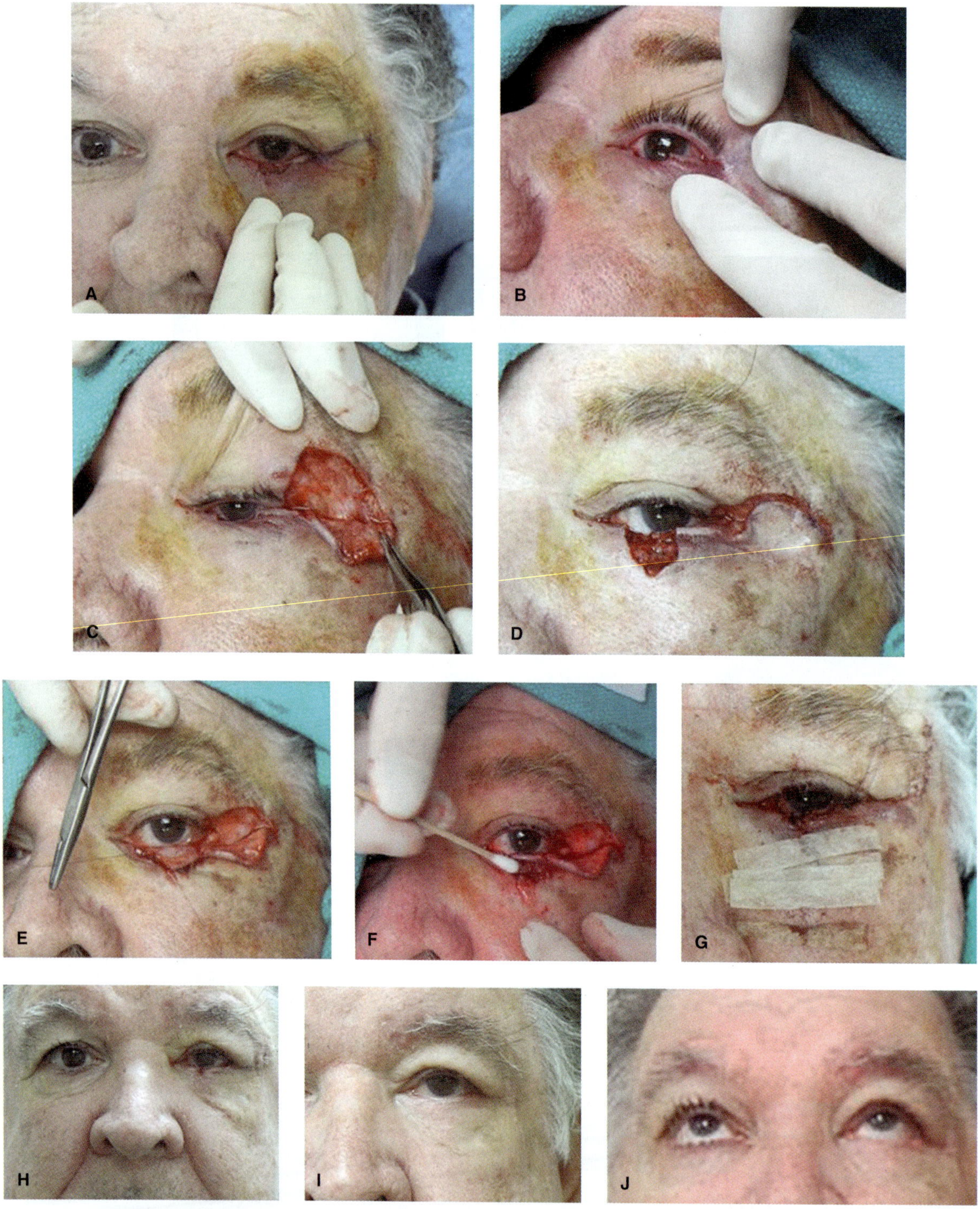

Figure 18-21 Tenzel semicircular rotation flap. **A.** Post Mohs defect on the lower eyelid margin. **B.** Lateral canthotomy to maximize movement of the flap. **C.** A semicircular incision is made from the lateral canthus, curving superolaterally to the temple. Undermine widely to the depth of the superficial temporalis fascia, careful not to damage the temporal branch of the facial nerve. **D.** Remove the redundant cone of tissue along the lower lid. **E.** Closure of the primary defect along the lower lid. Using a 6-0 silk suture, the lid margin should be reapproximated in a vertical mattress fashion to evert the edges. **F.** Closure of the secondary defect along the temple. **G.** Final wound closure. The suture along the lid margin should be left long and taped down with steri-strips to avoid contact with the cornea. **H.** Suture removal at 1 week. There is slight lid notching noted. **I, J.** One month follow-up with resolution of the lid notching. No ectropion is noted with the "Yawn test" – ask the patient to open his mouth and look up.

or infraorbital periosteum. A redundant cone of tissue is created and removed along the lower eyelid crease lateral to the defect. (Fig. 18-22A) Because the primary tension vector is directed vertically, the key stitch in this flap is a tacking or suspension suture which is critical to prevent ectropion.[9] Evaluation for ectropion should be performed during the repair by having the patient open his/her mouth and eyes and look upward (the "Yawn test"). Vertical tension on the lower eyelid necessitates replacement of the suspension suture. A crescentic modification of this flap places the incision line along the melolabial fold and nasofacial sulcus, avoiding the need to remove a standing cone on the inferior cheek (Fig. 18-22B).[10]

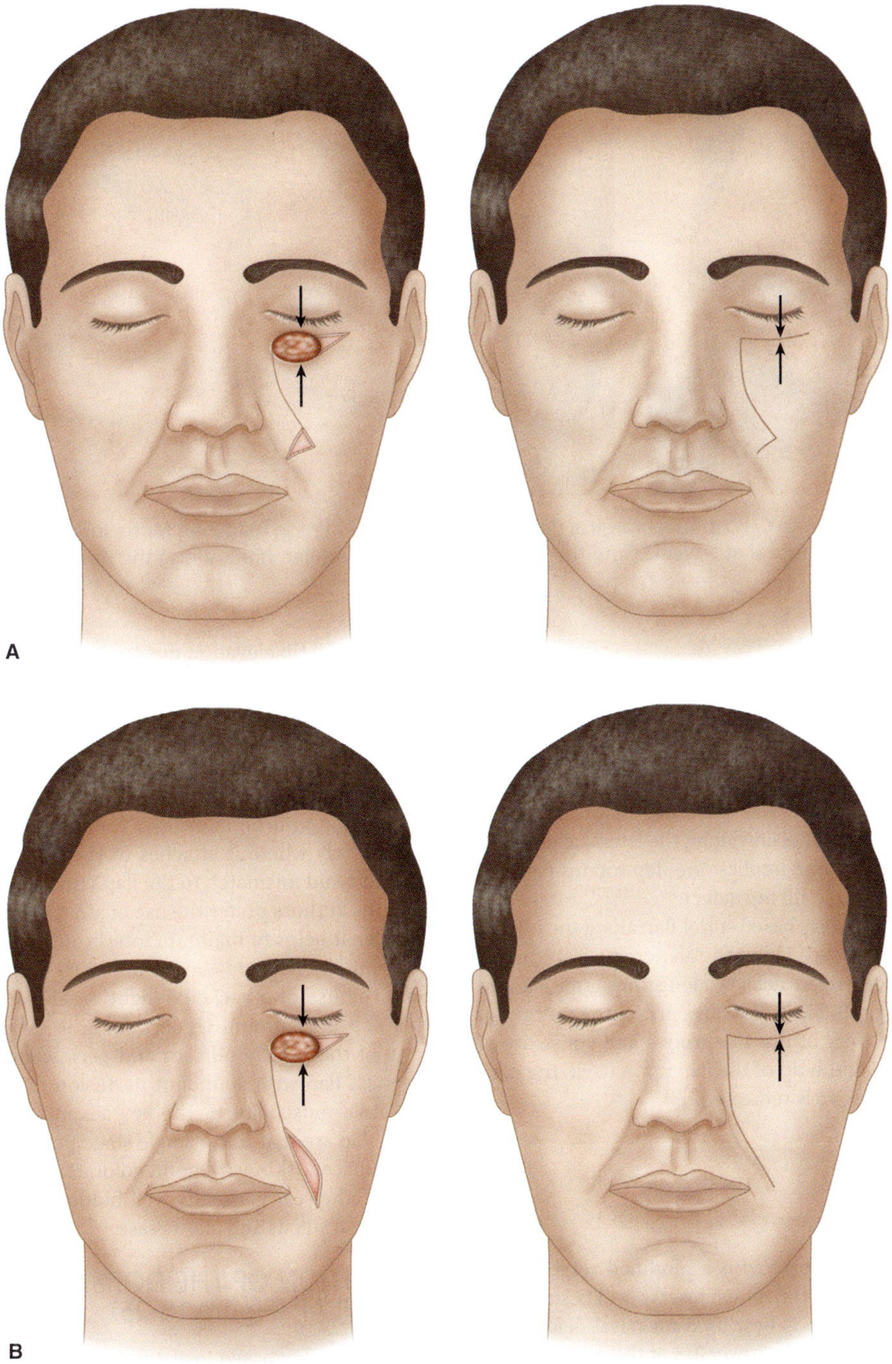

Figure 18-22 Medially based cheek rotation flap for short but wide defects. As the primary tension is vertically oriented, a tacking suture to the intraorbital periosteum is often required to prevent ectropion. **A.** Classic design. **B.** Crescentic modification to hide incision along the nasolabial fold and avoid removal of redundant cone. (*continued*)

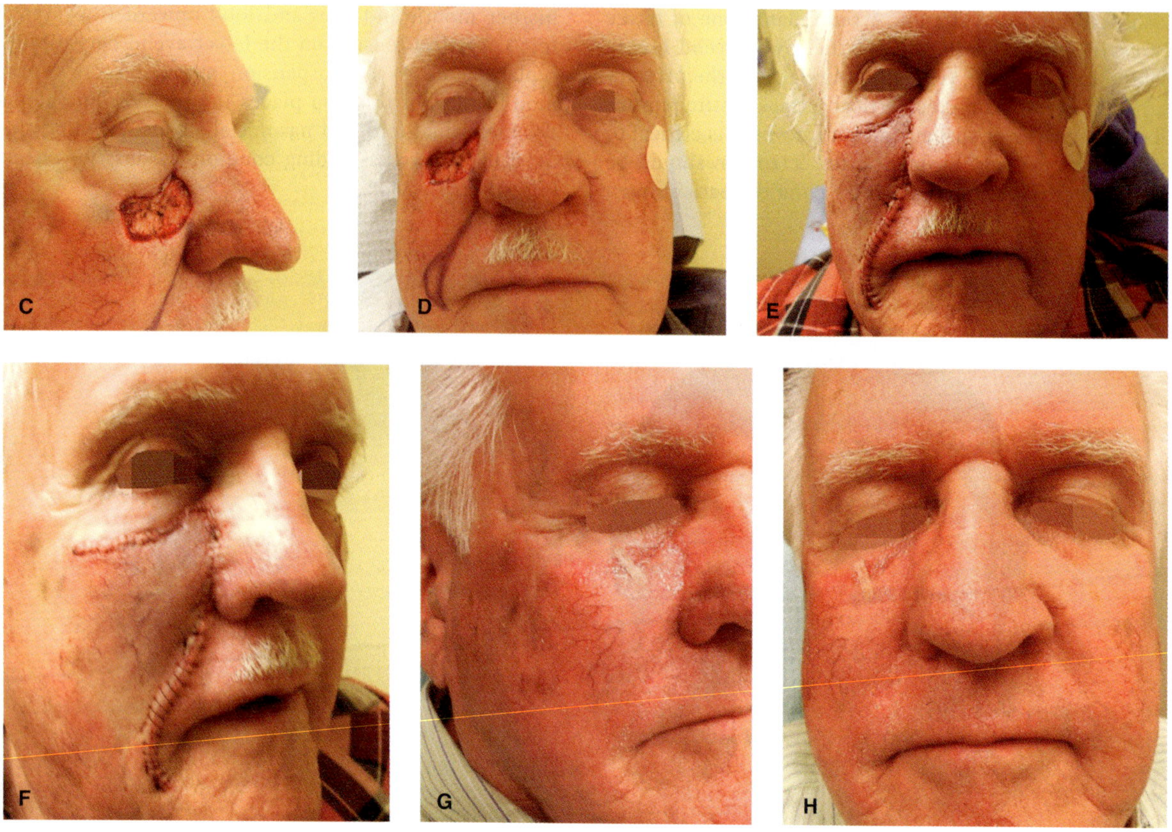

Figure 18-22 *(Continued)* **C.** Post-Mohs surgical defect. **D.** Preoperative design following Mohs surgery. **E, F.** Final wound closure. **G, H.** Suture removal at 1 week. Note the majority of the incision line hides along the nasolabial fold and lower lid crease.

NASAL SPIRAL FLAP

For small defects on the mid ala, a spiral flap designed along the alar groove allows closure of small defects involving no more than 50% of the anterior ala with perfectly matched skin. This flap prevents distortion of the alar rim and hides the incision along the lateral alar crease (Fig. 18-23). As its name implies, the flap rotates (spirals) upon itself at the tip to fill the defect.[11]

Similarly, a superiorly based spiral flap along the inferolateral nasal dorsum just above the alar crease is useful for small- to medium-sized defects along the nasal ala and alar groove (Fig. 18-24).[12] This flap prevents blunting of the natural concavity of the alar groove and convexity of the ala. By rotating the tip of the flap upon itself, the contour of the alar groove is recreated.

DORSAL NASAL ROTATION FLAP (REIGER/HATCHET FLAP)

The dorsal nasal rotation flap is a modified rotation flap that takes advantage of the robust reservoir of tissue in the glabellar area. This flap is best used for nasal defects less than 2.5 cm in width on the lower 2/3 of the nose, and can be contemplated when a defect on the distal third of the nose is too large for a bilobed flap and too small to warrant an interpolation flap. Ideally, the defect should be midline or paramedian and several millimeters away from the alar rim to avoid tip elevation due to flap shortening with rotation. However, some authors have reported good success repairing a full-thickness alar defect with the use of this flap.[13] The dorsal nasal flap is designed along the entire nasal dorsum/sidewall extending to the glabella. A backcut along the glabella results in a V-to-Y advancement, allowing the flap to drop inferiorly. The flap should be thinned aggressively where it attaches to the thinner medial canthus to avoid mismatch to the flap's thicker glabellar skin.

Some authors prefer the use of a Z-plasty at the glabella because it helps to maintain interbrow distance while still allowing for flap movement inferiorly (Fig. 18-25). Even with the use of a backcut, slight nasal tip elevation with this flap is common. Undermining is carried out at the level of the perichondrium and periosteum, making this a robust flap with abundant perfusion from the underlying nasal musculature. The key advantages of the dorsal nasal flap are that it is a single stage procedure and that it uses adjacent skin with good color, texture, and thickness match. The scar is usually well hidden along the glabella, nasofacial sulcus and alar crease.

EXECUTION OF THE DORSAL NASAL ROTATION FLAP (Figure 18-25)

1. Design a flap based ipsilateral to the defect to maximize flap rotation. Draw a curvilinear line from the inferior edge of the defect laterally to the nasofacial sulcus, extending upward to a point at least 5 mm medial to the medial canthus and

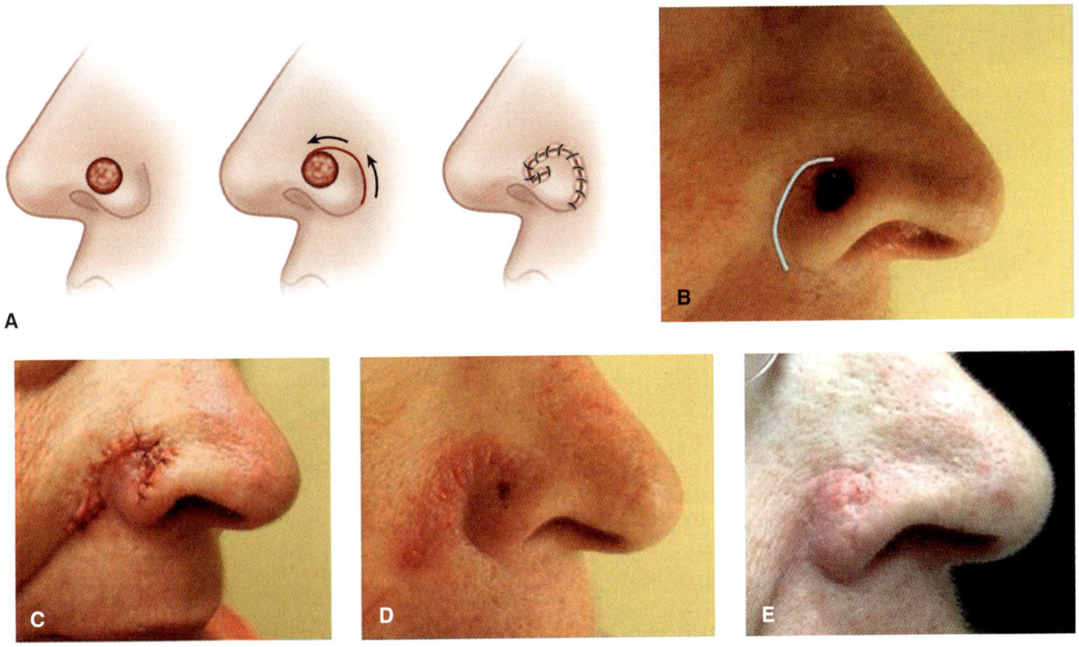

Figure 18-23 Spiral flap of the nose. **A.** Ala-based spiral flap for small defects on the ala. The incision hides along the alar crease. **B.** Mohs defect. **C.** Final wound closure. **D.** One week suture removal. **E.** One month follow-up. There is mild hypertrophic scarring present that resolved on its own over time. Occasionally, dermabrasion or laser resurfacing may be required to smooth out the scar.

into the glabellar crease. A backcut toward the contralateral medial canthus will improve flap mobility while hiding the scar in the glabellar crease.

2. The flap should be elevated in a submuscular plane above the periosteum and perichondrium on the nose to ensure a robust vascular supply. However, in the glabellar region, the flap should be harvested above the muscle and should include only skin, subcutaneous fat and a minimum of muscle. Further thinning of the flap may be necessary to prevent discrepancies in skin thickness, especially if the thick glabellar skin transfers to the medial canthal area.
3. The flap is broadly undermined across the entire nasal dorsum to the contralateral side prior to insetting. The surrounding tissue is also undermined to allow for secondary movement, especially at the nasal sidewall and the defect site. Minimal undermining occurs over the alar rim.
4. The donor site in the glabella should be closed first by V-to-Y advancement or Z-plasty. This will allow the flap to drop inferiorly into the defect.
5. Re-drape the flap and anchor it into place with deep sutures, making certain that there is no asymmetry or distortion of the nasal tip. Thereafter, inset the rest of the flap with buried sutures followed by epidermal sutures.

TRANSPOSITION FLAPS

Transposition flaps utilize a tissue reservoir adjacent to but not contiguous with the primary defect. By definition, the flap is lifted or transposed over a segment of intervening normal skin, and redirects and redistributes the tension vector for closure into a more desirable location within the secondary defect. Closure of the secondary defect effectively pushes the flap into the primary defect, leaving it relatively tension free. Thus, the main advantage of a transposition flap is displacement of the tension vector to a more acceptable location with mobilization of a noncontiguous adjacent skin reservoir for closure. Due to their geometric design, transposition flaps create multidirectional scars that may be less noticeable than the longer lines of rotation and advancement flaps. However, transposition flaps are more likely to produce a trap door deformity. This can be minimized with wide undermining of the defect and surrounding skin to create counterbalancing contractile forces that can help to flatten the flap.

Several important points should be considered when designing a transposition flap. First, these are pivotal flaps, much like rotation flaps, and one must therefore keep in mind the decrease in effective flap length that occurs with greater tissue movement. Lengthening of the flap may be required to account for this pivotal restraint. At the same time, one must avoid insetting oversized or bulky flaps, which are prone to pin-cushioning. The flap pedicle should ideally be oriented in an inferior direction to improve lymphatic drainage and reduce edema. Furthermore, the secondary defect should be closed first to reduce direct tension on the flap, to minimize free margin distortion, and to allow the flap to be pushed into the primary defect.

RHOMBIC FLAP

The classic Limberg rhombic flap redirects the tension vector by 90 degrees and creates a secondary defect perpendicular to the primary defect. Several variations of

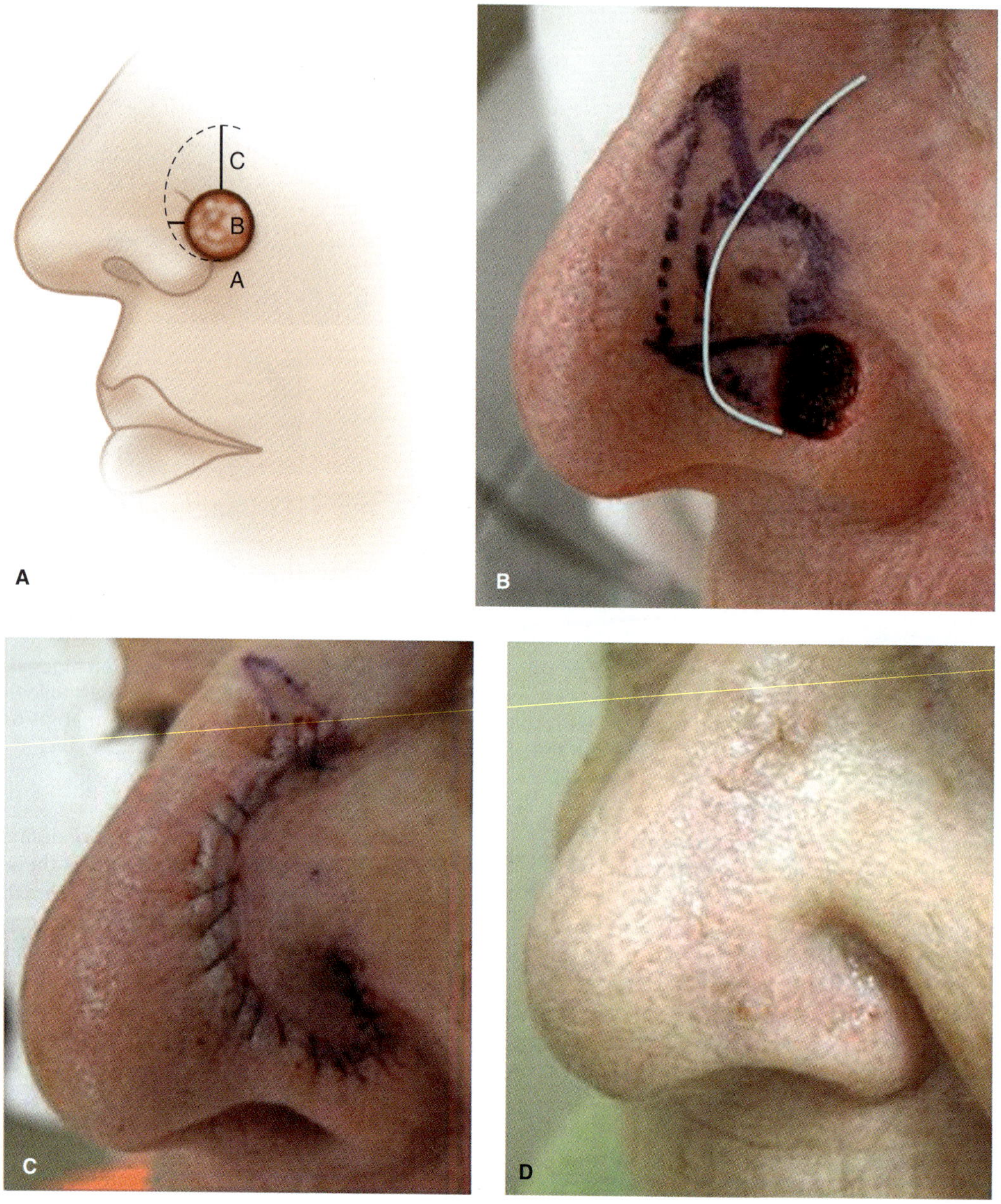

Figure 18-24 Superiorly based spiral flap along the lateral nasal dorsum for defects involving the ala and alar groove. **A, B.** Design of the spiral flap. Alternatives including a bilobed flap were considered but ultimately a spiral flap was chosen. **C.** Final wound closure. **D.** Suture removal 1 week.

rhombic flaps have been described, including the Dufourmental and Webster flaps. The classic Limberg flap starts with a rhombus-shaped defect with opposing tips at 60 degrees and 120 degrees. The flap is designed by extending a line from the short axis of the rhombus at a length of equal distance to the short axis. A second line is then drawn parallel to the side of the rhombus, creating a flap with a 60 degree tip. Closure of the secondary defect of the flap redirects the tension vector 90 degrees from the primary defect. With any rhombic flap, four possible flap designs can be created along the short axis (Fig. 18-26). The optimal flap design must take into account the local tissue reservoirs, free margins, and relaxed skin tension lines. These flaps are versatile and can be used in repairing defects along the nasal sidewalls, temple, and medial and lateral canthi. Large defects along the cheek and jawline can also be repaired with rhombic flaps (Fig. 18-27).

MODIFICATIONS TO THE RHOMBIC FLAP

Pivotal restraint limits movement of a rhombic flap and may create undue tip tension (Fig. 18-28A). This can be overcome by lengthening the leading edge of the flap to compensate for pivotal shortening (Fig. 18-28B). Alternatively, reducing the rotational arc of the flap also reduces pivotal restraint. The Dufourmental modification is designed by bisecting the angle between the extension of the short axis and the side of the defect to create the first

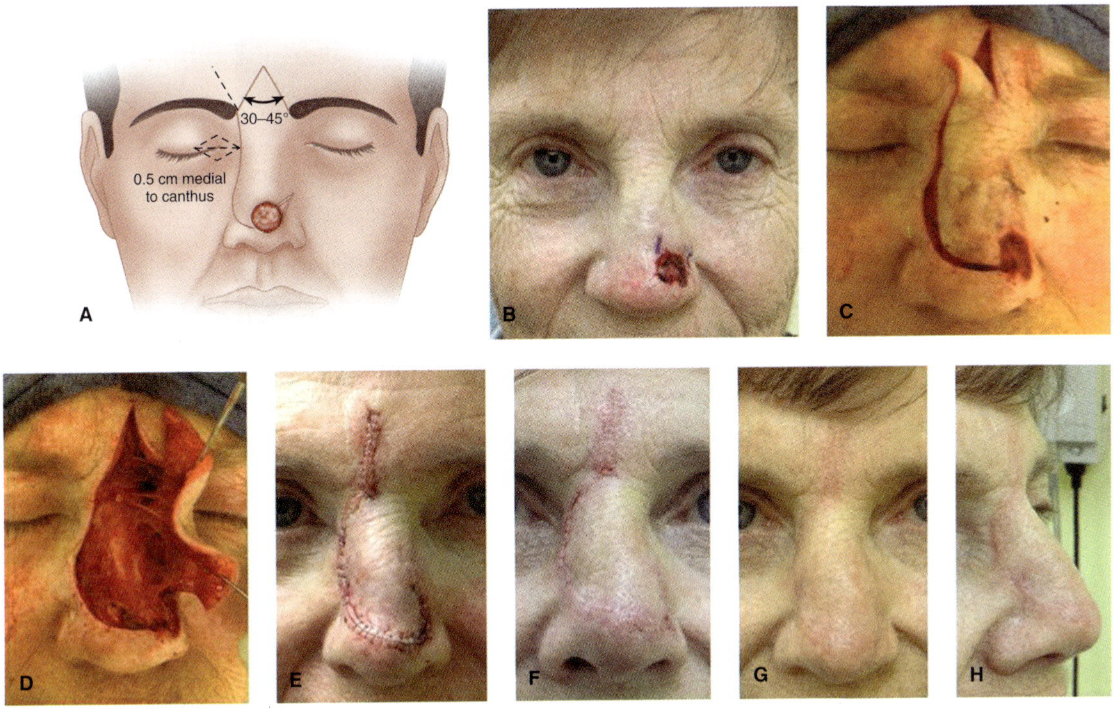

Figure 18-25 Dorsal nasal rotation (Reiger/hatchet) flap. **A.** Schematic drawing. Dotted line denotes optional Z-plasty at the glabella. **B.** Post Mohs defect. **C.** Design of the dorsal nasal flap with incision made from the inferior edge of the defect laterally to the nasofacial sulcus, extending upward along the nasofacial sulcus to the glabella. A backcut along the glabella allows the flap to drop inferiorly. **D.** Elevation of the flap in a submuscular plane above the periosteum and perichondrium on the nose. **E.** Final wound closure. **F.** Suture removal 1 week. **G, H.** Final result at 1 month. There is minor hypertrophic scar present by the medial canthus that resolved on its own over time. Occasionally, dermabrasion or laser resurfacing may be required to smooth out the scar.

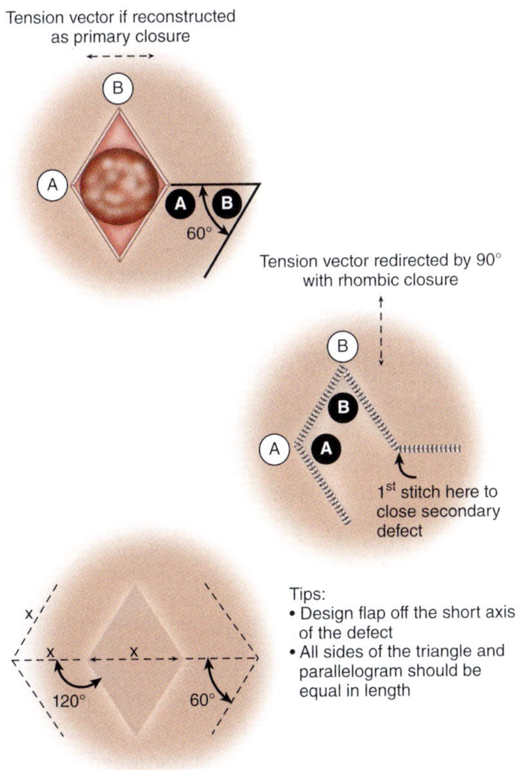

Figure 18-26 Classic Limberg rhombic flap.

limb of the flap (Fig. 18-28C). The second limb is then created parallel to the long axis of the rhombus. By reducing the arc of rotation, the flap more easily transposes into place with less tip tension (Fig. 18-29). However, the tension vector is no longer redirected at 90 degrees, rather more tension must be shared between the primary and secondary defect. Z-plasties can be used at the base of the rhombic flap to facilitate movement and closure of the secondary defect (Figs. 18-30 and 18-31).

NOTE FLAP

A modification to the rhombic flap, the note flap resembles the design of an eighth note. A tangential line is drawn from the primary defect with length 1.5 times the diameter of the defect. A second line is drawn at a 60 degree angle with a length equal to the diameter of the defect (Fig. 18-32).

BILOBED FLAP

Most commonly used for defects on the distal anterior nose, the bilobed flap utilizes adjacent skin laxity at the nasal sidewall and dorsum. It works well for defects less than 1.5 cm along the distal nasal sidewall, medial ala and nasal tip. It is also useful for larger defects on the lateral cheeks, temples, chin and submandibular area. The standard bilobed flap rotates along a 180 degree arc, while

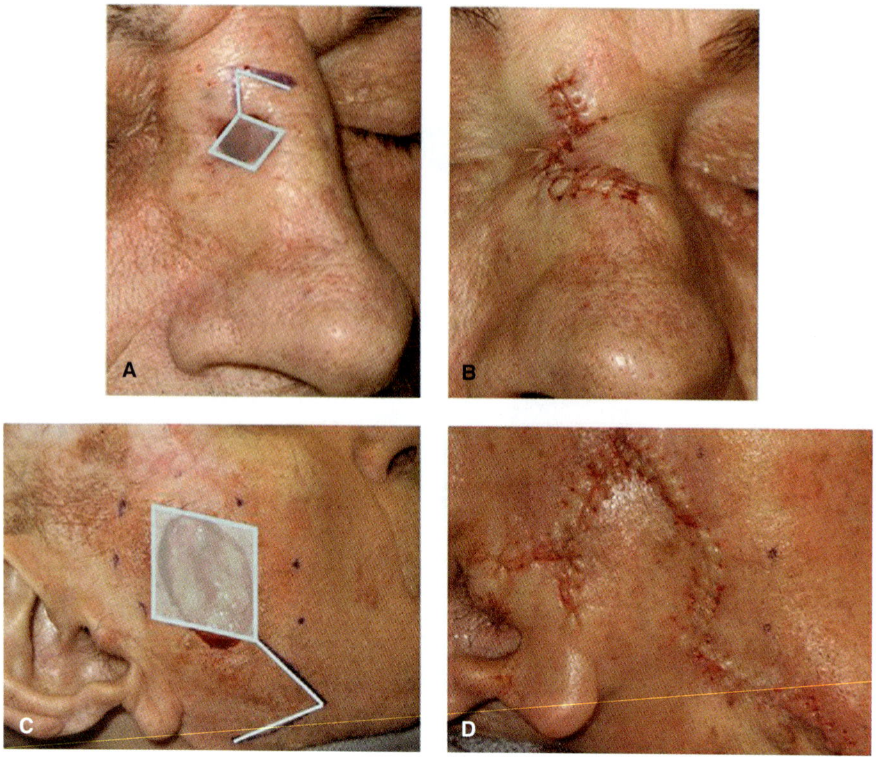

Figure 18-27 Classic rhombic flap on the nasal dorsum and lateral cheek.

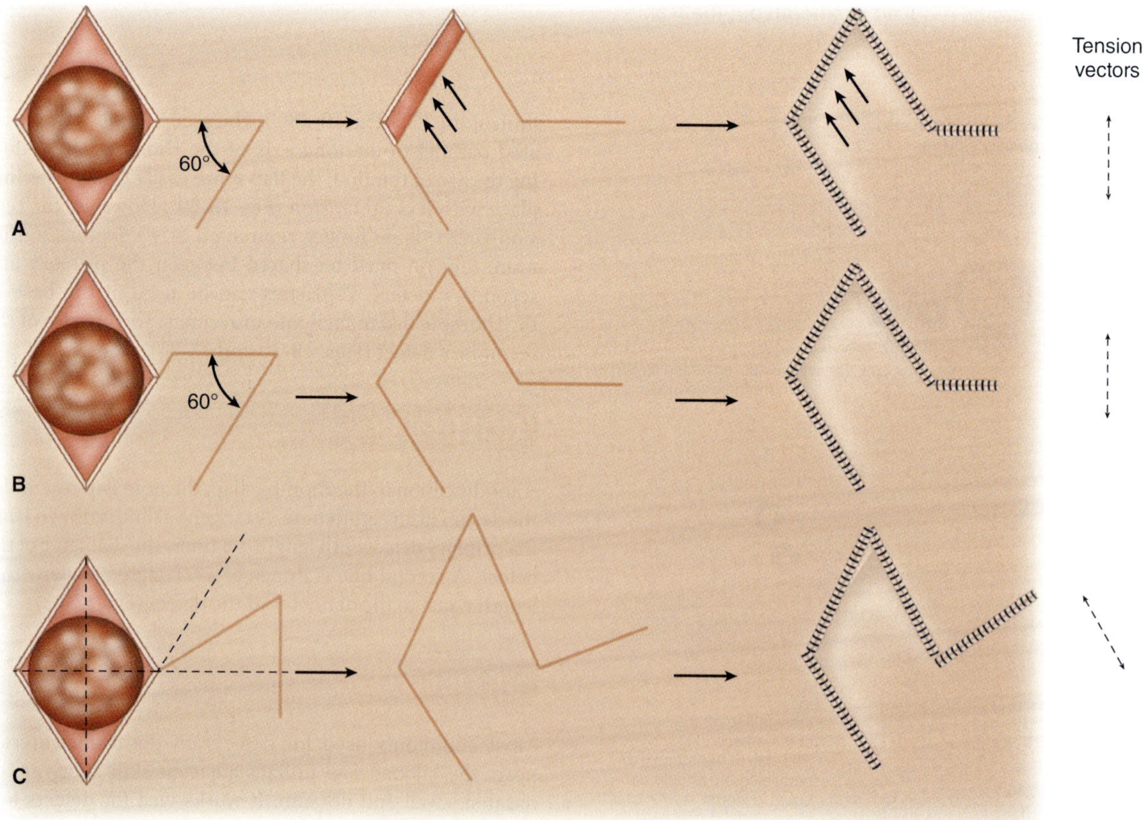

Figure 18-28 Modifications to the rhombic flap to compensate for pivotal restraints. **A.** Classically designed flap creates pivotal restraint and creating tip tension. **B.** Lengthening the flap compensates for flap shortening. **C.** Dufourmental modification reduces the arc of rotation and tip tension, but changes the tension vector as well.

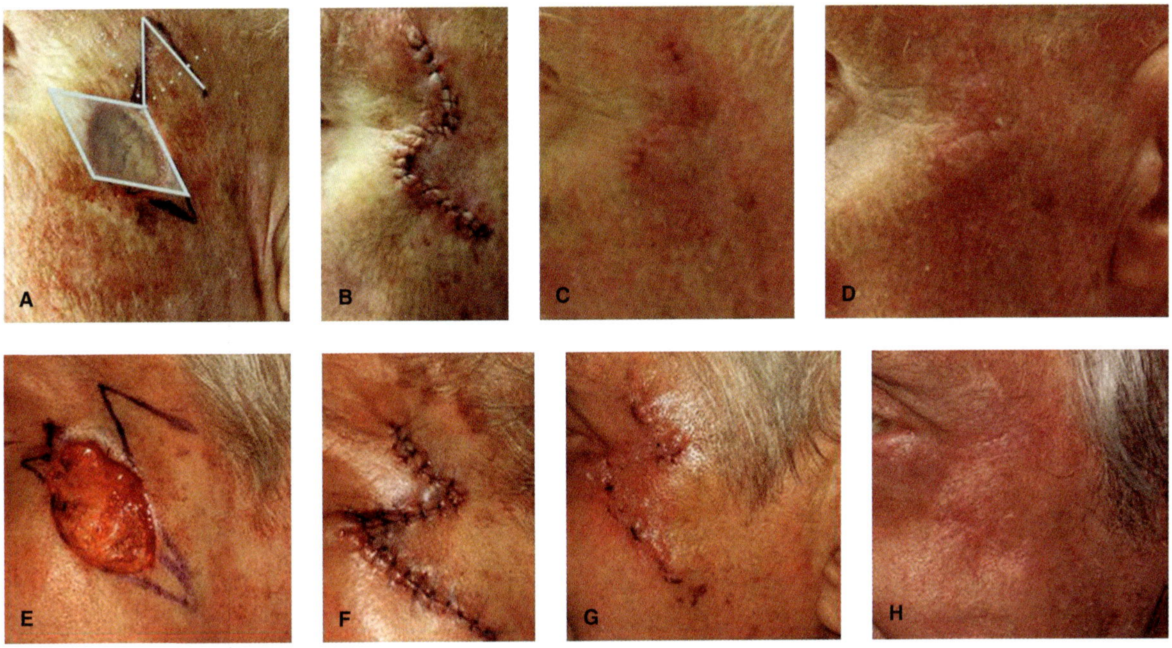

Figure 18-29 Two examples of Dufourmental modification to the rhombic flap. **A, E.** Post Mohs defect. **B, F.** Final wound closure. **C** and **G.** Suture removal at 1 week. **D, H.** One month follow-up.

the Zitelli modification only rotates along a 90 degree arc, which places the flap under less tension. (Fig. 18-33) The advantages of the Zitelli modification include reduction of pivotal restraint on the flap and incorporation of the Burow's triangle into the flap design. The bilobed flap offers significant advantages over other closures because it is a single-stage flap with perfect skin match and predictable viability. Proper design is critical, as small alterations in design can result in significant asymmetry and distortion of the nose. Meticulous suture technique is essential, as the curved incision lines do not always hide well within the sebaceous skin of the nose.

The bilobed flap can be thought of as a double transposition flap, which allows the surgeon to borrow tissue from the loose skin of the proximal nasal dorsum and transfer it to the less mobile nasal tip. The flap's primary lobe is transposed to cover the primary surgical defect. This in turn creates a secondary defect, which is covered by the secondary lobe. The tertiary defect is closed primarily. By closing the tertiary lobe first, the flap is effectively mobilized and rotated into place. Each lobe is designed at an approximately 45 degree angle of rotation.

Several important tips can reduce asymmetry of the nasal ala and tip when the bilobed flap is performed. Slight

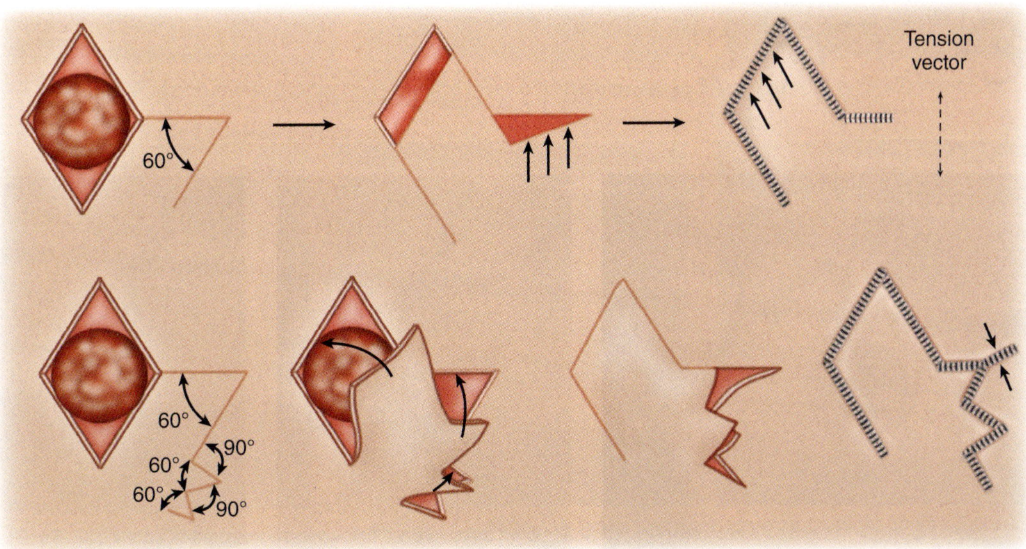

Figure 18-30 Z-plasty to the rhombic flap to facilitate movement of the flap and closure of the secondary defect.

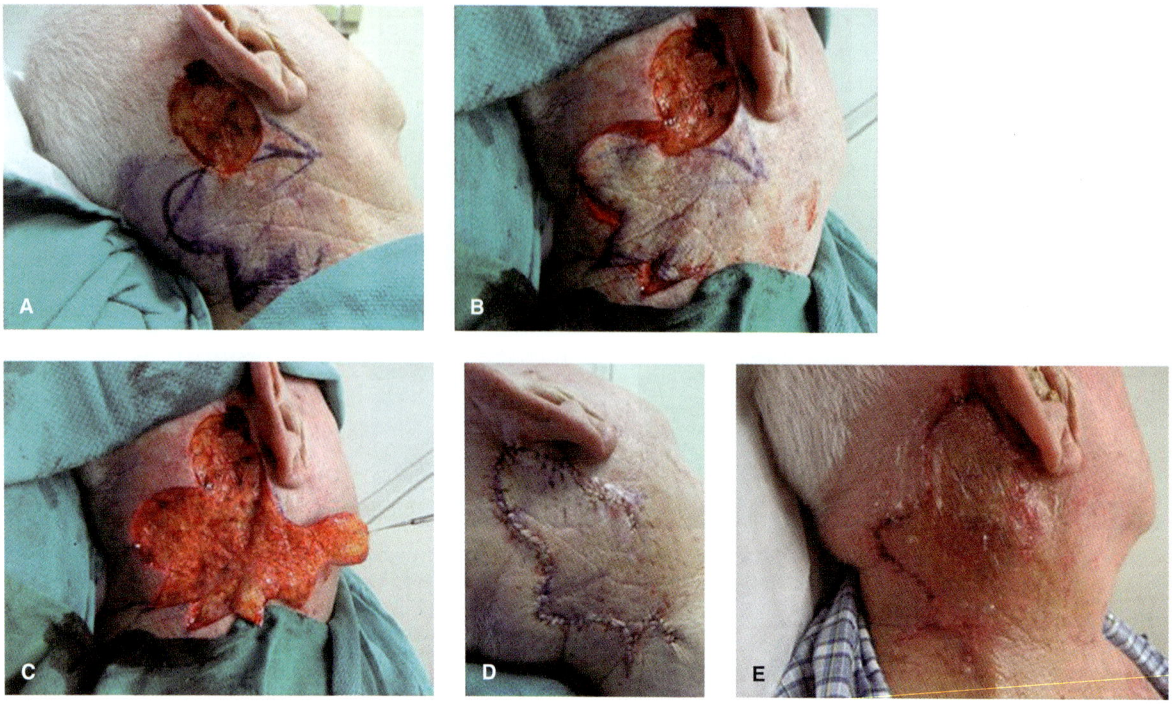

Figure 18-31 A large defect repaired with a transposition flap. This repair can be conceptually regarded as a rhombic flap with two Z-plasty or a trilobed flap. Z-plasty at the base of the flap facilitate movement and closure of the secondary defect. **A.** Post Mohs defect. **B.** Incision of the flap. **C.** Undermining in the subcutaneous plane. **D.** Final wound closure. **E.** Suture removal at 2 weeks.

tip depression and alar displacement can often occur on the ipsilateral side of the flap due to minor lengthening of the flap in a Z-plasty type manner as it is transposed into place. This "bulldozing" depression effect is more apparent when dealing with thicker sebaceous skin and only occurs when the flap is oversized with respect to the defect. Careful thinning of the inferior edge of the primary lobe reduces bulkiness of the flap and the tendency for the ala to be pushed downward. The Burow's triangle should therefore be angled superiorly, to place it in less sebaceous tissue. A more horizontally placed Burow's triangle will exaggerate the Z-plasty effect of the bilobed flap.[14]

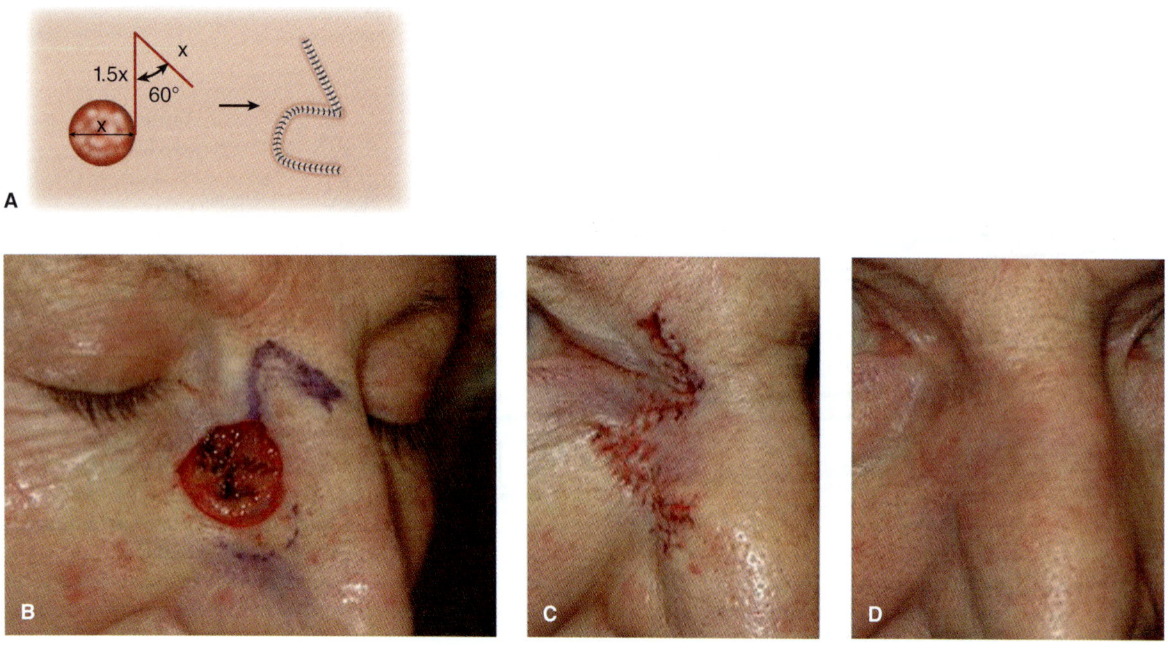

Figure 18-32 Note flap. **A.** Flap design. **B.** Post Mohs defect. **C.** Final wound closure. **D.** One month follow-up.

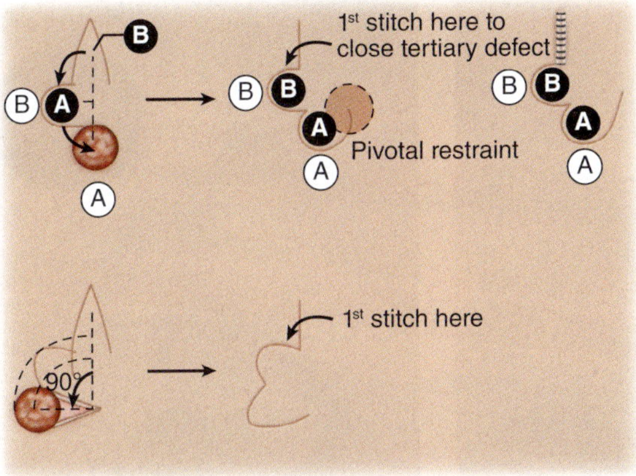

Figure 18-33 Bilobed flap. **A.** Traditional 180 degree bilobed flap with significant pivotal restraint. **B.** Zitelli 90 degree modification.

On the other hand, the alar margin can be displaced superiorly if the primary flap is undersized and does not adequately cover the defect, resulting in secondary upward motion. In general, the width of the primary lobe should be 90% to 100% of the primary defect diameter and the secondary lobe should be 80% to 85% of the primary lobe.[15] On thick sebaceous skin, however, the size ratio of the lobes should be closer to 1:1. The length of each lobe should also equal the length of the defect, especially in sebaceous or less elastic skin. As the flap rotates and transposes into place, pivotal restraint will result in minor shortening of the effective flap length. At the same time, care must be made to not oversize the lobes as this can result in trap-door deformity.

Proper placement of the secondary lobe is also critical in reducing asymmetry. When possible, the axis of second lobe should be oriented perpendicular to the alar rim. As the primary tension vector of the flap is along the tertiary defect, a closure oriented perpendicularly will result in the smallest amount of alar distortion.[16] If the second lobe cannot be placed along the perpendicular axis, a trilobed flap can be created to place a tertiary lobe along the vertical axis.[17]

EXECUTION OF THE BILOBED FLAP (Figs. 18-34 and 18-35)

1. Design of the flap
   a. Place the Burow's triangle at the base of the primary lobe. It should be angled superiorly and placed along the alar crease.

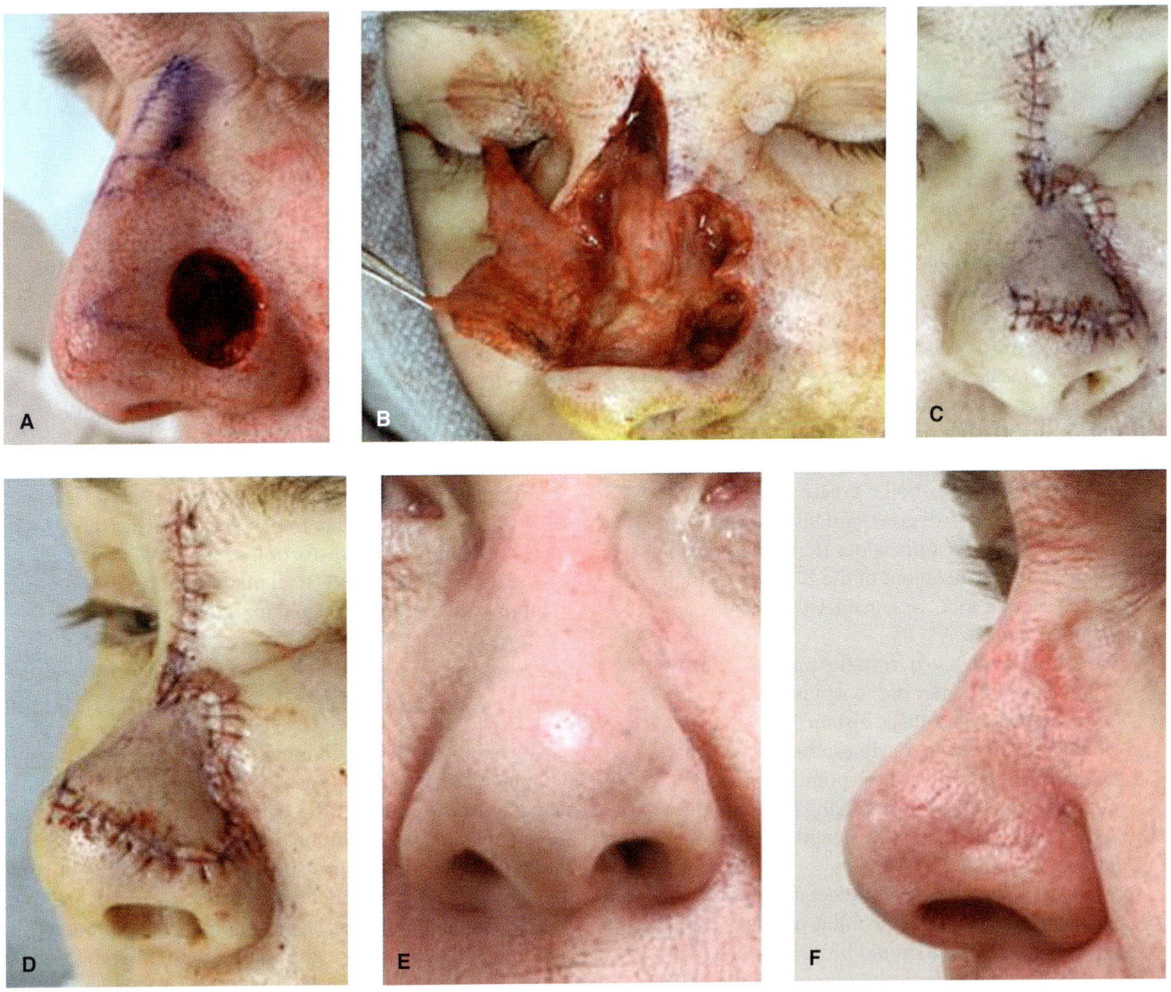

Figure 18-34 Bilobed flap. **A.** Post Mohs defect. **B.** Undermining in a submuscular plane above the periosteum and perichondrium. **C, D.** Final wound closure. **E, F.** Appearance at 3 months.

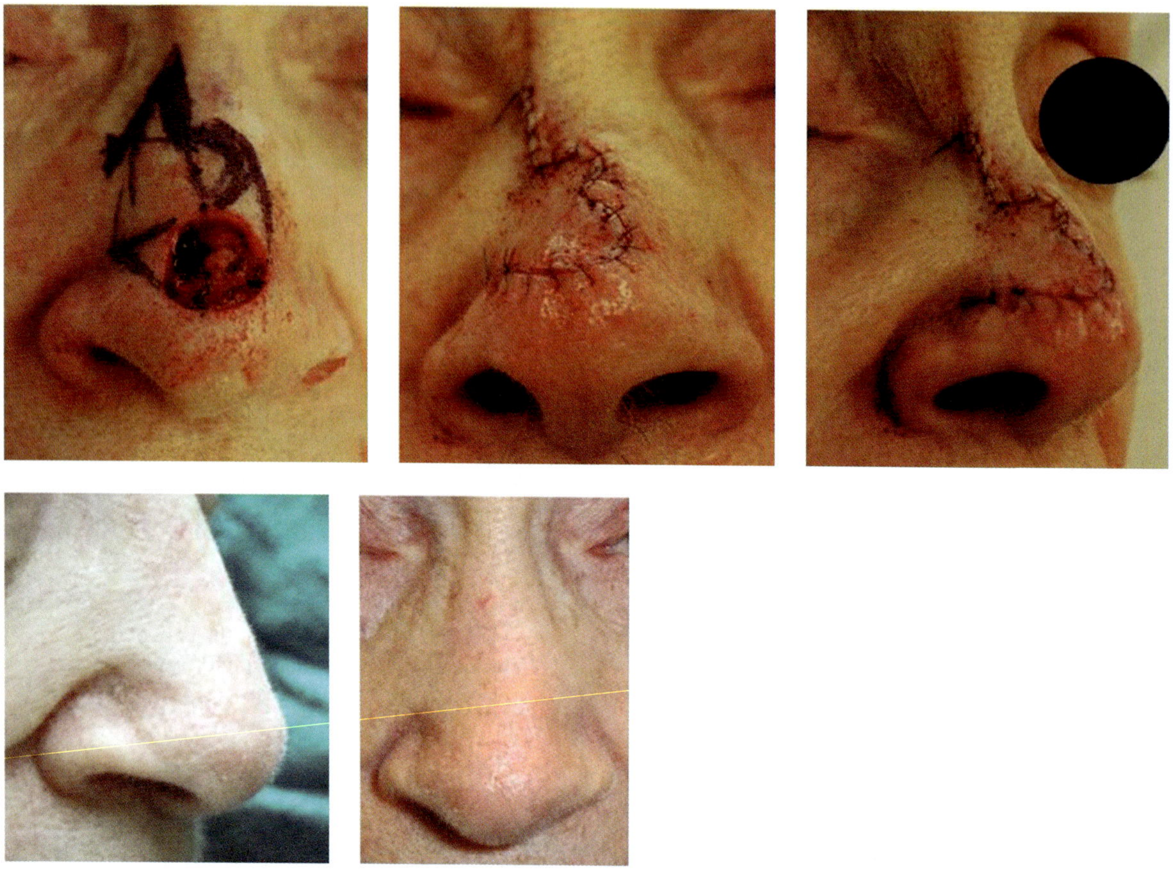

Figure 18-35 Bilobed flap. **A.** Post Mohs defect. **B, C.** Final wound closure. **D, E.** Appearance at 3 months.

b. Determine the placement of the second lobe. In most cases, it should be 90 degrees from the defect and oriented perpendicular to the alar margin to prevent alar distortion. Draw a line from the tip of the Burow's triangle to the center of the defect. Draw a second line to the center of the proposed second lobe. Draw a third line to bisect the two lines. The classic Zitelli bilobed flap should create angles at approximately 45 degrees and 90 degrees. If the angles are significantly wider than this, consider changing the placement of the Burow's triangle or the second lobe, or consider the use of a trilobed flap.

c. Measure the distance from the tip of the Burow's triangle to the center of the wound and the tip of the defect. Mark these distances along the 45 degree and 90 degree lines, then draw two parallel arcs based on these points. These arcs represent the tip and originating points of the lobes. This ensures that the lengths of the lobes are equal to that of the defect.

d. Measure the width of the defect and design the primary lobe to be 90% to 100% of this width. The secondary lobe should be 80% to 85% of the primary lobe. On more sebaceous skin, the ratio of the lobe to the defect should be close to 1:1.

e. Extend the second lobe into a triangular shape.

2. Sharply incise the flap at a 90 degree angle down to the submuscular plane below the nasalis muscle.
3. Undermine widely in a submuscular plane above the periosteum and perichondrium on the nose to ensure a robust vascular supply.
4. Remove the Burow's triangle prior to placement of the flap to reduce pivotal restraint.
5. Close the tertiary defect first to allow the flap to drop inferiorly into the defect.
6. While securing the flap in place, ensure that there is no asymmetry or distortion of the nasal tip. Inset the flap with buried vertical mattress sutures and approximate the epidermal margins.

BANNER FLAP

As its name implies, the banner flap is a long, thin triangle ("banner") shaped flap (Figs. 18-36 and 18-37). Its width is equal to the width of the defect and its length is equal to the distance from the pivot point to the length of the defect. The nasolabial transposition flap is a type of banner flap utilizing redundant skin along the nasolabial fold for defects along the nasal sidewall and ala. Although this is a one-stage flap with a good skin texture match, it often blunts the sidewall and alar subunits. Banner flaps from the pre- or postauricular area are useful for closure of defects on the superior helical rim.

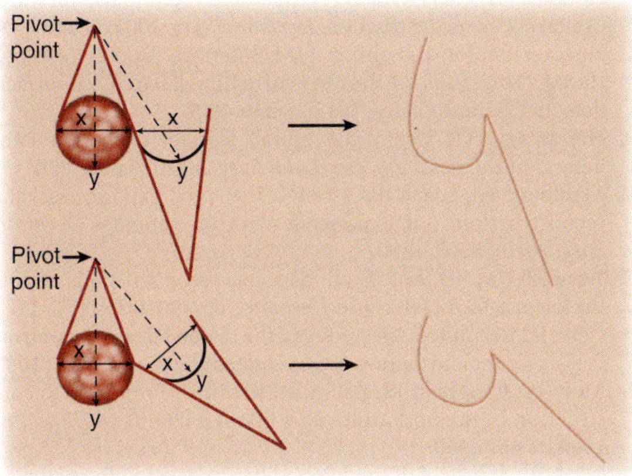

Figure 18-36 Banner flap design. The width of the flap should be equal to the width of the defect. The length of the flap should be at least the distance from the tip of pivot point to the tip of the defect.

CONCLUSION

When properly designed and executed, random pattern flaps are an ideal reconstructive option for a wide variety of defects. An understanding of the anatomy, blood supply, and tissue quality surrounding the defect will aid the surgeon in weighing the possible reconstructive options. It is important to be thoughtful and consider all options from simple closure to complex flaps, as there is often more than one reconstructive alternative for any one defect. It is also critical to remember that the main principles of reconstructive surgery must be obeyed for a successful aesthetic and functional repair, including avoiding distortion of anatomic landmarks and free margins, maintaining shape and symmetry, respecting cosmetic boundaries, hiding incisions along skin tension lines, repairing defects with skin of similar characteristics and minimizing tissue trauma. It is up to the surgeon to design and execute the closure that will provide the patient with the best possible aesthetic and functional outcome.

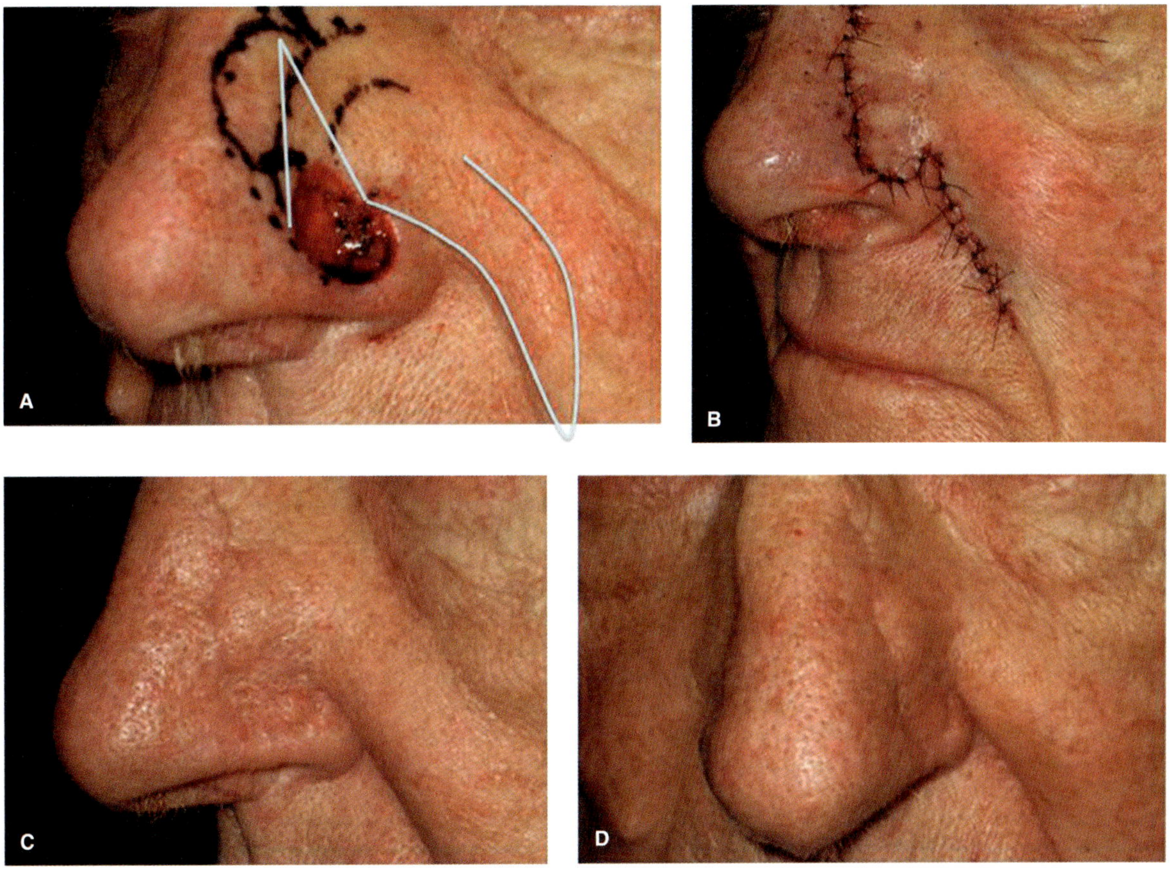

Figure 18-37 Melolabial transposition flap is one example of a banner flap. **A.** Design of the flap for a defect involving the ala and nasal sidewall. Alternatives including a bilobed flap were considered but ultimately a melolabial flap was chosen. **B.** Final wound closure. **C, D.** Suture removal 1 week. The nasolabial incision line is imperceptible, but there is loss of the alar groove which is common with this flap. There is also fullness of the left nasal sidewall superior to the alar groove. This trapdoor effect is not uncommon in transposition flaps on the nose. In some cases, the pin-cushioning may regress with time, and massage may help resolve congestion from lymphatic and venous obstruction. Direct injection of intralesional corticosteroid (usually triamcinolone acetonide 10–20 mg/cc every 4–6 weeks) may soften contracture of the scar and improve the trap-door effect. Occasionally, persistent deformity may require surgical correction to thin the flap.

REFERENCES

1. Moody BR, Sengelmann RD. Standing cone avoidance via advancement flap modification. *Dermatol Surg.* 2002;28:632–635.
2. Kaufmann AJ. Helical rim advancement flaps for reconstruction. *Dermatol Surg.* 2008;34:1229–1232.
3. Saleh DB, Tan J, Mohammed P, Majumder S. The lobular transposition flap: a useful adjunct to reconstruct helical defects. *J Plast Reconstr Aesth Surg.* 2012;65:963–965.
4. Braun M. The island pedicle flap. *Dermatol Surg.* 2005;31:995–1005.
5. Behan F. The Keystone design perforator island flap in reconstructive surgery. *ANZ J Surg.* 2003;73:112–120.
6. Hu M, Bordeaux JS. The Keystone flap for lower extremity defects. *Dermatol Surg.* 2012;38:490–493.
7. Goldman GD. Rotation flaps. *Dermatol Surg.* 2005;31:1006–1013.
8. Buckingham ED, Quinn FB, Calhoun KH. Optimal design of O-to-Z flaps for closure of facial skin defects. *Arch Facial Plast Surg.* 2003;5:92–95.
9. Honda K, Reichel J, Odland P. Anchored rotation flap for infraorbital cheek reconstruction. *Dermatol Surg.* 2007;33:516–520.
10. Hussain W, Tan E, Salmon PJM. Inferiorly based crescentic sliding cheek flaps for the reconstruction of paranasal surgical defects. *Dermatol Surg.* 2012;38:249–255.
11. Humphreys TR. Use of the "spiral" Flap for closure of small defects of the nasal ala. *Dermatol Surg.* 2001;27:409–410.
12. Mahlberg MJ, Leach BC, Cook J. The spiral flap for nasal alar reconstruction: our experience with 63 patients. *Dermatol Surg.* 2012;38:373–380.
13. Wentzell JM. Dorsal nasal flap for reconstruction of full-thickness defects of the nose. *Dermatol Surg.* 2010;36:1171–1178.
14. Cook JL. Reconstructive utility of the bilobed flap: lessons from flap successes and failures. *Dermatol Surg.* 2005; 31:1024–1033.
15. Moy RL, Grossfeld JS, Baum M, Rivlin D, Eremia S. Reconstruction of the nose utilizing a bilobed flap. *Int J Dermatol.* 1994;33:657–660.
16. Cook JL. A review of the bilobed flap's design with particular emphasis on the minimization of alar displacement. *Dermatol Surg.* 2000;26:354–362.
17. Albertini JG, Hansen JP. Trilobed flap reconstruction for distal nasal skin defects. *Dermatol Surg.* 2010;36:1726–1735.

CHAPTER 19

Axial Pattern and Interpolation Flaps

Christopher J. Miller, Joseph F. Sobanko, & John G. Albertini

INTRODUCTION

Facial symmetry correlates highly with facial attractiveness.[1] The symmetry of midline structures has the greatest impact on perception of beauty.[2] As the nose occupies the most central location on the face, its complex, symmetrical contours play a key role in how we perceive other people's faces. Observers normally focus their gaze on the central triangle of the eyes, nose, and mouth.[3] Asymmetric noses are perceived as less attractive, deformed noses attract excessive attention,[1,3] and even small nasal lesions are considered disfiguring, bothersome, and important to repair.[4] When local flaps are insufficient for coverage of a complex nasal defect, the surgeon may need to consider staged repair with a forehead or cheek interpolation flap. Similarly, the ear may require a postauricular interpolation flap (PIF) to repair a larger defect in an aesthetic fashion. Staged interpolation flaps present unique technical challenges. This chapter will discuss the planning and execution of: (1) the paramedian forehead flap for nasal reconstruction; (2) the melolabial interpolation flap (MIF) for alar reconstruction; and (3) the retroauricular interpolation flap for ear reconstruction.

ANATOMY OF THE EXTERNAL NOSE

The nose has subtle convexities and concavities resulting from the complex anatomy of the bone, cartilage, and soft tissue. The surgeon's task is to recreate or simulate the normal anatomy, restore the complex nasal topography and maintain airway patency. This section will focus on those aspects of external nasal anatomy essential to planning and executing the paramedian forehead flap and the MIF.

BONY FRAMEWORK OF THE NOSE

The pyriform aperture demarcates the boundary between the external and internal nasal cavities. It provides a stable frame for the cartilaginous framework of the nose and anchors most of the muscles of facial expression. The paired nasal bones form the superior border of the pyriform aperture, merging in the midline and projecting outward as the nasal dorsum. The maxilla forms the lateral and inferior borders of the pyriform aperture. The anterior nasal spine at the maxillary midline forms the most prominent inferior bony projection of the nose.

CARTILAGINOUS FRAMEWORK OF THE NOSE

Cartilage forms the nasal skeleton external to the pyriform aperture. The nasal cartilages determine nasal projection and support the airways. In contrast to the immobile bony skeleton, the flexible cartilaginous framework is vulnerable to distortion and compression, which can alter appearance and impair breathing. The external nasal framework consists of three primary structures: (1) the septal cartilage; (2) the paired upper lateral cartilages; and (3) the paired lower lateral cartilages. The septal and paired upper lateral cartilages are anchored to bone and therefore provide more resistance to compression.

The quadrilaterally shaped septal cartilage is rigid and flat, gaining stability through its articulations with the ethmoid bone, vomer, maxilla, and nasal bone. Its caudal margin slopes from the anterior nasal spine to the anterior septal angle, which is palpable at the supratip superior to the alar cartilage domes. The septal cartilage determines nasal projection and rotation, separates the two nasal cavities, and forms the medial boundary of the internal and external nasal valves. Surgical removal or compression of its distal aspect alters nasal projection. Septal deviation can compromise breathing by decreasing the size of the nasal valves.

The paired upper lateral cartilages support the lateral nasal sidewall and are relatively stable, due to articulation with the septum medially, attachment to the nasal bone's undersurface superiorly, and attachment to the pyriform aperture laterally. The upper lateral cartilage's caudal aspect forms the lateral border of the internal nasal valve, and attaches to the superior aspect of the lower lateral cartilages in a region termed the "scroll."

The lower lateral cartilages, or alar cartilages, provide structure to the nasal tip, contribute to its projection, and support the external nasal valve. They are subdivided into the medial, intermediate, and lateral crura. The medial crus stabilizes the ala and influences columellar appearance and projection. The intermediate crus forms the alar dome and defines anterior tip projection. The lateral crus projects laterally and provides support to the alar lobule and external nasal valve.

The alar cartilages are vulnerable to compression. Unlike the central septal and paired upper lateral cartilages, they do not articulate directly with bone, but derive their support from attachments to the septal and upper lateral cartilages, each other, and the pyriform aperture.[5] The footplate of the medial crus attaches to the septal cartilage. Its cephalic portion attaches to the upper lateral cartilages at the scroll. The interdomal ligament links the lower lateral cartilages at the midline. The lateral crus attaches to the pyriform aperture by the sesamoid complex ligament.[5,6] The upper and lower lateral cartilages gain strength from the pyriform ligament, which extends from the maxillary periosteum to the anterior nasal spine, and provides further stability to the nasal tip.[6]

SOFT TISSUE ANATOMY OF THE NOSE

The soft tissue of the external nose supports the underlying cartilage and adds to the subtle nasal surface contours. Except at the alar lobule, there are five distinct nasal soft tissue layers: the skin, subcutaneous fat, superficial musculoaponeurotic system (SMAS), deep areolar layer, and perichondrial or periosteal layer.[7] The SMAS is composed of the nasal muscles and fascia and is continuous with the facial SMAS.[7] Sharp dissection reveals the connection of the SMAS to the skin and cartilage, adhesions that add stability to the nasal framework and provide support to the skin, and help to preserve airway patency. Excluding the alar groove and lobule, subcutaneous dissection easily separates the skin from the underlying SMAS.

At the alar groove and lobule, the SMAS inserts into the dermis without a distinct subcutaneous layer. This connection between the muscle and dermis provides support to the external nasal valve; sharp dissection is necessary to separate the two. Dissection deep to the SMAS is also effortless for most areas on the nose, except at the internal valve, where the SMAS inserts, and the alar groove and lobule.

The anatomic layers of the alar lobule are unique. It does not contain cartilage, consisting of skeletal muscle and fat enveloped by dermis and epithelium on both sides.[8,9] The lack of an intrinsic framework and the absence of support at its free margin make it particularly susceptible to distortion. The dilator naris vestibularis muscle inserts directly into the dermis of the external and vestibular epithelia; sharp dissection is necessary to separate the two.[10]

The muscles ensheathed by the SMAS animate the nose and maintain airway patency.[10,11] They can be divided into four groups: the elevators, the depressors, the dilators, and the compressors. The elevators include the procerus, the levator labii superioris alaeque nasi, and the anomalous nasi, which rotate the tip in a cephalic direction and dilate the nostrils. The depressor muscles include the alar nasalis and the depressor septi, which lengthen the nose and dilate the nostrils. The dilator naris anterior is a pure nasal dilator. The compressor muscles include the transverse nasalis and the compressor narium minor, which rotate the tip in a caudal direction and narrow the nostrils. The muscles at the alar groove (i.e., the dilator naris anterior, the levator labii superioris alaeque nasi, and the dilator naris vestibularis) and alar-facial sulcus (i.e., the alar part of the nasalis) determine the shape of this landmark and contribute to airway patency.[10] The caudal part of the transverse nasalis defines the contour of the alar groove, which is challenging to recreate if the muscle is removed.

The nasal skin topography reflects its underlying structure. Its shadows and reflections define its subunits: the tip, dorsum, sidewalls, alae, and soft triangles.[12] Its concavities include the slight break at the supratip, the alar groove, the faint shadow at the soft triangles, and occasionally, bifidity of the nasal tip. Convex surfaces include the lobule, nasal tip, and dorsal nasal ridges. The dorsum and sidewalls have planar surfaces. Scars placed in the shadows of concavities or reflections at the peaks of the convexities are frequently inconspicuous, but preserving nasal contour is even more important in optimizing the aesthetic result.[13]

The nasal skin has varying textures and thickness, which also contribute to its topography. The dorsum and sidewalls have a thin dermis and few sebaceous glands. The midline dorsum has a scant layer of fat over the transverse nasalis aponeurosis. On the sidewall, a subcutaneous fat layer adds volume over the transverse nasalis muscle. The tip and alae have a thick dermis and dense sebaceous glands. The nasal root has a thick dermis, dense sebaceous glands, and a layer of fat over the procerus. The dermal thickness and pilosebaceous unit density are greater on the nose than in other facial areas, but the paramedian forehead and nasolabial folds are similar in color, thickness, and texture.[14]

THE EXTERNAL AND INTERNAL NASAL VALVES

The anatomic features of the nose help to serve its primary function: regulating airflow. Eighty-five percent of adults preferentially breathe through the nose, except when exercising or speaking.[15] The external and internal nasal valves are critical regulators of airflow and resistance, and are vulnerable to collapse from excessive tension, compression or loss of integrity. Nasal resistance is inversely proportional to the nasal passage radius raised to the fourth power (resistance = [viscosity × length]/radius^4).[16] Thus, small changes in nasal valve configuration, including removal or displacement of any individual component, can exponentially increase resistance to breathing, leading to airway compromise.[16]

The external valve controls air passage through the distal nostril, and is bounded by the upper lateral cartilage superiorly, the alar attachment of the lateral crus laterally, the septum and columella medially, and the nasal sill inferiorly.[8] The shape, size, and strength of the lower lateral cartilage determine the risk of external valve collapse. Patients with a flexible nasal tip, or whose ala collapses on forced inspiration, or whose breathing improves with lateral alar distraction are at higher risk for collapse.

The internal valve is located above the external valve, and its risk for collapse usually stems from septal deviation or caudal compression or weakening of the upper lateral cartilage.

This flow-limiting segment contributes approximately 50% of the total combined upper and lower airway resistance.[15] The angle between the septal and upper lateral cartilages is 10 to 15 degrees in Caucasians, and more obtuse and therefore more resistant to collapse in ethnic African Americans and Asians.[16]

THE PARAMEDIAN FOREHEAD FLAP

ASSESSING THE DEFECT

LOCATION. The paramedian forehead flap has sufficient length and a robust enough blood supply to repair nearly any nasal defect, although defect location influences both pedicle length and the risk of airway compromise. Distal defects lie further from the donor site and require a longer pedicle, potentially leading to the presence of scalp hair on the flap. These defects also pose a risk of airway compromise and are more likely to require cartilage grafts for support. More proximal defects of the nasal root, dorsum, and sidewall less commonly threaten airway function, as the septum and upper lateral cartilages gain support from their bony attachments. The paired lower lateral nasal tip cartilages provide only moderate resistance to compression and distortion. The lobule is especially vulnerable, frequently requiring nonanatomic cartilage to brace its rim against contraction and maintain external valve patency.

ASSESSING THE ANATOMIC DEPTH OF THE DEFECT AND INDICATIONS FOR CARTILAGE GRAFTING

Defect depth influences the required flap thickness and airway integrity. In general, soft-tissue loss without damage to cartilage poses little risk for airway compromise.[10] However, defects involving alar skin and muscle require special consideration because of the risk of airway compromise from defect instability or anticipated scar contraction, often requiring cartilage grafts for repair. Defects involving cartilage increase the complexity of reconstruction, as nasal projection may be decreased and airway stability compromised. Missing cartilage is usually replaced to restore nasal contour and projection and stabilize the airway. Preexisting cartilage should not be removed or its attachments violated unless absolutely necessary.

Full-thickness nasal defects present the greatest challenge, as they require repair of mucosal lining, cartilage, and skin. Such defects are most common on the lobule and soft triangle, where full-thickness excision is required if tumor involves the free margin. Such defects usually require a three-staged forehead flap for aesthetic repair and recreation of the mucosal lining.[17,18]

PRINCIPLES OF AESTHETIC DESIGN: DECIDING WHEN TO ENLARGE THE DEFECT

Although the surgeon cannot control the location, size, or depth of the defect, he or she may modify its size and depth to achieve a more aesthetic design. As noted above, soft-tissue defects not involving the ala or alar groove less commonly threaten the airway. Therefore, removing soft tissue to the level of the perichondrium or periosteum may be advantageous. The cartilaginous framework will appear more natural beneath a forehead flap of appropriate thickness, and the inset flap will have a better contour with decreased bulk. As the nasal lining lies immediately beneath muscle on the alar lobule, deepening the defect here requires caution to avoid an unnecessary full-thickness defect.

Enlarging a defect's breadth may also be desirable at times for better scar camouflage. The surgeon must weigh the benefits of defect extension against the risks of airway compromise and added donor site morbidity. Increasing defect size may make donor site closure more difficult. It also may increase pedicle length and the likelihood that the donor site will involve hair-bearing scalp.

Defect enlargement follows a few simple principles. Horizontal scars across subunits are conspicuous; extending the defect hides the scar at the free margin. If the defect involves the alar lobule or nasal tip, it should be extended distally to the free margin. Vertical scars on the ala tend to heal inconspicuously. If the defect does not involve the full alar height, its vertical aspect may be extended without hesitation. Caution must be observed with horizontal extension, because recreating the convex flare of the ala can be challenging. Even if cartilage grafts are placed, flattening of the alar margin (best seen from the swimmer's view) is common. As midline scars heal well, one may consider extending the defect to a "hemi-tip" subunit, rather than the entire tip, if it involves only one side. The smaller surface area will facilitate donor site closure with little or no compromise of the nasal scar (Fig. 19-1). Correct contour is more important than placing scars in subunit lines.[13] When the benefits of defect enlargement are uncertain, the focus should instead be on optimizing contour.

DESIGNING THE FLAP

MAKING THE TEMPLATE

Once the final nasal defect has been created, the surgeon must make a template that matches it exactly. It is therefore critical to heed the adage, "measure twice and cut once." An oversized template will result in a bulky flap with poor contour and occurs most commonly when the nasal wound has a surface area greater than that of the skin removed. Expansion occurs to a greater degree on the dorsum and sidewalls, where the skin is looser, and to a lesser degree on the tip and ala, unless the wound is deep or full thickness, or cartilage integrity has been damaged. No matter the location, the template should reflect the surface area of the tissue removed, not the size of the expanded wound. The contralateral side of the nose, if intact, can serve as a reference if estimating the true size of the removed tissue is difficult.

An undersized template will produce a forehead flap under excessive tension, and usually occurs when the template fails to reflect the three-dimensional surface of the defect's concavities and convexities. To avoid this error, it is useful to create the template with a flexible material that is stiff enough to retain a three-dimensional shape. Many surgeons use the aluminum foil of a suture package. Others create a soft cast of the nose by placing steri-strips over the wound and surrounding skin, then cutting out a precise template. Regardless of the material used, the surgeon will need to convert the three-dimensional template to a two-dimensional surface. The authors use a surgical marking pen to trace the defect's borders, then apply a nonstick gauze or suture package over it to conform to its three-dimensional contour. The resulting imprint allows precise determination of the wound edges. The template is cut out at the inside margin of the imprint and transferred back to the wound to confirm that the fit is precise.

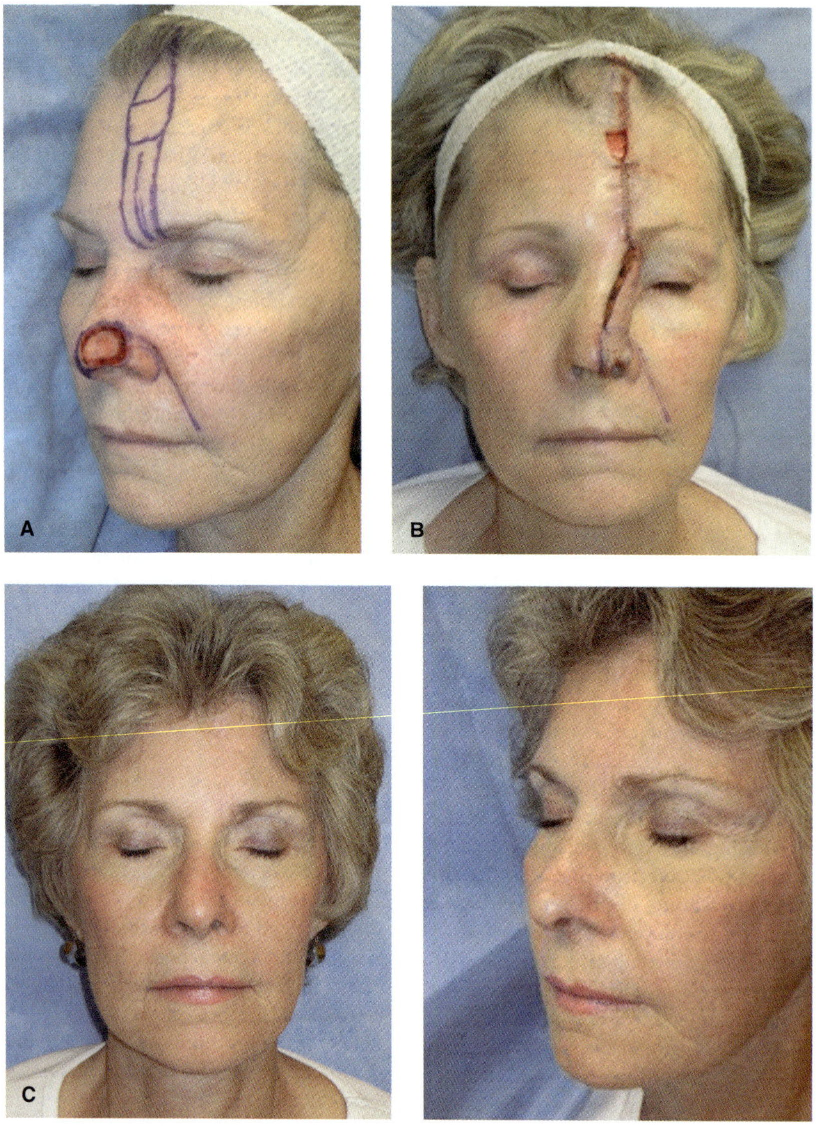

Figure 19-1 **A.** Defect involving the left hemitip and conforming to the surface area of the lower lateral cartilage. **B.** The wound was repaired as a hemitip subunit, rather than extending the defect to involve the entire nasal tip subunit. Appearance after paramedian forehead flap. Note that the donor site was too tight for primary closure. **C.** Appearance 6 months postoperatively. The midline scar is imperceptible, demonstrating that replacement of the entire cosmetic subunit is not always necessary. The small open wound at the forehead donor site has healed acceptably; no revision was performed.

TRANSFERRING THE TEMPLATE TO THE FOREHEAD DONOR SITE

After finalizing the template, the surgeon must identify a suitable donor site. The proposed site must be inspected for concerning lesions before surgery, so that these may be appropriately addressed. Previous surgery or traumatic scars can alter the flap's blood supply, so the surgeon must also look for scars that could threaten flap viability.

Determining the side on which to base the flap depends primarily on defect location. For laterally based wounds of the ala, distal sidewall, or hemitip, the surgeon will usually place the template on the ipsilateral forehead. The flap will then require less length to reach the wound and will be less likely to contain scalp hair. For laterally based wounds of the medial canthus and proximal nasal sidewall, contralateral flaps have less torque and still reach the defect without difficulty. Midline nasal wounds can use either side as the donor site.

After determining the side on which to base the flap, the surgeon maps the supratrochlear artery (STA), whose path determines template placement. Although the flap has axial flow from the STA, it also has blood flow from the angular, dorsal nasal, and supraorbital arteries via anastomoses in the superior orbital plexus.[19] A thorough understanding of anatomy helps to plan the flap appropriately. The STA is a terminal branch of the ophthalmic artery that exits the orbit by piercing the orbital septum at the superomedial orbital rim, travels superficial to periosteum and the corrugator supercilii muscle, then pierces the orbicularis oculi and frontalis muscles, and reaches the fat just above the eyebrow. On average, it reaches the subcutaneous plane 1 cm above the supraorbital rim.[20] On the lower forehead and brow, the artery and its branches may be found in the fat superficial to the frontalis muscle.[20] On the superior third of the forehead, the artery runs in the fat and continues in this plane beyond the junction of the sagittal and coronal sutures at the top of the skull.[19] Although its pulse is palpable in many patients, a Doppler probe can also be used to locate it and trace its path. If a probe is not available, the surgeon can use topographic landmarks to identify it. The most prominent glabellar frown line corresponds to the junction of the medial corrugator and procerus muscles, and can be accentuated by pushing the lateral forehead toward the midline. The STA is located anywhere from this glabellar frown line to 6 mm laterally.[21] The pedicle base should therefore be wide enough to include these landmarks.[20]

Once the STA is mapped, the surgeon transfers the template to the forehead. To orient it accurately, the 180 degree direction of flap rotation must be anticipated. We recommend placing the template on the nasal wound, then rotating it 180 degrees toward the side on which the flap will be based. The template is placed in line with the STA so that the portion corresponding to the distal wound lies just inferior to the hairline. Some patients have prominent vellus hairs on the upper forehead, and the template may therefore be placed lower to avoid hair transfer to the nose, assuming the pedicle has adequate reach. If the flap will not reach the defect, the template can be placed transversely instead, aiming at the contralateral forehead inferior to the hairline. Even without an axial blood supply, the flap will have sufficient perfusion via the subdermal plexus.[19]

Distal defects of the infratip and columella and patients with low hairlines present the greatest challenges for flap design. Ensuring adequate length is another instance where it pays to "measure twice and cut once." To avoid raising a flap that is not long enough, a gauze pad simulating its reach can be stretched from the most proximal part of the pedicle to the distal part of the template near the hairline. A surgical marking pen can be used to indicate the exact point at which the gauze meets the template's distal aspect. Keeping the gauze pressed against the pedicle base, its distal end is rotated 180 degrees toward the midline, avoiding excessive tension, so as not to overestimate pedicle length. If the marked area does not reach the distal defect, the flap may not be long enough. The surgeon should then place the template more superiorly on the forehead or extend the base more proximally toward the medial canthus. After assuring adequate length, the surgeon can finalize the design. The template is situated at its precise forehead location, and its border outlined, with the proximal pedicle centered on the STA. A width of 1.1 to 1.4 cm safely includes the STA and minimizes torque during flap transfer. The flap's template portion is usually wider than its base. To optimize its blood supply, the narrow portion should widen progressively until it meets the templated portion (Fig. 19-2).

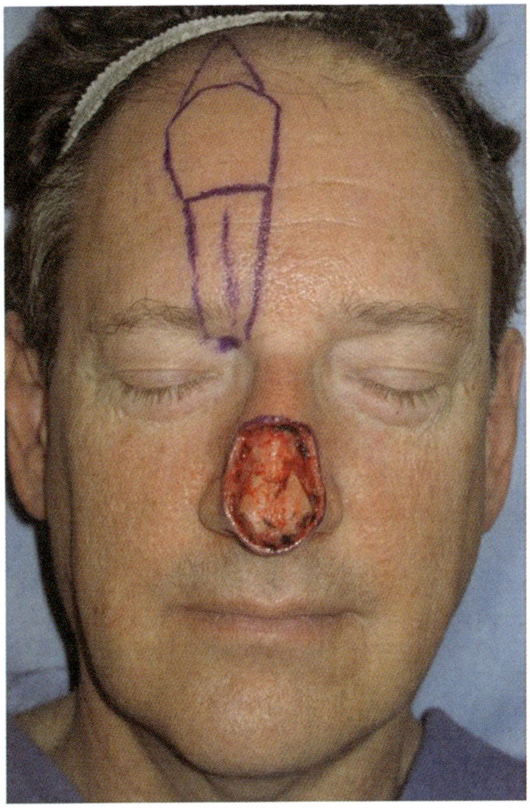

Figure 19-2 A template of the nasal defect has been transferred to the forehead donor site inferior to the hairline. The path of the supratrochlear artery (STA) has been mapped with a Doppler device, and the flap pedicle is based around the STA. The pedicle base has a width of 1.2 cm and fans out to meet the templated portion of the flap. As the defect is located in the midline, either side of the forehead would serve as a suitable donor site.

LIFTING THE FLAP

IDEAL ANATOMIC PLANES TO DETERMINE FLAP THICKNESS AND PRESERVE BLOOD SUPPLY

The anatomic plane in which the flap is lifted determines its thickness and blood supply. The layers of the mid to superior forehead include skin, subcutaneous fat, frontalis muscle, loose connective tissue, and periosteum. At the medial brow and suprabrow, the anatomy is more complex, including the skin, subcutaneous fat, orbicularis oculi, frontalis, and corrugator muscles, fat deep to the corrugator, and periosteum.[22,23] This discussion addresses dissection of the flap in three separate regions: (1) the distal flap (2) the mid-pedicle, or the mid-forehead portion of the flap, and (3) the base, or the most proximal portion at the medial brow. Each region requires unique strategies, but for all three, it is crucial to maintain exquisite hemostasis to maximize visibility and accuracy, as well as to improve the patient's physical and psychological comfort. When performing this flap under local anesthesia, bleeding flushes anesthesia rapidly, raising anxiety for the patient and the operating team.

DISSECTING THE TEMPLATED PORTION OF THE FLAP.

The plane of dissection of the templated portion of the flap depends on whether it has been planned as a two-stage or a three-stage process. Two-stage forehead flaps are indicated for partial-thickness defects or when cartilage graft placement is possible during the initial stage. Three-stage flaps are indicated when there is a full-thickness nasal tip defect requiring nasal lining and delayed cartilage grafting, or when the defect has complex contours that may require sculpting of the flap at an intermediate stage.

DISSECTING THE TEMPLATED PORTION OF THE FLAP FOR A PLANNED TWO-STAGE FOREHEAD FLAP

For two-stage flaps, the thickness of the templated portion should be a nearly perfect match for the defect, since aggressive thinning during pedicle division and inset may compromise blood supply. A two-stage flap that is too thick will require revision, which may be challenging due to fibrosis and scar contraction.

The templated portion of the flap should match the varying thicknesses of the nasal soft tissue. An incision is first made through dermis and fat along the lateral and distal template outlines. At the lateral margins, the incision should be vertical. Distally, a beveled angle can be used if the flap must match the thin skin of the columella, infratip, soft triangle, or alar rim. Sharp dissection can proceed subdermally for 2 to 3 mm to match the thin nasal skin. An incision is then made through the fat to reveal the frontalis muscle fibers or galea. Full-thickness forehead skin usually provides a good match for the proximal ala and nasal tip.

At this point, the surgeon can inspect the distal and lateral incision margins to identify the precise depth of the STA branches coursing through the fat. These vessels provide a visual landmark that guides the rest of the dissection. The dissection should proceed immediately superficial to frontalis for most, and preferably all, of the remaining templated portion of the flap (Fig. 19-3). As long as the dissection cleanly separates fat from frontalis, the STA branches, and therefore the flap's blood supply, will remain intact.[20] An accidental incision into the base of the fat can transect the vessels and compromise blood supply. With the surgeon at the head of the operating table (bird's-eye view), skin hooks at the distal flap can be held by an assistant to provide firm countertraction as the scalpel or scissors gently separates subcutaneous fat from frontalis. The tissue plane should separate effortlessly with almost no bleeding. If the wound or the flap undersurface demonstrates excessive bleeding or scalloped ridges corresponding to passes of the blade or cuts from the scissors, flap

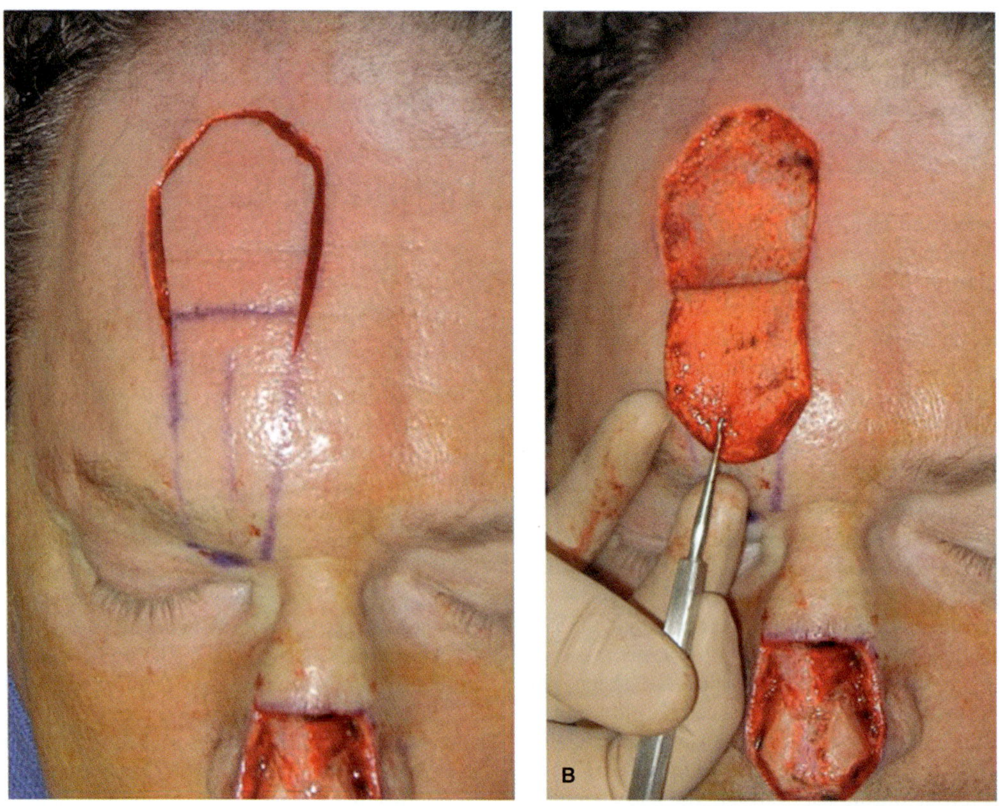

Figure 19-3 **A.** The incision is limited to the templated portion of the flap to minimize bleeding. **B.** For this planned two-stage flap, the entire templated portion is elevated superficial to the frontalis muscle. The absence of bleeding at the flap base indicates that the supratrochlear vessels are intact.

viability may be compromised and the surgeon should find a more precise dissection plane.

If the incision extends through frontalis or galea before reaching the proximal 10% to 20% of the templated portion of the flap, the flap will usually have more volume than the nasal defect. At the time of division and pedicle inset, efforts to excise muscle from the proximal flap will risk compromise to the blood supply. The flap should therefore be dissected from the muscle at the time of harvest, which requires intimate knowledge of the tissue planes. Although novice surgeons may prefer to lift a flap with frontalis fibers intact to protect the vessels in the fat, flap dissection at the desired level presents multiple advantages.[20] Defining tissue planes is easier when skin tension provides countertraction. When flap thickness is precisely defined from the beginning, less manipulation is required at division and inset, and its blood supply will be optimized. Finally, if tension on the forehead prevents primary donor site closure, the intact frontalis will accelerate second intention healing of the forehead wound.

DISSECTING THE TEMPLATED PORTION OF THE FLAP FOR A PLANNED THREE-STAGE FOREHEAD FLAP

The three-stage forehead flap includes an intermediate stage, usually 3 weeks after the primary inset, to lift and contour the flap. Perfect flap thickness at the time of primary inset is therefore neither necessary nor expected. The primary concept behind the three-staged flap is that minimal fibrosis occurs if the galea or frontalis muscle remains intact. The fat is then easier to manipulate during the intermediate procedure, and lifting the flap is effortless.[17] The indications for a planned three-stage flap include full-thickness defects requiring distal flap turnover to recreate lining; complex, multi-subunit defects requiring considerable contouring to restore symmetry; patients with a tenuous blood supply; and defects requiring delayed cartilage grafting. Unplanned three-stage flaps may be necessary if primary inset of an intended two-stage flap is too bulky. However, fibrosis after frontalis removal may make contouring more difficult.

Dissection of the templated portion of a planned three-stage flap is straightforward. The incision proceeds through galea and frontalis, and the flap is lifted in the plane deep to the muscle. The loose connective tissue creates excessive bulk so the flap should not include it. The flap thickness usually exceeds that of the defect, making it difficult to inset within the distal nasal skin. The flap edge may then be beveled to facilitate insetting.

DISSECTING THE MID-PEDICLE

Once the templated portion of the flap is elevated, the dissection should proceed through frontalis and continue in the plane of the loose connective tissue (Fig. 19-4). A scalpel or blunt-tipped scissors dissects the tissue away from muscle with minimal effort. This dissection strategy poses no risk to the STA and does not vary between a two-stage flap versus a three-stage flap.

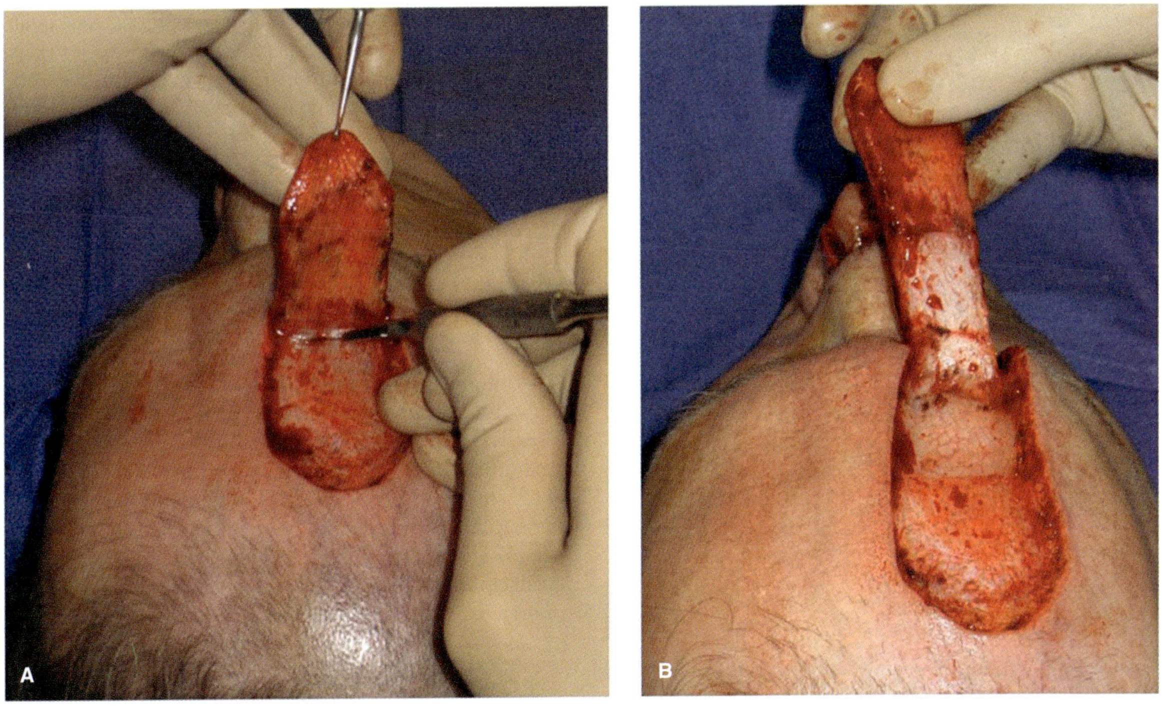

Figure 19-4 A. After elevating the templated portion of the flap superficial to frontalis, the muscle is incised and the dissection proceeds deeply in the loose connective tissue. This figure shows the surgeon's view from the head of the table while incising through frontalis muscle. **B.** The mid-pedicle is elevated deep to muscle in the loose connective tissue. The transition of surgical planes is visible on the flap undersurface and at the base of the forehead wound.

DISSECTING THE BASE OF THE PEDICLE

As dissection of the mid-pedicle approaches the brow, the surgeon will see yellow fat deep to the corrugator. At this point, an incision should be made through the fat to periosteum. The periosteum should not be incised, as it provides no lengthening of the flap and hemostasis may be complicated if a deep vein is transected.

Dissection at the pedicle base proceeds deep to the corrugator. Cotton-tipped applicators can be used to push away the corrugator muscle fibers without causing bleeding of the superior orbital plexus (Fig. 19-5). Vessels deep to the corrugator should be left intact, but can be precisely electrocauterized if necessary. Flap length should be assessed by rotating the flap toward the midline and stretching it toward the nasal wound. If it reaches the defect without tension, further dissection at the base can be avoided.

If the flap does not reach the distal defect, dissection can be carried proximally beyond the orbital rim. Incisions at the lateral edges of the pedicle are carried through the orbicularis oculi, frontalis, and corrugator muscles; a cotton-tipped applicator is used to push all soft tissue away from the periosteum. This blunt dissection should be deliberate and carried out with precise hemostasis. By carrying the dissection proximally, the flap gains considerable length. If the flap still does not reach the nasal defect, horizontal incisions may be made across the frontalis at its undersurface to gain additional movement, being careful to avoid transecting the STA by inadvertently extending the incisions into fat. Intraoperative stretching of the pedicle by an assistant while closing the donor site can also provide some "tissue creep."

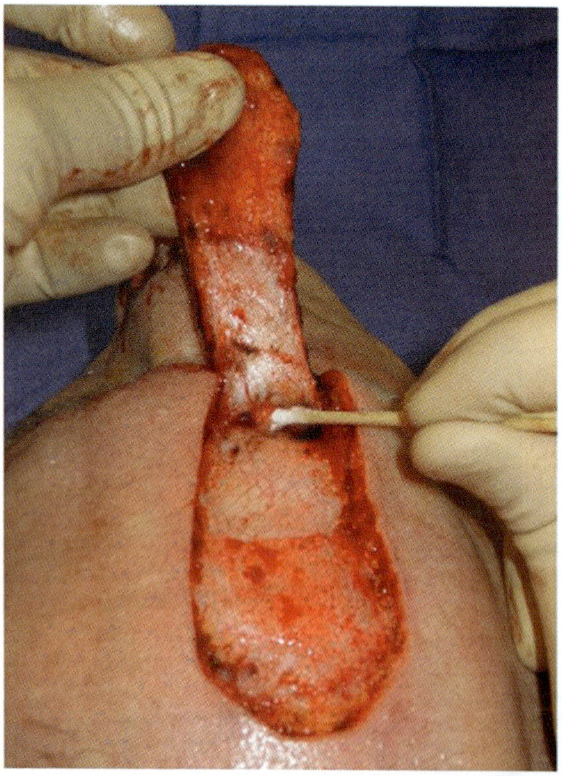

Figure 19-5 When the yellow fat deep to the corrugator muscle becomes visible, blunt dissection is used to push the muscle fibers away from the periosteum. The STA runs superficial to the corrugator, so incision through periosteum is not necessary to protect it. A cotton-tipped applicator is used to free the pedicle base from the periosteum.

INSETTING THE FLAP

PRIMARY INSET OF A TWO-STAGE FOREHEAD FLAP

If the template has been sized precisely and the flap and defect thickness match, inset should be straightforward. For a two-staged flap, cartilage grafts should be placed prior to inset. For a three-staged flap, they may be delayed until the nasal lining has been secured. Difficulty insetting will occur if the flap is undersized or oversized. Undersized flaps risk nasal cartilage compression and are difficult to fix. An oversized flap will result in poor contour, but the recovery is easier, since the flap can be trimmed to decrease its size.

The main objectives during flap inset are to align the templated portion with its corresponding nasal defect site. Undermining the defect margins prior to inset may help prevent pin-cushioning. The distal flap is anchored to the nasal wound; suturing proceeds proximally along its lateral aspects. For flaps that barely reach their intended site or cover asymmetric defects, the surgeon may secure the proximal flap edges to the skin overlying the upper lateral cartilages to prevent upward or lateral displacement of the lower lateral cartilages. The surgeon should make sure that the flap undersurface conforms properly to the base and eliminates dead space. For complex defects, quilting sutures can be used to recreate nasal concavities (Figs. 19-6 and 19-7). Some authors use cutaneous sutures alone for flap inset. We prefer to use a few deep sutures to prevent wound-edge inversion.

INTERMEDIATE STAGE OF A THREE-STAGE FOREHEAD FLAP FOR CONTOURING AND SECONDARY FLAP INSET

The intermediate stage of a three-stage flap provides the opportunity to improve contour (Figs. 19-8–19-10). Approximately 3 weeks after inset, the templated portion is incised and lifted in the plane beneath galea or frontalis. Cartilage grafts may be placed and the fibrotic tissue at the wound base sculpted, if needed. The elevated flap has a robust blood supply and can be thinned more aggressively than during primary inset, removing frontalis or galea and fat.[17] The contoured flap is sutured into place as described before.

CLOSING THE FOREHEAD DONOR SITE

The donor site is undermined in the loose connective tissue and closed in layers. Defect closure at the base and mid-pedicle is usually straightforward. However, there may be

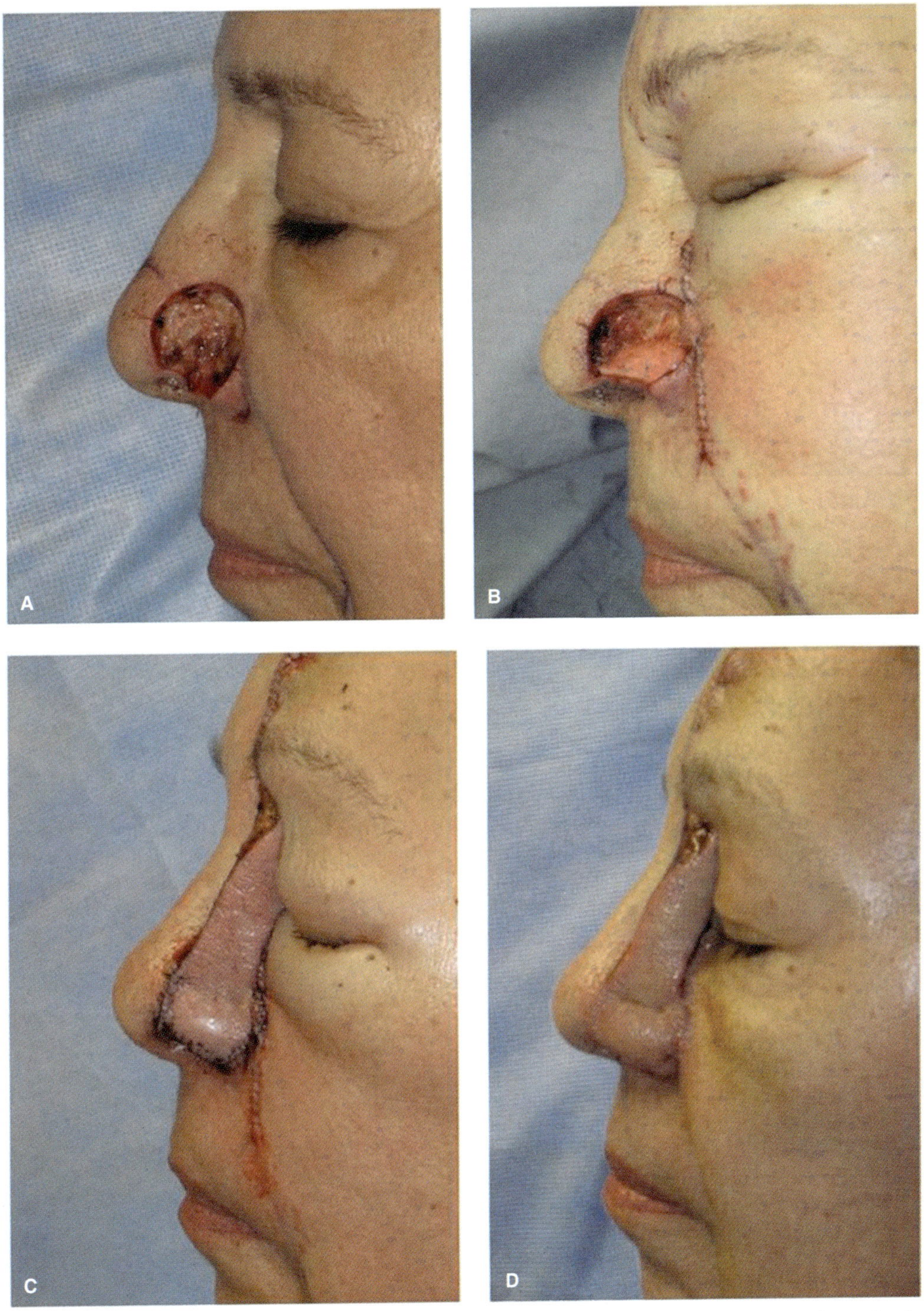

Figure 19-6 **A.** Distal nasal defect involving alar lobule, nasal sidewall, and premaxillary cheek. **B.** Intraoperative photo showing the free auricular cartilage graft supporting the alar margin and cheek advancement to prevent blunting of the nasofacial sulcus. **C.** Appearance after primary inset of a planned two-stage paramedian forehead flap. Tacking sutures from the flap base to the base of the wound were used to recreate the alar groove. The concavity from the tacking sutures is visible. **D.** Appearance 1 week after primary inset. Note the deep groove created by the tacking sutures. Edema around the sutures is common.

significant tension superiorly. If the wound is under tension, but closure is possible, excising the frontalis and loose connective tissue may be helpful. Excising a standing cone on the scalp is usually necessary. Any area too tight to close primarily should be left to granulate. The shiny scar from a wound left to heal by second intention will often be aesthetically acceptable (Fig. 19-1). Efforts to close the forehead site with rotation flaps or grafts lengthen the procedure, increase discomfort, and provide few long-term cosmetic benefits. If the forehead scar is unsatisfactory, serial excisions spaced several months apart will usually permit direct closure.

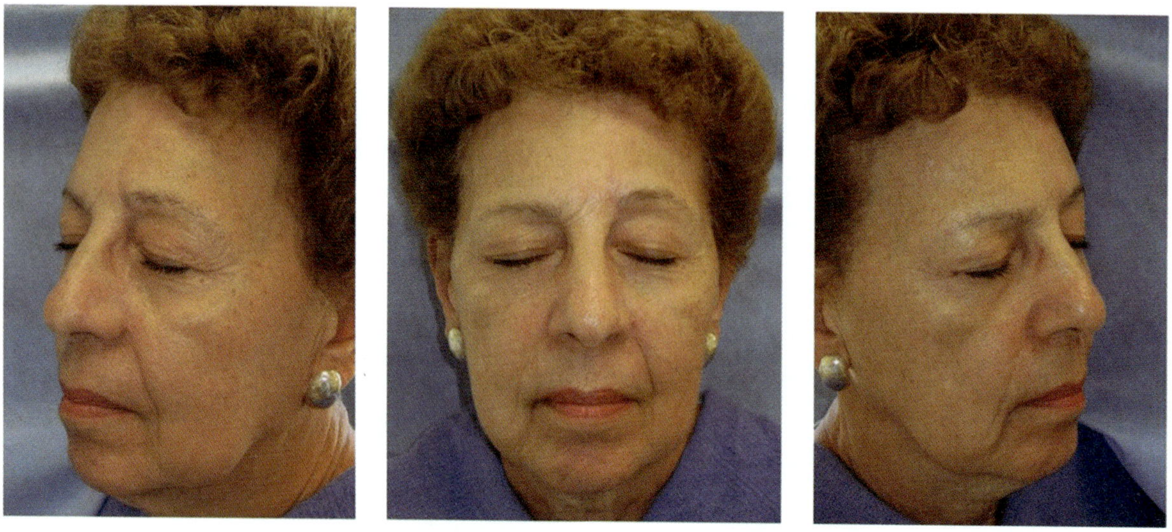

Figure 19-7 Postoperative appearance of the patient from Figure 19-6 10 months after division and inset of the two-stage paramedian forehead flap. The patient has retained concavity along the left alar groove as a result of the tacking sutures. No revision was performed.

DIVISION AND INSET OF THE PEDICLE

Once the flap is fully integrated with the nasal blood supply, the STA is no longer needed for its survival. Some authors successfully divide the pedicle as early as 1 week after primary inset.[24] However, most surgeons divide and inset the pedicle 3 weeks later, especially if cartilage grafts are used, the patient smokes, the flap is under tension, or if cosmesis would be optimized by refinement at pedicle division.

To begin the process, the flap's mid-pedicle is incised and hemostasis achieved on both ends. The cut end can be retracted with a skin hook and its proximal aspect bluntly dissected from the defect's proximal aspect. The exact defect margin is often not visible until the flap is elevated; it can be freshened by removing 1 to 2 mm of skin to the level of the perichondrium or periosteum. The freshened edge provides a target for sizing the flap in the horizontal and vertical dimensions. The pedicle's severed end is draped over the freshened proximal edge of the defect and trimmed. The proximal aspect of the flap is sculpted with a scalpel or tissue scissors to match the nasal skin thickness (Fig. 19-11). If the flap was too bulky at the time of inset, reshaping may be necessary. Because excessive thinning or flap elevation risks interruption of its newly formed blood supply, sculpting should be limited to the flap's proximal 10% to 20%. In most cases, the surgeon will need to remove any muscle left proximally at its base.

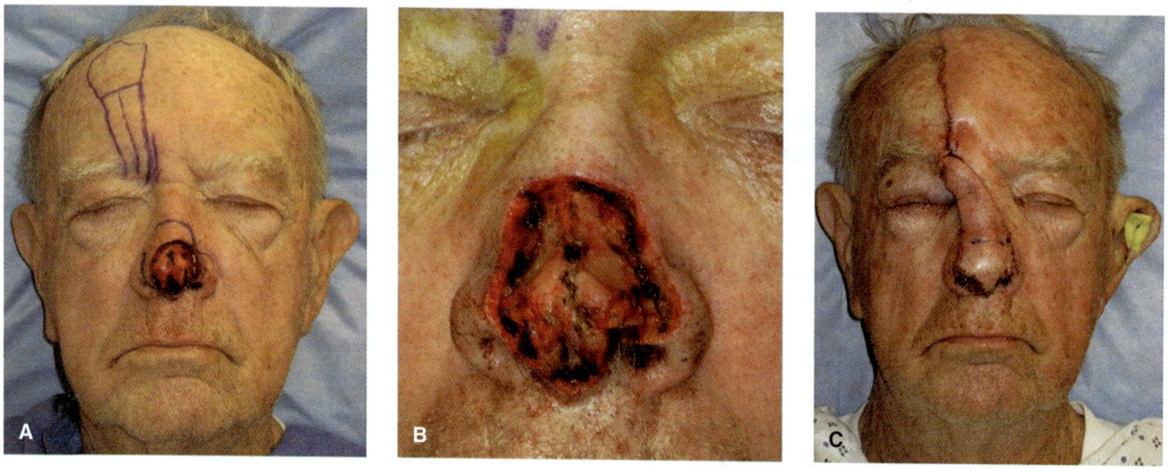

Figure 19-8 **A.** Defect involving the nasal tip, ala, and caudal margins of the lateral crura on both sides. **B.** Intraoperative photos demonstrating defect enlargement to include the entire tip subunit. Two small cartilage grafts have been sutured to the caudal remnants of the lateral crura. **C.** After primary inset of a planned three-stage paramedian forehead flap, the bulky flap lacks contour.

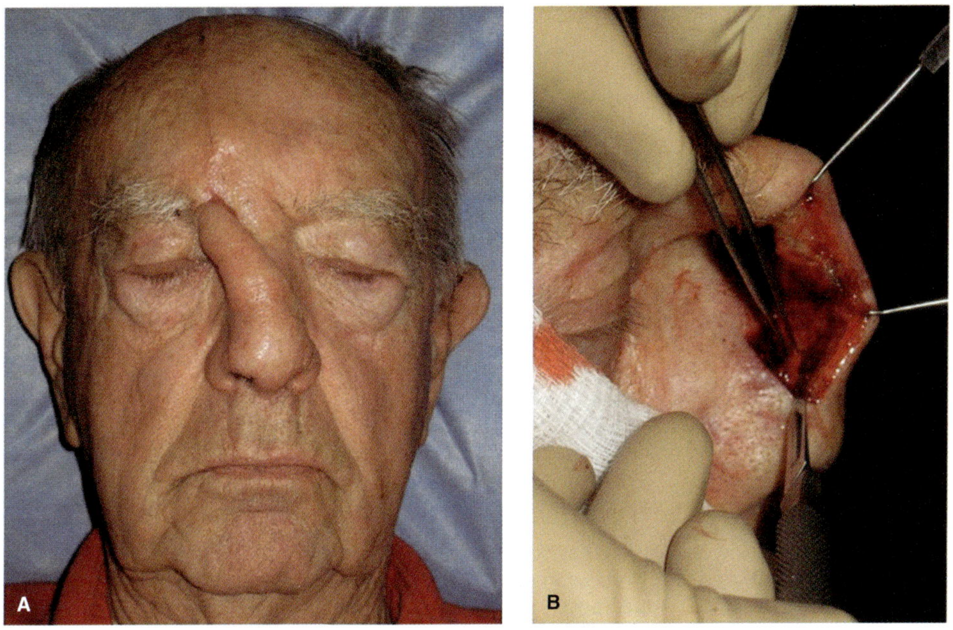

Figure 19-9 **A.** Appearance 3 weeks after primary inset. The flap remains bulky, especially at its proximal two-thirds. **B.** Intraoperative photo of flap thinning 3 weeks after primary inset. The proximal portion of the flap has been elevated, and a 15 blade scalpel is being used to excise frontalis muscle and sculpt the flap to the desired thickness. Elevation of the entire flap was not necessary in this case. The thinned flap was subsequently sutured back to the nose.

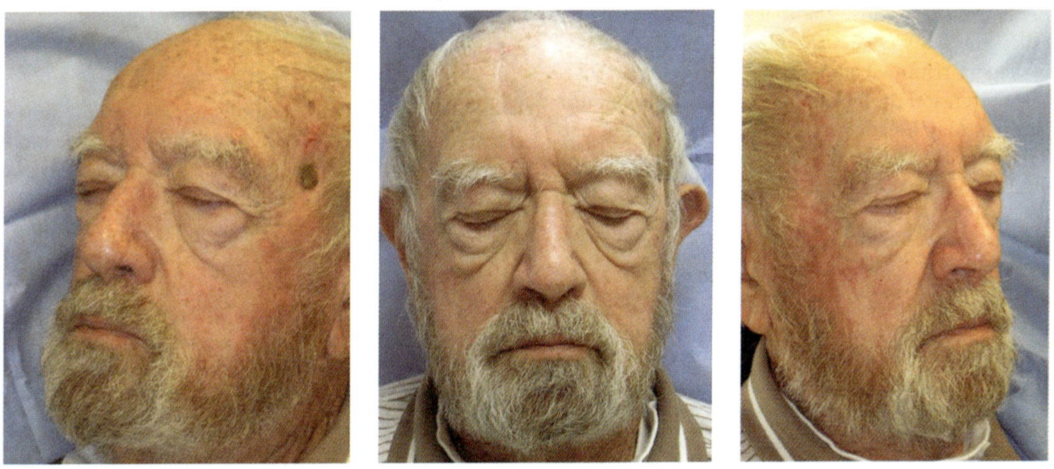

Figure 19-10 Appearance 6 months after division and inset of the three-staged flap. Contour is much improved.

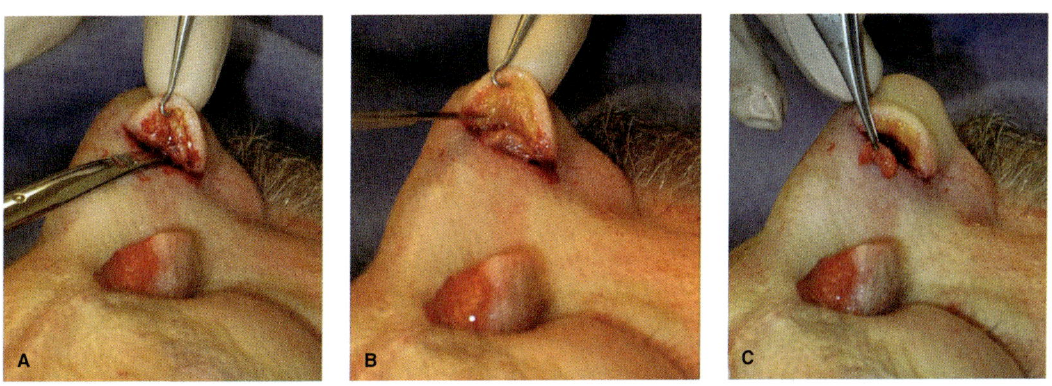

Figure 19-11 Surgeon's view from the head of the bed. **A.** The pedicle has been divided and blunt-tipped scissors are being used to elevate the flap from the proximal defect. **B.** Remnants of frontalis muscle and fibrous tissue are visible deep to the subcutaneous fat. A scalpel is used to excise the frontalis muscle and fibrous tissue from the base of the subcutaneous fat. **C.** A wedge of frontalis and fibrofatty tissue has been excised. The proximal flap now has appropriate thickness for inset.

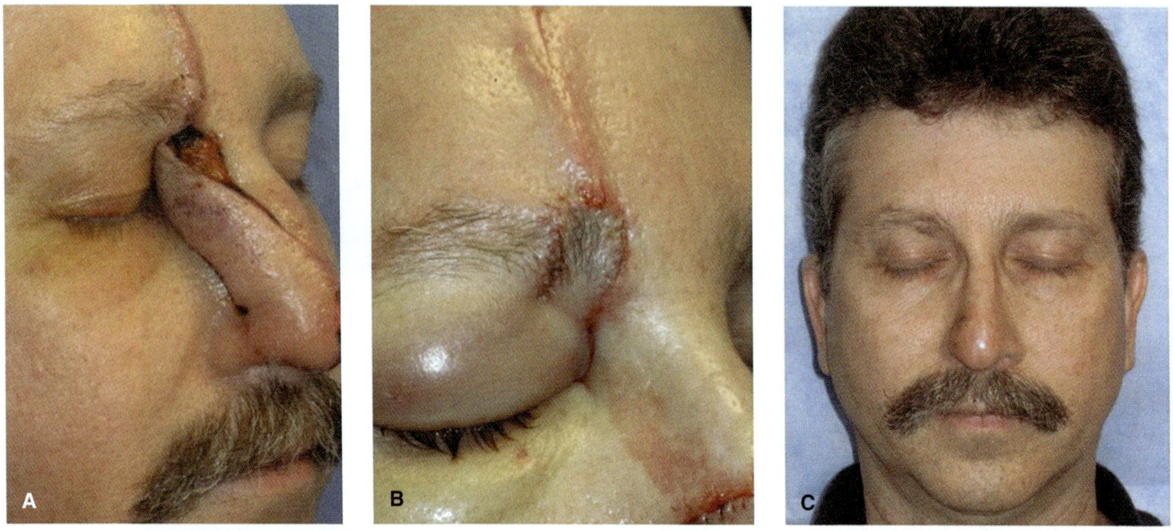

Figure 19-12 **A.** The pedicle of this two-stage flap has been dissected proximally through the brow to avoid hair transfer to the nose. Brow hair must be returned to restore symmetry. **B.** Inverted V-shaped suture line immediately after division of the pedicle and inset of the brow hair. **C.** Appearance 4 months after division and inset. Symmetry of brow hair has been restored. Ecchymosis on the nose is from a sculpting revision procedure 1 week previously.

The corners of the proximal defect require special attention. The pedicle's free edges have already begun to contract and reepithelialize. The nasal defect is typically most fibrotic at its corners, where the flap could not be sutured. A scalpel is used to remove the newly epithelialized skin and freshen the flap's edges. The fibrotic tissue is excised and the flap is trimmed and sutured into place. There should be no tension on the wound; a single layer of cutaneous sutures may be adequate. Strategically placed dermal sutures may help to minimize scar inversion. Excessive eversion should be avoided.

ADDRESSING THE DONOR SITE: INSETTING THE BASE OF THE PEDICLE

Insetting the pedicle at the brow begins by retracting its severed portion and bluntly dissecting the flap to reveal the edges of the wound, which will be in the shape of an upside down "V." The lateral margins of the pedicle base have contracted and reepithelialized. A scalpel is used to excise the epithelialized skin and to freshen its edges. Fibrotic tissue at the wound base should also be excised. The proximal pedicle is now rectangular. The severed end is draped over the proximal defect edge and cut to match the inverted "V" at the edge of the donor site. The pedicle is usually too thick, primarily due to fibrosis below the corrugator muscle. The fibrotic tissue can be excised, and the flap base sculpted to match the wound thickness at the donor site.

The surgeon must pay careful attention to the position of the eyebrow hairs. If the pedicle base was carried through the brow to increase flap reach, the hairs may have been pulled inferiorly and medially. To maintain symmetry, the surgeon may want to realign them, or tailor the wound at the donor site (Fig. 19-12). If insetting the hairs is not necessary, it may be possible to excise the base of the pedicle and repair the wound with a linear closure. Residual muscle at the flap base increases the risk of contraction. A carefully placed deep suture layer prevents pin-cushioning while cutaneous sutures approximate the epidermis, ideally with eversion.

COMMON PITFALLS AND SOLUTIONS

Each of the previous sections addresses common pitfalls and solutions, so this section will briefly review key points. First, the surgeon must take care to fashion a template that exactly fits the nasal defect contours. An undersized or oversized flap must be avoided. Second, it is important to map the STA's path, including the precise location at which it pierces the orbital septum. Careful mapping will increase the likelihood that the blood supply will remain intact, especially if the pedicle is dissected from the orbital rim to gain sufficient length to reach the nasal defect. The donor site is less likely to include scalp hair when the surgeon can mobilize the pedicle with confidence. Third, during primary inset of a two-stage flap, one should aim to match the thickness and contour of the nasal defect. A bulky flap frequently prevents perfect contouring at the time of pedicle division and inset. Fourth, meticulous hemostasis is critical to decrease the risk of postoperative bleeding, as well as to improve accuracy, efficiency, and patient comfort and confidence. Fifth, the surgeon should be patient with donor site repair. If the tension is too great for primary closure, the wound may heal by second intention. A suboptimal forehead scar can usually be revised later.

MELOLABIAL INTERPOLATION FLAP

The MIF is a random pattern pedicle flap based upon the muscular perforators branching from the facial, superior labial, and angular arteries in the nasolabial fold.[25] The fold provides a generous tissue reservoir with an excellent color and texture match for the ala. Previous authors have described multiple variants, such as a banner-type flap [26] and an interpolated paranasal flap from the hairless nasofacial sulcus.[27] In most cases, we prefer the traditional design.[28,29] Compared to one-stage melolabial flaps, the two-stage MIF has the advantage of preserving the alar-facial sulcus, the apical triangle, and the narrow isthmus between the melolabial fold and alar lobule.

ASSESSING THE DEFECT

LOCATION

The MIF is most suitable for reconstructing partial-thickness defects limited to the ala or the alar component of a defect involving multiple cosmetic subunits.[12] The natural contraction of the flap reliably recreates the alar convexity, especially when the scar's boundaries conform to the alar groove and distal free margin. The MIF may also repair columellar defects. While small tip defects can be resurfaced with an MIF, the blood supply to the distal portion of the flap is unpredictable. The paramedian forehead flap is a better choice for larger tip defects or multi-subunit nasal defects. The MIF can be turned over on itself to repair small full-thickness alar rim defects involving 2 to 3 mm of vestibular skin, but the forehead flap provides a better option for full-thickness defects with larger defects of the vestibular lining.

ASSESSING THE ANATOMIC DEPTH OF THE DEFECT AND INDICATIONS FOR CARTILAGE GRAFTING

The alar lobule does not contain cartilage.[8,9] Its lack of an intrinsic framework and the absent support at its free margin make it particularly susceptible to distortion. Loss of muscle decreases alar support, so defects involving more than 50% of the distal lobule usually require cartilage grafts to brace against contraction, support the airway, and provide convexity to the ala, to optimize cosmesis and function.[18] The concave antihelical cartilage at the lateral conchal bowl produces a C-shaped strut that preserves the flare of the lobule and provides a scaffold for the flap. With cartilage supporting the external valve and restoring alar projection, internal valve patency is ensured and airflow obstruction is minimized.

PRINCIPLES OF AESTHETIC DESIGN: DECIDING WHEN TO ENLARGE THE DEFECT

Circumferential scar contraction, known as "pin-cushioning" or "trapdooring," recreates the alar structure when the MIF is used for total alar defects. It is so predictable that nearly all partial alar defects may be expanded to the alar crease superiorly and the free margin of the rim inferiorly. However, horizontal expansion should be executed with caution and avoided if it risks external valve weakening or flattening of the alar flare. The alar base should be preserved, as its three-dimensional projection forms the alar foundation.[30] The lateral alar-facial sulcus is especially difficult to repair, so 1 to 2 mm of the ala should be preserved if possible.

As the MIF is best applied to the ala, portions of the defect beyond it may require separate closure. To identify the precise alar boundaries, the surgeon marks the cosmetic junction lines bilaterally and makes a template of the defect and the contralateral ala (Fig. 19-13). Defect components on the adjacent sidewall or extending onto the tip beyond the MIF's reach are best repaired separately. Superficial paranasal defects do not necessarily preclude MIF

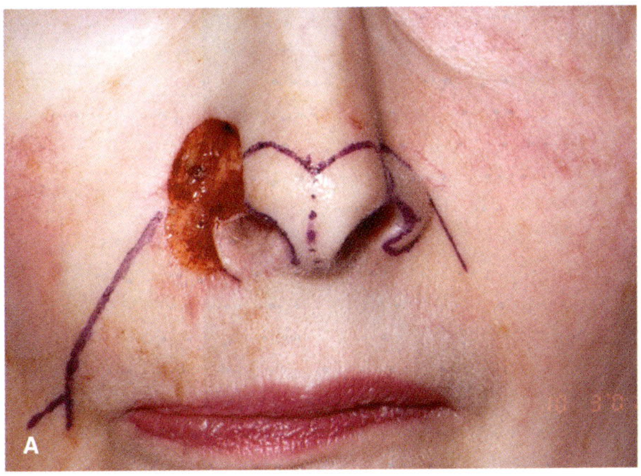

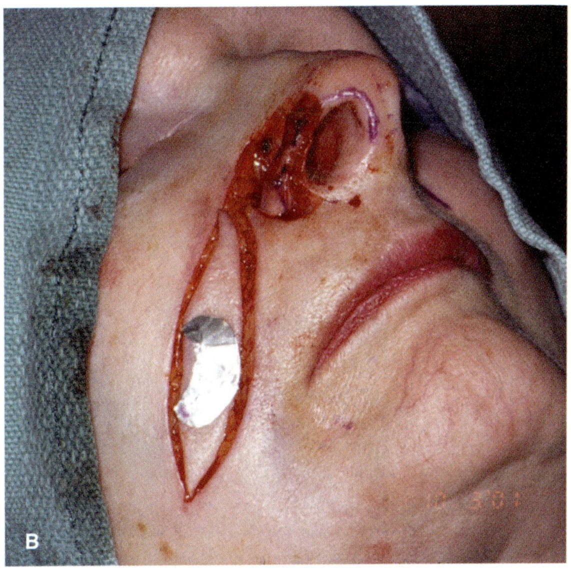

Figure 19-13 **A.** Cosmetic subunits have been defined bilaterally. As the defect extends beyond the cosmetic subunit of the alar lobule, the contralateral ala is used to create a template to match the portion of the defect corresponding to the alar lobule. **B.** The foil template from the contralateral alar subunit has been transferred to the donor site on the melolabial fold.

repair, because the muscular perforators that supply blood to the flap will still be intact. To avoid ablating the alar-facial sulcus and apical triangle, paranasal cheek defects are best allowed to heal by second intention if small, or can be repaired at the time of takedown with remnants from the pedicle. The alar crease heals well by second intention. A thinned flap margin can also be basted with curvilinear quilting sutures to recreate this concavity.[31,32] When the paranasal defect is large, other options may be preferable to avoid ablation of the alar-facial sulcus.[33]

DESIGNING THE FLAP

MAKING THE TEMPLATE

The majority of alar defects large and deep enough to require a MIF will also demand a cartilage strut. The surgeon must prepare templates for the cartilage graft and the MIF. The cartilage template is designed first. The ideal donor site is the ipsilateral conchal bowl-antihelix junction, which affords the patient a pain-free contralateral ear and cheek on which to rest. This cartilage maintains its elasticity, and rarely develops solar induced calcification or ossification, and its C-shape supports the MIF by recapitulating the alar flare. The template is transferred to the ear and the best matching location marked. The graft's vertical height should be 1/3 to 1/2 the alar height (generally 5–8 mm), as it provides sufficient support and allows easy suturing. The horizontal graft dimension may be longer than the defect's horizontal axis to allow insertion of the long ends of the cartilage into soft-tissue pockets, particularly at the alar base.

After determining the appropriate graft size, an incision is made along the antihelical rim, and the skin is dissected off the perichondrium. The template is transferred to the donor site to ensure appropriate size. The cartilage graft is excised with care (Fig. 19-14). Narrow donor defects can be reapproximated, but generally the skin is

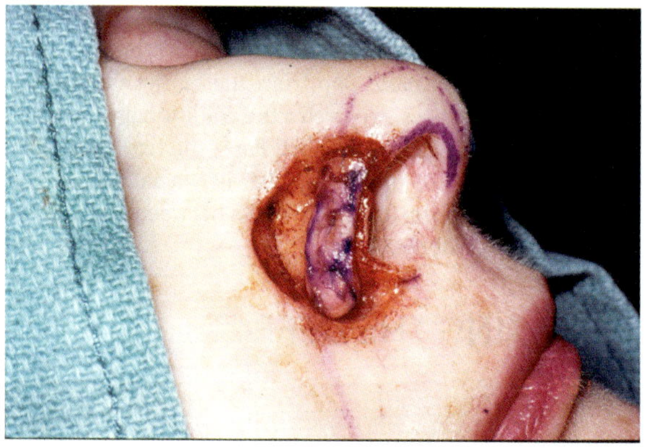

Figure 19-15 A nonanatomic free cartilage graft has been sutured to the base of the defect.

replaced, trimmed if needed, and sutured. A bolster may be placed for additional hemostasis. The cartilage graft is then secured to the defect (Fig. 19-15). Using the scalpel or the tips of a scissors, pockets between the alar muscle and vestibular mucosa are created along the defect margins to allow insertion of the graft ends. The cartilage may require additional trimming. Care must be taken to secure the graft inferiorly to support the alar rim. A common mistake is to set it too superiorly, which results in insufficient bulk and risks contraction, shortening the vertical height of the flap. Grafts less than 5 mm in height can be difficult to suture without fracturing. One or two 5-0 absorbable sutures can be lassoed around these narrow grafts to secure them; 6-0 sutures can be passed through larger grafts without fracturing. One must carefully pass the needle along its curvature to avoid fracturing the cartilage; it should pass through the defect base without interrupting the mucosal surface.

Once the cartilage graft is in place, attention is turned to making the MIF template. The subunit (or defect) borders are inked; light pressure imprints the outline. The goal is to transfer the ink without flattening the template, which would underestimate the three-dimensional size of the ala.

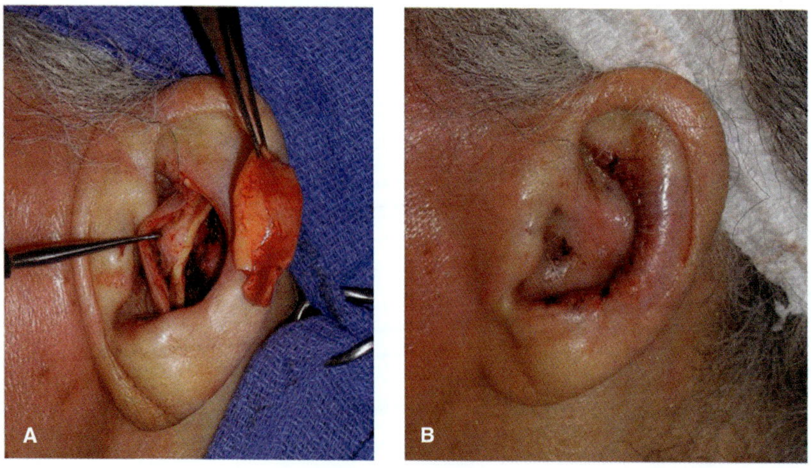

Figure 19-14 **A.** A generously sized free cartilage graft has been harvested from the concha via an antihelical incision. Cartilage from this location has a natural curvature that simulates the normal contour of the alar lobule. **B.** The auricular incision is sutured with a layer of running cutaneous sutures. Quilting sutures or a bolster dressing may be helpful to reduce dead space and decrease the risk of hematoma.

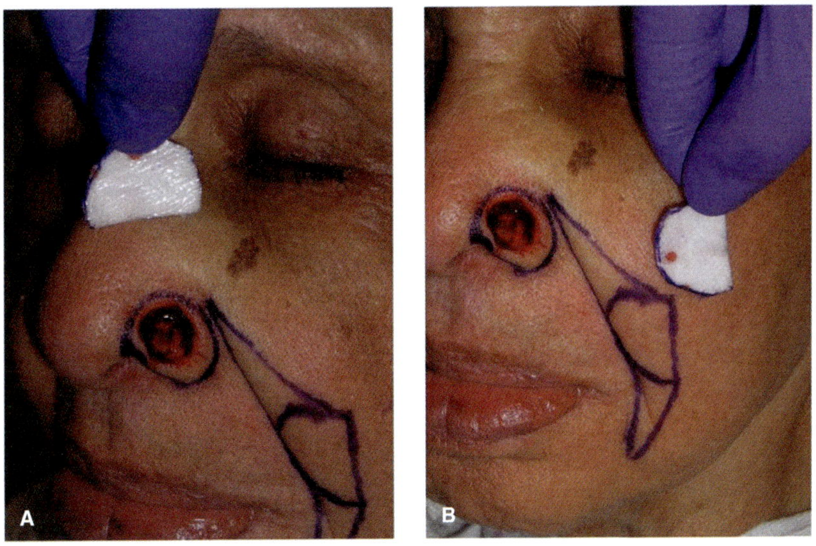

Figure 19-16 **A.** A Telfa pad has been used to make a template of the alar subunit. The defect will be enlarged to the boundaries of the subunit prior to flap transfer. **B.** The template has been rotated inferolaterally and transferred to the melolabial fold donor site. The fusiform design is completed by drawing a Burow's triangle on each side of the templated portion of the flap.

If the defect precludes accurate alar sizing, the contralateral ala should be used for the template, which is then transposed to the ipsilateral defect to define the subunit borders, retaining the three-dimensional shape and mirror image.

TRANSFERRING THE TEMPLATE TO THE DONOR SITE

The melolabial fold is traced with a marking pen prior to injecting anesthesia. The cheek skin superolateral to the melolabial fold is inspected for lesions or scars. In general, the donor site is located at the midpoint of the melolabial fold between the alar sill and labial commissure.

The donor location must allow sufficient length to reach the defect. To assess flap length, a 4″ × 4″ gauze is opened, rolled into a tube shape to approximate the MIF's caliber, and held at the planned pedicle base lateral to the ala. The gauze is rotated 110 to 120 degrees superomedially, simulating the anticipated flap rotation, and placed on the defect, where it is soiled with blood. If its stain is faint, a surgical pen may be used to mark the point at which the gauze crosses the defect margins. The gauze is rotated back to the donor area; the template location correlates with the marked areas on the gauze. This assessment should be repeated, with care not to stretch the gauze so the flap length will not be underestimated.

The template is placed onto the cheek donor site, relaxed, flattened, and outlined (Fig. 19-16), its orientation corresponding to the exact shape of the defect when the flap is in place. We recommend placing the template directly on the alar wound, then rotating it 110 to 120 degrees laterally. Its superior edge will lie against the melolabial fold with its anterior edge on the cheek. After ensuring proper orientation, the template margins are traced, and the fusiform design completed by drawing Burow's triangles along the melolabial fold and the nasofacial sulcus. The triangles should be long enough that their apical angles are 30 degrees or less.

It can be helpful to mark the skin overlying the flap's planned blood supply to ensure that dissection does not extend too far proximally during its elevation.[34] The axis of rotation lies at the base of the superior dog-ear, which is later excised. A triangular pedicle MIF is preferred over a banner configuration for this reason. The former design reduces torque, as removing the superior dog-ear frees the proximal margin to move laterally as the distal end rotates into the alar defect. Reducing torque on the flap base decreases tension and optimizes blood flow.

LIFTING THE FLAP

IDEAL ANATOMIC PLANES TO DETERMINE FLAP THICKNESS AND PRESERVE BLOOD SUPPLY

The MIF is incised through the skin into the superficial fat. The inferior dog-ear may be retained until after flap elevation, so that any length insufficiency can be accommodated. The flap is elevated from its distal to proximal aspect, and includes the layer of fat immediately adherent to the underside of the dermis. This plane is found most reliably along the melolabial fold. The angular artery lies deep to the zygomaticus major and levator labii superioris, and is protected by dissecting at the junction of the subcutaneous fat and lip elevators.[35] While elevating the lateral aspects of the flap, the surgeon must avoid the tendency to dive into the nasolabial fat pad.[36] Inclusion of the fat pad will result in excessive flap thickness and bulky contour.

Once the distal 80% to 90% of the flap has been dissected, the dissection transitions to a plane in the deeper fat, with care to preserve the perforators at the base. The

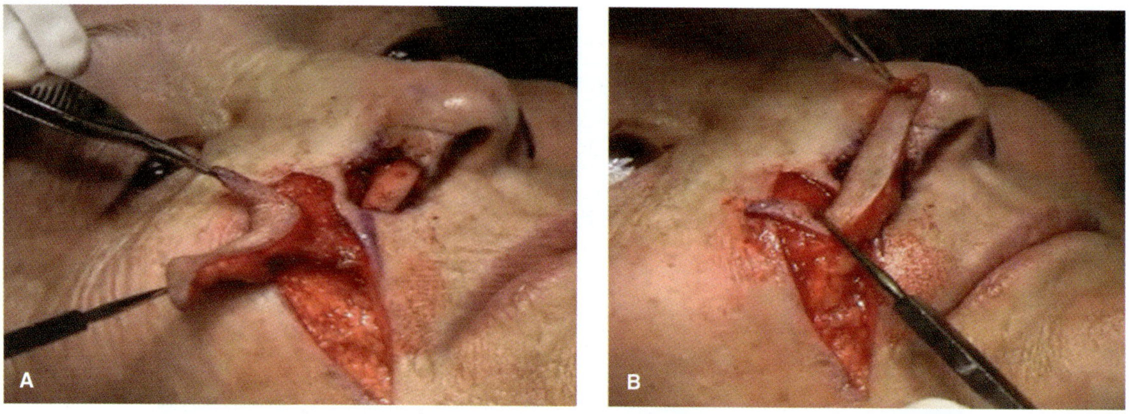

Figure 19-17 **A.** Intraoperative photo demonstrating elevation of the proximal and distal arms of the flap around the central muscular pedicle. The auricular cartilage graft has already been sutured to the alar defect. **B.** The flap freely rotates toward the defect. The proximal and distal paddles of the flap rotate like helicopter blades around the pedicle.

proximal flap should have the base of a finger-width over the paranasal perforators, and the dissection is performed with blunt scissor tips held parallel to the flap's long axis and spread 3 to 4 mm apart with a gentle forward pressing motion. This technique loosens the fibrous septae while preserving the vessels. One continues proximally until the flap can move freely into the defect. The same technique is used at its superior and lateral margins, although there are fibrous connections along the alar crease and isthmus that may need sharp scissor dissection in the plane above the muscle. Dissection continues until the flap freely rotates without tension or torque (Fig. 19-17).

The thickness of the flap is evaluated. If the initial dissection was too deep and the flap is bulky, the fat is thinned, being careful to preserve the dermal plexus. More fat can be retained if bulk is required, but deep defects will likely require a cartilage graft to fill this void. As cheek and alar thickness, texture, and sebaceous quality almost always match, and the flap tends to develop a convex structure, 2 to 3 mm of retained fat will likely produce a natural appearance. Rarely, if ever, does a MIF require additional bulk, although it may occasionally need thinning at takedown or later revision. The outer edges of the donor site are undermined to the degree needed for closure. Undermining is especially vital in the hairless triangle and paranasal areas, and is performed just under the dermis and above the muscle. This affords a broad-based pedicle of muscle at the origin of the MIF, with robust vascularization.

INSETTING THE FLAP

The flap should be inset with the tension that exists natively to prevent pin-cushioning or necrosis. The margins of the nasal defect are undermined above the lower lateral cartilage or superficial to the vestibular mucosa. The flap is inset using 5-0 buried sutures, most importantly at the nasal tip/alar junction and the alar base. The rim requires only epidermal sutures. 6-0 sutures are placed along the flap margins, with extra eversion along the free margin to prevent notching. To promote concavity, the crease is allowed to heal secondarily or cutaneous guiding sutures are placed. Eversion should be avoided along the alar groove (Fig. 19-18).

If the flap extends over the groove, horizontal mattress quilting sutures oriented along the alar crease will bend the flap to conform to the concavity at the inferior margin of the lower lateral cartilage (Fig. 19-19). The template or precise measurements should be used to ensure symmetry. The flap is trimmed distally only after the alar crease and rim are repaired and recreated. Tissue characteristics and flap dynamics frequently dictate that flap length is either shorter or longer than measured, despite meticulous planning.

TAKING DOWN THE FLAP

After 1 week, cheek and ear donor site sutures are removed. The alar sutures can be removed after 1 to 2 weeks, with crease sutures retained for longer. Mid-pedicle compression allows assessment of blood supply; the flap should remain pink by the third week. Takedown is accomplished by dividing the pedicle and excising the base as an ellipse in the melolabial fold and repairing with standard layered closure.

The proximal flap must be inset with appropriate tension to prevent pin-cushioning or excessive bulk. A template based upon the contralateral ala is used to define the exact lateral crease. The flap is gently stretched and incised along this mark. Using a skin hook and sharp dissection, fat and fibrotic tissues are thinned from the flap base to match the alar thickness. It is important to retain bulk at the alar base, as it is a structural landmark. Generally, thinning is performed along the flap rather than within the defect. The flap is sutured into the alar crease with simple or mattress cutaneous sutures, allowing the true margin to heal secondarily to recreate the concavity (Fig. 19-18). At the superior margin, the crease can be deepened with a V-shaped partial to full-thickness excision following a symmetric arc (Fig. 19-19).

COMMON PITFALLS AND SOLUTIONS

The most significant complication of the MIF is necrosis. Overly aggressive thinning of the pedicle base threatens survival. In our experience, necrosis more frequently

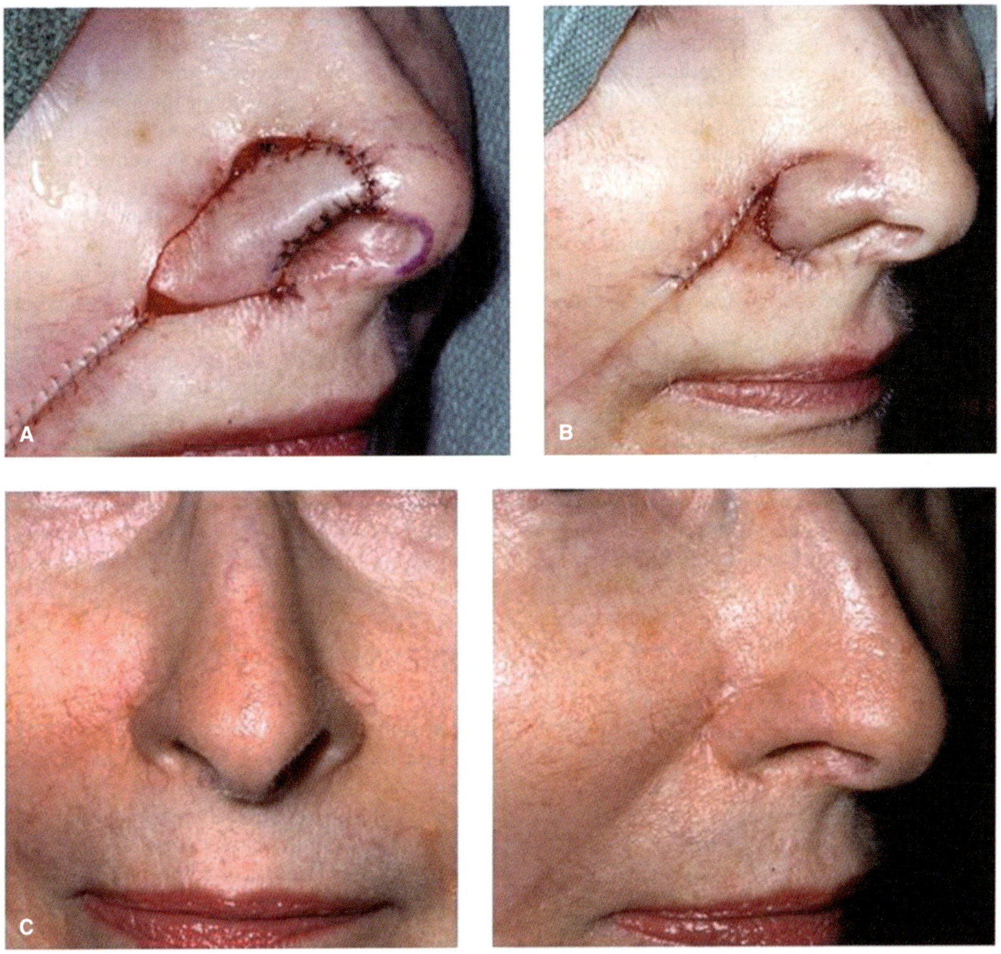

Figure 19-18 **A.** Melolabial interpolation flap immediately after placement of a nonanatomic free cartilage graft and primary inset of the flap. The original defect extended beyond the lobule into the alar groove. Note that the alar crease has been allowed to heal by second intention, rather than ablating the groove with the flap. **B.** Appearance immediately after division and inset of the flap. The cheek donor site has been repaired with a layered closure. The alar-facial sulcus has been allowed to heal by second intention to recreate the deep, natural concavity. **C.** Appearance 6 months after division and inset. The flap has restored symmetry of the alar subunits and second intention healing has recreated the alar groove.

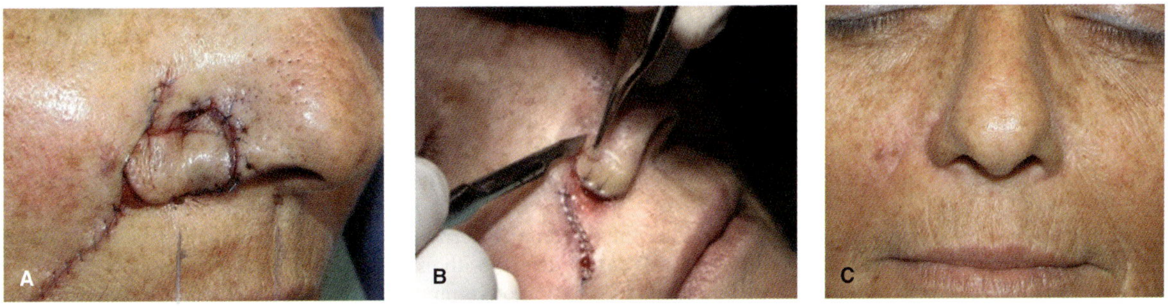

Figure 19-19 **A.** Melolabial interpolation flap after placement of free cartilage graft and primary flap inset. Vertical mattress sutures at the tip – alar junction accentuate eversion. Quilting sutures and second intention healing produce inversion along the alar groove. **B.** Intraoperative photo during division and inset. The cheek donor site has been repaired. A scalpel is used to sculpt the alar crease, and the alar-facial sulcus is left to heal by second intention to promote inversion. **C.** Appearance 6 months after division and inset demonstrating good contour and imperceptible scars.

results from an excessively thick pedicle, whose torque restricts blood flow. This torque is exacerbated by inadequate undermining, especially in the paranasal sulcus.

Flap elevation that is carried out too proximally or too deeply can sever vital perforating vessels. Overly conservative elevation or flap design with a pedicle that is based too inferiorly can cause flap buckling and inability to reach its intended site. A base designed too far laterally on the cheek can compromise blood supply and requires excessive length to reach the defect. In our experience, even the banner flap will have restricted movement and require a more challenging inset procedure.

Asymmetry is another common problem, often resulting from excessive size in any dimension relative to the normal ala. Intralesional steroid injections at concentrations of 5 to 20 mg/cc are helpful for mild to moderate pincushioning starting about 1 month after takedown and repeated monthly as needed. Edge irregularities, common in sebaceous skin, can be smoothed with dermabrasion 4 to 8 weeks after division and inset. Deepening of the alar crease can also be improved in this manner. Flap height may be reduced by excising tissue along the superior alar crease, and flap width reduced by excising tissue along the lateral alar crease. The rim may be thinned by excising excess bulk via an incision at the alar margin, while flap volume may be reduced by sharply debulking the fibrofatty tissue along the alar crease. These revisions are usually performed 2 to 4 months after division and inset, when the scar tissue has stabilized.

For flaps that lack bulk or develop a notched or unstable alar rim, cartilage struts can be placed. A stab incision can be made at the soft triangle or alar base to create a tunnel into which is placed a small cartilage graft. A flap can be raised to allow easier placement, but excessive elevation should be avoided to reduce the risk of necrosis.

THE POSTAURICULAR INTERPOLATION FLAP

ANATOMY

The external ear is a topographically complex structure that projects from the head at a 30 degree angle aligned between vectors drawn from the lateral eyebrow and the alar base.[37,38] It contains concavities and convexities that possess varying degrees of skin thickness and sebaceous gland density. Some subunits vary widely in size and shape, such as the antihelix, concha, scapha, and lobe, whereas others, like the helical rim and postauricular surfaces, vary less.

Cartilage provides unique structural nuances to the ear. A cross-sectional view of the upper two-thirds of the ear reveals an elastic cartilage substructure enveloped by skin. The thin anterior skin firmly adheres to the perichondrium without subcutaneous tissue interposed, and contains a high density of sebaceous glands, particularly in the scaphoid and conchal regions. The posterior skin is thicker and more loosely adherent, contains a 1 to 3 mm thick adipose layer, and is less sebaceous. A curl in the cartilage and a roll of subcutaneous tissue contribute to the size and shape of the helical rim.[39] A freely hanging lobule comprising the lower one-third of the ear consists of adipose tissue enveloped by skin and devoid of cartilage.

Ligaments and muscles connect the external ear to the skull. It projects slightly from the sides of the head with the superior portion slightly more visible than the inferior one from an anterior view,[40] and connects to the middle and inner ear via the external auditory canal. Patency of the canal during reconstruction is paramount as constriction can compromise hearing.

Tributaries of the external carotid system, including the postauricular artery and the superficial temporal artery, deliver blood to the ear. While the postauricular artery supplies the posterior surface, the anterior aspect is supplied by anastomosing vessel connections, which allow the ear to remain vascularized if one of the arterial systems is sacrificed.[41] In addition, occipital artery branches deliver blood to the posterior auricle and adjacent mastoid skin. Because of this robust blood supply, helical rim and anterior defects are often repaired with postauricular skin, as it possesses an easily mobilized subcutaneous layer and its surgical scars are inconspicuous.

ASSESSING THE DEFECT

Successful auricular reconstruction preserves contour. Because the ears cannot be appreciated simultaneously, minor height discrepancies rarely affect aesthetic outcomes.[42] Likewise, minor alterations to surface topography are not likely to distract from the lateral or anterior profiles. Ear positioning is important. Distances greater than 2 cm between the upper helix and temporal skin may be perceived as abnormal.[43] Malpositioning can arise when flaps cause ear shortening or "cupping," which can be avoided with distal tissue transfer in the form of a skin graft or interpolation flap.

The depth, site, and size of an ear defect define the approach to its repair. Medial anterior defects may granulate if perichondrium is intact. Granulation on the helical rim may be possible for shallow defects, but can lead to notching with deeper ones. Less than 2 cm helical rim or anterior surface defects may be repaired with flaps, grafts, or wedge resections.[44] Flaps mobilized from adjacent skin do well for defects less than 2 to 2.5 cm, but rarely is there a sufficient tissue reservoir for larger defects. Attempts at wedge repair or random flap closure can shorten the ear or deform its contour. Skin grafts may be an option if perichondrium is preserved.

The PIF is an ideal reconstructive option for most medium- to large-sized cutaneous defects of the helical rim and anterior ear, and provides sufficient tissue to cover large defects without distortion. Its abundant random pattern blood supply allows for reliable coverage of defects with exposed cartilage, and allows for reconstruction of composite defects. Cartilage grafts from the contralateral ear can restore the structural framework and preserve contour, and are necessary if the antihelical or helical cartilages have been sacrificed (Fig. 19-20). Because conchal bowl cartilage does not contribute to overall ear shape and size, cartilage grafts are usually not required for reconstruction in this location.[39] The plentiful reservoir of skin that PIFs provide also allows for repair of large lobular defects, with or without cartilage placement.

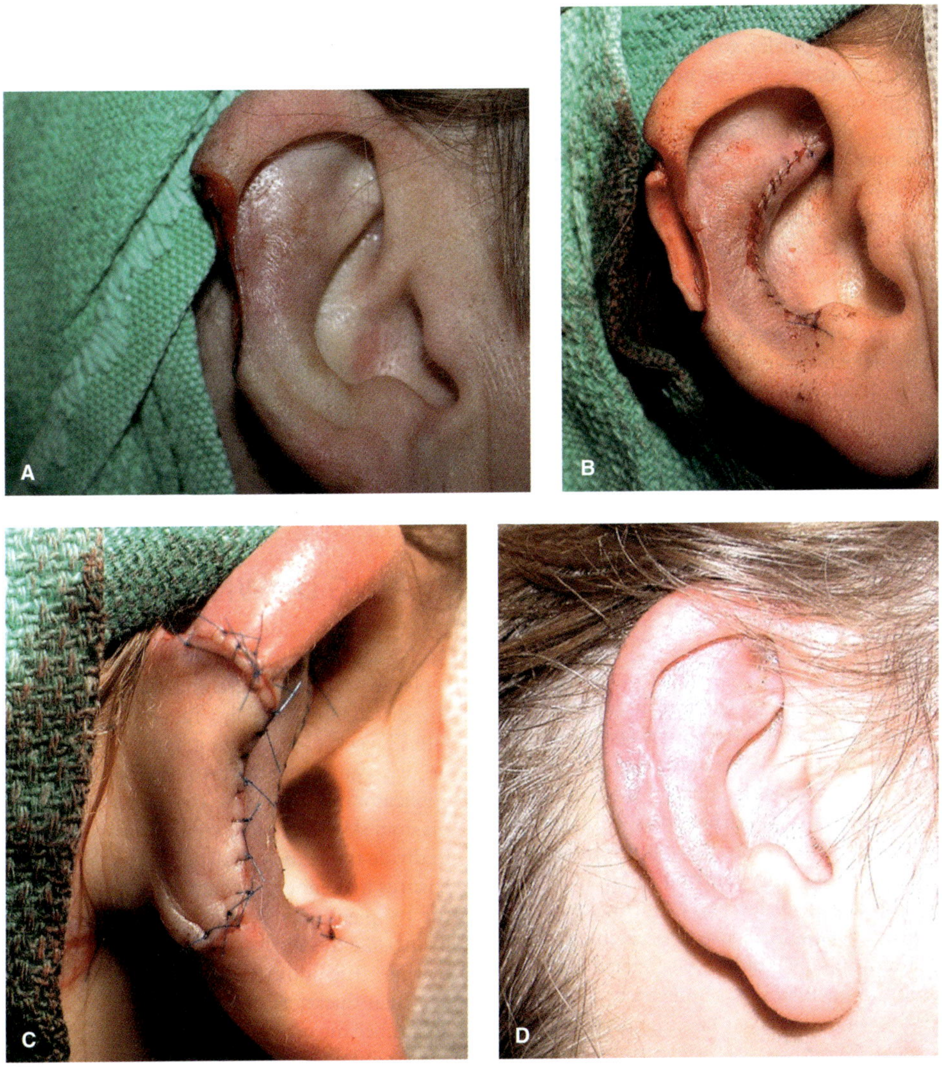

Figure 19-20 **A.** Composite defect of skin and cartilage along the mid helical rim. **B.** A free cartilage graft has been harvested from the ipsilateral antihelix. The donor site has been sutured with running cutaneous sutures. The cartilage graft has been sutured to the defect. **C.** Appearance of the postauricular interpolation flap immediately after primary inset. Note that it covers the anterior and posterior surfaces of the cartilage to optimize blood supply. **D.** Appearance 1 month after division and inset demonstrating restored helical rim contour.

DESIGNING THE FLAP

Once it has been determined that the PIF may repair a particular defect, one must decide whether cartilage support is necessary. If the ear's structural integrity or the helical rim convexity has been compromised, cartilage grafting should be considered. A PIF repair for helical or antihelical composite defects without cartilage can provide coverage but may not recreate the auricular contour. A contralateral conchal strut provides strength and a longitudinal substructure for the PIF, and is typically performed immediately prior to PIF transfer.

For both skin and composite defects, PIF design should precisely match the defect dimensions. Appreciation of the defect's three-dimensional nature will allow for successful repair. First, the vertical height must be measured, corresponding to the height of the PIF. A more challenging task is to precisely measure the horizontal dimension, dictated by whether the defect involves the rim or extends to the anterior or posterior surface. In these scenarios, the flap must reach the most anteromedial portion of the defect without tension. If the defect involves the helical rim and anterior ear, length must be added to account for the skin curving or bending around the rim into the scaphoid fossa. Incorrect flap design can lead to excessive tension or inability to reach the anteromedial aspect of the defect. Anteriorly rotated ears or large antihelical defects challenge the surgeon to develop a flap traversing the span from scalp to ear without excessive tension. Tacking the posterior ear to the mastoid area above and/or below the position of the anticipated flap bridge secures and pins back the pinna, reducing both the effective defect length, and its required length.

Marking the template will vary based upon the defect's anteromedial aspect. Typically, for defects restricted to the helical rim, the leading edge can be drawn within the postauricular sulcus, its vertical dimension mirroring the defect's vertical dimension. As the template extends toward the mastoid, these horizontal lines may be widened slightly and Burow's triangles added to increase flap movement. Placing the flap's leading edge in the sulcus for defects extending medially onto the antihelix may not provide sufficient reach. In these cases, postauricular skin can be used. The vertical flap is drawn as previously noted but its leading edge marked to the posterior angle of the helical rim. For wide defects extending onto the postauricular surface, the flap's leading edge may actually begin at the defect's posterior edge, which allows the PIF to be brought medially with minimal tension and ensures a width-flap ratio less than 3:1. A general guide for flap length can be estimated by pushing the ear against the mastoid skin. The proximal PIF base should stop just short of hair-bearing skin to avoid transferring hair to the ear.

LIFTING THE FLAP

The PIF is incised along the rectangular markings to the level between the subcutaneous tissue and fascia and elevated beginning at the leading edge of the flap. If template design begins on the postauricular surface, the flap should be raised at the level of perichondrium; dissection continues to the posterior sulcus, where there is a transition to mastoid fascia. The dissection is carried as far as needed to reach the distal defect. If necessary, Burow's triangles may be removed at the proximal base to assist in distal flap movement. Undermining should be performed but does not tend to mobilize mastoid skin significantly.

Because the PIF is not an axial flap, the surgeon must preserve its subcutaneous fat. The preserved subcutaneous tissue not only increases flap viability but also provides bulk to recreate the helical rim convexity. Even if cartilage has been placed, bulky flaps rarely present a problem, as they can be recontoured later. When the flap is in place, a small open pocket remains behind the ear, an issue because the mastoid fascia has perforators that can cause postoperative bleeding. Besides compromising flap viability, limited access may require flap take-down to allow hemostasis. To avoid this complication, hemostasis must be obtained before insetting.

INSETTING THE FLAP

The preceding steps should ensure that the flap is raised with sufficient subcutaneous tissue and can reach the defect with minimal tension. Posteromedial displacement of the ear toward the mastoid during inset can also decrease tension. The anterior ear skin is so thin that dermal suture placement can be difficult, although the more generous soft tissue at the helical rim can provide an anchor for buried sutures. Exaggerated eversion at the helical rim will decrease the risk of notching. The flap should reach without tension and can be approximated with a single layer of sutures, which may be left in place for 2 weeks to gain additional strength.

If the PIF extends over the scaphoid fossa, one may consider using horizontal mattress quilting sutures oriented along the scaphoid fossa to recreate its concavity (Fig. 19-21).[45] For large antihelical defects sparing the rim, a modified PIF may be chosen, performing a fusiform excision of cartilage along the scaphoid fossa concavity, through which the PIF can be pulled to preserve the helical rim.[46] There are instances in which postauricular skin may not be sufficient to resurface a large anterior defect. The surgeon should consider using skin grafts or an interpolated preauricular flap for these cases.

After the PIF is sutured into place, Xeroform gauze is generally placed around the raw pedicle and changed weekly. Excessive compression should be avoided. Inserting gel foam or Merocel nasal packing into the pocket behind the PIF can minimize the risk of bleeding.[47] The patient should limit compression of this site by sleeping on their back or contralateral side.

TAKING DOWN THE FLAP

At 1 week, sutures are removed and the Xeroform gauze replaced. Mid-pedicle compression allows assessment of the distal blood supply. Takedown is usually performed after 3 weeks, but delaying division for an additional week or two can improve the blood supply. A cotton-tipped applicator may be inserted in the pocket behind the PIF and mastoid skin to provide counterpressure and a scalpel used to divide the pedicle. Judicious selection of the incision site ensures that enough postauricular skin will be mobilized to the recipient area. A conservative approach may be taken by incising the vertical length of the flap at its base near the hairline. The additional skin can be thinned to match the auricular thickness. If the defect extends to the postauricular surface the excess flap skin is wrapped around the helical rim, and the proximal aspect sutured in a layered fashion.

Postauricular defects are sometimes too wide to be fully covered by the PIF, but are out of view and have healthy granulation tissue by the time of takedown. The PIF may therefore be wrapped around the postauricular surface as far as tension allows and sutured into place. The remaining defect may granulate without aesthetic penalty.

The skin edges of the mastoid defect should be freshened. This tissue may be mobilized and advanced to the postauricular sulcus. A layered repair may be performed if it reaches the sulcus. If the skin cannot be mobilized, the area may be left to heal or closed partially. Skin grafts are usually not necessary because of the hidden location and reliable cosmesis of second intention healing.

COMMON PITFALLS AND SOLUTIONS

Complications are rare and can usually be avoided by proper flap design and gentle tissue handling. To avoid postoperative bleeding, patients should have all nonessential anticoagulants discontinued preoperatively. The flap should be wrapped carefully with light pressure after the procedure. In certain instances, a hematoma may arise, which can compromise viability and cause flap necrosis.

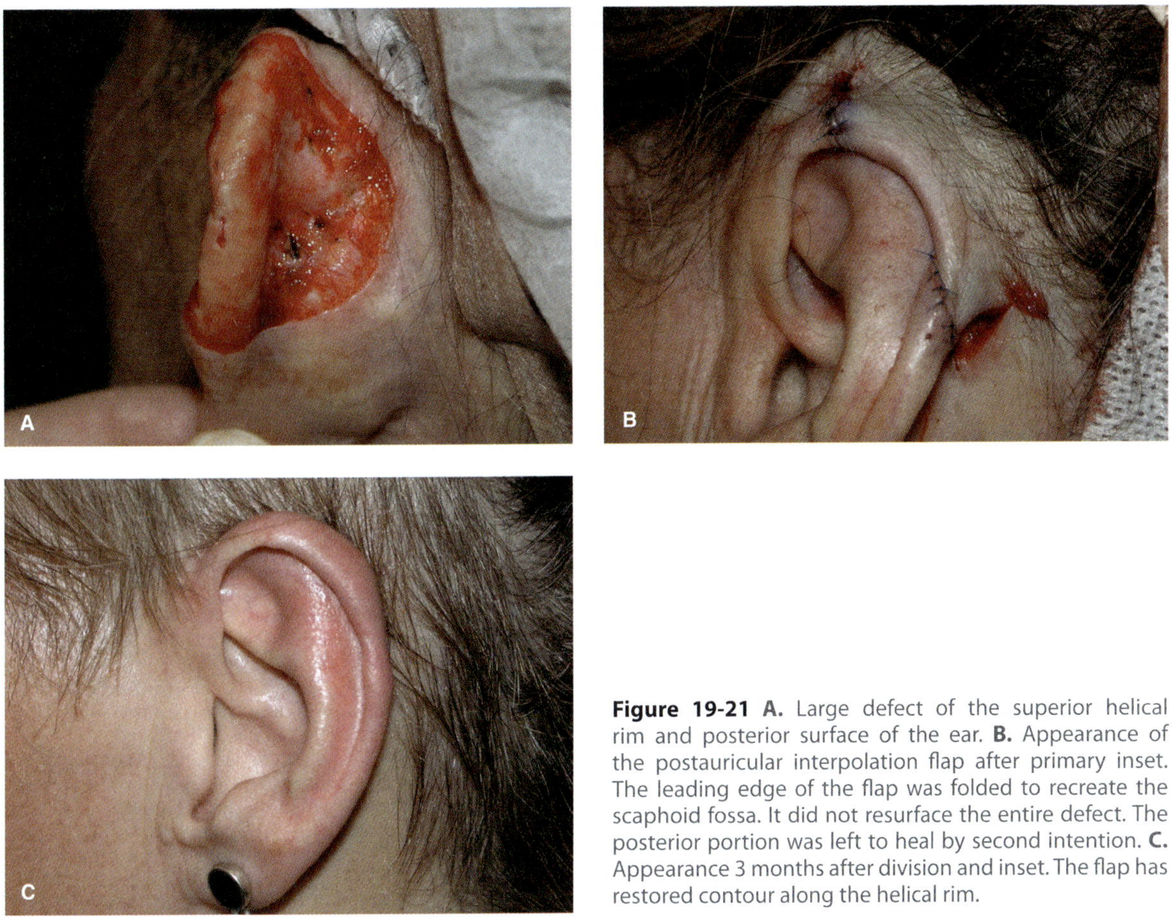

Figure 19-21 **A.** Large defect of the superior helical rim and posterior surface of the ear. **B.** Appearance of the postauricular interpolation flap after primary inset. The leading edge of the flap was folded to recreate the scaphoid fossa. It did not resurface the entire defect. The posterior portion was left to heal by second intention. **C.** Appearance 3 months after division and inset. The flap has restored contour along the helical rim.

A common error is to underestimate the distance that the PIF must travel to reach the anteromedial aspect of the defect. This can be avoided by marking its leading edge on the postauricular surface rather than within the sulcus. Necrosis can also occur if the flap is raised without subcutaneous fat or thinned too much at transfer. Raising the PIF at the mastoid fascia-fat junction and avoiding excessive thinning at takedown will help optimize viability. Infection and chondritis can complicate PIFs, usually presenting 3 to 5 days after flap transfer. Material available for culture should be sent for speciation and sensitivities, and patients may be placed on antibiotics. Nonsteroidal anti-inflammatory agents can minimize pain and inflammation.

Two common aesthetic complications seen with the PIF include helical rim notching and scaphoid fossa blunting. The former may result from inadequate skin transfer. The surgeon must carefully measure the defect and ensure that the flap markings on the postauricular surface are correct. The incision made at takedown should occur close to the hairline to provide more bulk if necessary. If large composite defects are not supported with cartilage prior to PIF transfer, notching or decreased helical rim projection can result. Notching may also occur if the wound edges are not everted when the flap is sutured into place. Vertical mattress sutures may be of some help. Scaphoid fossa blunting can be prevented with quilting sutures at PIF transfer.

CONCLUSION

"Form and function are a unity, two sides of one coin. In order to enhance function, appropriate form must exist or be created."

Ida P. Rolf

Optimal facial reconstruction realizes the dual goals of restoring both natural appearance and normal function. One needs masterful knowledge of facial anatomy, technical proficiency and artistic creativity. Staged flaps like the paramedian forehead flap, MIF, and PIF to repair complex defects of the nose and ear serve as perfect examples of this fundamental tenet.

REFERENCES

1. Roxbury C, Ishii M, Godoy A, et al. Impact of crooked nose rhinoplasty on observer perceptions of attractiveness. *Laryngoscope*. 2012;122(4):773–778.
2. Springer IN, Wannicke B, Warnke PH, et al. Facial attractiveness: visual impact of symmetry increases significantly towards the midline. *Ann Plast Surg*. 2007;59(2):156–162.
3. Godoy A, Ishii M, Byrne PJ, Boahene KD, Encarnacion CO, Ishii LE. The straight truth: measuring observer attention to the crooked nose. *Laryngoscope*. 2011;121(5):937–941.
4. Godoy A, Ishii M, Byrne PJ, Boahene KD, Encarnacion CO, Ishii LE. How facial lesions impact attractiveness and

perception: differential effects of size and location. *Laryngoscope.* 2011;121(12):2542–2547.
5. Han SK, Lee DG, Kim JB, Kim WK. An anatomic study of nasal tip supporting structures. *Ann Plast Surg.* 2004;52(2):134–139.
6. Rohrich RJ, Hoxworth RE, Thornton JF, Pessa JE. The pyriform ligament. *Plast Reconstr Surg.* 2008;121(1):277–281.
7. Saban Y, Andretto Amodeo C, Hammou JC, Polselli R. An anatomical study of the nasal superficial musculoaponeurotic system: surgical applications in rhinoplasty. *Arch Facial Plast Surg.* 2008;10(2):109–115.
8. Bruintjes TD, van Olphen AF, Hillen B, Huizing EH. A functional anatomic study of the relationship of the nasal cartilages and muscles to the nasal valve area. *Laryngoscope.* 1998;108(7):1025–1032.
9. Ali-Salaam P, Kashgarian M, Davila J, Persing J. Anatomy of the Caucasian alar groove. *Plast Reconstr Surg.* 2002;110(1):261–266; discussion 7–71.
10. Hur MS, Hu KS, Youn KH, Song WC, Abe S, Kim HJ. New anatomical profile of the nasal musculature: dilator naris vestibularis, dilator naris anterior, and alar part of the nasalis. *Clin Anat.* 2011;24(2):162–167.
11. Figallo EE, Acosta JA. Nose muscular dynamics: the tip trigonum. *Plast Reconstr Surg.* 2001;108(5):1118–1126.
12. Burget GC, Menick FJ. The subunit principle in nasal reconstruction. *Plast Reconstr Surg.* 1985;76(2):239–247.
13. Rohrich RJ, Griffin JR, Ansari M, Beran SJ, Potter JK. Nasal reconstruction–beyond aesthetic subunits: a 15-year review of 1334 cases. *Plast Reconstr Surg.* 2004;114(6):1405–1416; discussion 17–19.
14. Rahman M, Jefferson N, Stewart DA, Oliver R, Walsh WR, Gianoutsos MP. The histology of facial aesthetic subunits: implications for common nasal reconstructive procedures. *J Plast Reconstr Aesthet Surg.* 2010;63(5):753–756.
15. Lane AP. Nasal anatomy and physiology. *Facial Plast Surg Clin North Am.* 2004;12(4):387–395, v.
16. Lee J, White WM, Constantinides M. Surgical and nonsurgical treatments of the nasal valves. *Otolaryngol Clin North Am.* 2009;42(3):495–511.
17. Menick FJ. A 10-year experience in nasal reconstruction with the three-stage forehead flap. *Plast Reconstr Surg.* 2002;109(6):1839–1855; discussion 56–61.
18. Burget GC, Menick FJ. Nasal support and lining: the marriage of beauty and blood supply. *Plast Reconstr Surg.* 1989;84(2):189–202.
19. Reece EM, Schaverien M, Rohrich RJ. The paramedian forehead flap: a dynamic anatomical vascular study verifying safety and clinical implications. *Plast Reconstr Surg.* 2008;121(6):1956–1963.
20. Yu D, Weng R, Wang H, Mu X, Li Q. Anatomical study of forehead flap with its pedicle based on cutaneous branch of supratrochlear artery and its application in nasal reconstruction. *Ann Plast Surg.* 2010;65(2):183–187.
21. Vural E, Batay F, Key JM. Glabellar frown lines as a reliable landmark for the supratrochlear artery. *Otolaryngol Head Neck Surg.* 2000;123(5):543–546.
22. Janis JE, Ghavami A, Lemmon JA, Leedy JE, Guyuron B. The anatomy of the corrugator supercilii muscle: part II. Supraorbital nerve branching patterns. *Plast Reconstr Surg.* 2008;121(1):233–240.
23. Janis JE, Ghavami A, Lemmon JA, Leedy JE, Guyuron B. Anatomy of the corrugator supercilii muscle: part I. Corrugator topography. *Plast Reconstr Surg.* 2007;120(6):1647–1653.
24. Somoano B, Kampp J, Gladstone HB. Accelerated takedown of the paramedian forehead flap at 1 week: indications, technique, and improving patient quality of life. *J Am Acad Dermatol.* 2011;65(1):97–105.
25. Herbert DC. A subcutaneous pedicled cheek flap for reconstruction of alar defects. *Br J Plast Surg.* 1978;31(2):79–92.
26. Pharis DB, Papadopoulos DJ. Superiorly based nasolabial interpolation flap for repair of complex nasal tip defects. *Dermatol Surg.* 2000;26(1):19–24.
27. Fisher GH, Cook JW. The interpolated paranasal flap: a novel and advantageous option for nasal-alar reconstruction. *Dermatol Surg.* 2009;35(4):656–661.
28. Fosko SW, Dzubow LM. Nasal reconstruction with the cheek island pedicle flap. *J Am Acad Dermatol.* 1996;35(4):580–587.
29. Fader DJ, Baker SR, Johnson TM. The staged cheek-to-nose interpolation flap for reconstruction of the nasal alar rim/lobule. *J Am Acad Dermatol.* 1997;37(4):614–619.
30. Cook JL. The lateral ala's volume and position are critical determinants of aesthetically successful nasal reconstruction: a photographic case series. *Dermatol Surg.* 2009;35(4):667–673.
31. Zitelli JA. Secondary intention healing: an alternative to surgical repair. *Clin Dermatol.* 1984;2(3):92–106.
32. Zitelli JA. Wound healing by secondary intention. A cosmetic appraisal. *J Am Acad Dermatol.* 1983;9(3):407–415.
33. Fader DJ, Wise CG, Normolle DP, Johnson TM. The multidisciplinary melanoma clinic: a cost outcomes analysis of specialty care. *J Am Acad Dermatol.* 1998;38(5 Pt 1):742–751.
34. Karsidag S, Ozcan A, Sumer O, Ugurlu K. Single-stage ala nasi reconstruction: lateral nasal artery perforator flap. *J Craniofac Surg.* 2010;21(6):1887–1889.
35. Smit JM, Ruhe PQ, Acosta R, Kooloos JG, Hartman EH. The nasolabial fold as potential vascular receptor site: an anatomic study. *J Reconstr Microsurg.* 2009;25(9):539–543.
36. Rohrich RJ, Pessa JE. The fat compartments of the face: anatomy and clinical implications for cosmetic surgery. *Plast Reconstr Surg.* 2007;119(7):2219–2227; discussion 2228–2231.
37. Allison GR. Anatomy of the auricle. *Clin Plast Surg.* 1990;17(2):209–212.
38. Sclafani AP, Mashkevich G. Aesthetic reconstruction of the auricle. *Facial Plast Surg Clin North Am.* 2006;14(2):103–116, vi.
39. Park SS, Hood RJ. Auricular reconstruction. *Otolaryngol Clin North Am.* 2001;34(4):713–738, v–vi.
40. Brodland DG. Auricular reconstruction. *Dermatol Clin.* 2005;23(1):23–41, v.
41. Park C, Lineaweaver WC, Rumly TO, Buncke HJ. Arterial supply of the anterior ear. *Plast Reconstr Surg.* 1992;90(1):38–44.
42. Farkas LG. Vertical location of the ear, assessed by the Leiber test, in healthy North American Caucasians 6–19 years of age. *Arch Otorhinolaryngol.* 1978;220(1–2):9–13.
43. Adamson JE, Horton CE, Crawford HH. The growth pattern of the external ear. *Plast Reconstr Surg.* 1965;36(4):466–470.
44. Shonka DC Jr, Park SS. Ear defects. *Facial Plast Surg Clin North Am.* 2009;17(3):429–443.
45. Johnson TM, Fader DJ. The staged retroauricular to auricular direct pedicle (interpolation) flap for helical ear reconstruction. *J Am Acad Dermatol.* 1997;37(6):975–978.
46. Mellette JR, Ho DQ. Interpolation flaps. *Dermatol Clin.* 2005;23(1):87–112, vi.
47. Justiniano H, Eisen DB. Pearls for perfecting the mastoid interpolation flap. *Dermatol Online J.* 2009;15(6):2.

CHAPTER 20

Skin Grafting

Hillary Johnson-Jahangir & Kira Minkis

INTRODUCTION AND BACKGROUND

The origin of skin grafting dates back approximately 3000 years ago, when autologous grafts were used to repair mutilated noses, ears, and lips in India.[1] In the era of modern medicine, the first reports of successful skin grafting date from the mid to late 19th century, with Reverdin's report in 1869 presenting the use of pinch grafts to accelerate healing of granulating wounds. Currently, there are a multitude of applications utilizing skin grafting. These include reconstruction following surgery, tissue replacement in burn victims and patients with epidermolysis bullosa, treatment of chronic ulcers, and hair transplantation.

Free skin grafts are pieces of skin of variable thickness and size that are completely detached from their origin (donor site) to cover a defect (recipient site). Skin grafts can be subdivided into four types, including full-thickness skin grafts (FTSGs), split-thickness skin grafts (STSGs), composite grafts (CG), and free cartilage grafts (FCG). FTSGs are composed of the entire epidermis and the full thickness of dermis, including adnexal structures such as hair follicles and sweat glands. STSGs are composed of the full epidermis and partial dermis that vary by overall thickness. CGs are composed of at least two different tissue types, usually skin and cartilage in cutaneous surgery. FCGs consist of cartilage with its overlying perichondrium and are typically placed into a wound to provide structural support (Table 20-1).[2]

WOUND HEALING

The survival of a skin graft is dependent upon establishment of an adequate blood supply from the recipient site. Graft wound healing takes place through three phases. The first phase, plasmatic imbibition, takes place 24 to 48 hours after placement. During this phase, fibrin acts as an adhesive to help attach the graft to the recipient bed.[3] The graft is then able to absorb exudate from the recipient bed and becomes edematous, with its weight increasing up to 40%.[4] This allows graft hydration, provides a nutrient supply, and helps to temporarily preserve graft vessel patency. With time, granulation tissue replaces fibrin in the wound bed, allowing permanent attachment.

Inosculation follows 48 to 72 hours after grafting and is a process of revascularization. During this phase, vascular anastomoses are formed between the recipient bed and pre-existing vessels in the dermis of the graft.[5] Neovascularization and vascular proliferation constitute the final stage of graft survival, consisting of blood vessel budding and sprouting in the graft and the wound bed and the development of vascular connections allowing blood flow between them. The "bridging phenomenon" also allows for inosculation to occur in small avascular wound

TABLE 20-1
Comparison of Skin Graft Types Used in Reconstruction

Graft		Benefits	Risks
FTSG	Full-thickness skin	Optimal cosmesis, function, and healing for many defects	Defect size limited by donor tissue availability Requires vascular graft bed due to high metabolic demand
STSG	Partial-thickness skin	Greater survival on avascular graft bed due to lower metabolic demand Greater donor tissue availability permits coverage of larger defects	Suboptimal cosmesis Contracts more as it heals Donor site granulation and cosmesis
CG	Skin–cartilage–skin	One stage repair of full-thickness or deeper alar defects requiring cartilage	Greatest metabolic demand can limit survival and size of defect (<2 cm) Donor sites limited, more difficult to repair, possible donor site pain and chondritis Cartilage increases risk of infection or graft displacement
FCG	Cartilage-perichondrium	Structural/functional support for some alar, helical rim, or lower eyelid defects	Possible donor site pain and chondritis Cartilage increases risk of infection or graft displacement

beds through vascular reanastomoses that derive exclusively from the wound edges.[6] Revascularization requires adequate, healthy microvasculature in the recipient site. Within 4 to 7 days, full circulation is restored to the graft, the rate of which is determined by graft thickness as well as recipient bed vascularity. By 7 days, lymphatic circulation is also restored.[7] Reinnervation of the graft may begin in approximately 2 to 4 weeks, but recovery of full sensation may require months to years or may never return completely.

Establishment of a stable vascular supply is essential for graft survival. Factors that can decrease graft survival include prolonged ischemic periods as a result of disruption of vascular connections, usually due to mechanical shearing forces, seroma, hematoma, or infection. The most common infectious agents associated with graft failure include coagulase-positive staphylococci, β-hemolytic streptococci, and *Pseudomonas* species. The latter are especially common on the ears or near the feet since *Pseudomonas* flourishes in moist locations as normal flora or due to associated nosocomial infection.[8]

In addition, patient factors such as nicotine intake, nutritional deficiencies, and diabetes mellitus can limit graft nutrient or vascular supply. Moreover, certain medications may slow wound healing including corticosteroids, chemotherapeutic agents, immunosuppressive medication, and anticoagulants. A proper preoperative patient evaluation is, therefore, essential, as are meticulous operative technique and postoperative wound care.

FULL-THICKNESS SKIN GRAFTS

FTSGs are most commonly used to reconstruct facial defects after skin cancer excision. While FTSGs are more prone to necrosis than STSGs due to greater nutritional requirements, FTSGs tend not to contract as much and also display a superior color and texture match. The main requirements for use of FTSGs include a recipient bed with a sufficient vascular supply for neovascularization and nutritional support of the graft, as well as fibroblasts to supply collagen for graft adherence. The success of grafting avascular areas depends on the depth and vascular integrity of the recipient site as well as the size of the area, with small avascular areas less than 1 cm in diameter allowing reestablishment of the blood supply through the bridging phenomenon.[6] FTSGs may lack a sufficient blood supply if their wound bed features larger areas of avascular tissue (exposed cartilage, bone, nerve, or tendon lacking overlying perichondrium, periosteum, perineurium, or peritenon, respectively).

FTSGs contain epidermis and full-thickness dermis, making them good reconstructive options for repair of facial defects owing to their intact adnexal structures and superior color, texture, and thickness matches compared with partial-thickness grafts. Facial areas in which FTSGs are particularly useful include the lower eyelid, ear, or nasal sites (tip, dorsum, ala, or lateral sidewall).

PREOPERATIVE ASSESSMENT

As with any cutaneous surgery, a comprehensive preoperative patient evaluation can help assess the risk of bleeding and clot formation and gauge the potential success of skin grafting. Important questions that help predict challenges for intraoperative hemostasis or postoperative bleeding include anticoagulant medications, blood thinning herbal supplements, a history of bleeding tendencies, and hypertension.[9] Questions regarding the patient's general medical health may highlight factors that could impair wound healing due to a limited vascular supply. Compliance with postoperative wound care instructions is essential to graft survival. Physical activities or graft site manipulation resulting in shearing forces between the graft and its recipient bed may result in graft failure. A discussion regarding postoperative expectations including healing time, surgical scars, and potential complications is important for increased patient compliance and optimization of surgical outcomes.

TABLE 20-2
Characteristics for Determining FTSG Donor Sites

Color
Texture
Thickness
Sebaceous quality of the surrounding skin
Vascular pattern
History of sun exposure
Ability to camouflage donor scar

DONOR SITE SELECTION

The selection of an FTSG donor site depends on optimal matching of donor tissue to recipient site tissue based on the following characteristics: color, texture, thickness, sebaceous quality of the surrounding skin, vascular pattern, and history of sun exposure (Table 20-2).[7] FTSGs obtained from sun-exposed areas above the shoulders provide an optimal match for most facial defects. The thickness of the desired graft is one factor that determines the site of graft harvesting (Table 20-3). The thinnest grafts are usually harvested from the upper eyelid or the postauricular sulcus. The preauricular and cervical regions can provide donor tissue for medium-thickness grafts. Thicker grafts can be taken from the supraclavicular or clavicular region, conchal bowl, forehead, or nasolabial fold. However, patient variability in skin thickness, texture, sun exposure, and color preclude strict guidelines for

TABLE 20-3
FTSGs Donor Sites Based on Graft Thickness

Thinnest grafts	Upper eyelid or the postauricular sulcus
Medium-thickness grafts	Preauricular and cervical regions
Thickest grafts	Supraclavicular or clavicular region, conchal bowl, forehead, or nasolabial fold

TABLE 20-4
Potential Donor Sites for FTSG Based on Location of Defect

Defect location	Potential donor site location
Lower eyelid	Redundant upper eyelid skin
Eyelid and auricular defects	Postauricular skin
Nasal defects	Preauricular skin (graft should be obtained from the hairless area between the tragus and the lateral cheek)
Eyebrows or mustache area	Hair-bearing skin of the temporoparietal region or preauricular beard
Nasal tip	Nasolabial folds or forehead skin
Distal nose	Conchal bowl
Larger defects on sun-damaged skin (forehead and vertex scalp)	Supraclavicular region or lateral neck, inner upper arm

selection of donor sites. Rather, individual patients need to be examined carefully and their location for ideal graft harvesting will be determined by the characteristics of the recipient bed and donor tissue.

Obtaining a graft from skin in close proximity to the recipient site may potentially provide the best tissue match for a given defect (Table 20-4). Redundant upper eyelid skin can be used to graft lower eyelid defects, thus providing an optimal textural and color match. Using upper eyelid skin as donor tissue has the additional advantage of leaving an inconspicuous donor site scar.[10–12] Lax tissue adjacent to a facial defect can also be used a Burow's triangle as a partial FTSG. This usually occurs when there is sufficient skin mobility to permit partial closure of the wound, thereby allowing the adjacent skin to resurface the remaining defect. Postauricular skin provides ample donor tissue for repair of eyelid and auricular defects, and donor site scars in this area can be camouflaged easily, which can be advantageous. However, this skin may be a poor color match for sun-exposed facial defects because it is relatively less actinically damaged.

Preauricular skin can be used for repair of many nasal defects, owing to its thickness, numerous sebaceous glands, and similar degree of sun exposure.[13,14] One must take care to avoid harvesting preauricular hair-bearing skin to avoid unwanted hair growth within the graft, particularly on the nose. The graft should be obtained from the hairless area between the tragus and the lateral cheek, and all follicles should be trimmed from the underlying subcutaneous fat to ensure their removal. Conversely, if hair growth is desired within a graft, such as for repair of the eyebrows or mustache area in men, a graft may be harvested from the hair-bearing skin of the temporoparietal region or preauricular beard. The nasolabial folds or forehead skin can be used as donor sites to repair small defects of the nasal tip, although the donor scar may be somewhat conspicuous.[15,16] The conchal bowl can also provide a source for skin grafting the sebaceous distal nose. Perichondrial cutaneous grafts consisting of epidermis, dermis, scant subcutaneous tissue, and the thin perichondrium have been reported to result in less wound retraction and to provide greater lasting thickness and possibly reduced necrosis.[17] The success of conchal FTSGs without perichondrium has also been demonstrated; the donor site is allowed to heal secondarily.[16] These grafts should be slightly undersized to minimize bulkiness due to "trapdoor" or "pin-cushioning" effects.

The supraclavicular region or lateral neck may be potential donor sites for repair of larger defects on sun-damaged skin, such as the forehead and vertex scalp. Other areas that may be used as donor sites for FTSGs include areas with thin redundant skin including the upper inner arms, forearms, and inguinal area, although these tend to have a suboptimal color and texture match for facial skin.

TECHNIQUE

Multiple different techniques for performing FTSGs exist.[2,7,16,18,19] To plan for harvesting an FTSG, a template of the recipient defect may be used to recreate the dimensional needs for coverage, particularly when the defect's depth or contour requires accommodation (Fig. 20-1A–G). Any flexible material, including paper, gauze pads, or aluminum foil, can be used . The periphery of the defect is marked with a sterile marking pen. The material is pressed against the recipient site in order to outline the border drawn with the pen, thus creating a template that can be used to harvest an appropriate FTSG. The template can then be used to mark the donor site prior to injection of anesthetic to avoid sizing error resulting from tissue distortion. In many cases, the FTSG will have sufficient tissue stretch to properly cover the defect. Sometimes the FTSG may be resized to be larger than the template to allow for contraction and shrinkage of the graft after harvesting. When defects approach a free margin such as the lower eyelid or over joint surfaces, grafts should be oversized to avoid excess tension and dysfunction that may occur due to graft contraction. In addition, concave wounds and surfaces with complex surface contours require special sizing considerations to prevent tenting of the graft in the concavities of the recipient bed.[2] Standard surgical preparation using local anesthetic and application of antiseptic soap is performed. Epinephrine may be used without adversely impacting graft survival. During the harvesting of the FTSG, the recipient bed should be kept moist and may be covered with saline-soaked gauze.

The donor skin is excised to the level below the dermis and placed in a sterile container with normal saline while hemostasis of the donor site is achieved. The graft is usually used within 1 to 2 hours but may be used up to 24 hours after harvesting if refrigerated or kept on ice. Minimally delaying graft placement is optimal, however. The graft may need to be defatted prior to placement by trimming superfluous fat with sharp, curved, or serrated scissors from the dermal aspect of the graft until the undersurface has a white, shiny appearance (Fig. 20-1C). This step can improve direct contact between the graft dermis and recipient bed for nutritional requirements, establishment of anastomoses between blood

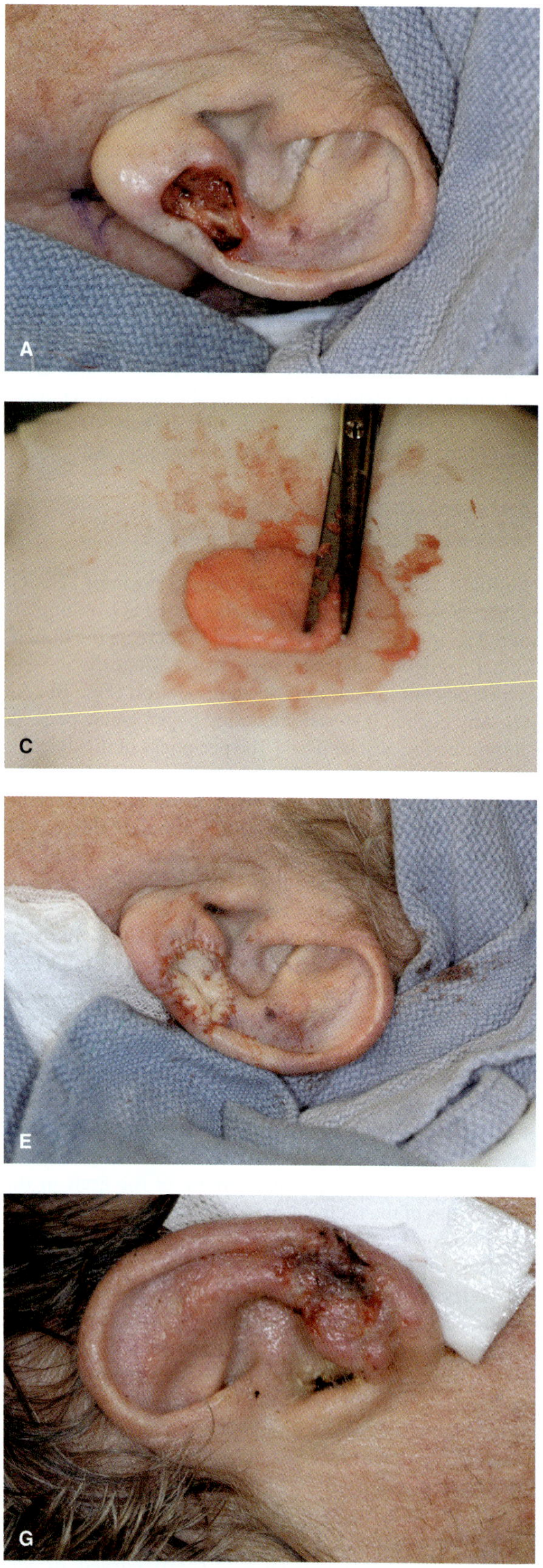

Figure 20-1 Placement of a full-thickness skin graft. **A.** A defect of the lower anterior ear is present after removal of a basal cell carcinoma with Mohs micrographic surgery. A postauricular donor site provided the best tissue match in this case. **B.** A template of the defect is made from a telfa pad by pressing it against the defect. The resulting outline of the blood-stained pad serves as a guide to cutting a precise template. **C.** The graft is carefully defatted so that only the white, glistening surface of the dermis remains. **D, E.** Full-thickness skin graft sewn into place with 6-0 fast absorbing gut sutures. **F.** Xeroform™ bolster sewn into place over full-thickness skin graft with 5-0 polypropylene tie-over sutures. **G.** One-week follow-up.

vessels, and new vessel growth. The dermis may be further trimmed if indicated to conform to beveled wound edges or differences in recipient site depth, or to recreate normal surface contours. Prior to graft placement, some authors advocate that the recipient site be further prepared. The recipient site edges of the defect may be undermined to minimize postoperative pin-cushioning, promote uniform wound contracture, and improve epidermal approximation of the recipient site and FTSG. However, undermining of the recipient site is not uniform practice and may not be necessary. Careful hemostasis of the recipient site should be obtained to prevent any barrier to good contact between the graft and its nutrient supplying bed. Caution to avoid excessive charring is also needed. Particularly when grafting auricular defects, portions of cartilage that are not needed for structural support should be removed to increase the chance of graft survival; this may be particularly useful for auricular defects, and may be accomplished using a punch device.[18,20,21]

The FTSG is then positioned in the recipient bed. To ensure adequate wound healing, FTSGs must make direct contact with the underlying wound bed and should be immobilized in the immediate postoperative period to prevent graft separation. Various methods accomplish anchoring of the FTSG, including perimeter sutures, basting sutures, support dressings, or a combination of these (Fig. 20-1E,F). Perimeter sutures reapproximate the edges of the graft with those of the recipient site. After the graft is placed in the recipient bed with the dermal side down, it may be secured with anchoring sutures so that apposing skin edges may be approximated (Fig. 20-1D). Suturing the full length of the skin edges can be carried out using a variety of suture materials, matching the caliber of the suture to the skin thickness. Absorbable sutures such as 6-0 fast-absorbing gut or 5-0 mild chromic gut have the advantage that they dissolve over several days to weeks and thereby reduce the potential for graft disruption during suture removal. Sutures are placed with the needle first passing through the graft side and exiting from the adjacent recipient tissue. The sutures should be placed deeply enough to approximate the epidermis, papillary dermis, and reticular dermis. Very superficial placement of sutures has been implicated as a potential etiology of graft pin-cushioning and hematoma formation, as well as a more depressed, prominent scar.[12] Sutures placed slightly higher in the dermis on the graft side and slightly deeper in the dermis of the recipient side, modestly insetting the graft relative to the recipient skin edges, may prevent graft edge tenting and enhance graft–recipient bed contact.[19] The full graft periphery may be sutured to the recipient defect using simple interrupted sutures placed a few millimeters apart or by placement of interrupted sutures at opposite edges of the graft periphery followed by a simple running suture (Fig. 20-1E). Additional graft trimming as needed during this stage generates an ideal shape.

Additional sutures, termed basting sutures, can be placed centrally, particularly for large or concave surfaces, to increase contact between the graft and recipient bed (Fig. 20-2A). These sutures are useful for grafts over concave surfaces to prevent tenting or for larger grafts to minimize movement. Basting sutures often extend through the central portion of the graft to the level of the recipient bed and back up to the graft surface; they may also extend through the full thickness of the recipient bed to the opposing epidermal surface and back to the graft surface in locations such as the pinna. Some authors recommend placement of the basting sutures prior to fully securing the perimeter of the graft to allow for direct visualization and to avoid injury to underlying structures such as blood vessels. Less commonly, fenestrations or small slits puncturing the graft may be placed to allow for drainage if there is concern for impending fluid collection beneath the graft.

SECURING THE GRAFT

Traditionally, the graft is immobilized with a tie-over bolster dressing that serves to keep the graft in place through application of direct, constant pressure (Fig. 20-1F). Bolstering the graft promotes neovascularization, prevents formation of hematoma or seroma, and prevents patient manipulation of the graft. A generous amount of emollient such as petrolatum is first applied over the graft. A nonadherent contact layer may be applied with a product such as petrolatum-impregnated gauze (Xeroform™ gauze: bismuth tribromophenate-petrolatum-impregnated gauze, Kendall; N-Terface, Winfield Laboratories, Dallas, TX; Adaptic, Johnson & Johnson Medical). An anchoring stent can be made of a variety of materials (petrolatum-impregnated gauze, cotton balls, foam rubber, sponges, plastic beads, or disks) and is normally sutured into place. Staples, adhesive wound closure tapes, or Steri-Strips™ can be used as an alternative. In a classic tie-over bolster, nonabsorbable sutures are placed on opposite sides of the periphery of the graft, cut long (3 to 6 cm), and tied tightly over the bolster to secure it in place. The number of sutures placed should be sufficient to prevent tangential movement of the bolster materials. Subsequently, a light dressing consisting of nonstick gauze and stretchable bandage tape (Telfa pad and Hypafix tape; Smith & Nephew, Inc., Largo, FL) may be placed. The donor site can be dressed with a standard pressure dressing. The utility of bolster dressings is a subject of debate and they may not be strictly necessary; no difference in graft survival has been reported with or without use of a bolster dressing.[22,23]

POSTOPERATIVE CARE

Pressure dressings from both donor–recipient and graft–recipient sites may typically be removed in 24 to 48 hours. Following removal of these, the donor site as well as the area surrounding the bolster dressing can be cleansed once or twice daily with hydrogen peroxide and a petrolatum-based emollient generously applied. The bolster dressing remains in place for 1 week. After removal of the bolster dressing and all tie-over sutures at about 1 week, the graft may not necessarily appear pink and well-vascularized and the patient should be counseled to expect this prior to suture removal to avoid alarm. The ideal graft should be light pink in color, but may be yellowish or range in color from dark pink to blue or purple, which may be

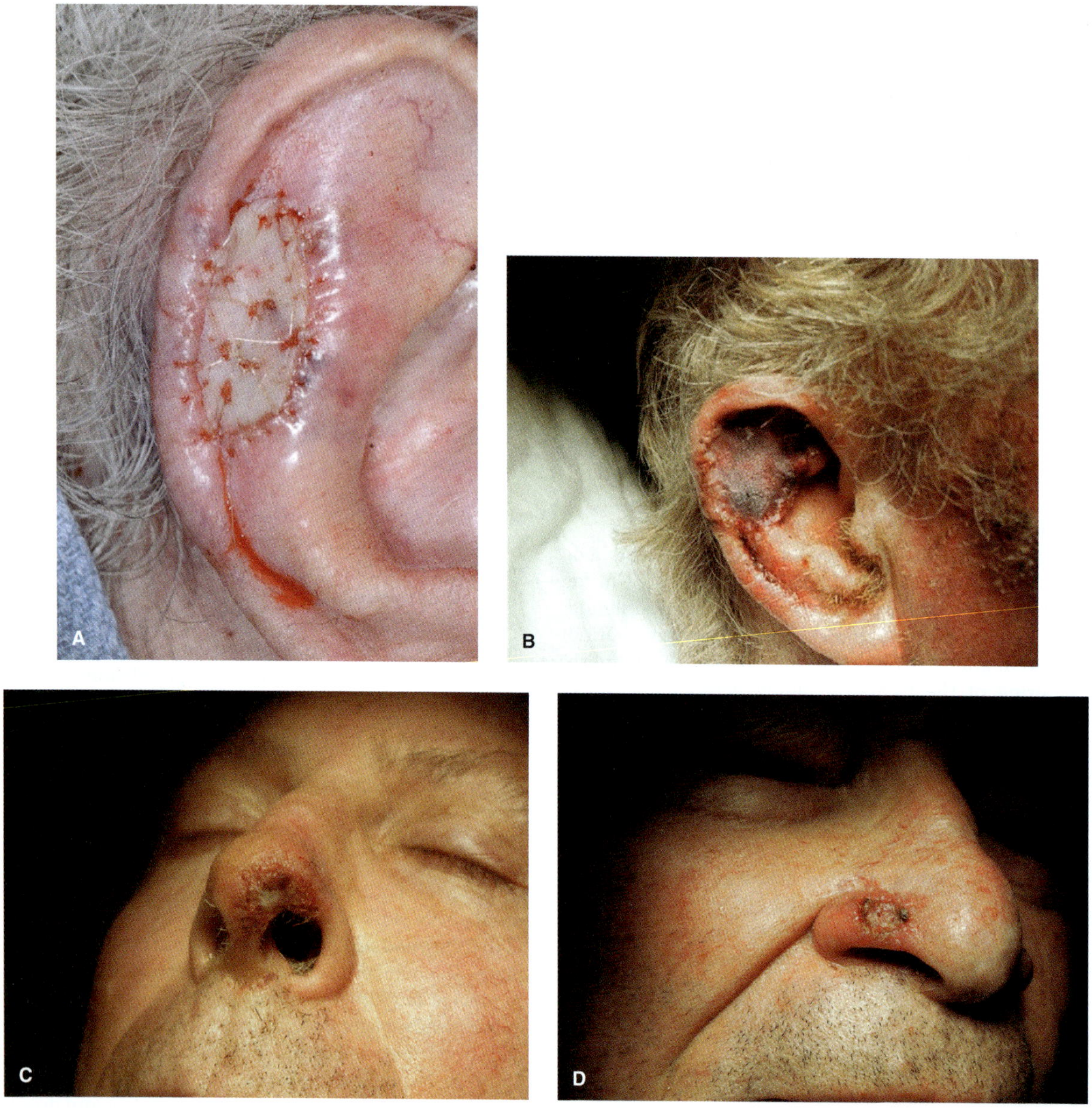

Figure 20-2 **A**. FTSG for repair of an ear defect. Note multiple quilting, or basting, sutures. **B–D**. FTSGs at time of suture removal. While grafts ideally are pink when the bolster is removed, they can be varying shades of pink, yellow, blue, or even purple, due to the presence of ecchymosis or crusting. (Figures 20-2B–D used with permission of Desiree Ratner, MD.)

secondary to ecchymosis (Fig. 20-2B–D). A graft that is black or white in color may be an indication of necrosis and graft failure. However, despite the possibility of epidermal necrosis, the graft dermis and appendages may remain viable and the necrosed epidermis can serve as a natural biologic dressing. For this reason, the eschar should not be debrided, but rather left to protect any remaining viable dermis and to allow for second-intention healing in the event of graft death.

Following suture removal, the graft can be cleansed gently with hydrogen peroxide to remove all crusts and loose debris, followed by a layer of emollient. It is also important to counsel patients that the vascular supply of the graft remains fragile for weeks. Patients should, therefore, avoid trauma, such as direct shower water to the area, as well as factors that could induce circulatory overload or swelling of the graft, such as excessive physical activity, for several additional weeks.

SPECIAL CONSIDERATIONS

DEFECT SIZE REDUCTION

If feasible, a purse-string suture may be placed around the periphery of the defect to make it smaller. The purse-string suture is commonly a nonabsorbable monofilament that is placed subcuticularly around the skin edges for a period of 3 weeks. After carefully cinching and tying the suture, the horizontal dimensions of the defect may be

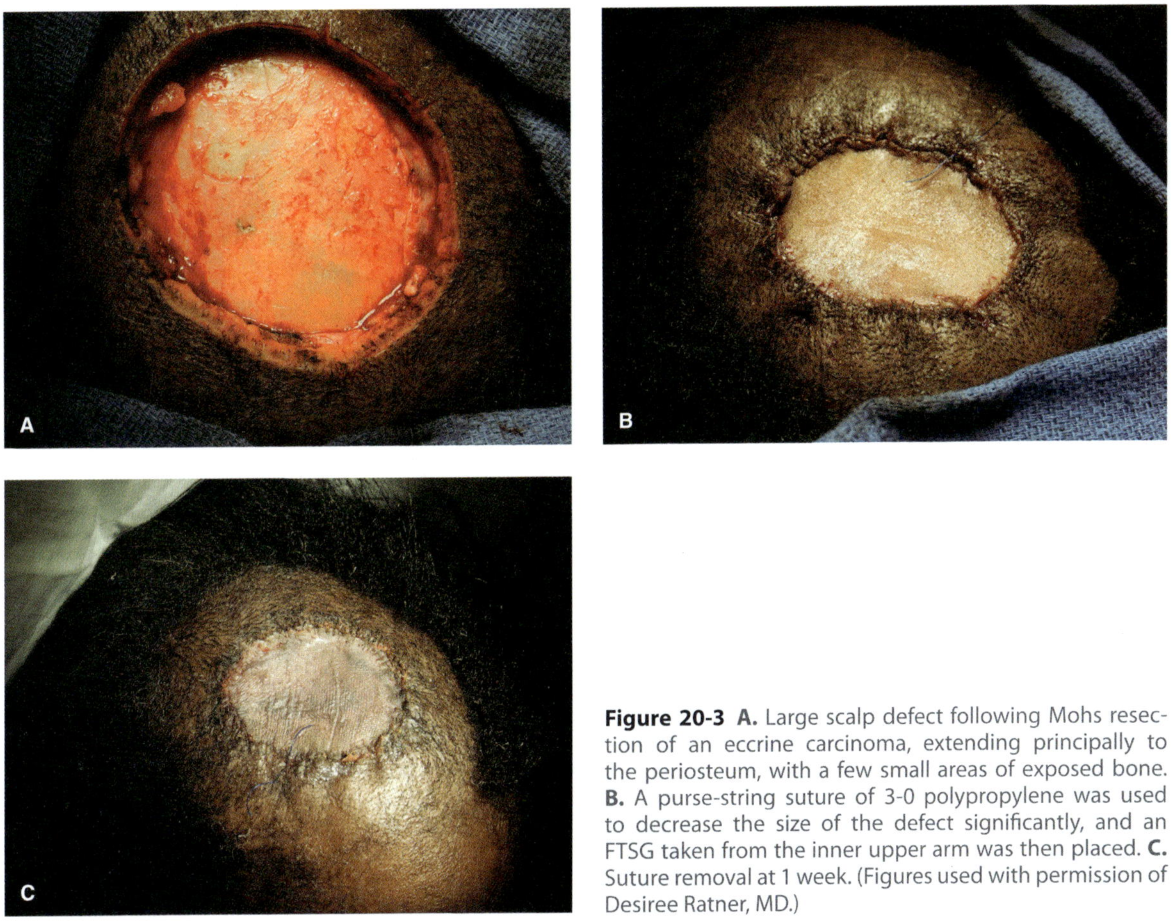

Figure 20-3 **A.** Large scalp defect following Mohs resection of an eccrine carcinoma, extending principally to the periosteum, with a few small areas of exposed bone. **B.** A purse-string suture of 3-0 polypropylene was used to decrease the size of the defect significantly, and an FTSG taken from the inner upper arm was then placed. **C.** Suture removal at 1 week. (Figures used with permission of Desiree Ratner, MD.)

evenly reduced in size depending on the surrounding tissue laxity (Fig. 20-3A–C).[24]

DEEP WOUNDS

To graft deep defects that cannot be effectively covered by FTSGs, several strategies can be undertaken. These include delayed graft placement to allow for granulation tissue growth over the recipient site base, dermal grafting, and hinge flaps. Delaying graft placement by 12 to 14 days may increase graft survival over areas with poor recipient bed vascularity such as defects of the nasal tip and ala with denuded cartilage. A prospective trial of immediate versus delayed FTSGs of the nasal tip and ala with denuded cartilage showed improved graft survival, decreased contraction and decreased graft depression with delayed FTSGs as opposed to immediate FTSGs.[25]

Dermal grafting is another method used to fill deep defects prior to placement of FTSGs. Dermal grafts are autologous and are generated by removing the epidermis and subcutaneous fat from harvested skin. One common source for these grafts consists of the Burow's triangles from the FTSG donor site or other primary defect closure. After harvesting this tissue, the epidermis is meticulously removed to prevent epidermoid cyst formation and the subcutis is also removed. The remaining dermis can then be inserted as a dermal graft under any contour irregularities in the recipient site or to fill in a deep recipient site to act as tissue filler. Small "pinch" dermal grafts can be used or larger strips may be harvested and placed in a grid-like pattern along the defect base.[26]

Hinge flaps offer another approach to filling sizeable defects by making use of nearby deep tissue. Subcutaneous hinge and myocutaneous hinge flaps both help to create a recipient bed that is well-vascularized and allow for immediate repair of deep wounds with an FTSG. These flaps borrow subcutaneous adipose and/or muscle tissue that lies adjacent to the defect. The borrowed tissue is hinged like the page of a book into the primary defect, thus reducing the depth of the defect, and resurfacing its base with vascular tissue. The FTSG can then be placed directly over the hinge flap.[27–29] The galeal hinge flap is a unique method for extending the partial thickness of adjacent galea aponeurotica on the scalp to cover exposed bone (Fig. 20-4A–C).[28] Yet another strategy for repair of deep nasal alar defects is the use of the "drumhead" graft repair. This graft was designed to prevent graft depression and the inward collapse of the nasal vestibule due to surgical loss of tissue. The graft involves application of an overlying rigid plastic suspension coupled with an undersized graft.[30]

Perichondrial cutaneous grafts (PCCGs) may also be used in the repair of deep nasal tip and alar defects, particularly in defects with exposed cartilage. These skin grafts are CGs harvested from the conchal bowl, and are composed of epidermis, dermis, a small amount of subcutaneous tissue, and underlying perichondrium. However, they do not include the cartilage. PCCGs are thicker, may offer better

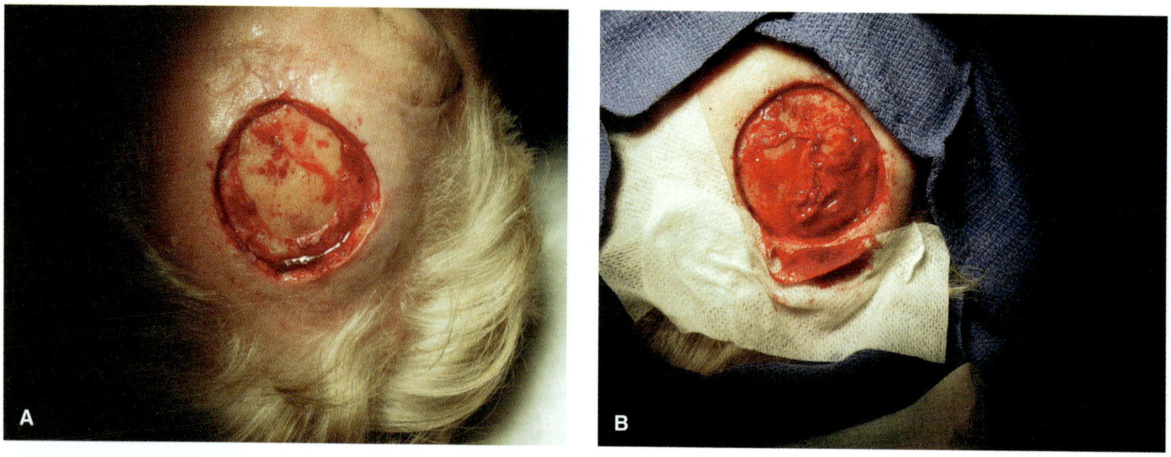
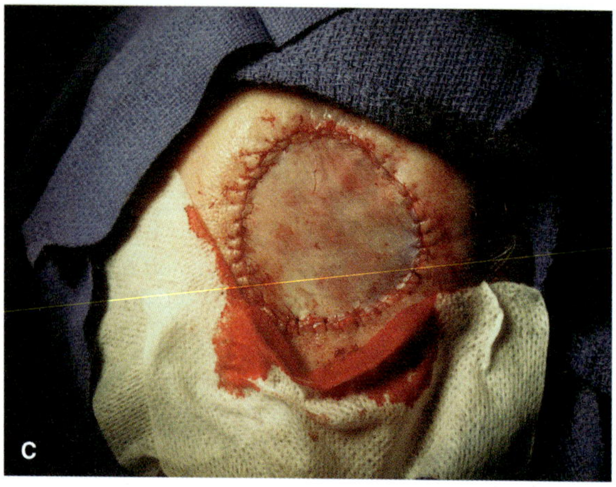

Figure 20-4 **A.** Scalp defect following Mohs resection of a large basal cell carcinoma, extending to bone. **B.** Galeal hinge flaps harvested from the adjacent scalp tissue were placed to cover the exposed bone. **C.** An FTSG harvested from the inner upper arm skin was placed thereafter. (Figures used with permission of Desiree Ratner, MD.)

survival under conditions of vascular compromise, and have a decreased tendency for contraction compared to FTSGs.[31]

BUROW'S GRAFTS

The Burow's graft is an FTSG whose donor site is the skin adjacent to a wound, usually consisting of Burow's triangles (Fig. 20-5A,B). The advantage of a Burow's graft is that it provides skin with a more closely matched color, texture, and thickness compared to grafts obtained from distant donor sites. Additional advantages include the proximity of the donor site to the recipient site, requiring a single bandage for the two, and the use of these grafts in hair-bearing areas given the close match of the type and direction of the hair with the recipient site hair. There are

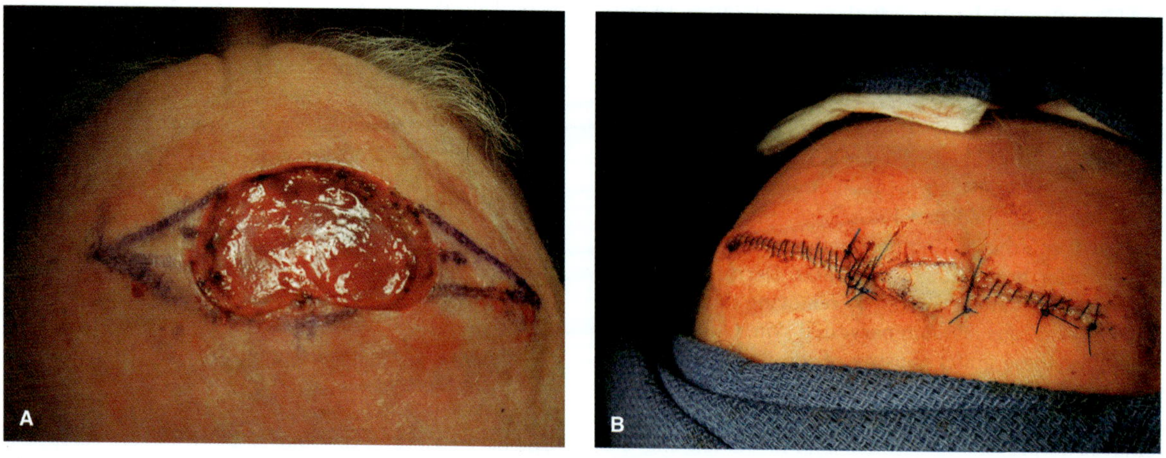

Figure 20-5 **A.** Large defect of central forehead after Mohs surgery. There was sufficient tissue laxity to close a significant portion of the wound. **B.** A Burow's FTSG from one of the Burow's triangles was used to repair the central portion of the defect, which could not be closed primarily. (Figures used with permission of Desiree Ratner, MD.)

several variations of the Burow's graft.[12] The classic technique consists of excising two Burow's triangles on either side of the wound. Primary linear closure of the ends of the wound results in narrowing of the central portion. The remaining wound is grafted with one or both of the the Burow's triangles as described above for FTSGs. One variation helpful in areas to avoid bidirectional lengthening of the scar (i.e., to avoid crossing cosmetic boundaries) is to use a single Burow's graft. Again, primary closure of the excised Burow's graft side of the wound causes narrowing of the defect to a teardrop-shape, which is then grafted using the Burow's triangle as above. A similar variation for wounds with immobile margins is the use of a larger Burow's triangle that results in a graft as wide as the original wound. Finally, a variation for wounds extending onto two cosmetic units makes use of one Burow's triangle as the FTSG for one cosmetic unit while the second portion of the defect is closed by tissue advancement.[12]

HAIR-BEARING GRAFTS

Although used less commonly than flaps in hair-bearing areas, grafts can be used in these areas with some special considerations. One important consideration is that the graft should be obtained from a location with hair characteristics similar to those of the recipient site, namely hair of the same caliber and density. It is important to anticipate a patient's propensity for developing androgenetic alopecia when determining the location from which to harvest an FTSG from the scalp. The occipital and temporal regions of the scalp are commonly used donor sites as these sites are less likely to develop androgenetic alopecia; however, these would not be ideal for grafting of the vertex scalp in a patient with androgenetic alopecia, as the grafted skin would likely retain terminal hairs whereas the hairs in the surrounding skin would miniaturize. When harvesting and preparing the hair-bearing FTSG, the graft should be minimally defatted, as the hair bulbs are contained in the subcutis and extensive defatting can result in loss of follicles. Defatting, therefore, should only be performed between the hair bulbs, if at all. In addition, proper orientation of the graft, taking into consideration the direction of hair growth, is important to maintain a uniform direction of hair shafts within the graft and the surrounding skin.

POSTOPERATIVE COMPLICATIONS. The complications of full-thickness grafting can be divided into two categories: short-term problems of graft failure and long-term problems of poor functional outcomes and cosmetic deficits. Of utmost importance in graft survival is uninterrupted direct contact between the graft and the recipient bed, which is key to neovascularization. Short-term causes of graft failure include infection, hematoma, seroma, and shearing forces of the graft over the wound bed.[19] Although infection is rare in grafts, care should be taken when handling the graft and electrocautery of the recipient bed should be avoided to minimize the presence of devitalized tissue. Antibiotics are not given routinely but may be considered in selected patients that are at higher risk for infection. When given, the antibiotics should cover *Staphylococcus* and *Streptococcus* species; for auricular grafts, anti-pseudomonal coverage may be necessary.

Hematoma and seroma formation can be avoided by meticulous intraoperative hemostasis, pressure dressings, and postoperative avoidance of physical activity, bending, and lifting for the first few weeks after surgery to minimize shearing forces of the graft over its bed. Preoperative avoidance of anticoagulants, pending consultation with the patient's cardiologist or primary care provider, is advisable only if these agents are not necessary for management of coagulopathy or prevention of blood clots and their sequelae. Nicotine-induced vasoconstriction is also associated with an increased risk of graft failure, and patients should, therefore, be encouraged to decrease cigarette or nicotine consumption for several days prior to and following surgery.

Long-term complications of FTSGs consist of cosmetic and functional problems. Extensive preoperative counseling is important in alleviating patient's postoperative concerns regarding graft appearance following surgery. It should be stressed that it may take 6 months or longer for grafts to heal and reach their ultimate cosmetic outcome. FTSGs may be depressed initially, but this depression tends to improve within 4 to 6 weeks. Camouflage make-up and sunblock can usually be applied 3 to 4 weeks after graft placement, thereby minimizing erythema and textural irregularities. Spot dermabrasion or laser resurfacing of the graft and the surrounding complete cosmetic unit can lead to improvement in color, consistency and elevation.[32] This can be performed at any time after 6 weeks to 6 months, although it is best performed 6 to 8 weeks following grafting. Hyperpigmentation of the graft can be treated with a brief course of topical hydroquinone and/or tretinoin combined with sunblock and usually resolves completely.

Functional complications of FTSGs occur primarily as a result of wound contraction. The degree of wound contraction depends in part on thickness of the FTSG and in part on location of the graft, with grafts applied to the periorbital or nasal areas contracting more than those applied to the scalp and temples. Therefore, grafts placed in defects with lax free margins (such as eyelids, lips, nasal ala) should be oversized to account for graft contraction.[19] Graft contraction usually increases as the thickness of the graft decreases. If poor functional or cosmetic outcomes result from wound contraction, secondary revisional surgery may be needed.

COMPOSITE GRAFTS

CGs are simply modified FTSGs composed of two or more tissue layers. Typically, within the scope of dermatologic surgery, these two layers are skin and cartilage, although they can likewise be composed of skin and perichondrium, or skin and adipose tissue.[31,33–35] Scenarios in which the use of CGs is most beneficial include repair of defects that require recreation of structural integrity such as full-thickness alar rim defects and nasal tip defects with cartilage loss (Fig. 20-6A–F).[36]

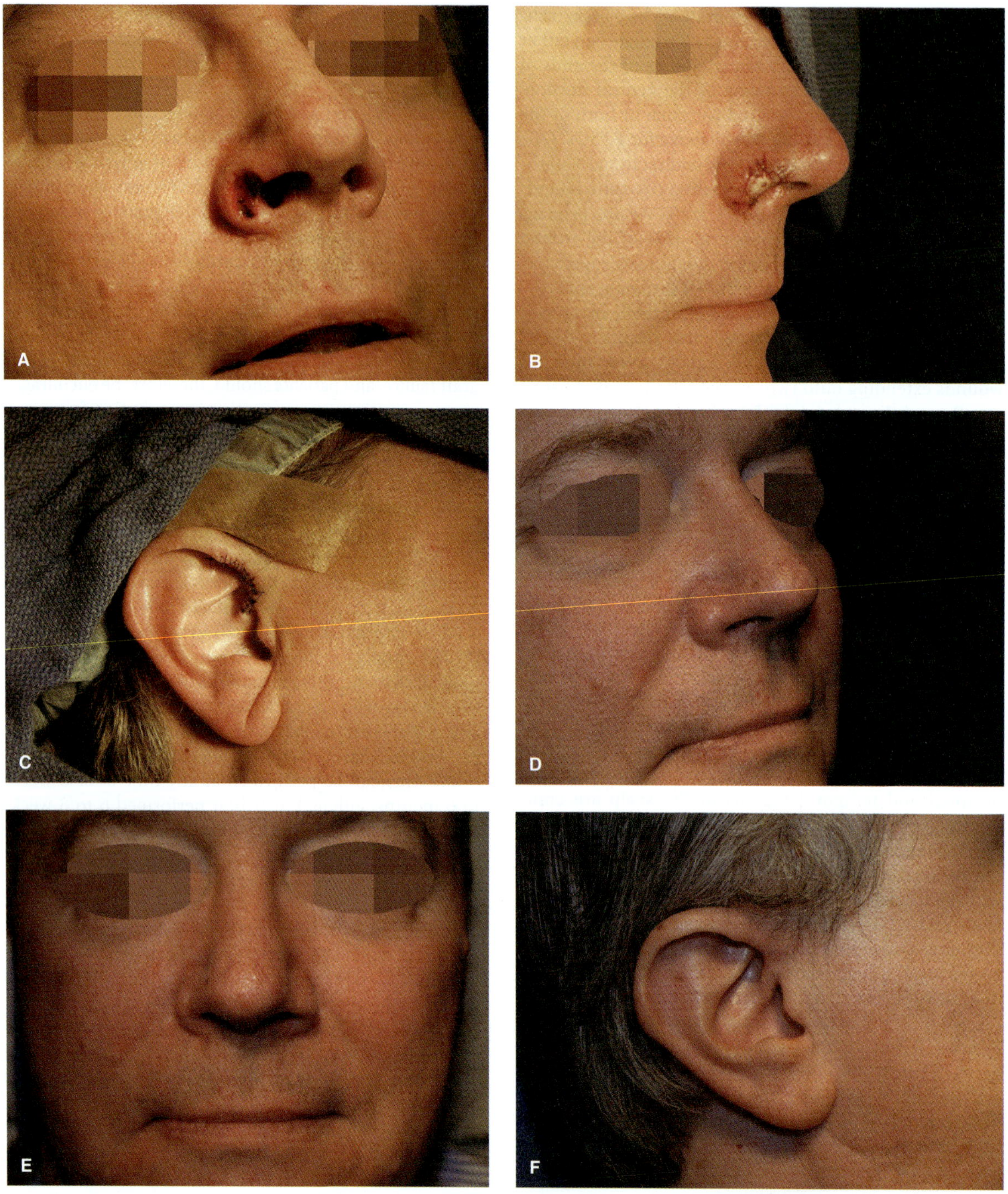

Figure 20-6 **A.** Deep partial-thickness defect of right nasal ala after Mohs surgery for basal cell carcinoma. **B.** Composite graft taken from right helical crus sewn into place with 6-0 fast absorbing gut sutures. **C.** Right helical donor site closed primarily. **D.** Follow-up view 4 years postoperatively (side view). **E.** Follow-up view 4 years postoperatively (front view). **F.** View of the donor site 4 years postoperatively. (Used with permission of Desiree Ratner, MD. Reproduced with permission from Kaporis HG, Carucci JA. Repair of a defect on the ala. In: Ratner DS, Cohen JL, Brodland DG, eds. *Reconstructive Conundrums in Dermatologic Surgery: The Nose*. Oxford: Wiley Blackwell;2014. Copyright © 2014 American Society for Dermatologic Surgery.)

Cartilage contributes significantly to maintaining the anatomic structure and function of the nose and ears. In instances when cartilage must be excised, a functional and structural deficit results, which necessitates repair with either a composite skin graft or an FCG.

Reinforcement of structural integrity of the nose using cartilage helps prevent alar notching and nasal valve dysfunction. Alar notching is a potential problem associated with deep wounds of the nasal ala. Contraction of a defect close to the rim can result loss of the smooth, continuous contour of the alar-free margin. Repair of full-thickness alar rim defects may involve a layered skin–cartilage–skin CG "sandwich" versus a combination of composite or FCGs with overlying flap reconstruction.[2,19] Alar and alar crease defects can also cause nasal valve dysfunction. The nasal valve lies at the upper end of the lateral crus of the alar cartilage. It provides resistance that controls the speed and volume of inspired air so that the nasal passages are kept patent. Problems with nasal valve function can result from loss of alar tissue or cartilaginous support, causing the passage of air to become occluded during inspiration with symptoms of reduced nasal airflow. This occurs when the remaining nasal tissue collapses inward toward the nasal septum due to lack of structural support. Cartilage can be used as part of the graft to reestablish the structural integrity of the ala, thereby reducing alar collapse during inspiration. Delayed nasal valve obstruction can also occur if a cartilage graft is not placed when needed, as scar contracture of existing cartilage can also cause a functional nasal obstruction.[37] Similarly, loss of cartilage from the ear canal may require replacement to maintain ear canal patency.

Other locations in which CGs are commonly utilized include the nasal sidewall and columella. Deeper nasal defects farther from the alar rim, particularly with exposed cartilage, can be repaired with either conchal bowl CGs using skin and cartilage or PCCGs, consisting only of skin and perichondrium.[31]

PREOPERATIVE CONSIDERATIONS

Survival of CGs depends on rapid revascularization. CGs have greater metabolic demands than simpler skin grafts and are dependent upon the bridging phenomenon for survival, as revascularization takes places through direct vessel anastomoses between the subdermal plexus of the graft and the subdermal plexus of the wound edge. Unlike FTSGs, in which reestablishment of blood flow occurs through direct contact of the graft base with the underlying wound bed, the primary establishment of CG circulation relies on wound edge vascular supply, which, therefore, limits the size of these grafts. CGs for defect diameters greater than 2 cm are contraindicated due to an increased risk of central necrosis. The ideal maximum size of CGs is, therefore, 1 to 2 cm with no more than 0.5 to 1 cm between any point of the graft and the wound edge.[34,38–40] Areas of limited size with a rich vascular supply, such as the ear or the nose, are the most useful sites for use of CGs. Surgical strategies to refurbish the recipient vascular bed include use of hinge flaps from the margins of the defect or delayed grafting for optimal granulation tissue growth.[41] Delay allows the defect to heal by second intention for several weeks with wound contraction and formation of granulation tissue that can better support a graft with a high nutritional demand. If this approach is undertaken, however, one must monitor for excessive wound contraction that can lead to functional or aesthetic impairment. The higher nutritional requirements of CGs may hamper wound healing, especially in patients with suboptimal health. Therefore, patients who have underlying risk factors for poor wound healing such as smokers, diabetics, and patients with vaso-occlusive disease, would not be ideal candidates for such repair options.

DONOR SITE SELECTION

The ear can typically serve as the donor site for CGs since it features multiple areas with variable cartilaginous contours with overlying skin. The most commonly used area of the ear for repair of nasal alar defects is the crus of the helix; other areas that can be used include the helical rim, tragus, antitragus, and concha.[36] The thin overlying skin and subcutis of the ear may provide a good tissue match for the alar skin, except for the most sebaceous areas in certain patients, typically located on the distal third of the nose. Repair of a highly sebaceous nasal tip is best performed using an auricular FCG in combination with a better matched FTSG or local skin flap instead of a CG. If a CG is deemed useful, the more sebaceous, thicker cartilaginous aspect of the concha serves as the preferred donor site. The concha can also be used for reconstruction of nasal sidewall, columella, and larger alar nasal defects.[42–44] Repair of donor sites on the ear varies by location. Helical rim donor sites are typically repaired with wedge excision; defects involving the crus of the helix can be closed either linearly or by use of a local flap; and defects of the triangular fossa, scapha, conchal bowl, or cymba heal well by secondary intention. Removal of conchal cartilage with a small punch (2–3 mm) can also help with more rapid secondary intention healing from the opposing dermal tissue.

TECHNIQUE

After appropriate surgical decontamination, scar tissue at the recipient site should be evaluated and debrided, if necessary, to optimize blood supply for the CG. A template conforming to the recipient site is prepared and the donor site marked using the template. The CG should be approximately 5% to 10% larger than the defect in order to compensate for the natural shrinkage of the graft that occurs during healing.[2] Both the cutaneous boundaries of the donor site as well as what will become the cartilaginous wings framing the graft should be drawn out. After the marking is complete, the areas may be anesthetized with 1% lidocaine with epinephrine. The CG is harvested by incising perpendicular to the surface of the skin, with the first pass of the scalpel blade cutting through the skin and the second pass through the cartilage. The harvested CG is thus excised en bloc as a skin–cartilage or skin–cartilage–skin "sandwich," depending on the coverage needs. The donor site can then be closed by the most appropriate method, as mentioned previously. During this time, the recipient site should be kept moist and the graft may be stored in saline.

The CG should be handled delicately to prevent any disruption of vasculature or detachment of skin or adipose tissue from the cartilage. For a typical CG, the cartilage may be secured using sutures of 5-0 polyglactin. The cutaneous wound edges are reapproximated using 5-0 or 6-0 absorbable or nonabsorbable sutures. Meticulous suturing technique helps to minimize strangulation of blood vessels and facilitates anastomoses between graft and recipient vascular beds.

To prepare a CG for placement near a free margin, a design using interlocking cartilaginous pegs may be considered to enhance graft adherence without the need for placement of sutures within the cartilage. The skin overlying the cartilaginous wings of the graft may need to be trimmed. The remaining cartilaginous pegs with overlying perichondrium frame the lateral aspects of the graft.[2] The recipient site is prepared by undermining pockets using a hemostat or scissors parallel to the alar or helical rim on each side of the defect. The cartilaginous pegs are carefully inserted into these pockets so that the graft interlocks with its recipient bed. The interlocking of the graft with its recipient bed aids in increasing the surface area for revascularization as well as minimizing shearing forces. Once the graft is interlocked, the intranasal and cutaneous skin edges are sutured into place; the cartilage does not require suturing.[45]

Finally, a dressing is placed, which can consist of support in the nasal vestibule using petrolatum-impregnated dressing and antibiotic ointment with an overlying nonstick dressing placed on the external surface of the graft. Given the high rate of colonization of the nares with bacteria, oral antibiotics are typically prescribed. Sutures are removed in 1 week. Postoperatively, the patient should be advised to apply ice packs to the area for several days.

COMPLICATIONS

Similar to other types of grafts, CGs may incur textural, color, and contour irregularities. These can be treated if desired using spot dermabrasion or laser resurfacing. Due to their high nutritional demands, CGs can also fail. Revision can be accomplished using a two-stage melolabial interpolation flap or by attempting a second CG procedure.

Potential complications at the donor site include pain and an increased risk of bleeding from conchal bowl donor sites healing by secondary intention. Therefore, auricular donor sites should be covered both anteriorly and posteriorly with a pressure dressing. Addition of hemostatic foam can also be considered. Another potential complication of surgery involving the ear results from its propensity toward infection with *Pseudomonas spp.* Measures that can be undertaken to decrease this risk include cleansing the area with dilute vinegar solution, applying topical gentamicin ointment, or prophylactic oral fluoroquinolone antibiotics.[8] Perichondritis or chondritis due to either cartilaginous inflammation or infection (suggested by additional presence of fever or purulent drainage) can occur at the surgical site, causing redness and pain. If an inflammatory etiology is suspected, use of NSAIDs as indicated may reduce the symptoms.[46]

FREE CARTILAGE GRAFTS

FCGs are used to restore structural or functional deficits due to tissue loss, particularly near free margins of the nose, ears, or eyelids (Fig. 20-7A–C).[2,35,47] While most commonly performed along the alar rim, cartilage grafts

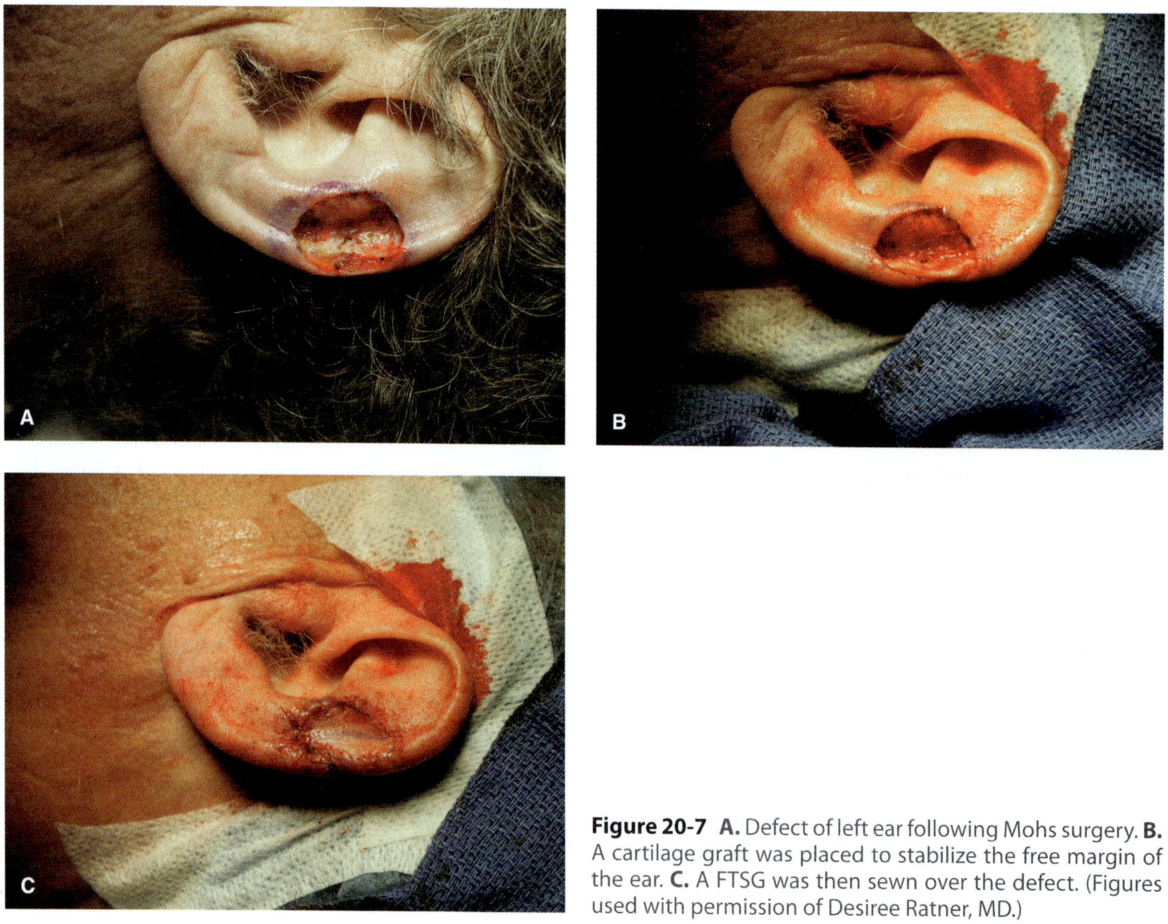

Figure 20-7 **A.** Defect of left ear following Mohs surgery. **B.** A cartilage graft was placed to stabilize the free margin of the ear. **C.** A FTSG was then sewn over the defect. (Figures used with permission of Desiree Ratner, MD.)

are also used at times in repairing defects of the distal nasal tip, lower eyelid margin, or along the helical rim to optimize both cosmetic and functional results.[35] In the context of dermatologic surgery, FCGs derive most commonly from the elastic auricular cartilage as it is more pliable, and often more easily accessible, than nasal septum or rib cartilage.[2,35]

Removal of a sizable portion of the conchal bowl cartilage can be achieved without significant aesthetic or functional compromise at the donor site. Antihelical cartilage grafts can also serve as useful alternatives and tend to be less brittle.[48] Potential complications of FCGs include donor site morbidity such as chondritis, infection, hematoma, or distortion of the helical rim. FCGs are avascular and depend on a nutrient supply from the subdermal vascular plexus of their recipient bed wound edges. Patients who are smokers or have an impaired vascular supply are at higher risk for cartilage graft failure. Graft displacement or resorption is thought to be more likely following mechanical trauma or unmet nutritional demand.

Placement of a flat strip of cartilage, also termed a batten, along the nasal alar rim or supra-alar crease can provide a rigid framework for prevention of nasal valve collapse, maintaining airway patency and protecting against contraction during healing.[49–51] Tissue loss resulting from excisional surgery on the nasal ala or supra-alar crease can cause functional obstruction due to nasal valve collapse. During inspiration, the remaining nasal tissue is pulled inward toward the septum, creating airway obstruction. A delayed nasal valve obstruction can also occur from scar contracture and stenosis if a cartilage graft is not placed or if an existing graft is resorbed. When FCGs are combined with flaps and FTSGs, the risk of scar contraction and airway collapse is greatly reduced. Before and after FCG placement, airway patency can be tested and confirmed by comparing the patient's ability to inspire through the affected nostril with inspiration on the contralateral side.

DONOR SITE SELECTION

Several different donor sites can be used for harvesting FCGs including the conchal bowl, antihelix, nasal septum, or ribs.[35] Conchal and antihelical cartilage more closely approximate the contours and elasticity of nasal cartilage and serve most readily as donor sites.[2,35,52] Cartilage that is inflamed or diseased should not be harvested.[8]

TECHNIQUE

Different techniques for harvesting conchal cartilage have been described, including both anterior and posterior approaches.[2,52] To obtain the graft, the area is first prepped in a sterile fashion and local anesthesia is achieved with infiltration of both the anterior and posterior aspects of the donor site to ensure that removal of the graft is painless.[2] First, the amount of cartilage desired is estimated by measuring the length of the surgical defect at the free margin and adding an extra 2 to 5 mm on either side to provide enough excess tissue to interlock with the peripheral edges of the defect.[53] The width of the free cartilage batten may range from 3 to 6 mm. Once the size is determined, the skin overlying the donor site is sharply incised, then undermined to expose the perichondrium.[2,35] If only a strip of cartilage is needed, a curvilinear incision may be performed. For larger-sized FCGs, greater access to the bulk of the conchal bowl can be obtained by lifting a curved flap of skin from the conchal bowl skin via an anterior approach.[52] The desired shape of the cartilage graft is then outlined and incised with a scalpel blade, after which the cartilage with its overlying perichondrium is carefully removed by sharp dissection. The FCG should be placed in a sterile moist environment, such as sterile saline, until ready for use. Buried sutures to reapproximate the cartilage or dermal wound edges are not required at the donor site. The cutaneous surface of the donor site may be reapproximated simply using a variety of superficial suturing techniques; a running locked suture may be helpful if bleeding risk is a concern.[2]

Several techniques may be used to secure the FCG. One of the most commonly used techniques involves creating a pocket in the recipient bed by undermining medially and laterally beneath the skin edges, tucking the peripheral edges of cartilage into these soft-tissue pockets sequentially, and securing the cartilage with absorbable sutures to the underlying soft tissue.[2,53] This pocket increases the graft contact with the rich vascular network of the recipient bed. Buried polyglactin sutures encircling the cartilage strip may also be used to secure it to the underlying soft tissue. Larger grafts may require absorbable suture placement through or around the full thickness of the cartilage to optimize their inset. Once the graft is secured, an FTSG or flap can be performed to complete the wound closure (Fig. 20-8A–C).[2,54] Given its vascularity, it is possible that a flap's additional blood supply may help to enhance survivability of the FCG.

In those circumstances when a less complex repair is preferred, FCG placement with secondary intention healing thereafter can yield acceptable, although perhaps not aesthetically ideal, wound healing for nasal wound defects.[55,56] Likewise, correction of lower eyelid retraction may involve placement of an FCG with secondary intention healing on the conjunctival surface to provide structural support, or a conchal bowl-derived chondrocutaneous CG to further enhance the contour of the cutaneous surface.[57,58]

Conchal cartilage is commonly used to repair helical rim defects. A partial wedge closure of the helical rim defect may be used to decrease the size of the cartilage graft required, and can help to minimize the helical rim collapse that can occur with wound contraction. The FCG is then secured with sutures as mentioned previously, and may be covered with a pedicled retroauricular advancement flap.

POSTOPERATIVE CARE

Appropriate postoperative care is imperative for the success of cartilage grafts.[2,9] A bolster dressing may be applied to the wound surface at the discretion of the surgeon. A non-adherent pressure dressing is typically used to give added support and help prevent bleeding complications. Using intermittent ice packs for the first 2 to 3 days after surgery can help to minimize edema and may help to increase

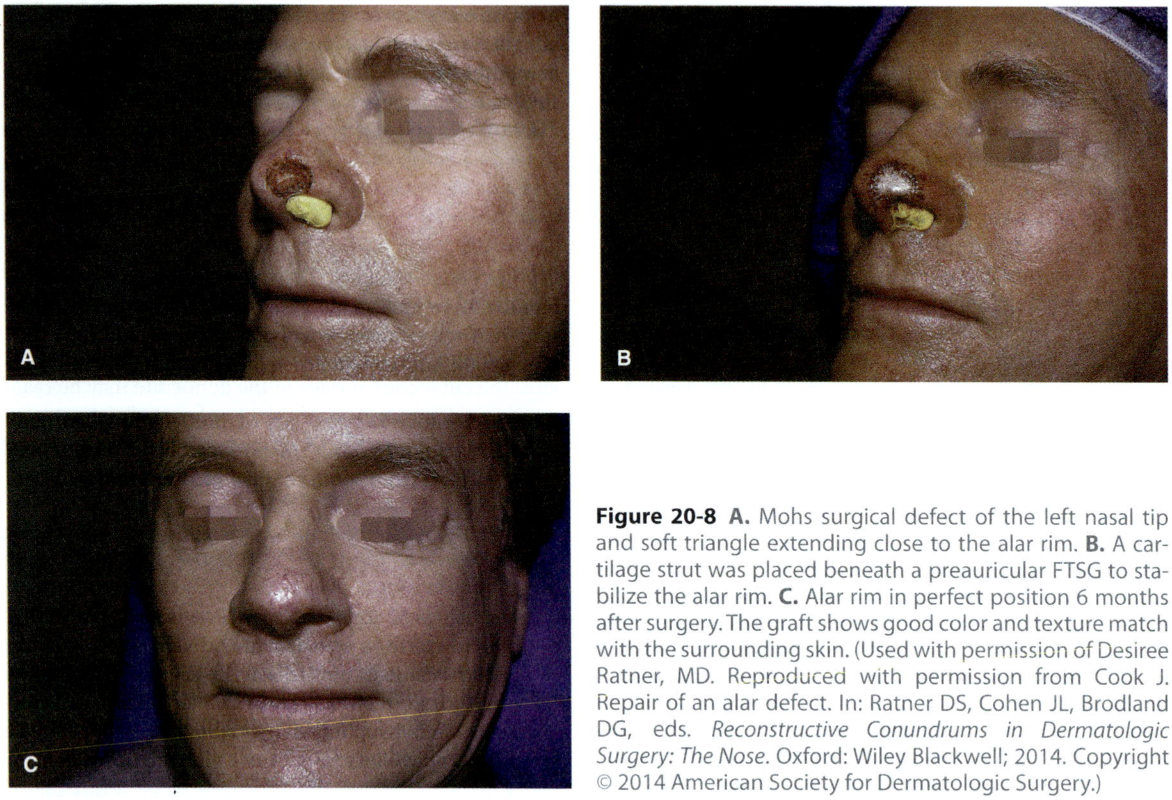

Figure 20-8 **A.** Mohs surgical defect of the left nasal tip and soft triangle extending close to the alar rim. **B.** A cartilage strut was placed beneath a preauricular FTSG to stabilize the alar rim. **C.** Alar rim in perfect position 6 months after surgery. The graft shows good color and texture match with the surrounding skin. (Used with permission of Desiree Ratner, MD. Reproduced with permission from Cook J. Repair of an alar defect. In: Ratner DS, Cohen JL, Brodland DG, eds. *Reconstructive Conundrums in Dermatologic Surgery: The Nose*. Oxford: Wiley Blackwell; 2014. Copyright © 2014 American Society for Dermatologic Surgery.)

graft survival.[2] Prescription of postoperative broad-spectrum oral antibiotics is variably practiced and lacks specific evidence-based guidance. While topical antibiotic application has not generally been shown superior to petrolatum in routine wound care, it is possible that its use near the nares may help to reduce the risk of impetiginization.[59]

COMPLICATIONS

As with any skin surgery, risks of infection are present at both the donor and the recipient sites. Gram-negative bacteria are commonly the culprit at auricular donor sites.[46] If any exudate is present, empiric fluoroquinolones can be considered while wound culture is in progress. If the patient is not improving with antibiotics, a fungal culture should be considered.[2] Chondritis at auricular donor sites presents as erythema, edema, and tenderness without an exudate.[60] Treatment often requires several weeks to months of cold compresses and nonsteroidal anti-inflammatory drugs.[2,19]

Late complications that might require surgical revision include graft resorption or extrusion, which can lead to deformation of the site.[2,35] Securing a cartilage graft of the appropriate thickness and stiffness is important.[35] To avoid complications, it is critical to minimize trauma to the site or movement of the graft with respect to its recipient bed.

SPLIT-THICKNESS SKIN GRAFTS

STSGs contain the entire epidermis and variable amounts of dermis. Unlike FTSGs, they usually lack adnexal structures including hair follicles, eccrine glands, and sebaceous glands. STSGs can range in thickness from 0.125 mm to 0.75 mm. Typically thinner grafts from 0.3 to 0.4 mm are used in the head and neck region whereas 0.5 to 0.6 mm grafts are used on the trunk.[9]

There are many advantages to using STSGs. STSGs are able to cover very large defects. They heal faster and can survive better than FTSGs, especially in areas of vascular compromise as these thinner grafts have reduced nutritional requirements compared to FTSGs.[2,9] Trophic ulcers on the lower legs are a good example of an instance in which an STSG can cover a large defect and survive despite the poor vascularity of the recipient bed.[7,9,61] Since they are thin and semitransparent, STSGs allow for improved surveillance for recurrence of high-risk tumors.[2] STSGs can also be fenestrated to enable a smaller graft to cover a larger defect. Their donor sites do not require primary closure and heal secondarily.

The most recognized disadvantage of STSGs is their suboptimal color and texture match with the surrounding skin, which is partly due to their lack of adnexal structures.[2,7] Another disadvantage of STSGs is that harvesting them requires specialized equipment. The donor site wound requires further care and tends to heal with a noticeable outline. Finally, STSGs may contract as much as 70%, and if placed near the free margins of the eyelids, oral commissures, or nasal alae, such contraction can lead to both functional and cosmetic compromise.[7]

STSGs are harvested from broad areas of skin that are hidden by clothing, whether manually with a freehand device, or with a power-driven dermatome.[62] Many donor sites are possible, including the thighs, upper arms, inner forearms, lower back, and abdomen, with the anteromedial thigh being the most common. Large grafts needed to

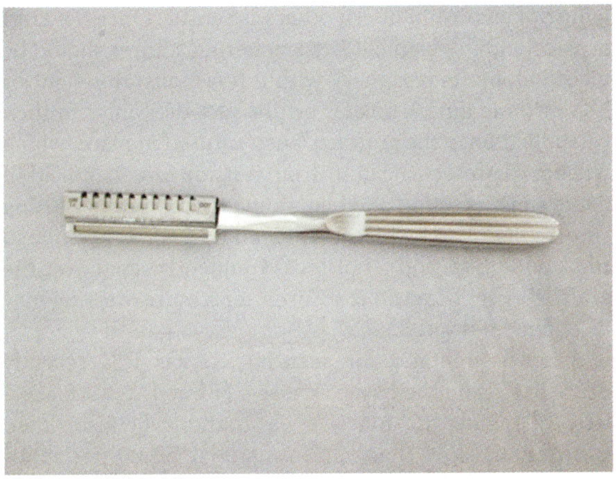

Figure 20-9 Weck blade.

cover a substantial defect should be harvested from broad, flat surfaces, usually with a power-driven dermatome. Smaller grafts can be quickly harvested with a freehand #10 or #15 scalpel blade from a variety of different donor sites, including the mastoid processes and upper lateral arms.[2,63] The difficulty in harvesting STSGs manually lies in obtaining a graft with uniform dermal thickness, which is highly technique dependent.[64] A Weck blade can provide a solution to this problem; these are freehand blades with templates that allow the physician to choose the desired graft thickness, although there is a learning curve associated with use of these devices as well (Fig. 20-9).[2]

Several recent studies have advocated harvesting STSGs from the posterior scalp as a donor site due to its rapid wound healing, low risk of complications, and excellent cosmetic results.[65,66] The scalp is thought to contain a large number of epidermal stem cells due to its significant number of hair follicles, which may explain why it tends to heal so well. In addition, the color and texture of scalp STSGs tend to match those of facial recipient sites more closely, leading to improved cosmesis.[65,66]

HARVESTING THE STSG

After the donor site is anesthetized and prepped in a sterile fashion, a freehand STSG can be performed with a #10 or #15 blade by orienting the blade parallel to the skin, and gently harvesting the graft by making superficial incisions just below and parallel to the epidermis (Fig. 20-10A–C).[2] A Weck blade can also be used for harvesting of STSGs. The presence of pinpoint bleeding from the donor site is generally a good indication that the graft is the appropriate thickness, and that the papillary dermis has been reached.[67] Multiple blades may be required to harvest a single STSG, as they tend to dull quickly during harvesting.[19]

For power-driven dermatomes, it is important to lubricate the skin with mineral oil or normal saline to enable the dermatome to glide gently over the skin surface. The

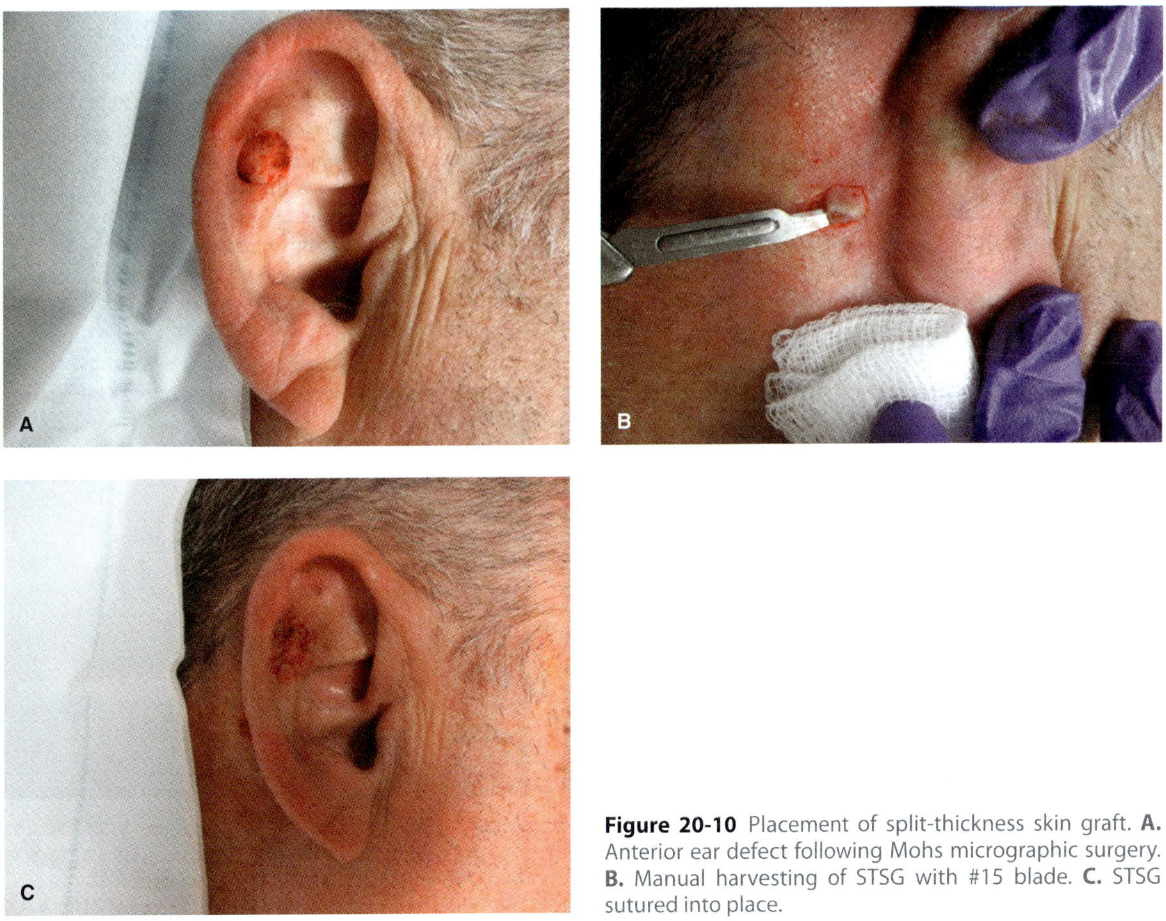

Figure 20-10 Placement of split-thickness skin graft. **A.** Anterior ear defect following Mohs micrographic surgery. **B.** Manual harvesting of STSG with #15 blade. **C.** STSG sutured into place.

handpiece is then held at a 30 degree angle with steady pressure oriented downward and forward.[7,67] An assistant applies traction to create a flat, even surface while the surgeon applies pressure to the dermatome as it starts to cut. In the absence of adequate surrounding traction and a broad flat surface for harvesting, it is likely that an uneven graft will result. The graft is then gently removed from the pocket area of the dermatome with forceps. It is then placed on sterile saline-soaked gauze or directly onto the recipient site, at which point it can be trimmed to match the defect.[2] It is important to remember that the STSG will tend to curl on itself, which helps the surgeon to distinguish between the dermal and epidermal surfaces, and minimizes the risk of the graft being placed upside down. If the edges of the graft are not perfectly approximated with the wound edges, the overlapping skin will slough without affecting the cosmetic outcome. The donor site is later covered with mupirocin 2% ointment, petrolatum ointment, gelfoam, or a nonadherent dressing of the surgeon's choice.[68]

Power-driven dermatomes are used to harvest large STSGs, which may be up to 4 in wide, and can easily create grafts with a uniform dermal thickness, up to 0.75 mm thick.[2] An adjustable dial allows the operator to increase or decrease the thickness of the graft, enabling grafts between 0.05 and 0.76 mm thick to be easily harvested.[68]

Another distinct advantage of STSGs is their ability to be enlarged with a meshing device, which can increase their coverage by 25% to 35%.[2] Most meshing devices compress STSGs on a plastic grid with a steel roller, thereby creating uniform fenestrations. The fenestrations allow the graft to increase its coverage size, and allow for drainage of serosanguinous material that could inhibit graft healing. For larger grafts, a meshing device can be quite helpful, while simple fenestrations can be made with a #11 or #15 blade in smaller grafts to increase their size.[2]

SECURING THE STSGS

Before securing the STSG, it is important to prepare the recipient bed to receive the graft. Hemostasis must be achieved before attaching the graft, since a hematoma and failure of engraftment can otherwise ensue. Once the graft is placed on its recipient site, anchoring sutures should be placed along its periphery with 6-0 fast absorbing gut or 5-0 chromic gut. A bolster or pressure dressing can then be applied once the graft has been sutured in place, which will act to protect the graft from outside forces and aid in decreasing infection and hematoma formation.[2,7,9] Basting sutures may also be placed to facilitate graft adherence to the wound bed, and a bolster is frequently sewn over the graft.[9,68] After the graft is secured, a pressure dressing may be applied if desired.

A newer method for securing STSGs was recently described using the tissue adhesive N-butyl-2-cyanoacrylate.[69] Applying the adhesive was found to be faster than suturing, cheaper than suture material ($2.00 per application), and seemed to have no higher rates of infection than securing a graft with sutures. The adhesive is simply applied to the periphery of the graft, and allowed 60 seconds to fully set. Afterward a bolster may be applied.

For the donor site, a moist occlusive dressing with petrolatum is recommended.[2,70] Moist dressings decrease postoperative pain and promote re-epithelialization.[70,71] The donor site usually heals over 1 to 3 weeks, although postoperative erythema at the site may last for months before fading. Ultimately, a hypo- or hyperpigmented donor site scar will likely result.[2]

POSTOPERATIVE CARE AND COMPLICATIONS

Despite meticulous wound care, complications can sometimes occur. Early complications of STSGs include failure of engraftment, which can result from hematoma or seroma formation, infection, or trauma to the graft site. Within the first day or two after placing the graft, a large amount of serosanguinous fluid can accumulate beneath it, potentially compromising its survival. Placement of a bolster dressing can help to minimize this risk. If this complication does occur, the fluid should be drained with a sterile needle and syringe, and a new pressure dressing

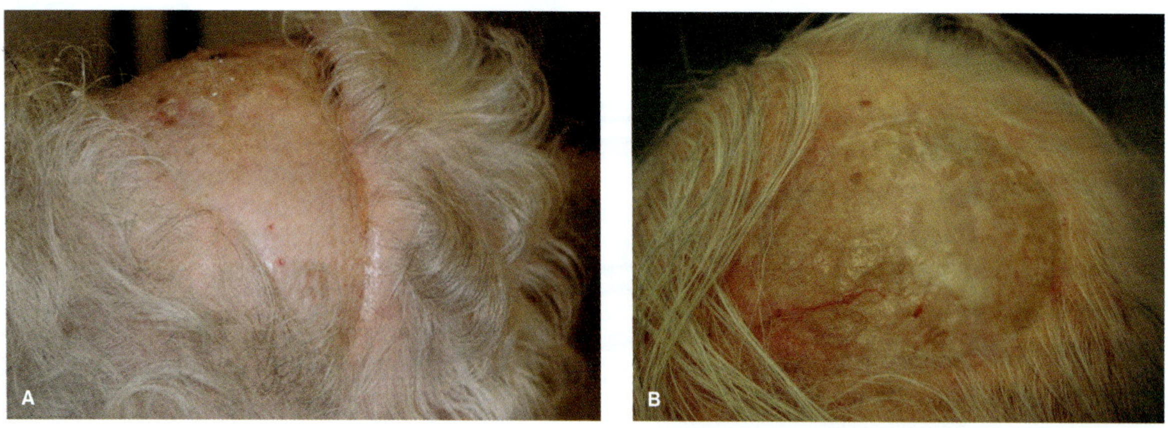

Figure 20-11 A. Three-month follow-up of STSG placed on scalp after large scalp rotation flap for large forehead and frontal bone defect following melanoma resection. Note the hypopigmentation and smooth, shiny, hairless surface of the STSG in contrast to the hair-bearing scalp. **B.** One-year follow-up of STSG placed on scalp after resection of large SCC. Note the poor color and texture match with the surrounding skin. (Figure 20-11B used with permission of Desiree Ratner, MD.)

applied. Patients should be educated to avoid trauma to their grafts, especially in the early healing phase.

Late complications typically include color and texture mismatch or functional problems with the graft itself.[2,19] Once STSGs have healed, their color may vary significantly, but they rarely match the surrounding skin (Fig. 20-11A,B). Some remain erythematous to light pink, whereas others may become hyperpigmented, hypopigmented, or largely depigmented. To minimize the risk of hyperpigmentation, especially in darker-skinned individuals, patients should limit sun exposure and wear sunscreen. Other STSG complications include graft scaling and dryness, likely due to the presence of decreased adnexal structures resulting in decreased sweating and desquamation, but this problem can be reduced with frequent emollients.

Functional problems with the grafts are another late complication. These problems are usually due to STSG contraction, which can cause joint contractures if placed near or overlying a joint, ectropion near the free eyelid margin or upper cheek, eclabium near the free margin of the lip, or distortion of the nose if placed near the free margin of the alar rim. Significant hypertrophic scarring of graft sites and donor sites has also been reported.[2] If recognized early, this complication may be successfully treated with intralesional steroids. If it persists, treatment with the pulsed dye laser may be helpful.

CONCLUSIONS

As the incidence of skin cancers continues to rise, and the population continues to age, an increasing number of skin grafts will be required to repair a variety of facial and non-facial defects. A working knowledge and complete understanding of the indications, donor site considerations, techniques, and complications of all types of skin grafts is, therefore, essential for the practicing reconstructive surgeon.

REFERENCES

1. Hauben DJ, Baruchin A, Mahler A. On the history of the free skin graft. *Ann Plast Surg.* 1982;9(3):242–245.
2. Adams DC, Ramsey ML. Grafts in dermatologic surgery: review and update on full- and split-thickness skin grafts, free cartilage grafts, and composite grafts. *Dermatol Surg.* 2005;31(8 Pt 2):1055–1067.
3. Converse JM, Smahel J, Ballantyne DL Jr, Harper AD. Inosculation of vessels of skin graft and host bed: a fortuitous encounter. *Br J Plast Surg.* 1975;28(4):274–282.
4. Converse JM, Uhlschmid GK, Ballantyne DL Jr. "Plasmatic circulation" in skin grafts. The phase of serum imbibition. *Plast Reconstr Surg.* 1969;43(5):495–499.
5. Clemmesen T, Ronhovde DA. Restoration of the blood-supply to human skin autografts. *Scand J Plast Reconstr Surg.* 1968;2(1):44–46.
6. Gingrass P, Grabb WC, Gingrass RP. Skin graft survival on avascular defects. *Plast Reconstr Surg.* 1975;55(1):65–70.
7. Johnson TM, Ratner D, Nelson BR. Soft tissue reconstruction with skin grafting. *J Am Acad Dermatol.* 1992;27(2 Pt 1):151–165.
8. Unal S, Ersoz G, Demirkan F, Arslan E, Tutuncu N, Sari A. Analysis of skin-graft loss due to infection: infection-related graft loss. *Ann Plast Surg.* 2005;55(1):102–106.
9. Ratner D. Skin grafting. *Semin Cutan Med Surg.* 2003; 22(4):295–305.
10. Kaufman AJ. Adjacent-tissue skin grafts for reconstruction. *Dermatol Surg.* 2004;30(10):1349–1353.
11. Silapunt S, Peterson SR, Alam M, Goldberg LH. Clinical appearance of full-thickness skin grafts of the nose. *Dermatol Surg.* 2005;31(2):177–183.
12. Zitelli JA. Burow's grafts. *J Am Acad Dermatol.* 1987;17(2 Pt 1):271–279.
13. Breach NM. Pre-auricular full-thickness skin grafts. *Br J Plast Surg.* 1978;31(2):124–126.
14. Corwin TR, Klein AW, Habal MB. The aesthetics of the preauricular graft in facial reconstruction. *Ann Plast Surg.* 1982;9(4):312–315.
15. Beare RL, Bennett JP. The naso-labial full thickness graft. *Br J Plast Surg.* 1972;25(3):315–317.
16. Rohrer TE, Dzubow LM. Conchal bowl skin grafting in nasal tip reconstruction: clinical and histologic evaluation. *J Am Acad Dermatol.* 1995;33(3):476–481.
17. Stucker FJ Jr, Shaw GY. The perichondrial cutaneous graft. A 12-year clinical experience. *Arch Otolaryngol Head Neck Surg.* 1992;118(3):287–292.
18. Palkar VM. Full-thickness skin grafting. *J Surg Oncol.* 2000;73(1):31.
19. Ratner D. Skin grafting. From here to there. *Dermatol Clin.* 1998;16(1):75–90.
20. Hill TG. Contouring of donor skin in full-thickness skin grafting. *J Dermatol Surg Oncol.* 1987;13(8):883–888.
21. Mellette JR Jr, Swinehart JM. Cartilage removal prior to skin grafting in the triangular fossa, antihelix, and concha of the ear. *J Dermatol Surg Oncol.* 1990;16(12):1102–1105.
22. Langtry JA, Kirkham P, Martin IC, Fordyce A. Tie-over bolster dressings may not be necessary to secure small full thickness skin grafts. *Dermatol Surg.* 1998;24(12):1350–1353.
23. Shimizu I, MacFarlane DF. Full-thickness skin grafts may not need tie-over bolster dressings. *Dermatol Surg.* 2013;39(5):726–728.
24. Brady JG, Grande DJ, Katz AE. The purse-string suture in facial reconstruction. *J Dermatol Surg Oncol.* 1992;18(9):812–816.
25. Robinson JK, Dillig G. The advantages of delayed nasal full-thickness skin grafting after Mohs micrographic surgery. *Dermatol Surg.* 2002;28(9):845–851.
26. Meyers S, Rohrer T, Grande D. Use of dermal grafts in reconstructing deep nasal defects and shaping the ala nasi. *Dermatol Surg.* 2001;27(3):300–305.
27. Fader DJ, Wang TS, Johnson TM. Nasal reconstruction utilizing a muscle hinge flap with overlying full-thickness skin graft. *J Am Acad Dermatol.* 2000;43(5 Pt 1):837–840.
28. Halpern M, Adams C, Ratner D. Galeal hinge flaps: a useful technique for immediate repair of scalp defects extending to periosteum. *Dermatol Surg.* 2009;35(1):127–130.
29. Johnson TM, Baker S, Brown MD, Nelson BR. Utility of the subcutaneous hinge flap in nasal reconstruction. *J Am Acad Dermatol.* 1994;30(3):459–466.
30. Draper BK, Wentzell JM. The "drumhead" graft repair of deep nasal alar defects. *Dermatol Surg.* 2007;33(1):17–22.
31. Gloster HM Jr, Brodland DG. The use of perichondrial cutaneous grafts to repair defects of the lower third of the nose. *Br J Dermatol.* 1997;136(1):43–46.
32. Nehal KS, Levine VJ, Ross B, Ashinoff R. Comparison of high-energy pulsed carbon dioxide laser resurfacing and dermabrasion in the revision of surgical scars. *Dermatol Surg.* 1998;24(6):647–650.
33. Geyer AS, Pasternack F, Adams C, Ratner D. Use of a skin-fat composite graft to prevent alar notching: an alternative to delayed postoperative repair. *Dermatol Surg.* 2005;31(5):602–607.
34. Haas AF, Glogau RG. A variation of composite grafting for reconstruction of full-thickness nasal alar defects. *Arch Dermatol.* 1994;130(8):978–980.
35. Otley CC, Sherris DA. Spectrum of cartilage grafting in cutaneous reconstructive surgery. *J Am Acad Dermatol.* 1998;39(6):982–992.
36. Field LM. Nasal alar rim reconstruction utilizing the crus of the helix, with several alternatives for donor site closure. *J Dermatol Surg Oncol.* 1986;12(3):253–258.

37. Robinson JK, Burget GC. Nasal valve malfunction resulting from resection of cancer. *Arch Otolaryngol Head Neck Surg.* 1990;116(12):1419–1424.
38. Mc LC. Composite ear grafts and their blood supply. *Br J Plast Surg.* 1954;7(3):274–278.
39. Ruch MK. Utilization of composite free grafts. *J Int Coll Surg.* 1958;30(2):274–275.
40. Weisberg NK, Becker DS. Repair of nasal ala defects with conchal bowl composite grafts. *Dermatol Surg.* 2000;26(11): 1047–1051.
41. Teltzrow T, Arens A, Schwipper V. One-stage reconstruction of nasal defects: evaluation of the use of modified auricular composite grafts. *Facial Plast Surg.* 2011;27(3):243–248.
42. Keck T, Lindemann J, Kuhnemann S, Sigg O. Healing of composite chondrocutaneous auricular grafts covered by skin flaps in nasal reconstructive surgery. *Laryngoscope.* 2003; 113(2):248–253.
43. Meade RJ. Composite ear grafts for construction of columella; composite ear grafts for the correction of nasal deformities associated with cleft lip and other congenital and post-traumatic deficiencies of the columella. *Plast Reconstr Surg Transplant Bull.* 1959;23(2):134–147.
44. Raghavan U, Jones NS. Use of the auricular composite graft in nasal reconstruction. *J Laryngol Otol.* 2001;115(11):885–893.
45. Ratner D, Katz A, Grande DJ. An interlocking auricular composite graft. *Dermatol Surg.* 1995;21(9):789–792.
46. Cummings CW, Flint PW, Haughey BH, et al., eds. Infections of the external ear. Chapter 137. *Otolaryngology: Head & Neck Surgery.* 5th ed. Philadelphia, PA: Mosby Elsevier; 2010.
47. Andreassi A, Bilenchi R, Biagioli M, D'Aniello C. Classification and pathophysiology of skin grafts. *Clin Dermatol.* 2005; 23(4):332–337.
48. Sage RJ, Leach BC, Cook J. Antihelical cartilage grafts for reconstruction of mohs micrographic surgery defects. *Dermatol Surg.* 2012;38(12):1930–1937.
49. Cervelli V, Spallone D, Bottini JD, et al. Alar batten cartilage graft: treatment of internal and external nasal valve collapse. *Aesthetic Plast Surg.* 2009;33(4):625–634.
50. Millman B. Alar batten grafting for management of the collapsed nasal valve. *Laryngoscope.* 2002;112(3):574–579.
51. Toriumi DM, Josen J, Weinberger M, Tardy ME Jr. Use of alar batten grafts for correction of nasal valve collapse. *Arch Otolaryngol Head Neck Surg.* 1997;123(8):802–808.
52. Byrd DR, Otley CC, Nguyen TH. Alar batten cartilage grafting in nasal reconstruction: functional and cosmetic results. *J Am Acad Dermatol.* 2000;43(5 Pt 1):833–836.
53. Ratner D, Skouge JW. Surgical pearl: the use of free cartilage grafts in nasal alar reconstruction. *J Am Acad Dermatol.* 1997;36(4):622–624.
54. Zopf DA, Iams W, Kim JC, Baker SR, Moyer JS. Full-thickness skin graft overlying a separately harvested auricular cartilage graft for nasal alar reconstruction. *JAMA Facial Plast Surg.* 2013;15(2):131–134.
55. Ibrahimi OA, Campbell T, Youker S, Eisen DB. Nonanatomic free cartilage batten grafting with second intention healing for defects on the distal nose. *J Drugs Dermatol.* 2012;11(1): 46–50.
56. van der Eerden PA, Verdam FJ, Dennis SC, Vuyk H. Free cartilage grafts and healing by secondary intention: a viable reconstructive combination after excision of nonmelanoma skin cancer in the nasal alar region. *Arch Facial Plast Surg.* 2009;11(1):18–23.
57. Marks MW, Argenta LC, Friedman RJ, Hall JD. Conchal cartilage and composite grafts for correction of lower lid retraction. *Plast Reconstr Surg.* 1989;83(4):629–635.
58. Matsuo K, Hirose T, Takahashi N, Iwasawa M, Satoh R. Lower eyelid reconstruction with a conchal cartilage graft. *Plast Reconstr Surg.* 1987;80(4):547–552.
59. Campbell RM, Perlis CS, Fisher E, Gloster HM Jr. Gentamicin ointment versus petrolatum for management of auricular wounds. *Dermatol Surg.* 2005;31(6):664–669.
60. Kaplan AL, Cook JL. The incidences of chondritis and perichondritis associated with the surgical manipulation of auricular cartilage. *Dermatol Surg.* 2004;30(1):58–62; discussion 62.
61. Anderson JJ, Wallin KJ, Spencer L. Split thickness skin grafts for the treatment of non-healing foot and leg ulcers in patients with diabetes: a retrospective review. *Diabet Foot Ankle.* 2012;3:1–7.
62. Ameer F, Singh AK, Kumar S. Evolution of instruments for harvest of the skin grafts. *Indian J Plast Surg.* 2013;46(1):28–35.
63. Snow SN, Stiff M, Lambert D, Tsoi C, Mohs FE. Freehand technique to harvest partial-thickness skin to repair superficial facial defects. *Dermatol Surg.* 1995;21(2):153–157.
64. Johnson T, Ratner D. Skin grafts. In: Ratz J, ed. *Textbook of Dermatologic Surgery.* Philadelphia, PA: Lippincott-Raven; 1998.
65. Quilichini J, Benjoar MD, Hivelin M, Lantieri L. Split-thickness skin graft harvested from the scalp for the coverage of extensive temple or forehead defects in elderly patients. *Arch Facial Plast Surg.* 2012;14(2):137–139.
66. Weyandt GH, Bauer B, Berens N, Hamm H, Broecker EB. Split-skin grafting from the scalp: the hidden advantage. *Dermatol Surg.* 2009;35(12):1873–1879.
67. Foroozan M, Pouaha J, Truchetet F. Simple method for harvesting split-thickness skin grafts. *Dermatol Surg.* 2010;36(11):1743–1745.
68. Housewright CD, Lenis A, Butler DF. Oscillating electric dermatome use for harvesting split-thickness skin grafts. *Dermatol Surg.* 2010;36(7):1179–1182.
69. Sterling JB, Skouge JW. Surgical glue to secure small split-thickness skin grafts: a cost-effective and time-saving technique. *Dermatol Surg.* 2008;34(2):246–247; discussion 247–248.
70. Karlsson M, Lindgren M, Jarnhed-Andersson I, Tarpila E. Dressing the split-thickness skin graft donor site: a randomized clinical trial. *Adv Skin Wound Care.* 2014;27(1):20–25.
71. Rakel BA, Bermel MA, Abbott LI, et al. Split-thickness skin graft donor site care: a quantitative synthesis of the research. *Appl Nurs Res.* 1998;11(4):174–182.

CHAPTER 21

Surgical Scar Revision

Lee M. Miller & Seaver L. Soon

INTRODUCTION

Scar formation is vital to the wound healing process. As surgeons, we spend much of our day creating wounds in the skin, and as a result, scarring is an inherent reality of surgical practice. Many patients may present with reconstructive challenges, resulting in scars that are cosmetically or functionally unsatisfactory to the patient, physician, or both. As such, a comprehensive understanding of scar revision and the various modalities by which scars may be managed is essential. While a plethora of techniques are available to improve both functional and cosmetic outcomes, this chapter focuses specifically on "cold steel" surgical scar revision techniques. With proper preoperative analysis of the scar and surrounding tissue, as well as skilled execution of an appropriately planned surgical revision, optimal results may be consistently attained.

PREVENTION

Proper planning and attention to detail during the initial reconstruction may obviate the need for scar revision in many cases. This goal is attained by adhering to basic principles of surgical reconstruction, specifically avoiding unnecessary trauma to the surrounding tissues, successfully accessing available tissue reservoirs, careful planning of reconstruction to camouflage incision lines along junctions of cosmetic subunits and within relaxed skin tension lines (RSTL), and flawless suturing technique with meticulous reapproximation, eversion, and avoidance of epidermal strangulation. When successful, reconstructive surgeons may achieve their goal of creating a scar that is nearly imperceptible. This scar is level with and similar in texture and color to the surrounding skin, is under minimal tension, follows underlying structural contours, aligns with RSTL or the junctions of cosmetic subunits, and is not straight, but favorably broken up to scatter reflected light. These features minimize any negative functional or aesthetic impact of the scar.

SCAR CLASSIFICATION

As wound repair and new collagen formation proceed, the aforementioned criteria may be compromised, and result in an unsatisfactory scar. There are four main ways in which this may occur, conveniently dividing scars into the following etiologic categories: (1) traumatic; (2) poor design; (3) poor healing; and (4) disease-related.[1] Table 21-1 summarizes scar characteristics, possible etiologies, and recommended approaches to revision.

TIMING

Once the decision is made to proceed with surgical scar revision, the surgeon should wait until the appropriate time to act. In general, scar revision should be deferred until the final phase of wound healing (6–12 months), when mature collagen makes up most of the scar bed.[2–6] In the meantime, patients should continue to practice good wound care and may begin massaging their scar 1 month postoperatively to minimize scar hypertrophy and contracture. A few exceptions exist to this general rule. First, scars perpendicular to RSTL or that cross the boundary between adjacent cosmetic subunits are obvious and often lead to deformity during animation. This deformity tends to worsen with time, and should therefore be corrected earlier to re-establish proper anatomic contours and margins.[2,3] Second, dermabrasion and debulking of hypertrophic flaps should be considered at 6 to 9 weeks due to the greater intrinsic fibroblastic activity during this time frame.[3,6] In contrast, when considering surgical revision in a child, the surgeon should wait as long as possible, as childhood scars are likely to improve substantially over time.[2]

OPTIMIZATION

To ensure the best result the surgeon must optimize the patient's healing ability, which includes assuring that the patient is receiving good nutrition, has discontinued medications that may adversely affect healing, avoiding surgery in heavily irradiated areas and controlling acute or chronic inflammatory skin conditions. Insufficient caloric intake or nutritional deficiencies in vitamin A, vitamin C, ferrous iron, and zinc may ultimately retard the skin's ability to heal by decreasing protein production, collagen synthesis, or impairing the immune system. Likewise, medications such as systemic corticosteroids, immunomodulators, and chemotherapy may alter healing either via a direct antimetabolic effect or by immune alteration. If possible, these medications should be withheld during the period of surgical scar revision. Tissues receiving greater than 50 Gy of radiation may display basilar fibrosis, dermal plexus obliteration, atrophy of the subcutaneous and surface epithelium, and loss of dermal appendages, all of which may adversely affect the healing potential of the skin. However, patients who have received less than 50 Gy of radiation and who are otherwise healthy may predictably

TABLE 21-1
Scar Abnormalities and Surgical Treatment Approaches [1,5]

Scar Abnormality	Etiology	Surgical Correction Techniques	Alternate Therapies
Elevated	Poor approximation of wound edges Excess wound tension Oversized grafts or flaps	Re-excision Shave excision Scalpel sculpting	Intralesional steroids Dermabrasion Laser resurfacing
Depressed	Deep shave biopsy Electrodesiccation/curettage Inadequate wound-edge eversion Prior hematoma or infection	Re-excision Subcision/ Subdermal undermining	Soft tissue augmentation Laser resurfacing
Hypertrophic scars/ Keloids	Excess inflammation (infection, foreign body reaction, etc.) Excess tension Genetic predisposition	Re-excision Shave excision scalpel sculpting	Intralesional immunomodulators Radiation Cryosurgery Lasers Compression therapy
Widened scars	Excess tension (inadequate undermining) Poor suturing technique	Re-excision	Lasers
Long straight scars	Laceration Poor surgical planning: Crossing RSTL or adjacent cosmetic subunits Distortion of free margins Long linear design Poor suturing technique (lack of eversion, inadequate approximation, etc.)	Z-plasty W-plasty Geometric broken line closure Repositioning	Dermabrasion
Contracted scars/ webbing	Traversing concavities	Z-plasty	Intralesional steroids
Free margin deviation	Poor surgical planning Proximity to free margins	Z-plasty V–Y advancement	Lasers
Icepick/Pitted scars	Prior acne Trauma	Punch excision	Punch grafting Dermal pocket grafting Dermabrasion
Boxcar scars	Prior acne Varicella	Punch excision Punch elevation	Lasers
Rolling scars	Prior acne	Subcision	Soft-tissue augmentation Lasers

undergo successful surgical scar revision.[2] Finally, avoiding unnecessary cutaneous inflammation assists in the healing process. For instance, if an area is actively infected, treatment with systemic antibiotics and delaying surgery for at least 6 weeks should allow for the inflammation to subside.[2] Patients with chronic inflammatory skin conditions may benefit substantially from appropriate medical therapy; for example, surgical candidates with active acneiform or eczematous eruptions should receive appropriate medical therapy to optimize the outcome of their scars. Finally, the importance of skin hygiene to minimize inflammation should be emphasized to patients. Taking the preceding factors into account while planning for surgical scar revision will increase the likelihood of superior patient outcomes.

EXCISIONAL TECHNIQUES

RE-EXCISION

Perhaps the simplest form of scar revision is to remove the abnormal scar in its entirety. This is accomplished by excising the existing scar with narrow margins and carefully reapproximating each layer of the normal surrounding tissues with attention paid to wound-edge eversion and tension. Re-excision of scars is particularly useful for relatively small irregular or hypertrophic linear scars that are aligned within 30 degrees of the surrounding RSTL.[1,2] Buried vertical mattress sutures will help achieve adequate wound-edge eversion (Fig. 21-1). As with any standard

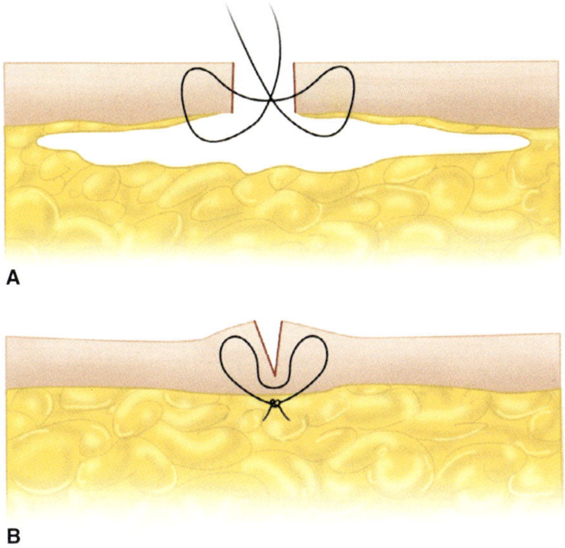

Figure 21-1 Buried vertical mattress suture. **A.** The suture is placed such that the free ends exit the dermis on the undermined surface of the wound. **B.** Once tied, this suture technique promotes wound-edge eversion.

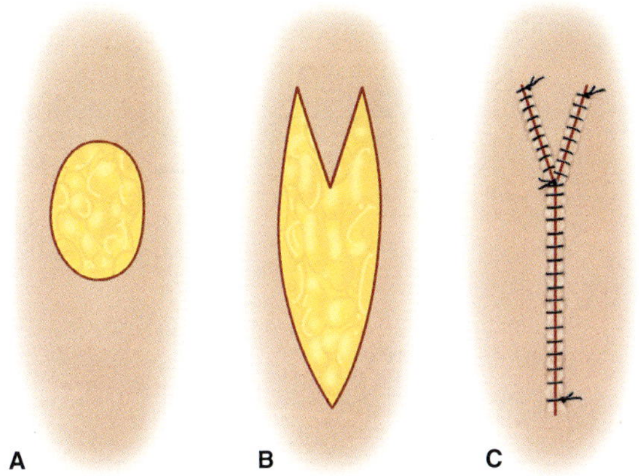

Figure 21-2 M-Plasty. **A.** The M-Plasty is a useful technique that shortens the length of the incision. The traditional 30 degree apex inferiorly and the tip are inverted for the M-plasty at the superior tip. **B.** The excess tissue is excised, revealing an "M-shaped" wound at the superior apex. **C.** The wound edges are reapproximated and sutured in place.

lentiform excision, the angles of the apices of the excised tissue should not exceed 30 degrees to avoid standing cone deformities. If the angle of the apex exceeds 30 degrees and there is insufficient tissue to lengthen the scar, one may consider M-plasty revision (Fig. 21-2). Although re-excision may be effective, patients should be informed that the re-excised scar will be longer than the original (Fig. 21-3A,B).

Surgical incisions under tension or in areas of high mobility, particularly on the trunk and proximal extremities, often spread over time, resulting in a wide, depressed scar. These scars are amenable to re-excision; however, to avoid a similar problem in the future, one may consider leaving a plate of scar tissue behind to serve not only as a base onto which deep tissues may be anchored, but also to add bulk to fill the depressed area of the scar. This may be accomplished using either bilateral or unilateral tissue mobilization resembling a tongue in groove structure (Fig. 21-4A,B). In either case, the scar is first de-epithelialized. In the unilateral mobilization technique (Fig. 21-4A), a full-thickness incision is made along only one side of the de-epithelialized scar tissue. The skin is then undermined in one direction, away from the bed of scar tissue. The resultant flap edge is then thinned to match the depth and width of the bed of scar tissue. The thinned skin edge is then advanced over the bed of scar tissue and the deep portion of the skin edge is anchored to the scar tissue while the two skin edges are reapproximated

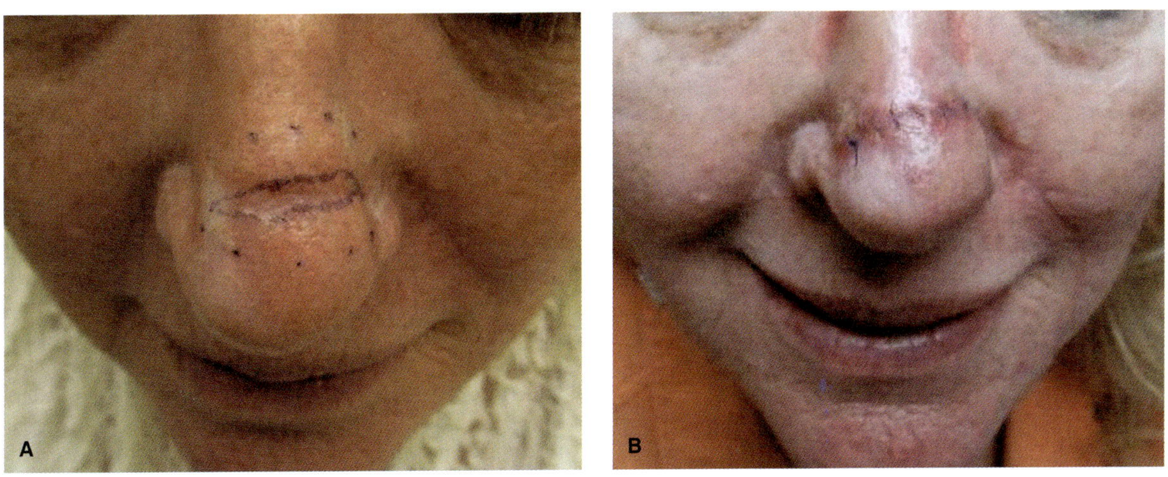

Figure 21-3 Re-excision. **A.** Depressed scar of the nasal supra-tip. Dotted outline shows planned area of undermining to sufficiently mobilize tissue. **B.** Re-excision results in a longer scar and a more aesthetic contour of the nasal tip. (Photos reprinted by permission of Nicole M. Annest, MD, MS.)

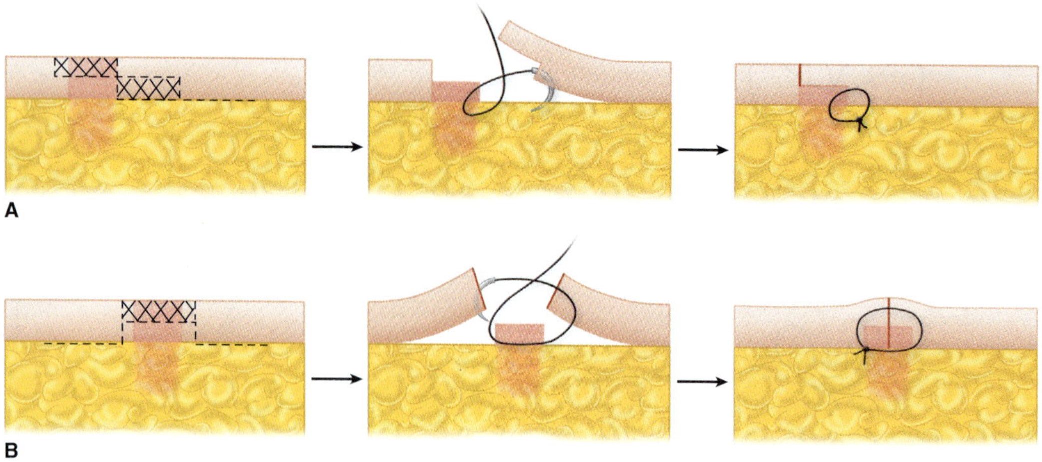

Figure 21-4 Re-excision with anchoring to scar tissue for revision of depressed scars. **A.** Unilateral technique: a full-thickness incision is made on one side of the scar and flap is undermined unilaterally. The scar is deepithelialized and the underside of the flap is thinned to match (crosshatched areas are removed). The deep suture is then placed from the deepithelialized scar to the corresponding location on the deep surface of the flap. This deep suture buries the tension, anchoring the flap and allowing for fine reapproximation of the epidermal edges. **B.** Bilateral technique: full-thickness incisions are made on either side of the scar and both sides are undermined. Area undermined should be at least twice the width of the defect or scar. The scar is deepithelialized by removing its top portion (crosshatched). The two sides are anchored to the bed of scar tissue using a buried vertical mattress suture placed through the scar tissue. The scar may be variably thinned depending on the need for bulk.

with a subcuticular suture to avoid suture marks.[2,7] For the bilateral mobilization technique (Fig. 21-4B), the scar is de-epithelialized in a similar fashion. A full-thickness incision is then made along both sides of the bed of scar tissue. The skin edges are undermined bilaterally, advanced, and anchored to the bed of scar tissue. The mobilized skin overlying the scar tissue may or may not need to be thinned, depending on the amount of tissue needed to correct the depressed component of the scar. Temporary fullness may develop, although it generally flattens with pressure and time.[2]

Several surgical pearls may be helpful in context where re-excision may be appropriate. For example, to reduce tension on the revised surgical incision, the wound margins should generally be undermined to a distance at least twice the width of the scar and the subsequent defect (Fig. 21-4B). For cases in which the defect will close, but is under some tension, a slight "S" shape or wavy ellipse will close more easily with a smaller standing tissue cone deformity.[2] In order to maintain the curvature of the S-shaped excision, it is helpful to suture from the ends first, working toward the middle to avoid sewing out the curvature, as would occur by using the rule of halves. Re-excision and repositioning is useful for scars aligned parallel to a distinct RSTL or near the boundary between cosmetic subunits, and consists of excising normal tissue between the scar and the desired location of scar placement within the RSTL or at the junction between cosmetic subunits. The surgeon can use this technique to move scars to areas that camouflage the scar, such as the hairline, nasolabial fold, preauricular crease, glabellar crease, or forehead rhytides.[3]

TISSUE EXPANSION

When there is insufficient surrounding tissue to excise and close the deformity in one session, a staged excision technique or use of a tissue expander may be considered.[5] Tissue expanders consist of a high-grade silicone bag with a reinforced backplate, and may have an injection port within the wall, or a remote injection port connected via a silicone tube. These devices are implanted in the skin adjacent to the area to be excised and slowly filled to gradually expand the normal surrounding tissues, taking advantage of the viscoelastic properties of the skin. In areas where tissue mobility is limited and excellent tissue match is important, such as the scalp, a tissue expander may expand the adjacent tissue reservoir to provide perfect tissue texture and color match.

Tissue expanders offer the ability to predictably repair large defects with excellent match of tissue color and texture by increasing the available reservoir of surrounding normal tissues. However, their use is fraught with unique disadvantages, including the need for multiple stages and frequent visits for reinjection. Patients also experience progressive deformity during expansion. Each injection may be accompanied by discomfort. Typically this is minimal and limited to the first 24 to 48 hours following injection.[8] Finally, as with any surgery, tissue expanders may be subject to such complications as infection, hematoma, pressure-induced necrosis, wound dehiscence, and exposure or perforation of the implant.

During consultation, the area to be removed should be measured and the tissue expander should be sized to

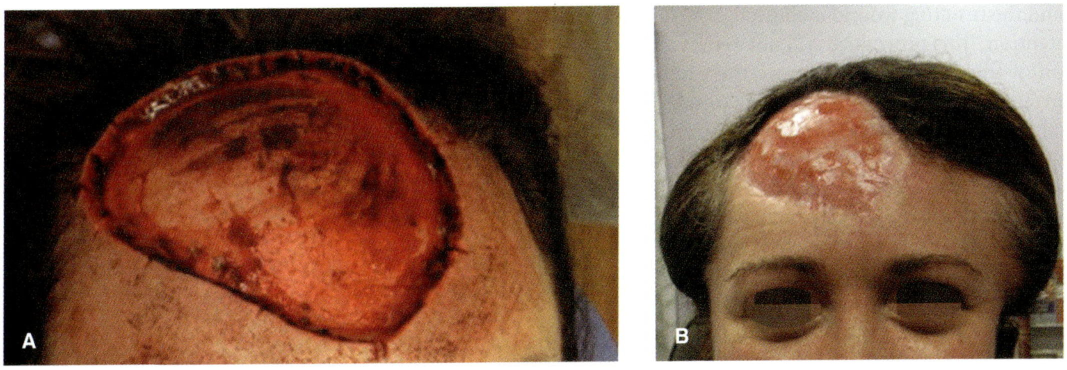

Figure 21-5 Tissue expander. **A.** Large surgical defect following Mohs excision of a dermatofibrosarcoma protuberans. **B.** Tissue expanders inserted bilaterally adjacent to the surgical wound and volumized such that the apical circumference is two to three times the width of the defect. (Photos reprinted by permission of Rachael L. Moore, MD.)

match. The expander should be capable of holding enough volume to reach an apical circumference two to three times the width of the planned defect to allow sufficient tissue to cover the defect and the donor area (Fig. 21-5A,B).[8] The device is implanted and filled minimally with sterile saline. Once the wound has healed sufficiently, the device is slowly expanded by injecting sterile saline on a weekly basis (frequency may range from 3 to 10 days depending on location and tolerability). The volume injected at each visit will depend on the overlying skin tension, wound strength, and patient discomfort. If the overlying skin blanches following injection, some saline should be withdrawn to avoid ischemic necrosis and subsequent exposure of the tissue expander, which is the most common complication.[8] As the dermis expands, neovascularization occurs around the device, resulting in a bluish discoloration that resolves following final reconstruction. Once an apical circumference two to three times the defect width is reached, the surgeon drains the saline, removes the tissue expander, and performs the final reconstruction, which may consist of a primary closure, broad-based rotation, advancement, or "jigsaw puzzle" design. During the process of tissue expansion, a capsule forms around the device, and should be left intact whenever possible as it improves the blood supply and viability of the flap, and provides a strong foundation to hold buried sutures.

KELOIDS

In those patients prone to hypertrophic or keloid scarring, one must proceed with caution. Although adjuvant treatments such as intralesional steroids, topical imiquimod, or postoperative radiotherapy may minimize an exuberant scarring response, this process may recur and result in a similar or possibly worse outcome. Excisional techniques should be avoided when dealing with keloid scars in high-tension areas. Persistent sources of inflammation should be removed as these may promote exuberant scarring.

SCULPTING

SHAVE AND FEATHERING TECHNIQUES.

A shave excision may address elevated or pedunculated scars, using a flexible razor blade or a #15 blade to shave the elevated portion of the scar level with the surrounding

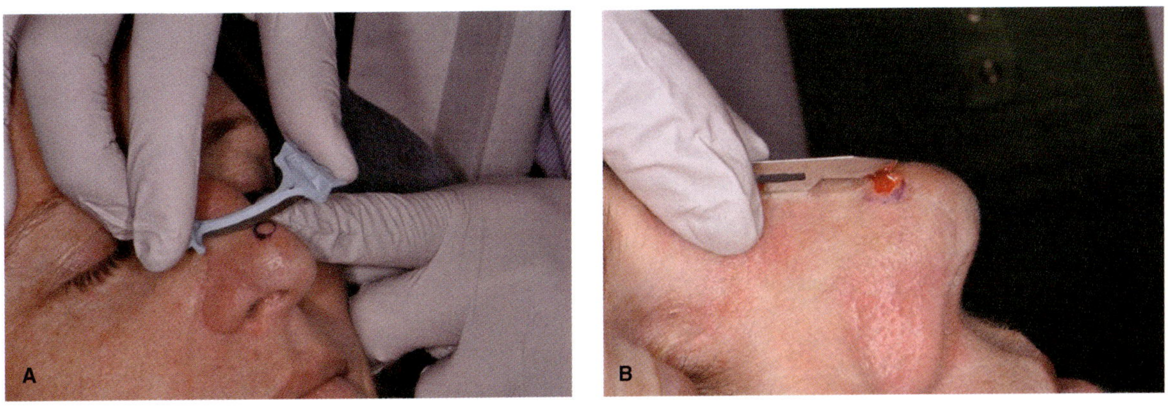

Figure 21-6 **A.** Exophytic component of transposition flap scar shaved flush with adjacent skin using a flexible blade. **B.** Feathering the wound with a #15 scalpel blade applied perpendicular to the skin surface minimizes the line of demarcation. (Photos reprinted by permission of Seaver L. Soon, MD.)

skin, and the resulting wound is allowed to heal by secondary intention. This procedure will not remove the deeper portion of the scar, but will remove the exophytic component and its associated shadowing, resulting in substantial benefit in properly selected situations. The deep portion may be excised later if necessary. Dermabrasion may also be considered for such cases, but often entails longer set-up times and relative biohazards.[9] For irregular scars with a depressed component, the proper sculpting plane is determined by selecting the skin height midway between the plane of the surrounding skin and the lowest plane of the abnormality, in an effort to remove the elevated portions and create a homogeneous plane that blends into the surrounding skin. Once the bulk of a scar is removed and is level with the surrounding tissue, the edges can be feathered to blend the scar by scraping a #15 blade perpendicularly across the skin's surface to remove the epidermis to the level of the superficial papillary dermis, with the clinical endpoint being pinpoint bleeding (Fig. 21-6A,B).[9]

The surgeon must exercise caution when considering scalpel sculpting or feathering in abnormal skin, such as that subjected to prior radiation therapy or steroid therapy, or skin with extensive sun damage or atrophy. In general, shave and feathering techniques are useful for correcting discrepancies in contour, but will do little for other scar abnormalities. In addition, one must refrain from excessively deep sculpting to avoid surpassing the regenerative properties of the scar tissue, which may be limited.[9]

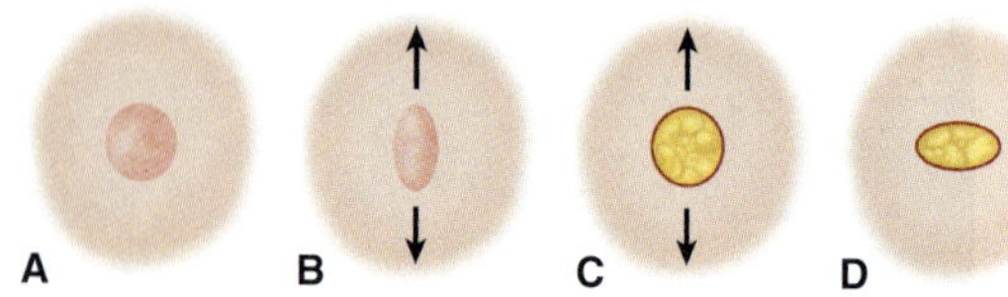

Figure 21-7 Punch excision technique. **A.** Small circular scar. **B.** Constant tension is applied perpendicular to the relaxed skin tension lines with the nondominant hand. **C.** The scar is removed via a punch excision. **D.** As tension is relieved, the defect is found to be oriented parallel to the relaxed skin tension lines.

PUNCH TECHNIQUES

PUNCH EXCISION AND ELEVATION

For small boxcar or ice-pick scars, a punch excision may be considered. In this case, a small punch is used to remove the entire scar. If tension is applied perpendicular to the RSTL while the lesion is excised, the result is an elliptical defect oriented parallel to the RSTL, which will facilitate closure (Fig. 21-7A–C). Another option for treatment of depressed or boxcar scars is the punch elevation. In this procedure, the punch is sized to match the diameter of the deepest portion of the scar. The deepest portion is then incised, lifted slightly with forceps, and fixed in place with medical grade skin adhesive.[1]

DERMAL POCKET GRAFTING

Dermal pocket grafting may be used to correct depressed rolling or boxcar acne scars, as well as deep rhytides, using postauricular dermal donor tissue. In this technique, the desired site of correction should be undermined approximately 10 to 14 days before. At the time of the procedure, the donor site is first dermabraded to de-epithelialize the tissue. The dermal tissue is then harvested as punches or strips. The autologous dermal grafts are placed into dermal or subdermal pockets in the desired location to assist in elevating the depressed tissue. Advantages to this technique include reliability, long-lasting effect, and the ability to tailor the tissue for a precise correction.[5]

SUBCISION

Subcision is a useful technique for depressed scars, particularly of the rolling type, as seen in acne scars. The area is anesthetized locally and an 18 gauge needle or other suitable blade is inserted into the superficial subcutaneous

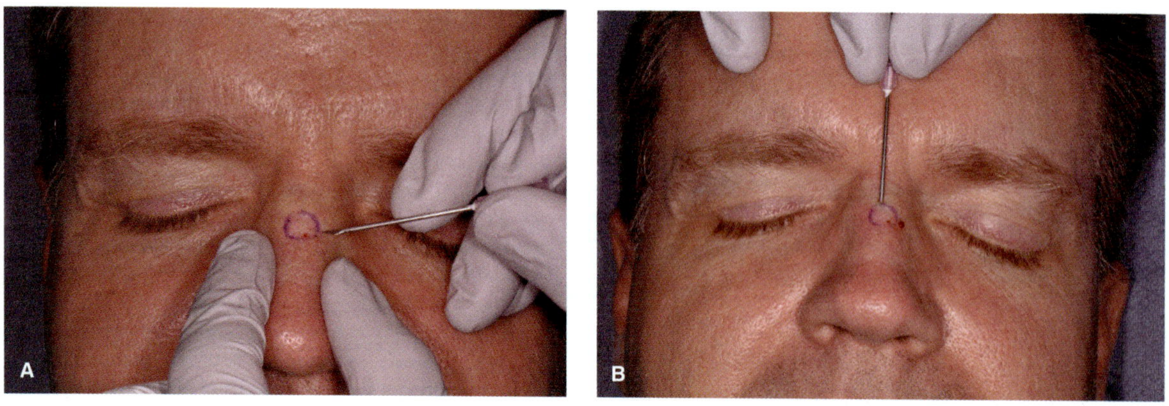

Figure 21-8 **A.** An 18 gauge subcision needle is used to subcise a depressed scar on the nasal dorsum from a deep shave biopsy. **B.** Fanning subcision in multiple directions allows for adequate tissue separation of the depressed scar from the underlying dermis. (Photos reprinted by permission of Seaver L. Soon, MD.)

tissue at a shallow angle. The needle or blade is then fanned out as it is advanced and retracted. The tissue is stabilized with the opposite hand, while the underlying fibrous adhesions are released (Fig. 21-8A,B).

SCAR IRREGULARIZATION

Noticeable scars often disturb the normal facial contours, resulting in an undesirable appearance. Scars that are long and straight often cross adjacent cosmetic subunits, distort anatomic relationships, or cause webbing. In such situations, one must devise a plan to break up or irregularize the scar in an effort to make the defect less noticeable. These irregularization techniques may be followed by adjunctive scar treatment techniques such as fractionated laser or dermabrasion to optimize the final result.[5] It must be noted that while these procedures have the potential to improve the final outcome, they are time consuming and if not precisely executed, may worsen a scar's appearance.

Z-PLASTY

Although conceptually difficult, the Z-plasty may be considered a workhorse of surgical revision for contracted or misoriented scars. Scar contracture places tension on adjacent tissue, and results in either webbing across tissue concavities or in sites of free margin deviation. Incisions are sometimes placed unfavorably across RSTL due to other concerns at the time of reconstruction. As mentioned previously, scars less than 30 degrees from the RSTL may be re-excised. However, when scars cross RSTL at angles greater than 30 degrees simple re-excision is no longer feasible.[10] The Z-plasty offers the ability to easily reorient such scars. In addition, the Z-plasty results in a relative recruitment of tissue laterally, culminating in lengthening along the original axis of the scar and removing tension on adjacent tissue concavities and free margins (Figs. 21-9A–C and 21-10A,B). Many cosmetic and/or functional deformities from suboptimal scars may be ameliorated by reorientation, lengthening, or creating irregular scar lines, which may all be accomplished with a Z-plasty.

To perform the Z-plasty, the original healed incision line is marked. The central limb of the Z-plasty is placed within or parallel to the long axis of the scar. Alternatively, the scar may be excised with narrow margins with the new fusiform defect serving as the central incision of the Z-plasty.[11] Two parallel limbs are then drawn, each originating from opposite ends of the original incision. For any given Z-plasty, there are two ways in which the limbs may be oriented. Generally one of the arrangements will blend more naturally into the RSTL, which results in a less noticeable scar (Fig. 21-11A). To conceptualize the approximate final orientation, one may simply leave the orientation of the limbs unchanged and

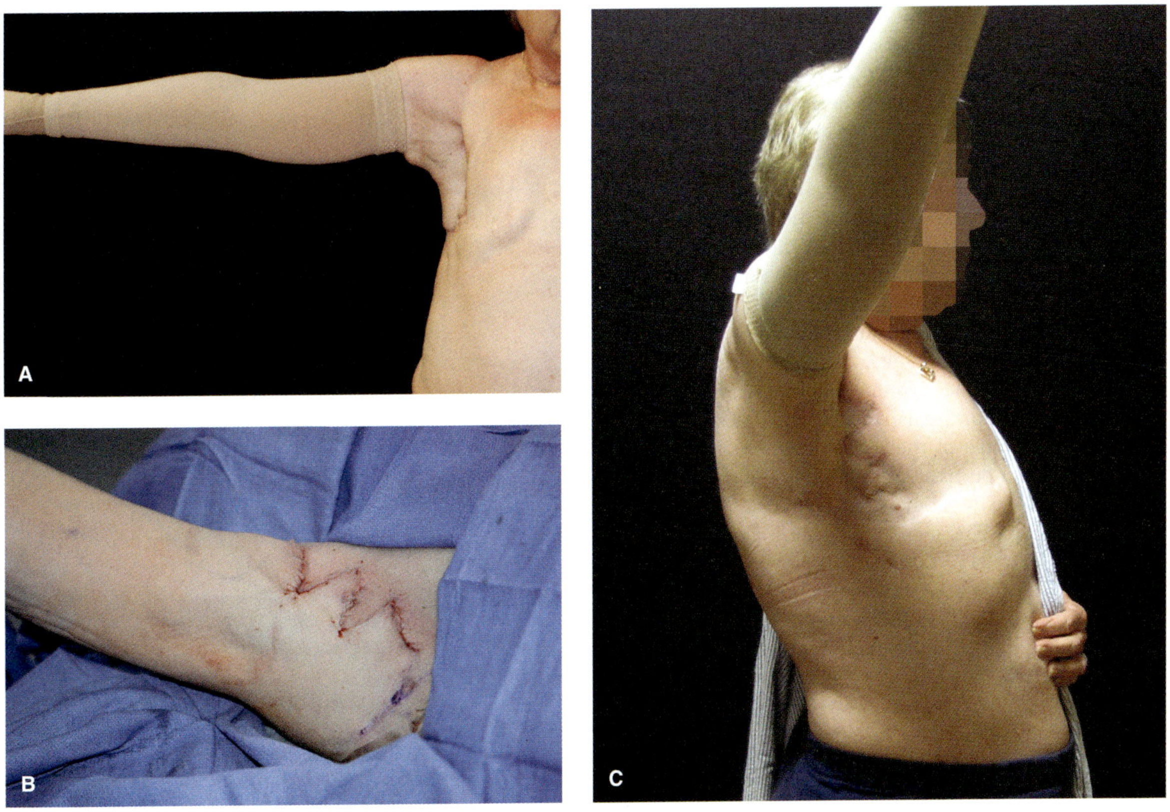

Figure 21-9 Z-plasty. **A.** Scar contracture following right mastectomy and axillary lymph node dissection results in decreased maximal abduction of the right arm. **B.** Serial Z-plasty revision oriented to lengthen the long axis of the axillary scar contracture. **C.** Successful lengthening of the axillary scar via serial Z-plasty revision results in a substantial increase in range of motion. (Photos reprinted by permission of Jyoti Arya, MD.)

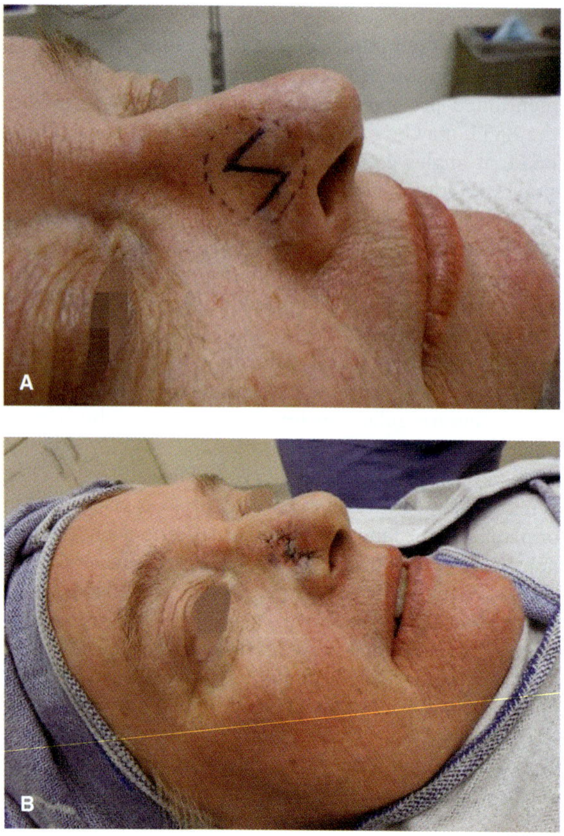

Figure 21-10 Z-plasty to correct alar elevation. **A.** Postoperative elevation of the right alar rim, with Z-plasty revision designed to depress the free margin by lengthening the longitudinal axis of the scar. **B.** Following Z-plasty revision, right alar margin assumes a more anatomic position. (Photos reprinted by permission of Nicole M. Annest, MD.)

connect the free tips of the two limbs with a new imaginary central incision (Fig. 21-11B).[11] Once the appropriate "Z" is determined, incisions are placed along these lines. The two triangular flaps and surrounding skin are undermined and elevated. As tension is applied to the tips of the "Z," the triangular flaps are transposed and sutured into position (Fig. 21-11C–E). To optimize results, the triangles must be completely released and the surrounding tissues must be widely undermined to maximize flap movement.

Varying the angle of the diagonal limbs of the Z has substantial effect on tissue recruitment and the degree of lengthening along the original axis. Classically a 60 degree angle results in a 75% increase in length along the original axis (Fig. 21-11F). As the angle between the diagonal limbs and the original axis becomes more acute, less lateral tissue is recruited, such that a 45 degree angle results in a 50% increase in length and a 30 degree angle results in a 25% increase in length along the original axis.[11] These calculations are based upon theoretical and mathematical models; the actual gain in length in vivo is less than these theoretical gains due to tissue elasticity.[10] Variations of the Z-plasty, including the double-opposing Z-plasty, the unequal triangle Z-plasty, the four-flap Z-plasty, the planimetric Z-plasty, and the compound Z-plasty provide distinct advantages. For longer linear scars, the compound Z-plasty is useful, as the larger flaps of a single Z-plasty

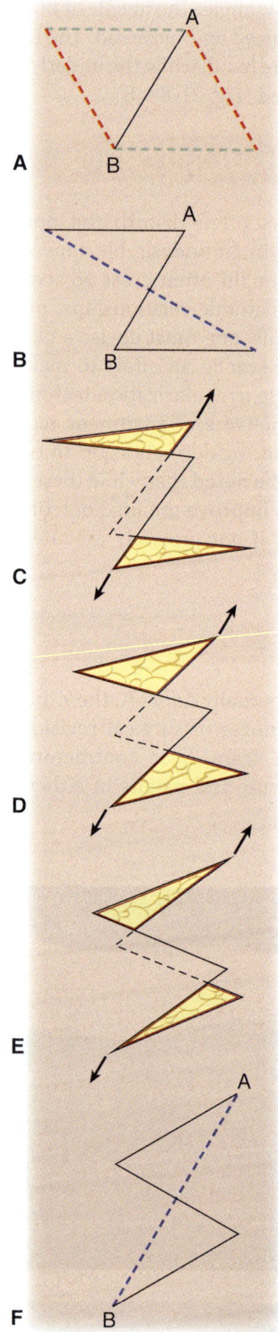

Figure 21-11 Classic 60 degree Z-plasty. **A.** For any scar running from A to B, there are two orientations in which any Z-plasty may be planned. Orienting the two limbs parallel to the RSTL is desirable (*green*). **B.** The two limbs are drawn at a 60 degree angle with respect to the central limb and with the same length as the central limb. Although not geometrically accurate, one can visualize the approximate orientation of the final outcome by connecting the free ends of the two limbs with an imaginary new central limb (*blue line*). **C–E.** The Z is incised, undermined, and the two flaps are elevated. As gentle tension is applied to the ends of the original scar, the two flaps are transposed, fall into place naturally, and the original scar (**A–B**) is lengthened. **F.** The flaps are sutured into place, and the final outcome of a classic 60 degree Z-plasty results in a 75% increase in the distance from **A** to **B** (the original scar axis) while reorienting the central limb of the Z.

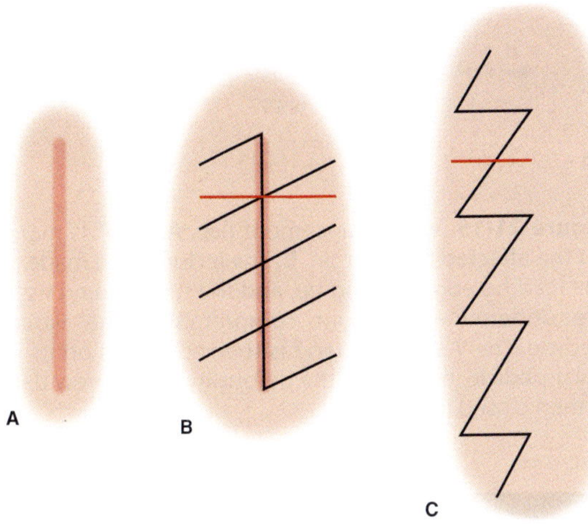

Figure 21-12 Multiple Z-plasty. **A.** Original scar. **B.** Multiple Z-plasties marked. Red line isolates one Z-plasty for demonstration purposes. **C.** The flaps are transposed and sutured into place. Increase of 75% in the original axis length.

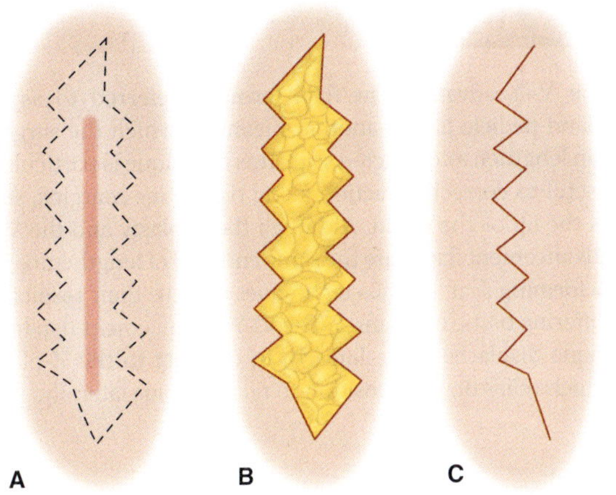

Figure 21-13 W-plasty. **A.** A pattern of 5 to 8 mm interlocking "Ws" is marked on either side of the scar. Care must be taken not to exceed 30 degrees at the apices in order to avoid tissue redundancy. **B.** The scar with its pattern of "Ws" is excised. **C.** The interlocking patterns are sutured into place.

may result in additional distortion of surrounding cosmetic subunits. In this technique, the scar is divided into segments and multiple smaller Z-plasties are linked together along the length of the scar (Fig. 21-12A–C). Hove et al.[11] published an excellent review of Z-plasty techniques that details the benefits of the variations listed earlier.

W-PLASTY

Both the W-plasty and the Geometric Broken Line Closure (GBLC) rely on the principle that an irregular line is less visible than a straight line. The W-plasty is a useful technique to break up a long, linear scar with relatively consistent width that may cross RSTL. This technique is particularly well-suited to assist in camouflaging those scars on convex surfaces.[2] To perform a W-plasty, the original scar is narrowly excised with a pattern of interlocking "Ws" on each side (Fig. 21-13A–C). Ideally, half of the limbs should be aligned with the RSTL. In addition, the limbs should be approximately 5 to 8 mm in length with angles of 60 to 90 degrees to allow for adequate tissue interposition, optimal vascularity with minimal tip edema, and crosslinking of healed tissues to resist tension and contracture.[2] Deep sutures should principally be used to avoid tip ischemia and venous congestion. Tissue tapes may be helpful for up to 6 weeks.[2] In contrast to the transposition component characteristic of the compound Z-plasty, the W-plasty is composed of interposition flaps. Thus, there is no added length or decrease in wound tension as observed in a compound Z-plasty. In fact, this procedure will increase tension slightly as a small amount of normal tissue is excised from either side of the wound, which must be considered in areas with minimal tissue laxity.

GEOMETRIC BROKEN LINE CLOSURE

The GBLC is a variant of the W-plasty more suited to long, irregular scars, as the regular zigzag pattern of the W-plasty may become more noticeable as scar length increases.[2,10] Rather than interlocking "Ws," GBLC is composed of a random pattern of interlocking geometric shapes (triangles, squares, and semicircles) on each side of the scar (Fig. 21-14A–C). Each excised geometric shape should range from 3 to 7 mm in size and may extend 3 to 6 mm from the margin of the wound.[1] While technically more difficult, the GBLC is thought to have enhanced ability to camouflage the scar, particularly in cases where the scar crosses the RSTL at angles greater than 30 degrees. Apex angles less than 30 degrees (Fig. 21-13A) and wide undermining are necessary for optimum cosmetic result with both the W-plasty and the GBLC.

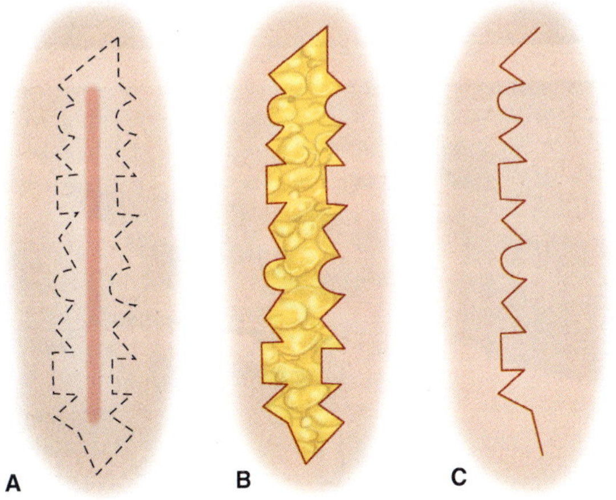

Figure 21-14 Geometric broken line closure (GBLC). **A.** A pattern of randomly arranged interlocking geometric shapes ranging from 3 to 7 mm in size is marked on either side of the scar. **B.** The scar and pattern on either side are excised. **C.** The two patterns are interposed and sutured into place.

V–Y ADVANCEMENT FLAP

The V–Y advancement flap, formerly referred to as the island pedicle flap, is another means by which the surgeon can lengthen a contracted scar. This technique is particularly useful to correct retraction along tissue-free margins, such as the lip or the eyelid. Although the Z-plasty and the V–Y advancement flap share the same end goal of lengthening the deforming scar, the two techniques achieve their results via differing tissue mechanics. The V–Y advancement flap technique displaces tissue linearly, in contrast to the Z-plasty, which relies on transposition to recruit tissue laterally.

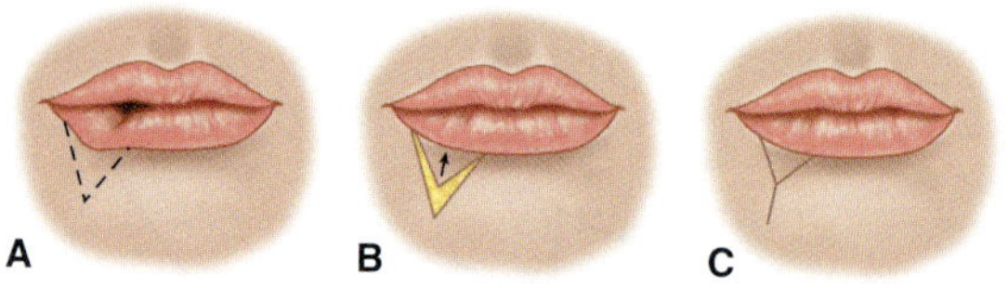

Figure 21-15 V–Y advancement flap. **A.** A "V" is marked on the affected free margin. **B.** The incisions are made and the leading edge, trailing tip, and the surrounding tissues are undermined without compromising the vascular pedicle. The V-shaped island is then advanced on its vascular pedicle, correcting the deformity. **C.** The new defect is then closed linearly.

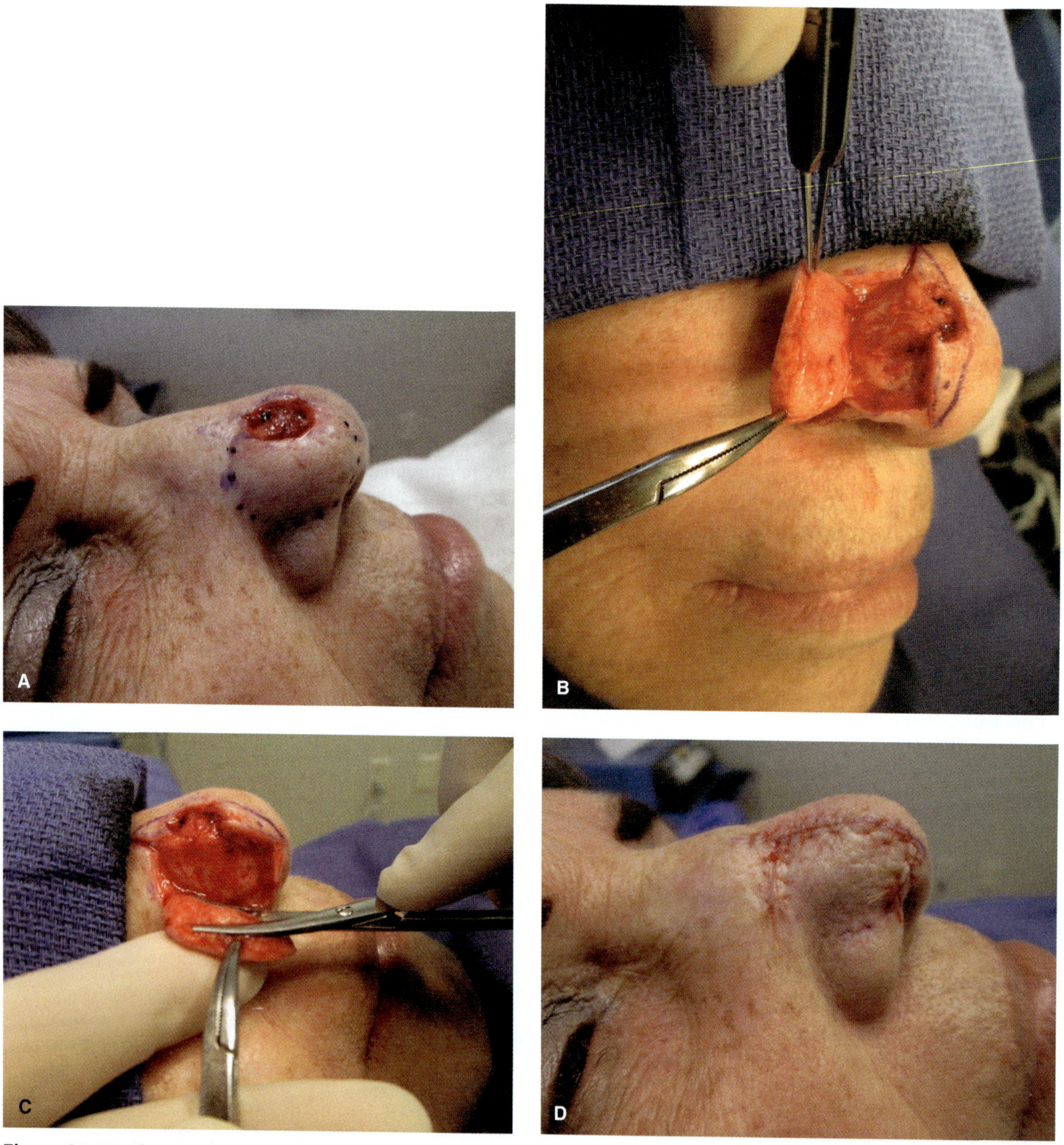

Figure 21-16 Flap revision. **A.** Bulky, protuberant scar following paramedian forehead flap repair on the right nasal tip. **B.** Bulky flap is incised along the previous scar line and reflected to expose excess fibrofatty tissue. **C.** Excess fibrofatty tissue is excised to allow for a more anatomic contour. **D.** The flap is reset and sutured in place. (Photos reprinted by permission of Seaver L. Soon, MD.)

To perform this technique, a V-shaped incision is placed, and the surrounding tissues are undermined widely. The skin edges of the flap may then be undermined with care so as to avoid compromising the vascular supply from the base. The V is then displaced along its central axis, and the newly created defect from the displaced tip of the V is closed in a linear fashion (Fig. 21-15A–C). This technique is generally restricted to smaller corrections, as movement is limited by the deep tissues that provide the vascular supply to the tissue being advanced.[4] This technique may also be reversed to shorten the length of a scar as the Y-V advancement flap.[12]

FLAP REFINEMENT

FLAP HYPERTROPHY/TRAPDOOR DEFORMITY

The trapdoor deformity is a relatively common complication that tends to occur in rounded flaps on noses characterized by highly sebaceous skin. The trapdoor effect can be minimized by proper sizing of the flap, wide undermining, squaring the edges of the defect, and meticulous surgical technique.[4,12] Despite these precautions, trapdoor deformity may still occur and must be corrected to achieve the optimal cosmetic outcome.

If the flap is mildly hypertrophic and the incision scar blends into the surrounding tissue, intralesional corticosteroid injections may provide improvement. However, for cases of moderate-to-severe hypertrophy or for those with flap hypertrophy and a recessed incision scar, surgical correction may be indicated.[12]

After the area is anesthetized, a portion of the flap is reincised. If the original incision is depressed or retracted, the scar may be excised narrowly, leaving precise, squared-off edges. The entire incision need not be reincised, only that part of it which is necessary to gain access to the hypertrophied area. Generally the surgeon should choose the most uneven, raised, or spread section of the incision that provides the necessary exposure.[4] The flap is then reflected to gain access to the area of hypertrophy, and both the flap and/or the wound base can be debulked

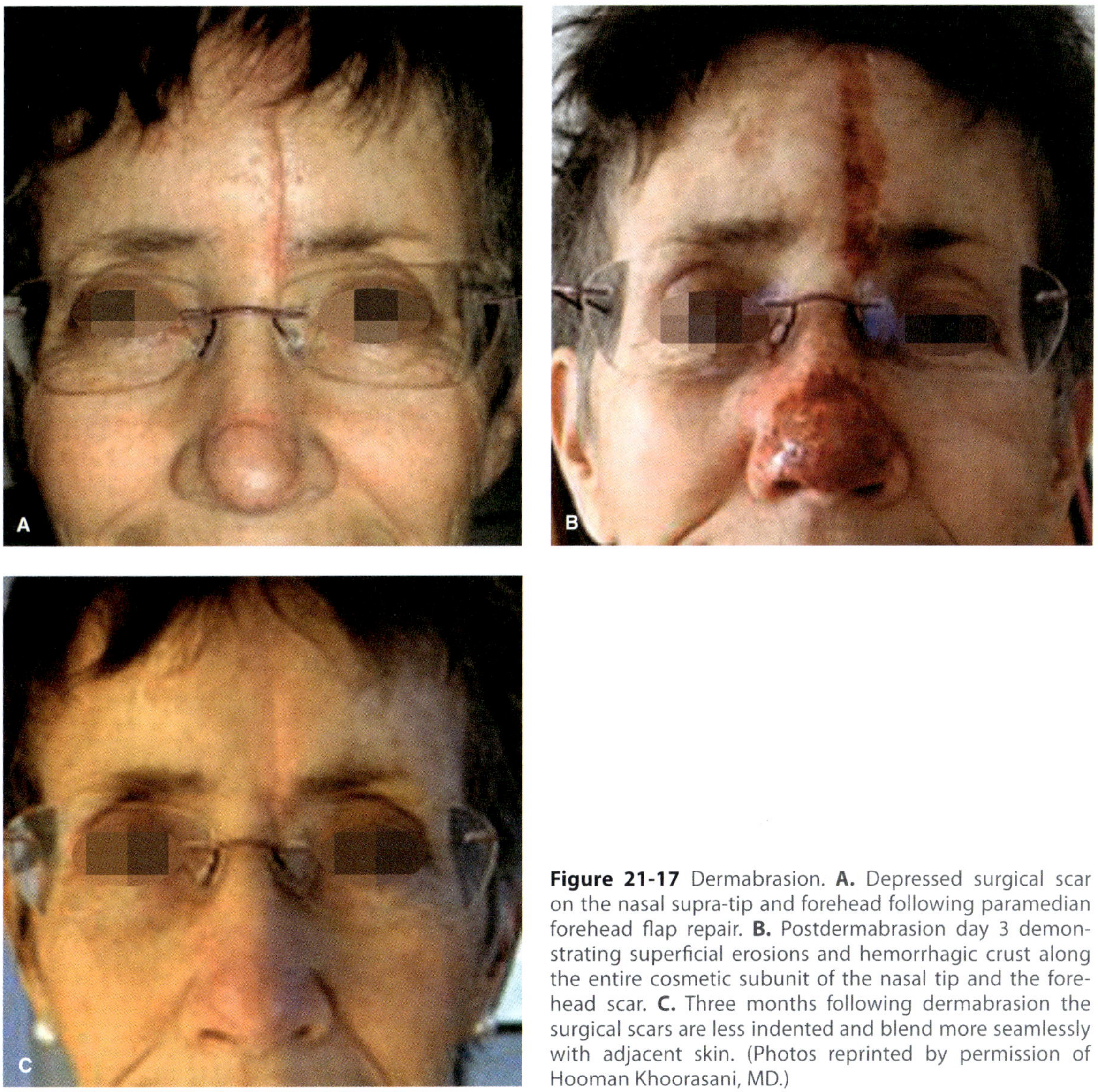

Figure 21-17 Dermabrasion. **A.** Depressed surgical scar on the nasal supra-tip and forehead following paramedian forehead flap repair. **B.** Postdermabrasion day 3 demonstrating superficial erosions and hemorrhagic crust along the entire cosmetic subunit of the nasal tip and the forehead scar. **C.** Three months following dermabrasion the surgical scars are less indented and blend more seamlessly with adjacent skin. (Photos reprinted by permission of Hooman Khoorasani, MD.)

of excess fibrofatty tissue. The goal is to remove a uniform disc of excess tissue, flattening the flap and correcting the deformity. The newly thinned flap may require additional trimming of redundant skin from the edges to precisely fit the defect, and is then sutured into place (Fig. 21-16A–D).

POSTOPERATIVE CARE

Following surgical scar revision, proper wound care will optimize outcomes. The area should be kept well-hydrated with topical emollients. Regular sunscreen use may prevent postinflammatory hyperpigmentation. Massage is encouraged after approximately 1 month to aid collagen fiber realignment and to prevent adhesions to deeper structures.[3,10] Following repair, surface taping at bedtime for 3 to 6 months, may help to smooth scar lines.

ADJUVANT TREATMENT

Following surgical scar revision, subtle irregularities may remain. These may be amenable to a variety of adjuvant techniques such as dermabrasion, chemical peels, and laser resurfacing as described elsewhere in this text (Fig. 21-17A–C). Most adjuvant techniques should be performed approximately 4 to 12 weeks following the surgical revision.[2,6] Although cumbersome for the patient, silicone sheeting on a daily basis for 2 to 6 months promotes fibroblast modification through wound hydration and may help improve color, texture, thickness, and size.[6,13] Patient education and individualization of their postoperative wound care regimen based on their ability and competence will ensure consistent compliance.

CONCLUSION

There are a variety of "cold steel" surgical techniques that may be useful in revising unsatisfactory scars. A working knowledge of these techniques is essential to obtain the best aesthetic and functional results for our patients. Although much of the end result relies on our skill as surgeons, it is important to keep patients' expectations in mind. Patients should be counseled prior to any attempt at revision that a scar can never be completely removed, but rather modified to achieve a more aesthetic and functional result. Although any scar with suboptimal appearance can be revised, the greatest satisfaction is achieved in those patients with realistic expectations. Therefore it is critical to be honest with patients regarding the level of possible improvement. With thorough planning and meticulous execution, we can improve many of the unacceptable scars encountered in surgical practice, thereby positively influencing our patients' quality of life.

REFERENCES

1. Batra RS. Surgical techniques for scar revision. *Skin Therapy Lett.* 2005;10(4):4–7.
2. Horswell BB. Scar modification: techniques for revision and camouflage. *Atlas Oral Maxillofac Surg Clin North Am.* 1998; 6(2):55–72.
3. Thomas JR, Prendiville S. Update in scar revision. *Facial Plast Surg Clin North Am.* 2002;10(1):103–111.
4. Lee KK, Mehrany K, Swanson NA. Surgical revision. *Dermatol Clin.* 2005;23(1):141–150.
5. Kaplan B, Potter T, Moy RL. Scar revision. *Dermatol Surg.* 1997;23:435–442.
6. Brenner MJ, Perro CA. Recontouring, resurfacing, and scar revision in skin cancer reconstruction. *Facial Plast Surg Clin North Am.* 2009;17:469–487.
7. Wilson AL. Widening of scars: foe coaxed into a friend? The Millard technique revisited. *Plast Reconstr Surg.* 2000;106(7): 1488–1493.
8. Roenigk RK, Wheeland RG. Tissue expansion in dermatologic surgery. *Dermatol Clin.* 1987;5(2):429–436.
9. Snow SN, Stiff MA, Lambert DR. Scalpel sculpturing techniques for graft revision and dermatologic surgery. *J Dermatol Surg Oncol.* 1994;20:120–126.
10. Shockley WW. Scar revision techniques: z-plasty, w-plasty, and geometric broken line closure. *Facial Plast Surg Clin North Am.* 2011;19(3):455–463.
11. Hove CR, Williams EF, Rodgers BJ. Z-Plasty: a concise review. *Facial Plast Surg.* 2001;17(4):289–294.
12. Isenhath SN, Swanson NA, Lee KK. Scar revision. In: Robinson JK, Hanke CW, Siegel DM, Fratila A, eds. *Surgery of the Skin: Procedural Dermatology.* 2nd ed. Philadelphia, PA: Elsevier Mosby; 2010:chap 20.
13. Chang CW, Ries WR. Nonoperative techniques for scar management and revision. *Facial Plast Surg.* 2001;17(4):283–288.

CHAPTER 22

Nail Surgery

Joshua W. Trufant, John A. Carucci, Nathaniel Jellinek, & Chris G. Adigun

ANATOMY

Nail procedures require a detailed knowledge of the anatomy and physiology of the distal digit. A thorough understanding of nail unit structures and their functions will allow the surgeon to maximize diagnostic and therapeutic results while minimizing patient discomfort and postoperative deformity. A comprehensive anatomic review is beyond the scope of this text, but a brief primer will allow for better understanding of the procedures described subsequently.

The nail unit is composed of the nail matrix, nail bed, nail plate, and their bordering structures (Fig. 22-1). The nail matrix is the germinative epithelium that produces the keratinized nail plate on the dorsal aspect of the distal digit.[1] A portion of the matrix is visible through the proximal nail plate as the pink–white, semicircular lunula. The lateral horns of the crescent-shaped matrix extend approximately 6 mm proximally from the visible edge of the nail plate. The proximal portion of the matrix forms the dorsal – or most superficial – portion of the nail plate, while the distal portion produces the ventral portion (Fig. 22-2). As the predominant germinative structure, the nail matrix is an irreplaceable component of the nail unit, and extreme care must be taken to minimize trauma. Procedures affecting the proximal matrix, responsible for up to 80% of the nail plate, are more likely to result in noticeable postoperative split-nail deformity.[2]

The matrix makes up the inferior and proximal portion of a cul-de-sac from which the nail plate emerges. The superior portion or "roof" of the cul-de-sac is formed by the proximal nail fold (PNF). Its ventral aspect, in contact with the nail plate, is often referred to as the eponychium. The most distal aspect of the PNF is the cuticle, a translucent rim of stratum corneum that seals the proximal fold to the nail plate, thereby preventing microorganisms and irritants from entering the cul-de-sac. The sides of the nail plate are bordered by the lateral nail folds (LNF), which are anatomically similar to the PNF but do not form a cuticle.

Abutting the matrix and comprising the majority of the base of the nail plate is the nail bed. Characterized by linear, parallel rete ridges, this highly vascular tissue lends a pink color to the nail. The nail bed is firmly adherent to the plate, to which it may contribute a small number of cells.[2,3] The bed extends from the lunula to the hyponychium, which seals the potential subungual space and is the point at which the nail separates from the underlying epithelium. The distal nail groove marks

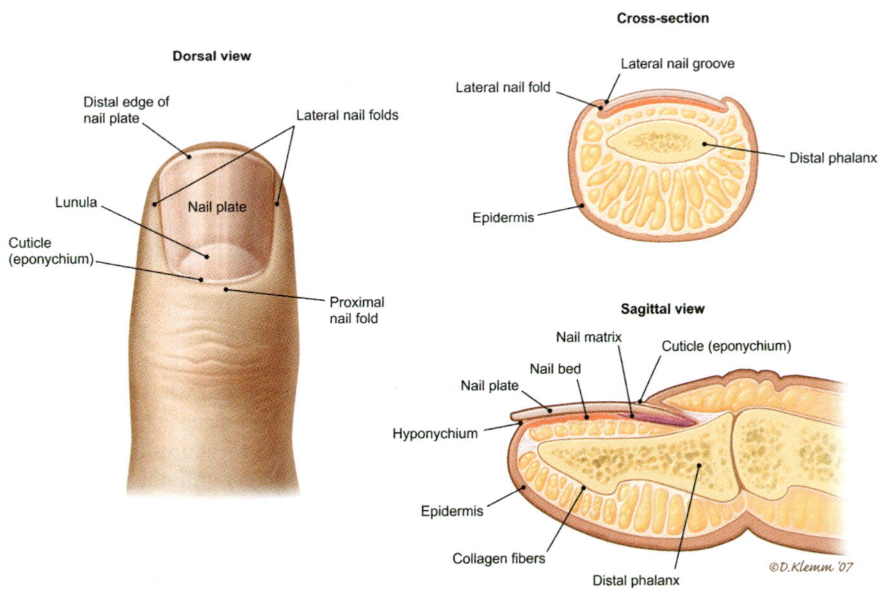

Figure 22-1 Anatomy of the nail. (Reproduced with permission from Dave Klemm. © 2007 Dave Klemm.)

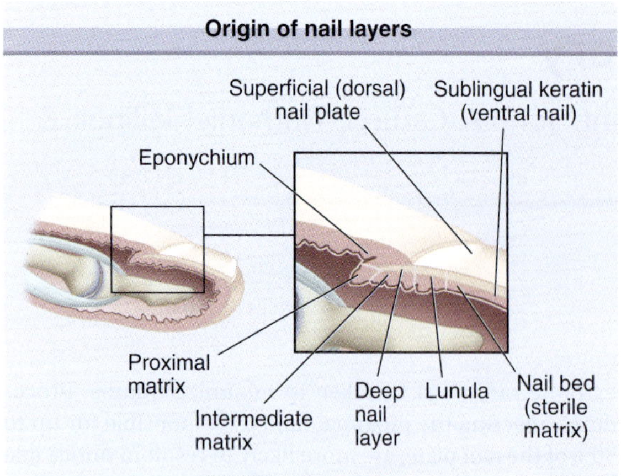

Figure 22-2 Origin of nail layers. (Used with permission from P. Kechijian, MD.)

the convex distal edge of the hyponychium, separating it from the fingertip. The nail bed dermis sits directly atop the periosteum of the distal phalanx without any intervening subcutaneous tissue. Flexor and extensor tendons cross the distal interphalangeal (DIP) joint and attach to the distal phalanx, while lateral tendons attached to the distal ungual process further stabilize the joint.

The blood supply to the nail unit is provided by the proper dorsal and palmar digital arteries, which course down the lateral aspects of each digit and anastomose to form an arcade of smaller vessels and capillaries (Fig. 22-3). They are branches of the common palmar digital arteries radiating from the superficial palmar arch, with the exception of the radial artery of the lateral index finger and the princeps pollicis artery of the thumb, which branch from the deep palmar arch. Venous drainage generally mirrors arterial architecture, with the exception of collecting veins in the LNF that form an arch over the PNF.[3] Innervation of the nail apparatus is provided by the dorsal and ventral lateral digital nerves, which course alongside the blood vessels.

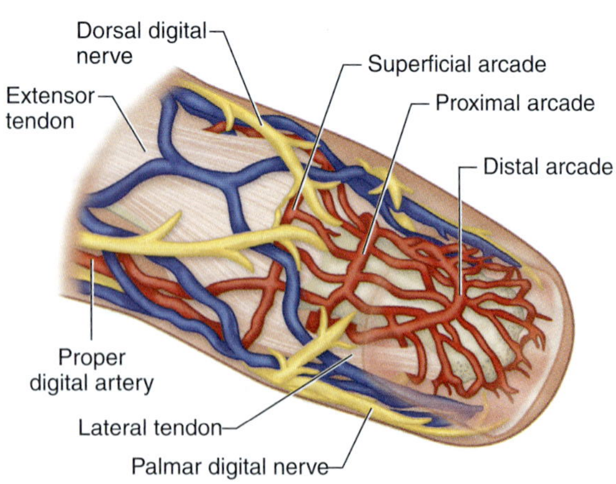

Figure 22-3 Vessels, nerves, and tendons of the nail unit. (Adapted with permission from Fleckman P, Allan C. Surgical anatomy of the nail unit. *Dermatol Surg*. 2001;27:257.)

KEY ASPECTS OF PREOPERATIVE EVALUATION

The preoperative evaluation should inform the surgical approach and allow for better anticipation and/or preemption of surgical and postoperative complications. Occasionally, it may reveal contraindications for surgery. Important items in the past medical history include: factors predisposing to infection, such as a history of diabetes or other immunocompromised states, as well as the presence of artificial heart valves, joints, or prostheses; bleeding diatheses or coagulopathies; a history of coronary artery disease, arrhythmias, hypertension, peripheral vascular disease, Raynaud's disease, or other vasospastic disorders; connective tissue diseases; arthritides; and psychological disorders that may affect the patient's ability to tolerate a procedure. For patients with multiple comorbidities or advanced age, it may be advisable to request preoperative clearance from a primary medical doctor.

A thorough medication history must be completed, with special emphasis on agents that may increase bleeding risk (antiplatelet and anticoagulant agents, particularly when used in combination),[4] predispose to infection (chemotherapeutic, steroidal, or other immunosuppressive agents), inhibit wound healing (corticosteroids), or interfere with anesthesia or analgesia (anxiolytics, opiates, or other analgesics). There are no data concerning the effect of herbals or vitamins on intra- or postoperative bleeding in the dermatologic literature, and studies of the effects of nonsteroidal anti-inflammatory drugs (NSAIDs) are equivocal.[5,6] In general, antithrombotic agents should not be stopped prior to dermatologic procedures, despite an increased risk of bleeding. Any further consideration of stopping prescribed medications perioperatively should be discussed with the patient's primary doctor or appropriate specialty physician. Medication allergies – particularly to anesthetics, antibiotics, or analgesics – must also be documented carefully.

Key aspects of the social history include substance use, employment, and social support network. Casual alcohol users may be counseled to abstain from consuming alcoholic beverages prior to surgery due to its vasodilatory and blood-thinning effects, although there is no data to support this. For misusers, abstaining from alcohol at least 1 month before elective surgery has been shown to decrease postoperative morbidity.[7] Patients who smoke should be made aware of tobacco's detrimental effects on wound healing and composite graft survival following digital amputation.[8,9] It is also important to be familiar with a patient's living situation and potential care givers, as well as their form of employment. Procedures temporarily affecting ambulation or use of a hand may be particularly burdensome for those whose jobs involve manual labor, computers, or prolonged standing or walking. As the vast majority of nail procedures are nonemergent, it is advisable to delay surgery until the patient can arrange for time off from work or home responsibilities.

In addition to close inspection of all 20 nails, preoperative physical examination should include palpation of peripheral pulses and assessment of vital signs. Plain films help to define the extent of any underlying bony abnormalities. Magnetic resonance imaging (MRI) provides optimal tumor localization for select neoplasms (glomus tumors, myxoid cysts), but is rarely necessary.[10]

ANXIOLYSIS

Adequate management of patient discomfort involves more than local anesthesia, particularly when performing surgeries on fully conscious patients. Patients with a prior history of anxiety disorder may require preoperative dosing of anxiolytics. Even those without a history of anxiety may be apprehensive about nail procedures. In addition to being unpleasant for the patient, anxiety may also cause elevated blood pressure and heart rate, potentially resulting in greater intra- and postoperative bleeding. During the surgical consultation visit, the physician should inquire directly about any anticipated emotional discomfort, and a prescription for an anxiolytic agent to be taken preoperatively should be offered when appropriate. Oral midazolam has been demonstrated to be helpful in both pediatric and adult patients undergoing dermatologic surgery.[11,12] Patients who elect to premedicate with an anxiolytic must be reminded to bring a companion who is able to escort or drive the patient home following the procedure. On the day of the surgery, patients should be seated comfortably in a reclined or supine position. Attention to ambient temperature, lighting, and background noise will help to ensure a more comfortable experience for patient and surgeon.

ANESTHESIA

Lidocaine is the most commonly used local anesthetic agent in nail procedures due to its low allergenicity, rapid onset, and 1 to 2 hours' duration of action. Bupivacaine or prilocaine may be used for longer procedures or in particularly pain-sensitive patients.[13] Traditionally, the addition of epinephrine for hemostasis was not recommended in hand and finger surgeries due to concerns for digital necrosis. However, more recent studies do not support this long-held surgical dogma. A retrospective study of 1111 cases and another prospective study of 3110 cases of hand or finger surgeries employing 1% lidocaine with epinephrine (typically 1:100,000) found no instances of digital ischemia or tissue loss.[14,15] Earlier reports implicating epinephrine in digital gangrene have since been attributed to other causes such as the use of older anesthetic compounds (many of which had an abnormally low pH), excessive tourniquet pressure, "ring-block" technique, high-volume injection, and thermal burns from hot soaks.[14,16] On the contrary, by enhancing and prolonging the effects of lidocaine, epinephrine may decrease the number of lidocaine injections required, prolong post-procedure pain relief, and decrease the need for a digital tourniquet.[16–18] Some authors advise caution when using epinephrine in patients with hyperthyroidism, severe hypertension, cardiac disease, Raynaud's disease, peripheral vascular disease, or tobacco use.[17,19] Recently, some have proposed the use of ropivacaine as a long-acting, rapid-onset anesthetic that may have some inherent vasoconstrictive properties.[20]

To minimize patient discomfort, anesthesia should be administered slowly via a 30 gauge needle.[21] Topical cryogen spray applied for 1 to 2 seconds immediately prior to needle insertion also lessens the pain of injection.[19] Buffering lidocaine–epinephrine mixtures with 7% to 8% sodium bicarbonate in a 5:1 or 10:1 ratio has been reported to reduce the burning sensation associated with administration, as has the use of room-temperature anesthetic.[22,23] Patients should always be placed in a reclined or supine position during administration to prevent negative sequelae in the event of a vasovagal reaction.

There are several effective approaches to anesthetizing the nail unit. The two most commonly used techniques are the proximal and distal (or "wing") blocks. The traditional proximal digital block is considered less painful, but requires up to 10 minutes for complete anesthesia. In addition, it is contraindicated in the setting of bacterial infection.[24] The proximal block is achieved by two injections laterally at the base of the involved finger or toe (Fig. 22-4). The hand is typically laid flat, palm down, with fingers spread. The foot is also approached dorsally, but in a neutral position with the patient's leg extended. After cleaning the injection site with an alcohol pad, the needle is inserted tangentially at the web space on either side of the proximal bony phalanx, between the metacarpophalangeal (or metatarsophalangeal) joints and the proximal interphalangeal (PIP) joints, and advanced into the subcutaneous fat. After pulling back briefly on the syringe to ensure no blood reflux, between 1 and 2 mL is administered with each injection. The use of greater than 5 mL risks creating a tourniquet effect that could cause ischemia. Similarly, a "ring-block," in which multiple injections are used to create a tumescent ring of anesthetic encircling the base of the digit, is unnecessary and may be associated with increased risk of digital necrosis.[16] If the anticipated scope of the procedure involves only one side of the nail unit, a block of the ipsilateral nerve only may be used. The surgeon should allow 10 minutes for the anesthetic to take full effect. Additional injections may be required, depending on the length of the procedure.

The distal "wing" block has the advantage of being nearly instantaneous. The rapid effect likely has more to do with tumescence than with chemical properties of the lidocaine itself. Hemostasis resulting from tumescence may be sufficient to preclude the need for epinephrine or

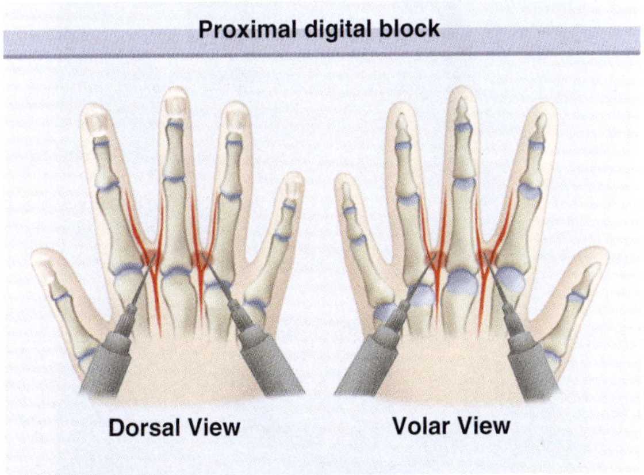

Figure 22-4 Proximal digital block. (Reproduced with permission from Goldsmith LA, Katz SI, Gilchrest BA, Paller AS, Leffell DJ, Wolff K. *Fitzpatrick's Dermatology in General Medicine*. 8th ed. McGraw-Hill, Inc.; 2012. Fig. 245-2. Copyright © McGraw-Hill Education LLC.)

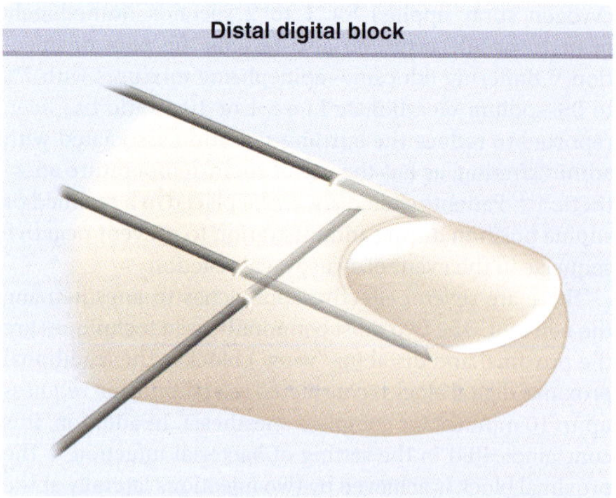

Figure 22-5 Distal digital block. (Reproduced with permission from Goldsmith LA, Katz SI, Gilchrest BA, Paller AS, Leffell DJ, Wolff K. *Fitzpatrick's Dermatology in General Medicine*. 8th ed. McGraw-Hill, Inc.; 2012. Fig. 245-3. Copyright © McGraw-Hill Education LLC.)

a digital tourniquet.[25] The wing block has been reported to be more painful than the proximal block, but the use of topical cryogen spray can significantly lessen patient discomfort.[19] The needle is first inserted superficially into the superficial PNF, 2 to 4 mm inferolaterally from the junction of the PNF and LNF (Fig. 22-5). A dermal wheal is created by the injection of a small amount of anesthetic. Additional anesthetic is then slowly injected, creating a gradual blanching of the LNF that resembles the unfolding of a wing (Fig. 22-6). The process is then repeated at the opposite lateral edge of the PNF. Some authors advise repositioning the needle without withdrawing after the first injection and injecting transversely across the PNF as well.[24] Care should be taken to limit injections to the dorsal half of the digit, as the pulp of the volar surface of the digit could serve as an unintended reservoir for the injected anesthesia. Additional injections of the distal digit may rarely be needed. A total of 1 to 3 mL of anesthetic is typically required to anesthetize the dorsal digital tip, which should appear blanched upon completion.

In an alternative medial approach to the distal wing block, the needle is introduced at a 30 degree angle between the DIP joint and PNF, then angled toward one junction of the PNF and LNF. Approximately 1 to 2 mL of anesthetic is slowly injected.[26] The procedure is then repeated using the same insertion point but with the needle pointing to the opposite LNF. A simplified, single-injection median distal administration may also be used for procedures involving only the proximal half of the nail unit. In this technique, the needle is introduced at a 30 degree angle into the middle of the PNF, and anesthetic is injected slowly but continuously as the needle is advanced distally through the soft, subcutaneous nail plate, the matrix, and the proximal nail bed.[24]

Other less commonly used techniques include the transthecal digital block, in which 2 mL of anesthetic is injected into the potential space of the flexor tendon sheath at the level of the palmar flexion crease.[27] Although some advocate its use in selected procedures involving the middle three fingers, this method has been shown to be no more effective, and yet significantly more painful, than volar subcutaneous single-injection techniques or the traditional two-injection proximal digital block.[26,28–31] Both volar injection techniques may risk inadequate anesthesia of the dorsal digit, particularly in surgeries of the thumb and little finger.[29] Wrist blocks are rarely used for nail procedures, except in cases involving extensive flap reconstruction.

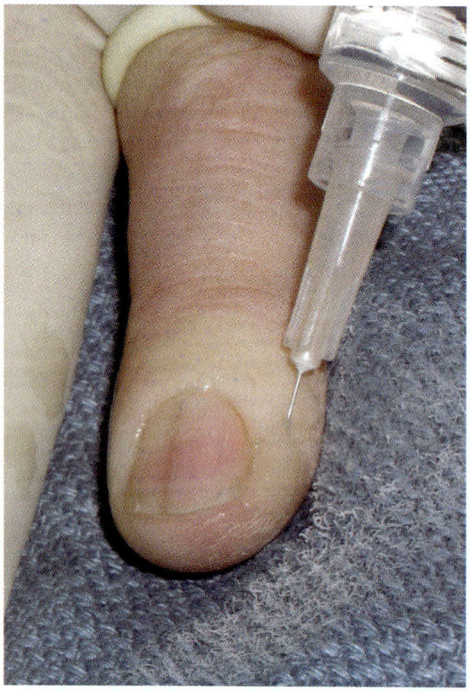

Figure 22-6 Wing block anesthesia.

POSTOPERATIVE ANALGESIA

Postoperative pain after nail surgery can be significant, and the surgeon should not shy away from prescribing strong analgesics when appropriate. It is advisable for the patient to take an analgesic agent immediately after surgery in anticipation of increased pain when the anesthesia wears off.[32] Although data are scarce in the dermatologic literature, one randomized controlled trial comparing postoperative analgesia regimens after Mohs micrographic surgery (MMS) found that the combination of acetaminophen and ibuprofen provided better pain control than acetaminophen alone or acetominophen plus codeine.[33] This regimen was also better tolerated and associated with fewer side effects, including bleeding, than the other regimens. Importantly, studies from other surgical specialties have similarly shown that NSAIDs, in combination with other analgesics, provide superior postoperative pain control and are not associated with an increased risk of bleeding.[5,33] For smaller procedures, acetaminophen alone may provide adequate pain relief. The addition of codeine or oxycodone to acetaminophen prolongs relief of acute postoperative pain, but may also increase the incidence of adverse events such as gastrointestinal distress.[34,35] As mentioned earlier, the use of longer-acting bupivacaine anesthesia may lessen the need for analgesics in the first 24 hours postoperatively, during which time pain tends to peak.[33] Regardless of the choice of analgesic, the patient should be educated about the intensity, quality, and duration of pain to be expected, as well as signs of a potential complication. Pulsating pain that develops 36 to 48 hours after nail surgery may indicate an infection.[24]

SURGICAL PREPARATION, INSTRUMENTS AND SUTURE OPTIONS, HEMOSTASIS, POSTOPERATIVE DRESSINGS

Nail surgery is ideally performed under sterile conditions. The involved hand or foot is cleansed with an antiseptic such as chlorhexidine, isopropyl alcohol, or povidone–iodine solution, or a combination of several agents. For fingernail procedures, a sterile surgical glove with the corresponding fingertip cut off is then placed over the hand and the glove finger rolled down to the base of the digit.[36] This technique serves the dual purpose of a sterile surgical field and an effective tourniquet. Some authors advise preoperative antiseptic foot soaks to reduce bacterial colonization, although it is unclear whether decreased flora leads to a reduction in clinically significant postoperative infections.[37,38] At the least, soaking softens the nail plate and facilitates cutting a thickened nail plate. Antibiotic prophylaxis is generally not recommended in dermatologic surgery, although there is a paucity of large-scale, prospective studies. A recent advisory statement incorporating American Heart Association recommendations provides helpful guidance.[39]

Most instruments required for nail procedures can be found on a standard dermatologic surgery tray, with a few notable exceptions. A Freer septum elevator or dental spatula is useful for nail avulsion and for protecting the matrix during nail fold biopsies. An English anvil-action nail splitter, or rarely a bone rongeur, is helpful for partial nail avulsion. A dual-action nail clipper is a versatile instrument for cutting through hard nail plate. Frequently used standard instruments include fine skin hooks, pointed curved scissors, small-nosed hemostats, #11 and #15 scalpel blades, a fine-tipped needle holder, and punch biopsy tools. Monofilament, nonresorbable 5-0 or 6-0 sutures are typically used for closure. It is also advisable to have 6-0 resorbable suture material available for nail bed closure or vessel ligation if necessary.

HEMOSTASIS

A bloodless field is essential for successful nail surgery. Traditionally, intraoperative hemostasis was achieved with a digital tourniquet, although in practice this is rarely necessary. Standard surgical teaching prohibited the use of epinephrine for hemostasis in hand and finger surgeries due to isolated reports of digital necrosis. However, as mentioned previously, more recent studies have challenged that traditional wisdom and demonstrated the relative safety and advantages of using standardized mixtures of lidocaine with epinephrine.[14,15] One potential disadvantage of epinephrine is that its vasoconstrictive effects may mask inadequate hemostasis until after the patient has left the surgeon's office. The tumescent effect of lidocaine alone during a distal digital block may provide sufficient hemostasis for smaller procedures. There are several digital tourniquet options, should the use of one be deemed necessary. An adjustable metal ring with a screw that is turned to regulate pressure may be applied at the base of the digit. A flat Penrose drain or catheter wrapped around the digit and clamped may also serve as an improvised tourniquet. Perhaps the best solution is the use of a sterile surgical glove with the tip of the involved finger cut off and then rolled back to the base of the digit, as mentioned earlier. Studies have shown that this technique provides safe, effective, steady pressure.[40–42] Prolonged tourniquet time (i.e., >30 minutes) should be avoided, although studies evaluating digital tourniquet time sequelae are lacking. Pressure may be applied manually over the proper digital arteries at the sides of the digit as needed. Although pressure alone usually proves to be sufficient, in rare cases, electrosurgery, ferric subsulfate (Monsel's solution), or oxidized cellulose (Gelfoam) may be used prior to wound closure.

POSTOPERATIVE DRESSINGS

A pressure dressing applied by the surgeon can help to reduce postoperative throbbing pain and bleeding. However, care should be taken not to apply the dressing too tightly to allow for anticipated postoperative edema and to prevent the formation of a postoperative tourniquet. Petrolatum or antibiotic ointment is first applied to the wound, followed by a nonadherent dressing and a bulky gauze wrap to protect against incidental trauma. The nail plate is sometimes used as a biologic dressing or splint following avulsion or nail bed punch biopsy.[43] An alternative, novel technique for splinting following nail avulsion is the use of a piece of aspiration tubing cut to fit the nail bed.[44] A bolster dressing sutured to the surgical site may be used after more complex repairs involving flaps or grafts. Elevation of the operated extremity reduces pressure on the surgical wound and further decreases pain and bleeding. Wearing a sling on the operated arm for 48 hours serves this purpose, although this is usually not necessary. Patients undergoing toenail procedures should be advised to wear open-toed sandals on the day of the surgery. A meta-analysis of other postoperative interventions after ingrown toenail surgery – such as the use of antibiotics, honey, or paraffin dressings – did not show any decrease in the risk of postoperative infection, pain, or healing time.[45]

TECHNIQUES IN NAIL SURGERY: NAIL BED AND MATRIX EXPOSURE OPTIONS

TOTAL AVULSION

Avulsion, the process of removing all or a portion of the nail plate, is one of the most fundamental nail procedures. It is also one of the most traumatic, and should be performed only when absolutely necessary for diagnosis or treatment of disease. Avulsion facilitates visualization of the nail bed and matrix, allowing for matrix biopsies and other more complex procedures. Traditionally, the total nail plate was avulsed by either distal or proximal approach to maximize exposure of underlying structures, but partial transverse or longitudinal avulsion often provides sufficient exposure and results in less trauma.[43] Total avulsion eliminates important counterpressure provided by the nail plate, which can result in nail bed hypertrophy and distal embedding of the new nail plate.[46] It may also be complicated by postoperative paronychia and increased throbbing pain. Some authors suggest that total avulsion may increase physiological transverse nail plate curvature, predisposing to pincer-nail deformity, a condition that avulsion was once proposed to treat.[47] However, there are definite indications for total avulsion, such as large tumors, frank melanoma or squamous cell carcinoma (SCC), and onychomatricomas that project into the nail plate.

In distal total nail avulsion, the Freer septum elevator or a dental spatula is first inserted between the PNF and nail plate and moved firmly with a lifting–lowering motion to disrupt attachments (Fig. 22-7).[48] This is repeated across the entire proximal fold to completely free the dorsal nail plate. The instrument is then reinserted at the hyponychium between the ventral nail plate and nail bed and advanced toward the proximal edge of the nail plate. A sudden decrease in resistance signals proximity to the matrix; further advancement increases the risk of trauma and residual nail dystrophy. At this point the plate should be easily removed with the elevator, or if needed, by gently pulling and rotating a hemostat clamped to the distal nail plate. Some authors maintain that use of the straight mosquito hemostat alone is preferable for avulsion, as recommended in earlier surgical textbooks.[49]

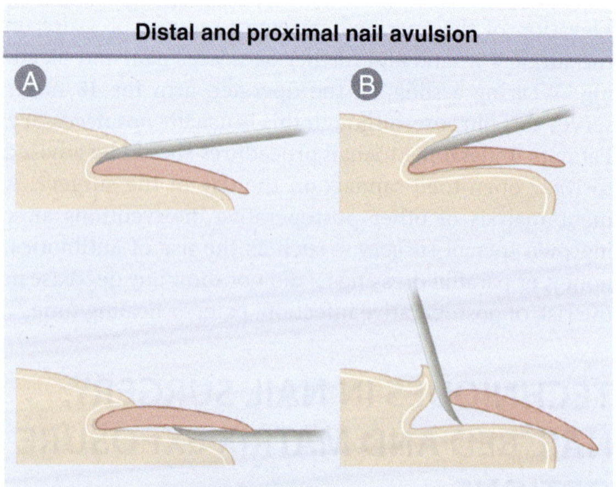

Figure 22-7 **A.** Distal nail avulsion. **B.** Proximal nail avulsion. (Reproduced with permission from Goldsmith LA, Katz SI, Gilchrest BA, Paller AS, Leffell DJ, Wolff K. *Fitzpatrick's Dermatology in General Medicine.* 8th ed. McGraw-Hill, Inc.; 2012. Fig. 245-5A and B. Copyright © McGraw-Hill Education LLC.)

The proximal approach may be the less traumatic of the two classic total avulsion techniques, particularly if there is very tight adhesion between nail plate and bed at the hyponychium.[26] It is also employed if there is no distal nail edge due to dystrophy. Proximal avulsion begins similarly to the distal approach with the septum elevator inserted between the PNF and nail plate and moved gently back and forth. However, rather than reinserting at the hyponychium, the tip of the elevator is kept in place while the handle of the instrument is rotated end-over-end toward the patient's wrist, gently reflecting the PNF. The nail plate is then lifted at its proximal edge with the elevator or a hemostat. If necessary, the elevator can be advanced distally beneath the nail plate to sever any remaining attachments to the nail bed.[50] In practice, the proximal approach is only rarely used and is a more traumatic and less elegant technique.

PARTIAL AND TRAPDOOR AVULSIONS

As noted earlier, partial avulsion provides adequate exposure for many nail procedures and may be associated with less postoperative morbidity. Importantly, it preserves some of the counterpressure provided by the nail plate that is lost with total avulsion. Partial avulsion also facilitates replacement of the removed portion of the nail plate when histologic evaluation is not required. The avulsed segment can be sutured or secured with Steri-Strips to act as a biological dressing to protect the defect and promote healing. There are a variety of partial avulsion techniques, well described in a recent review, and several of these may be effective for a given clinical indication. In selecting the most appropriate approach, the surgeon must consider lesion size, localization, and suspected anatomic origin, as well as the overall surgical objective (i.e., biopsy vs. removal of the whole lesion).[43]

Partial distal plate avulsion is useful for investigating lesions involving the distal nail bed or hyponychium. It may also facilitate the topical treatment of distal subungual onychomycosis or allow drainage of subungual purulent material in the setting of acute bacterial infection. After anesthesia, the nail plate is transected with a nail clipper or English nail splitter and then avulsed using a septum elevator or hemostat. Soaking the nail in warm water prior to the procedure can ease cutting. Partial lateral avulsion may be performed to evaluate a neoplasm, foreign body, or hematoma abutting the LNF. It also has a role in the treatment of chronic paronychia (CP) and ingrown nails prior to chemical matricectomy. A longitudinal incision is made using an English nail splitter (with the flat, anvil-like portion beneath the nail plate), and the lateral portion of the nail plate avulsed by one of the approaches described previously.

When examination of the proximal matrix is required, as in cases of longitudinal melanonychia (LM), a partial proximal nail plate avulsion can be performed (Fig. 22-8). The PNF is first incised obliquely at its lateral aspects, then undermined with a Freer elevator and reflected using either fine skin hooks or sutures. An English nail splitter is then inserted from the lateral edge of the nail plate and a transverse cut is made approximately 4 mm

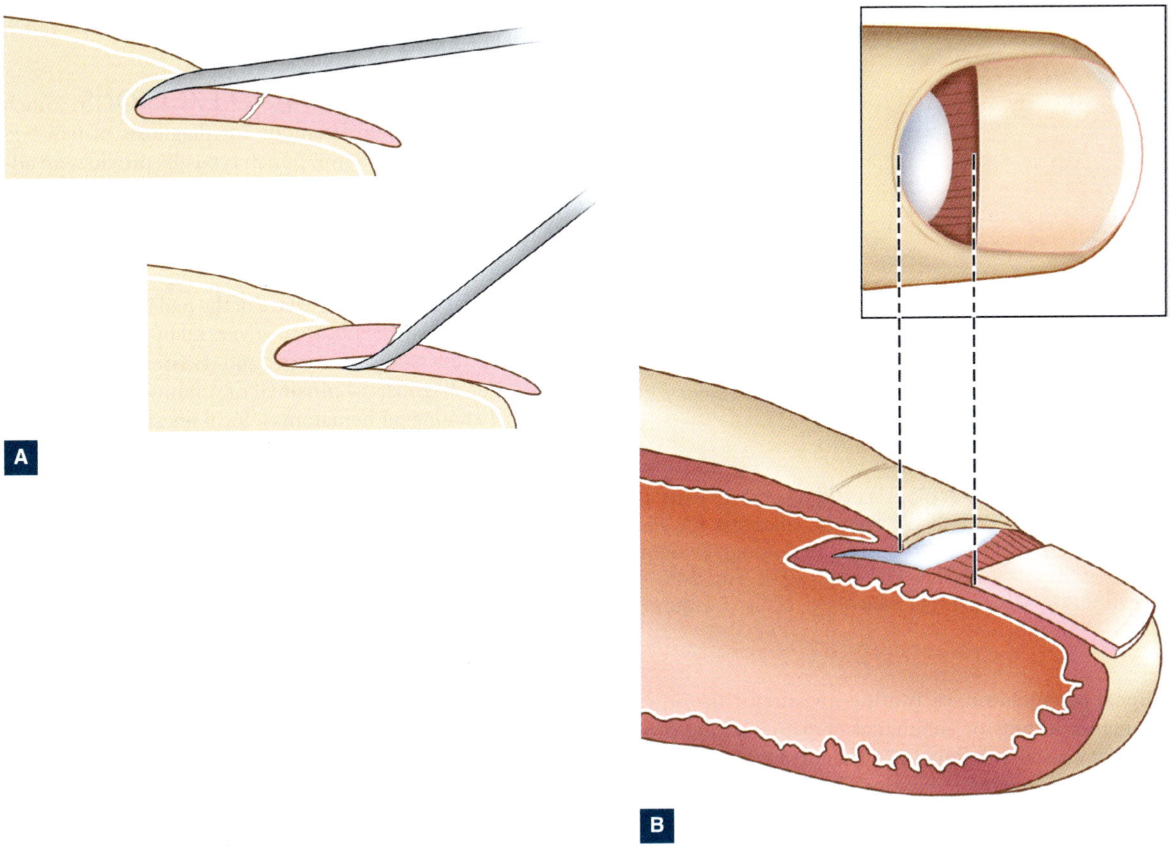

Figure 22-8 **A.** Partial avulsion of the proximal nail plate. **B.** Resulting exposure of the distal matrix and proximal nail bed. (Reproduced with permission from Goldsmith LA, Katz SI, Gilchrest BA, Paller AS, Leffell DJ, Wolff K. *Fitzpatrick's Dermatology in General Medicine*. 8th ed. McGraw-Hill, Inc.; 2012. Fig. 245-6A and B. Copyright © McGraw-Hill Education LLC.)

from the former site of the cuticle. A hemostat is used to remove the proximal portion of the nail plate, which can be reinserted after the procedure. If the lesion of interest is confined to the lateral nail unit, the lateral plate curl technique also provides exposure of the proximal matrix. After oblique incision and reflection of the involved LNF, a hemostat or Freer elevator is inserted beneath the lateral free edge of the nail plate and advanced proximally with steady dorsal pressure on the ventral surface of the plate. Once freed, the lateral plate is grasped with a hemostat and rolled or peeled medially, exposing the underlying nail bed, nail fold, and proximal matrix. At the close of the procedure, the plate may be rolled back and sutured to the LNF.[43]

Another alternative to total avulsion is the "trapdoor" technique, which exposes the distal matrix, nail bed, and hyponychium without removing the nail plate.[43] In this approach, the Freer elevator or a hemostat is inserted between the free nail edge and nail bed and advanced proximally to the lunula. The nail plate is then reflected superiorly in trapdoor fashion from the distal edge. Two oblique incisions of the lateral PNF afford greater proximal exposure if needed. This approach can be used to avulse the full width of the nail plate, or only the lateral or medial segments by first longitudinally incising with an English nail splitter. An abbreviated version of the trapdoor avulsion involves the use of a #11 blade to cut three sides of a small "window" in the nail plate that is then elevated to expose underlying nail bed. This technique is useful in the case of small, well-demarcated lesions, foreign bodies, or to allow drainage of blood or purulent material. Alternatively, a fourth cut can be made and the entire "window" removed, or a circular window can be created with a punch biopsy tool.

NONSURGICAL AVULSION

Ablative carbon dioxide (CO_2) laser treatment is effective but potentially damaging to the nail bed and matrix, and should only be performed if total matricectomy is planned.[51] Chemical avulsion with 40% urea paste or nail lacquer may be useful in the treatment of onychomycosis.[52]

NAIL UNIT BIOPSIES AND EXCISIONS

INDICATIONS. Biopsies of the nail unit are performed to diagnose neoplastic, infectious, or inflammatory conditions that cannot be diagnosed by history,

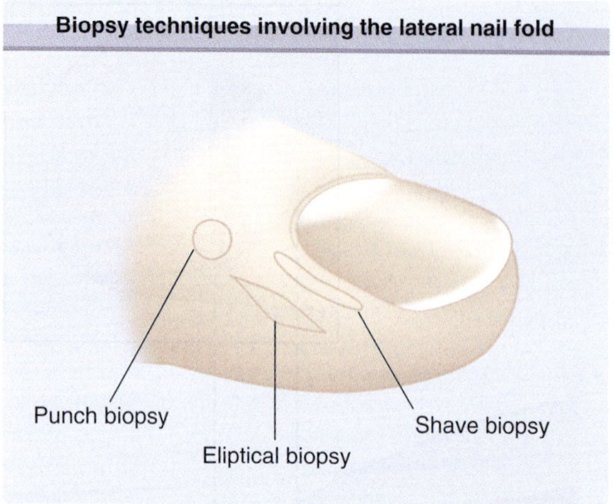

Figure 22-9 Nail fold biopsies. (Reproduced with permission from Goldsmith LA, Katz SI, Gilchrest BA, Paller AS, Leffell DJ, Wolff K. *Fitzpatrick's Dermatology in General Medicine*. 8th ed. McGraw-Hill, Inc.; 2012. Fig. 245-15.2. Copyright © McGraw-Hill Education LLC.) (E-Figure on AccessMedicine).

clinical examination, or routine mycology.[1] In the case of smaller lesions or subungual hematomas, the procedure may also be therapeutic. The most commonly used techniques are punch, elliptical, longitudinal, and shave biopsies. The nail unit is first anesthetized as described previously, and the biopsy technique and orientation tailored to the anatomic structure involved. The goal, as with all nail procedures, is to maximize diagnostic or therapeutic effect while causing as little pain and residual nail dystrophy as possible.

NAIL FOLD BIOPSIES. Lesions of the PNF and LNF may be biopsied using a shave, punch, or elliptical technique in a similar fashion to other cutaneous biopsies (Fig. 22-9). Small spindle-shaped excisions are particularly well-suited to this region. A Freer elevator with the curved tip angled ventrally can be inserted under the nail fold during PNF biopsies to protect the underlying matrix from trauma (Fig. 22-10).[1] Even large defects of the PNF heal well by second intention, with an exaggerated, lengthened nail plate as a sequela.

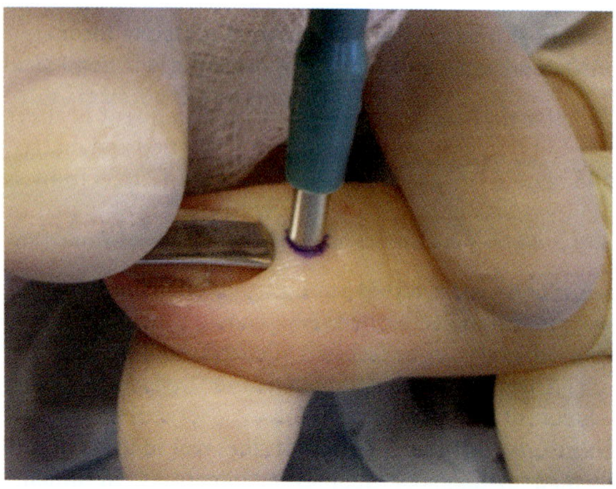

Figure 22-10 Punch biopsy of proximal nail fold, with elevator to protect matrix.

NAIL BED BIOPSIES AND EXCISIONS. Punch biopsy is a versatile technique for diagnosis of nail bed and plate lesions. A 3 mm punch typically provides an adequate tissue sample and is less likely to result in residual dystrophy than larger diameter punches.[19] Soaking the digit in warm water for 10 minutes prior to the procedure will soften the plate and facilitate cutting. The punch tool may be used to score the surface of the nail plate to confirm optimal localization. It is then advanced by simultaneously applying downward pressure and twisting the circular blade. For diagnosis of proximal onychomycosis or evacuation of subungual hematomas, local anesthesia is not always required. The punch tool is advanced only as far as the ventral portion of the plate, signaled by a decrease in resistance. The severed disk of nail plate may be removed with fine-tipped scissors or a #11 blade and submitted for periodic acid-Schiff (PAS) staining if indicated. The surgeon should also take care to examine the punch before discarding it, as the sample may remain attached to the blade.

If a nail bed sample is desired, as in the diagnosis of neoplasms or inflammatory conditions such as lichen planus or psoriasis, punch or elliptical biopsy techniques may be used (Fig. 22-11). Elliptical biopsy necessitates at least partial avulsion of the overlying nail plate by one of the techniques described previously. A longitudinal fusiform incision through to the periosteum is then made around the lesion with a #11 blade. Resorbable sutures are used to close defects larger than 3 mm.[1] Avulsion may be performed prior to punch biopsy, or, alternatively, the punch may be advanced through the plate and nail bed until bone is reached. The punch is then withdrawn, and the sample extracted gently using fine-tipped scissors or #11 blade. Forceps tend to damage the tissue and are not recommended. The punch should be carefully examined to ensure that a part or all of the sample has not been retained. A variation on this technique involves the use of a larger, 6 mm punch to remove the overlying nail plate, followed by a 3 mm or 4 mm punch biopsy of the nail bed (Fig. 22-12). This facilitates visualization of the nail bed and eases extraction of the tissue sample while avoiding the discomfort and morbidity associated with total avulsion.[43] If needed, hemostasis may be assured with Monsel's solution or Gelfoam. Sutures are not required. If not of

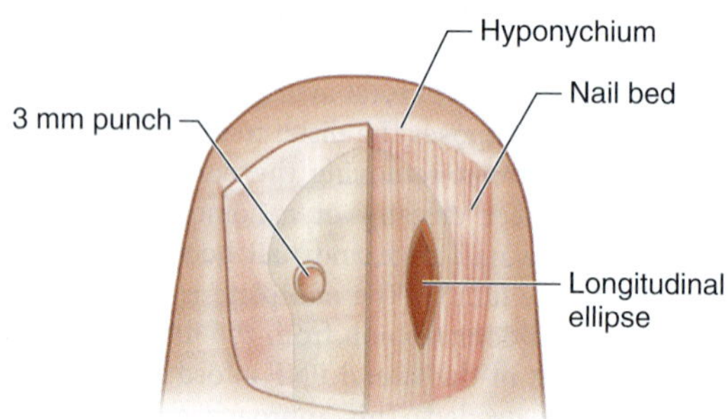

Figure 22-11 Nail bed biopsies. (Adapted with permission from Rich P. Nail biopsy: indications and methods. *Dermatol Surg*. 2001;27:229.)

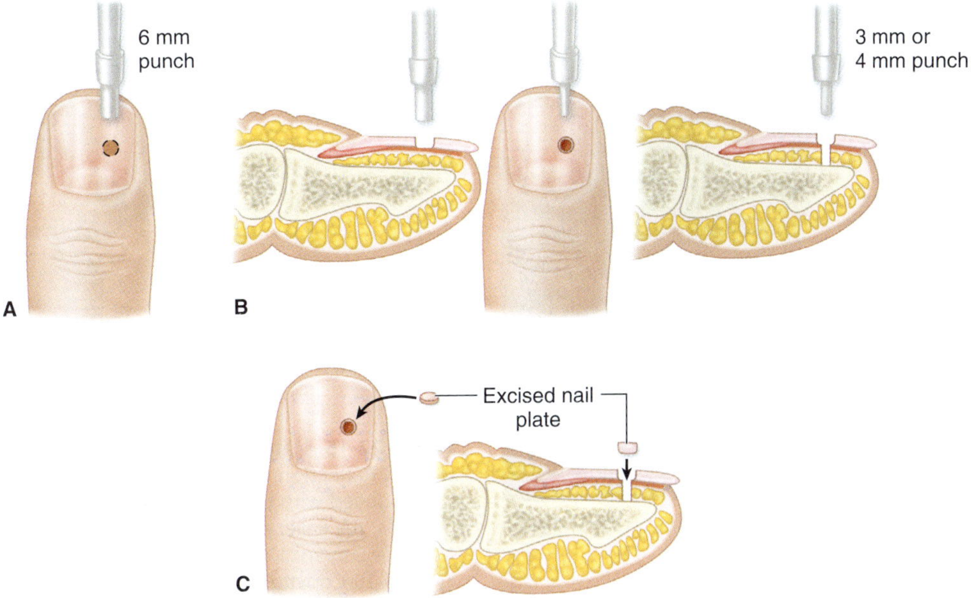

Figure 22-12 Telescope "two-punch" technique for punch biopsy of nail bed. **A.** 6 mm punch device through nail plate only, and this portion of plate is set aside **B.** A 3 or 4 mm punch device is used to sample the nail bed through the defect in the nail plate created by the 6 mm punch device **C.** The removed 6 mm portion of the nail plate is then used to cover the defect. (Adapted with permission from Richert B. Basic nail surgery. *Dermatol Clin*. 2006;24:313. Copyright © Elsevier.)

diagnostic importance, the avulsed nail plate is replaced over the resulting defect. The nail bed typically heals without scarring, although a small focus of onycholysis may persist after surgery.[53]

NAIL MATRIX BIOPSIES AND EXCISIONS.

The primary indication for nail matrix biopsy is to rule out malignant melanoma in a patient with a pigmented nail lesion. Longitudinal nail excision and punch, elliptical, and shave biopsies all have a role in diagnosis (Fig. 22-13). The surgeon's chosen approach must be informed by a thorough history and physical examination. Proximal matrix biopsies in particular carry a high risk of permanent postoperative split nail, and less traumatic approaches may be indicated for less clinically concerning lesions. However, excisional biopsy is recommended when clinical suspicion for melanoma is high. An excision that reduces matrix length will generally result in a thinner nail plate, while one that reduces matrix width will result in a narrower plate.

Lateral longitudinal excision is most useful for diagnosis of LM of the lateral one-third of the nail. Partial avulsion may be performed first, but is not required and may alter the histologic appearance of the specimen. Following local anesthesia, an incision to bone is made beginning at the distal crease of the dorsal DIP joint. It is then carried distally through the PNF, matrix, nail bed, and plate (if not previously avulsed) 1 to 2 mm parallel to the LNF, ending at a point 2 to 3 mm beyond the hyponychium.[54] An English nail splitter may be used for cutting through particularly resistant nail plate. A second incision is then made through the LNF. Complete excision of the lateral matrix horn prevents formation of postoperative spicules or cysts.[55] In cases involving the great toe, whose matrix horns extend more laterally, the second excision should be made 1 to 2 mm beyond the LNF to ensure complete excision.[54] Drawing the planned incisions with a surgical marker will help to ensure an adequate specimen. Dissection can be completed using fine scissors, and the sample inked for orientation during processing and histologic interpretation. The defect is then closed by reapproximating the skin edges and using resorbable simple interrupted

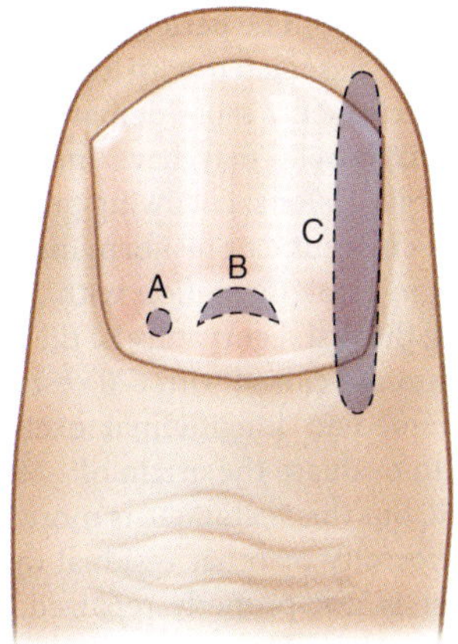

Figure 22-13 Nail matrix biopsies. **A.** Punch biopsy may be used for pigmented bands less than 3 mm in diameter. **B.** Transverse biopsy of distal nail natrix may be used for pigmented bands in the middle of the nail plate. **C.** Longitudinal nail biopsy may be used for lateral pigmented nail lesions. (Adapted with permission from Braun RP, Baran R, Le Gal FA, et al. Diagnosis and management of nail pigmentations. *J Am Acad Dermatol*. 2007;56:835. Copyright © Elsevier.)

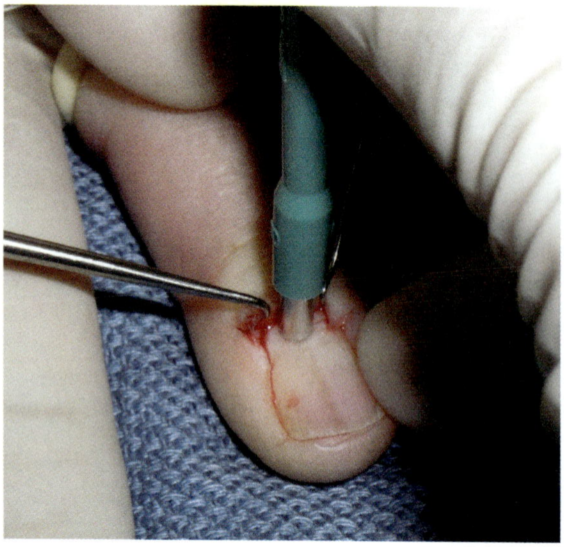

Figure 22-14 Punch biopsy of longitudinal melanonychia.

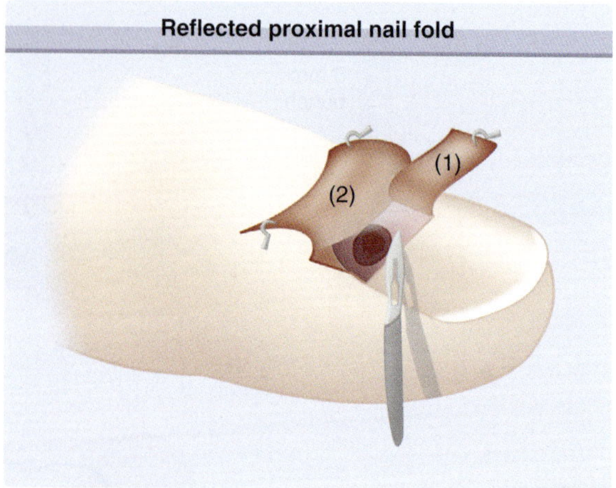

Figure 22-15 Matrix shave biopsy. (1) Partial Lateral Avulsion (2) Reflection of the dorsal fold with fine skin hooks. (Reproduced with permission from Goldsmith LA, Katz SI, Gilchrest BA, Paller AS, Leffell DJ, Wolff K. *Fitzpatrick's Dermatology in General Medicine*. 8th ed. McGraw-Hill, Inc.; 2012. Fig. 245-10. Copyright © McGraw-Hill Education LLC.)

or horizontal mattress sutures passed from skin to nail to recreate the LNF.[54,56] This "back-stitch" technique helps to avoid implantation of nail plate fragments in the nail bed, which can result in keratin granuloma formation. Bipedicle flap or partial closure with second intention healing of the remaining defect may be employed in cases of high tension.

Punch biopsy, with or without preceding avulsion, can also be used to evaluate matrix lesions.[25] Following reflection of the PNF, a 3 mm punch excision is made perpendicularly to the skin through to the underlying periosteum (Fig. 22-14). The punch should be immediately inspected to see if it contains the sample. If not, fine-tipped scissors are then gently inserted around the specimen to snip at the base.[57] Forceps should not be used due to the risk of crush artifact. Sutures are not required for matrix defects of 3 mm or less. Two 3 mm punches or a single larger punch can be performed for larger lesions, but are frequently associated with residual nail dystrophy. Although technically more demanding, elliptical or crescentic matrix biopsy may have improved cosmetic outcomes for larger lesions. Following proximal nail avulsion, transverse crescentic or fusiform incisions are made around the origin of pigmentation with 1 to 2 mm margins, paralleling the distal curvature of the lunula. Defects larger than 3 mm are closed with 6-0 resorbable sutures. A midline/paramedian longitudinal excision may also be performed to evaluate the origin of LM in the middle third of the nail, but this technique is more likely to result in split-nail deformity or other residual dystrophy if the resulting defect is not properly repaired.[58] Several nail matrix flaps have been described to address these surgical challenges.

Another useful approach for diagnosing LM wider than 3 mm with minimal residual dystrophy is the tangential matrix excision or matrix shave biopsy.[56] If the PNF or cuticle is pigmented, a shave biopsy of the involved area can be performed prior to obliquely incising and reflecting the PNF.[56,57,59] A proximal nail plate avulsion is then performed and the plate reflected to one side, exposing the proximal matrix and allowing identification of the origin of melanonychia. Using a #15 blade, the surgeon scores 1 to 2 mm margins around the origin and then shaves the lesion tangentially (Figs. 22-15 and 22-16). Although resulting specimens are less than 1 mm thick, this technique has been shown to yield adequate tissue for histologic diagnosis and to have excellent aesthetic outcomes.[60,61] Placement of the specimen on a piece of wet paper or cardboard will prevent it from curling, which can complicate subsequent processing.[56] To repair the defect, the proximal nail plate and nail fold are laid back in place. Trimming the free lateral edge of the avulsed plate by a few millimeters will help prevent lateral embedding.[57] The plate can then be secured with a horizontal mattress suture. Alternatively, sutures closing the oblique incisions of the PNF may be sufficient to hold it in place.

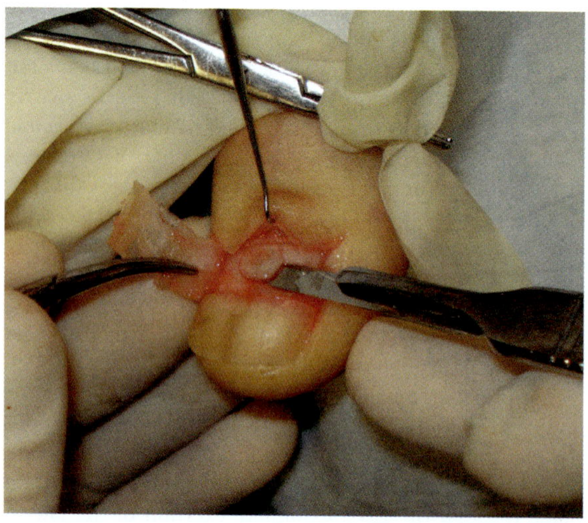

Figure 22-16 Matrix shave biopsy following partial proximal nail plate avulsion and retraction of proximal nail fold.

DESTRUCTIVE TECHNIQUES: MATRICECTOMY AND TOTAL NAIL ABLATION

Treatment of recalcitrant nail hypertrophy or extensive benign and malignant neoplasms may necessitate matricectomy or total ablation of the nail unit. There are a variety of techniques at the surgeon's disposal. If histopathologic examination is required, surgical excision must be performed. Otherwise, chemical, laser, or electrocautery ablation are acceptable and effective destructive methods.

MATRICECTOMY. The first steps in surgical matricectomy are oblique lateral incision and reflection of the PNF, followed by avulsion of the proximal one-third of the nail plate (Fig. 22-17). The nail bed is then incised 1 to 2 mm distal to the lunula and the matrix carefully dissected from the periosteum with blunt-tipped scissors. Incomplete excision of the matrix lateral horns will result in postoperative cysts or spicules.[55] Care should be taken to avoid trauma to the extensor digitorum tendon, which inserts in the distal phalanx just proximal to the matrix. The ventral epithelium of the PNF is tangentially excised as well, completely eliminating all germinative lining of the nail cul-de-sac.

If no histologic specimen is required, chemical matricectomy is effectively and safely carried out using liquefied phenol, a protein-denaturing alcohol that causes tissue necrosis.[62] This technique is commonly used for treatment of ingrown nails. Following proximal plate avulsion, 88% phenol solution is vigorously applied to the entire matrix – paying particular attention to the lateral horns – using a cotton-tipped swab (Fig. 22-18). Success rates generally exceed 98%, although recommendations for the necessary application time to achieve permanent effect vary from 2 to more than 4 minutes.[63,64] Adjoining nail structures can be protected using petrolatum, and the destructive action of phenol neutralized with isopropyl alcohol. Recent data suggest that trichloroacetic acid and 10% sodium hydroxide show promise in chemical matricectomy.[65,66]

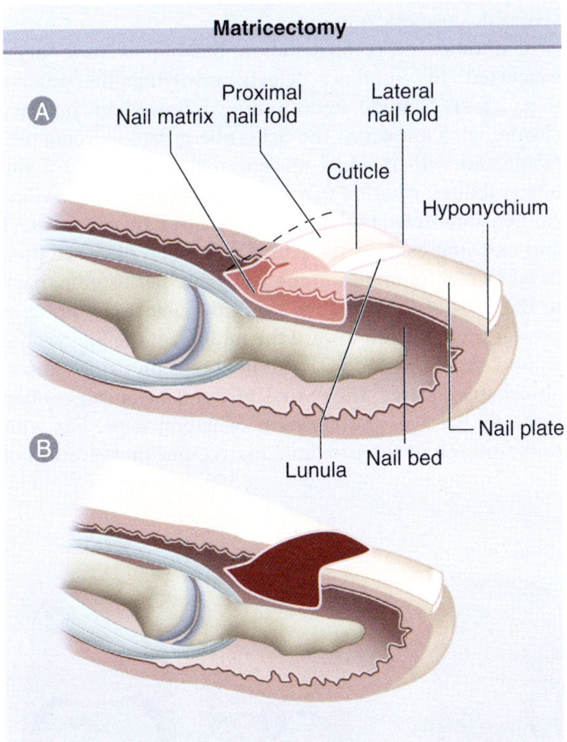

Figure 22-17 Surgical matricectomy. (Reproduced with permission from Goldsmith LA, Katz SI, Gilchrest BA, Paller AS, Leffell DJ, Wolff K. *Fitzpatrick's Dermatology in General Medicine*. 8th ed. McGraw-Hill, Inc.; 2012. Fig. 245-12.1A and B. Copyright © McGraw-Hill Education LLC.) (E-Figure on AccessMedicine).

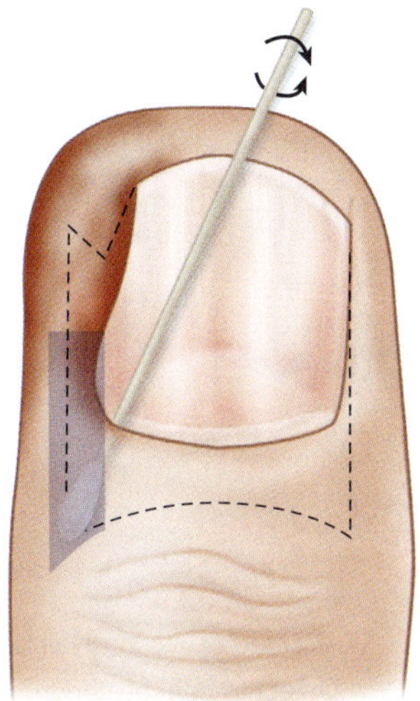

Figure 22-18 Chemical matricectomy of the lateral matrix horn. (Adapted with permission from Haneke E. Controversies in the treatment of ingrown nails. *Dermatol Res Pract.* 2012;2012:783924. Copyright © 2012 Eckart Haneke.)

CO_2 laser or curettage with electrocautery are also effective options for partial or complete matricectomy. The CO_2 laser has the advantage of creating a bloodless field, and may be associated with less postoperative pain and faster healing times.[67,68]

TOTAL NAIL ABLATION. Total nail ablation, also known as "en bloc" excision, is an alternative to amputation for the treatment of malignant neoplasms of the nail unit (Fig. 22-19). Avulsion is not necessary, but if performed, some authors recommend staining the matrix with methylene blue to allow for better visualization during dissection.[69] After anesthesia, an incision to bone is made around the periphery of the nail unit. The most proximal transverse cut should be made approximately three-quarters of the distance from the cuticle to the dorsal DIP joint, a point proximal to the matrix but distal to the insertion of the extensor digitorum tendon.[70,71] The transverse incision is continued to the midlateral line of the digit on each side, then carried longitudinally paralleling the LNF and across the fingertip, 2 to 5 mm from the hyponychium. Proceeding in a distal-to-proximal direction, the tissue is carefully dissected from the periosteum using blunt-tipped scissors. Complete excision of the matrix lateral horns prevents postoperative cysts or

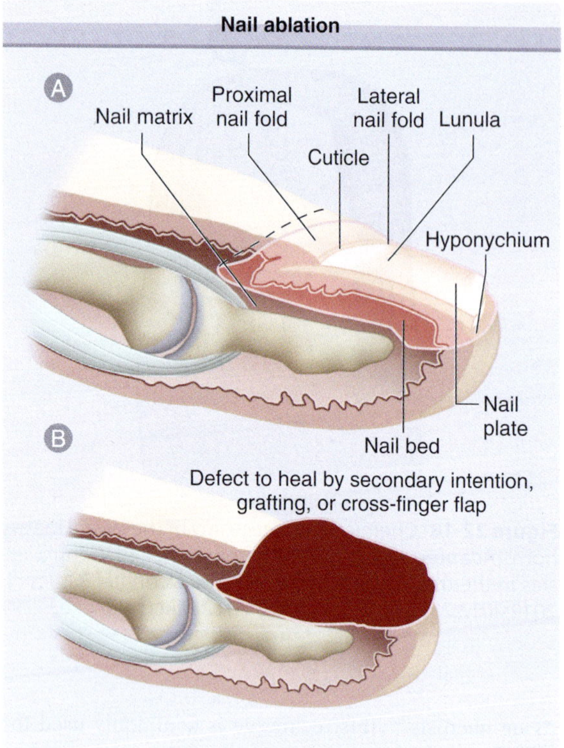

Figure 22-19 Total nail ablation. (Reproduced with permission from Goldsmith LA, Katz SI, Gilchrest BA, Paller AS, Leffell DJ, Wolff K. *Fitzpatrick's Dermatology in General Medicine*. 8th ed. McGraw-Hill, Inc.; 2012. Fig. 245-12A and B. Copyright © McGraw-Hill Education LLC.)

spicules.[55] The surgical defect may be allowed to heal by second intention or repaired with a skin graft, described in greater detail in the following paragraphs.

NAIL DEFECT REPAIRS

The repair of surgical and traumatic nail unit defects ranges in complexity from healing by second intention to skin grafts and flaps. There is no one correct repair for each type of defect. As with all other nail procedures, repairs call upon the surgeon's detailed knowledge of the anatomy and physiology of affected structures, familiarity with previously described approaches, and ability to improvise and tailor the chosen approach to the specific needs of each individual patient.

PROXIMAL NAIL FOLD REPAIRS. Smaller PNF defects resulting from trauma or surgical excisions can often be closed primarily. However, wider defects may require relaxing incisions to facilitate wound closure (Fig. 22-20). A midline or paramedian defect can be easily closed by first making incisions at each side of the nail fold, then undermining the nail fold to the level of the nail plate. The PNF flaps are then rotated toward the midline and sutured without tension. For particularly wide medial defects, flaps employing skin from the lateral digit can be mobilized by creating two arcing incisions from the midlateral line of the digit to the medial cuticle. In both cases, the relaxing incisions are left to heal by second intention. For more lateral defects, the creation of one or two relaxing incisions on the contralateral side followed by undermining achieves a similar effect.[61]

NAIL MATRIX REPAIRS. Matrix defects are associated with a high risk of permanent nail dystrophy, and the surgeon must make every effort to repair them meticulously while minimizing wound tension. Second intention healing is a less than optimal choice given that any scarred tissue will be incapable of producing normal nail plate. The inelastic quality of the dermal matrix makes primary closure of defects more challenging than in other cutaneous surgeries. In some cases, thorough yet delicate undermining of surrounding tissue enables primary repair, but a flap is often required to close matrix defects to achieve favorable cosmetic outcomes.

A number of reconstruction techniques have been suggested for midline defects involving the matrix (Fig. 22-21).[58] Wide undermining followed by primary closure, also known as the Schernberg flap, is frequently associated with residual midline nail dystrophy.[72,73] The bilateral distal rotation flap involves creating two curvilinear incisions down to the bone at the distal tip of the defect and carrying each to the lateral sulci. The flaps are then freed by careful undermining above the periosteum, back to the level of the proximal tip of the defect, resulting in greater mobilization toward the midline of the digit.[74] The wound can be closed with minimal tension using simple, absorbable sutures. The A-to-T bilateral advancement flap similarly involves mobilization of lateral flaps, but with undermining of the proximal matrix and preservation of

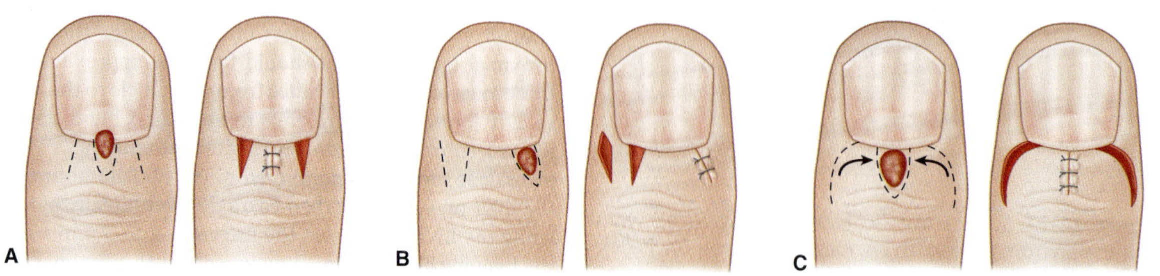

Figure 22-20 Proximal nail fold repairs. **A.** Small medial defect repair facilitated by lateral relaxing incisions. **B.** Lateral defect depair facilitated by two contralateral relaxing incisions. **C.** Larger medial defect repaired with bilateral rotational flaps.

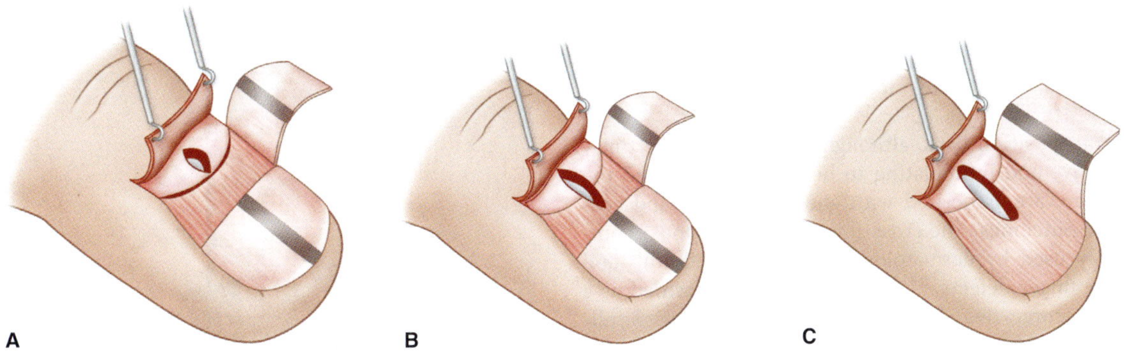

Figure 22-21 Matrix defect repairs. **A.** Bilateral distal rotation flap. **B.** A-to-T bilateral advancement flap. **C.** Bilateral bipedicle flap. (Adapted with permission from Collins SC, Cordova KB, Jellinek NJ. Midline/paramedian longitudinal matrix excision with flap reconstruction: alternative surgical techniques for evaluation of longitudinal melanonychia. *J Am Acad Dermatol*. 2010;62:627. Copyright © Elsevier.)

the matrix–nail bed junction. After reflecting the PNF, arcing incisions are made down to the bone beginning at the midline of the defect at the most proximal point of the matrix and carried to the LNF sulci. The flaps are then sharply undermined above the periosteum, completely freeing the proximal matrix and facilitating midline closure with absorbable sutures.[58]

The widest medial defects involving the nail matrix and bed can be repaired using a flap or graft. The bipedicled bilateral matrix advancement flap exploits the relative laxity of skin from the lateral digit.[58,75] Deep relaxing incisions are made longitudinally at both sides of the PNF, in line with the LNF. The matrix flaps are then sharply undermined with a scalpel at the level of periosteum in a medial-to-lateral direction, taking care to preserve the proximal and distal attachments. The medial edges of the flaps can then be approximated and sutured in a tension-free fashion. Alternatively, a free matrix graft employing a thin slice of matrix harvested from the intact big-toenail can be placed in the defect.[61] If the recipient nail plate has been totally avulsed, the toenail plate can be trimmed down and placed in the recipient nail bed to act as a splint.

Narrow lateral defects of the nail matrix and bed can be closed with a Schernberg flap, but, for larger defects, a bipedicled lateral nail wall flap may result in better cosmesis and functionality (Fig. 22-22).[61] This technique is most useful after lateral longitudinal excision or excisional biopsy of erythro- or melanonychia. The lateral wall of the defect is first undermined and dissected from bone. A relaxing incision is then made in the pulp of the fingertip to facilitate greater movement of the flap into the defect. Back-stitches (passed from nail bed to nail plate) are used to raise the flap above the remaining nail plate, thereby reconstructing the lateral nail wall. The secondary defect heals by second intention.[61]

LARGER DEFECTS OF THE DISTAL DIGIT

The surgeon has several options for reconstruction of the distal digit following conservative excision of subungual malignancy. Second intention healing is a viable option, but may require several months to restore functionality. Full-thickness skin grafting, probably the most common technique, is associated with good functionality and acceptable cosmesis.[70,76,77] Grafts are typically harvested from the inner arm or groin, and may be performed immediately or delayed until a final pathology report confirms complete excision.[78,79] A bolster dressing sutured to the surgical site and left in place for 1 week helps promote apposition and protects the healing wound from injury. A less frequently used technique is the reversed dermal graft, in which a donor graft is stripped of its epidermis and sutured into place on the defect upside-down, allowing the richly vascularized superficial dermis to improve the chances for successful take. The exposed deep dermis is left to heal by second intention or split-thickness skin graft.[61] Split-thickness skin grafts alone do not provide much protection for the distal digit, and color and texture matching can be problematic.[70] Split-thickness toenail bed grafts, free nail grafts and free vascularized nail transfers, more

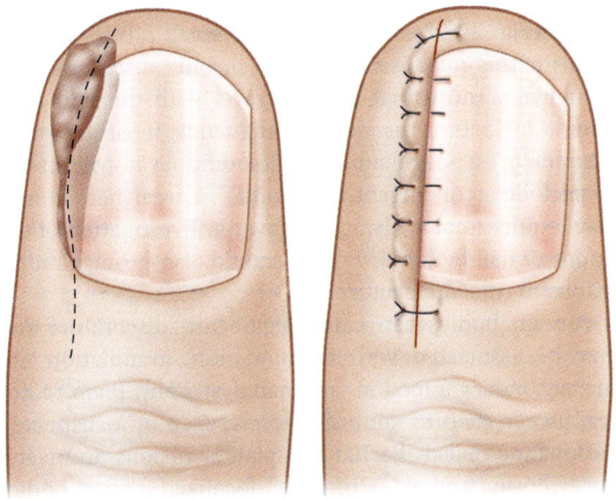

Figure 22-22 Bipedicled lateral nail wall flap.

commonly described in the plastic surgery literature for repair of congenital or traumatic defects, require considerable technical expertise and are associated with significant donor-site morbidity and variable success rates.[80–82]

Transposition flaps, although potentially more time-intensive and intimidating to both the patient and the surgeon, are associated with good functional and cosmetic outcomes. The cross-finger flap is the most commonly used by dermatologic surgeons for thumb and index finger defects.[70,83,84] It is typically performed as a two- or three-staged interpolation flap procedure. A full-thickness flap of appropriate size is incised in the volar aspect of an adjacent digit. It is left in place for up to 10 days to "train" the flap, and then transposed to cover the primary defect. Takedown of the pedicle is performed 2 to 3 weeks after the transposition, and a full-thickness skin graft used to repair the secondary defect.[61] The flag flap[85] and Foucher island flap[86] are single-stage procedures favored by some hand surgeons for distal digit reconstruction.

INDICATIONS FOR SURGERY

The most common indications for surgery of the nail unit are to diagnose and treat benign or malignant neoplasms, to relieve patient discomfort and to improve cosmesis. The nail unit is a compact anatomical space bound on one side by a relatively hard, keratinized nail plate. Any space-occupying lesion, particularly of the nail bed, can be extremely painful and lead to deformity of the nail plate by exerting pressure on the matrix or the plate itself.

TRAUMA AND HEMORRHAGE

Subungual hematomas resulting from injury to the nail bed appear as red to purple or black discolorations beneath the nail plate. Typically, the patient can provide a history of recent trauma. Hematomas can be exquisitely painful in the acute setting. Trephination, the creation of a small opening in the nail plate to relieve pressure and allow escape of subungual material, is the treatment of choice (Fig. 22-23). A #11 blade or small punch may be used for this purpose. For more chronic discolorations, particularly those that do not travel with the nail as it grows, melanoma or other malignancy must be ruled out. The presence of subungual blood does not necessarily exclude a concurrent melanoma.[87] Larger hematomas may require total avulsion to allow for investigation of the extent of nail bed injury. They should also prompt radiographs to rule out fracture.

Foreign bodies can cause significant discomfort and may be associated with inflammation, granulation tissue, secondary infection, and nail dystrophy. Plain radiographs can help to confirm the presence of a suspected radiopaque object. Partial nail plate avulsions are useful for exploring and extracting well-localized foreign bodies in the nail bed.[43] The surgeon must take care when suturing the nail plate not to implant foreign bodies in the form of keratin fragments in the nail bed, which may result in granuloma formation.

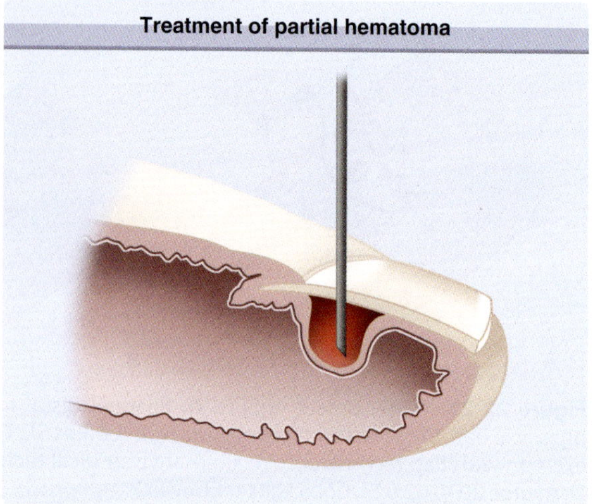

Figure 22-23 Trephination of subungual hematoma. (Reproduced with permission from Goldsmith LA, Katz SI, Gilchrest BA, Paller AS, Leffell DJ, Wolff K. *Fitzpatrick's Dermatology in General Medicine.* 8th ed. McGraw-Hill, Inc.; 2012. Fig. 245-14. Copyright © McGraw-Hill Education LLC.)

INFECTIONS AND PARONYCHIA

Nail unit infections are frequently preceded by trauma to the nail fold or cuticle, which enables microorganism inoculation. Acute paronychia, an inflammatory reaction of the nail folds, is most commonly caused by *Staphylococcus* species. Incision and drainage is indicated if an abscess is present. Trephination or partial avulsion can help to relieve pain and allow drainage of infections unresponsive to oral antibiotics alone.[88] A culture should be performed to guide oral antibiotic coverage, if indicated. Twice-daily antimicrobial soaks are also recommended.

CP is often associated with nail dystrophy. It is commonly seen in people whose jobs involve wet work, such as dishwashers, launderers, and bartenders. *Candida* species may be isolated from the nail, but their role in the pathogenesis of CP is unclear.[89,90] In one double-blind study, topical steroids were found to be a more effective treatment than systemic antifungals, suggesting that CP may be more correctly thought of as a type of hand dermatitis caused by environmental exposures rather than a form of onychomycosis.[91] Intralesional corticosteroids may also be beneficial.[19] En bloc excision of the PNF with nail avulsion is an effective treatment for recalcitrant cases.[92]

True onychomycosis is caused by dermatophyte infection. It is frequently characterized by subungual hyperkeratosis, onycholysis, dystrophy, and dyschromia of the nail plate. A simple nail clipping with subungual keratotic material submitted for PAS staining is the most sensitive diagnostic test.[93] Occasionally, partial avulsion or punch biopsy may be required for diagnosis of more proximal infections. Topical treatment is extremely challenging, and avulsion does not appear to improve success rates.[94] Dark brown to black pigmentation due to pigmented mycoses or reactive melanocytes occasionally mimics the LM caused by melanoma or benign melanocytic neoplasms.

INFLAMMATORY DISEASES

Intralesional corticosteroid injections are an effective treatment for nail dystrophy associated with inflammatory conditions like psoriasis, lichen planus, and CP.[95] A 30 gauge needle is introduced into the PNF, angled toward the nail plate, and 0.05 to 0.1 mL of corticosteroid (usually triamcinolone, 2.5–10 mg/mL) is injected to create a dermal wheal over the matrix. This may be repeated two or three times per nail to cover the entire PNF. The use of a refrigerant spray immediately before injection reduces patient discomfort.[19] Injections are continued monthly for a few months until normal nail begins to form, then tapered in frequency.

INGROWN NAILS

Ingrown nails, also known as onychocryptosis, are a common problem, particularly among adolescents and young adults. The most common variety is the "distal–lateral" ingrowing nail, in which the obliquely-trimmed lateral edges of the nail plate become embedded in the distal–lateral nail grooves (Fig. 22-24). This results in a foreign body reaction characterized by inflammation, granulation tissue, and secondary infection. The choice of treatment depends on the degree of inflammation and induration of the LNF.[96] Taping the LNF is a common conservative approach effective in mild cases, but requires excellent patient adherence.[97] Surgical tape is applied obliquely in a proximal–lateral direction to the LNF, thereby pulling it away from the lateral edge of the nail plate (Fig. 22-25). Packing the lateral nail groove with a small wisp of cotton is another conservative modality for separating the LNF and nail plate.[98] The "gutter treatment," performed under local anesthesia, entails the placement of a piece of sterile plastic tubing, cut lengthwise, over the entire length of the lateral nail margin.[99] The tubing is secured with stitches, tape, or acrylic glue and left in place for 6 to 12 weeks. Steel, plastic, or alloy nail braces to flatten the nail plate are sometimes used by podiatrists, based on the theory that over-curvature is a major etiologic factor.[96,100]

Surgical treatment of ingrown nails is generally associated with lower recurrence rates, particularly in more severe cases.[45] The prevailing approach is excision or chemical destruction of the lateral matrix, which results in a narrowing of the nail plate (Figs. 22-18 and 22-26). Phenol matrix cauterization, described in detail previously, may be more effective than excision in preventing recurrence.[101,102] Particular care must be taken to completely excise or destroy the lateral matrix horns to prevent recurrence or nail spicule formation. Isolated reports of high rates of infection and other complications associated with phenolization have not been supported by meta-analysis.[45] Partial matricectomy by CO_2 laser ablation, with or without concomitant LNF vaporization, is an increasingly popular treatment modality, although reported recurrence rates vary widely.[67,103,104] Other surgeons eschew matricectomy in favor of resection of the overgrown lateral borders of the nail.[105] Proponents of this technique, which leaves the nail width unaltered, cite improved cosmesis and fewer complications.[106] However, this approach may be associated with higher recurrence rates, perhaps due to a failure to address the primary etiology of the ingrowing nail.[64,96]

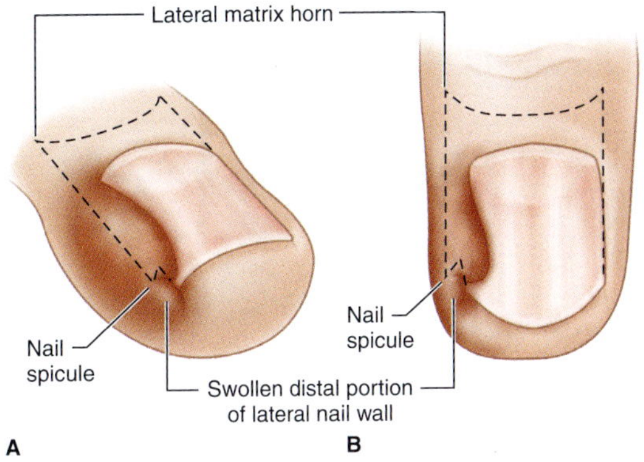

Figure 22-24 Distal–lateral ingrowing nail. **A.** Nail spicule embedded in swollen distal lateral nail fold **B.** Nail spicule almost completely engulfed by swollen lateral nail fold tissue. (Adapted with permission from Haneke E. Controversies in the treatment of ingrown nails. *Dermatol Res Pract.* 2012;2012:783924. Copyright © 2012 Eckart Haneke.)

SPLIT NAILS

Split-nail deformity most commonly results from sharp or blunt trauma to the matrix, resulting in a scarred segment unable to produce normal nail plate.[107] Neoplasms of the distal phalanx, nail bed, matrix, or plate may also lead to

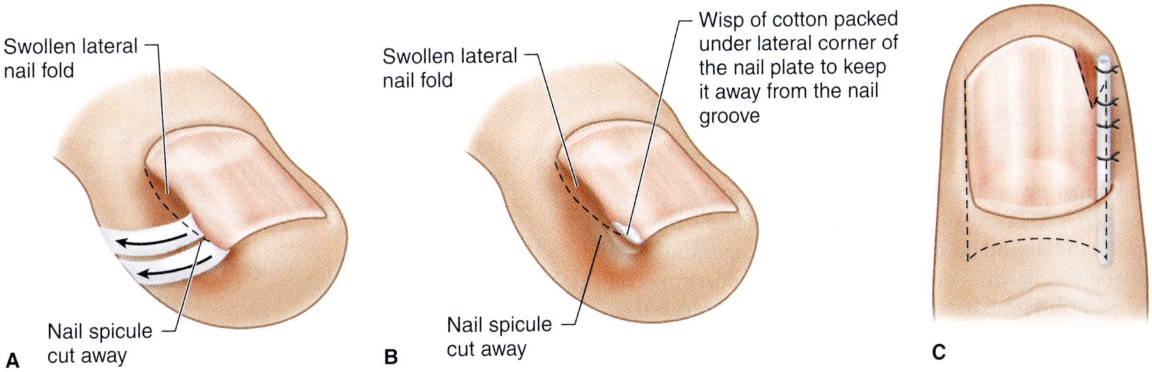

Figure 22-25 Conservative management of ingrown nails. **A.** Taping. **B.** Cotton packing. **C.** Gutter treatment. (Adapted with permission from Haneke E. Controversies in the treatment of ingrown nails. *Dermatol Res Pract.* 2012;2012:783924. Copyright © 2012 Eckart Haneke.)

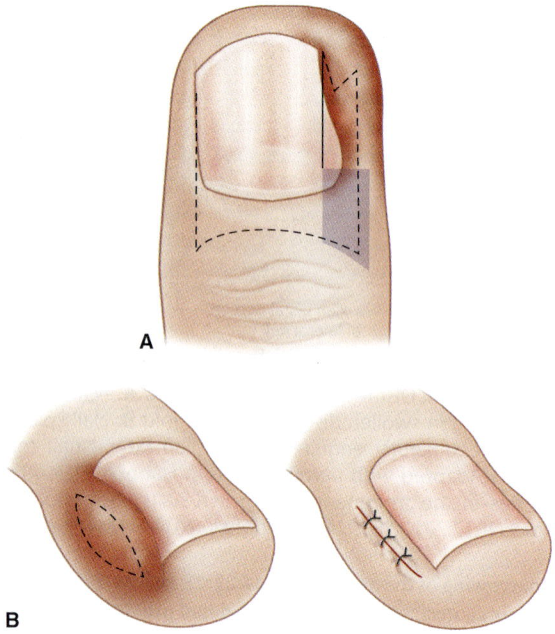

Figure 22-26 Surgical management of ingrown nails. **A.** Selective lateral matrix horn resection. **B.** Reduction of the lateral nail fold by fusiform incision. (Adapted with permission from Haneke E. Controversies in the treatment of ingrown nails. *Dermatol Res Pract.* 2012;2012:783924. Copyright © 2012 Eckart Haneke.)

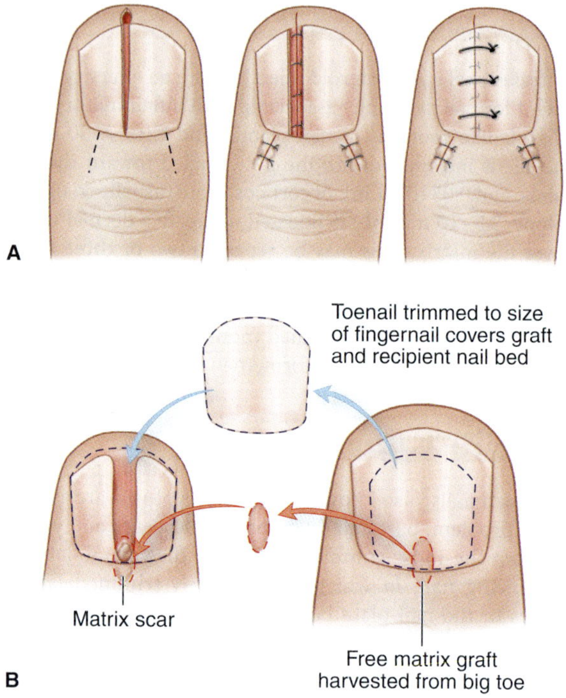

Figure 22-27 **A.** Classical method of split nail repair. **B.** Free matrix graft from the big-toenail may be used for wider defects.

a split nail, as can biopsy or other iatrogenic manipulation of the matrix. An understanding of the specific etiology of the deformity in each case is absolutely essential to reduce the risk of recurrence. Optimal surgical repair, described in more detail previously, hinges on careful excision of the scarred portion of matrix and meticulous reconstruction (Fig. 22-27). The narrowest matrix defects may be closed primarily with absorbable sutures. However, the creation of matrix flaps may be necessary to eliminate tension on the wound and reduce the risk of additional scarring.[58] Wide undermining of the nail bed just above the periosteum facilitates reapproximation and suturing of the bed and the two remaining nail plate fragments (if not avulsed). For wider defects on the fingernail, a free matrix graft from the big-toenail can be performed.[61] If the recipient nail plate has been totally avulsed, the trimmed toenail plate or a piece of surgical tubing can be used as a splint.

PINCER NAILS

Pincer-nail deformity describes a transverse over-curvature of the nail plate most frequently affecting the toenails of young adults. In the "common" variety, the aperture of the curving nail narrows distally, pinching the underlying nail bed and causing inflammation and often severe pain (Fig. 22-28). Symmetric congenital pincer nails are due to inherited anomalies of the distal phalanges, while acquired disease is commonly due to deformation of the foot with deviation of the phalanges due to ill-fitting shoes, chronic conditions such as psoriasis and osteoarthritis, or neoplasms of the nail unit such as exostoses or cysts.[47] Recurrence following surgical or conservative treatment is all but assured if the underlying abnormality is not corrected. Plain radiographs can be helpful in identifying causative bony anomalies. One effective surgical approach involves bilateral partial avulsion of the nail plate followed by permanent excision or chemical destruction of the lateral matrix horns.[19,47] This may also be achieved with CO_2 laser.[51] The nail plate is then shortened to allow dissection of the nail bed from the phalanx and removal of osteophytes with a bone rongeur prior to closure. Reverse-tie sutures in the LNF help

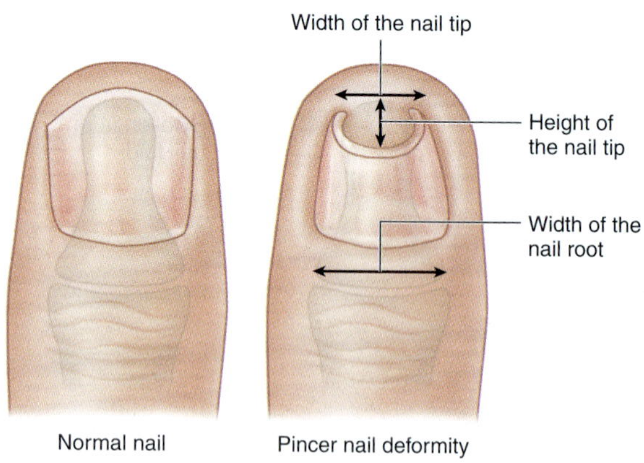

Figure 22-28 Pincer-nail deformity. (Adapted with permission from Mutaf M, Sunay M, Isk D. A new surgical technique for the correction of pincer nail deformity. *Ann Plast Surg.* 2007;58:496.)

to stretch the nail bed. An alternate, matrix-preserving approach includes total avulsion followed by insertion of dermal grafts under the lateral edges of the dissected nail bed and matrix to widen and flatten the nail unit.[108] The use of a modified five-flap Z-plasty technique to correct the nail bed shape has also been described.[109] In most instances, simple lateral matrix horn chemical matricectomy is used, with predictable success.

ONYCHAUXIS AND ONYCHOGRYPHOSIS

Onychauxis, or thickening of the nail plate, and onychogryphosis, or gross hyperkeratosis coupled with increased curvature of the nail, are common among the elderly. They are frequently associated with neglect, poor nail grooming, and ill-fitting footwear, as well as trauma, onychomycosis, and psoriasis. Idiopathic, congenital, and acquired cases involving the toenails are not uncommon. Fingernail involvement is rare. Periodic nail grinding can provide symptomatic relief, but recurrence is common. The most effective, lasting treatment of nail thickening that originates in the matrix is surgical shortening of the matrix length. Following proximal avulsion, the distal one-third of the matrix is removed with a crescentic excision that parallels the curvature of the lunula.[110] Severe onychogryphosis may require complete matricectomy.[111]

RACQUET NAILS

Racquet nails, or brachyonychia, is an autosomal-dominant inherited deformity characterized by wide nail plates. It most commonly affects the thumbs in women, and may be associated with conditions such as the Rubinstein–Taybi syndrome.[112] Surgical treatment options are similar to those for other causes of ingrown nails: partial matricectomy to narrow the plate or resection of the LNFs.

BENIGN TUMORS

Benign tumors of the nail unit can cause nail deformity and significant discomfort. Surgical excision or destruction is indicated to relieve pain, improve cosmesis, and prevent recurrence of the deformity. The surgical approach will depend upon the nail structure(s) involved. Benign tumors of the nail folds can generally be excised by the same approaches used in other cutaneous surgeries. Small spindle-shaped excisions performed in this region heal well by second intention. When excising PNF tumors, a Freer elevator inserted under the nail fold can protect the underlying matrix from trauma.[1] Excision of nail bed and matrix tumors is more challenging. A few of the more commonly encountered benign neoplasms of the nail bed are glomus tumors, periungual warts, pyogenic granulomas, epidermal cysts, myxoid cysts, onychopapillomas, fibromas, and exostoses. Rarer tumors include enchondromas and osteochondromas. Some benign tumors, like pyogenic granulomas, can mimic subungual melanoma.[113] Periungual warts may be impossible to distinguish clinically from SCC. Plain radiographs can aid in the diagnosis of bony neoplasms, whereas MRI may help to differentiate soft tissue and cystic lesions and better define the contours of a tumor prior to surgery.[10] Partial and trapdoor avulsions are helpful conservative techniques that facilitate treatment of localized nail bed tumors. Punch biopsy is often sufficient to remove smaller lesions, whereas elliptical, crescentic, or wedge excisions may be required for larger lesions. A bone rongeur is useful for removal of bony or cartilaginous tumors. Repair of associated deformities such as split nails, pincer nails, or ingrown nails may be required. Destructive modalities such as CO_2 laser and cryotherapy should be used with caution as they do not permit histopathologic exclusion of malignancy.

NONMELANOMA SKIN CANCERS

SCC and Bowen's disease are the most common malignancies affecting the nail folds, hyponychium, and most commonly, nail bed. Clinically, SCC may be indistinguishable from HPV-associated periungual and subungual warts, which can delay diagnosis for years if destructive treatment modalities are repeated without biopsy (Fig. 22-29).[114] Subungual tumors may also present with erythronychia, leukonychia, melanonychia, hyperkeratosis, paronychia, mild onycholysis, or nail

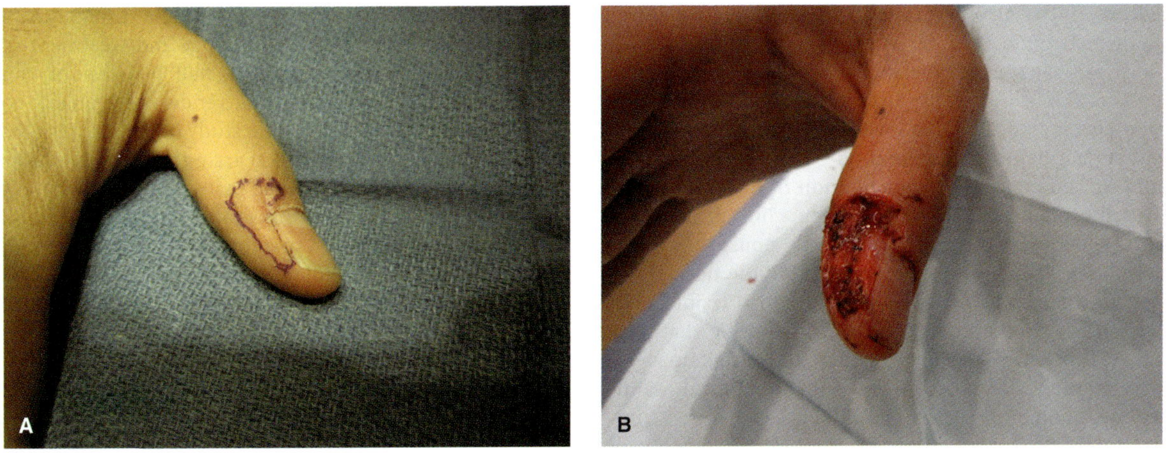

Figure 22-29 Periungual SCC (**A**) before and (**B**) after excision.

plate destruction. Most cases are invasive at the time of diagnosis, including up to 60% of longstanding cases with bony involvement requiring amputation of the distal phalanx.[115,116] Unfortunately, the sensitivity of radiographic evaluation for bony involvement is unclear.[117,118] MMS, one of the preferred treatment modalities, may reduce amputations by enabling histopathologic examination of the deep and peripheral margins of a tumor.[119] Reported cure rates with MMS approach 96% for tumors not involving the bone.[120] However, long-term follow-up data is lacking, and reported recurrence rates approach 20% (compared to 3% for other cutaneous SCC).[114] If MMS is not available, wide surgical excision is associated with a low risk of relapse.[116] Radiation therapy has been proposed as a possible alternative to distal phalanx amputation, but experience and follow-up is limited.[121–123] Data is also lacking on the efficacy of photodynamic therapy (PDT) and topical therapies such as 5-fluorouracil and imiquimod.

Basal cell carcinoma (BCC), the most common malignancy worldwide, is exceedingly rare in the nail unit. It frequently presents with ulceration, but like SCC, may clinically resemble a number of benign neoplasms, inflammatory conditions, and infections.[124] Shave biopsy is typically adequate for diagnosis.[125] MMS is the most common treatment modality. Repairs described in the literature include second intention healing and full-thickness skin grafts.[126] Other rare malignancies of the nail unit include Kaposi's sarcoma, Merkel cell carcinoma, and metastases, most commonly from lung, kidney, and breast cancers. In nearly half of reported cases, subungual metastases were the presenting sign of the primary malignancy.[127] Once confirmed by biopsy, excision may theoretically be performed for symptomatic solitary lesions. However, metastases typically involve the bone, affect multiple digits, and portend a very poor prognosis.

MELANOCYTIC LESIONS AND LONGITUDINAL MELANONYCHIA

Subungual melanoma is a rare form of acral lentiginous melanoma arising from the nail matrix. It makes up less than 4% of all melanoma subtypes, but up to 20% of melanomas in Black, Asian, and Native American populations.[76] It is also associated with a poorer prognosis than melanoma of other sites, likely due to delays in diagnosis. Subungual melanoma most commonly presents as LM, a sign with a broad differential diagnosis that also includes benign melanocytic lesions as well as subungual hemorrhage, mycotic or bacterial infection, and Bowen's disease.[56] Pigmentation of the nail fold, or Hutchinson's sign, should heighten clinical suspicion for melanoma, but is also a relatively nonspecific finding.[59] Several algorithms exist to guide the dermatologist in the management of pigmented nail lesions (Fig. 22-30).[57,128] However, it is also worth noting that anywhere from 15% to 65% of subungual melanomas are amelanotic.[129] Dermoscopy can enhance clinical examination, but a biopsy is required if there is the least clinical suspicion for malignancy. Longitudinal, punch, and shave techniques have been described. Each of these techniques may be used to excise the lesion completely at the time of biopsy for complete histopathologic evaluation. Punch or shave biopsies may be associated with less residual nail dystrophy.[56,57]

Current trends in the surgical management of nail melanoma favor conservative, tissue-sparing approaches over traditional wide surgical excision or amputation when possible. "En bloc" excisions and MMS are most commonly performed for nail melanoma in situ (MIS). Recommendations for appropriate margins in "en bloc" excisions vary from 2 to 10 mm around all nail structures.[70,76] MMS has the advantage of complete margin analysis, but is not as well-studied.[83,130] Amputation at the PIP or DIP joint (or interphalangeal joint of the thumb) is still the predominant treatment for invasive nail melanoma, but some authors have begun to cast doubt on any survival benefit over local excision.[70,85,131–133] In every case, but particularly in those with tumors located on the thumb and index finger, a detailed discussion of treatment options, including digit-sparing versus amputation surgeries, should be initiated with the patient and family. Excision with clear margins remains the most important goal of surgery, and patients must guide the surgeon's decision, with an understanding of the pros and cons of each technique, as well as postoperative sequelae.

COMPLICATIONS

Complications of nail surgery are infrequent, but similar to those associated with other dermatologic surgeries, namely pain, bleeding, infection, scarring, and recurrence. A recent patient survey identified sensory disturbance, including paresthesias and cold intolerance, as a potentially under-recognized complication.[134] Reports of digital necrosis due to epinephrine, well-enshrined in surgical lore, are exceedingly rare to nonexistent in more recent large-scale retrospective studies.[14,15] Preoperative and postoperative hygienic soaks for ingrown toenail surgery, while commonly practiced, are of unclear benefit in reducing postoperative infection, and oral antibiotics are not routinely indicated, except in immunosuppressed patients or those with artificial heart valves or prosthetic joints.[39,45]

Nail dystrophy caused by iatrogenic trauma is a unique aspect of nail surgery. Biopsy and treatment of nail matrix, and less frequently, nail bed lesions can result in scarring of the matrix, rendering it unable to produce normal nail plate. One study of nail procedures cited a 22% rate of residual scarring and dystrophy.[135] Split nails, pincer nails, hooked nails, or misaligned nails have all been reported.[55] Surgical corrections of these deformities are discussed previously. Nail dystrophy can cause significant psychological distress, which may be lessened by preoperative discussion of risks and patient expectations.[135,136]

Incomplete excision or destruction of the lateral matrix horns during matricectomy can result in postoperative spicules or cysts.[55] This risk is increased in cases involving the big toe, where the matrix horns extend more

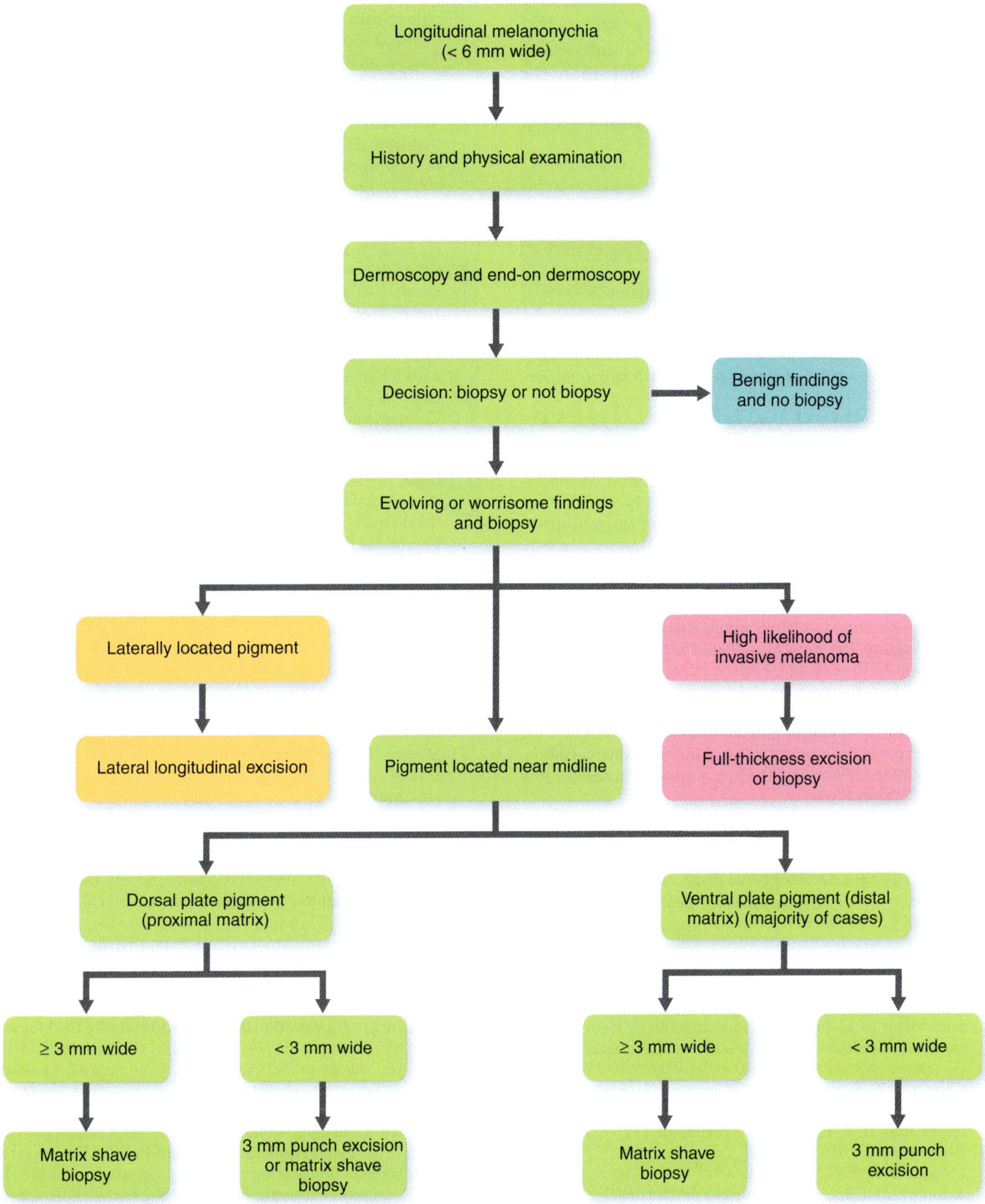

Figure 22-30 A proposed algorithm for approach to biopsy of longitudinal melanonychia. (Adapted with permission from Jellinek N. Nail matrix biopsy of longitudinal melanonychia: diagnostic algorithm including the matrix shave biopsy. *J Am Acad Dermatol*. 2007;56:803. Copyright © Elsevier.)

laterally.[54] Phenol cauterization has rarely been associated with excessive tissue necrosis, persistent exudative drainage, and periostitis.[137] Other potential surgical complications include injury to the extensor tendon during en bloc nail excision, which can be avoided if the surgeon is aware of its relationship to the proximal matrix.[70] Excess thermal damage to the nail matrix or bed from a CO_2 laser can cause the same nail dystrophies as the cut of a scalpel.

CONCLUSION

Surgical procedures are an essential component of the diagnosis and treatment of neoplastic, infectious, and inflammatory conditions of the nail unit. A detailed understanding of nail anatomy, thorough preoperative evaluation, and thoughtful attention to patient comfort allow the surgeon to maximize results while minimizing postoperative deformity and dysfunction. Procedures involving the germinative matrix must be approached with particular care. Nail unit repairs pose an interesting and potentially gratifying challenge, drawing upon the surgeon's familiarity with previously described approaches and ability to improvise to suit the specific needs of each individual patient.

REFERENCES

1. Rich P. Nail biopsy: indications and methods. *Dermatol Surg.* 2001;27:229.
2. de Berker D, Mawhinney B, Sviland L. Quantification of regional matrix nail production. *Br J Dermatol.* 1996;134:1083.
3. Fleckman P, Allan C. Surgical anatomy of the nail unit. *Dermatol Surg.* 2001;27:257.
4. Bordeaux JS, Martires KJ, Goldberg D, Pattee SF, Fu P, Maloney ME. Prospective evaluation of dermatologic surgery complications including patients on multiple antiplatelet and anticoagulant medications. *J Am Acad Dermatol.* 2011;65:576.
5. Billingsley EM, Maloney ME. Intraoperative and postoperative bleeding problems in patients taking warfarin, aspirin, and nonsteroidal antiinflammatory agents. A prospective study. *Dermatol Surg.* 1997;23:381.
6. Lewis KG, Dufresne RG Jr. A meta-analysis of complications attributed to anticoagulation among patients following cutaneous surgery. *Dermatol Surg.* 2008;34:160.
7. Tonnesen H, Rosenberg J, Nielsen HJ, et al. Effect of preoperative abstinence on poor postoperative outcome in alcohol misusers: randomised controlled trial. *BMJ.* 1999;318:1311.
8. Sorensen LT. Wound healing and infection in surgery: the pathophysiological impact of smoking, smoking cessation, and nicotine replacement therapy: a systematic review. *Ann Surg.* 2012;255:1069.
9. Heistein JB, Cook PA. Factors affecting composite graft survival in digital tip amputations. *Ann Plast Surg.* 2003;50:299.
10. Goettmann S, Drape JL, Idy-Peretti I, et al. Magnetic resonance imaging: a new tool in the diagnosis of tumours of the nail apparatus. *Br J Dermatol.* 1994;130:701.
11. Ravitskiy L, Phillips PK, Roenigk RK, et al. The use of oral midazolam for perioperative anxiolysis of healthy patients undergoing Mohs surgery: conclusions from randomized controlled and prospective studies. *J Am Acad Dermatol.* 2011;64:310.
12. Otley CC, Nguyen TH, Phillips PK. Anxiolysis with oral midazolam in pediatric patients undergoing dermatologic surgical procedures. *J Am Acad Dermatol.* 2001;45:105.
13. Haneke E. Nail surgery. *Eur J Dermatol.* 2000;10:237.
14. Chowdhry S, Seidenstricker L, Cooney DS, Hazani R, Wilhelmi BJ. Do not use epinephrine in digital blocks: myth or truth? Part II. A retrospective review of 1111 cases. *Plast Reconstr Surg.* 2010;126:2031.
15. Lalonde D, Bell M, Benoit P, Sparkes G, Denkler K, Chang P. A multicenter prospective study of 3,110 consecutive cases of elective epinephrine use in the fingers and hand: the Dalhousie Project clinical phase. *J Hand Surg Am.* 2005;30:1061.
16. Krunic AL, Wang LC, Soltani K, Weitzul S, Taylor RS. Digital anesthesia with epinephrine: an old myth revisited. *J Am Acad Dermatol.* 2004;51:755.
17. Wilhelmi BJ, Blackwell SJ, Miller JH, et al. Do not use epinephrine in digital blocks: myth or truth? *Plast Reconstr Surg.* 2001;107:393.
18. Firoz B, Davis N, Goldberg LH. Local anesthesia using buffered 0.5% lidocaine with 1:200,000 epinephrine for tumors of the digits treated with Mohs micrographic surgery. *J Am Acad Dermatol.* 2009;61:639.
19. Jellinek NJ. Nail surgery: practical tips and treatment options. *Dermatol Ther.* 2007;20:68.
20. Keramidas EG, Rodopoulou SG. Ropivacaine versus lidocaine in digital nerve blocks: a prospective study. *Plast Reconstr Surg.* 2007;119:2148.
21. Watts AC, McEachan J. The use of a fine-gauge needle to reduce pain in open carpal tunnel decompression: a randomized controlled trial. *J Hand Surg Br.* 2005;30:615.
22. Tomlinson PJ, Field J. Warm or refrigerated local anaesthetic for open carpal tunnel release: a single blind randomized controlled study. *J Hand Surg Eur Vol.* 2010;35:232.
23. Vossinakis IC, Stavroulaki P, Paleochorlidis I, Badras LS. Reducing the pain associated with local anaesthetic infiltration for open carpal tunnel decompression. *J Hand Surg Br.* 2004;29:399.
24. Baran R. Nail surgery. In: Wolff K, Goldsmith LA, Katz SI, et al., eds. *Fitzpatrick's Dermatology in General Medicine.* 7th ed. New York, NY: McGraw-Hill; 2008:2320.
25. Scher RK. Biopsy of the matrix of a nail. *J Dermatol Surg Oncol.* 1980;6:19.
26. Haneke E. Surgical anatomy of the nail apparatus. *Dermatol Clin.* 2006;24:291.
27. Chiu DT. Transthecal digital block: flexor tendon sheath used for anesthetic infusion. *J Hand Surg Am.* 1990;15:471.
28. Low CK, Vartany A, Engstrom JW, Poncelet A, Diao E. Comparison of transthecal and subcutaneous single-injection digital block techniques. *J Hand Surg Am.* 1997;22:901.
29. Yin ZG, Zhang JB, Kan SL, Wang P. A comparison of traditional digital blocks and single subcutaneous palmar injection blocks at the base of the finger and a meta-analysis of the digital block trials. *J Hand Surg Br.* 2006;31:547.
30. Keramidas EG, Rodopoulou SG, Tsoutsos D, Miller G, Ioannovich J. Comparison of transthecal digital block and traditional digital block for anesthesia of the finger. *Plast Reconstr Surg.* 2004;114:1131.
31. Williams JG, Lalonde DH. Randomized comparison of the single-injection volar subcutaneous block and the two-injection dorsal block for digital anesthesia. *Plast Reconstr Surg.* 2006;118:1195.
32. De Berker DA, Langtry J. Treatment of subungual exostoses by elective day case surgery. *Br J Dermatol.* 1999;140:915.
33. Sniezek PJ, Brodland DG, Zitelli JA. A randomized controlled trial comparing acetaminophen, acetaminophen and ibuprofen, and acetaminophen and codeine for postoperative pain relief after Mohs surgery and cutaneous reconstruction. *Dermatol Surg.* 2011;37:1007.
34. Toms L, Derry S, Moore RA, McQuay HJ. Single dose oral paracetamol (acetaminophen) with codeine for postoperative pain in adults. *Cochrane Database Syst Rev.* 2009;(1):CD001547.
35. Gaskell H, Derry S, Moore RA, McQuay HJ. Single dose oral oxycodone and oxycodone plus paracetamol (acetaminophen) for acute postoperative pain in adults. *Cochrane Database Syst Rev.* 2009;(3):CD002763.
36. McGinness JL, Parlette HL III. Versatile sterile field for nail surgery using a sterile glove. *Dermatol Online J.* 2005;11:10.
37. Ng AB, Adeyemo FO, Samarji R. Preoperative footbaths reduce bacterial colonization of the foot. *Foot Ankle Int.* 2009; 30:860.
38. Becerro de Bengoa Vallejo R, Losa Iglesias ME, Alou Cervera L, Sevillano Fernández D, Prieto Prieto J. Preoperative skin and nail preparation of the foot: comparison of the efficacy of 4 different methods in reducing bacterial load. *J Am Acad Dermatol.* 2009;61:986.
39. Wright TI, Baddour LM, Berbari EF, et al. Antibiotic prophylaxis in dermatologic surgery: advisory statement 2008. *J Am Acad Dermatol.* 2008;59:464.
40. Hixson FP, Shafiroff BB, Werner FW, Palmer AK. Digital tourniquets: a pressure study with clinical relevance. *J Hand Surg Am.* 1986;11:865.
41. Naim S, Srinivasan MS. Digital tourniquets: a comparative analysis of pressures and pain perception. *Acta Orthop Belg.* 2008;74:195.
42. Smith IM, Austin OM, Knight SL. A simple and fail safe method for digital tourniquet. *J Hand Surg Br.* 2002;27:363.
43. Collins SC, Cordova K, Jellinek NJ. Alternatives to complete nail plate avulsion. *J Am Acad Dermatol.* 2008;59:619.
44. Ozawa T, Yabe T, Ohashi N, Harada T, Muraoka M, Ishii M. A splint for pincer nail surgery: a convenient splinting device made of an aspiration tube. *Dermatol Surg.* 2005;31:94.

45. Eekhof JA, Van Wijk B, Knuistingh Neven A, van der Wouden JC. Interventions for ingrowing toenails. *Cochrane Database Syst Rev.* 2012;4:CD001541.
46. Arai H, Arai T, Nakajima H, Haneke E. Formable acrylic treatment for ingrowing nail with gutter splint and sculptured nail. *Int J Dermatol.* 2004;43:759.
47. Baran R, Haneke E, Richert B. Pincer nails: definition and surgical treatment. *Dermatol Surg.* 2001;27:261.
48. Albom MJ. Surgical gems: avulsion of a nail plate. *J Dermatol Surg Oncol.* 1977;3:34.
49. Boyce S, Huang CC. Surgical Pearl: hemostat-assisted nail avulsion revisited. *J Am Acad Dermatol.* 2001;45:943.
50. Miller PK, Roenigk RK. Diagnostic and therapeutic nail surgery. *J Dermatol Surg Oncol.* 1991;17:674.
51. Lane JE, Peterson CM, Ratz JL. Avulsion and partial matricectomy with the carbon dioxide laser for pincer nail deformity. *Dermatol Surg.* 2004;30:456.
52. Baran R, Tosti A. Chemical avulsion with urea nail lacquer. *J Dermatolog Treat.* 2002;13:161.
53. Scher RK. Punch biopsies of nails: a simple, valuable procedure. *J Dermatol Surg Oncol.* 1978;4:528.
54. Jellinek NJ, Rubin AI. Lateral longitudinal excision of the nail unit. *Dermatol Surg.* 2011;37:1781.
55. Moossavi M, Scher RK. Complications of nail surgery: a review of the literature. *Dermatol Surg.* 2001;27:225.
56. Haneke E, Baran R. Longitudinal melanonychia. *Dermatol Surg.* 2001;27:580.
57. Jellinek N. Nail matrix biopsy of longitudinal melanonychia: diagnostic algorithm including the matrix shave biopsy. *J Am Acad Dermatol.* 2007;56:803.
58. Collins SC, Cordova KB, Jellinek NJ. Midline/paramedian longitudinal matrix excision with flap reconstruction: alternative surgical techniques for evaluation of longitudinal melanonychia. *J Am Acad Dermatol.* 2010;62:627.
59. Baran R, Kechijian P. Hutchinson's sign: a reappraisal. *J Am Acad Dermatol.* 1996;34:87.
60. Di Chiacchio N, Loureiro WR, Michalany NS, Kezam Gabriel FV. Tangential biopsy thickness versus lesion depth in longitudinal melanonychia: a pilot study. *Dermatol Res Pract.* 2012;2012:353864.
61. Haneke E. Advanced nail surgery. *J Cutan Aesthet Surg.* 2011;4:167.
62. Siegle RJ, Harkness J, Swanson NA. Phenol alcohol technique for permanent matricectomy. *Arch Dermatol.* 1984;120:348.
63. Becerro de Bengoa Vallejo R, Losa Iglesias ME, Viejo Tirado F, Serrano Pardo R. Cauterization of the germinal nail matrix using phenol applications of differing durations: a histologic study. *J Am Acad Dermatol.* 2012;67:706–711.
64. Rounding C, Bloomfield S. Surgical treatments for ingrowing toenails. *Cochrane Database Syst Rev.* 2005;(2):CD001541.
65. Kim SH, Ko HC, Oh CK, Kwon KS, Kim MB. Trichloroacetic acid matricectomy in the treatment of ingrowing toenails. *Dermatol Surg.* 2009;35:973.
66. Bostanci S, Kocyigit P, Gurgey E. Comparison of phenol and sodium hydroxide chemical matricectomies for the treatment of ingrowing toenails. *Dermatol Surg.* 2007;33:680.
67. Yang KC, Li YT. Treatment of recurrent ingrown great toenail associated with granulation tissue by partial nail avulsion followed by matricectomy with sharpulse carbon dioxide laser. *Dermatol Surg.* 2002;28:419.
68. Serour F. Recurrent ingrown big toenails are efficiently treated by CO_2 laser. *Dermatol Surg.* 2002;28:509.
69. Haneke E. Nail surgery. In: Robinson J, Hanke CW, Siegel D, et al., eds. *Surgery of the Skin.* Edinburgh: Elsevier; 2010.
70. Jellinek NJ, Bauer JH. En bloc excision of the nail. *Dermatol Surg.* 2010;36:1445.
71. Reardon CM, McArthur PA, Survana SK, Brotherston TM. The surface anatomy of the germinal matrix of the nail bed in the finger. *J Hand Surg Br.* 1999;24:531.
72. Schernberg F, Ameil M. [Local rotational flap of the nail]. *Handchir Mikrochir Plast Chir.* 1987;19:259.
73. Bali D, Casanova D, Aharoni C, Mutaftschiev N, Cilirie K, Legré R. [Longitudinal melanic nail bands (melanonychia): report of 22 cases]. *Chir Main.* 2002;21:225.
74. Antony AK, Anagnos DP. Matrix-periosteal flaps for reconstruction of nail deformity. *Plast Reconstr Surg.* 2002;109:1663.
75. Johnson RK. Nailplasty. *Plast Reconstr Surg.* 1971;47:275.
76. Sureda N, Phan A, Poulalhon N, Balme B, Dalle S, Thomas L. Conservative surgical management of subungual (matrix derived) melanoma: report of seven cases and literature review. *Br J Dermatol.* 2011;165:852.
77. Clarkson JH, McAllister RM, Cliff SH, Powell B. Subungual melanoma in situ: two independent streaks in one nail bed. *Br J Plast Surg.* 2002;55:165.
78. Lazar A, Abimelec P, Dumontier C. Full thickness skin graft for nail unit reconstruction. *J Hand Surg Br.* 2005;30:194.
79. Puhaindran ME, Cordeiro PG, Disa JJ, Mehrara BJ, Athanasian EA. Full-thickness skin graft after nail complex resection for malignant tumors. *Tech Hand Up Extrem Surg.* 2011;15:84.
80. Lille S, Brown RE, Zook EE, Russell RC. Free nonvascularized composite nail grafts: an institutional experience. *Plast Reconstr Surg.* 2000;105:2412.
81. Shepard GH. Nail grafts for reconstruction. *Hand Clin.* 1990;6:79.
82. Endo T, Nakayama Y, Soeda S. Nail transfer: evolution of the reconstructive procedure. *Plast Reconstr Surg.* 1997;100:907.
83. High WA, Quirey RA, Guillen DR, Munõz G, Taylor RS. Presentation, histopathologic findings, and clinical outcomes in 7 cases of melanoma in situ of the nail unit. *Arch Dermatol.* 2004;140:1102.
84. Brown RE, Zook EG, Russell RC. Fingertip reconstruction with flaps and nail bed grafts. *J Hand Surg Am.* 1999;24:345.
85. Rayatt SS, Dancey AL, Davison PM. Thumb subungual melanoma: is amputation necessary? *J Plast Reconstr Aesthet Surg.* 2007;60:635.
86. Foucher G, Khouri RK. Digital reconstruction with island flaps. *Clin Plast Surg.* 1997;24:1.
87. Bormann G, Marsch WC, Haerting J, Helmbold P. Concomitant traumas influence prognosis in melanomas of the nail apparatus. *Br J Dermatol.* 2006;155:76.
88. Keyser JJ, Littler JW, Eaton RG. Surgical treatment of infections and lesions of the perionychium. *Hand Clin.* 1990;6:137.
89. Rigopoulos D, Larios G, Gregoriou S, Alevizos A. Acute and chronic paronychia. *Am Fam Physician.* 2008;77:339.
90. Hay RJ, Baran R, Moore MK, Wilkinson JD. Candida onychomycosis–an evaluation of the role of Candida species in nail disease. *Br J Dermatol.* 1988;118:47.
91. Tosti A, Piraccini BM, Ghetti E, Colombo MD. Topical steroids versus systemic antifungals in the treatment of chronic paronychia: an open, randomized double-blind and double dummy study. *J Am Acad Dermatol.* 2002;47:73.
92. Grover C, Bansal S, Nanda S, Reddy BS, Kumar V. En bloc excision of proximal nail fold for treatment of chronic paronychia. *Dermatol Surg.* 2006;32:393.
93. Lawry MA, Haneke E, Strobeck K, Martin S, Zimmer B, Romano PS. Methods for diagnosing onychomycosis: a comparative study and review of the literature. *Arch Dermatol.* 2000;136:1112.
94. Grover C, Bansal S, Nanda S, Reddy BS, Kumar V. Combination of surgical avulsion and topical therapy for single nail onychomycosis: a randomized controlled trial. *Br J Dermatol.* 2007;157:364.
95. de Berker DA, Lawrence CM. A simplified protocol of steroid injection for psoriatic nail dystrophy. *Br J Dermatol.* 1998;138:90.
96. Haneke E. Controversies in the treatment of ingrown nails. *Dermatol Res Pract.* 2012;2012:783924.
97. Nishioka K, Katayama I, Kobayashi Y, Takijiri C, Nishioka K. Taping for embedded toenails. *Br J Dermatol.* 1985;113:246.
98. Senapati A. Conservative outpatient management of ingrowing toenails. *J R Soc Med.* 1986;79:339.
99. Wallace WA, Milne DD, Andrew T. Gutter treatment for ingrowing toenails. *Br Med J.* 1979;2:168.
100. Harrer J, Schoffl V, Hohenberger W, Schneider I. Treatment of ingrown toenails using a new conservative method: a pro-

spective study comparing brace treatment with Emmert's procedure. *J Am Podiatr Med Assoc.* 2005;95:542.

101. Bos AM, van Tilburg MW, van Sorge AA, Klinkenbijl JH. Randomized clinical trial of surgical technique and local antibiotics for ingrowing toenail. *Br J Surg.* 2007;94:292.
102. Mitchell S, Jackson CR, Wilson-Storey D. Surgical treatment of ingrown toenails in children: what is best practice? *Ann R Coll Surg Engl.* 93:99, 2011.
103. Orenstein A, Goldan O, Weissman O, et al. A comparison between CO_2 laser surgery with and without lateral fold vaporization for ingrowing toenails. *J Cosmet Laser Ther.* 2007;9:97.
104. Lin YC, Su HY. A surgical approach to ingrown nail: partial matricectomy using CO_2 laser. *Dermatol Surg.* 2002;28:578.
105. Aksakal AB, Oztas P, Atahan C, Gurer MA. Decompression for the management of onychocryptosis. *J Dermatolog Treat.* 2004;15:108.
106. Noel B. Surgical treatment of ingrown toenail without matricectomy. *Dermatol Surg.* 2008;34:79.
107. Desciak EB, Eliezri YD. Split nail deformities: a surgical approach. *Dermatol Surg.* 2001;27:252.
108. Brown RE, Zook EG, Williams J. Correction of pincer-nail deformity using dermal grafting. *Plast Reconstr Surg.* 2000;105:1658.
109. Mutaf M, Sunay M, Isk D. A new surgical technique for the correction of pincer nail deformity. *Ann Plast Surg.* 2007; 58:496.
110. Baran R. An effective surgical treatment for nail thickening in Darier's disease. *J Eur Acad Dermatol Venereol.* 2005;19: 689.
111. Baran R, Haneke E. Matricectomy and nail ablation. *Hand Clin.* 2002;18:693.
112. Richert B, Choffray A, de la Brassinne M. Cosmetic surgery for congenital nail deformities. *J Cosmet Dermatol.* 2008; 7:304.
113. O'Leary JA, Berend KR, Johnson JL, Levin LS, Seigler HF. Subungual melanoma. A review of 93 cases with identification of prognostic variables. *Clin Orthop Relat Res.* 2000;(378):206.
114. Riddel C, Rashid R, Thomas V. Ungual and periungual human papillomavirus-associated squamous cell carcinoma: a review. *J Am Acad Dermatol.* 2011;64:1147.
115. McHugh RW, Hazen P, Eliezri YD, Nuovo GJ. Metastatic periungual squamous cell carcinoma: detection of human papillomavirus type 35 RNA in the digital tumor and axillary lymph node metastases. *J Am Acad Dermatol.* 1996;34:1080.
116. Dalle S, Depape L, Phan A, Balme B, Ronger-Savle S, Thomas L. Squamous cell carcinoma of the nail apparatus: clinicopathological study of 35 cases. *Br J Dermatol.* 2007;156:871.
117. Peterson SR, Layton EG, Joseph AK. Squamous cell carcinoma of the nail unit with evidence of bony involvement: a multidisciplinary approach to resection and reconstruction. *Dermatol Surg.* 2004;30:218.
118. Dika E, Piraccini BM, Balestri R, et al. Mohs surgery for squamous cell carcinoma of the nail: report of 15 cases. Our experience and a long-term follow up. *Br J Dermatol.* 2012; 167:1310–1314.
119. De Berker D. Hold on the amputation. *Br J Dermatol.* 2003; 148:1077.
120. de Berker DA, Dahl MG, Malcolm AJ, Lawrence CM. Micrographic surgery for subungual squamous cell carcinoma. *Br J Plast Surg.* 1996;49:414.
121. Rosen LR, Powell K, Katz SR, Wu HT, Durci M. Subungual squamous cell carcinoma: radiation therapy as an alternative to amputation and review of the literature. *Am J Clin Dermatol.* 2010;11:285.
122. Yaparpalvi R, Mahadevia PS, Gorla GR, Beitler JJ. Radiation therapy for the salvage of unresectable subungual squamous cell carcinoma. *Dermatol Surg.* 2003;29:294.
123. Grootenboers DA, Poortmans PM, Haas RL. Radiotherapy preserves fingers in the management of subungual squamous cell carcinoma, obviating the need for amputation. *Radiother Oncol.* 2007;85:473.
124. Martinelli PT, Cohen PR, Schulze KE, Dorsey KE, Nelson BR. Periungual basal cell carcinoma: case report and literature review. *Dermatol Surg.* 2006;32:320.
125. Baran R, Sayag J. Nail biopsy–why, when, where, how? *J Dermatol Surg.* 1976;2:322.
126. Forman SB, Ferringer TC, Garrett AB. Basal cell carcinoma of the nail unit. *J Am Acad Dermatol.* 2007;56:811.
127. Cohen PR. Metastatic tumors to the nail unit: subungual metastases. *Dermatol Surg.* 2001;27:280.
128. Braun RP, Baran R, Le Gal FA, et al. Diagnosis and management of nail pigmentations. *J Am Acad Dermatol.* 2007;56:835.
129. Levit EK, Kagen MH, Scher RK, Grossman M, Altman E. The ABC rule for clinical detection of subungual melanoma. *J Am Acad Dermatol.* 2000;42:269.
130. Brodland DG. The treatment of nail apparatus melanoma with Mohs micrographic surgery. *Dermatol Surg.* 2001;27:269.
131. Moehrle M, Metzger S, Schippert W, Garbe C, Rassner G, Breuninger H. "Functional" surgery in subungual melanoma. *Dermatol Surg.* 2003;29:366.
132. Cohen T, Busam KJ, Patel A, Brady MS. Subungual melanoma: management considerations. *Am J Surg.* 2008;195:244.
133. Martin DE, English JC, Goitz RJ. Subungual malignant melanoma. *J Hand Surg Am.* 2011;36:704.
134. Walsh ML, Shipley DV, de Berker DA. Survey of patients' experiences after nail surgery. *Clin Exp Dermatol.* 2009;34:e154.
135. de Berker DA, Dahl MG, Comaish JS, Lawrence CM. Nail surgery. an assessment of indications and outcome. *Acta Derm Venereol.* 1996;76:484.
136. Alam M, Moossavi M, Ginsburg I, Scher RK. A psychometric study of patients with nail dystrophies. *J Am Acad Dermatol.* 2001;45:851.
137. Gilles GA, Dennis KJ, Harkless LB. Periostitis associated with phenol matricectomies. *J Am Podiatr Med Assoc.* 1986;76:469.

CHAPTER 23

Ear Piercing and Ear Lobe Repairs

Steven S. Greenbaum, Charles H. Greenbaum, &
Joshua M. Greenbaum

The external ear is made up of the pinna or auricle, and the auditory canal, or meatus. The pinna serves to collect the sound waves that travel through the air, and the meatus guides these vibrations to the middle ear. The concave outer surface of the pinna consists of a series of depressions and convexities that result from the folding of its fibrocartilaginous structure. Specifically, the lobule (commonly known as the ear lobe), located below the antitragus, is composed of tough areolar and adipose tissue, and lacks the developed structure of the rest of the pinna[1] Fig. 23-1.

The auditory canal or meatus, extends approximately 1 inch from the bottom of the concha to the tympani or middle ear. The meatus forms an S-shaped curve and is composed of cartilage, membrane and bone, and is lined by skin.[1]

In analyzing the aesthetic variations of the ear, it is important to understand the anatomic variations of the human ears. Ears may be categorized into specific types, "hyper-," "hypo-," and "meso-"based on their appearance. In "hyper"- ear types, the helix is pressed down toward the head, the anti-helix protrudes beyond the helix, the lower helix and lobule bend toward the head, and the tragus and anti-tragus protrude and turn outward. In "hypo"- ear types, the helix is protruding, the anti-helix is pressed in toward the head, the lower helix and lobule point outward almost horizontally, and the tragus and anti-tragus press inward in comparison to the surrounding parts of the ear. In "meso"- ear types both the helix and anti-helix protrude from the head, the lower helix and lobule evert from the head at an angle slightly less than the horizontal angle of the hypo-type, and the tragus and anti-tragus are in an intermediate position.[2]

Understanding different ear types can aid in more accurate and aesthetic auricular reconstruction. A study conducted at Tulane University compared specific attributes of the human ear observed among 67 Caucasian men and 120 African American men, both living and deceased. In analysis of the measurements of total ear length, ear width, ear base, and concha length and width, it was observed that Caucasians generally have long, narrow ears and Americans of African descent have shorter, broader ears. The average length and width of the ear respectively were 64.18 mm and 37.19 mm for Caucasian men, and 58.58 mm and 37.43 mm for African American men. Americans of African descent had minimal-to-no hair on the ear in comparison to Caucasian ears. The helix was observed to be broader in African Americans, whereas the antihelix was more prominent in Caucasians.[2] As the blending of races, cultures, and ethnicities has become more common, such differences have become less pronounced. When doing surgery on a given individual, there is no better comparison than the contralateral ear!

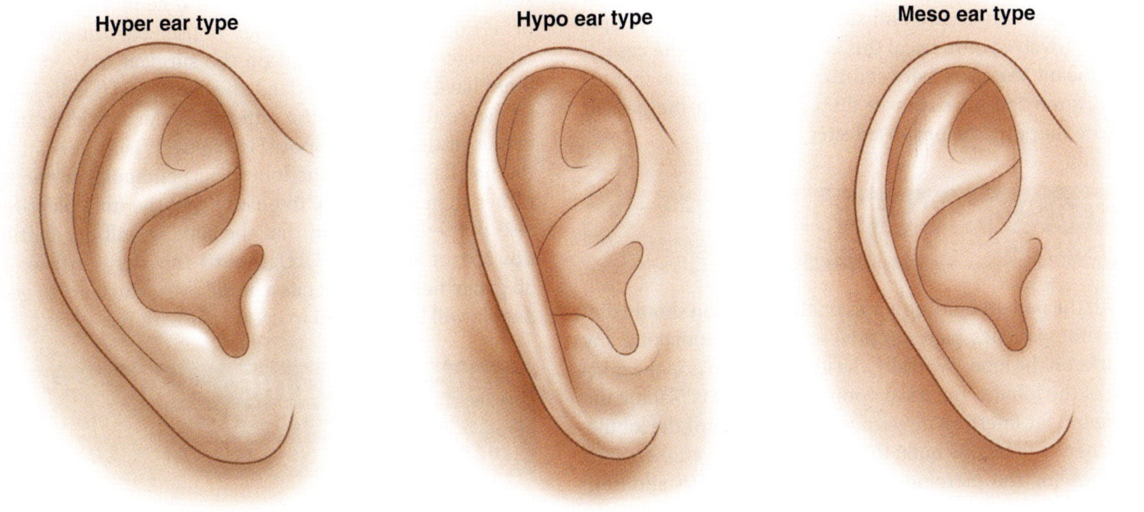

Figure 23-1 Variations in the basic structure of the external ear.

EAR LOBE PIERCING

Many individuals have their initial ear piercing done in a non-medical setting, such as a shopping mall, by relatively untrained personnel under varying conditions. There are people who prefer to have their piercing done in a more controlled environment such as a physician's office. Sometimes, this is for the initial piercing but in many cases it is after a prior complication. Certainly, many patients and physicians prefer that a physician perform a secondary piercing if there has been previous earlobe surgery. There are many advantages of doing earlobe piercings in a doctor's office, most notably its sterile, controlled environment. Precise hole placement can be discussed and the procedure can be done carefully and skillfully. Although the vast majority of piercings done in a commercial setting occur without complications, bleeding, vasovagal response, equipment malfunction, improper positioning, and infection are possible. The medical office environment is prepared to handle these possibilities. As with any technique or procedure, there are many approaches and methods. We describe the technique that we have found to be effective, safe, and reproducible over a period of many years.

STEP 1: CONSULTATION WITH THE PATIENT

Consultation with the patient is of paramount importance. A discussion regarding the exact location in which the piercing (s) will be placed is critical. There is an inherent advantage if the ears have not been previously pierced. Ideally, the patients' desired location and the physician's idea of optimum position intersect. If not, the ramifications of "improper" placement should be explained to the patient. If the physician is not comfortable with the patient's desires, an impasse may be reached and the doctor may not feel comfortable proceeding. Fortunately, this is rare as most patients respect the judgment of the doctor with whom they have chosen to consult.

In deciding upon the proper location, the patient should be handed a large mirror so that an interactive, informed discussion can take place. Each individual's ear lobes have a slightly different size and shape. Although most people are relatively symmetrical this is not invariably the case. If significant variation between the ears exists, it is incumbent upon the physician to discuss this with the patient before marking the proposed sites.

STEP 2: MARKING THE EAR LOBES BEFORE PIERCING

With the patient holding a mirror, the physician should discuss the patient's piercing preferences before making any marks on the lobe. Typically, the ideal position is in the middle of the lobule. The most common mistake is placing the hole too far inferiorly toward the free margin of the lobule. As there will be less bulk, this often results in an increased chance for the piercing to elongate or tear. In addition, heavier earrings will not have the soft-tissue support to allow them to lay perpendicular to the lobe, resulting in a downward tilt, which may be aesthetically unacceptable. If the hole is placed too far anteriorly, the earlobe symmetry may be disrupted, and the diameter of the earring that the patient can wear may be limited due to reduced space. Once the necessary discussion has occurred, the physician can mark the mutually agreed upon location.

Before doing this, the ear should be cleaned. Although infection is extremely rare, meticulous preparation can reduce this risk even further. We typically use chlorhexidine gluconate due to its antiseptic, antimicrobial, and bactericidal effectiveness, although other antibacterial agents can be used. Once the ear has been cleaned, marking can proceed, typically with a fine point surgical pen. Alcohol pads should be available to remove the marking if it is deemed unacceptable. For initial piercings, the marking is straightforward. If there has been prior surgery on that ear or the contralateral one, this must be taken into account. Similarly, if there is already one hole in the lobule and the patient desires a second piercing, careful evaluation of the appropriate location is paramount. The new ostium should be placed far enough away from the prior hole so as not to compromise the strength or integrity of either piercing site.

Once the first ear has been marked, attention is shifted to the other side. As earlobes are not identical even in the same person, strictly measuring for a location can be inadequate. Aesthetic evaluation to ensure that the eventual appearance will be pleasing is critical. Open communication is especially important during this phase. Once the sites have agreed upon and the other ear has been similarly cleansed, it can be marked. The patient is given the opportunity to view both markings before piercing.

STEP 3: ANESTHETIZING THE EAR AND UTILIZING A 30 GAUGE NEEDLE AS A GUIDE

After marking has been satisfactorily accomplished, the ears must be anesthetized.[3] Typically we use 1% lidocaine mixed with epinephrine 1:200,000. The procedure is so quick that epinephrine is not required, but there may be an advantage to having its hemostatic effect. As so little anesthetic is used, any adverse effect is negligible. A 30 gauge needle attached to a 1.0 cc luer lock syringe or a 1.0 cc tuberculin syringe is utilized. An additional 30 gauge needle is placed on the surgical tray. After the lobes have been anesthetized, the additional needle is used to pierce the lobe on the anterior surface directly in the center of the marked spot (Fig. 23-2). It is important that the needle penetrate the lobule perpendicular to the skin rather than at an angle to ensure that the final piercing is also perpendicular and that the earring will not be tilted upward or downward relative to the skin surface. The 30 gauge needle will act as a guide over which an 18 gauge needle will later be slid to create the ostium.

STEP 4: SLIDING THE 18 GAUGE NEEDLE OVER THE 30 GAUGE GUIDE TO CREATE THE OSTIUM

Once the 30 gauge needle has been used to puncture the lobule from anteriorly to posteriorly, the positioning should

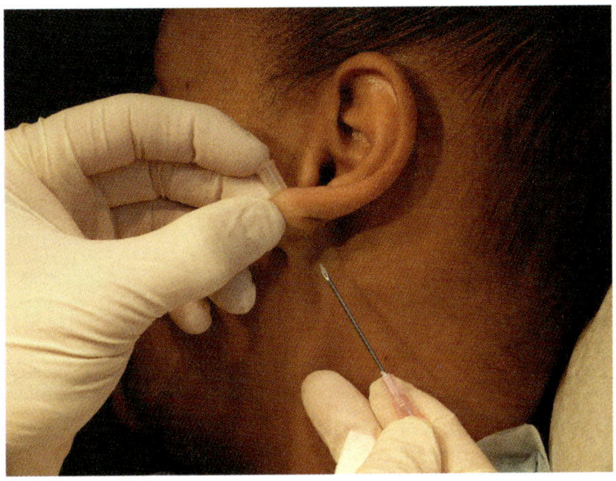

Figure 23-2 After the lobes have been anesthetized the additional needle is used to pierce the lobe on the anterior surface directly in the center of the marked spot.

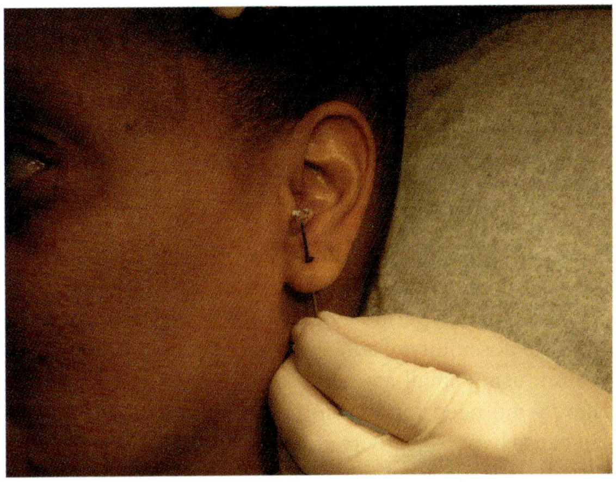

Figure 23-4 The post of the earring (must be smaller than the lumen of the 18 gauge needle) is placed into the lumen of the 18 gauge needle.

once again be checked. A sterile 18 gauge needle can then be slid over the tip of the 30 gauge needle that protrudes from the posterior surface of the lobe. Care must be taken to avoid needle sticks while sliding the larger needle over the smaller needle. Once this has been accomplished, the 18 gauge needle should be advanced from posterior to anterior as the 30 gauge needle is withdrawn (Fig. 23-3).[4] Care must be taken not to withdraw it too quickly, as its guidance will then be lost. The 18 gauge needle should perforate the skin perpendicular to the lobe's surface and through the center of the mark drawn on the anterior surface of the ear.

STEP 5: INSERTION OF THE EARRING

Typically, we ask the patient to bring an earring with them, specifying that it be a "stud" made of gold, sterling silver, stainless steel, titanium, or other material unlikely to cause an allergic reaction. We specifically ask them not to bring a hoop or an earring with a fine wire post because these are more likely to cause damage to the lobe. It should be determined prior to the procedure whether the earring post fits inside the lumen of the 18 gauge needle. If the post is too thick a slightly lower gauge must be used.

The post should be placed into the lumen of the 18 gauge needle while holding the ear and the needle steady (Fig. 23-4) to minimize the chance of an inadvertent needle stick. Once the post is inserted, the earring is gently pushed from anterior to posterior as the 18 gauge needle is simultaneously withdrawn from the posterior surface. A slow synchronous movement is desired so that the earring emerges from the posterior lobe at the same time that the tip of the 18 gauge needle is removed (Fig. 23-5). Once the earring has been positioned, its backing can be placed. Care should be taken not to press too tightly, as the lobule may be swollen from the anesthesia and could swell even more in the ensuing hours if manipulation is excessive.

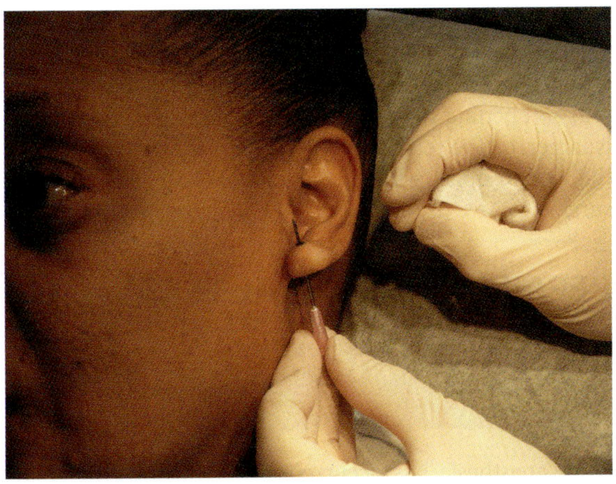

Figure 23-3 The 18 gauge needle is gently and precisely pushed anteriorly as the 30 gauge guide needle is simultaneously slowly pulled out of the lobule.

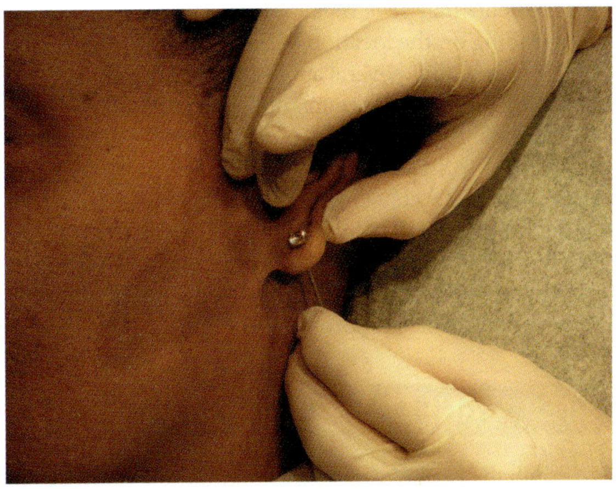

Figure 23-5 The earring is slowly pushed from anteriorly to posteriorly as the 18 gauge needle guides it through the ostium.

STEP 6: POSTOPERATIVE WOUND CARE

Once the earring(s) have been placed, wound care instructions are given. Typically the new ostium will epithelialize within 6 to 10 weeks, although there is some variability. Patients should be instructed to cleanse the area once or twice a day with soap and water, alcohol or hydrogen peroxide. It is important that the patient not over manipulate the earring or remove it prematurely. We advise gentle periodic rotation of the earring to minimize the possibility of adherence to the inner lining of the ostium, using small amounts of Vaseline for lubrication. There is no need for antibiotic ointment as these agents can cause hypersensitivity and allergic contact dermatitis. We advise the patient that they may change their earring in 6 to 8 weeks barring any unforeseen complications, and to call if any pain, swelling, redness, drainage, or other symptoms arise.

EAR LOBE REPAIR

Ear lobes can sustain injury in many ways.[5–9] They can be lacerated due to trauma or as a consequence of piercing. A hoop-shaped earring can pull through the ear causing a full split or leading to elongation of the ostium. Keloids may develop due to piercing or an inflammatory process. Improper healing may lead to tissue overgrowth that can extend significantly beyond the actual piercing site. As the ear protrudes from the side of the head and the lobe itself is unique, this site is difficult to reconstruct. The paucity of appropriate adjacent donor tissue in this location limits the options for repair.

DILATED OR STRETCHED EARRING HOLE

A dilated or stretched hole usually results either from an acute injury, as when an earring is pulled partially through the lobule, or from chronic stress on the ostium from heavy earrings. Inappropriate ostium placement, especially inferiorly, can exacerbate the problem. In either event patients may seek repair.

Depending on the location of the piercing as well as the extent of stretching, several approaches are available.[10–14] If the dilated hole is in the center of the lobule it may be possible to de-epithelialize the ostium and repair it. A scalpel can be used to incise around the old hole, although this can be technically challenging because often the area to be incised is quite small. Sometimes a Beaver blade and handle can be utilized (Fig. 23-6). In other instances a round or elliptical surgical punch can be used. A punch slightly larger than the hole is appropriate.

STEP 1: ANESTHETIZE THE EAR

We numb the ear before selecting our punch as the size of the ostium changes from the turgor of the anesthetic. We typically wait several minutes before initiating surgery so that the beneficial effects of the epinephrine occur.

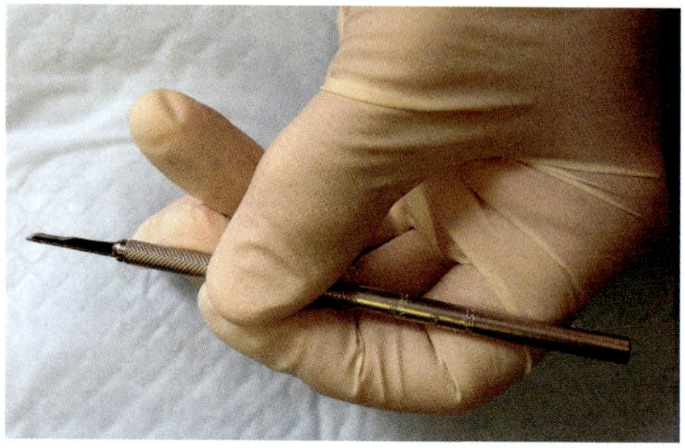

Figure 23-6 Beaver handle and blade—useful for delicate, precise surgical control.

STEP 2: PUNCH OUT THE LINING OF THE OLD HOLE

Once the area is anesthetized we select the size of the punch to be used. We stretch the skin in the direction perpendicular to the long axis of the dilated hole. In this way, we create a more elliptical wound, which will be easier to close, and minimize standing cone deformities (Figs. 23-7 and 23-8). A tongue blade or chalazion clamp can be used to stabilize the lobe and act as a "backstop" for the punch as it pierces the skin. A combination of pressure and rotation are used to create as precise a cut as possible, minimizing tissue fraying and irregular edges.

STEP 3: REPAIRING THE WOUND

If the wound is small and under minimal tension, simple interrupted sutures can be placed. We use nylon or polypropylene because rapidly absorbable suture may lose its integrity before the wound gains sufficient strength. We commonly leave the sutures in for 10 days. If they are placed properly and are not under undue tension, suture marks rarely occur. We utilize the smallest caliber suture on the smallest needle to minimize additional trauma, which can be especially important in patients prone to keloid formation. If the wound is significantly larger than a typical earring hole, consideration must be given to using buried sutures. When the wound is small we close it entirely rather than closing part of it to maintain an opening for a newly placed earring. If the wound is larger, or the tear more complete, we can leave part of the wound open, while placing an earring at the time of surgery to save the step of re-piercing later (Fig. 23-9).

REPAIRING A PARTIAL TEAR

STEP 1: DE-EPITHELIALIZATION OF THE TEAR

Once anesthesia has occurred the lobe should be stabilized in preparation for removal of the opposing epithelium (Fig. 23-10). Depending on the defect's location and extent, extending the tear to completion is often preferred,

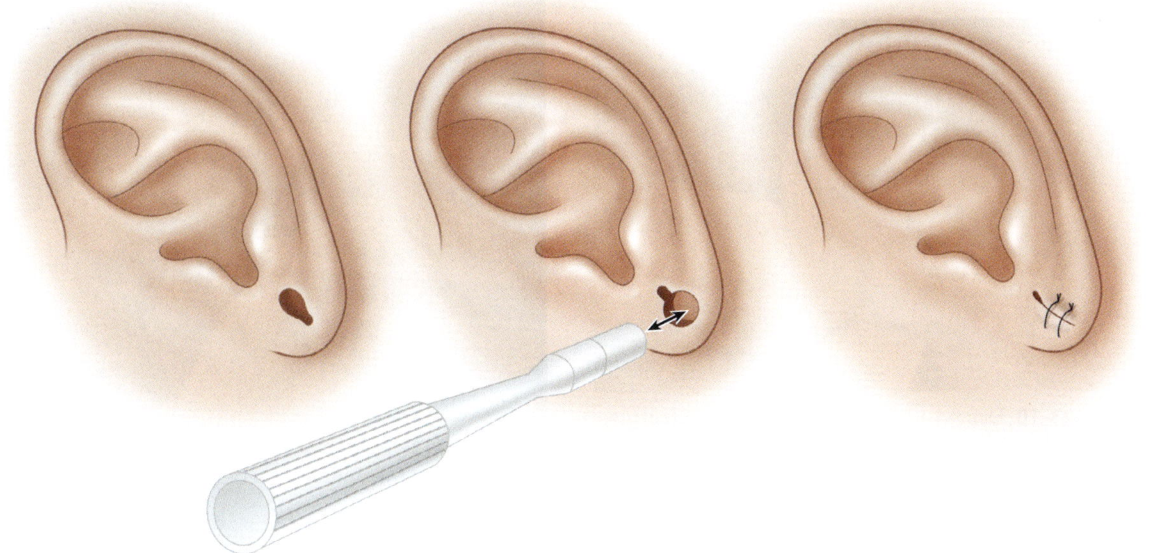

Figure 23-7 Drawing demonstrating "punch technique" in repairing a dilated hole while preserving an opening at the superior aspect of the incision for an earring. (Reproduced with permission from Amer M, Greenbaum S, Lask GP, Parish LC. Ear piercing and repair. In: Parish LC, Lask GP, eds. *Aesthetic Dermatology*. New York: McGraw-Hill;1991:187. Copyright © McGraw-Hill Education LLC.)

as reapproximation of the opposing edges of a fully split lobule is easier than opposing those of a partially split one.

Prior to de-epithelialization and conversion of the partial tear to a full tear, the lobe must be stabilized. We employ one of two methods. A tongue blade can be placed posterior to the lobule by the "non-cutting" hand of the surgeon, who can then manipulate the lobe with that hand, or by a surgical assistant, although it can be difficult to have too many hands in this confined space (Fig. 23-11). Alternatively, a chalazion clamp can be utilized (Fig. 23-12). The advantage of this approach is that it frees the surgeon's hands and provides compression hemostasis.[15] Once the lobule is stabilized the edges of the ostium can be de-epithelialized, usually with a scalpel (Figs. 23-13 and 23-14). Alternatively, a scissors, carbon dioxide laser or other modality may be used.[16–17]

STEP 2: SUTURING THE DEFECT

Depending on the size of the defect either one or two absorbable (and in certain instances nonabsorbable) buried sutures may be used to take tension off the final closure and add strength to the repair. If the wound appears almost to close on its own without tension, this step can be eliminated and the wound can be repaired simply with cutaneous sutures. We typically use 6-0 nylon or polypropylene sutures and leave them in for 7 to 14 days.[18,19] We recommend that the patient cleanse the area twice a day with hydrogen peroxide and apply a thin coating of Vaseline as needed until the sutures are removed to keep the wound moist and facilitate healing. We do not recommend that patients bandage the ear as it may be difficult to dress and over manipulation can disrupt the repair.

REPAIRING A COMPLETE TEAR

Complete ear lobe tears can occur anywhere although they tend to be centrally located. As trends and fashions change, some individuals choose to have multiple piercings. A complete tear can occur at any of these sites, but repair of all of these tears is similar (Figs. 23-15 to 23-17).

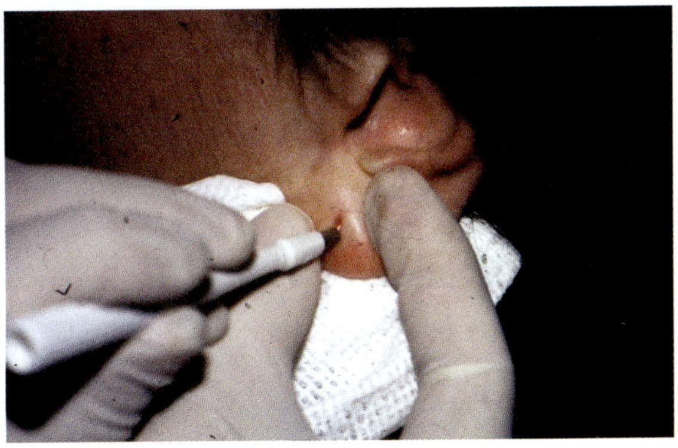

Figure 23-8 Punch being used to de-epithelialize the lining of the dilated ostium.

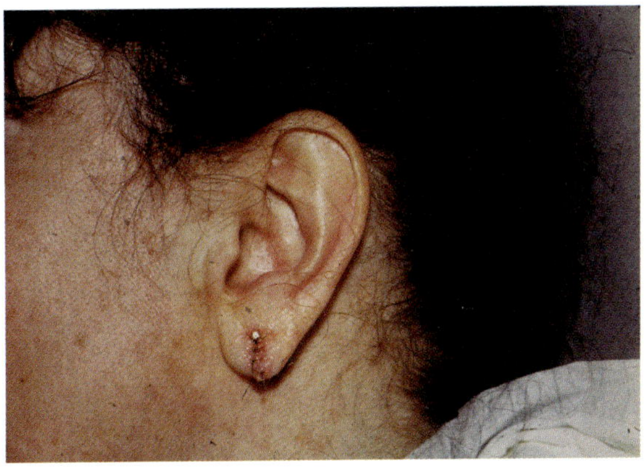

Figure 23-9 Result showing repaired enlarged hole with earring in place.

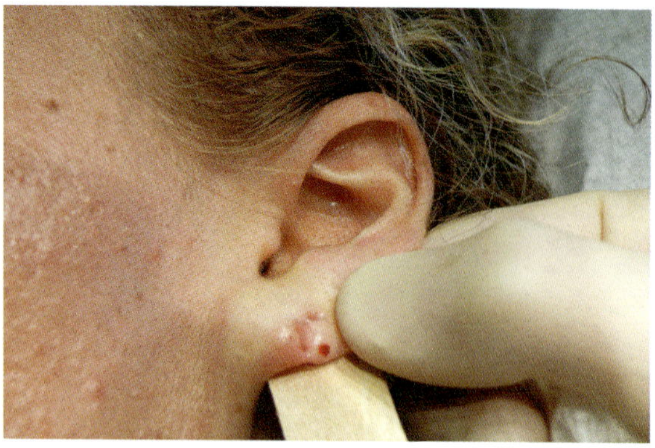

Figure 23-10 Dilated (partially torn) earring hole with posteriorly placed tongue blade being used for stabilization and ease of incision.

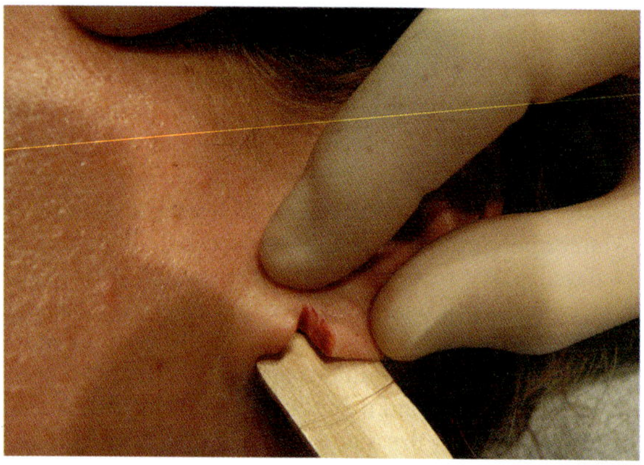

Figure 23-11 Conversion of partial tear to complete tear.

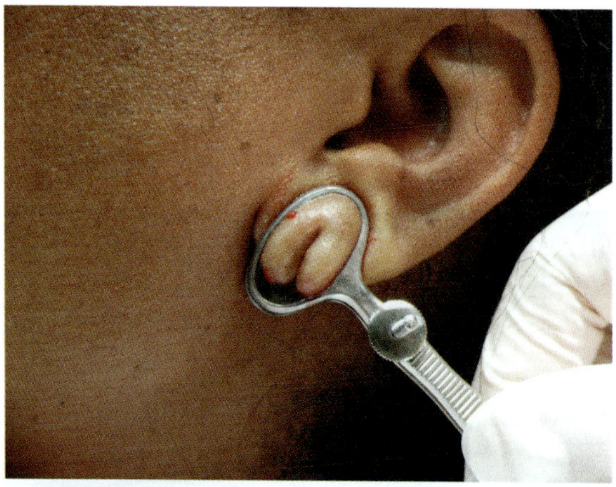

Figure 23-12 Example of chalazion clamp positioned allowing for stabilization and hemostasis.

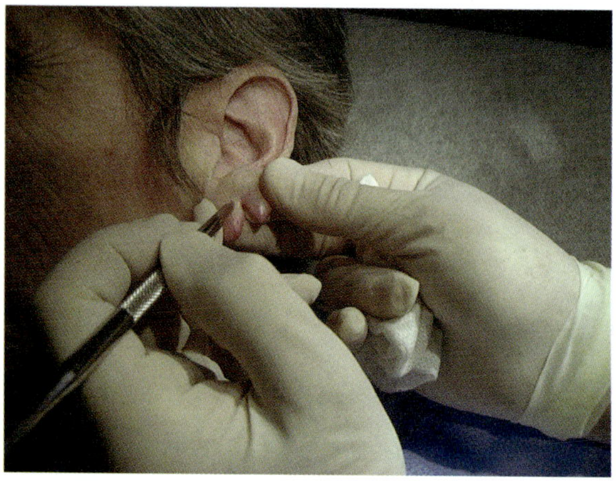

Figure 23-13 Scalpel positioned such that it is being pulled toward the operator for best control of incision.

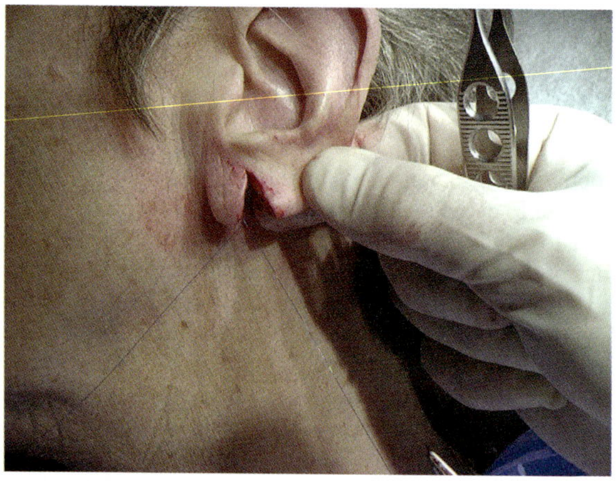

Figure 23-14 Fully de-epithelialized wedge.

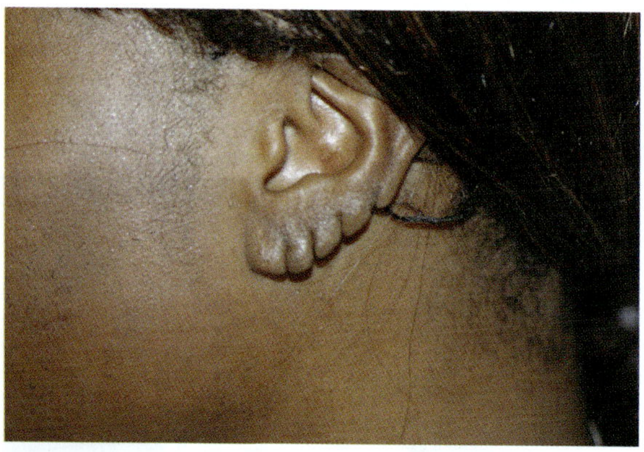

Figure 23-15 Ear lobe with multiple complete tears.

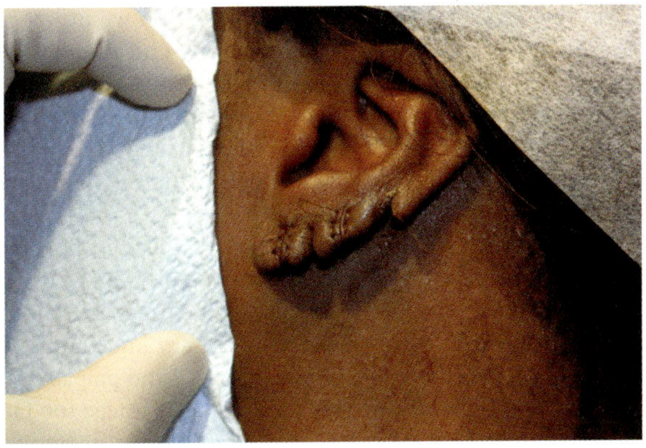

Figure 23-16 Technique showing repair of alternate defects. Attempts to fix all tears at the same time can be technically difficult and can also leave several thin, poorly vascularized flaps that can have tenuous healing.

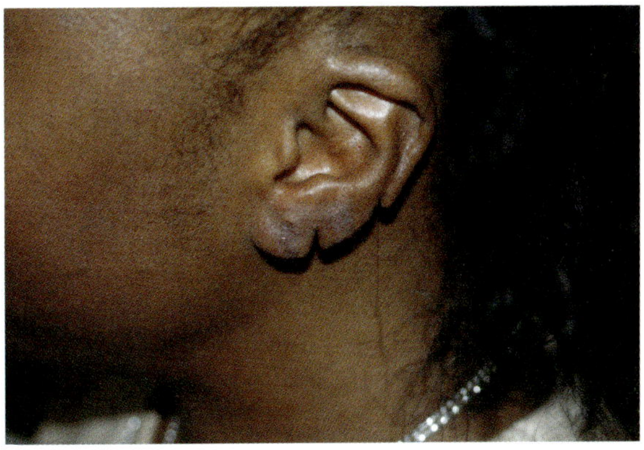

Figure 23-17 Follow-up showing healing of the repaired tears before fixing the remaining ones.

STEP 1: STABILIZE THE LOBULE

After the earlobe has been anesthetized, a waiting period ensues to allow the epinephrine to take effect. As discussed previously, we stabilize the lobe before incising it to allow for more precise surgery. Depending on the defect's position, we either use a tongue blade placed posteriorly to act as a backstop for the scalpel, or a chalazion clamp, which is available in various sizes. If the clamp is too small, it can get in the way and make surgery awkward. For this reason we tend to use the larger clamp sizes.

STEP 2: INCISION OF THE EPITHELIAL EDGES

With the earlobe stabilized, the lobe is incised by pulling the scalpel superiorly from the free edge of the lobule toward the vertex of the defect. If the surgeon chooses to incise in the opposite direction, he or she must be positioned so as to "pull" the scalpel toward them rather than "pushing" it away. As little normal tissue as possible is removed when de-epithelializing the split, because the less tissue removed, the greater the symmetry with respect to the contralateral side. Sometimes it is more effective to begin the incision with a scalpel and complete it with fine scissors. In either case the tissue to be discarded should be grasped with forceps to reduce trauma to the remaining tissue.

STEP 4: SUTURING THE DEFECT

Once incision of the edges is complete the clamp is removed to facilitate approximation of the wound edges. We also minimize thermal injury to optimize the cosmetic result. As there are no major blood vessels in the lobe, significant bleeding is rarely a problem; simple pressure is often all that is needed. Once hemostasis has been obtained the actual repair can begin.

In nearly all instances at least one buried suture is necessary to give prolonged strength to the wound. Traditionally, absorbable sutures have been used for this purpose. However, we often use a nonabsorbable suture. As a repaired laceration only regains at most 85% of its original strength there will always be inherent weakness along the suture line. This may be unimportant if another piercing hole is not planned along the line of closure.[20] However, in patients with small lobes or multiple piercings in the same lobe, it may be necessary to re-pierce in essentially the same location as the original hole and thus along the line of closure. In these cases a buried permanent suture not only gives prolonged strength to the wound but if placed properly can also provide a supportive sling under a newly pierced hole. To accomplish this, the buried suture must be located slightly inferior to where the new piercing site would be. We use polypropylene due to its relative inertness and ease of use. Although it may eventually degrade, it gives prolonged strength to the wound. We typically place the suture with the needle oriented vertically rather than horizontally to keep the suture "buried" in the lobule and farther from the skin surface, thereby minimizing the chance of suture "spitting" and palpability. We also leave an approximately 1 mm tag after cutting it to help minimize the chance of the knot untying. If multiple intradermal sutures are needed we often use one permanent suture to act as the sling among the other absorbable sutures to decrease the chance of a granulomatous reaction causing added earlobe bulk.

Once the buried suture(s) have been placed the skin may be closed. The most important consideration is to ensure that the opposing edges are properly aligned to give continuity to the smooth, even contour of the lobule's surface. After placement of the buried sutures the lobe should be relatively well aligned, although we typically place a key suture at its inferior aspect to guarantee that this is the case. We also try to achieve good wound-edge eversion with this suture to minimize the chance of notching or developing a groove along the incision line. If we cannot achieve proper eversion with an interrupted suture we may elect to place a vertical mattress suture instead. The selection of suture material varies depending on the wound size, the lobe size, and the skin texture. Use of nonabsorbable suture allows us to control how long the sutures remain in place. Rapidly absorbable gut suture can be used but typically loses tensile strength quickly and does not maintain the same degree of integrity as a nonabsorbable suture. We utilize a running suture or multiple closely spaced interrupted sutures to enhance eversion. If more "fine-tuning" of lobe contour is needed, multiple interrupted sutures may be more appropriate. In most instances both the anterior and posterior surfaces align readily. However, in a minority of cases there may be a slight discrepancy between the anterior and posterior surfaces. In these cases it is important to first align the anterior surface as it is most visible. If a Burow's triangle needs to be removed it should be done from the posterior aspect to optimize the final result. We leave the sutures in place for 7 to 10 days depending on the age of the patient and their skin type and texture. Wound care includes cleaning twice a day, typically with hydrogen peroxide, water or isotonic saline. The area is then blotted dry and coated with a thin layer of Vaseline. We rarely utilize antibiotic ointments and have found the incidence of postsurgical infection to be extremely low. If an infection develops we manage it with appropriate systemic antibiotics.

TONGUE AND GROOVE CLOSURE OF THE EAR LOBE

The tongue and groove closure is a modification of the standard side-to-side closure.[21–23] It is technically more difficult and requires greater precision. The inherent beauty of this technique, and thus its main advantage, is that it allows for avoidance of a full-thickness defect along the line of closure. By creating two overlapping "tongues" of tissue, each flap maintains 50% of its bulk (Fig. 23-18). This advantage becomes particularly valuable when a re-piercing is planned along the line of closure.

The preoperative evaluation and anesthesia remain unchanged. When designing the repair it must be decided which side of the split will be the overlying flap and which the underlying flap. Once this has been decided the surgery can begin. Again stabilization of the lobe with a tongue blade or a chalazion clamp facilitates the procedure. Simply put, half of each flap's bulk is removed. On one flap, the anterior half is removed. For the complementary flap the posterior half is removed. When the two flaps are brought together they interlock to give the line of closure 100% of its needed bulk.

As this technique requires great precision we utilize a Beaver blade and handle. The fine blade and ergonomically designed handle enable removal of the thin tissue strips required. Flap symmetry is paramount. If a 5 mm wide strip is removed from the left flap, then an equally sized reciprocal strip must be removed from the right flap for proper approximation.

Because each flap is only one-half of the thickness of the lobe, placement of buried sutures becomes more difficult. The smallest caliber suture should be used. The knots should be secure. More than the necessary knot number increases the likelihood of suture "spitting" and palpability. The superficial layer of sutures should not be placed too far from the incision edge. Each needle bite should penetrate the overlying and underlying complementary flaps to ensure stability and to prevent sliding of the flaps during healing.

It is often technically more difficult to align the free margin of the lobe when utilizing this repair method because more surfaces must be approximated, adding to the complexity of the closure. Again, careful attention is paid first to the free margin of the lobule, as even a minor step-off is readily apparent. If done properly this repair can elegantly lead to a strong wound that can more confidently be re-pierced along its incision line.

FIXING ATTACHED (PIXIE) EAR LOBES

Occasionally, a dermatologic surgeon may be consulted regarding complications resulting from previous surgery. It is, therefore, important to be familiar with the many ways of treating scars, hypertrophic scars, and keloids. Not all complications can be avoided nor do they necessarily indicate improper or poorly performed surgery. After a rhytidectomy, a combination of scar contraction and aggressive skin excision can sometimes cause the healing tissue to pull the earlobe taut and downward. This contributes to formation of a "pixie" ear, which is a tell-tale sign of cosmetic facial surgery, at times providing an aesthetically displeasing result.[24,25] As the free floating lobule is converted to a stretched, tight, elongated, fixed lobe, it

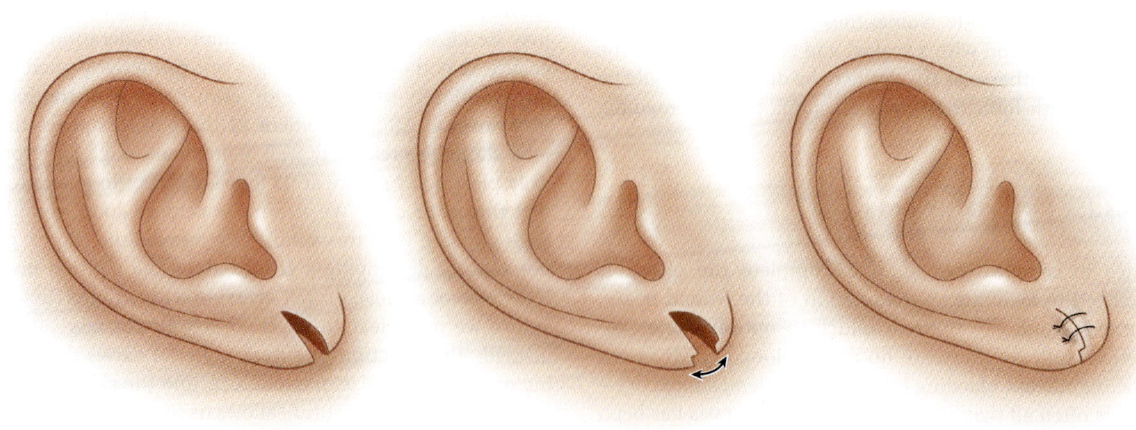

Figure 23-18 Drawing showing "tongue and groove" method of ear lobe repair. (Reproduced with permission from Amer M, Greenbaum S, Lask GP, Parish LC. Ear piercing and repair. In: Parish LC, Lask GP, eds. *Aesthetic Dermatology.* New York: McGraw-Hill;1991:188. Copyright © McGraw-Hill Education LLC.)

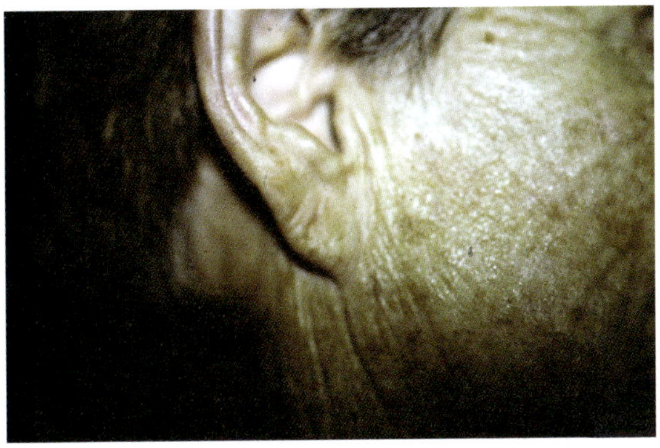

Figure 23-19 Pixie ear deformity prior to surgery.

appears unnatural and at times unusual. The repair of such a problem can make a difference in how the individual views their overall cosmetic result (Figs. 23-19 and 23-20).

STEP #1: ANESTHETIZE THE EAR AND SURROUNDING AREA

- We typically use enough anesthetic to render the lobule insensate but not so much as to distort the anatomy. We also anesthetize the cheek tissue that directly abuts the lobule.

STEP #2: FREEING THE EARLOBE

- An incision is made at the junction of the taut, elongated lobule where it joins the face. The incision proceeds superiorly from the anterior surface of the lobe in an inferior direction toward the bottom of the lobule. It then sweeps posteriorly and superiorly with care taken to keep the blade and the incision parallel to the anterior incision. This will create wounds of equal lengths that can be approximated without the need for standing cone deformity repairs or other "fine-tuning."
- Detaching the lobule from its attachment along the face creates a secondary defect. Minimizing this defect, to the extent possible, will enhance cosmesis.

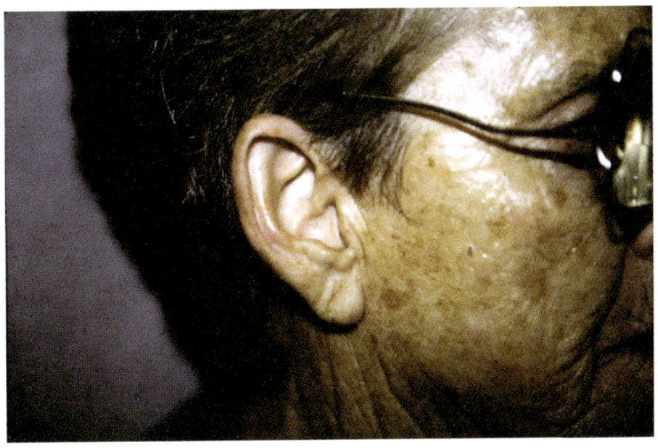

Figure 23-20 Pixie ear deformity following revision.

STEP #3: SUTURING THE SECONDARY DEFECT

- The secondary defect needs to be sutured as meticulously as possible, although it may also be allowed to granulate. However, unless healing proceeds perfectly, a widened scar can result. For this reason we usually choose to suture the wound.
- If the wound edges are not at 90 degree angles to one another, they are modified to enable optimal wound-edge apposition, leading to a less perceptible scar.
- Typically we use 5-0 buried absorbable suture to decrease wound tension as much as possible. We then use a running 6-0 nylon or polypropylene suture or 6-0 fast absorbing gut.

REJUVENATION OF THE AGING EAR LOBE

The ears are typically sun-exposed and often as sun-damaged as the rest of the face. The lobe is the only part of the ear with a substantial adipose and connective tissue component. Due to its unique composition the lobe can age similarly to the rest of the face, developing rhytides, lentigines, and sagging due to intrinsic and extrinsic aging. Individuals who are less consistent in applying sunscreen to the ears can exacerbate this problem. When cosmetic surgery is performed on the aging face and neck it does not usually address the ear lobes. To render the appearance of the ear lobes consistent with the newly rejuvenated face and neck the surgeon can utilize several approaches.

#1: CHEMICAL PEELING. Chemical peels have been utilized for many years to rejuvenate the aging, sun-damaged face.[26,28] The same technique is useful when applied to the ear lobes. Superficial peeling agents such as glycolic acid, salicylic acid and dilute trichloroacetic acid can be applied to the lobes when the face is treated. With superficial peeling the results are less dramatic and multiple, sequential treatment sessions are needed.

Deeper peeling agents such as more concentrated trichloroacetic acid and phenol can restore the lobes to a more youthful appearance. As is the case when using these agents on any type of skin, care must be taken to avoid creating an injury deep enough to cause visible scarring. Injuries extending into the lower one-third of the dermis have a significant chance of causing such scarring. It is also possible, and often recommended, to treat different parts of the ear with different peeling agents. Since the lobule is endowed with a greater blood supply and looser connective tissue, it may be treated with a deeper peeling agent while the rest of the ear is peeled more conservatively.

#2: LASER RESURFACING. The morphologic changes that occur in the aging ear lobe can be addressed with lasers as well to create a depth of injury commensurate with the degree of photodamage. The ability to use lasers in a controlled fashion may be easier for some surgeons than applying a chemical that must be neutralized or is self-neutralizing.[28–31] Fully ablative carbon dioxide and erbium YAG lasers were once utilized for resurfacing. More recently the advent of fractionated ablative and nonablative lasers has given dermatologic surgeons a larger repertoire of tools from which to choose. The primary principle behind use of these techniques is awareness of the depth of injury being created. The fractionated lasers leave interstices of normal tissue between the columns of lasered skin. As the entire skin surface is not destroyed, wound repair and reepithelialization occur more rapidly. Caution must still be utilized as scarring is possible. As with chemical peeling, the surgeon can use lasers to destroy tissue to different depths on different regions of the ear. To effectively reduce deeper rhytides on the lobe, the depth of injury should be carried at least into the mid dermis. Not only will the rhytides be improved but the tissue contraction will enhance the skin's appearance as well.

#3: FILLING AGENTS. Prolonged exposure to ultraviolet irradiation can lead to solar elastosis with dermal thinning as well as atrophy of the underlying adipose tissue, which contributes to wrinkled, sagging, deflated ear lobes. The same tenets that allow us to utilize dermal "fillers" on the face hold true for the ear lobe.[32–34] If a feather pillow loses too many of its feathers, the pillowcase that once was taut becomes large, wrinkled, and creased. The same analogy holds true with the ear lobe. To give the overlying skin a tighter appearance, some skin has to be removed, or more volume has to be put into the lobe. It is simpler, more effective, and more conservative to plump up the lobe with a filling agent. Many of the newer agents are composed mainly of hyaluronic acid, which tends to last significantly longer than older collagen derived materials. In addition, there is a smaller chance of developing an allergic reaction.

Hyaluronic acid or similar agents are injected deep into the adipose tissue of the earlobe. Injections are done slowly, initially as a bolus. Once a significant amount has been injected it is massaged firmly to evenly distribute it. As these agents are hydrophilic some normal swelling will occur. After observing the site for several minutes it can be decided whether it is necessary to inject more filler. It is often surprising about how much needs to be injected to achieve the desired degree of correction. The amount required varies according to the amount of damage the ear lobes have sustained. The varying size of lobes amongst individuals is also a determining factor. Care should be taken to not over inject, which could lead to vascular compression, decreased blood flow and possible necrosis. It is always easier to add filler than to remove it.

As the ear lobe is injected and the skin becomes more taut, piercing sites will be affected. A hole that was slightly dilated can become tighter as the lobe becomes "volumized." Whereas the hole itself does not become smaller, its effective size is smaller as the filler compresses the ostium circumferentially. Similarly, a piercing site located too inferiorly can be supported by injecting filler beneath the hole, thus bolstering the tissue supporting the earring.

Temporary filling agents such as poly-L lactic acid and calcium hydroxylapatite are used in a similar fashion. As the ear lobes are static, in contradistinction to mobile areas on the face, the fillers tend to persist for a longer period of time. The fact that hyaluronic acid can be dissolved using hyaluronidase should be kept in mind, especially for those just gaining experience with ear lobe rejuvenation.[35,36]

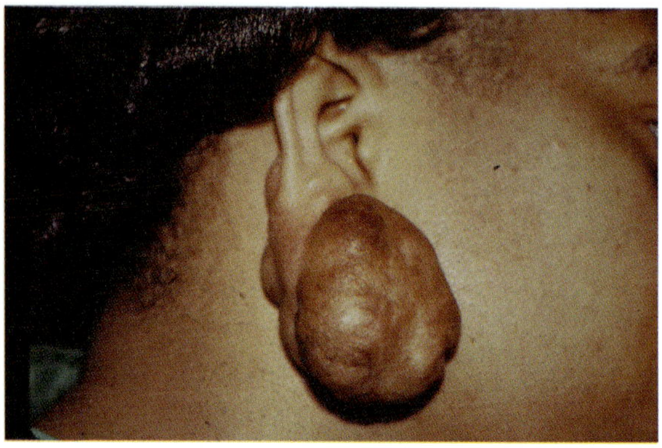

Figure 23-21 Extensive ear lobe keloid.

TREATMENT OF EAR LOBE KELOIDS

Keloid, a term derived from the Greek word for crab-claw-like, refers to an abnormal response of the skin to trauma. The response consists of an aggressive proliferation of fibrous connective tissue at the site of trauma, with extension beyond the immediate area. Keloids, unlike hypertrophic scars, rarely regress spontaneously, and often recur after treatment (Fig. 23-21).

Simple excision of keloids results in a recurrence rate of 55%, while irradiation with heavy filtration following surgery lowers the recurrence rate by 70% to 90%.[37] With decreased use of radiation for benign lesions, other adjuvants to surgery have been studied. It is known that intralesional corticosteroids decrease collagen synthesis and inhibit fibroblast proliferation. Intralesional corticosteroid injection after surgery, repeated every 2 weeks for five injections, accompanied by topical application of a steroid ointment twice daily for 6 months, yielded a 14.3% recurrence rate over a study period of 24 to 57 months. Side effects included reversible purpura (100%), atrophy (50%), and telangiectasia. A number of chemotherapeutic agents, known for their ability to suppress fibroblastic activity, have also been studied, with significant reduction of recurrences. Surgery with adjuvant therapy remains the treatment of choice.

Ear lobe keloids are a source of annoyance and frustration for patient and surgeon alike. They are a cosmetic issue as well as symptomatic, and can be susceptible to cyst formation and infection. They can present a significant challenge not only in their removal and repair but perhaps more importantly their risk of recurrence (Fig. 23-21). For all of these reasons patients seek the attention of a dermatologic surgeon.[7,37,38]

In the initial consultation it is important to stress the need for realistic expectations. Several key points as the following should be emphasized:

- Nonsurgical approaches should be tried first.[39–43]
- Surgery has limitations
    - Perfection is nearly impossible to achieve
    - Recurrence is common and typically not caused by faulty surgical technique or poor wound management

- Although symmetry and complete eradication are the primary goals of keloid surgery, both may be difficult if not impossible to achieve.
- Postsurgical treatment is critical to prevent recurrence. If the patient is unwilling to return it is incumbent upon the surgeon to reconsider whether surgery is appropriate because recurrence rates following surgery alone are high.[44–49]
- As many patients who seek surgical treatment for keloids are minors, it is important that a clear understanding of the procedure and subsequent treatment exists between surgeon, patient, and parent. The parent must be willing to support the process to achieve optimal results.

As is the case with almost all surgery, the best type of surgery is no surgery at all. If a patient presents with an incipient keloid or hypertrophic scar, it should be managed nonsurgically if possible. This is especially true for keloids that are small and rather soft. Conservative approaches such as high-potency intralesional corticosteroid injections should be offered. As keloids are by nature hypertrophic, the side effect of atrophy works to the patient's advantage. The anti-inflammatory attributes of the steroid are also advantageous. We typically start with intralesional triamcinolone acetonide at a minimum concentration of 20 mg/cc. As keloidal tissue is firm and difficult to inject, instead of using a 30 gauge needle in a tuberculin syringe we use a 27 gauge needle attached to a 1.0 cc luer-lock syringe. If a "slip" type of needle/syringe combination is used the needle and syringe may disconnect during injection due to retrograde pressure, posing significant danger to the surgeon, assistants, and patient. In addition, the spraying of steroid and blood is to be avoided.

We typically inject directly into the keloid to optimize the therapeutic benefits of the injection. Because the injected material seeks the point of least resistance there is a tendency for it to flow around the keloidal tissue rather than into it. This may lead not only to ineffective treatment but may also lead to unintended atrophy of the surrounding tissue. If injection is difficult it can be aborted or in some instances facilitated by spraying the injection site and keloid with fluoroethyl to ease injections and minimize discomfort. Typically we inject the keloid approximately 5 to 10 seconds after spraying the area. If injection is attempted too early, it can be even more difficult due to the firmness of the formed "ice-ball." We stress to the patient that multiple injections over time are the rule rather than the exception, and typically space them at 4 week intervals. If we see no improvement after two to three sessions, we abandon the approach. If the patient is noncompliant in returning, we seriously evaluate whether they will comply with postsurgical instructions and postoperative steroid injections.

SURGICAL APPROACH TO KELOID REMOVAL

No two keloids are exactly the same. However, there are certain patterns of keloid development that are more common than others. The type of repair and the options available depend to a certain degree on the morphology of the keloid.[50–53]

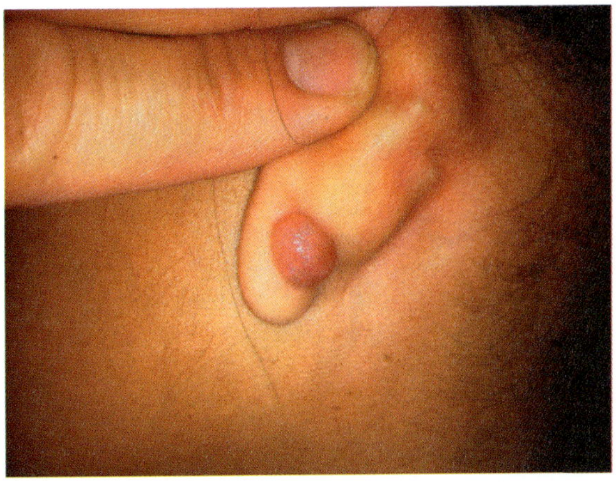

Figure 23-22 Posterior lobule "marble"-type keloid, presaucerization removal.

One of the most common types of keloids is the "marble" type, which typically presents as a round, firm keloid on the anterior or posterior surface of the lobule. The etiology of the keloid can to a certain extent determine its morphology. If it is the direct result of piercing, the keloid can extend onto the anterior and posterior surfaces of the lobe. In these instances the tract or ostium is usually involved and can act as a conduit through which the keloid develops. If a keloid is the result of an inflammatory lesion such as a cyst, it may be confined to one surface or the other.

"MARBLE"-TYPE KELOID

The simplest type of keloid to remove is the posterior surface "marble"-type that does not extend into a piercing ostium (Fig. 23-22). In these cases, there are several approaches that can be utilized:

POSTERIOR SURFACE INVOLVEMENT ONLY

1. If after palpation of the keloid and lobe it is felt that there is "normal" tissue between the base of the keloid and the anterior surface of the ear, a simple keloidectomy can be performed (Figs. 23-23 to 23-27).
2. A scalpel, scissors, electrosurgical cutting current, or a cutting laser can be used to dissect the keloid free from the surrounding tissue (Figs. 23-25 and 23-26). It is wise in these instances to extend the dissection 1 to 2 mm lateral to the keloid so as not to inadvertently leave behind any keloid that could serve as a nidus for recurrence. Each modality of removal has its advantages. Electrosurgery or a laser creates a bloodless surgical field, improving visibility and often obviating the need for postsurgical hemostasis (Figs. 23-28 and 23-29). Whether or not the heat generated in the tissue can act as sufficient trauma to induce recurrence is unclear. Cold steel surgery such as a scalpel or scissors allows for direct

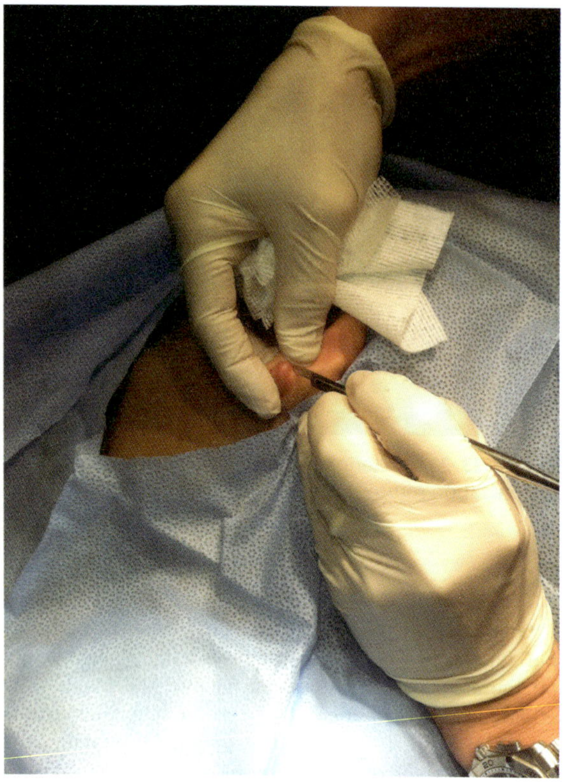

Figure 23-23 Incision around the base of the keloid into fatty tissue.

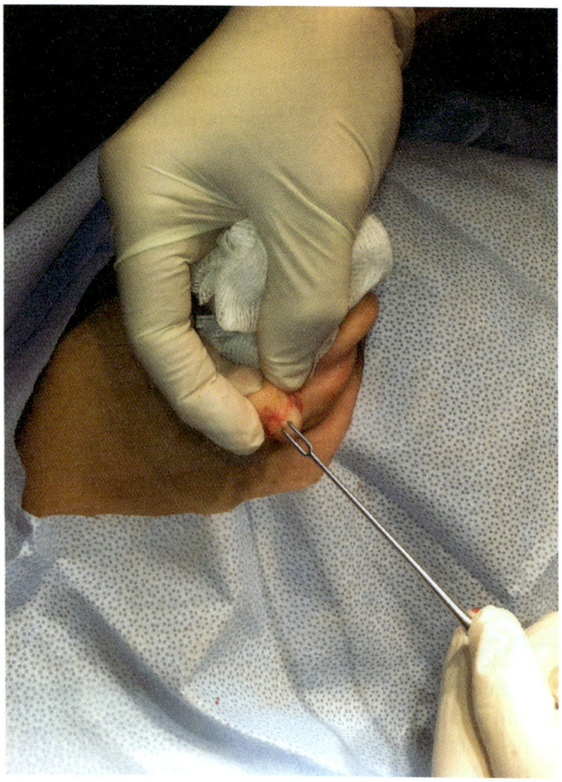

Figure 23-24 Skin hook being used to grasp the keloid for better surgical manipulation and control.

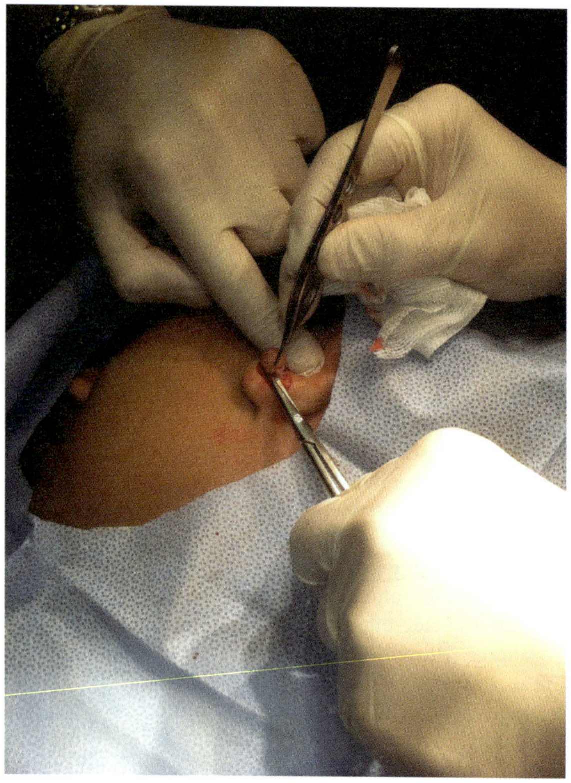

Figure 23-25 Dissecting scissors being used to remove the keloidal mass from the underlying tissue.

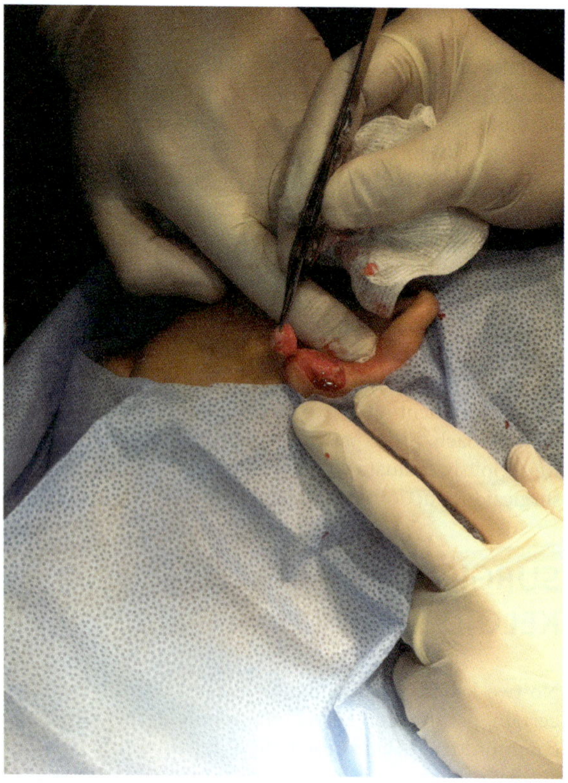

Figure 23-26 Keloid being completely removed.

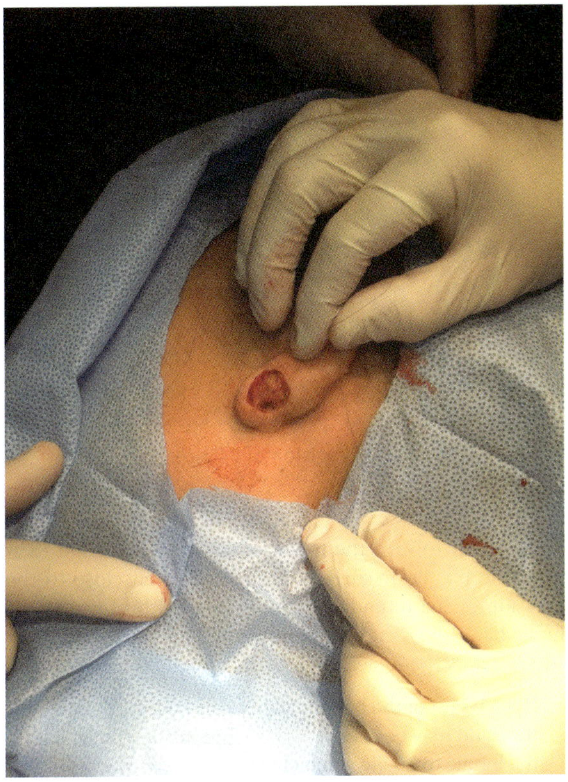

Figure 23-27 Resultant defect after aluminum chloride was applied to the base of the wound for hemostasis.

tactile "feel" of the tissue, which can in certain instances help guide the surgeon more precisely. It is typically thought best to remove all, or as much as possible, of the keloid. In many cases there will be a variably sized layer of tissue separating the base of the dissection from the anterior surface of the ear. The greater the thickness of that layer, the less contraction will occur if the wound is left to heal secondarily. If the surgical defect is wide and deep, contraction can lead to distortion with

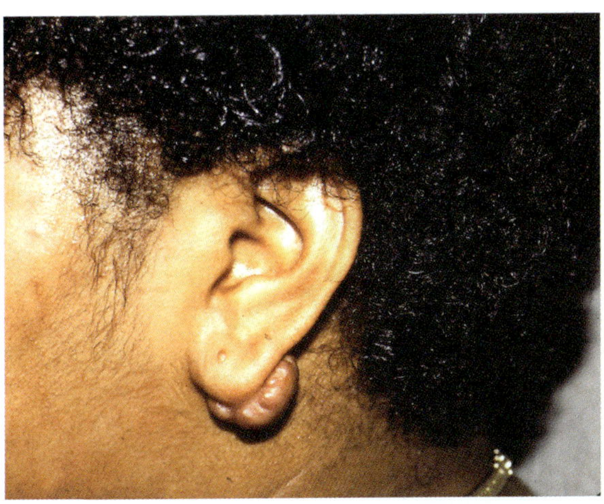

Figure 23-28 Posterior surface ear lobe keloid prior to carbon dioxide laser removal.

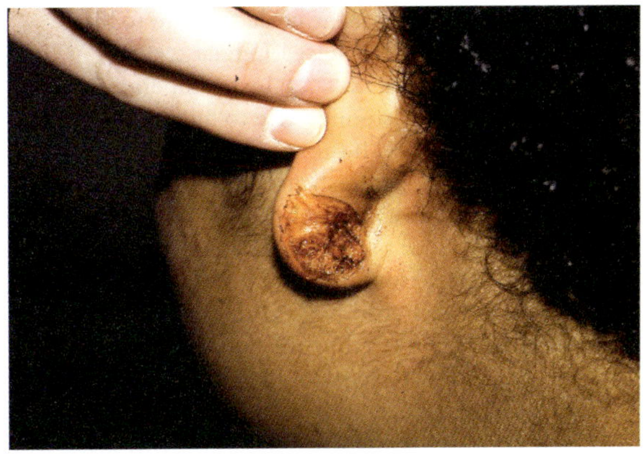

Figure 23-29 Posterior surface of lobe immediately following carbon dioxide laser removal.

possible lobe asymmetry. As the posterior surface of the ear is not visible, second intention healing in these cases is often a good option, as it offers the least manipulation of the skin. As the wounds heal, they can be injected with corticosteroids to retard collagen formation and possibly reduce the chance of recurrence. Once the wound is healed, close follow-up and sequential corticosteroid injections are advised to prevent new keloid growth. We advise patients to be meticulous in their wound care. As applying a bandage to the area may be logistically difficult, we advise patients to recoat the base of the wound with Vaseline multiple times during the day to facilitate reepithelialization.

3. If the original keloid was small but deep, it may be preferable to simply suture the wound. In these cases, as few buried sutures as possible should be used. Suturing may lead to a more aesthetically pleasing cosmetic outcome.

ANTERIOR SURFACE INVOLVEMENT ONLY

When the anterior surface of the lobe is the only area involved, the cosmetic consequences of removal and repair are more critical. Care should be taken to utilize an approach that maximizes the chance of successful removal and aesthetic healing and minimizes recurrence.

1. The width of the base of the keloid is critical in determining an approach. If the pedicle is relatively thin, and the keloid sessile, an excellent approach is to incise the ear lobe in a "V" formation extending from the base of the keloid into the lobe itself. The operator should palpate the keloid to determine the angle of incision so as to remove the entire base.
2. Once the keloid has been removed, the defect is closed using buried absorbable suture and a 6-0 rapidly absorbable or nonabsorbable cuticular stitch.
3. If the base of the keloid is too wide to make this approach possible, there are several alternatives. The wound can be left to heal by second intention. The results can be good although in darker

skin, the tendency is for the healed wound to be hyperpigmented with a more irregular texture than the surrounding skin. Again, postoperative intralesional corticosteroids help to minimize the chance of recurrence. If the secondary defect is deep and broad a "purse-string" can be utilized.[54–57] In this scenario, an absorbable material such as 5-0 or 6-0 Monocryl or a similar permanent material can be utilized to close the wound. We prefer Monocryl to other absorbable materials for this purpose because it is a monofilament, and creates minimal inflammatory response. The surgeon should be aware that knot security is decreased with this type of suture as its coefficient of friction is less, and it may be necessary to add an extra "throw" to maintain the integrity of the closure.

Another possibility in dealing with "marble"-type keloids on the anterior or posterior surface of the ear is to "shell" them out.[54,58–60] With this approach, the surgeon dissects the keloid free while creating a superficial flap, which is then used to repair the resultant defect. We typically incise along the base of the keloid in an arc of 180 to 220 degrees. We prefer cold steel to laser or electrosurgery for these dissections. Depending on the size of the keloid, either a #15 scalpel blade or a Beaver blade is used to dissect it free from the overlying skin, which is peeled from the underlying keloid to be used as a flap. We leave the flap intact and only trim it once we see the size of the defect. At that point, the flap is laid over the wound and trimmed to size with a sharp scissors. It should be cut precisely to minimize tension, and should not be oversized because when normal wound contraction occurs, it will not lay flat. Once the flap has been loosely but precisely laid over the wound, it is sutured into place using either 6-0 nylon or polypropylene sutures or 6-0 rapidly absorbable gut. We typically do not employ buried sutures here. If nonabsorbable sutures are used, they are removed in 7 days.

REMOVAL OF INFERIORLY POSITIONED SEMI-LUNAR KELOIDS

Sometimes, especially after an inferiorly placed piercing, a keloid can develop in such a way as to extend from the anterior ear toward the free margin of the lobe and then onto the posterior surface of the ear, often close to the location of the intended ostium. The width of this semi-lunar band of tissue can vary (Figs. 23-30 to 23-32). The thinner it is, the easier the repair.

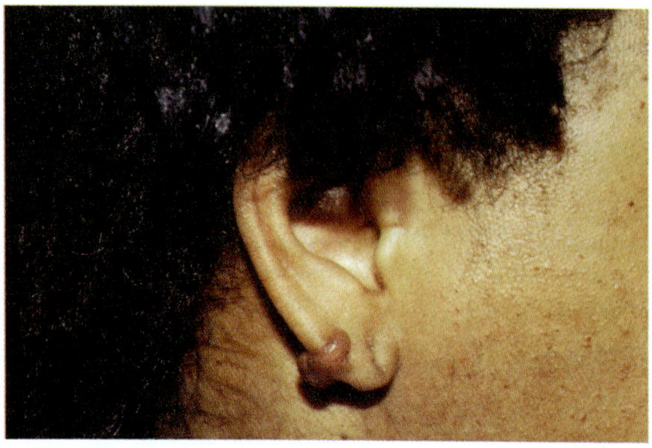

Figure 23-30 Semi lunar inferiorly based keloid prior to surgery.

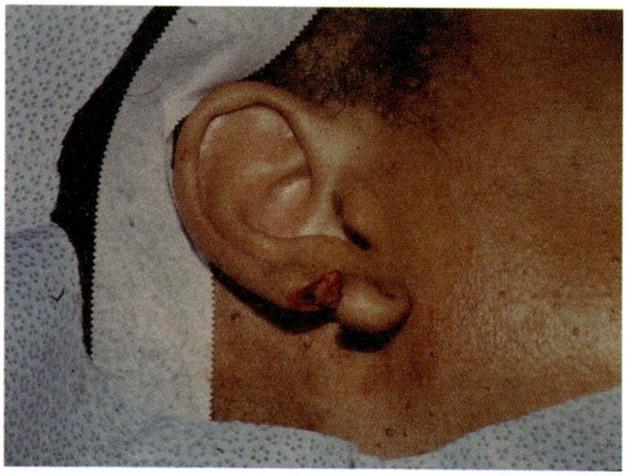

Figure 23-31 Wedge excision of keloid.

1. If the width of the band is narrow and the lobe large, the band may be excised as a wedge, cutting through the lobule to create a defect that can be easily closed. Depending on the exact location of the defect we can repair it as if we were repairing a traumatically torn or enlarged piercing. Buried absorbable or nonabsorbable suture is used to close the subcutaneous tissue followed by closure of the skin edges.
2. As the width of the band increases and or the size of the lobe decreases, there is more of a disparity in lobe symmetry. However, it may still be advantageous to use this approach because rarely are both lobes viewed simultaneously.

REMOVAL OF MORE COMPLICATED KELOIDS

Unfortunately, many keloids are neither of the "marble" or "semi-lunar band" types, and can assume many sizes and shapes. As the keloid becomes larger and involves a greater

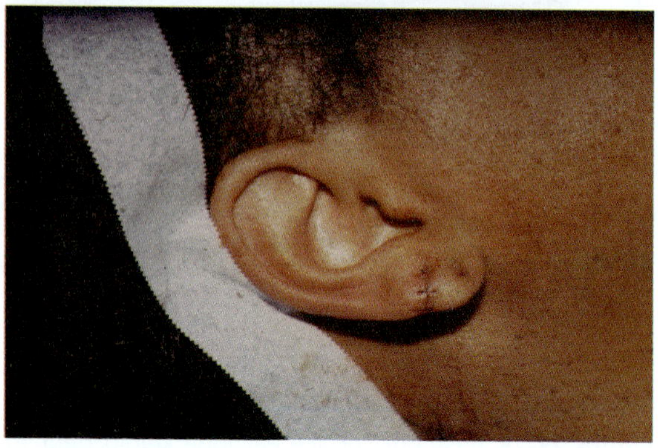

Figure 23-32 Closed wound.

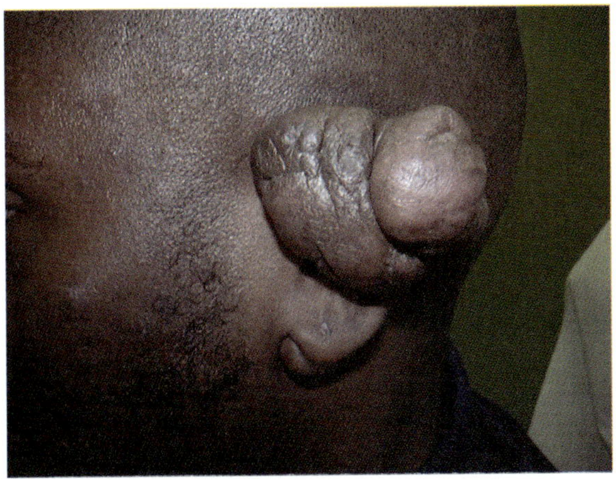

Figure 23-33 In the case of complex keloids, it is often necessary to combine multiple techniques to achieve the best result.

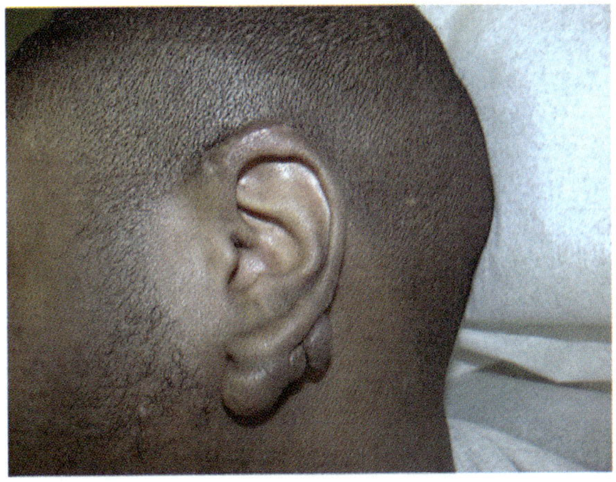

Figure 23-35 Result at 3 months following initial surgery before repairing large posterior lobe keloid.

portion of the ear, the challenge for the surgeon increases accordingly. Sometimes the keloid can occupy a large portion (if not all) of the ear lobe. In these cases, preservation of as much normal tissue as possible is required to facilitate reconstruction. Creativity and an artistic sense are needed to form a lobule that appears "normal" and is as similar as possible to the contralateral side. As described previously, there are multiple methods of removing keloids, including wedge excision, a "shelling out" approach, or saucerization. For complex keloids, it is often necessary to combine techniques to achieve the best result (Figs. 23-33 to 23-37). As the keloid extends from the lobule onto surrounding structures, it is even more critical to preserve as much tissue as possible. Once the helical rim is affected, through and through removal carries with it reconstructive challenges. Decreasing the size of the rim appreciably will lead to asymmetry. In these cases, we often will try to shell out the keloid as described previously, maintaining as much of the overlying uninvolved covering as possible. In certain instances, this additional tissue may be utilized to reconstruct portions of the ear that had to be sacrificed in removing the keloid. There is no "cookbook" formula or algorithm to removal and repair, and it is helpful to have an image of the opposite ear as a guideline for comparison. Perhaps the simplest way to do this is to take a photograph of the opposite ear using 1:1 magnification, which can be printed and placed near the surgical field for easy reference. If the affected ear is the "right" ear, a photo can be taken of the normal "left" ear using a 1:1 magnification lens. That image can be flipped horizontally in a photo editing program and printed out to make the image

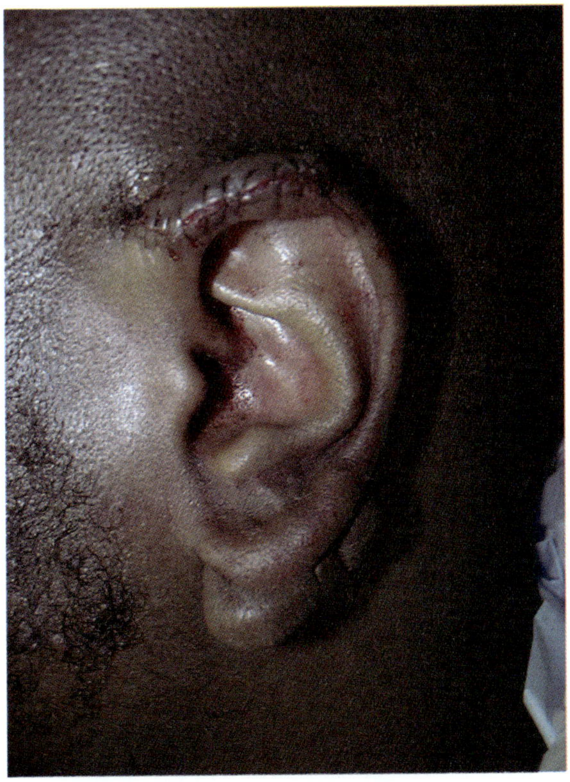

Figure 23-34 Superior component of the keloid has been removed. "Normal" skin overlying the keloid has been preserved after shelling out the keloid and is used to cover the defect and help recreate a more normal appearing rim.

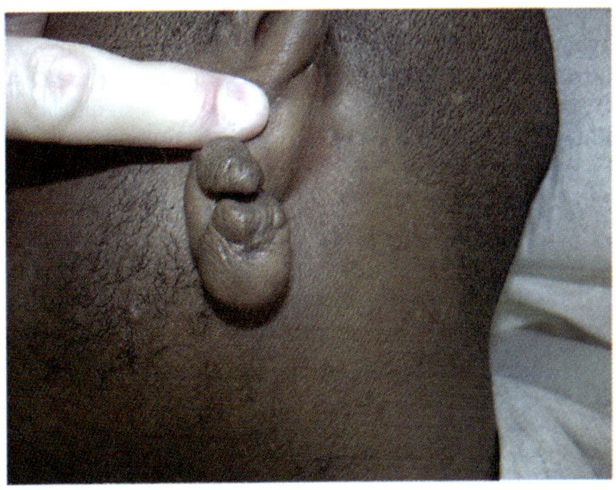

Figure 23-36 Posterior view of lobule keloid.

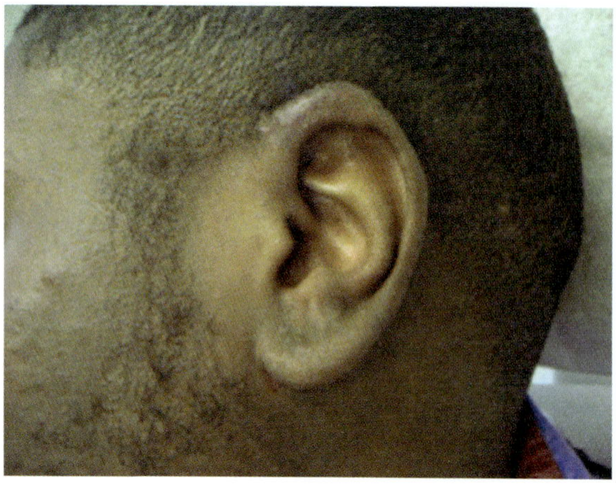

Figure 23-37 Results following staged repair of complex keloid.

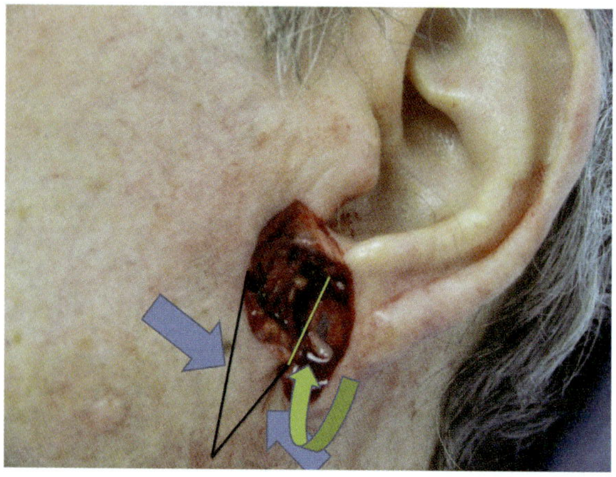

Figure 23-38 Preauricular subunit closed primarily (*blue arrows*). Ear lobule recreated utilizing a "foldover flap" (*green arrow*).

appear as if it is the "right" ear for use as a template or model for reconstruction. The ability to do this is built into most photo-editing software programs, although the details vary from program to program. As surgery itself is a risk factor for keloids, we try to do as much as possible during the initial surgery to minimize the necessity for subsequent revisions. As has been stressed previously, return visits for intralesional corticosteroid injections are often necessary to minimize the chance of recurrence.

The patient may inquire about re-piercing the ear after lobe repair. Although it is best to discourage this as piercing may induce keloid formation, sometimes patients are insistent. Rather than have them do it in a poorly controlled environment, we will offer to do it in our office. Our hope is that careful surgical technique and sterile conditions will minimize the chance of keloid formation due to re-piercing. We stress to the patient that this cannot be guaranteed and that they are taking a risk by having the lobe re-pierced.

TUMORS OF THE EAR LOBE

The ear lobes are subject to various benign and malignant growths in addition to keloids. Cysts of various types are common due to the density of sebaceous and apocrine glands. When they are relatively new, intralesional corticosteroids can be utilized in an attempt to obviate the need for surgery. When this approach is unsuccessful, surgery is indicated. Whenever possible, removing the cyst via a posterior approach is preferable, most significantly to conceal the incision. When cysts are 1.0 to 3.0 mm in size, a punch excision may be easiest. When utilizing this technique, the cyst should be immobilized with the thumb on the posterior surface and the second and third fingers spanning the cyst anteriorly. The punch is then pushed directly into the lobe surrounding the cyst. Care should be taken not to inadvertently perforate the skin on the anterior surface. A chalazion clamp can also be utilized for stabilization, although a disadvantage to this technique is that the operator loses direct tactile sensation of the size, location, and relative position of the cyst. If it is relatively close to the posterior skin surface, the stretching and compression from the clamp can make the cyst readily visible. When it is larger, the punch technique becomes less practical. We utilize the smallest incision possible overlying the cyst, which is then carried deeper into the lobe in a pyramidal fashion. The cyst is dissected free from the surrounding stroma using scissors. Once it has been isolated, we often use a hemostat to grasp the cyst wall to optimize control. If grasped indelicately, the cyst can rupture, making complete removal more difficult and the chance for recurrence greater. If the cyst is large and has been present for a long time the "tissue expansion" that has occurred over it will leave excess skin. The size of the overlying ellipse should vary accordingly.

Common skin tumors such as basal cell, squamous cell carcinoma, and melanoma can occur on the ear lobe. If the lesions are small, primary closure may be easily accomplished. If they occupy a larger portion of the lobule, reconstruction becomes more challenging. Adjacent periauricular skin can sometimes be used to recreate portions of the lobe (Figs 23-38 to 23-40). Full-thickness or split-thickness skin grafts are seldom used, although the posterior lobule can be an excellent donor source for small full-thickness grafts. Depending on the size and shape of the recipient defect a "punch" graft may be the best option. The donor defect on the lobe can be sutured or left to heal by second intention.

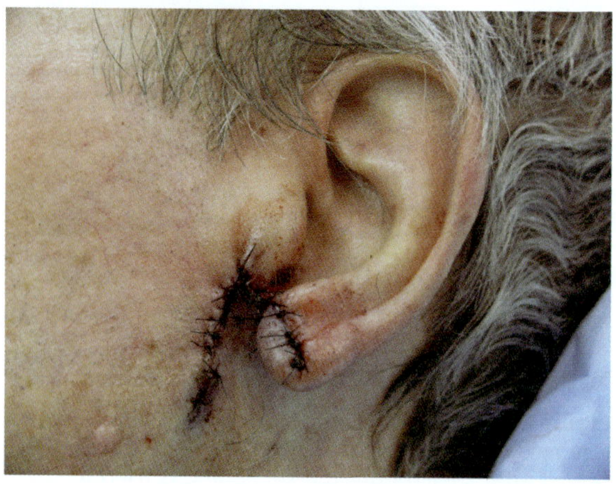

Figure 23-39 Sutured infra-tragal subunit and lobe flap.

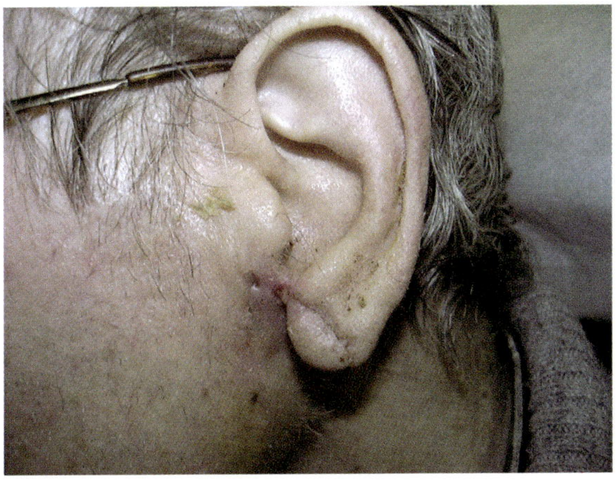

Figure 23-40 Result at suture removal.

As the lobule is relatively thick, significant graft thinning will be required before suturing it into position.

"Friends, Romans, countrymen—lend me your ears."[1] Our external ears are valuable for a number of reasons. The outer ear helps to collect sound waves and funnel them toward the inner ear, where they can be processed. Because the ears are among our most prominent facial features, they may be a source of adornment from a very early age. Piercing and placement of jewelry on the ears are meant to call attention to them. When they are malformed, torn, asymmetrical or affected by disease, the ears can be a source of consternation and self-consciousness. Whether the task is to pierce an ear, remove a keloid, fix a laceration or reconstruct a defect of the skin and cartilage after tumor removal, the outcome is often of great importance to the patient. It is incumbent upon us to use our skills as dermatologic surgeons in such a way as to meet or exceed our patients' expectations, and to provide them with the best possible aesthetic and functional results.

[1] Shakespeare, William. *Julius Caesar.* Act III, scene II.

REFERENCES

1. Gray H. Organs of special sense: The ear. In: *Gray's Anatomy.* 15th ed. New York, NY: Barnes & Noble Books; 1995:830–834.
2. Bean RB. Some ears and types of men. *American Anthropologist* 1915;17:529–533.
3. Greenbaum SS, Greenbaum CH. *Aesthetic Dermatology.* New York, NY: McGraw- Hill; 1991:19–29
4. Amer M, Greenbaum SS, Lask GP, Parrish LC. *Aesthetic Dermatology.* New York, NY: McGraw-Hill; 1991:185–189.
5. Hwang K, Hwang PJ. Which type of earring and which piercing point is safest with regards to tearing through the ear by an external force? *Dermatol Surg.* 2012;38:772–777.
6. Hendricks WM. Complications of ear piercing: treatment and prevention. *Cutis.* 1991;48:386–394.
7. Wolfram D, Tzankov A, Pulzl P, Piza-Katzer P. Hypertrophic scars and keloids—a review of their pathophysiology, risk factors, and therapeutic management. *Dermatol Surg.* 2009;35:171–181.
8. Murray JC. Scars and keloids. *Dermatol Clin.* 1993;11: 697–707.
9. Nemeth AJ. Keloids and hypertrophic scars. *J Dermatol Surg Oncol.* 1993;19:738–746.
10. Nikko A, Hsu S, Quan LT, Greenbaum SS. Surgical pearl: repair of partially torn earlobes—punch technique versus conversion to complete tear. *J Am Acad Dermatol.* 2000;43: 99–101.
11. Niamtu J. Eleven pearls for cosmetic earlobe repair. *Dermatol Surg.* 2002;28:180–185.
12. Zilinsky I, Tessone A, Winkler E, Mendes D, Alon L. Partially torn ear lobe repair using a cross-stitching technique. *Dermatol Surg.* 2009;35:987–989.
13. Kalimuthu R, Larson BJ, Lewis N. Earlobe repair: a new technique. *Plast Reconstr Surg.* 1984;74:299–300.
14. Pardue AM. Repair of torn earlobe with preservation of the perforation for an earring. *Plast Reconstr Surg.* 1973;51: 472–473.
15. Smith C, Glaser DA. Surgical pearl: repair of split or deformed ear lobe with a tongue depressor blade for stabilization during surgery. *J AM Acad Dermatol.* 1998;38: 990–991.
16. Dessy KA, Buccheri EM. Modified punch technique for incomplete earlobe cleft repair. *Aesthetic Plast Surg.* 2006;30: 731–732.
17. Robinson JK. Split earlobe repair. In: Robinson JK, Arndt KA, LeBoit PE, Wintroub BU, eds. *Atlas of Cutaneous Surgery.* Philadelphia, PA: W.B. Saunders; 1996:207–209.
18. Greco JF, Stanko CS, Greenbaum SS. Use of a deep polypropylene suture during earlobe repair: A method to provide permanent reinforcement in the prevention of recurrent earlobe tract elongation. *Dermatol Surg.* 2005;31:1442–1443.
19. Bennett RG. Selection of wound closure materials. *J Am Acad Dermatol.* 1988;18:619–637.
20. Zoltie N. Split earlobes: a method of repair preserving the hole. *Plast Reconstr Surg.* 1987;80:619–621.
21. Argamaso RV. The lap-joint principle in the repair of the cleft earlobe. *Br J Plast Surg.* 1978;31:337–338.
22. Amer M, Greenbaum SS, Lask GP, Parrish LC. *Aesthetic Dermatology.* New York, NY: McGraw-Hill; 1991:187–188.
23. Harahap M. Repair of split earlobes. A review and a new technique. *J Dermatol Surg Oncol.* 1982;8:187–190.
24. Mowlavi A, Meldrum DG, Wilhelmi BJ, Russell RC, Zook EG. The "pixie"ear deformity following face lift surgery revisited. *Plast Reconstr Surg.* 2005;115(4):1165–1171.
25. Man D. Reducing the incidence of ear deformity in facelift. *Aesthet Surg J.* 2009;29(4):264–271.
26. Rubin MG. *Manual of Chemical Peels Superficial and Medium Depth.* Philadelphia, PA: JB Lippincott Co; 1995.
27. Brody HJ, Monheit GD, Resnik SS, Alt TH. A History of chemical peeling. *Dermatol Surg.* 2000;26:405–409.
28. Kauvar AN, Dover JS. Facial skin rejuvenation: Laser resurfacing or chemical peel: choose your weapon. *Dermatol Surg.* 2001;27:209–212.
29. Reddy KK, Brauer JA, Geronemus RG. Evidence for fractional laser treatment in the improvement of cutaneous scars. *J Am Acad Dermatol.* 2012;66(6):1005–1006.
30. Brightman LA, Brauer JA, Anolik R, et al. Ablative and fractional ablative lasers. *Dermatol clin.* 2009;27(4):479–489.
31. Greenbaum SS, Rubin MG. Surgical pearl: The high-energy pulsed carbon dioxide laser for immediate scar resurfacing. *J AM Acad Dermatol.* 1999;40:988–990.
32. Tzikas TL. A 52-Month summary of results using calcium hydroxylapatite for facial soft tissue augmentation. *Dermatol Surg.* 2008;34:S9–S15.
33. Alam M, Gladstone H, Kramer EM, et al. ASDS Guidelines of care: Injectable fillers. *Dermatol Surg.* 2008;34:S115–S148.
34. Redbord KP, Busso M, Hanke CW. Soft-tissue augmentation with hyaluronic acid and calcium hydroxyl apatite fillers. *Dermatol Ther.* 2011;24:71–81
35. Lee A, Grummer SE, Kriegel LD, Marmur E. Hyaluronidase. *Dermatol Surg.* 2010;36:1071–1077.
36. Brody HJ. Use of hyaluronidase in the treatment of granulomatous HA reactions or unwanted hyaluronic acid misplacement. *Dermatol Surg.* 2005;31:893–897.

37. Vivas AC, Tang JC, Maderal AD, Viera MH. Hypertrophic scars and keloids, part 1: conventional treatments. *Cos Dermatol.* 2012;25:309–316.
38. Shaffer JJ, Taylor SC, Cook-Bolden F. Keloidal scars: a review with a critical look at therapeutic options. *J Am Acad Dermatol.* 2002;46:S63–S97.
39. Tziotzios C, Profyris C, Sterling J. Cutaneous scarring: pathophysiology, molecular mechanisms, and scar reduction therapeutics: part II. Strategies to reduce scar formation after dermatologic procedures. *J Am Acad Dermatol.* 2012;66:13–24.
40. Atkinson JA, McKenna KT, Barnett AG, McGrath DJ, Rudd M. A randomized, controlled trial to determine the efficacy of paper tape in preventing hypertrophic scar formation in surgical incisions that traverse Langer's skin tension lines. *Plast Reconstr Surg.* 2005;116:1648–1658.
41. Shih R, Waltzman J, Evans GR. Review of over-the-counter topical scar treatment products. *Plast Reconstr Surg.* 2007;119:1091–1095.
42. Morganroth P, Wilmot AC, Miller C. Over-the-counter scar products for postsurgical patients: disparities between online advertised benefits and evidence regarding efficacy. *J Am Acad Dermatol.* 2009;61:e31–e47.
43. Mustoe TA, Cooter RD, Gold MH, et al. International clinical recommendations on scar management. *Plast Reconstr Surg.* 2002;110:560–571.
44. Berman B, Flores F. Recurrence rates of excised keloids treated with postoperative triamcinolone acetonide injections or interferon alfa-2b injections. *J Am Acad Derm.* 1997;5:755–757.
45. Fulton JE. Silicone gel sheeting for the prevention and management of evolving hypertrophic and keloid scars. *Dermatol Surg.* 1995;21:947–951.
46. Klumpar DI, Murray JC, Anscher M. Keloids treated with excision followed by radiation therapy. *J Am Acad Dermatol.* 1994;31:225–231.
47. Darzi MA, Chowdri NA, Kaul SK, Khan M. Evaluation of various methods of treating keloids and hypertrophic scars: a 10 year follow-up study. *Br J Plast Surg.* 1992;45:374–379.
48. Berman B, Bieley HC. Adjunct therapies to surgical management of keloids. *Dermatol Surg.* 1996;22:126–130.
49. Alster TS, Williams CM. Treatment of keloid scars with 585 nm flashlamp-pumped pulsed-dye laser. *Lancet.* 1995;345:1198–1200.
50. Park TH, Seo WS, Kin K, Chang CH. Earlobe keloids: classification according to gross morphology determines proper surgical approach. *Derm Surg.* 2011;38:406–412.
51. Music EN, Engel G. Earlobe keloids: a novel and elegant surgical approach. *Dermatol Surg.* 2010;36:395–400.
52. Rosen DJ, Patel M, Freeman K, Weiss P. A primary protocol for management of ear keloids: results of excision combined with intraoperative and post-operative steroid injections. *Plast Reconst Surg.* 2007;120:1395–1400.
53. Lee Y, Minn K, Baek R, Hong J. A new surgical treatment of keloid: keloid core excision. *Ann Plast Surg.* 2001;46:135–140.
54. Greenbaum SS, Radonich MA. The purse-string closure. *Dermatol Surg.* 1996;22:1054–1056.
55. Brady JG, Grande DJ, Katz AE. The purse-string suture in facial reconstruction. *J Dermatol Surg Oncol.* 1992;18:812–816.
56. Vujevich J, Obagi. Repair of partial earlobe cleft using a "purse-string"repair. *Derm Surg.* 2006;32:969–971.
57. Kontos AP, Ozog DM. (2006), Use of purse-string suture technique in closure of flesh tunnel defects of the bilateral earlobes. *Dermatologic Surgery*, 32:1070–1071
58. Qi Z, Liang W, Wang Y, et al. X"-shaped incision and keloid skin-flap resurfacing: a new surgical method for auricle keloid excision and reconstruction. *Dermatologic Surgery.* 2012;38:1378–1382.
59. Field LM. Subtotal keloid excision – a preferable preventative regarding recurrence. *Dermatol Surg.* 2001;27:323–324.
60. Kim DY, Kim ES, Eo SR, Kim KS, Lee SY, Cho BH. A surgical approach for earlobe keloid: keloid fillet flap. *Plast Reconstr Surg.* 2004;113:1668–1674.

CHAPTER 24

Surgical Complications and Their Management

Milène K. Crispin, Erik S. Cabral, & Sumaira Z. Aasi

INTRODUCTION

Complications, defined as any adverse and unexpected events, are inevitable in surgery. The recent increase in the number of outpatient surgical procedures has led to a critical appraisal of its safety. Yet several studies have demonstrated the overwhelming safety of dermatologic surgery.[1,2] In a 10 year prospective study of office-based surgeries in Florida, where there is mandatory reporting of surgical complications, there were 309 reported adverse incidents, out of which dermatologists accounted for just 1.3% of all complications (no deaths).[3] The first comprehensive prospective study documenting the relative incidence of postoperative complications in dermatologic surgery, specifically Mohs surgery, found the overall incidence to be 1.6%.[4] In a recent multicenter prospective study of 20,821 Mohs procedures, there were 149 adverse events (0.72%), including four serious events (0.02%), and no deaths reported.[5] The most common adverse events were infections (61.1%), dehiscence and partial or full necrosis (20.1%), and bleeding and hematoma (15.4%). This chapter will review some common complications associated with dermatologic surgery and provide strategies for the prevention, assessment, and management of these complications.

PREOPERATIVE ASSESSMENT

Preoperative assessment, particularly of pre-existing medical conditions and medications, can help the surgeon identify patients at higher risk for intra- and postoperative complications such as bleeding, infection, and poor wound healing. A preoperative evaluation, discussed thoroughly in other parts of this text, includes guidelines on identifying the correct surgical site, reviewing pertinent medical history, prior surgeries including any problems with wound healing, medications (including anticoagulants), allergies, social history (including the use of tobacco and alcohol), and anticipating the postoperative care of the wound in the patient's particular social supportive setting.

IDENTIFYING THE CORRECT SURGICAL SITE

Identifying and confirming the correct surgical site prior to surgery is axiomatic. In a survey that included 300 Mohs surgeons, wrong-site surgery was the most frequent cause of medical lawsuits.[6] A photograph of the prebiopsy site is crucial for avoiding wrong-site surgery, as evidenced in a study by McGinness and Goldstein, in which all surgical sites were identified correctly with a preoperative biopsy-site photograph. Without the photograph, 16% of patients and 5.9% of physicians incorrectly identified the site, and in 4.4% of cases, both the patient and physician incorrectly identified the site despite having access to the pathology report listing the anatomic site.[7] Once the surgical site has been identified with a prebiopsy picture, the physician should have the patient mark the site to confirm the area with a pen and mirror.

PACEMAKERS

It was previously thought that the use of electrosurgical devices in dermatologic surgery could cause pacemaker and implantable cardiac defibrillator (ICD) malfunction; however, it is now known that patients with these devices have a low overall risk of cardiac complications in dermatologic surgery,[8] and that the types of interference reported have not led to any significant morbidity or mortality.[9] It is recommended that these devices be kept on during dermatologic surgery, and that surgeons exercise precautions to minimize interference such as utilizing short bursts of less than 5 seconds, using minimal power, avoiding the area directly around the device, using bipolar forceps, and, if necessary, true electrocautery to achieve hemostasis.

ALLERGIES

A history of allergies is important to obtain in dermatologic surgery, particularly allergies to local anesthetics, topical antibiotics, cleansers, tape/adhesives, and latex. Allergic reactions include type I (IgE-mediated, causing anaphylaxis) and type IV (delayed-type) hypersensitivities. Local anesthesia typically used in dermatologic surgery includes esters and amides, and amides are almost universally tolerated. When an allergy is reported, it is usually to the preservative compounds such as methylparaben, and not the anesthetic compound itself. Some patients mistakenly believe that they have an "allergy" to epinephrine due to the physiological side effect of palpitations and rapid heartbeat. Education and reassurance regarding this side effect often allays any misapprehension. Regardless, a careful history of any "allergic" episode to local anesthesia should be elicited and clarified, and in the rare cases of true allergy to local anesthetics a referral to an allergist prior to surgery would be prudent.

The most common allergy to topical antibiotics is a type IV hypersensitivity to neomycin (15%). Of note, bacitracin

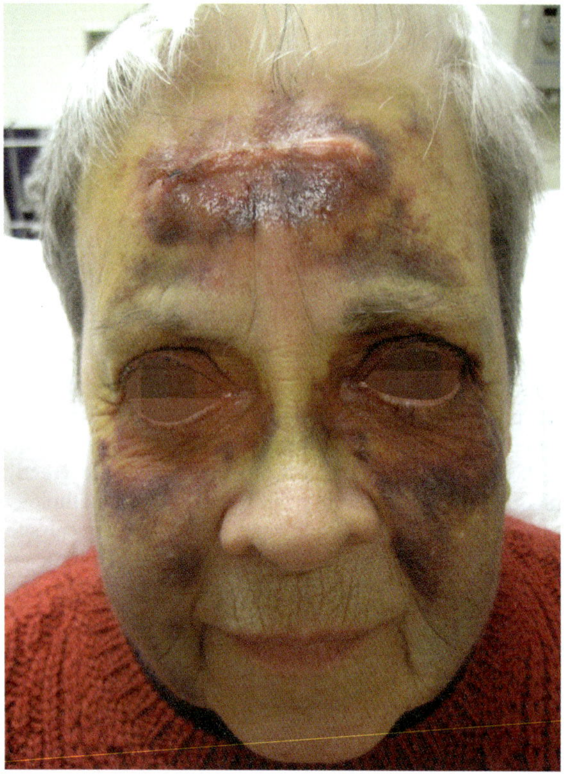

Figure 24-1 Ecchymosis: Extensive bruising developed bilaterally inferior to the surgical site on this patient's face.

can cross-react with neomycin and it is generally recommended to use topical mupirocin or erythromycin if a topical antibiotic is preferred. Eliciting allergies to oral antibiotics is important in the event that the patient needs pre- or postsurgical antibiotic prophylaxis or develops a postsurgical wound infection.

An allergic contact dermatitis (ACD) may result from preservatives in emollients or bacitracin or neomycin, which are key components of over-the-counter antibiotic ointments such as Polysporin or from any components of the wound dressing. The morphology of an ACD is typically bright erythema surrounding the wound with discrete margins, reflecting the distribution in which the offending agent came into contact with the skin. An ACD with a geometric shape is suggestive of an allergy to a tape adhesive component such as colophony. The patient will often complain of pruritus in an ACD rather than pain, which is more commonly associated with infection.

TOBACCO

Smoking tobacco has been associated with a higher incidence of postoperative complications including infections, impaired wound healing, wound dehiscence, and graft/flap necrosis.[10] Case series have shown a higher rate of flap failure in smokers who smoked even one pack per day compared with those who smoked fewer cigarettes and abstainers.[11] The consensus recommendations for smoking cessation before dermatologic surgery are to stop or decrease (as much as possible) smoking at least 2 weeks before and 1 week after surgery. Surgeons should minimize undermining in the deep subcutaneous plane and limit tissue dissection during the procedure, and avoid large flap reconstructions, if possible. In cases necessitating flaps, a delayed flap may have an improved outcome.[12]

BLEEDING AND HEMATOMA

Bleeding is usually the first postoperative complication that occurs in dermatologic surgery, and it can often initiate the other dreaded complications: wound tension and necrosis, infection, and dehiscence. Increased intraoperative and postoperative bleeding can be multifactorial in nature. Abnormal hemostasis can occur due to an acquired or inherited bleeding disorder, thrombocytopenia, platelet dysfunction, or pharmacologic interference. Assessment of anticoagulants and medical comorbidities can help a surgeon identify patients at higher risk for adverse events such as bleeding and hematoma.

ANTICOAGULATION

Dermatologic surgeons used to routinely recommend the discontinuation of anticoagulation and antiplatelet therapies prior to surgery in order to avoid bleeding complications. Prospective and meta-analysis studies have shown the relative paucity of serious complications with the continuation of multiple antiplatelet and anticoagulant medications.[13] Otley et al.[14] found the rate of serious complications in anticoagulated patients to be 1.6% as compared with 0.7% for controls. Moreover, Billingsley et al.[15] studied the bleeding risk with Mohs micrographic surgery in a prospective fashion and showed that there was no significant increase in postoperative hematoma, although there was a slight increase without statistical significance in anticoagulated patients. In the largest prospective study of Mohs micrographic surgeries, most bleeding and wound-healing complications occurred in patients receiving anticoagulation therapy[5]; however, the incidence of complications related to bleeding and wound healing was very low (0.11% and 0.14%, respectively) and none of the bleeding complications were life-threatening. Despite the insignificantly increased risk of bleeding in patients on anticoagulants, ironically, a study showed that when dermatologic surgeons were blinded to the use of anticoagulants in their surgical patients, they were unable to identify which patients were taking them.[16]

Although there is no official consensus statement regarding the discontinuation of anticoagulant and antiplatelet therapy prior to dermatologic surgery, it is now generally accepted that patients should continue these medications if they are being used for primary stroke prevention. There have been several reports of life-threatening adverse events such as ischemic strokes in patients who have discontinued their anticoagulants prior to dermatologic surgery.[17–20] As there been no reports of life-threatening hemorrhagic events in the setting of anticoagulant therapy, anticoagulation therapy used for primary prevention may be continued before and after dermatologic surgery.

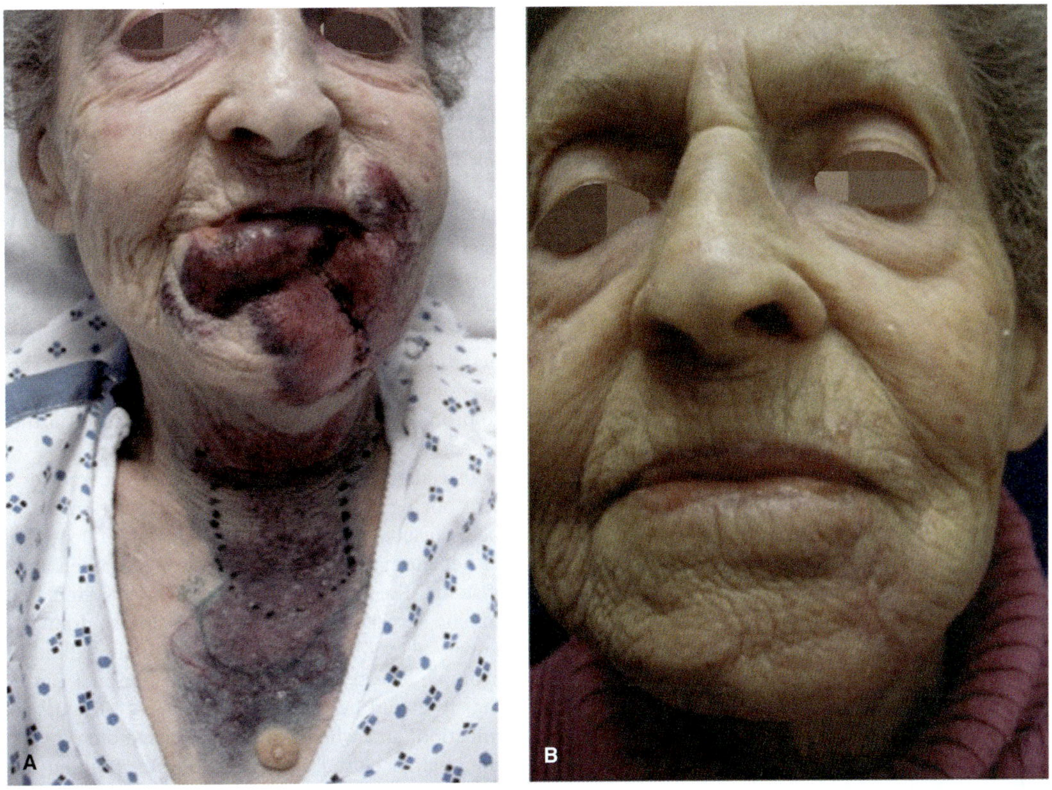

Figure 24-2 **A.** Hematoma: This patient developed a hematoma and persistent oozing from her surgical wound on the lip and chin. **B.** Hematoma resolved without any functional or aesthetic consequences.

The most commonly used anticoagulants are aspirin, clopidogrel, NSAIDs, warfarin, and heparin. Aspirin and clopidogrel irreversibly inhibit platelet function by inactivating cyclooxygenase (COX). It is recommended to discontinue these medications 10 to 14 days prior to surgery if they are not being taken for primary prevention. NSAIDs also inhibit COX, but reversibly. These can be substituted with acetaminophen if taken for pain control, and should also be discontinued 10 to 14 days prior to surgery. Warfarin inhibits the synthesis of serum anticoagulation proteins II, VII, IX, and X, and is thought to increase thrombotic risk in the setting of discontinuation by its compensatory increase in the synthesis of proteins C and S. Warfarin interferes with wound healing by inhibiting the formation of a fibrin plug, which typically occurs 72 to 96 hours post surgery. It is recommended to check a patient's international normalized ratio (INR) before surgery if a large surgical procedure such as a complex two-staged flap is anticipated. The INR should ideally be kept between 2 and 3. Two newer anticoagulants approved for the prevention of systemic emboli are dabigatran (Pradaxa) and rivaroxaban (Xarelto). Both of these medications inhibit the coagulation cascade; dabigatran is a direct thrombin inhibitor whereas rivaroxaban is a direct factor Xa inhibitor. There have been reports of bleeding complications with both of these drugs.[21] Multiple studies have compared the overall risk of bleeding between multiple agents. The risk of complications was higher in patients taking warfarin rather than aspirin as compared with controls.[22] In terms of antiplatelet agents, clopidogrel posed a higher complication risk than aspirin monotherapy.[23]

Patients will often fail to report nonprescription medications and may even be hesitant about reporting herbal remedies. Because of the growing list of herbal products that affect hemostasis, it is important to specifically question a patient about all nonprescription medications and supplements as well. It is generally recommended that these herbal supplements be discontinued 10 to 14 days prior to surgery.

MEDICAL COMORBIDITIES THAT AFFECT HEMOSTASIS

Preoperative assessment should include a screening for bleeding disorders, including prior surgeries and family history. If the patient's personal or family history is suspicious for a bleeding disorder, the surgeon should check the platelet count, a functional in vitro bleeding time assay, PT (extrinsic pathway) and aPTT (intrinsic pathway). A review of medical comorbidities should include assessing for chronic hepatic or renal disease, which can affect clearance of local anesthesia, bleeding risk, and coagulation compromise. Hypertension is also a risk factor for bleeding complications,[24] and blood pressure measurement is a vital component of the preoperative visit and immediately prior to surgery. Finally, alcohol consumption has been shown to inhibit platelet function, decrease coagulation, and increase fibrinolysis.[25] Therefore, it is crucial for dermatologic surgeons to elicit history of alcohol consumption and advise patients to abstain from alcohol at least 48 hours prior to and following surgery.

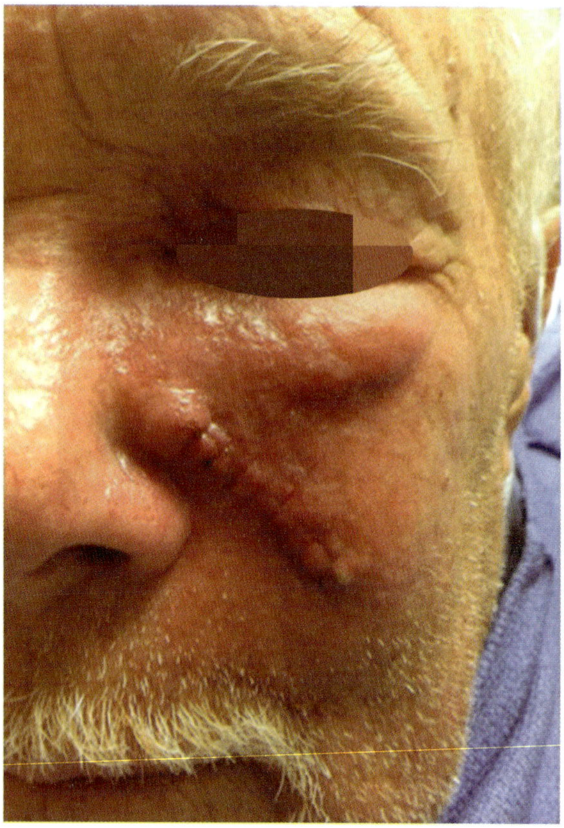

Figure 24-3 Surgical wound infection on the cheek demonstrates redness, swelling, and increased tension upon the superficial sutures. The patient complained of increasing pain despite analgesics.

INTRAOPERATIVE BLEEDING

The addition of epinephrine to the local anesthetic causes local vasoconstriction and helps minimize intraoperative bleeding. Managing intraoperative bleeding efficiently involves proper patient positioning, adequate lighting, and meticulous surgical technique. Vessels and nerves can be damaged or severed during undermining. Although adequate undermining is crucial for decreasing wound tension, it does increase the risk of bleeding and creates potential spaces for hematoma formation and thus should not be excessive. With any surgical procedure, a careful, methodical inspection underneath all wound edges using skin hooks before the wound is sutured is good practice. Once the source vessel has been identified, electrosurgery is appropriate for achieving hemostasis of small arteriolar and venular hemorrhages, whereas ligation is preferred for large vessels. A horizontal figure-of-eight tie with an absorbable suture is preferable for vessel ligation. Absorbable sutures should also be used to close potential dead space to minimize the risk of hematoma formation.

Often, oozing rather than frank bleeding occurs at the surgical site. Goldman[26] has described the approach to intraoperative oozing, and offers varying approaches for the management of superficial (dermal) oozing and deep (musculature) oozing. Superficial oozing may be managed by manual pressure, chemical agents such as aluminum chloride or ferric subsulfate, or cauterization (electrodesiccation, electrocoagulation, or disposable heat cautery). For deeper or muscular oozing, the aforementioned methods of manual pressure and cautery may be used. In addition, absorbable hemostatic agents or drains may be used if the persistent oozing and bleeding cannot be controlled, so as to prevent the development of a hematoma. Hemostatic agents include gelatin foams (Gelfoam®), oxidized cellulose (Oxycel®, Surgicel®), and microfibrillar collagen (Avitene®, Collastat®).[27] Of note, the application of excessive oxidized cellulose has been shown to result in a postsurgical foreign body granulomatous reaction, and caution should be used with this agent.[28] Topical thrombin can also be used to promote a more rapid coagulation cascade at the site of bleeding/oozing.

Placement of a drain should be considered for persistent oozing or with large, complex repairs more likely to be associated with dead space and subsequent formation of hematomas. Drains are classified into open and closed systems. The most commonly used open system in dermatologic surgery is placement of a Penrose drain, whereby gravity allows for the passive movement of fluid through a simple fenestrated drain for collection in a gauze dressing. It should be removed after 24 to 48 hours to avoid infection, and when the risk for hematoma formation is minimal. A closed system includes a draining tube that connects the wound's interior to an outer, sealed container, creating a vacuum with suction, allowing for collection of fluid generated inside the wound. Examples of a closed system include the Jackson–Pratt drain and the mini-flap wound suction drain.[29]

POSTOPERATIVE BLEEDING AND HEMATOMA

Postoperative bleeding most frequently occurs within the first 24 hours, and usually within the first 6 hours after surgery (Fig. 24-1). During this period, epinephrine dissipates, and the subsequent vasodilation can lead to oozing or bleeding of small vessels (Fig. 24-2). Newly formed clots are also sensitive to movement, and can be easily dislodged. Minimizing the risk of postoperative bleeding and hematoma formation begins in the surgical suite, with the application of an adequate pressure dressing and clear, detailed patient instructions. The pressure dressing is usually kept in place for at least 24 hours and should provide pressure without causing ischemia. The dressing typically includes ointment with an overlying nonadherent contact film (Telfa®, Release®), followed by at least one absorbent layer of cotton, sponges, or gauze. It should be secured by an outer layer of adhesive tape and/or a stretchable covering (Ace Wrap®, Coban®).

Written and verbal instructions should be provided to the patient to minimize bleeding, as well as what to do if bleeding or hematoma formation occurs. These instructions include avoidance of movement, bending over, or lifting weight heavier than 10 lb. Patients should also avoid alcohol for at least 48 hours. If the surgical site is perioral, the patient should minimize talking, eat soft foods, and take precautions when inserting or removing dentures. Patients should also be counseled about the

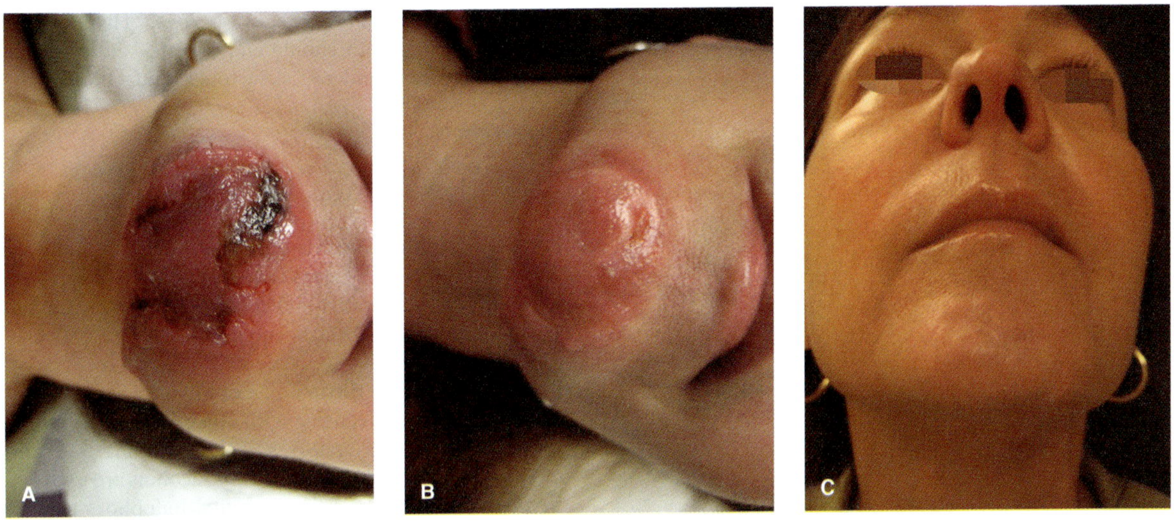

Figure 24-4 **A.** Increased tension on the distal portion of this bilobed transposition flap caused superficial necrosis and dehiscence. **B.** With conservative wound management, the dehisced area heals by second intention. **C.** The bilobed flap has healed without significant scarring.

inevitable development of ecchymoses following surgery. These bruises can extend beyond the surgical wound, especially onto dependent areas of the face, and patients should be counseled to minimize alarm as well as to differentiate this from postoperative bleeding.

MANAGEMENT OF HEMORRHAGE OR HEMATOMA FORMATION

When a hematoma occurs, the patient often experiences increasing pain or pressure at the site. If the patient is concerned about persistent bleeding or hematoma formation, he/she should be instructed to remove the pressure dressing and visualize the wound to ascertain whether there is a specific area that is the source of bleeding. The patient should apply direct pressure for 15 to 20 minutes, while watching a clock. In many cases, minor postoperative bleeding or oozing will cease with this intervention. However, if bleeding persists then the patient needs to be evaluated by the surgeon.

A hematoma is a localized collection of blood and its evolution can be divided into four stages: early (stage I), gelatinous (stage II), organized (stage III), and liquefaction (stage IV).[30] Within the first 48 hours of surgery, the surgeon is confronted with early stage or expanding hematomas. These have the potential to cause wound ischemia and necrosis, and are a nidus for infection. If an early or expanding hematoma is found on evaluation, the surgeon should reanesthetize the wound (with or without epinephrine), evacuate the hematoma, visualize the source(s) of bleeding, achieve hemostasis, and irrigate the wound bed. If a source cannot be ascertained or oozing persists, a drain may be placed. The wound may be left open to heal by secondary intention or partially sutured or completely reclosed, depending on the surgeon's confidence that adequate hemostasis has been achieved. Due to the increased risk of infection in this case, many surgeons advocate initiating a course of empiric antibiotics.

A later stage hematoma, in the gelatinous or organized stage, often cannot be easily extracted without opening the wound. If a gelatinous or organized hematoma is not expanding, evacuation can be delayed until 7 to 10 days postoperatively, when the hematoma is in the liquefactive stage and can be evacuated with simple needle aspiration. In many instances, a nonexpanding gelatinous hematoma will liquefy and be resorbed by the body and does not necessarily need evacuation.

ANTIBIOTIC PROPHYLAXIS AND WOUND INFECTIONS

The efficacy of prophylactic oral antibiotics in dermatologic surgery is unclear, and the current guidelines are not based on multiple, large-scale, prospective trials.[31] It is generally accepted that patients at high risk for developing infective endocarditis or a joint infection (as defined by the American Heart Association and American Academy of Orthopaedic Surgeons, respectively) who are undergoing dermatologic surgery involving the breach of a mucosal barrier or infected skin should receive antibiotic prophylaxis. The guidelines and rationale are discussed in the chapter on preoperative evaluation.

Most surgical wounds in dermatologic surgery are categorized as clean or clean-contaminated. In general surgery, where sterile technique is practiced in all aspects of surgery, the risks of infection for these wounds are +/− 2% and 10%, respectively. In cutaneous surgery, the rates are much lower than expected, and are estimated at less than 1% to 3%.[32–34] These rates are even lower in Mohs micrographic surgery (0.44%–0.91%), after which wounds often may be left open for prolonged periods of time and sterile technique may only be practiced during reconstruction.[5,35] Not surprisingly, more complex repairs such as flaps have been associated with the highest risk of infection (2.4%–2.67%).[34] In a study of 5091 skin surgery cases, there

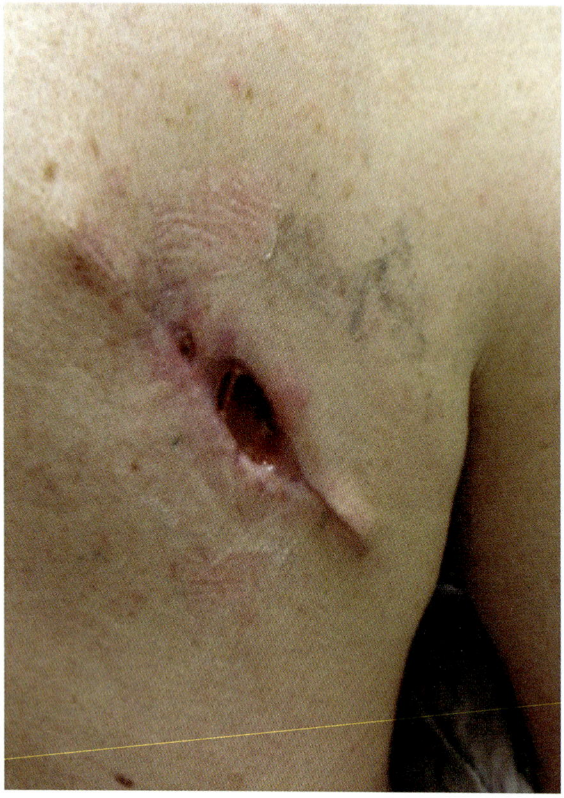

Figure 24-5 Extensive suture reaction causing a dehiscence.

was an overall infection rate of 1.47%, with increased risk in specific sites, including below the knee (6.92%), groin area (10%), wedge excisions of the lip and ear (8.57%), and grafts (8.7%).[32] In contrast, the Mohs micrographic surgery prospective studies showed no increase in the rate of infection in cases involving skin graft repairs, or having surgical defects on the lips, ears, or below the knee.[34] Hemorrhagic complications in both simple and complex dermatologic surgeries are independent risk factors for infection.[32,36]

PREVENTION OF SURGICAL SITE INFECTIONS

Preventive measures such as antibiotic prophylaxis and the use of sterile surgical gloves have been shown to correlate with fewer postoperative infections in some studies, but these measures have not been shown to be causative.[5,37] Most Mohs surgeons use sterile gloves during reconstruction, but not during the removal of Mohs layers.[5] In addition, preoperative cleansing with one or more antiseptics, including alcohol, iodophors, and chlorhexidine, is recommended for prevention of infection. Alcohols are used less frequently due to their flammability. Iodophors provide antimicrobial protection, but are inactivated by serum or blood. They should not be used in patients with iodine or shellfish allergies. Chlorhexidine provides broad-spectrum antibiotic activity, but should be used with caution around the eyes and ears due to potential corneal irritation and ototoxicity. Shaving the skin has been shown to increase the risk of infection,[38] and surgeons should clip hair in lieu of shaving when possible.

TREATMENT OF SURGICAL SITE INFECTIONS

Although postoperative infections are rare in dermatologic surgery, they will typically present 4 to 7 days following surgery with symptoms of increasing pain, swelling, warmth, erythema, and/or purulent drainage (Fig. 24-3). When an infection is suspected, a wound culture should be obtained and empiric antibiotics initiated that are appropriate to the surgical site (Table 24-1) and probable microorganism.

TABLE 24-1

Antibiotic Management of Postsurgical Infections According to Microorganism and/or Surgical Site

Agent	Regimen	Duration	Microorganism/Site
Cephalexin	250–500 mg PO BID-QID	7–10 d	*S. aureus*, first-line agent
Dicloxacillin	250–500 mg PO BID-QID	7–10 d	*S. aureus*, first-line agent
Azithromycin	250 mg	2 tabs on day 1 and 1 tab on days 2–5	*S. aureus*, first-line alternative in penicillin-allergic patients
Amoxicillin/Clavulanate	500 mg PO TID or 875 mg PO TID	7–10 d	*S. viridans* coverage for oral mucosal site, first-line agent
Ciprofloxacin	500 mg PO BID	7–10 d	*S. aureus* and *Pseudomonas* coverage for ear or genitourinary site
Clindamycin	300 mg PO QID	7–10 d	*S. aureus* and *S. viridans* coverage for skin or oral surgery
Erythromycin	500 mg PO BID	7–10 d	*S. viridans* coverage for oral mucosal site, second-line agent
Trimethoprim/Sulfamethoxazole	1 DS tab PO BID	7–10 d	*S. aureus* and *E. coli* coverage for skin and genitourinary sites

Source: Reproduced with permission from Wood LD, Warner NM, Billingsley EM. Infectious complications of dermatologic procedures. *Dermatol Ther.* 2011;24:558–570.

Depending on the severity of infection and the amount of purulence, some, if not all, of the percutaneous sutures should be removed to allow for drainage and healing by secondary intention. Abscesses always require drainage. In rare cases, if patients report fever or other worsening systemic symptoms, hospital admission and intravenous antibiotics may be indicated. Most surgical site infections result from the presence of bacteria on the patient's skin and accordingly, their frequency is as follows, in descending order: *Staphylococcus aureus*, coagulase-negative staphylococci, enterococcus spp., *Escherichia coli*, *Pseudomonas aeruginosa* and streptococci. Certain pathogens follow a time course of presentation following cutaneous surgery. Streptococcal infections usually present early, in the first 1 to 2 days after surgery, and typically appear as rapidly spreading, painful erythema. Staphylococcal infections appear 2 to 5 days postoperatively and are usually associated with a collection of purulent material. In the later postoperative period, such as 2 to 4 weeks after surgery, infections with *Mycobacterium* can present with nonhealing ulcers and recurrent papulonodules. Surgeons should also be aware of the prevalence of methicillin-resistant *S. aureus* (MRSA) and initiate appropriate antibiotic therapy if there is a high suspicion for a MRSA infection prior to return of the culture results. Viral, fungal, and mycobacterial infections are much less common but when they do occur, the culprit is usually HSV-1, HSV-2, *Candida* species, and multiple species of *Mycobacterium*.[39] Of note, contact allergies and inflammatory response to sutures often mimic infection in their presentations.

TISSUE ISCHEMIA AND NECROSIS

Tissue ischemia and necrosis occur due to inadequate blood supply, often in relation to other complications such as edema, increased wound tension secondary to bleeding or poor operative design and execution, infection, underlying medical conditions that impair wound healing, or patient noncompliance, such as inappropriate postoperative physical activity. Tissue ischemia can lead to wound necrosis and even dehiscence (Fig. 24-4). In order to avoid ischemia and necrosis, surgeons should minimize direct tissue injury and excessive wound tension intraoperatively.

Direct tissue injury can occur intraoperatively due to traumatization of wound edges. Surgeons and their assistants should take care not to crush the wound edges when handling them with skin hooks or forceps, or grasp them for excessive periods of time. Sutures should not be tied too tightly, especially superficial sutures. Excessive electrocautery can also cause direct tissue injury, and charred and necrotic tissue can serve as a nidus for infection after wound closure. Vascular compromise of the wound can also occur if blood vessels are traumatized either by electrocautery or excessive undermining.

Excessive wound tension not only leads to wound necrosis, but can also result in wound dehiscence, scar widening, and an undesirable cosmetic result. Excessive tension can be avoided by adequate undermining, proper placement of buried sutures to avoid surface tension, and the appropriate use of flaps and grafts to minimize tension when surgical defects cannot be repaired linearly. As excessive wound tension is often the result of poor design, every effort should be made to carefully plan a closure that is appropriate to the surgical site. If it becomes apparent that the closure is burdened by excessive tension, the surgeon can attempt to alleviate this by placing relaxing incisions 2 to 3 cm from the wound bed, using tissue expanders, or opting for a partial closure with healing by secondary intention, depending on the site of the surgical defect.

Flaps and grafts are subject to relative ischemia and are therefore more susceptible to necrosis and infection. Complications of flaps can arise from a variety of causes: poor reconstructive design, traumatic tissue handling, inappropriate dog-ear correction at the vascular base of the flap, aggressive control of bleeding, and excessive wound tension. Grafts are especially vulnerable in certain sites with poor blood supply such as exposed bone, exposed cartilage, and at sites of previous radiation. Adequate contact between the graft and the wound bed must be established, as poor placement or accumulation of blood may lead to inadequate contact. Methods to maximize graft viability include achieving a balance between adequate hemostasis while minimizing electrocautery of the wound bed and proper apposition of graft to the wound bed. Fenestrations in the graft can minimize the accumulation of blood or a seroma and a pressure dressing can help keep the graft in place, minimizing shearing forces over the wound bed. Neither a necrotic graft nor a flap should be removed or debrided, unless there is an obvious infection. In many instances, the necrotic tissue serves as a biologic dressing, and avoiding aggressive debridement may lead to an unexpected amount of tissue survival beneath the necrotic areas. Reassuring the patient and seeing them regularly throughout the healing process, however, is critical.

DEHISCENCE

Wound dehiscence can occur due to excessive tension, infection, hematoma, or necrosis (Fig. 24-5). It typically occurs at the time of suture removal, but can occur at any time in the first few months following surgery. The tensile strength of scar tissue is approximately 80% of the tensile strength of the uncut skin, and 2 weeks following surgery it is 10% or less than normal.[40] It is therefore important to instruct patients regarding which activities should be avoided after surgery (exercise, no lifting more than 10 lb of weight, stair climbing, long walks) and to verbally reinforce the lack of tensile strength of the wound. If dehiscence occurs due to a complication such as infection or hematoma, those conditions should be treated. If dehiscence occurs without evidence of infection, necrosis, or hematoma, it may be appropriate to resuture the wound as long as there is no excessive tension.

TRAPDOOR DEFORMITY

Transposition flaps with curvilinear borders and V-Y advancement flaps become susceptible to trapdoor deformity. Trapdoor deformity may also result from flap lymphedema, excess subcutaneous fat beneath the flap or a failed connection between the flap base and the recipient bed. Scar tissue around the border of the flap contracts in a concentric fashion. This concentric contractile force pushes the skin of the flap upward and leads to a pin-cushion appearance. Properly sizing the flap as well as wide undermining to create an even plate of scar contraction that extends beyond the flap help to minimize the risk of trapdoor deformity.[41] Some of the trapdoor appearance of the flap may improve with time. Steroid injection into the scar and subcutaneous tissue or scar revision helps in those cases that do not resolve.

NERVE INJURY

In dermatologic surgery, there is a risk of motor or sensory nerve injury, which may or may not be reversible. During the preoperative evaluation, the surgeon should perform a focused neurologic examination to identify any pre-existing deficits or asymmetries, and make the patient aware of such anatomical variations. The types of nerve injury that occur include neurapraxia, axonotmesis, and neurotmesis. Neurapraxia is the least severe form of nerve injury, and occurs when there is a temporary interruption of nerve conduction due to compression or ischemia. Axonotmesis occurs when there is structural damage to the axon and its myelin sheath, with preservation of the encapsulating tissue, epineurium, and perineurium, and restoration of nerve conduction requires axon regeneration. This type of injury usually occurs due to crushing trauma or severe stretching of the nerve. Neurotmesis is transection of the nerve and is the most severe form of nerve injury. This disruption in the architecture of the nerve makes recovery from this type of injury the least likely of all.

Injury to superficial cutaneous sensory nerves is common, and may result in hypoesthesia, anesthesia, paresthesia, or dysesthesia. Dysesthesia and hypoesthesia are extremely common at sites of primary closure or over graft sites. The digits, forehead, and scalp are most susceptible to sensory nerve injury. Motor nerve injury results in deficits that correspond to the associated proximal nerve root. If motor or sensory nerve injury occurs after surgery, the surgeon should counsel the patient that the nerve injury is often temporary, and that function may return in a matter of days to months. Patients should wait at least 9 to 12 months prior to seeking cosmetic or functional repair.

There are well-known anatomic "danger zones" that are at higher risk for nerve injury, and the dermatologic surgeon should exercise caution when performing surgery at these sites. The temporal branch of the facial nerve is most superficial where it crosses the zygomatic arch in the temporal region. The anterior branches supply the frontalis, orbicularis oculi, and corrugator supercilii, and the temporal branch serves as the efferent limbs of the corneal reflex. Injury results in the inability to raise the eyebrows on the affected side, resulting in flattening of the forehead. The marginal mandibular branch of the facial nerve is located at the mid-mandible, approximately 2 cm posterior and inferior to the oral commissure. It supplies the muscles of the lower lip and chin, including the depressor labii inferioris, the depressor anguli oris, and the mentalis. Injury results in drooping and inward retraction of the mouth on the affected side. Finally, the spinal accessory nerve is most vulnerable to injury at Erb's point, which is located 6 cm below the mastoid process or 2 to 3 cm above the clavicle, along the border of the sternocleidomastoid muscle. The spinal accessory nerve provides motor innervation to the sternocleidomastoid and trapezius muscles, and injury results in winging of the scapula, adduction of the arm and inability to elevate the shoulder.

SUTURE GRANULOMA

Suture reactions may take the form of small granulomas or abscesses. Anticipatory guidance regarding the time frame for suture absorption should be provided to patients for suture granulomas. Dermal sutures may emerge from the deep layer and break through the epidermis 4 to 6 weeks after surgery as a result of foreign body reaction to the absorbable sutures. Protruding sutures can be removed with forceps or left to dissolve if the surrounding tissue is friable. Removing the extruding suture can facilitate wound healing. Deeper placement of buried sutures usually helps to prevent suture granuloma formation.

KELOIDS AND HYPERTROPHIC SCARS

Keloids and hypertrophic scars are dreaded, poorly understood complications for both patients and surgeons. They have a predilection for the extremities, neck and trunk, and are thus thought to occur secondary to increased wound tension in areas with constant dynamic movement. They are more common in higher Fitzpatrick skin types and individuals of Asian descent. A hypertrophic scar is characterized as a firm, smooth, elevated scar at the site of cutaneous surgery or injury, whereas a keloid is a smooth elevated scar that extends beyond the site of injury or surgery. Both hypertrophic scars and keloids can be treated with multiple rounds of intralesional corticosteroids with varying success.

CONCLUSION

Even the most scrupulous surgeon will encounter operative complications. Fortunately the overall incidence and morbidity of complications in dermatologic surgery are low. Many complications can be anticipated and avoided by performing a comprehensive preoperative assessment, as well as thoughtful operative design and meticulous execution. Recognizing and appropriately managing complications early can often minimize adverse long-term surgical outcomes.

REFERENCES

1. Merritt BG, Lee NY, Brodland DG, Zitelli JA, Cook J. The safety of Mohs surgery: a prospective multicenter cohort study. *J Am Acad Dermatol.* 2012;67(6):1302–1309.
2. Elliott TG, Thom GA, Litterick KA. Office based dermatologic surgery and Mohs surgery: a prospective audit of surgical procedures and complications in a procedural dermatology practice. *Australas J Dermatol.* 2012;53:264–271.

3. Starling JS, Thosani MK, Coldiron BM. Determining the safety of officed-based surgery: what 10 years of Florida Data and 6 years of Alabama data reveal. *Dermatol Surg.* 2012;38:171–177.
4. Cook JL, Perone JB. A prospective evaluation of the incidence of complications associated with Mohs micrographic surgery. *Arch Dermatol.* 2003;139(2):143–152.
5. Alam M, Ibrahim O, Nodzenski M, et al. Adverse events associated with Mohs micrographic surgery. *JAMA Dermatol.* 2013;149(12):1378–1385. doi:10.1001/jamadermatol.2013.6255.
6. Perlis CX, Campbell RM, Perlis RH, Malik M, Dufresne RG Jr. Incidence of and risk factors for medical malpractice lawsuits among Mohs surgeons. *Dermatol Surg.* 2006;32(1):79–83.
7. McGinness JL, Goldstein G. The value of preoperative biopsy-site photography for identifying cutaneous lesions. *Dermatol Surg.* 2010;36(2):194–197.
8. Matzke TJ, Christenson LJ, Christenson SD, Atanashova N, Otley CC. Pacemakers and implantable cardiac defibrillators in dermatologic surgery. *Dermatol Surg.* 2006;32(9):1155–1162.
9. El-Gamal HM, Dufresne RG, Saddler K. Electrosurgery, pacemakers and ICDs: a survey of precautions and complications experienced by cutaneous surgeons. *Dermatol Surg.* 2001;27(4):385–390.
10. Gill JF, Yu SS, Neuhaus IM. Tobacco smoking and dermatologic surgery. *JAMA Dermatol.* 2013;68:167–172.
11. Goldminz D, Bennett RG. Cigarette smoking and flap and full-thickness graft necrosis. *Arch Dermatol.* 1991; 127(7):1012–1015.
12. Reus WF 3rd, Colen LB, Straker DJ. Tobacco smoking and complications in elective microsurgery. *Plast Reconstr Surg.* 1992;89(3):490–494.
13. Bordeaux JS, Martires KJ, Goldberg D, Pattee SF, Fu P, Maloney ME. Prospective evaluation of dermatologic surgery complications including patients on multiple antiplatelet and anticoagulant medications. *J Am Acad Dermatol.* 2011; 65(3):576–583.
14. Otley CC, Fewkes JL, Frank W, Olbricht SM. Complications of cutaneous surgery in patients who are taking warfarin, aspirin, or nonsteroidal anti-inflammatory drugs. *Arch Dermatol.* 1996;132(2):161–166.
15. Billingsley EM, Maloney ME. Intraoperative and postoperative bleeding problems in patients taking warfarin, aspirin, and nonsteroidal anti-inflammatory agents. A prospective study. *Dermatol Surg.* 1997;23(5):381–383.
16. West SW, Otley CC, Nguyen TH, et al. Cutaneous surgeons cannot predict blood-thinner status by intraoperative visual inspection. *Plast Reconstr Surg.* 2002;110(1):98–103.
17. Schanbacher CF, Bennett RG. Postoperative stroke after stopping warfarin for cutaneous surgery. *Dermatol Surg.* 2000; 26(8):785–789.
18. Alam M, Goldberg LH. Serious adverse vascular events associated with perioperative interruption of antiplatelet and anticoagulant therapy. *Dermatol Surg.* 2002;28(11):992–998.
19. Kovich O, Otley CC. Thrombotic complications related to discontinuation of warfarin and aspirin therapy perioperatively for cutaneous operation. *JAMA Dermatol.* 2003; 48(2):233–237.
20. Kimyai-Asadi A, Jih MH, Goldberg LH. Perioperative primary stroke: is aspirin cessation to blame? *Dermatol Surg.* 2004;30(12 Pt 2):1526–1528.
21. Schmitt AR, Zender CA, Bordeaux JS. A new oral anticoagulant in the setting of dermatologic surgery. *J Am Acad Dermatol.* 2013;68(5):869–870.
22. Lewis KG, Dufresne RG Jr. A meta-analysis of complications attributed to anticoagulation among patients following cutaneous surgery. *Dermatol Surg.* 2008;34(2):160–164.
23. Cook-Norris RH, Michaels JD, Weaver AL, et al. Complications of cutaneous surgery in patients taking clopidogrel-containing anticoagulation. *J Am Acad Dermatol.* 2011;65(3):584–591.
24. Straith RE, Raju DR, Hipps CJ. The study of hematomas in 500 consecutive face lifts. *Plast Resconstr Surg.* 1977;59(5): 694–698.
25. Salem RO, Laposata M. Effects of alcohol on hemostasis. *Am J Clin Pathol.* 2005;123(suppl):S96–S105.
26. Goldman G. Surgical complications and optimizing outcomes. In: Bolognia JL, Jorizzo JL, Schaffer JV, eds. *Dermatology*, 3rd ed. China: Elsevier Limited; 2012:2464.
27. Achneck HE, Sileshi B, Jamiolkowski RM, Albala DM, Shapiro ML, Lawson JH. A comprehensive review of topical hemostatic agents. *Ann Surg.* 2010;251:217–228.
28. Billingsley EM, Maloney ME. Considerations in achieving hemostasis. In: Robinson JK, Arndt KA, Leboit PE, Wintroub BU. *Atlas of Cutaneous Surgery.* Philadelphia, PA: WB Saunders; 1996:67–73.
29. Nasser NA. The use of the Mini-Flap wound suction drain in maxillofacial surgery. *Ann R Coll Surg Engl.* 1986;68(3): 151–153.
30. Nguyen TH, Erickson QL. Hemostasis. In: Robinson JK, Hanke CW, Siegel DM, Fratila A, eds. *Surgery of the Skin,* 2nd ed. New York, NY: Mosby Elsevier; 2010:225–238.
31. Wright TI, Baddour LM, Berbari EF. Antibiotic prophylaxis in dermatologic surgery: advisory statement 2008. *J Am Acad Dermatol.* 2008;59:464–473.
32. Futoryan T, Grande D. Postoperative wound infection rates in dermatologic surgery. *Dermatol Surg.* 1995;21:509–514.
33. Dixon AJ, Dixon MP, Askew DA, Wilkinson D. Prospective study of wound infections in dermatologic surgery in the absence of prophylactic antibiotics. *Dermatol Surg.* 2006;32:819–827.
34. Rogues AM, Lasheras A, Amici JM, et al. Infection control practices and infectious complications in dermatological surgery. *J Hosp Infect.* 2007;65:258–263.
35. Maragh SLH, Brown MD. Prospective evaluation of surgical site infection rate among patients with Mohs micrographic surgery without the use of prophylactic antibiotics. *J Am Acad Dermatol.* 2008;59:275–278.
36. Amici JM, Rogues AM, Lasheras A, et al. A prospective study of the incidence of complications associated with dermatological surgery. *Br J Dermatol.* 2005;153:967–971.
37. Xia Y, Cho S, Greenway HT, Zelac DE, Kelley B. Infection rates of wound repairs during Mohs micrographic surgery using sterile versus non-sterile gloves: a prospective randomized pilot study. *Dermatol Surg.* 2001;37(5):651–656.
38. Cruse PJ, Foord R. A five-year prospective study of 23,649 surgical wounds. *Arch Surg.* 1973;107:206–210.
39. Wood LD, Warner NM, Billingsley EM. Infectious complications of dermatologic procedures. *Dermatol Ther.* 2011;24:558–570.
40. Stasko T. Complications of cutaneous procedures. In: Roenigk RK, Roenigk HH Jr, eds. *Dermatologic Surgery Principles and Practice.* 2nd ed.. New York, NY: Marcel Dekker; 1996:149–175.
41. Kaufman AJ, Kiene KL, Moy RL. Role of tissue undermining in the trapdoor effect of transposition flaps. *J Dermatol Surg Oncol.* 1993;19(2):128–132.

SECTION 3

Skin Tumors

CHAPTER 25

Benign Subcutaneous Tumors

Paul X. Benedetto & Allison T. Vidimos

OVERVIEW

There are a variety of benign dermal and subcutaneous tumors that present to the procedural dermatologist for management. We provide an overview of the epidemiology, clinical presentation, differential diagnosis, histopathology, and surgical management of each of these tumors, and discuss the surgical management of these lesions.

FAT TUMORS

LIPOMA (AND VARIANTS)

Lipomas are a common benign neoplasm composed predominantly of lobules of mature adipocytes and fibrous stroma.[1] They are found most often in the subcutaneous tissue and less frequently in internal organs. They are often delineated from surrounding normal hypodermis by fibrous septa. There are numerous subtypes of benign lipomas. At the malignant end of the spectrum is the liposarcoma, which likely arises de novo, rather than from malignant transformation of benign lipomas.[2] Specific variants of benign lipomas (e.g., angiolipoma, spindle cell lipoma, lipoblastoma, fibrolipoma, adenolipoma) are largely histopathologic distinctions, as their clinical presentations are often quite similar. For the purposes of surgical management, these lesions will be considered together, with special mention made of any identifying or exceptional features.

EPIDEMIOLOGY

Lipomas are the most common soft tissue tumor, occurring in between 0.1% and 1% of the population.[3]

CLINICAL PRESENTATION

Lipomas present as soft or rubbery nodules or masses located within the subcutaneous tissue. They are poorly defined and freely mobile, unless trapped beneath skeletal muscle or galea, which limits their lateral mobility. The overlying epidermis appears clinically unremarkable. Lipomas commonly present as slow-growing tumors with a size range of approximately 1 to 10 cm. They are most often confined to the hypodermis but may achieve substantial mass if left intact for many years. Most lipomas are painless and asymptomatic, but anatomic locations with restricted room for expansion (e.g., forehead and scalp), and histologic subtype (e.g., angiolipoma) may predispose the patient to developing pain with these lesions. Common anatomic locations include the back, shoulders, neck, and proximal upper and lower extremities.[3,4] Lipomas that occur on the forehead are often buried underneath the frontalis muscle or galea.[5]

Lipomas most often present as a solitary lesion, but multiple lesions can occur in certain circumstances, such as familial lipomatosis and genodermatoses such as Gardner's syndrome, Proteus syndrome, neurofibromatosis, Cowden syndrome, Bannayan–Riley–Ruvalcaba syndrome, and others.[6]

Furthermore, certain lesions can mimic lipomas. In some cases, the alternative diagnosis may not be known or suspected until the tumor is assessed intraoperatively. For example, a liposarcoma may be brighter yellow and greasier than a typical lipoma. A lesion that felt rubbery and was clinically consistent with a lipoma, may have the appearance of a vascular tumor intraoperatively. In such cases, it may be advisable to remove a smaller biopsy sample, terminate the case prematurely, and plan a more definitive approach once the results of histopathology are known. Certain unexpected tumors, such as a liposarcoma or dermal metastases, may require preoperative imaging with CT or MRI scans to assess the extent of involvement of underlying tissue prior to surgical excision.

HISTOPATHOLOGY

Lipomas appear histologically as sheets of adipocytes forming fat lobules of varying sizes dissected by fibrous septa and often enclosed by a thin fibrous capsule within the subcutaneous space. Varying degrees of angiogenesis may be appreciated, with angiolipomas displaying numerous small- to medium-sized blood vessels throughout the lobules and septa. Lipomas with relatively increased fibrous tissue are referred to as fibrolipomas. Adenolipomas are a rare variant with prominent eccrine glands. Spindle cell, sclerotic, ossifying fibromyxoid, and chondrolipomas are other rare variants that have been characterized histologically.[7]

TREATMENT/SURGICAL MANAGEMENT OF LIPOMAS

Treatment of lipomas is undertaken for a variety of reasons, and most often is achieved surgically. Tumors that grow unabated warrant excision and histopathologic examination. The clinical diagnosis of a lipoma cannot always be made with complete certainty, and excision for the purpose of histologic examination is a reasonable step in the diagnosis. Removal of lipoma variants such as an angiolipoma may be necessitated by patient discomfort or pain.

PREOPERATIVE ASSESSMENT

As with any other surgical excision, careful preoperative planning will result in the most optimal surgical outcome. It is important to conduct a review of the patient's past medical and surgical histories, social history including tobacco use and alcohol intake, current medications and allergies, and obvious contraindications to surgery.[8]

Regarding the medical history, it is critical to review comorbidities that may impact the surgical procedure. Hypertension may lead to intraoperative or postoperative bleeding. Diabetes may contribute to suboptimal wound healing or higher risk of postoperative infection. Patients may have underlying conditions associated with prolonged bleeding times, such as hemophilia, or abnormal coagulation, such as factor V Leiden deficiency.[9]

A review of the patient's surgical history may uncover issues previously encountered with other surgical procedures, such as keloid formation or hypertrophic scarring, allergies or sensitivities to local anesthetic or epinepherine, allergies or irritation from bandage adhesive, and a history of postoperative infection. A patient who actively smokes tobacco should be warned of the risks of poor wound healing and skin necrosis, especially with larger excisions or tight closures.[10] Heavy alcohol consumption may decrease platelet aggregation and increase the risk of developing a hematoma.[9,11] A thorough review of the patient's medication list is important. Antiplatelet and anticoagulant therapy obviously increases the patient's bleeding risk, but it is not advisable to stop these medications for minor surgery in most cases.[12,13] Likewise, a review of all over-the-counter medications, herbal supplements, and vitamins is important because of the clinically significant side effect profile of many of these medications.[14]

Regarding contraindications to surgery, active infection overlying or near the surgical site should be considered an absolute contraindication for routine elective surgery. Although pregnancy does not absolutely preclude surgical excision of benign lipomas, the excision will need to be conducted with plain lidocaine, as epinephrine is pregnancy category C. Proceeding with excision during pregnancy should be reserved for smaller or problematic lesions, or for lesions for which the diagnosis is not entirely clear.

SURGICAL PLANNING

The next step in planning the excision involves the evaluation of the lesion itself, and any anatomic or functional considerations that may impact the procedure.

When marking the overlying skin to plan the surgical removal, it is helpful to palpate the tumor and mark out the clinically perceived peripheral margins. This will give a rough estimate of the overall size of the lesion. Depending on the size of the tumor, and how long it has been present, the overlying epidermis may exhibit varying amounts of redundancy. For smaller nodules, or lesions without excessive overlying skin, a linear incision may be planned over the center of the lipoma after carefully marking out the borders (Fig. 25-1). For larger lesions, or for tumors that have expanded the overlying skin creating significant redundancy, it is helpful to draw out a conservative ellipse overlying the tumor to remove some of the excess skin. As with any excision, the ellipse should be oriented in the direction of the relaxed skin tension lines. Once the surgical site is marked with ink, anesthetized with local anesthetic, and prepped with a surgical scrub such as chlorhexidine or betadine, the initial incision can be made.

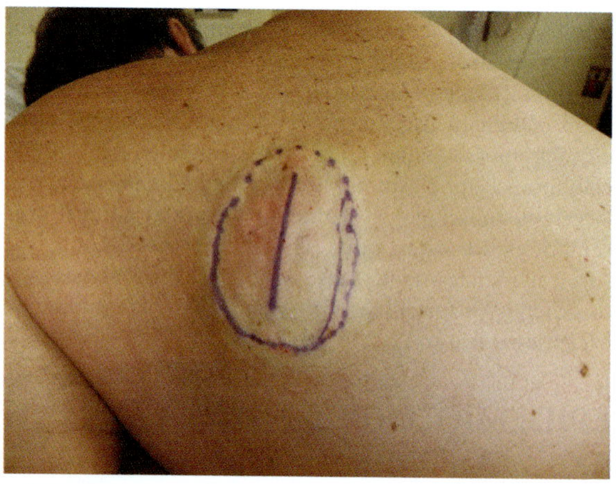

Figure 25-1 Lipoma with peripheral margin and central incision marked.

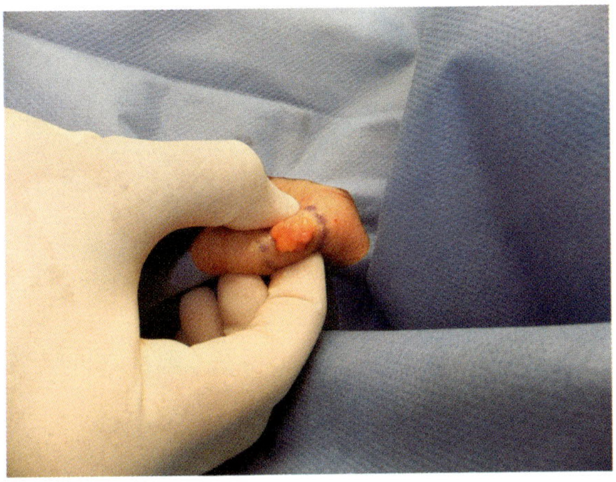

Figure 25-2 Squeezing lipoma through a small incision.

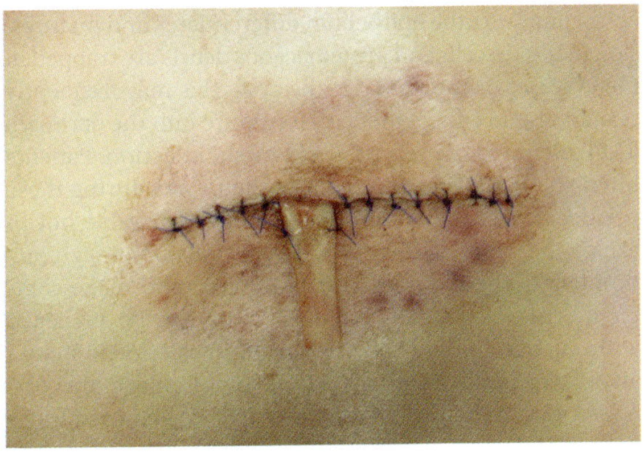

Figure 25-3 Penrose drain placed after lipoma excision.

SURGICAL REMOVAL

The incision should be carried down through the epidermis and dermis into the subcutaneous plane. At this point, firm pressure can be applied circumferentially around the incision site to gently express the lipoma through the skin surface. In the event of a small, superficial lipoma without many fibrous adhesions, this technique may sufficiently deliver the tumor through the skin surface, where it may be cut away from the surrounding adipose tissue with the operating scissors. (Fig. 25-2).[15,16] This technique has been reported to be successful a varying percentage of the time, but is most useful for lipomas of the extremities with adequate overlying soft tissue, and in which the underlying muscle is not involved.[3]

However, in the event of a larger lipoma, or one with more abundant fibrous adhesions, skin hooks may be used to open the incision and expose the depth of the surgical wound. Using a blunt-tipped, curved surgical scissors (e.g., curved Metzenbaums), the lipoma with its associated fibrous septa can be dissected from the surrounding adipose tissue. The fat lobules and adherent fibrous stroma can often be palpated between the surgeon's index finger and thumb, helping to delineate the borders of the tumor. Once the lipoma is dissected from the surrounding adipose tissue and the dissection is carried to a plane beneath the lipoma, the tumor can be sharply transected at the base with the operating scissors. Some authors have described techniques to use tumescent anesthesia to help hydrodissect the lipoma from the surrounding adipose tissue, facilitating surgical removal.[17]

Removal of a large lipoma may result in a defect with significant dead space. This problem must be addressed to prevent the formation of a postoperative seroma or hematoma. One technique that is helpful is to plicate the base of the wound with deep sutures in successive layers of fibroadipose tissue and deep reticular dermis before placing dermal sutures to approximate the skin. In the event that the plicating sutures do not keep the fat well approximated, or if the dead space is too large, placement of a surgical drain, such as a Penrose drain, for several days after the procedure can help prevent fluid collection (Fig. 25-3).

DISTANT INCISION

In the case of a lipoma located in a more conspicuous anatomic location (e.g., forehead), or one approximating a cosmetic unit, the surgical incision can be planned remote from the actual site of the tumor.[18] The incision can be made up to several centimeters from the site of the lipoma, and the dissection carefully carried out around the tumor mass, so that the scar will be hidden (e.g., within the hairline for a forehead lesion). The surgeon is cautioned that such a removal is technically more difficult, and careful technique is required to minimize excess trauma and bleeding. Knowledge of the local surgical anatomy is paramount and meticulous hemostasis is imperative.

LIPOSUCTION TECHNIQUE

Liposuction may be considered a reasonable alternative to surgical excision for the removal of lipomas. This method may be advisable in the case of very large lipomas that may produce excessive surgical scars, lesions that have grown in conspicuous anatomic locations, or in special situations, such as in the case of benign symmetric lipomatosis.[19] The benefits of suction lipectomy relate to its improved cosmesis for smaller surgical scars and overall diminished trauma from less invasive surgical technique.[20] The obvious drawback is the significantly higher rate of recurrence, owing to the fact that the fibrous septa are not always sufficiently removed with this technique. However, some cases may warrant the risk of a higher rate of recurrence to obtain a significantly diminished scar line. Some authors have also described techniques for removing the fibrous capsule through the small liposuction incision as well.[21]

CYSTS

EPIDERMAL INCLUSION CYSTS

Epidermal inclusion cysts (a.k.a. sebaceous cysts, epidermoid cysts, wens) are common benign dermal nodules that frequently present for removal. These lesions consist of a cystic wall composed of stratified squamous epithelium.[7] As the epithelium differentiates and matures, sloughed skin cells and proteinaceous debris are trapped in the cystic cavity and enlarge the cyst. This may frequently result in rapid enlargement, cyst rupture into the dermis, a local inflammatory reaction, and rarely, infection. Patients often present for management of their cysts during these periods of inflammation. It is, however, advisable not to excise the cysts at this time, as the inflammatory reaction will obscure the borders of the cyst and make complete removal difficult. Inflamed cysts can be managed with injection of a small amount of intralesional steroid and warm compresses, or incision and drainage plus oral antibiotics in the case of a potentially infected cyst. Once the inflammatory reaction has resolved, the patient can be scheduled for definitive excision. As long as the entire cystic structure is removed, the chance of recurrence is very small. It is important to note that some authors have argued that it is more economical, and produces less morbidity, to excise acutely inflamed cysts preemptively.[22] Rare development of squamous cell carcinomas arising in epidermal inclusion cysts has been reported.[23] It is, therefore, advisable to send all excised specimens for histologic examination.

PLANNING THE EXCISION

In most cases, the surgical removal of an epidermal inclusion cyst is a fairly straightforward procedure. Once the area is cleaned with alcohol, one can mark out the clinically palpable borders of the cyst with a marking pen and draw out an ellipse over the center of the lesion. For small cysts, the ellipse may be drawn around the entire nodule, but for larger cysts, the ellipse overlies the center of the lesion. It is important to draw the ellipse around the central punctum, as failure to remove the punctum may leave remnants of the epithelium in the dermis and result in a recurrence of the cyst. The area can then be anesthetized with local anesthetic such as lidocaine, and prepped with a surgical scrub such as chlorhexidine or betadine.

EXCISING THE CYST

Smaller epidermal inclusion cysts can be excised *in toto*, either by removing an ellipse around the entire cyst, or by doing a larger punch excision that encompasses the cyst. However, for larger nodules, the ellipse is drawn over the center of the lesion. The scalpel incision may be carried down to the mid dermis until the cyst wall is visualized, taking care not to rupture the cyst during the excision (Fig. 25-4). At this point, the use of surgical hooks to retract the skin edges is helpful to better visualize the field. The ellipse and superficial skin overlying the cyst may be grabbed with Brown-Adson forceps, or a curved hemostat. Alternatively, a suture can be placed through the superficial skin paddle overlying the cyst, so that it can be manipulated easily without obstructing the view of the surgical field (Fig. 25-5). The dissection is then carried down around the cyst using a curved pair of surgical scissors, such as curved iris or small Metzenbaum scissors. This will allow for sharp dissection of the fibrous adhesions tethering the cyst, as well as blunt dissection around the cyst wall to the deep margin. Once all adhesions between the lateral cyst wall and the surrounding tissue have been removed, a cut may be made at the base to transect the cyst from the underlying fibroadipose tissue.

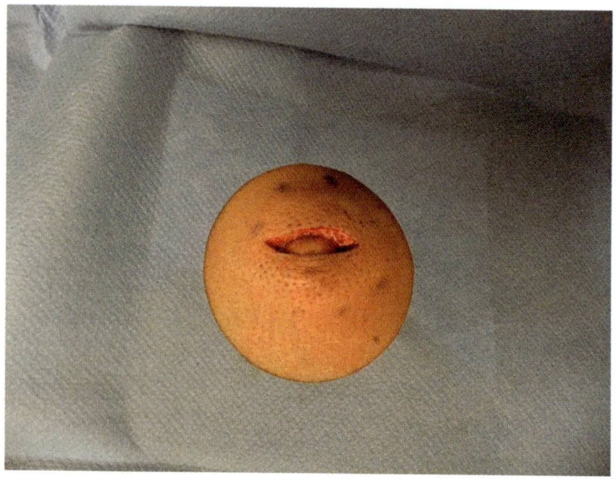

Figure 25-4 Cyst wall visualized.

If the cyst should rupture during the procedure, the cavity should be flushed with sterile normal saline. If the keratinous debris is left in the wound upon closure, it will provoke an inflammatory reaction in the dermis that will inhibit wound healing and may lead to a delayed infection of the surgical site.

ALTERNATIVE TECHNIQUES

In situations that require minimization of the scar, one may use a punch removal technique. After marking out the peripheral borders of the cyst and identifying the overlying punctum, a small (3–4 mm) punch incision can be made directly into the cyst. This will allow the surgeon to collapse the cyst by extruding the contents with gentle manual pressure on either side of the incision. Once the cyst contents have been removed, it is often possible to remove the cyst wall with a 2 to 3 mm curette, or by grasping the wall with a small hemostat and gently pulling it away from the surrounding dermis and subcutis.[24] Once

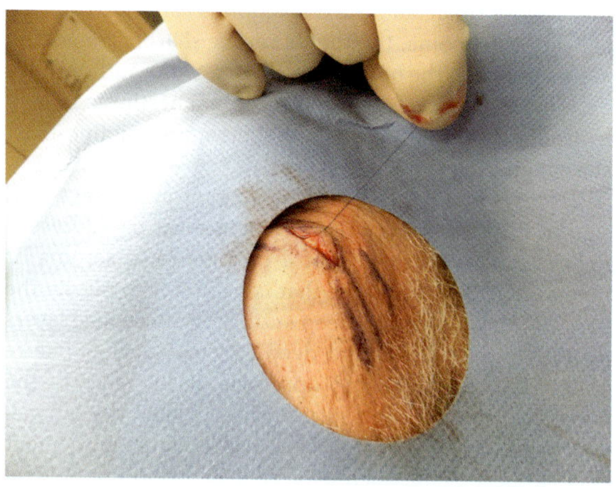

Figure 25-5 Suture tied to skin paddle overlying cyst to aid manipulation of the cyst.

the cyst is removed, the cavity will need to be flushed with a generous amount of normal saline. When this technique works properly, the cyst removal can be conducted very quickly through a small incision and can lead to a very nice cosmetic outcome. This technique should not be used in cases of larger cysts in which there is overlying skin laxity, as it will likely not remove a sufficient amount of redundant skin.

PILAR CYSTS

Pilar cysts (a.k.a. trichilemmal cysts) are benign growths that commonly occur on the scalp in areas of dense hair follicle distribution. In contrast to epidermal inclusion cysts, the epithelium that makes up pilar cysts resembles that of the outer root sheath of the hair follicle and undergoes more rapid trichilemmal keratinization. The stratified squamous epithelium lacks a granular cell layer, and the rapidly produced keratin is more compact within the cyst giving a more firm structure to the cyst itself.[7] Furthermore, there is no punctum connecting the cyst to the overlying epidermis. This lack of punctum and firm cystic structure often allows for the cyst to be extracted intact through a small incision overlying the cyst. Given the common scalp location of most pilar cysts, and the fact that the underlying skull does not permit much tissue expansion for the cyst, the pressure exerted by the cyst on the overlying scalp and hair follicles frequently produces a localized area of alopecia overlying the cyst.

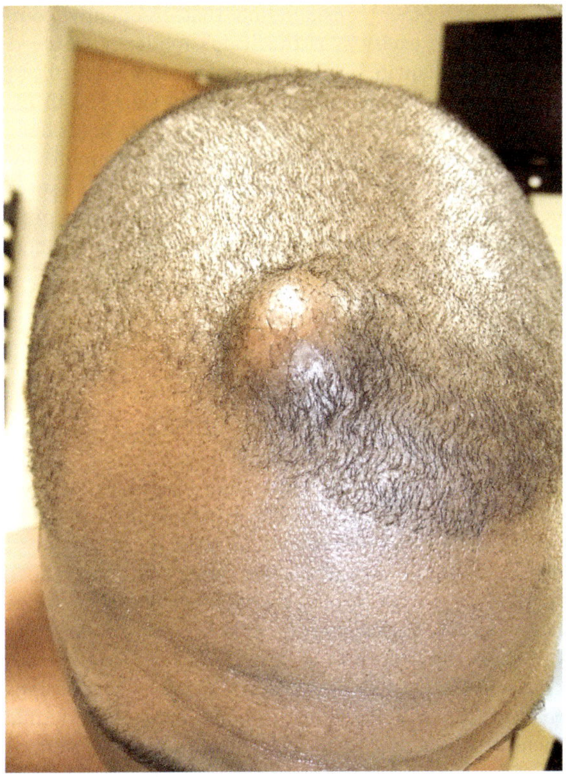

Figure 25-7 Large pilar cyst with overlying alopecia.

EXCISING A PILAR CYST

Planning the excision of a pilar cyst often depends on the clinical appearance of the scalp overlying the lesion. Relatively small cysts that do not have significant overlying skin laxity or alopecia can be removed through a small linear incision over the center of the cyst (Fig. 25-6). Because there is no punctum connecting the cyst to the skin surface, its wall is firm and resistant to rupture, and there are relatively few fibrous adhesions tethering it to the surrounding soft tissue, often the cyst can be extracted *in toto* through a small incision by applying gentle pressure to the scalp circumferentially around the cyst. If the cyst does not release easily, it can be grasped with an Allis clamp or Adson–Brown forceps and extracted through the small incision with gentle pressure and blunt undermining with curved tissue scissors.

In the case of larger or longer-standing cysts that have clinically significant alopecia overlying the cyst, the redundant skin will likely need to be removed to achieve an acceptable cosmetic outcome (Fig. 25-7). In such cases, a small ellipse may be excised overlying the lesion to reduce the area of alopecia and redundant skin (Fig. 25-8). Once the excision is carried out through the full thickness of the dermis and subcutis, the cyst should be easily extracted.

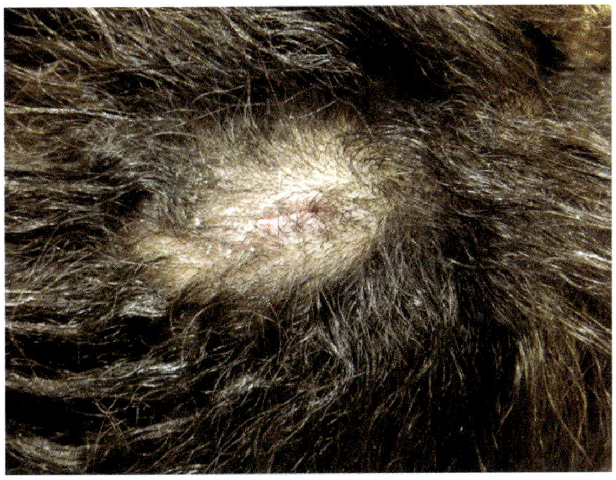

Figure 25-6 Healing linear incision from pilar cyst extraction.

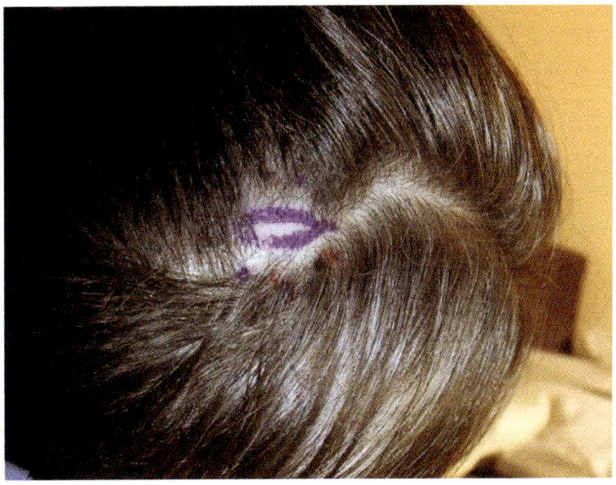

Figure 25-8 Ellipse drawn over pilar cyst to remove alopecic redundant skin.

The only other consideration that frequently complicates these excisions is the scalp's tendency to bleed. Achieving adequate hemostasis is made more difficult by the retraction of the thick fibrous scalp skin due to the underlying action of the scalp muscles, which holds open the perforating vessels. Waiting a full 10 to 15 minutes for the epinephrine to work, and using a running locked stitch in the wound closure, as well as applying an adequate pressure dressing for 24 to 48 hours can help provide the necessary hemostasis.

CONCLUSIONS

In this chapter, we present some of the more common benign dermal tumors, and several approaches to their surgical management. When planning excisions of cysts and lipomas, as with any condition, it is important to give preoperative consideration to the differential diagnosis, factors that may complicate the surgery, and alternative methods of management. It is also important to recognize that even lesions that are presumed to be classic examples of benign tumors have the capacity to surprise the clinician when the tissue is examined histologically. Lesions that are clinically presumed to be lipomas or epidermal inclusion cysts may turn out to be liposarcomas, desmoplastic melanomas, proliferating trichilemmal tumors or a variety of other tumors masquerading as benign lesions. As such, it is advisable to send any surgical specimen for histopathologic examination.

REFERENCES

1. Mentzel T, Fletcher CD. Lipomatous tumours of soft tissues: an update. *Virchows Arch.* 1995;427(4):353–363.
2. Weiss SW, Goldblum JR, eds. *Enzinger and Weiss's Soft Tissue Tumors.* 5th ed. Mosby Elsevier; 2008.
3. Rydholm A, Berg NO. Size, site and clinical incidence of lipoma. Factors in the differential diagnosis of lipoma and sarcoma. *Acta Orthop Scand.* 1983;54(6):929–934.
4. Truhan AP, Garden JM, Caro WA, Roenigk HH Jr. Facial and scalp lipomas: case reports and study of prevalence. *J Dermatol Surg Oncol.* 1985;11(10):981–984.
5. Worle B, Kunte C, Schaller M, Konz B. Lipoma of the forehead. *Hautarzt.* 2000;51(9):661–665.
6. Spitz J. *Genodermatoses: a Clinical Guide to Genetic Skin Disorders.* 2nd ed. Lippincott Williams and Wilkins; 2005.
7. Weedon D. *Weedon's Skin Pathology.* 3rd ed. Churchill Livingstone Elsevier; 2010.
8. Otley CC. Perioperative evaluation and management in dermatologic surgery. *J Am Acad Dermatol.* 2006;54(1):119–127.
9. Bunick CG, Aasi SZ. Hemorrhagic complications in dermatologic surgery. *Dermatol Ther.* 2011;24(6):537–550.
10. Delaney A, Diamantis S, Marks VJ. Complications of tissue ischemia in dermatologic surgery. *Dermatol Ther.* 2011;24 (6):551–557.
11. Salem RO, Laposata M. Effects of alcohol on hemostasis. *Am J Clin Pathol.* 2005;123(suppl):S96–S105.
12. Otley CC. Continuation of medically necessary aspirin and warfarin during cutaneous surgery. *Mayo Clin Proc.* 2003; 78(11): 1392–1396.
13. Kovich O, Otley CC. Thrombotic complications related to discontinuation of warfarin and aspirin therapy perioperatively for cutaneous operation. *J Am Acad Dermatol.* 2003; 48(2):233–237.
14. Dinehart SM, Henry L. Dietary supplements: altered coagulation and effects on bruising. *Dermatol Surg.* 2005;31(7 Pt 2): 819–826; discussion 826.
15. Rao SS, Davison SP. Gone in 30 seconds: a quick and simple technique for subcutaneous lipoma removal. *Plast Reconstr Surg.* 2012;130(1):236e–238e.
16. Kenawi MM. 'Squeeze delivery' excision of subcutaneous lipoma related to anatomic site. *Br J Surg.* 1995;82(12):1649–1650.
17. Capriotti K, Humphreys TR. A novel technique for the extraction of larger lipomas. *Dermatol Surg.* 2009;35(3):493–495.
18. Funayama E, Minakawa H, Oyama A. Forehead lipoma resection via a small remote incision using a surgical raspatory. *J Am Acad Dermatol.* 2007;56(3):458–459.
19. Coleman WP 3rd. Noncosmetic applications of liposuction. *J Dermatol Surg Oncol.* 1988;14(10):1085–1090.
20. Pinski KS, Roenigk HH Jr. Liposuction of lipomas. *Dermatol Clin.* 1990;8(3):483–492.
21. Al-basti HA, El-Khatib HA. The use of suction-assisted surgical extraction of moderate and large lipomas: long-term follow-up. *Aesthetic Plast Surg.* 2002;26(2):114–117.
22. Jun GB, Qi H, Golap C. One-stage excision of inflamed sebaceous cyst versus the conventional method. *S Afr J Surg.* 2010; 48(4):116–118.
23. Anton-Badiola I, San Miguel-Fraile P, Peteiro-Cancelo A, Ortiz-Rey JA. Squamous cell carcinoma arising on an epidermal inclusion cyst: a case presentation and review of the literature. *Actas Dermosifiliogr.* 2010;101(4):349–353.
24. Yang HJ, Yang KC. A new method for facial epidermoid cyst removal with minimal incision. *J Eur Acad Dermatol Venereol.* 2009;23(8):887–890.

CHAPTER 26 Mohs Micrographic Surgery: Indications and Technique

Nicholas B. Countryman & C. William Hanke

INTRODUCTION

Developed by a meticulous, pioneering general surgeon and refined by a host of forward-thinking dermatologists, Mohs micrographic surgery (MMS) represents the standard of care today for treatment of many cutaneous tumors. With cure rates unparalleled by standard destructive and excisional surgeries and the innate ability to preserve healthy surrounding tissue, MMS should be considered for large, aggressive, or recurrent carcinomas as well as those in functionally or cosmetically sensitive areas. In utilizing the serial staged excisional process as illustrated subsequently, the Mohs surgeon is able to immediately repair ensuing wounds as necessary. Due to the safety and cost-effective nature of the procedure, MMS appropriately represents the gold standard for treatment of many cutaneous tumors.

HISTORY AND EVOLUTION

As a sophomore medical student at the University of Wisconsin, Frederic Mohs, while experimenting with the injection of zinc chloride and other chemicals into rat tumors, noted excellent preservation of the microscopic features of the treated tissue. After shaving the tumor nodules horizontally with respect to the skin surface, he made the observation that zinc chloride acted as an in situ fixative. The in situ fixation along with the concept of horizontal sectioning initiated a series of experiments that has eventually led to modern MMS. In 1936, the first patients were treated with chemosurgery, and in 1941, Dr. Mohs reported success using microscopic surgery on 440 patients.[1] Initially termed "chemosurgery" to indicate that the tissue was chemically treated and surgically excised, early chemosurgery procedures were initiated by the application of a paste composed primarily of zinc chloride applied to malignant tissue. After a period of 4 to 24 hours, saucerized surgical excision ensued followed by microscopic examination of the horizontal sections. Accordingly, Mohs confirmed tumor removal or precisely identified remaining tumor, repeating the staged excision as necessary.

Traditional medicine proved slow to adopt Mohs' chemosurgery technique. The early days of the procedure were met with great skepticism and hostility. With meticulous records and eventually adequate patient data revealing extremely high cure rates, chemosurgery began to gain acceptance. Despite being trained as a general surgeon, Dr. Mohs recognized that dermatologists represented the most interested group of physicians in his technique. Thus, following the creation of American College of Chemosurgery in 1967, the college's first meeting was held that year, and consisted of 23 attendees of the American Academy of Dermatology Annual Meeting.[2]

Chemical fixation used in the initial chemosurgery posed several challenges, namely the time consuming nature of the standard 24 hour fixation, the pain associated with chemical fixation, and the limited reconstruction options following the final excision of tissue. These were all overcome upon the development of the fresh tissue technique using horizontal frozen sections without zinc chloride fixation. Although Dr. Mohs first used the technique in 1953, a presentation by Dr. Theodore Tromovitch at the American College of Chemosurgery Annual Meeting in 1970 reporting his success using the fresh tissue technique changed the future of the specialty.[3,4] With the evolution of the use of frozen section pathology, the title of the procedure, Mohs' chemosurgery, was altered, and became "microscopically controlled excision" (MCE). Other names suggested at the time included a mnemonic by Dr. Walter Shelley who suggested MOHS, microscopically oriented histographic surgery.[5]

There are several advantages to the technique of MCE. The main advantage is the decreased pain with elimination of the zinc chloride paste. The usual 24 hour paste fixation caused significant pain, which often required narcotic management. With repeat excisions, pain often increased. With the advent of MCE, the pain of the zinc chloride paste was exchanged for the brief discomfort associated with the injection of local anesthetic. MCE is also faster and allows for multiple layers of tissue to be removed in a single day. The final and unexpected advantage is that once the borders of the wound are tumor free, the fresh wound can be closed by any number of surgical reconstructive methods. With the classic chemosurgery wound, approximately 7 to 10 days were required for the remaining fixed tissue to slough. The patient would then wait for healing by second intention or a split thickness skin graft could be applied. The new technique has encouraged the development of reconstruction options, many of which have been advanced by Mohs surgeons.

In their 8 year retrospective study, Stegman and Tromovitch reported an overall cure rate of 98.4% for basal cell carcinoma (BCC), confirming that the modified technique is capable of achieving results comparable to those reported with zinc chloride paste chemosurgery.[6,7] More recent literature confirms similarly high cure rates for primary BCC.[8] MMS for recurrent BCC reveals slightly lower but still superior cure rates when compared to those standard excisional surgery.[9] In addition, squamous cell carcinoma (SCC), both primary and recurrent, is amenable to MMS with cure rates superior to all other methods of removal.[10] Dr. Mohs successfully documented high cure rates using chemosurgery for melanoma[11] and current evidence has confirmed that modern MMS can also be successful in the treatment of melanoma.[12]

In the first randomized trial concerning MMS, Muller et al. demonstrated that it is a tissue-sparing treatment. The median area of the surgical defect following surgical excision was 1.6 times that of the defect obtained after MMS.[13] The smaller defect size subsequently allowed for the simplest repair, which often consisted of healing by second intention. A recent study of national Mohs surgery practices found that 18% of Mohs defects are allowed to heal by second intention.[14] Primary closure techniques can also be utilized to repair a significant number of MMS defects, minimizing the need for more complex flaps and grafts.

In addition to the advantages of providing the highest cure rates and having an inherent tissue-sparing nature, MMS is also safe and cost-effective. Recent evidence confirms anecdotal accounts that MMS is an extremely safe outpatient procedure performed under local anesthesia with extremely low complication rates.[15] Despite the staged nature and length of MMS, documented rates of surgical site infections with MMS are equal to or below those of similar procedures performed in operating rooms.[16] Several studies also illustrate the cost-effective nature of MMS. It is lower in cost than surgical excision, which often includes an ambulatory surgery center (ASC) facility fee.[17,18] MMS has high intrinsic value, which is cost-effective in comparison to traditional surgical excision.[19] Cost-effectiveness analysis demonstrating the outcomes based efficiency of MMS are critical in the current health care climate, as heightened sensitivity to financial pressures and declining reimbursements may challenge patients' ability to receive optimal treatment for nonmelanoma skin cancer (NMSC).

In 1985, the term "micrographic surgery" was first used to indicate unambiguously the use of the microscope and the drawing of maps to achieve complete MCE.[20] That same year, the American College of Chemosurgery decided to change the name of the procedure to Mohs micrographic surgery and the name of the organization to American College of Mohs Micrographic Surgery and Cutaneous Oncology (ACMMSCO). More recently, this name was changed to the American College of Mohs Surgery (ACMS). Until the recent transition to the American Council for Graduate Medical Education (ACGME), the ACMS served as the accreditation organization for fellowship training in MMS. Fellowship training in MMS currently consists of a 1 to 2 year training program encompassing teaching of MMS, cutaneous oncology, and reconstructive surgery in addition to other dermatologic surgery and procedural dermatology.[21] As of 2012, the ACGME had accredited 56 procedural dermatology fellowship training programs.[22] The ACMS continues to approve a small number of international programs. Completion of an accredited fellowship qualifies applicants for membership in the ACMS.

INDICATIONS

MMS is a technique for the removal of complex or ill-defined skin tumors. NMSC represents the vast majority of cutaneous tumors treated with MMS. In the United States in 2006, there were an estimated 3.5 million NMSC diagnosed, and it is projected that there will be nearly 4 million new cases of NMSC diagnosed in the United States each year.[23] In general, cutaneous tumors with aggressive histologic subtypes, that are recurrent, located in functionally or cosmetically sensitive areas, located in areas known to have higher rates of recurrence or metastasis, tumors in immunocompromised patients or in areas of previous radiation, should be considered for MMS. BCC and SCC comprise greater than 95% of all NMSC. A review of long-term cure rates of over 10,000 cases of primary BCC treated with standard excision and traditional margin assessment as opposed to MMS showed a 10.1% recurrence rate for standard excision compared to 1.0% for MMS.[8] Similarly, the long-term recurrence rate utilizing MMS for recurrent BCC was 5.6% compared to 9.8% for radiation therapy and 17.4% or standard surgical excision.[9] Another review of treatments for SCC revealed equally superior results for MMS when compared to standard surgical excision. MMS yielded a long-term recurrence rate of 3.1% while standard surgical excision yielded a 10.9% recurrence rate. Similarly superior results for recurrent SCC were noted with MMS resulting in a 10.0% recurrence versus a 23.3% recurrence rate with standard surgical excision.[24]

Another indication for MMS is lentigo maligna (LM) or melanoma in situ (MIS). The incidence of MIS continues to increase with an estimated 55,560 cases to be newly diagnosed in 2012.[25] Although considerable controversy persists in relation to the use of MMS for melanoma and MIS, ample evidence suggests that it is safe and effective.[26] MMS may be particularly useful to conserve tissue for melanomas on the head, neck, hands, or feet or for melanomas with indistinct clinical margins.[12] Many Mohs surgeons now use immunohistochemical staining (see below) to optimally visualize melanoma on frozen section histology.[27,28]

Superior cure rates utilizing MMS compared to standard excision for other rare cutaneous tumors have also been demonstrated. These include dermatofibrosarcoma protuberans (DFSP),[29] sebaceous carcinoma,[30] atypical fibroxanthoma (AFX),[31] malignant fibrous histiocytoma (MFH),[32] microcystic adnexal carcinoma (MAC),[33] extramammary Paget's disease (EMPD),[34] leiomyosarcoma,[35] desmoplastic trichoepithelioma,[36] angiosarcoma,[37] mucinous carcinoma,[38] and Merkel cell carcinoma (MCC).[39]

In 2012, a consensus statement was published addressing the appropriate use of MMS for cutaneous tumors.[40] This statement did not compare MMS with other treatments; rather it provides a framework to assess the appropriateness of MMS for individual cutaneous tumors. Use of MMS in various clinical scenarios was rated as appropriate, uncertain, or inappropriate. As pointed out in this statement, uncertain indications often require individual physician judgment and understanding of the patient and other clinical factors to better determine the appropriateness of MMS for a particular scenario. The authors note that the ranking of uncertain should not be viewed as limiting the use of MMS for patients and in appropriate settings. Treatment of tumors with an uncertain ranking with MMS should be reimbursable when determined appropriate by the clinician. Tables 26-1 to 26-3 summarize the recommendations of this statement for the use of MMS for BCC, SCC, and LM/MIS. In this consensus statement, area "H" includes the central face and eyelids including inner and outer canthi, eyebrows, nose, lips, chin, ear and periauricular skin, temple, genitalia including perineal and perianal

TABLE 26-1

Summary from a Consensus Statement Addressing the Appropriate Use of MMS in Area "H" Comprising the Central Face and Eyelids, Including Inner and Outer Canthi, Eyebrows, Nose, Lips, Chin, Ear and Periauricular Skin, Temple, Genitalia Including Perineal and Perianal Regions, Hands, Feet, Nail Units, Ankles, and Nipples and Areolae

Area H	Appropriate	Uncertain
BCC	Primary or recurrent: Aggressive, nodular, superficial	
SCC	Primary or recurrent: Aggressive, nonaggressive,[a] verrucous, KA-type, in situ/Bowen's	
LM and MIS	Primary or recurrent: Lentigo maligna, melanoma in situ	

[a]SCC without aggressive features, <2 mm depth without other defining features, ≤Clark level III; listed indications are for both healthy and immunocompromised (IC) patients, and tumors of any size unless otherwise specified.

Source: Modified with permission from Connolly SM, Baker DR, Coldiron BM, et al. AAD/ACMS/ASDSA/ASMS 2012 Appropriate Use Criteria for Mohs Micrographic Surgery: A Report of the American Academy of Dermatology, American College of Mohs Surgery, American Society for Dermatologic Surgery Association, and the American Society for Mohs Surgery. *J Am Acad Dermatol.* 2012; 67(4);531–550. Copyright Elsevier.

TABLE 26-2

Summary from a Consensus Statement addressing the Appropriate Use of MMS in Area "M" Including the Cheeks, Forehead, Scalp, Neck, Jawline, Pretibial Surface

Area M	Appropriate	Uncertain
BCC	Primary or recurrent: Aggressive, nodular, superficial (IC) Primary: Superficial ≥0.6 cm	Primary: Superficial ≥0.6 cm
SCC	Primary or recurrent: Aggressive, nonaggressive,[a] verrucous, KA-type, in situ/Bowen's	
LM and MIS	Primary or recurrent: Lentigo maligna, melanoma in situ	

[a]SCC without aggressive features, <2 mm depth without other defining features, ≤Clark level III; listed indications are for both healthy and immunocompromised (IC) patients, and tumors of any size unless otherwise specified.

Source: Modified with permission from Connolly SM, Baker DR, Coldiron BM, et al. AAD/ACMS/ASDSA/ASMS 2012 Appropriate Use Criteria for Mohs Micrographic Surgery: A Report of the American Academy of Dermatology, American College of Mohs Surgery, American Society for Dermatologic Surgery Association, and the American Society for Mohs Surgery. *J Am Acad Dermatol*. 2012;67(4);531–550. Copyright Elsevier.

TABLE 26-3

Summary from a Consensus Statement Addressing the Appropriate Use of MMS in Area "L" Including the Trunk and Extremities Excluding Pretibial Surface, Hands, Feet, Nail Units, and Ankles

Area L	Appropriate	Uncertain
BCC	Recurrent: Aggressive, nodular Primary: Aggressive ≥0.6 cm, nodular >2 cm, nodular (IC) ≥1.1 cm	Primary: Aggressive ≤0.5 cm, nodular 1.1–2 cm, nodular (IC) 0.6–1 cm, superficial (IC) ≥1.1 cm
SCC	Primary or recurrent: Aggressive, KA-type (IC) ≥0.6 cm Recurrent: Non aggressive,[a] KA-type Primary >2 cm: Non Aggressive,[a] In situ/Bowen's Primary ≥1.1 cm: Non aggressive,[a] KA-type, in situ/Bowen's (IC)	Recurrent: In situ/Bowen's Primary 1.1–2 cm: Non aggressive,[a] in situ/Bowen's Primary ≤1 cm: Non aggressive[a] (IC) Primary 0.6–1 cm: In situ/Bowen's Primary ≤0.5 cm: KA-type (IC)
LM and MIS	Recurrent: Lentigo maligna, melanoma in situ	Primary: Lentigo maligna, melanoma in situ

[a]SCC without aggressive features, <2 mm depth without other defining features, ≤Clark level III; listed indications are for both healthy and immunocompromised (IC) patients, and tumors of any size unless otherwise specified.

Source: Modified with permission from Connolly SM, Baker DR, Coldiron BM, et al. AAD/ACMS/ASDSA/ASMS 2012 Appropriate Use Criteria for Mohs Micrographic Surgery: A Report of the American Academy of Dermatology, American College of Mohs Surgery, American Society for Dermatologic Surgery Association, and the American Society for Mohs Surgery. *J Am Acad Dermatol.* 2012;67(4);531–550. Copyright Elsevier.

regions, hands, feet, nail units, ankles, and nipples and areolae. Area "M" includes the cheeks, forehead, scalp, neck, jawline, and pretibial surface. Area "L" indicates the trunk and extremities excluding pretibial surface, hands, feet, nail units, and ankles.

In the consensus statement, MMS was also deemed appropriate for adenocystic carcinoma, adnexal carcinoma, apocrine/eccrine carcinoma, AFX, DFSP, EMPD, leiomyosarcoma, MFH (undifferentiated pleomorphic sarcoma), MAC, also known as sclerosing sweat duct carcinoma, mucinous carcinoma, and sebaceous carcinoma in all locations regardless of patient type. MCC was determined to be appropriate in areas "H" and "M" with MMS as monotherapy. Angiosarcoma in all locations, desmoplastic trichoepithelioma in areas "H" and "M," and MCC in area "L" were deemed uncertain.

TECHNIQUE

Today, MMS is a technique for the removal of complex or ill-defined skin cancers with histologic examination of

100% of the surgical margins. It is a combination of surgical excision and surgical pathology that requires a single physician to act in two integrated but separate and distinct capacities: surgeon and pathologist. The Mohs surgeon removes the tumor tissue, prepares a map, and divides the tumor specimen into pieces. Each piece is embedded into an individual tissue block for histopathologic examination. An outline of the technique of MMS is depicted later.

Achieving superior cure rates utilizing MMS in the removal of cutaneous tumors requires a standardized, precise, and exacting technique. Appropriate staffing with capable assistants trained in surgical technique as well as proper local anesthesia is paramount in creating an optimal patient and surgeon experience. Virtually all MMS is performed under local anesthesia utilizing the fresh tissue technique. After informed consent is obtained, the area is marked with a surgical marker to delineate the edges of the tumor to be treated. The patient is positioned in a prone position with unobstructed access to the operative site. The area is sterilely prepped and is anesthetized most commonly with 1% lidocaine with 1:100,000 epinephrine buffered with sodium bicarbonate. If necessary, the tissue to be removed may be remarked with gentian violet if preoperative markings are obscured.

Many Mohs surgeons utilize debulking of the obvious tumor to decrease false positives as well as to better delineate the extent of the tumor. Methods include curettage or sharp scalpel debulking. Removal of central tumor by any method allows for thinner, more flexible specimens.[41] Many surgeons prefer curettage although sharp debulking with a scalpel blade may be more effective in morpheaform BCC and other sclerotic cutaneous tumors that are not as amenable to curettage. Both methods are dependent on the ability of the surgeon to see or feel the difference between cancerous and noncancerous skin. Many Mohs surgeons feel that debulking represents an unnecessary step and move directly to removing the first layer of tissue. An added benefit of debulking the tumor is that the debulked tissue can be processed. Although processing this tissue may add a small amount of time, it serves several purposes: It helps in verifying the location of the tumor, provides visual cues as to the histology of the tumor being excised and can justify reimbursement when the tumor is cleared on the first stage. Disadvantages of processing the debulked tissue include the potential confusion of stray tumor that can attach to other specimens and the fact that handling more tissue can increase processing time and expense. Overly vigorous debulking may also necessitate an unnecessarily deep or wide stage.[42]

The first layer of tissue is most commonly removed using a #15 scalpel blade. Exceptionally large cutaneous tumors or those on the trunk or extremities may be more amenable to removal with a #10 blade. Generally, the first layer of tissue encompasses a 2 to 3 mm margin of normal appearing skin around and underneath the visible tumor or debulked area. Orienting the tissue in relation to the patient is accomplished using one of several different methods. The most common is superficial asymmetric nicking of the skin including the excised tissue. For example, two hatch marks at the 12 o'clock epidermal margin and one at the 6 o'clock margins are shown in Figure 26-1. Additional hatch marks are added as per need for large specimens (e.g., at 3 o'clock and 9 o'clock). Marking with gentian violet or other inks on the patient in the area from which the tissue is excised is an alternative approach to orienting the tissue. Other methods include stapling, wooden grids, and digital or Polaroid photographs.[43–46] Forty-five-degree incisions have traditionally been used to easily allow for the excised tissue to be flattened and processed into horizontal frozen sections, as they allow lateral and deep edges to be examined in one section. Some have referred to these sections as oblique rather than tangential, horizontal, or beveled.[47] Others have advocated 90 degree sections during removal of the first layers of tissue to minimize defect size and spare normal tissue, although this presents challenges in sectioning the entire tissue specimen.[42] Figure 26-2 illustrates the typical 45 degree-angle lateral incisions through the epidermis, dermis, and into the superficial fat typically employed during the first layer of MMS. Once the incisions

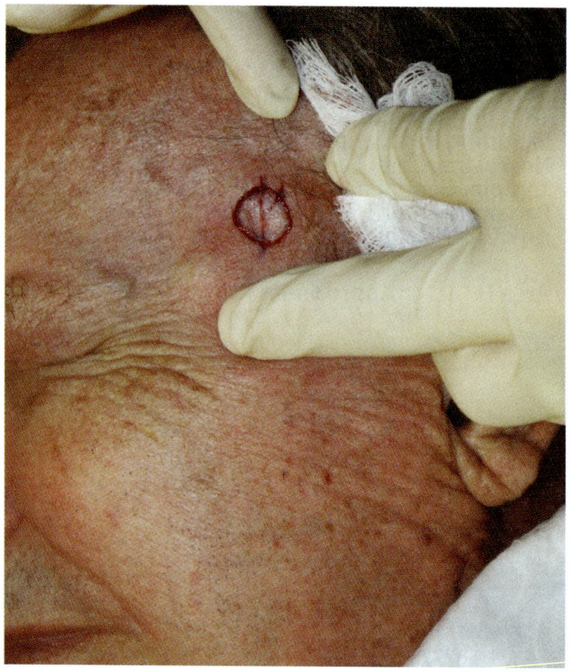

Figure 26-1 Photograph demonstrates asymmetric superficial nicking of epidermis to orient Mohs layer. Patient has an infiltrating basal cell carcinoma on the left temple.

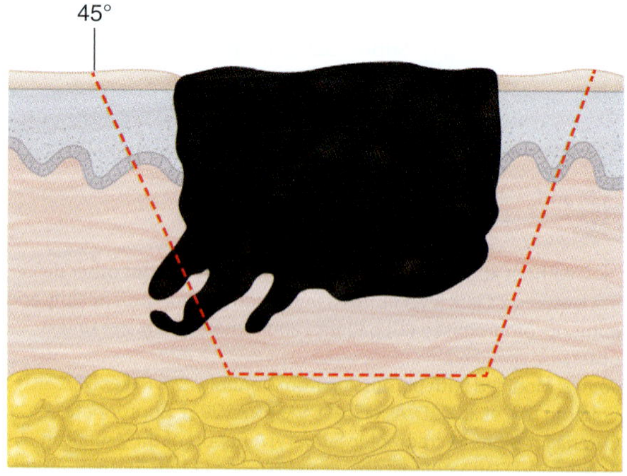

Figure 26-2 Diagram showing two-dimensional view of a typical 45 degree angle carried out in the first Mohs layer. In this circumstance, the first stage transects the asymmetric tumor pictured by the dark black area.

on the lateral margins of the tissue are made, the first layer is completed by incising the tissue in a horizontal plane, generally through the superficial fat with either the scalpel blade or sharp tissue-cutting scissors.

Once the tissue has been removed, pinpoint hemostasis is obtained and the patient is bandaged and returned to the reception area during processing of the tissue. Long-acting anesthetics or topical anesthetics (such as a compound of lidocaine, epinephrine, and tetracaine) may be employed to extend the local anesthetic effect and improve patient comfort.[48] Depending on tissue processing time, the anesthetized area will remain numb during the waiting period and require less anesthesia on subsequent Mohs layers and during reconstruction, thereby minimizing the risk of lidocaine toxicity. This is particularly essential when treating large cutaneous tumors.

Accurate mapping and inking of the excised tissue represents the next step in the process. Using stock body diagrams encompassing the involved area, a two-dimensional map approximating the shape and size of the excised tissue is drawn for future reference. Figure 26-3 shows a map of the excised tissue from the first Mohs layer. Although various methods are employed to maintain orientation of the tissue, use of 2- to 4-color tissue marking inks is most often used. Commonly used ink colors include red, blue, green, yellow, and black. Every Mohs surgeon uses various conventions to accomplish appropriate mapping. Two-ink systems are sufficient in virtually all cases as seen in Figure 26-4. Alternatives exist but are not as readily used.[49] The hand-drawn map is likewise marked to represent the location of the various tissue inks for orientation when interpreting the histologic specimens, as shown by the dotted and solid circles around the 12 o'clock and 6 o'clock hatch marks in Figure 26-3.

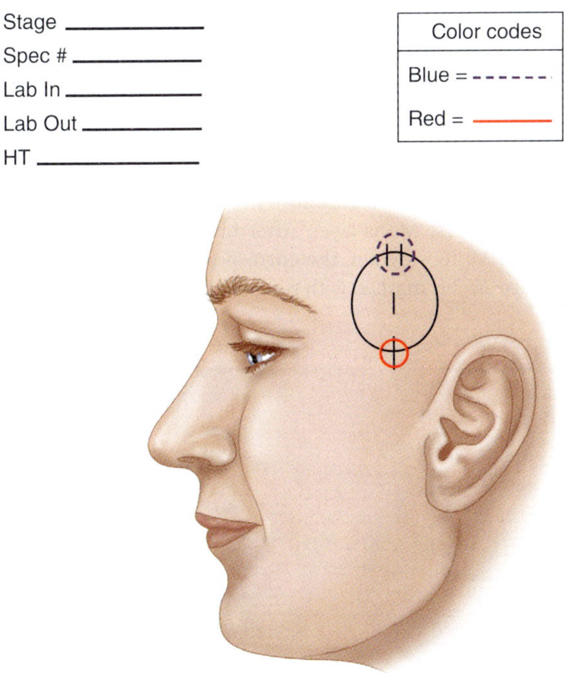

Figure 26-3 Map corresponding to tissue excised during the first Mohs layer. As the legend indicates, the dotted line around the two hatch marks at 12 o'clock corresponds with blue ink and the solid line around the hatch mark at 6 o'clock corresponds with the red ink.

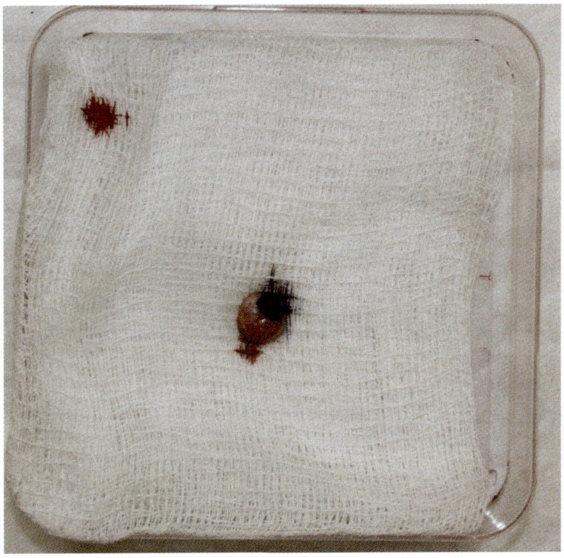

Figure 26-4 Excised tissue from first Mohs layer is transported to the laboratory and shown here on a "4 × 4" gauze in a petri dish with the two hatch marks at 12 o'clock inked with blue and the single hatch mark at 6 o'clock inked with red. Notice how the map from Figure 26-3 precisely matches the inked tissue.

After mapping and inking the tissue, the tissue is taken to the CLIA certified laboratory and the histotechnician (HT) prepares the tissue for processing. Most HTs proficient in sectioning excised tissue from MMS require extensive training and mentoring. Though formal training is available, most of the training takes place on the job. The first step in processing the tissue is grossing. The purpose of grossing tissue for MMS is to transform a three-dimensional piece of tissue from the patient into two dimensions on the slide thus providing complete margin control. This is accomplished using relaxing incisions when necessary. Depending on the size and shape of the tissue, it may be necessary to subdivide it into sections to allow for horizontal sectioning.

The next step is to mount and embed the tissue. This amounts to placing the tissue upside down on an appropriately sized cryostat chuck and embedding in OCT compound (Optimum Cutting Temperature: Tissue-Tek, Miles Inc., Diagnostics Division, Elkhart, IN). Figure 26-5 shows the embedded tissue mounted on the cryostat chuck. Again, numerous methods exist to accomplish this step. Some of the most commonly utilized include the Floating Method and Cryomold.[50,51] Embedding larger specimens with a membrane and vacuum system embedding machine may enhance efficiency.[52] These various techniques all aim to expose the lateral and deep margins of the tissue in a two-dimensional plane for cutting.

Once embedded, the tissue is frozen and mounted in the cryostat where the tissue is sectioned horizontally in 4 to 8 μm sections. After mounting on slides, the tissue is stained. Hematoxylin and eosin (H&E) staining is the most commonly used stain for this application. Although less frequently used, toluidine blue is another simple, useful stain, with an ability to metachromatically stain the mucopolysaccharide stroma of BCC a characteristic pink or magenta color. This signals the Mohs surgeon to carefully inspect the corresponding area for tumor. It is also a more rapid stain.[53]

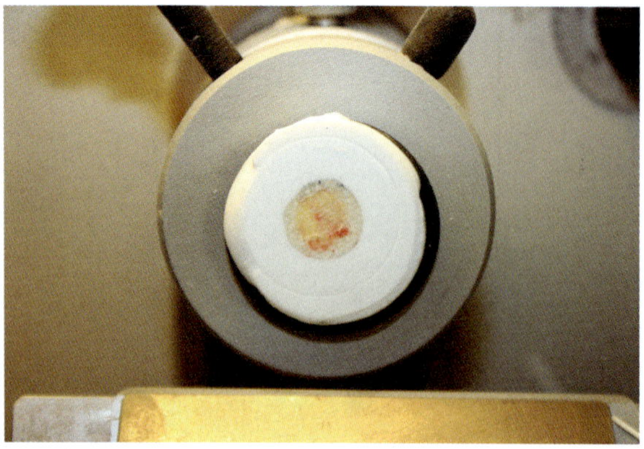

Figure 26-5 Mohs layer is mounted on a cryostat chuck embedded in OCT compound ready for horizontal sectioning.

The use of immunohistochemical staining is definitely on the rise, particularly in cases of LM and malignant melanoma. Immunostains can be an effective method of enhancing the accuracy of assessing the surgical margins of common and rare tumors, thereby maximizing tissue sparing and minimizing recurrence. The use of frozen tissue provides a template in which antigen preservation is maximized, allowing for better staining and improved localization of tumor.[54,55] Disadvantages and limitations of incorporating immunohistochemistry into a Mohs surgery practice include the additional processing time and cost involved, as well as more time-consuming slide interpretation. The antibodies most commonly used in conjunction with MMS are HMB-45 (50% of laboratories), S-100 (42%), and Melan-A and Mel-5 (42%) for melanoma; antikeratin for BCC and SCC (42%); and anti-CD34 for DFSP (33%).[56] Antikeratinocyte immunoperoxidase stains contain antikeratin cocktails useful in identifying carcinoma obscured by a dense lymphocytic infiltrate, nerve, or vessel.[57,58] In the case of EMPD, immunostaining with cytokeratin 7 can be helpful in delineating disease.[34] As immunohistochemical stains improve, the use of these stains in MMS will continue to improve efficiency and cost and will likely become more widespread.

The final step is the interpretation of the stained slides. High-quality frozen section slides and accurate interpretation by the Mohs surgeon provide the core of tumor extirpation during MMS. Extensive mentoring during an ACMS certified training program with at least 500 cases of proctored MMS cases affords the Mohs surgeon the expertise to accurately interpret frozen section histology.[59] Numerous pitfalls in interpreting horizontal frozen sections exist. Missed microscopic tumor cells can lead to higher recurrence rates. Alternatively, misinterpretation of benign entities as malignant leads to inappropriate removal of noncancerous tissue and unnecessarily large defects.[10,60] Utilizing the hatch marks and ink in the sections, microscopic findings of residual tumor are marked on the corresponding map with red ink in preparation for subsequent stages. Figure 26-6 shows a representative slide from the first Mohs layer. After histologic interpretation by the Mohs surgeon, the corresponding map as seen in Figure 26-7 is marked with red pencil indicating persistent

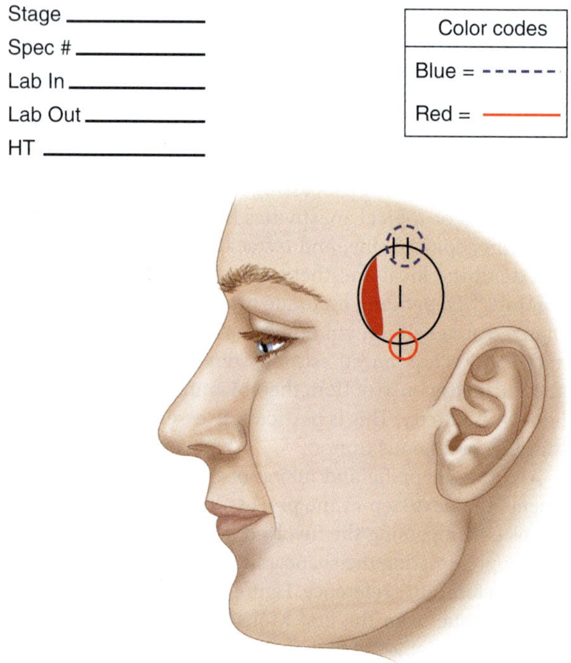

Figure 26-7 Using the hatch marks and tissue ink for orientation, the Mohs surgeon uses red pencil on the Mohs map to indicate where persistent tumor is seen on histologic interpretation of slide.

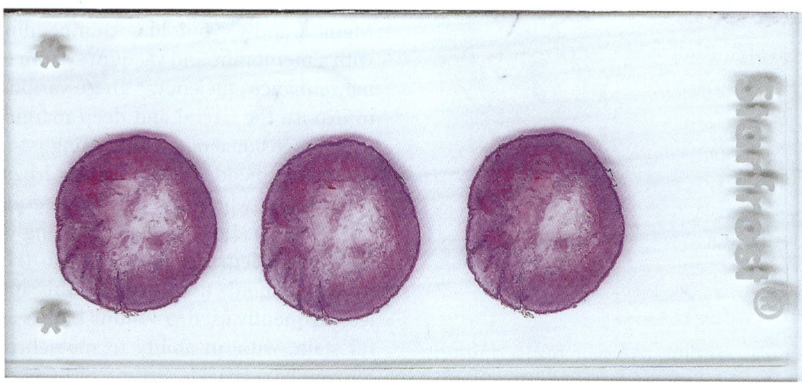

Figure 26-6 Representative slide from first Mohs layer demonstrating the horizontal section encompassing the entire lateral and deep margin.

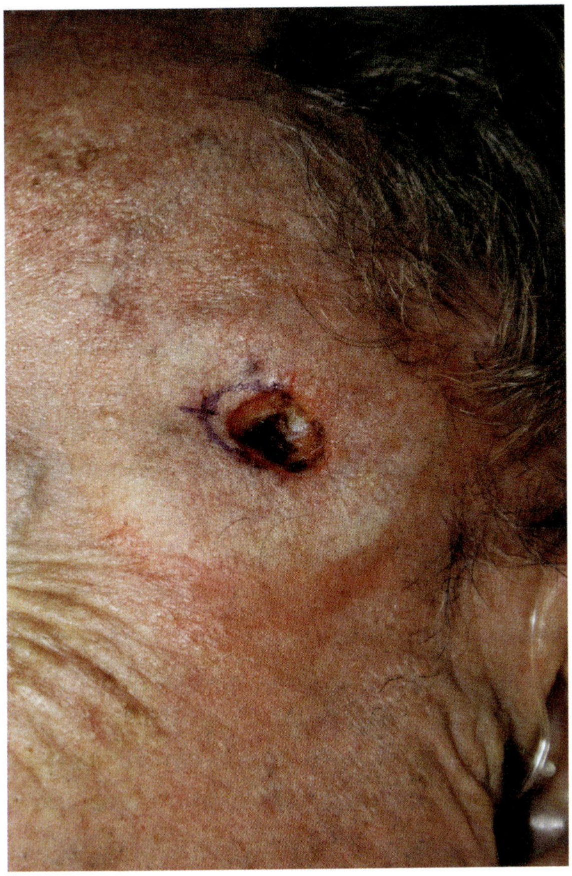

Figure 26-8 Using the map from the first Mohs layer, an area encompassing the persistent tumor with a 2 mm margin is marked indicating the tissue to be excised in the second Mohs layer. Note the hatch mark made centrally on the tissue and patient that will be used for orientation should further tissue need to be excised.

tumor. The hatch marks and tissue ink are employed to precisely map the persistent tumor.

During subsequent excisions, the entire area should be anesthetized to ensure that the patient remains as comfortable as possible between stages and to minimize total anesthetic used during the entire procedure. Subsequent Mohs stages are removed only around precisely mapped

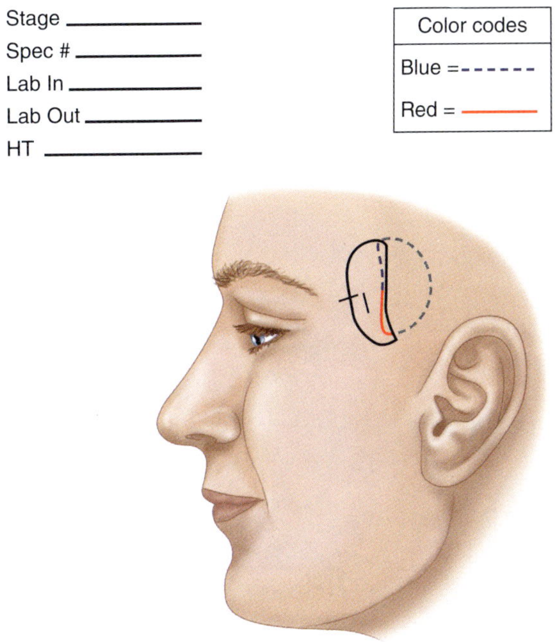

Figure 26-9 After excision of the second Mohs layer, a map corresponding to the excised tissue is drawn. Again, red and blue tissue inks are employed to orient the tissue during histologic interpretation.

tumor after the first and subsequent stages. In Figure 26-8, the patient is marked encompassing a 2 mm margin around the area from the first Mohs layer that contained persistent tumor. This represents the tissue to be excised during the second Mohs layer. Again, a superficial hatch mark centrally on the excised tissue and carried onto the patient assists in orientation. Ninety-degree incisions on subsequent stages are acceptable in most cases as the transformation from three-dimensions to two is more easily accomplished during embedding. Figure 26-9 shows the hand-drawn map corresponding to the excised tissue from the second Mohs layer. A slide showing stained vertical sections from a representative second Mohs layer can be seen in Figure 26-10. In this fashion, by utilizing the map and hatch marks on the patient, persistent tumor on the patient is marked and excised serially until the section

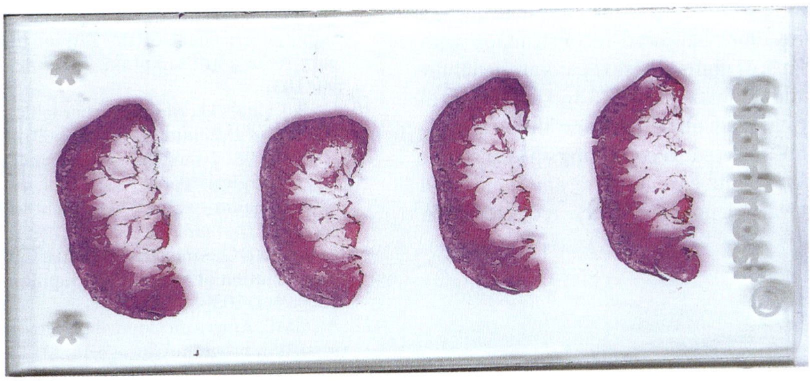

Figure 26-10 Representative slide from the second Mohs layer demonstrating the horizontal section again encompassing the entire lateral and deep margin of the excised tissue.

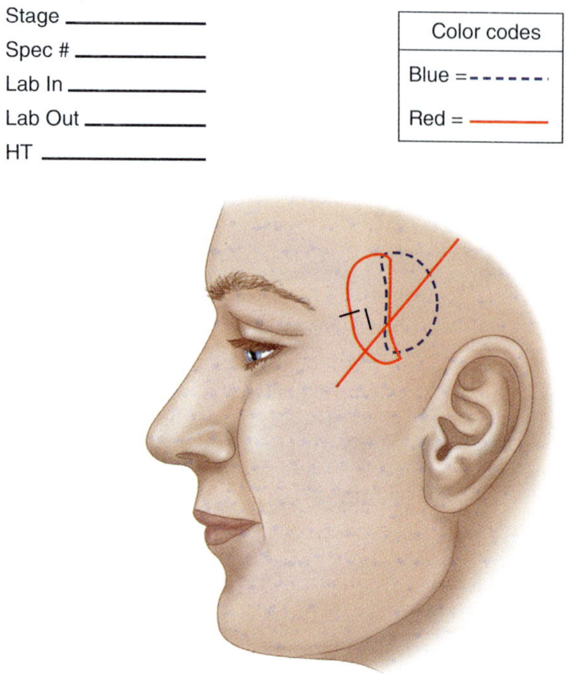

Figure 26-11 A red pencil line drawn through the Mohs map indicates that the margins on the second Mohs layer were free of persistent tumor. The patient can now be prepared for reconstruction of the wound.

confirms clear margins. Once histologic interpretation confirms clear margins, a red pencil line drawn through the Mohs map as seen in Figure 26-11 indicates that the tumor has been removed and the patient can be prepared for repair of the wound. The average number of Mohs stages is approximately 1.76 stages per case.[18]

Taking Mohs layers from specific locations at times provides additional challenges. One particular challenge arises when the perichondrium of the ear is involved by an overlying cutaneous tumor. In these situations, a Goulian knife with a Weck blade can be utilized to remove an adequate layer of tissue while sparing as much of the unaffected cartilage as possible.[61]

Once the tumor has been cleared microscopically, the Mohs surgeon evaluates the wound for reconstruction options. As previously mentioned, due to the tissue-sparing nature of MMS, many wounds can appropriately be allowed to heal by second intention. Alternatively, the wound may require more advanced reconstruction with primary closure, flaps, or grafts. These repairs are generally undertaken immediately following MMS and performed in the outpatient setting, again under local anesthesia. Exceptionally, patients are referred to consulting specialists for reconstruction. Postoperative wound care, antibiotics, and pain management vary depending on the reconstruction that is executed.

CONCLUSION

Its cost-effective and safe nature, superior cure rates and tissue-sparing properties make MMS the gold standard for the treatment of many cutaneous tumors. Histologically aggressive tumors, large and recurrent tumors, and tumors in cosmetically sensitive and functionally important locations should be considered for treatment with MMS.

REFERENCES

1. Mohs FE. Chemosurgery, a microscopically controlled method of cancer excision. *Arch Surg.* 1941;42:279–295.
2. Mohs FE. History of Mohs micrographic surgery. In: Roenigk RK, Roenigk HH, eds. *Dermatologic Surgery: Principles and Practice.* New York: Marcel Dekker; 1989:783–789.
3. Tromovitch TA, Stegman SJ. Microscopically controlled excision of skin tumors. *Arch Dermatol.* 1974;110(2):231–232.
4. Swanson NA, Taylor WB, Tromovitch TA. The evolution of Mohs surgery. *J Dermatol Surg Oncol.* 1982;8:650–654.
5. Shelley WB. Mohs: microscopically oriented histographic surgery. *Arch Dermatol.* 1978;114(7):1097–1098.
6. Stegman SJ, Tromovitch TA. Modern chemosurgery-microscopically controlled excision. *West J Med.* 1980;132:7–12.
7. Mohs FE. Chemosurgery for skin cancer. *Arch Dermatol.* 1976;112:211–215.
8. Rowe DE, Carroll RJ, Day CL Jr. Long-term recurrence rates in previously untreated (primary) basal cell carcinoma: implications for patient follow-up. *J Dermatol Surg Oncol.* 1989;15:315–336.
9. Rowe DE, Carroll RJ, Day CL Jr. Mohs surgery is the treatment of choice for recurrent (previously treated) basal cell carcinoma. *J Dermatol Surg Oncol.* 1989;15:424–431.
10. Mohs FE. *Chemosurgery: Microscopically Controlled Surgery for Skin Cancer.* Springfield, IL: Charles C. Thomas; 1978:1–356.
11. Mohs FE. Chemosurgery for melanoma. *Arch Dermatol.* 1977;113:285–291.
12. Zitelli JA, Brown C, Hanusa BH. Mohs micrographic surgery for the treatment of primary cutaneous melanoma. *J Amer Acad Dermatol.* 1997;37(2):236–245.
13. Muller FM, Dawe RS, Moseley H, Fleming CJ. Randomized comparison of Mohs micrographic surgery and surgical excision for small nodular basal cell carcinoma: tissue-sparing outcome. *Dermatol Surg.* 2009;35(9):1349–1354.
14. Casey AS, Kennedy CE, Goldman GD. Mohs micrographic surgery: how ACMS fellowship directors practice. *Dermatol Surg.* 2009;35(5):747–756.
15. Merritt BG, Lee NY, Brodland DG, Zitelli JA, Cook J. The safety of Mohs sugery: a prospective multicenter cohort study. *J Am Acad Dermatol.*2012;67(6):1302–1309.
16. Rogers HD, Desciak EB, Marcus RP, Wang S, MacKay-Wiggan J, Eliezri YD. Prospective study of wound infections in Mohs micrographic surgery using clean surgical technique in the absence of prophylactic antibiotics. *J Am Acad Dermatol.* 2010;63(5):842–851.
17. Tierney EP, Hanke CW. Cost effectiveness of Mohs micrographic surgery: review of the literature. *J Drugs Dermatol.* 2009;8(10):914–922.
18. Rogers HW, Coldiron BM. A relative value unit-based cost comparison of treatment modalities for the nonmelanoma skin cancer: effect of the loss of the Mohs multiple surgery reduction exemption. *J Am Acad Dermatol.* 2008;61:96–103.
19. Cook J, Zitelli JA. Mohs micrographic surgery: a cost analysis. *J Am Acad Dermatol.* 1998;39(5):698–703.
20. Hanke CW, Temofeew RK, Miyamoto RT, Lingeman RE. Chemosurgical report: basal cell carcinoma involving the external auditory canal—treatment with Mohs micrographic surgery. *J Dermatol Surg Oncol.* 1985;11(12):1189–1194.
21. Brodland DG, Amonette R, Hanke CW, Robins P. The history and evolution of Mohs micrographic surgery. *Dermatol Surg.* 2000;26(4):303–307.
22. ACGME. American Council for Graduate Medical Education reports by program. Chicago, IL; 2012. http://www.acgme.org/adspublic/. Accessed August 15, 2012.
23. Rogers HW, Weinstock MA, Harris AR, et al. Incidence estimate of nonmelanoma skin cancer in the United States, 2006. *Arch Dermatol.* 2010;146(3):283–287.

24. Rowe DE, Carroll RJ, Day CL. Prognostic factors for local recurrence, metastasis, and survival rates in squamous cell carcinoma of the skin, ear, and lip. Implications for treatment modality selection. *J Am Acad Dermatol.* 1992;29:976–990.
25. Society AC. Cancer Facts and Figures 2012. Atlanta, GA; 2012. http://www.cancer.org/acs/groups/content/@epidemiology surveilance/documents/document/acspc-031941.pdf. Accessed August 15, 2012.
26. Zitelli JA, Moy RL, Abell E. The reliability of frozen sections in the evaluation of surgical margins for melanoma. *J Am Acad Dermatol.* 1991;24:102–106.
27. Kelley LC, Starkus L. Immunohistochemical staining of lentigo maligna during Mohs micrographic surgery using MART-1. *J Am Acad Dermatol.* 2002;46:78–84.
28. Bricca GM, Brodland DG, Zitelli JA. Immunostaining melanoma frozen sections: the 1 hour protocol. *Dermatol Surg.* 2004;30:403–408.
29. Ratner D, Thomas CO, Johnson TM, et al. Mohs micrographic surgery for the treatment of dermatofibrosarcoma protuberans: Results of a multiinstitutional series with an analysis of the extent of microscopic spread. *J Am Acad Dermatol.* 1997;37(4):600–613.
30. Ratz JL, Duong SL, Kulwin DR. Sebaceous carcinoma of the eyelid treated with Mohs surgery. *J Am Acad Dermatol.* 1986;14:668–673.
31. Ang GC, Roenigk RK, Otley CC, Kim Phillips P, Weaver AL. More than 2 decades of treating atypical fibroxanthoma at Mayo Clinic: what have we learned from 91 patients? *Dermatol Surg.* 2009;35:765–772.
32. Hollmig ST, Kirkland EB, Henderson MT, Tang JY, Gladstone HB. The evolving conception and management challenges of malignant fibrous histiocytoma. *Dermatol Surg.* 2012;38(12):1922–1929.
33. Fleischmann HE, Roth RJ, Wood C, Nickoloff BJ. Microcystic adnexal carcinoma treated by microscopically controlled excision. *J Dermatol Surg Oncol.* 1984;10:873–875.
34. O'Connor WJ, Lim KK, Zalla MJ, et al. Comparison of Mohs micrographic surgery and wide excision for extramammary Paget's disease. *Dermatol Surg.* 2003;29:723–727.
35. Starling J, Coldiron BM. Mohs micrographic surgery for the treatment of cutaneous leiomyosarcoma. *J Am Acad Dermatol.* 2011;64(6):1119–1122.
36. Behroozan DS, Goldberg LH, Glaich AS, Kaplan B, Kaye VN. Mohs micrographic surgery for deeply penetrating, expanding benign cutaneous neoplasms. *Dermatol Surg.* 2006;32(7):958–965.
37. Goldberg DJ, Kim YA. Angiosarcoma of the scalp treated with Mohs micrographic surgery. *J Dermatol Surg Oncol.* 1993;19(2):156–158.
38. Marra DI, Schanbacher CF, Torres A. Mohs micrographic surgery of primary cutaneous mucinous carcinoma using immunohistochemistry for margin control. *Dermatol Surg.* 2004;30(5):799–802.
39. O'Connor WJ, Roenigk RK, Brodland DG. Merkel cell carcinoma: comparison of Mohs micrographic surgery and wide excision in 86 patients. *Dermatol Surg.* 1997;23:929–933.
40. Connolly SM, Baker DR, Coldiron BM, et al. AAD/ACMS/ASDSA/ASMS 2012 Appropriate Use Criteria for Mohs Micrographic Surgery. A Report of the American Academy of Dermatology, American College of Mohs Surgery, American Society for Dermatologic Surgery Association, and the American Society for Mohs Surgery. *J Am Acad Dermatol.* 2012;38(10):1582–1603.
41. Ratner D, Bagiella E. The efficacy of curettage in delineating margins of basal cell carcinoma before Mohs micrographic surgery. *Dermatol Surg.* 2003;29:899–903.
42. Davis DA, Pellowski DM, Hanke CW. Preparation of frozen sections. *Dermatol Surg.* 2004;30:1479–1485.
43. Cottel WI, Proper S. Mohs surgery, fresh-tissue technique: our technique with a review. *J Dermatol Surg Oncol.* 1982;8:576–587.
44. Larson PO. Staple and double-stable method of tissue orientation in Mohs micrographic surgery. *J Dermatol Surg Oncol.* 1987;13:732–734.
45. Lang PG Jr. Mohs micrographic surgery: fresh-tissue technique. *Dermatol Clin.* 1989;7:613–626.
46. Alcalay J. Digital computerized mapping in Mohs micrographic surgery. *Dermatol Surg.* 2000;26:692–693.
47. Rapini RP. Comparison of methods for checking surgical margins. *J Am Acad Dermatol.* 1990;23(2 Pt 1):288–294.
48. Albertini J. Mohs micrographic surgery pearls. *Semin Cut Med Surg.* 2004;23:184–195.
49. Grabski WJ, Salasche SJ. Mapping and orienting tissue during Mohs micrographic surgery: an alternative approach. *J Dermatol Surg Oncol.* 1991;17:865–868.
50. McCulloch M, Geddis C, Hetzer MR, et al. Embedding techniques. In: Fish FS, ed. *Manual of Frozen Section Processing for Mohs Micrographic Surgery.* Milwaukee, WI: American College of Mohs Surgery; 2008:601.
51. Leshin B, Cook SR, Frye D. Cryomold: Technique for tissue embedding in Mohs micrographic surgery. *J Dermatol Surg Oncol.* 1991;17:234–236.
52. Hanke CW, Leonard AL, Reed AJ. Rapid preparation of high-quality frozen sections using a membrane and vacuum system embedding machine. *Dermatol Surg.* 2008;34(1):20–25.
53. Todd MM, Lee JM, Marks VJ. Rapid toluidine blue stain for Mohs micrographic surgery. *Dermatol Surg.* 2005;31:244–245.
54. Thosani MK, Marghoob A, Chen CS. Current progress of immunostains in Mohs micrographic surgery: a review. *Dermatol Surg.* 2008;34(12):1621–1636.
55. Kader El Tal A, Abrou AE, Stiff MA, Mehregan DA. Immunostaining in Mohs micrographic surgery: a review. *Dermatol Surg.* 2010;36:275–290.
56. Robinson JK. Current histologic preparation methods for Mohs micrographic surgery. *Dermatol Surg.* 2001;27:555–560.
57. Jimenez FJ, Grichnik JM, Buchanan MD, Clark RE. Immunohistochemical techniques in Mohs micrographic surgery: their potential use in the detection of neoplastic cells masked by inflammation. *J Am Acad Dermatol.* 1995;32:89–94.
58. Zachary CB, Rest EB, Furlong SM, Arcedo PN, McGeorge BC, Kist DA. Rapid cytokeratin stains enhance the sensitivity of Mohs micrographic surgery for squamous cell carcinoma. *J Dermatol Surg Oncol.* 1994;20:530–535.
59. Murphy ME, Brodland DG, Zitelli JA. Errors in the interpretation of Mohs histopathology sections over a 1-year fellowship. *Dermatol Surg.* 2008;34(12):1637–1641.
60. Leshin B, White WL. Folliculocentric basaloid proliferation. *Arch Dermatol.* 1990;126:900–906.
61. Countryman NB, Leshin B. Use of a Goulian knife and Weck blade for Mohs layers when tumor extends to the perichondrium of the ear. *Dermatol Surg.* 2012;38(4):670–672.

CHAPTER 27

Practical Management of Atypical Nevi

June J. Park, Clara Curiel-Lewandrowski, & Caroline C. Kim

INTRODUCTION

Atypical nevi (AN) are melanocytic nevi that may exhibit ABCD features similar to those of melanoma, and patients with AN have an increased risk of developing melanoma. Since their first description over 30 years ago, confusion persists about the definition, as well as the clinical and surgical management, of AN. Patients with AN account for a significant percentage of patients seen in general dermatology practices and specialized pigmented lesion clinics, as well as in dermatologic surgical clinics for excision. It is, therefore, imperative that all general and procedural dermatologists understand the complexities of this diagnosis and the challenges of care for these patients. This chapter will review the diagnosis, clinical evaluation, approach for management and skin biopsies, and future directions in the care of patients with AN, including advanced imaging technologies.

BACKGROUND

In 1978, Wallace H. Clark and colleagues first reported the AN (termed "B-K" nevus by Clark) as a clinicopathologic entity and described particular nevi on individuals at risk for melanoma.[1] Several names are used in the literature to refer to such nevi, including AN, dysplastic nevus (DN), and Clark's nevus. In 1992, the US National Institutes of Health Consensus Conference recommended that AN refer to clinically atypical appearing nevi, while "nevus with architectural disorder" be used for pathologically evaluated nevi with dysplasia. To date, some clinicians use the terms AN and DN interchangeably. For the purpose of this chapter, we will use the term AN for clinically AN, and DN for lesions that have been biopsied with pathologically confirmed dysplasia.

Several definitions and criteria for the Familial Atypical Mole and Melanoma (FAMM) syndrome have been proposed, including one by the aforementioned 1992 conference that defined it by (1) occurrence of melanoma in one or more first- or second-degree relatives, (2) large numbers of moles (often greater than 50), some of which are atypical and often variable in size, and (3) moles that demonstrate certain distinct histologic features of dysplasia defined by the consensus conference. In addition, others have proposed FAMM syndrome as the presence of two or more family members with AN and at least one family member with melanoma.[2] The atypical mole syndrome has also been described as the presence of 50[3] to 100[4] or more melanocytic nevi including one or more 8 mm or larger in greatest diameter and one or more with clinically atypical (ABCD) features. In 1980, the term dysplastic nevus syndrome (DNS) was termed to describe the association of sporadic DN with nonfamilial melanoma.[5]

EPIDEMIOLOGY

Clinically, AN have been reported in up to 17% of the Caucasian population.[6] Histopathologically, DN are reported at a prevalence of approximately 10%.[7,8] AN are reported at a much higher frequency ranging from 34% to 59% among patients with a history of melanoma.[9–12] The prevalence of AN is positively associated with fair-skinned populations, presence of common melanocytic nevi,[13] and chronic sun exposure. A decrease in prevalence is seen with increasing age.[14] AN typically appear in childhood and can appear throughout adulthood.[15]

PATHOPHYSIOLOGY

AN can be inherited or occur sporadically. Molecularly, AN have been shown to exhibit altered gene expression patterns including p16 and p53, a higher proliferation index, and greater microsatellite instability compared to benign nevi.[16] Clark originally described AN as part of a tumor progression lineage toward melanoma.[1] However, as opposed to models of dysplasia progressing to carcinoma in other diseases such as colon cancer, there is no evidence that AN progress to melanoma at a rate greater than that of common nevi. Multiple studies have investigated pathologic associations between melanoma and preexisting nevi and have suggested similar rates of melanoma associated with preexisting banal nevi as with preexisting DN.[17–21] This would suggest that DN in general have no greater risk of malignant transformation than banal nevi and may not need to be treated more aggressively.[17–21]

Although AN is primarily sporadic in etiology, when inherited, the mode of inheritance of AN is thought to be autosomal dominant. Germline mutations in three genes have been linked to melanoma-prone families: CDKN2A,[22] CDK4,[23] and CMM1.[24] Up to 40% of FAMM harbor a mutation in the CDKN2A locus, exhibiting altered gene expression for p16 and ARF tumor suppressor proteins.[25]

RISK FOR MELANOMA IN PATIENTS WITH ATYPICAL NEVI

AN identify patients at slightly increased risk for melanoma. While the risk for melanoma in the general population is around 1.93%, patients with AN have been estimated to have a twofold to 12 fold increased relative risk depending on the number of nevi.[26,27] Furthermore, patients with atypical mole syndrome have been reported to have a 10 year cumulative risk of 10.7% for developing melanoma.[28] However, as described earlier, there is no evidence that individual AN progresses to melanoma any more frequently than common nevi. The majority of melanomas—around 75%—develop *de novo*.[19,29] Removal of AN as a means of preventing melanoma is not a viable approach, and biopsy of every atypical mole should not be considered the standard of practice. Patients with AN need to be monitored closely for suspicious lesions, given their higher risk for melanoma, and the decision to biopsy an individual lesion is based on suspicion for melanoma after a comprehensive and integrative evaluation of each individual patient.

CLINICAL PRESENTATION

Clinically, AN have been described as melanocytic lesions measuring 5 mm or more in diameter with variable pigmentation, poorly defined borders, and asymmetry.[12] They are typically larger than banal nevi, and their pigmentation can vary from pink and tan, to dark brown with patients often having their own particular "signature patterns" of one or more different types of AN.[30] AN may clinically exhibit the ABCDs described for melanoma (Asymmetry, Border irregularity, Color variegation, and larger Diameters), and, therefore, can look suspicious for melanoma. Although ultraviolet rays may affect the distribution of AN, with a higher prevalence in sun-exposed areas, AN can occur anywhere on the body including sun-protected areas.[31] One can generally diagnose AN based on the aforementioned features, but there can be discordance between the clinical impression of atypia and histopathologic dysplasia.[32,33] Therefore, if symptoms concerning for melanoma arise, including pruritus, bleeding, growth, or other worrisome clinical changes, one should consider removal to exclude the possibility of melanoma with minimal clinical features. The correlation between clinical atypia and histologic dysplasia has been reported to be 27% for small nevi (3~5 mm) and 70% for larger nevi (greater than 5 mm) in one study.[33]

MANAGEMENT

Early detection of melanoma while minimizing unnecessary biopsies is the primary goal of dermatologists for patients with AN. To date, most dermatologists rely on their clinical impression alone to differentiate AN versus melanoma. In several instances, the diagnosis of AN can be made clinically, without the need for a biopsy, using the characteristics described earlier. Many dermatologists use dermoscopy (epiluminescence microscopy) or total body photography (TBP) to assist in their clinical examination of patients with AN, which will be discussed later. When possible, clinicians should perform an excisional biopsy of any pigmented lesion with features suspicious for melanoma.

EDUCATING THE PATIENT

Patients' knowledge regarding AN may range from lack of awareness to extreme anxiety surrounding a fear of melanoma and the need for numerous surgical excisions. Providing education during visits is crucial in the care of patients with AN. Patients should be educated about the nature of AN, and offered reassurance that the great majority of lesions are not pre-cancerous, and, therefore, are not destined to progress to malignant melanoma (MM). However, patients should be aware of the need to be alert for any new or preexisting lesions that suddenly change to exhibit worrisome features. Clinicians can teach patients the self-skin examination including how to monitor their skin, the ABCDs of melanoma, and the identification of an "ugly duckling" lesion. Patients should be familiar with the warning signs of itching and bleeding and know when to call for an urgent evaluation. Clinicians can advise patients to use adequate sun protection (hats, cover-ups, sunscreen with sun protective factor 30 or higher, shade, and avoiding mid-day sun). The following facts concerning AN should be considered when discussing the clinical relevance of this entity with patients:

- AN are a kind of nevus associated with a slightly increased risk of developing melanoma.
- The majority of melanomas arise *de novo*; although it is important to follow one's nevi for any suspicious changes, it is also very important to monitor for new suspicious lesions arising in the normal skin.
- AN can be monitored clinically and do not need to be removed unless there are changes concerning for melanoma.
- Systematic removal of AN has not been shown to decrease one's risk of melanoma; therefore, the goal of management is careful and close observation instead of a "molectomy."
- The "ugly duckling" rule of melanoma for self-monitoring: look for any outlier pigmented lesions that display features not seen in other AN.
- The importance of sun protection and the self-skin examination.

CLINICAL EXAMINATION

Some patients may have a few AN, whereas others may have hundreds. When evaluating AN, the primary goal is to rule out melanoma. If the clinical and dermoscopic features of a lesion display symmetry and homogeneity of pigmentation, and lack dermoscopic warning signs, the clinician can choose to monitor the lesion by documenting its measurements, any particular clinical/dermoscopic features, and/or photograph it for short-term monitoring. The patient should also be asked to follow the lesion on self-skin examinations and to notify the clinician of any changes.

CLINICAL EXAMINATION OF PATIENTS WITH NUMEROUS ATYPICAL NEVI

For patients with numerous AN, a systematic approach becomes very useful. One technique that has been described is similar to the way in which a pathologist evaluates a slide. The clinician can first screen the patient at "low power" to assess that patient's typical mole patterns and their "signature" nevi, noting typical size, shape, and color ranges of those nevi.[34] Any pigmented lesions not fitting into these patterns (ugly ducklings), or of concern to the patient or clinician for any other reason can then be further evaluated at "higher power" through dermoscopic evaluation.[30]

CURRENT TOOLS FOR EVALUATION OF ATYPICAL NEVI

DERMOSCOPY. Dermoscopy is a technique that uses a handheld luminescing magnifier lens to visualize deep pigmentation and stromal and vascular structures below the skin surface. It is the most widely used diagnostic tool to examine a melanocytic lesion in vivo.[35] Traditional dermoscopy contains a nonpolarized light source and requires direct skin contact with a liquid interphase to cancel out light reflecting from the skin surface. Modern dermoscopy dispenses polarized light to allow inspection of subsurface structures. Dermoscopy is useful in examining underlying pigment patterns, ruling out malignant features, and monitoring AN clinically over time. The ability to diagnose melanoma accurately improves significantly when trained dermatologists use dermoscopy as opposed to the naked eye.[36–39] Accuracy has been shown to decrease when dermoscopy is used by untrained care providers.[40] It is, therefore, recommended that clinicians seek training and courses to properly learn dermoscopy, thereby optimizing the results of implementing this technique in clinical practice.

TOTAL BODY DIGITAL PHOTOGRAPHY. TBP is another tool currently used to aid in the management of patients with AN. A series of total body photographs in standardized positions to maximize viewing of nevi are taken of patients by a professional photographer trained in this technique. Close-up and dermoscopic photographs of individual nevi of concern may also be performed. During subsequent follow-up visits, clinicians are able to examine patients' skin with the ability to reference the baseline photographs to assess for clinical stability of nevi and any new or concerning changes. TBP is particularly useful for patients with numerous, clinically complex AN, or patients who are at a high risk for melanoma, as TBP has been shown to identify early, subtle changes for the detection of early melanoma.[41] In addition, TBP has been shown to reduce the number of unnecessary biopsies[42,43] and to reduce patient anxiety.[44] Some challenges to TBP include the cost and logistics of setting up imaging technology and increased time in performing complete skin examinations. However, TBP can greatly enhance the management of particularly complex and/or anxious AN patients. Even without having TBP in their own practices, clinicians can educate patients about TBP, refer them to clinics that utilize TBP, and collaborate with those clinics in the management of these high-risk individuals.

BIOPSY

If the clinician identifies a lesion concerning for melanoma, a biopsy should be performed, as histopathology is the gold standard for diagnosing melanoma. If feasible, an excisional biopsy is preferred so as to provide the pathologist with the complete lesion for histologic evaluation, and to avoid sampling error that could lead to a missed melanoma, while also allowing for accurate microstaging in the case of a melanoma.[45] Furthermore, complete removal of an AN with an excisional biopsy avoids concerns about recurrence and potential upgrading in atypia, described as "pseudomelanoma."[46] Another consideration for performing an excisional biopsy is to remove suspicious lesions in areas that are difficult for the patient to self-monitor.

Methods of biopsy include scoop/shave biopsy, punch biopsy, and elliptical excisions; their indications vary based on the clinical judgment and preference of the clinician. A previous study has shown that melanocytic lesions may microscopically extend laterally as much as 1.2 mm.[47] Therefore, when performing an excisional biopsy of a DN, clinicians should aim for biopsies with 1–2 mm peripheral margins if feasible regardless of the technique used.

Depending on the size of the pigmented lesion, punch and elliptical excisions can allow for 1–2 mm clinically clear lateral margins and will extend to the subcutis, thereby removing the entire depth of the lesion in question. For lesions that are highly suspicious for melanoma, this method ensures that one does not transect the melanoma and allows for the most accurate microstaging. It is important to be forward-thinking and to design the closure of the excisional biopsy along skin tension lines (parallel to the length of limbs for arms and legs, for example) in case a wider excision is needed. If scoop shave excisional biopsies are performed, in addition to aiming for 1–2 mm peripheral margins, one should aim for a depth of at least 1 mm and perhaps deeper depending on the clinical lesion to avoid transecting the lesion and to allow for complete histologic removal. Shallow shave biopsies should be avoided in lesions concerning for the diagnosis of melanoma.[29] Scoop/shave biopsies have been shown to be associated with a higher recurrence rate of DN, suggesting that it may be more difficult to achieve histologic clearance of a lesion with the shave technique.[29] In addition, because of a higher incidence of transecting melanomas with shave procedures, shave biopsies have also been associated with higher rates of sentinel node procedures due to uncertain definitive tumor depths at the time of initial biopsy.[48] However, shave/scoop biopsies may be preferred under certain circumstances. Clinicians may consider shave/scoop procedures for lesions without worrisome atypical features, lesions that are flat and large, lesions in anatomic locations under high skin tension that may not close well, and lesions on patients who may not tolerate more invasive procedures.[29]

HISTOPATHOLOGIC ASSESSMENT AND MANAGEMENT OF DYSPLASTIC NEVI

Histologically, DN are characterized by architectural disorder and cytologic atypia that include a basilar proliferation of atypical melanocytes in a lentiginous or epithelioid-cell pattern associated with at least two of the following criteria: (1) the presence of lamellar fibrosis or concentric eosinophilic fibrosis, (2) neovascularization, (3) inflammatory response, and (4) fusion of rete ridges.[49] Reporting of biopsied DN varies depending on the individual pathologist and/or institution. Some dermatopathologists differentiate high-grade (severe) DN only, while others will grade the degree of dysplasia as mild, moderate or severe, or levels in between (i.e., mild-moderate, moderate-focal severe, etc.). Because grading of DN has a significant subjective component depending on the pathologist's interpretation of the biopsy specimen, substantial discordance amongst pathologists has been reported in grading.[49] For challenging melanocytic lesions, it is not uncommon for second opinions to be requested of dermatopathologists experienced in interpreting melanocytic lesions.

RE-EXCISIONS

When DN are biopsied and removed with clear histologic margins, no further re-excision is needed since there are no data to suggest that fully excised DN can evolve into melanoma. However, some clinicians may recommend re-excision of severely DN with 5 mm margins so as to treat them as malignant melanoma in situ (MMIS). This stems from the fact that grading of DN can differ from pathologist to pathologist and often there can be discrepancies about what constitutes a severe DN vs. MMIS. Until further studies are performed addressing appropriate margins for severely DN, and markers are identified to predict which severe DN have malignant potential, many institutions are erring on the side of caution and re-excising them.

The clinical management of DN biopsied with positive histologic margins varies, as there are currently no formal guidelines for re-excision of DN. Some clinicians may choose to perform a re-excision of DN with positive margins to rule out sampling error and avoid recurrence, depending on the degree of dysplasia noted. A recent survey of 101 Chicago dermatologists[50] showed that the decision to re-excise or observe nevi depended on the histologic grade of dysplasia and margin status. Twenty-one percent of those surveyed reported that they would re-excise mild DN with positive biopsy margins, 81% would re-excise moderately DN, and 95% would re-excise severely DN. With biopsy margins that were clear, 9% would re-excise moderately DN, and 55% reported re-excising severely DN. However, given that recent studies suggesting AN and common banal nevi have similar rates of recurrence after biopsy and a similar risk of progression to melanoma, it is unclear whether re-excision of incompletely biopsied mild and moderately DN is necessary to prevent melanoma.[29,51] A few studies have examined the role of observation of mild and moderately DN with positive margins. One study showed no evolution to melanoma in a small study sample (26 DN) followed for a mean follow-up time of 6.12 years, and low rates of clinical recurrence (3.6% of 195 DN compared to 3.3% of 61 benign nevi) with at least 2 years' follow-up.[29,51] These data suggest that observation can be a safe alternative to re-excision for incompletely removed mild and moderately DN; however, large-scale studies are needed to develop data-driven guidelines for DN management.

FOLLOW-UP

Existing AN and new lesions should be carefully monitored by the clinician for concerning features during follow-up and by the patient regularly between visits. The risk of melanoma remains lifelong; regular self-skin examinations and examinations by a dermatologist are imperative. The frequency of follow-up usually varies from every 6 to 12 months based on the complexity of nevi, the patient's history, and their level of risk for melanoma.

FUTURE DIRECTIONS OF MANAGEMENT OF ATYPICAL NEVI: EMERGING TECHNOLOGIES

Multispectral imaging is an advanced technology that may be considered in the management of pigmented lesions. Multispectral imaging utilizes different wavelengths of light (400–1000 nm) to produce images of a pigmented lesion at different depths below the skin surface, up to 2 mm deep. Two multispectral imaging devices for spectrophotometric intracutaneous analysis, SIAscope (developed by Astron Clinica, Toft, Cambridgeshire, UK, and marketed by Biocompatibles since 2009) and MelaFind (MELA Sciences, Inc., Irvington, NY), are available. SIAscope emits eight different wavelengths of light between 400 to 1000 nm to obtain information regarding a lesion's color, epidermal and dermal melanin, blood, and collagen that is then interpreted by the clinician.[35] A preliminary investigation performed by Moncrieff et al. found that the presence of dermal melanin, collagen holes, and blood displacement with erythematous blush correlated with an 83% sensitivity and 80% specificity for melanoma detection in a study.[52] Glud et al.[53] performed a prospective study examining SIAscope's utility in diagnosing melanoma compared to dermoscopy in 2009. The authors found that the sensitivity of dermoscopy was 92%, compared to 100% for SIAscopy, while the specificity of dermoscopy was 81% compared to 59% for SIAscopy. The authors concluded that, overall, dermoscopy remains the best approach to diagnosing pigmented lesions, but SIAscope could produce dermoscopic images and thereby help train clinicians to recognize specific lesions. MelaFind, which is FDA-approved, emits 10 different wavelengths between 430 and 940 nm. By using a lesion classification algorithm, it provides a binary output of whether a pigmented lesion has a high or low degree of disorganization, which helps determine whether to biopsy a lesion.[35] To assist in making this decision, MelaFind compares the lesion's features to a pigmented lesion database and uses a lesion classification algorithm that has been shown to have a sensitivity of greater than 95% for melanoma detection.[54] MelaFind is not currently designed to evaluate amelanotic lesions, lesions on certain anatomical sites (acral, mucosal, subungual), lesions within areas of scarring, and pigmented lesions <2 mm in diameter. Preliminary studies utilizing MelaFind for melanoma diagnosis found that it had a sensitivity ranging from 98% to 100%, and specificity ranging from 44% to 85%.[55,56] Most recently, a 2010 prospective, multicenter, blinded study comparing MelaFind to clinician performance in detecting melanoma found that MelaFind had a biopsy sensitivity of 98.4%, while clinicians' biopsy sensitivity was 78%.[57] MelaFind's biopsy specificity was 9.9%, compared to the clinicians' specificity of 3.7%. The authors concluded that MelaFind may be a useful device for dermatologists evaluating pigmented lesions and that further studies are warranted to investigate its specific applications in patient care.

Other emerging technologies include confocal microscopy, which provides high-resolution horizontal section images of tissue using point illumination; optical coherence tomography, which provides sagittal section images of tissue using infrared light; electrical impedance, which detects electrical differences in malignant and benign cell/tissue structure[58]; and epidermal genetic information retrieval, which allows noninvasive sampling of stratum corneum with adhesive tape stripping.[59] Ultrasound, magnetic resonance imaging, dynamic infrared imaging, photoacoustic microscopy, and other advancements are expected to be incorporated for earlier and more accurate detection of melanomas.[35] Although many of these technologies are still undergoing investigation, an ideal diagnostic modality would improve clinicians' sensitivity and specificity for melanoma detection while also being a practical and cost-efficient bedside tool that could easily be integrated into clinical practice.

CONCLUSION

AN are melanocytic nevi that may exhibit ABCD features similar to those of melanoma and identify patients who may be at an increased risk for developing melanoma. It is imperative that all general and procedural dermatologists understand the complexities of this diagnosis in order to educate patients about the significance of AN as well as the need for regular monitoring to provide them with optimal care. Future investigations on imaging technology for patient monitoring and surgical management of AN, including biopsy techniques and re-excisions, will further enhance care for patients with AN.

REFERENCES

1. Clark WH Jr, Elder DE, Guerry D IV, Epstein MN, Greene MH, Van Horn M. A study of tumor progression: the precursor lesions of superficial spreading and nodular melanoma. *Hum Pathol.* 1984;15:1147–1165.
2. Greene MH, Clark WH Jr, Tucker MA, Kraemer KH, Elder DE, Fraser MC. High risk of malignant melanoma in melanoma-prone families with dysplastic nevi. *Ann Intern Med.* 1985;102:458–465.
3. Slade J, Marghoob AA, Salopek TG, Rigel DS, Kopf AW, Bart RS. Atypical mole syndrome: risk factor for cutaneous malignant melanoma and implications for management. *J Am Acad Dermatol.* 1995;32(3):479–494.
4. Kopf AW, Friedman RJ, Rigel DS. Atypical mole syndrome. *J Am Acad Dermatol.* 1990;22:117–118.
5. Elder DE, Goldman LI, Goldman SC, Greene MH, Clark WH Jr. Dysplastic nevus syndrome: a phenotypic association of sporadic cutaneous melanoma. *Cancer.* 1980;46(8):1787–1794.
6. Munro DD. Multiple active junctional naevi with family history of malignant melanoma. *Proc R Soc Med.* 1974;67(7):594–595.
7. Steijlen P, Bergman W, Hermans J, Scheffer E, Van Vloten WA, Ruiter DJ. The efficacy of histopathological criteria required for diagnosing dysplastic naevi. *Histopathology.* 1988;12(3):289–300.
8. Piepkorn MW, Barnhill RL, Cannon-Albright LA, et al. A multiobserver, population-based analysis of histologic dysplasia in melanocytic nevi. *J Am Acad Dermatol.* 1994;30:707–714.
9. Augustsson A, Stierner U, Rosdahl I, Suurküla M. Common and dysplastic naevi as risk factors for cutaneous malignant melanoma in a Swedish population. *Acta Derm Venereol.* 1991;71:518–524.
10. Grob JJ, Gouvernet J, Aymar D, et al. Count of benign melanocytic nevi as a major indicator of risk for nonfamilial nodular and superficial spreading melanoma. *Cancer.* 1990;66:387–395.
11. Garbe C, Buttner P, Weiss J, et al. Risk factors for developing cutaneous melanoma and criteria for identifying persons at risk: multicenter case-control study of the Central Malignant Melanoma Registry of the German Dermatological Society. *J Invest Dermatol.* 1994;102:695–699.
12. Tucker MA, Halpern A, Holly EA, et al. Clinically recognized dysplastic nevi: a central risk factor for cutaneous melanoma. *JAMA.* 1997;277:1439–1444.
13. Piepkorn M, Meyer LJ, Goldgar D, et al. The dysplastic melanocyric nevus: a prevalent lesion that correlates poorly with clinical phenotype. *J Am Acad Dermatol.* 1989;20:407–415.
14. Lasithiotakis KG, Kokolakis A, Giannikaki E, Krasagakis K, Tosca A. Factors associated with the prevalence of atypical nevus in a Mediterranean pigmented skin lesion clinic. *Melanoma Res.* 2011;5:469–473.
15. Halpern AC, Guerry DT IV, Elder DE, Trock B, Synnestvedt M, Humphreys T. Natural history of dysplastic nevi. *J Am Acad Dermatol.* 1993;29:51–57.
16. Duffy K, Grossman D. The dysplastic nevus: from historical perspective to management in the modern era: Part II. Molecular aspects and clinical management. *J Am Acad Dermatol.* 2012;67:19e1–19e12.
17. Skender-Kalnenas TM, English DR, Heenan PJ. Benign melanocyric lesions: risk markers or precursors of cutaneous melanoma? *J Am Acad Dermatol.* 1995;33:1000–1007.
18. Sagebiel RW. Melanocytic nevi in histologic association with primary cutaneous melanoma of superficial spreading and nodular types: effect of tumor thickness. *J Invest Dermatol.* 1993;100:322–325.
19. Bevona C, Gogins W, Quinn T, Fullerto J, Tsao H. Cutaneous melanomas associated with nevi. *Arch Dermatol.* 2003;139:1620–1624.
20. Lucas CR, Sanders LL, Murray JC, Myers SA, Hall RP, Grichnik JM. Early melanoma detection: nonuniform dermoscopic features and growth. *J Am Acad Dermatol.* 2003;48:663–671.
21. Goodson AG, Florell SR, Boucher KM, Grossman D. A decade of melanomas: identification of factors associated with delayed detection in an academic group practice. *Dermatol Surg.* 2011;37:1620–1630.
22. Cannon-Albright LA, Goldgar DE, Meyer LJ, et al. Assignment of a locus for familial melanoma, MLM, to chromosome 9p13-p22. *Science.* 1992;258(5085):1148–1152.
23. Nobori T, Miura K, Wu DJ, Lois A, Takabayashi K, Carson DA. Deletions of the cyclin-dependent kinase-4 inhibitor gene in multiple human cancers. *Nature.* 1994;368(6473):753–756.
24. Bale SJ, Dracopoli NC, Tucker MA, et al. Mapping the gene for hereditary cutaneous malignant melanoma-dysplastic nevus to chromosome 1p. *N Engl J Med.* 1989;320(21):1367–1372.
25. Chin L. The genetics of malignant melanoma: lessons from mouse and man. *Nat Rev Cancer.* 2003;3:559–570.
26. SEER Database. http://www.seer.cancer.gov/statfacts/html/melan.html
27. Greene MH. Genetics of cutaneous melanoma and nevi. *Mayo Clin Proc.* 1997;72:467–474.
28. Marghoob AA, Kopf AW, Rigel DS, et al. Risk of cutaneous malignant melanoma in patients with 'classic' atypical-

mole syndrome. A case-control study. *Arch Dermatol.* 1994; 130(8):993–998.
29. Goodson AG, Florell SR, Boucher KM, Grossman D. Low rates of clinical recurrence after biopsy of benign to moderately dysplastic melanocytic nevi. *J Am Acad Dermatol.* 2010; 6:591–596.
30. Bolognia JL. Too Many Moles. *Arch Dermatol.* 2006;142:508.
31. Stierner U. Melanocytes, moles and melanoma—a study on UV effects. *Acta Derm Venereol Suppl (Stockh).* 1991;168:1–31.
32. Meyer LJ, Piepkorn M, Goldgar DE, et al. Interobserver concordance indiscriminating clinical atypia of melanocytic nevi, and correlations with histologic atypia. *J Am Acad Dermatol.* 1996;34:618–625.
33. Annessi G, Cattaruzza MS, Abeni D, et al. Correlation between clinical atypia and histologic dysplasia in acquired melanocytic nevi. *J Am Acad Dermatol.* 2001;45:77–85.
34. Suh KY, Bolognia JL. Signature nevi. *J Am Acad Dermatol.* 2009;60:508–514.
35. O'Donneel AT, Kim CC. Update and clinical use of imaging technologies for pigmented lesions of the skin. *Semin Cutan Med Surg.* 2012;31(1):38–44.
36. Grin CM, Kopf AW, Welkovich B, Bart RS, Levenstein MJ. Accuracy in the clinical diagnosis of malignant melanoma. *Arch Dermatol.* 1990;126:763–766.
37. Miller M, Ackerman AB. How accurate are dermatologists in the diagnosis of melanoma? Degree of accuracy and implications. *Arch Dermatol.* 1992;128:559–560.
38. Wolf IH, Smolle J, Soyer HP, Kerl H. Sensitivity in the clinical diagnosis of malignant melanoma. *Melanoma Res.* 1998; 8:425–429.
39. Mayer J. Systematic review of the diagnostic accuracy of dermatoscopy in detecting malignant melanoma. *Med J Aust.* 1997;167:206–210.
40. Binder M, Puespoeck-Schwarz M, Steiner A, et al. Epiluminescence microscopy of small pigmented skin lesions: short-term formal training improves the diagnostic performance of dermatologists. *J Am Acad Dermatol.* 1997;36 (2 Pt 1):197–202.
41. Kelly JW, Yeatman JM, Regalia C, Mason G, Henham AP. A high incidence of melanoma found in patients with multiple dysplastic naevi by photographic surveillance. *Med J Aust.* 1997;167(4):191–194.
42. Goodson AG, Florell SR, Hyde M, Bowen GM, Grossman D. Comparative analysis of total body and dermatoscopic photographic monitoring of nevi in similar patient populations at risk for cutaneous melanoma. *Dermatol Surg.* 2010; 36(7):1087–1098.
43. Rhodes AR. Intervention strategy to prevent lethal cutaneous melanoma: use of dermatologic photography to aid surveillance of high-risk persons. *J Am Acad Dermatol.* 1998;39:262–267.
44. Rice ZP, Weiss FJ, DeLong LK, Curiel-Lewandrowski C, Chen SC. Utilization and rationale for the implementation of total body (digital) photography as an adjunct screening measure for melanoma. *Melanoma Res.* 2010;20(5):417–21.
45. Balch CM, Gershenwald JE, Soong SJ, et al. Final version of 2009 AJCC melanoma staging and classification. *J Clin Oncol.* 2009;27(36):6199–6206.
46. Kornberg R, Ackerman AB. Pseudomelanoma: recurrent melanocytic nevus following partial surgical removal. *Arch Dermatol.* 1975;111:1588–1590.
47. Rigel DS, Friedman RJ, Kopf A. Surgical margins for removal of dysplastic nevi. [abstract]. *J Dermatol Surg Oncol.* 1985; 11:745.
48. Lowe M, Hill N, Page A, Chen S, Delman KA. The impact of shave biopsy on the management of patients with thin melanomas. *Am Surg.* 2011;77(8):1050–1053.
49. Clemente C, Cochran AJ, Elder DE, et al. Histopathologic diagnosis of dysplastic nevi: concondance among pathologists convened by the World Health Organization Melanoma Programme. *Hum Pathol.* 1991;22:313–319.
50. Duffy KL, Mann DJ, Petronic-Rosic V, Shea CR. Clinical decision making based on histopathological grading and margin status of dysplastic nevi. *Arch Dermatol.* 2012;148: 259–260.
51. Kmetz EC, Sanders H, Fisher G, Lang PG, Maize JC. The role of observation in the management of atypical nevi. *Southern Med J.* 2009;102:45–48.
52. Moncrieff M, Cotton S, Claridge E, Hall P. Spectrophotometric intracutaneous analysis: a new technique for imaging pigmented skin lesions. *Br J Dermatol.* 2002;146: 448–457.
53. Glud M, Gniadecki R, Drzewiecki KT. Spectrophotometric intracutaneous analysis versus dermoscopy for the diagnosis of pigmented skin lesions: prospective, double-blind study in a secondary reference centre. *Melanoma Res.* 2009;19: 176–179.
54. Monheit G, Cognetta AB, Ferris L, et al. The performance of MelaFind: a prospective multicenter study. *Arch Dermatol.* 2011;147:188–194.
55. Elbaum M, Kopf AW, Rabinovitz HS, et al. Automatic differentiation of melanoma from melanocytic nevi with multispectral digital dermoscopy: a feasibility study. *J Am Acad Dermatol.* 2001;44:207–218.
56. Friedman RJ, Gutkowicz-Krusin D, Farber MJ, et al. The diagnostic performance of expert dermoscopists vs a computer-vision system on small-diameter melanomas. *Arch Dermatol.* 2008;144:476–482.
57. Langley RG, Rajadhyaksha M, Dwyer PJ, Sober AJ, Flotte TJ, Anderson RR. Confocal scanning laser microscopy of benign and malignant melanocytic skin lesions in vivo. *J Am Acad Dermatol.* 2001;45:365–376.
58. Glickman YA, Filo O, David M, et al. Electrical impedance scanning: a new approach to skin cancer diagnosis. *Skin Research and Tech.* 2003;9:262–268.
59. Wachsman W, Morhenn V, Palmer T, et al. Noinvasive genomic detection of melanoma. *Br J Dermatol.* 2011; 164: 797–806.

CHAPTER 28

Surgical Management of Melanoma

Peter L. Mattei, Elizabeth K. Jones, & Hensin Tsao

In the past several decades, the incidence of melanoma has steadily risen. In the United States, as of 2012, it is estimated that 76,250 new cases of melanoma will develop and 9,180 patients will die of the disease.[1] Data from 2006 to 2008 projects that 1 in 36 males and 1 in 55 females will develop invasive melanoma during their lifetime.[1] The median age of diagnosis is 59 years. Furthermore, the projected increase in the incidence of melanoma may be underestimated due to unreported outpatient treatments of superficial and in situ melanomas. Melanoma is one of the leading cancers in terms of average years of life lost per death from disease.[2] Melanoma has higher incidence rates in lightly pigmented Caucasians than in Hispanics, Asians, and African Americans.[2] Estimates indicate that 82% to 85% of patients present with localized disease, 10% to 13% with regional disease, and 2% to 5% with distant metastatic disease.[3] Melanoma is responsible for the majority of skin cancer-related deaths but is often cured when detected early. Outcome depends on the stage at presentation.

Strong evidence supports three histologic features of the primary tumor to be of high prognostic value: tumor (Breslow) thickness, the presence or absence of microscopic ulceration, and mitotic rate. All three are required components of the biopsy specimen's pathology report.[4] Maximum Breslow thickness is measured from the granular layer of the epidermis or the base of a superficial ulceration to the deepest depth of invasion by malignant cells to the nearest 0.1 mm, excluding extension into the adnexal adventitia. Microscopic ulceration is defined as tumor-induced full-thickness epidermal loss with subjacent dermal tumor and reactive dermal changes. Mitotic rate is measured as the number of dermal mitoses per square millimeter.

In 2010 the American Joint Committee on Cancer (AJCC) defined an updated staging system in which tumor (Breslow) thickness and mitotic rate were identified as the two major factors that predict melanoma survival in tumors ≤ 1 mm in thickness.[4] This change stemmed from the finding that a dermal mitotic rate ≥ 1 mitosis/mm^2 is independently associated with a worse disease-specific survival. As a result, in the 2010 AJCC staging guidelines, the dermal mitotic rate was used to upstage patients with melanoma ≤ 1 mm from stage IA to stage IB, replacing the anatomic (Clark) level of invasion. The impact of tumor thickness on prognosis is underscored by variations reported in survival outcomes. In patients with localized disease and primary tumors ≤ 1.0 mm in thickness, over 90% of patients achieve 5 year survival. For patients with localized melanomas thicker than 1.0 mm, survival ranges from 50% to 90%.[3] When the disease extends to regional nodes however, survival rates decrease by half.

BIOPSY OF A PRIMARY MELANOMA

The first step for definitive diagnosis of a cutaneous melanoma is to obtain a biopsy. A biopsy may be incisional and sample part of the lesion or excisional and encompass the entire lesion. If melanoma is suspected, the most appropriate approach is a narrow excisional biopsy with 1 to 3 mm margins. Most atypical melanocytic lesions are cleared by this approach.[4] The goal of a narrow excisional biopsy is to achieve clinically negative margins and an adequate depth while avoiding transection of the specimen. Wider margins should be avoided to allow subsequent wide local excision and accurate lymphatic mapping by sentinel lymph node biopsy (SLNB) if necessary.[2,3] Elliptical, disk, or punch excisions are often employed. A partial shave biopsy should generally be avoided and only used when the suspicion for melanoma is low, as tangential removal may result in transection of the tumor and complicate determination of the true Breslow depth.

An incisional biopsy is best reserved for cosmetically sensitive or anatomically difficult locations (palm/sole, digit, face, or ear), and is also appropriate in cases of exceptionally large lesions, a low clinical suspicion for melanoma, or diagnostic uncertainty. An incisional biopsy should encompass the full thickness of the skin to the level of the adipose tissue and should be taken from the darkest or most elevated portion of the lesion. Partly due to the difficulty in clinically predicting the thickest portion of the lesion, an incisional biopsy is less likely to guarantee accurate representation of the lesion's Breslow depth and a repeat biopsy may be required.[4] If the incisional biopsy indicates a cutaneous melanoma <1 mm thick and a clinically apparent lesion remains, a narrow margin excisional biopsy should follow. This subsequent narrow excisional biopsy allows microstaging if the patient requires SLNB, as well as histologic evaluation for upstaging, which could result in a change in treatment plan.[2] In one study of lesions with $\geq 50\%$ residual tumor postincisional biopsy, about one-fifth were upstaged and one-tenth required SLNB.[5] There is no evidence that incisional biopsy of a primary melanoma can "seed" tissue and negatively impact survival.[2] Regardless of the biopsy approach, after the histologic confirmation of a cutaneous melanoma, a wider and deeper excision is usually warranted. Melanoma cells can extend several millimeters to centimeters beyond the clinically detectable lesion.[4]

A HISTORICAL PERSPECTIVE ON SURGICAL MANAGEMENT OF MELANOMA

Despite research efforts toward nonsurgical management of primary melanomas, surgery continues to be the standard for primary lesions. Until the 1970s, surgical dogma opted for an aggressive approach with wide surgical margins extending 5 cm beyond the primary lesion.[6] Despite this historical, rather than evidence-based approach, an increasing incidence of melanoma established the need for better-defined surgical guidelines, early diagnosis, and identification of prognostic factors. Subsequent clinical trials led to the evolution of a more tailored approach linked to prognostic factors and risk of recurrence.[6] The identification of tumor thickness as a prognostic factor greatly influenced the evolution of narrower excision margins. Studies in the 1980s suggested that narrower excision margins were acceptable in many cases, particularly for thin melanomas, and did not adversely affect survival. Studies also indicated that narrow margins used in the treatment of thicker tumors often led to increases in local recurrence rates. Data from retrospective studies in the 1980s and 1990s continued to weigh the influence of narrow margins versus primary tumor characteristics on outcome. Ultimately, researchers determined that local recurrence is both a function of biologic factors and the extent of excision.[6] A paradigm emerged that dictated that wider margins were necessary for higher risk or thicker lesions.[6] These conclusions led to the conduction of various prospective randomized trials to establish more definitive guidelines for treatment.

Current surgical margin recommendations are based largely on conclusions from randomized controlled trials and consensus opinion. An algorithm to guide the management of cutaneous melanoma is available in Figure 28-1.[2]

BASIC CONCEPTS FOR EXCISION OF PRIMARY MELANOMA

The goals of excision for a primary cutaneous melanoma are to achieve negative margins on histology and prevent recurrence caused by residual disease. Wide excision is the standard of surgical therapy for primary cutaneous melanoma.[4] This practice is based on early findings that a wider excision is associated with a reduced risk of local recurrence due to disease persistence despite histopathologically confirmed tumor-free margins.[2,4] Outcomes of wide and narrow excision in the treatment of melanoma continue to be assessed.

To determine appropriate surgical margins for tumors less than 2 mm thick, the French Cooperative Group, the World Health Organization, and the Swedish Melanoma Study Group conducted various trials in the late twentieth and early twenty-first century. These trials varied in regard to sample size, margin width, and tumor thickness cutoff for patient inclusion, yet they ultimately reported similar conclusions.[6] Collectively, they demonstrated that in tumors less than 2 mm thick, wider margins did not significantly impact local and regional recurrence or long-term survival compared to narrow (1 cm) margins.

EXCISION MARGINS FOR TUMORS LESS THAN OR EQUAL TO 1.0 MM

Limited data exist on excision of primary invasive melanoma ≤1.0 mm in thickness. Wide excision with a 1 cm margin to the level of the fascia is recommended based on the WHO randomized trial.[4,6] The WHO trial studied 612 melanoma patients with tumors ≤2.0 mm (305 patients with 1 cm margin vs. 307 with ≥3 cm margins). This trial ultimately concluded that thin melanomas (≤1.0 mm thick) could be safely excised with a 1 cm margin (vs. a 3 cm margin). The use of a 1 cm margin in these tumors provides a good cosmetic outcome and functionality without adversely impacting therapeutic efficacy. In melanomas thicker than 1.0 mm, the WHO trial demonstrated a trend toward increased incidence of local recurrence in the narrow excision group. This trend was not statistically significant due to the small number of observed events.[7,8] As a result, the WHO trial did not reach a definitive conclusion for melanomas thicker than 1.0 mm.

EXCISION MARGINS FOR TUMORS 1 TO 2 MM IN THICKNESS

The margin recommendations for melanomas 1 to 2 mm in thickness are implemented based on conclusions from the WHO Melanoma Program and the Intergroup Melanoma Surgical Trial (IMST).[9] The IMST was initiated as a randomized controlled trial in the early 1980s to assess the margin approach to patients with intermediate-thickness melanomas (1–4 mm).[6,9–11] The study randomized 740 patients with melanomas 1 to 4 mm thickness into (a) 486 patients with melanomas on the trunk or proximal extremity to compare outcomes of 2 versus 4 cm margins and (b) 272 patients with melanomas on the head, neck, or distal extremity who underwent a 2 cm excision. Overall, 28 patients (3.8%) experienced a local recurrence associated with a high mortality rate, with a 5 year survival rate of 9% (first relapse) or 11% (any time) versus 86% survival for patients who did not experience a local recurrence ($p < 0.0001$). Comparing 2 versus 4 cm margin outcomes, no significant difference in 10 year survival (70% vs. 77%, respectively), incidence of local recurrence, or risk of in-transit disease was observed between treatment arms. This report indicated that survival of intermediate-thickness tumors (1–4 mm) was not influenced by the extent of excision (2 vs. 4 cm).[11] A 2 cm margin of excision was concluded to be safe for tumors 1 to 4 mm in thickness.

Guidelines for 1 to 2 mm thickness tumors have been established by findings of the IMST and WHO trials in this subset of melanomas. As noted earlier, the WHO trial detected a trend toward an increased incidence of local recurrence in the narrow excision group (1 vs. 3 cm margin). However, the IMST reported a lower incidence of local recurrence in 1.0 to 2.0 mm thickness lesions compared to the WHO trial (0.6% vs. 4.5%) and no advantage in local control or survival with a 4 versus 2 cm margin.

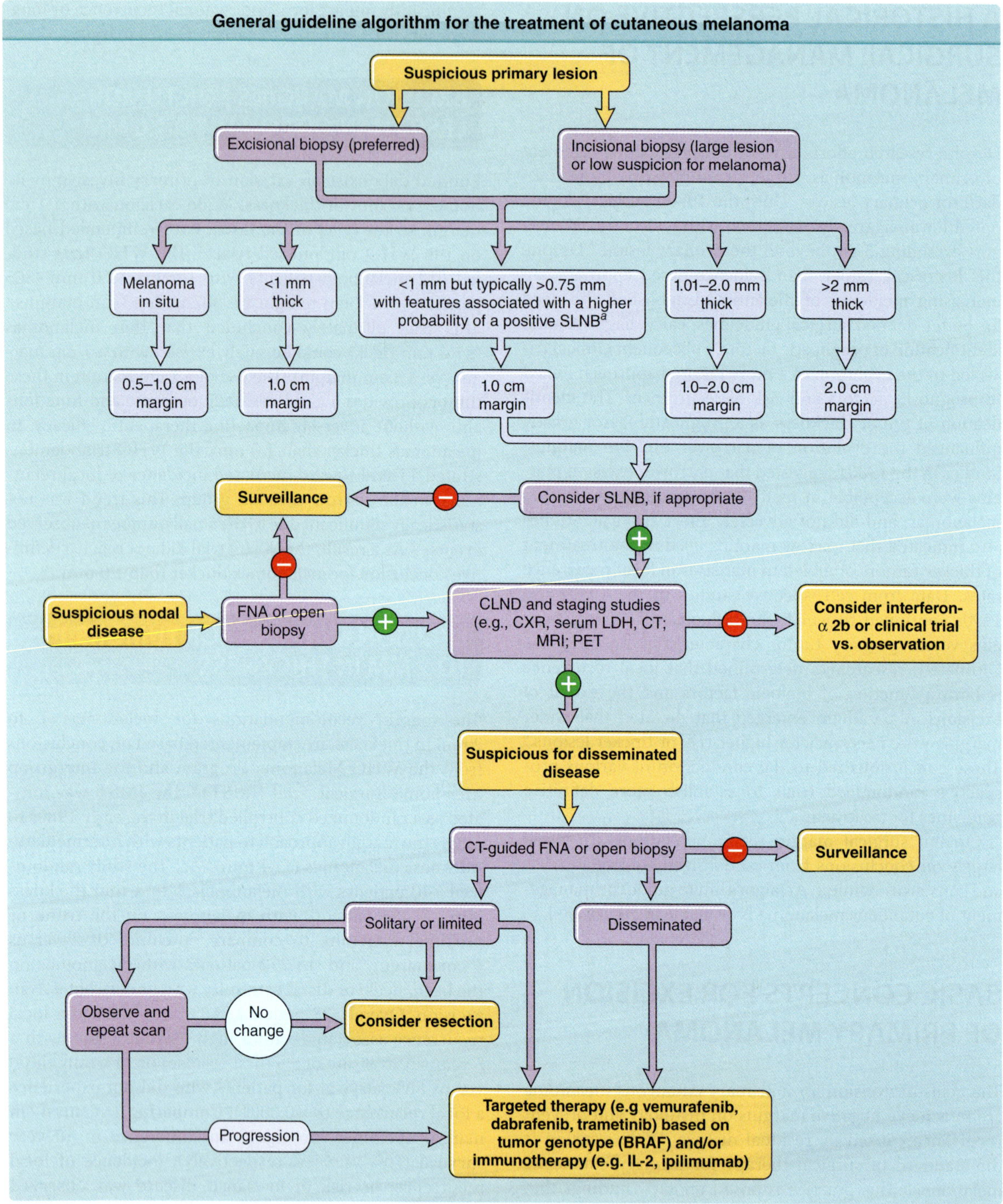

Figure 28-1 General guideline algorithm for the treatment of cutaneous melanoma. [a]Ulceration, extensive vertical regression to at least 1 mm thick, young patient age, high mitotic rate, especially in younger persons, shave biopsy with positive deep margin, presence of angiolymphatic invasion, and Clark level IV. CLND, completion lymph-node dissection; CNS, central nervous system; CT, computed tomography; CXR, chest X-ray; FNA, fine-needle aspiration; LDH, serum lactate dehydrogenase; MRI, magnetic resonance imaging; PET, positron emission tomography; and SLNB, sentinel lymph node biopsy. A minus sign indicates no evidence of disease, and a plus sign evidence of metastasis. Patients who are candidates for SLNB should be referred to a surgeon experienced in performing the procedure so that the benefits and complications can be fully discussed. (Reproduced with permission from Goldsmith LA, Katz SI, Gilchrest BA, Paller AS, Leffell DJ, Wolff K. *Fitzpatrick's Dermatology in General Medicine.* 8th ed. New York, NY: McGraw-Hill, Inc; 2012. Fig. 124-18. Copyright © McGraw-Hill Education LLC.)

Of note, the IMST detected a trend toward 10 year disease-specific survival seen in the wider margin group.[11] Regardless, consensus opinion agrees that according to these findings, in tumors 1 to 2 mm thick, if 2 cm margins are comparable to 4 cm margins, no additional advantage would be gained with a 3 cm margin.[6]

Many experts recommend a 2 cm margin as the standard of care for tumors 1 to 2 mm in thickness whenever anatomically feasible. No study to date has directly compared 1 with 2 cm surgical margins in these lesions.[6] Historically, the use of a 1 cm margin for 2 mm thick lesions has been met with resistance by some surgeons and dermatologists. The overall survival data from prospective clinical trials demonstrate no apparent benefit for a wider excision.[6] Following this guideline, a margin ranging from 1 to 2 cm may be adjusted for functional or cosmetic reasons for lesions up to 2 mm thick.

EXCISION MARGINS FOR TUMORS 2 TO 4 MM IN THICKNESS

For thick primary melanomas, 2 to 4 mm thick, most studies have failed to show a benefit of surgical margins greater than 2 cm.[4] The United Kingdom Melanoma Study Group (UKMSG) Trial randomly assigned 900 patients with melanomas 2.0 mm or thicker to two groups with excision margins of 1 and 3 cm. The study showed no significant difference in the rate of local recurrence or in overall survival between the groups, although the group with 1 cm margins had more combined locoregional recurrences. This finding provides evidence against use of a 1 cm margin for lesions of 2 to 4 mm thickness, and does not support a benefit of 3 versus 2 cm margins. In addition, the IMST data determined that a 4 cm margin is not superior to a 2 cm margin and ultimately established the adequacy of a 2 cm margin for 2 to 4 mm thick lesions. Summarizing the conclusions from both trials for tumors 2 to 4 mm thickness, if a 4 cm margin is not superior to a 2 cm margin, it follows that a 3 cm margin would not confer superiority. To date, no survival differences have been demonstrated with greater than 2 cm margins for thick tumors. This holds true for tumors thicker than 4 mm as well. A recent retrospective series of 632 patients with tumors greater than 4 mm showed that patients with histopathologic margins 16 mm or less had worse local disease-free survival (HR, 2.41; p = 0.01) than those with histopathologically determined primary tumor excision margins greater than 16 mm (i.e., corresponding to a 2 cm surgical margin), suggesting that a 2 cm surgical margin is both necessary and likely sufficient for local control of thick melanomas.[12] As a result, current recommendations hold that primary melanomas greater than 2 mm in thickness should undergo a wide excision with 2 cm margins. Of note, the large clinical trials to date have demonstrated a trend toward survival favoring wide excisions. Due to lack of power in trial design, these trends have not demonstrated significance. In the future, larger clinical trials are required to address the evolving hypothesis of equivalence between wide and narrow excision rather than the traditional hypothesis of the inferiority of the latter.

SUMMARY OF CURRENT RECOMMENDATIONS

Evidence for thin melanomas (≤1.0 mm) does not suggest that margins greater than 1 cm offer an improvement in survival or local recurrence rate. Accordingly, the current recommendation for stage IA melanoma (≤1.0 mm thickness) is wide excision with a 1.0 cm margin.

For thicker melanomas, the current recommendation for a surgical margin for invasive melanoma is at least 1 cm to no more than 2 cm around the primary tumor. Several large randomized controlled trials have failed to demonstrate a difference in survival rates or local recurrence between narrow (1–2 cm) versus wide (3–5 cm) margins.[2,7,11–17] Overall, greater than 2 cm margins for a primary melanoma of any thickness have not been shown to improve overall survival or local recurrence.[4] For 1.01 to 2.0 mm in thickness, wide excision with a 1.0 to 2.0 cm margin as large as anatomically possible is recommended. For melanomas greater than 2.0 mm in thickness, wide excision with 2.0 cm margins is recommended. Despite well-defined recommendations, the surgical approach must be decided on an individual basis. Margins may be modified according to anatomic or cosmetic considerations, and a 1 to 2 cm margin may be acceptable in certain circumstances where a 2 cm margin is difficult to achieve anatomically. Nonetheless, reconstruction concerns are secondary to achieving tumor clearance. Traditionally, the recommended depth of a therapeutic excision extends to muscle fascia when possible.[4] Many experts believe that in regions with a thicker adipose layer, extension to deep adipose tissue is adequate.

MELANOMA IN SITU

The appropriate excision margin for melanoma in situ remains an area of controversy. Clinical trials on this topic are lacking. As a result, margin recommendations for melanoma in situ are based on consensus of available experience. The current consensus is to perform a wide excision with a 0.5 to 1.0 cm margin for melanoma in situ, nonlentigo maligna subtype.[4] With these margins, most in situ melanomas are completely and easily excised and repaired with a primary closure.

Recently, the adequacy of a 0.5 cm margin for excision of melanoma in situ has been challenged. A prospective study of 1072 patients with 1120 melanomas in situ compared excision by Mohs micrographic surgery using 6 versus 9 mm margins and determined a clearance rate of 86% and 98.9% respectively (p < 0.001).[18] Investigators ultimately recommended 9 mm margins for standard excision of melanoma in situ and deemed 5 mm margins to be inadequate.

Careful consideration of the primary lesion's defining characteristics must be taken into account. For example, the melanoma in situ, lentigo maligna subtype, warrants concern for large subclinical extension of atypical junctional melanocytic hyperplasia.[3] In this subtype, histologically positive margins may be encountered, necessitating sequential excisions to clear the margins histopathologically.[6] Larger lesions on the head and neck may also require wider than 0.5 cm margins. Examination by Wood's lamp may be of benefit in identifying subclinical disease.[3]

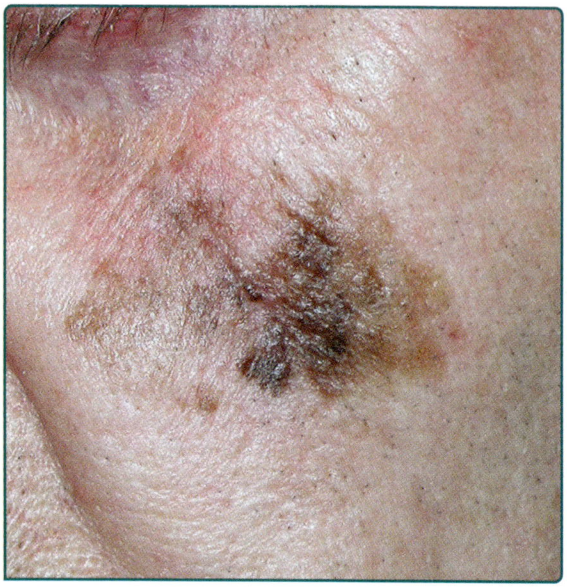

Figure 28-2 Lentigo maligna and lentigo maligna melanoma (LMM). Lentigo maligna (in situ) displays prominent asymmetry, poorly defined irregular borders, and pigment variegation. (Reproduced with permission from Goldsmith LA, Katz SI, Gilchrest BA, Paller AS, Leffell DJ, Wolff K. *Fitzpatrick's Dermatology in General Medicine*. 8th ed. New York, NY: McGraw-Hill, Inc.; 2012. Fig 124-4A. Copyright © McGraw-Hill Education LLC.)

Lentigo maligna melanoma (LMM) in situ and invasive LMM can be particularly difficult to manage because of their predilection for the face and scalp and their tendency to exhibit extensive clinical and microscopic extension (Fig. 28-2). Performing a complicated flap on such lesions, only to later discover that the margins are positive, is not ideal for the surgeon or the patient. As a result, accurate delineation of the clinical and histologic margins to the greatest degree possible is essential prior to closure.

LOCAL RECURRENCE

The risk of local recurrence has important implications for follow-up surveillance. If detected, treatment is required, and the nature of that treatment depends on the nature of the recurrence. Local recurrence may occur as a result of persistence of the primary lesion due to inadequate primary excision, or from underlying dermal lymphatic disease near the excision scar despite apparently adequate primary excision. Re-excision of a persistent primary lesion portends a better prognosis and should be performed according to the Breslow depth of the tumor.

The prognosis of a recurrence due to dermal lymphatic disease is akin to that of recurrent regional disease. Baseline imaging is utilized for further evaluation and staging. Lymphatic mapping and sentinel node biopsy may be performed if dermal lymphatic disease is suspected, and should be considered on an individual basis since the anatomy may have been altered by prior surgery. After excision of the recurrence, observation or adjuvant treatments, such as interferon-alpha or other agents administered through clinical trials, may be employed.[3]

IN-TRANSIT METASTASIS

A variety of treatment approaches are available for patients with Stage III, or in-transit metastasis. When possible, regional in-transit or satellite disease should be surgically excised with histologically confirmed clear margins, particularly in patients with one or a small number of in-transit metastases. Of note, in-transit metastases confer TNM staging status of N2c in the absence of metastatic lymph nodes and confer TNM staging status of N3 when present in conjunction with metastatic lymph nodes.[19]

Nonsurgical options tend to be considered for a greater number of in-transit metastases or multiple dermal lesions. Isolated limb perfusion (ILP) can be considered for control of this type of disease when it is limited to an extremity. ILP allows chemotherapy to be delivered in high doses to the limb, reducing systemic toxicity.[2] Melphalan is the typical chemotherapeutic agent used in ILP under hyperthermic conditions in patients with a risk of substantial morbidity; the goal is to achieve locoregional disease control rather than to improve overall survival.[2] For patients ineligible for ILP, a newer, less invasive, and simpler alternative with demonstrated efficacy is isolated limb infusion (ILI) with melphalan and actinomycin D.[2,20]

REGIONAL NODAL RECURRENCE

Regional nodal recurrence should be confirmed with FNA biopsy. The diagnostic workup involves FNA biopsy (preferred) or lymph node biopsy, chest radiograph and/or CT, LDH, and pelvic CT if inguinofemoral nodes are clinically positive. Abdominal/pelvic CT, MRI of the brain, and PET scan may be indicated depending on clinical presentation.[3] Patients who have not yet undergone prior lymph node dissection should undergo a complete lymph node dissection. If a complete lymph node dissection has already been performed, excision of the recurrence to achieve clear margins is appropriate. In patients with completely resected nodal recurrence and additional risk factors, the risk of further regional nodal recurrences may be decreased by postoperative adjuvant radiotherapy. Patients with distant recurrence are treated similarly to patients with stage IV metastasis.[3]

FOLLOW-UP

Follow-up depends on a patient's individual risk factors, including recurrence risk, family history, and previous primary melanoma. Patient disposition, skin type, dysplastic nevi, and history of other skin cancers also have an impact on the recommended follow-up regimen. Most recurrences are detected within the first 5 years after treatment of the primary melanoma. Nonetheless, recurrence greater than 10 years following the initial treatment is not uncommon.

The lifetime risk for developing a second primary melanoma is 4% to 8%.[3] According to expert opinion, lifetime dermatologic surveillance for melanoma patients is recommended and justified.[3] Closer surveillance may be preferable for patients at risk of regional recurrence who have not undergone sentinel node biopsy or for those with a positive lymph node who have not undergone a complete lymphadenectomy. Skin examination and surveillance at least once a year is recommended for all patients with melanoma, including those with in situ melanoma. Patients with stage IA melanoma should be evaluated every 3 to 12 months for 5 years and annually thereafter as indicated. Patients with stage IB to stage IV melanomas and no further evidence of disease should undergo follow-up every 3 to 6 months for 2 years, every 3 to 12 months for 3 years, and annually thereafter.[3] For patients with low and even intermediate risk tumors, routine radiographic and blood tests are considered low yield and generally not recommended. If a careful review of systems reveals a localizing symptom or sign, targeted evaluation with CTs or MRIs may be warranted. In patients with high-risk disease (e.g., greater than stage IIC), medical oncology follow-up is usually indicated.[3,4]

SPECIAL MELANOCYTIC LESIONS

Aside from common melanoma pathologic categories, atypical melanocytic lesions are not infrequently encountered. They may represent a diagnostic and management dilemma as these lesions may demonstrate a natural history that is different from typical melanoma lesions. Whenever pathologic uncertainty exists, conservative management according to the pathologic impression with the worst prognosis is the rule.

Desmoplastic melanoma is one atypical melanoma variant that displays some special characteristics. These lesions have a different natural history relative to other melanomas of the same Breslow thickness. They are more common in males and often are initially interpreted as benign at first biopsy. These lesions also clinically do not exhibit classic features of melanoma such as asymmetry, border irregularity, and color variation. Clinical and pathologic difficulty in recognition of desmoplastic melanoma may account for the increased thickness of these lesions at the time of diagnosis. Despite the frequently observed higher thickness of these lesions, they do not have as high a rate of regional lymph node metastasis at initial presentation as do typical melanomas of similar thickness. These lesions do, however, have a higher rate of local recurrence, particularly lesions that demonstrate perineural invasion.[21] Such neurotropism is more frequently observed in lesions of the head and neck. Lesions demonstrating neurotropism may benefit from adjuvant radiation therapy.

Once the clinically apparent lesion has been excised, frozen section processing does not accurately examine the margin of these lesions, as there may be a lack of melanocyte cytoplasmic vacuolization as well as other tissue fixation artifacts. In addition, these lesions frequently occur on a background of severely photodamaged skin that may contain baseline atypical melanocytes, making border delineation more difficult. To ensure complete removal, reconstruction can be delayed until formal pathologic evaluation can be completed utilizing paraffin embedded tissue, often with special stains such as immunohistochemistry. Studies using rush permanent slides[22,23] and immunohistochemistry[24] have demonstrated very low recurrence rates (0%–1.2%) and this practice is preferable to frozen sections for melanocytic lesions. Although this may result in a slower staged excision, it may save an unnecessary re-excision of inadequately excised tumor. During this waiting period, the patient can be covered with a temporary hydrocolloid dressing. Pharmacologic management of lentigo maligna with topical imiquimod has also been utilized in elderly patients and in poor surgical candidates. This is currently controversial with variable response rates in published studies and should be approached with caution.

SPECIAL BODY SITES

Although the guidelines for the excision of primary melanoma of varying thickness are usually fairly straightforward on body sites such as the trunk, adequate excision with acceptable cosmetic impact may be less easily achieved on other body sites, including the head, perineum, and acral sites. These areas require special considerations and necessitate particular techniques.

As discussed earlier, melanomas of the face may be difficult to manage as they may be near, or involve, vital structures. The cosmetic implications of lesions involving the eyes, nose, ears, and mouth require extensive planning and a specialized reconstructive effort. Standard excisional removal of such lesions to achieve an optimal aesthetic result may result in less than ideal margins and adjuvant radiotherapy may be indicated in such cases. Mohs micrographic surgery can be a useful technique for lentigo maligna on the face when combined with rush permanent sections or immunohistochemistry. The delicate ear area can be managed with wedge excision for smaller lesions with excellent cosmetic results (Fig. 28-3). More extensive lesions may necessitate partial or full amputation (Fig. 28-4).

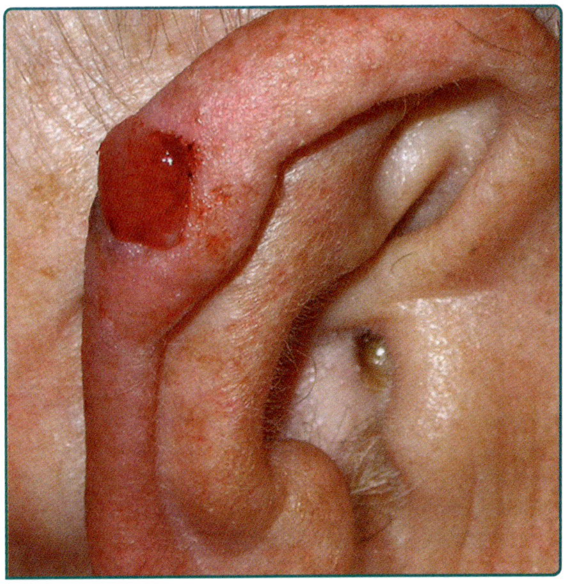

Figure 28-3 Nodular melanoma (NM). Amelanotic NM, Breslow depth 2.37 mm, 32 mitoses/mm^2, vertical growth phase, ulceration present. (Reproduced with permission from Goldsmith LA, Katz SI, Gilchrest BA, Paller AS, Leffell DJ, Wolff K. *Fitzpatrick's Dermatology in General Medicine.* 8th ed. New York, NY: McGraw-Hill, Inc.; 2012. Fig 124-3C. Copyright © McGraw-Hill Education LLC.)

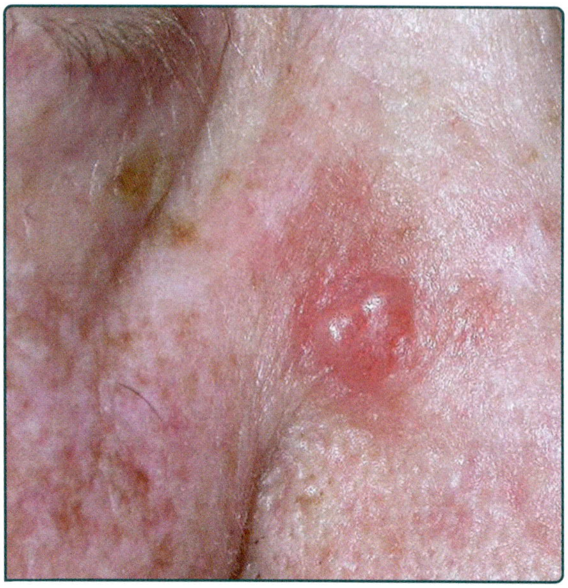

Figure 28-4 Lentigo maligna and lentigo maligna melanoma (LMM). Amelanotic LMM with nodular component initially suspected to be a basal cell carcinoma, nose, Breslow depth 2.2 mm, 5 mitoses/mm^2, ulceration present. (Reproduced with permission from Goldsmith LA, Katz SI, Gilchrest BA, Paller AS, Leffell DJ, Wolff K. *Fitzpatrick's Dermatology in General Medicine*. 8th ed. New York, NY: McGraw-Hill, Inc.; 2012. Fig 124-4C. Copyright © McGraw-Hill Education LLC.)

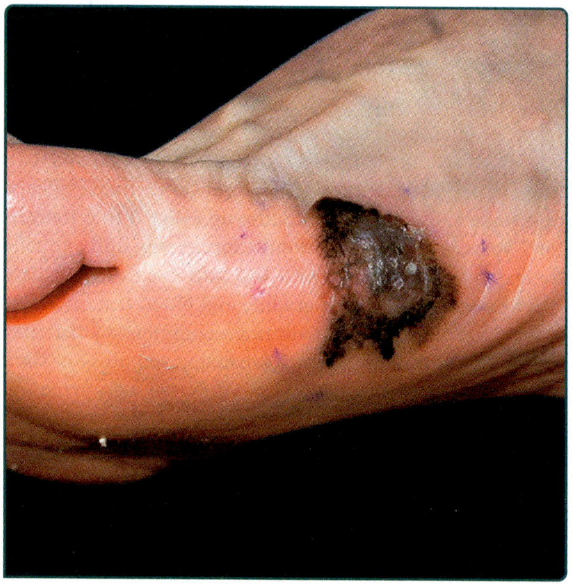

Figure 28-6 Acral lentiginous melanoma (ALM). Classic ALM demonstrating asymmetry, border, color, diameter/difference, elevation/evolving (ABCDs), left foot, Breslow depth 1.72 mm, ulceration present. (Reproduced with permission from Goldsmith LA, Katz SI, Gilchrest BA, Paller AS, Leffell DJ, Wolff K. *Fitzpatrick's Dermatology in General Medicine*. 8th ed. New York, NY: McGraw-Hill, Inc.; 2012. Fig 124-5A. Copyright © McGraw-Hill Education LLC.)

Acral sites present a particular challenge because of their geometry and functional implications. When the distal digits are affected by melanoma, adequate margins can be often achieved by amputation. While this is frequently performed on the toes, amputation of fingers (especially the thumb) carries a more significant functional deficit. Melanomas of the distal thumb may be treated with amputation proximal to the distal interphalangeal joint to maintain function if possible (Fig. 28-5). Adequate soft-tissue excision is usually achievable in proximal areas of the fingers.

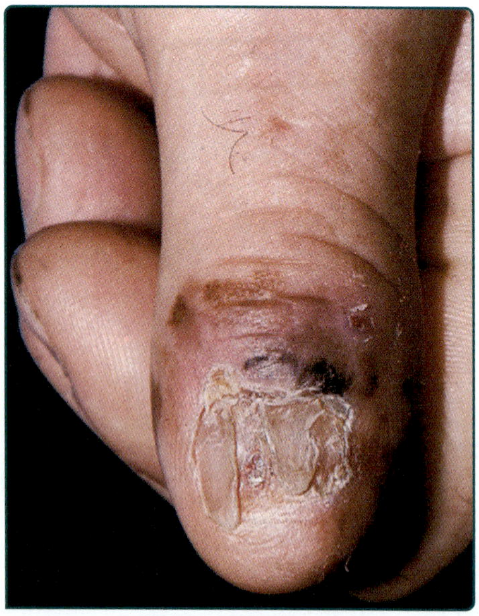

Figure 28-5 Subungual acral lentiginous melanoma (ALM). Extensive involvement of periungual skin (Hutchinson's sign) with dystrophy and loss of the nail plate secondary to the tumor. (Reproduced with permission from Goldsmith LA, Katz SI, Gilchrest BA, Paller AS, Leffell DJ, Wolff K. *Fitzpatrick's Dermatology in General Medicine*. 8th ed. New York, NY: McGraw-Hill, Inc.; 2012. Fig 124-6A. Copyright © McGraw-Hill Education LLC.)

Melanomas of the foot may present different types of dilemmas based on whether they involve weight-bearing or non–weight-bearing areas (Fig. 28-6). Non–weight-bearing sites are usually adequately closed with a split-thickness graft. However, weight-bearing areas may require full-thickness skin grafting in order to maintain viability and function of tissue.

SENTINEL LYMPH NODE BIOPSY (SLNB)

A full discussion of the utility and practice of lymphoscintography/selective lymphadenectomy (i.e., SLNB) is beyond the scope of this chapter. Furthermore, in the United States, the procedure is most commonly performed by nondermatologic surgeons. Therefore, only the rudiments of this procedure will be discussed in this chapter.

In addition to the body site involved, a common management consideration is whether to perform a SLNB. SLNB is a valuable prognostic tool and the presence of melanoma in the lymph nodes draining the primary tumor site is the strongest predictor of overall survival and risk of recurrence.[25,26] Despite the prognostic value of SLNB, removal of the regional lymph nodes among which

TABLE 28-1
Recommendations for Sentinel Lymph Node Biopsy[19,46]

Guideline	Sentinel Lymph Node Biopsy Not Recommended	Sentinel Lymph Node Biopsy Should be Considered	Sentinel Lymph Node Biopsy Should Be Discussed and Offered
2011 AAD	Stage 0 Stage IA Stage IB (≤0.75 mm unless angiolymphatic invasion, + deep margin, young age)	Stage IB (0.76–1 mm)	>1 mm Breslow depth
NCCN Guideline version 1.2013 to 4.2014	Stage IA with adverse features (lymphovascular invasion, ulceration, >0.75mm, mitosis >1/mm^2)	Stage IA with adverse features (lymphovascular invasion, >0.75 mm, young age)	Stage IB Stage II Stage III (with resectable solitary in transit disease)
2012 ASCC/SSO	<1 mm (without ulceration or mitosis)	<1 mm (with ulceration, mitosis >1/mm^2, 0.75–0.99 mm)	1–4 mm >4 mm (may recommend for staging and local disease control)

a positive node has been found has not been shown to improve outcomes in patients with melanoma.

Prior to development of the SLNB technique, elective lymph node dissection was commonly performed in the anatomic site predicted to be most likely to drain a particular lesion. This practice often resulted in significant morbidity and did not offer any survival benefit. SLNB was developed in 1990 using radio-labeled colloid, which could be injected at the tumor site.[27] The advantage of this technique is its ability to identify the afferent lymph node that would be predicted to first receive lymphatic drainage from the tumor site. This concept presumes orderly spread from the primary site to an afferent lymph node and does not account for hematogenous spread. When performed by an experienced team, SLNB offers greater than 95% probability of identification of the sentinel lymph node.[28,29]

When identified, melanoma in a sentinel node is a strong predictor for poor outcome.[30,31] In fact, a recent study examining disease confined to sentinel lymph nodes versus extension to nonsentinel lymph nodes prognosticated better outcomes in patients with sentinel lymph node involvement only.[32] Despite this prognostic value, removal of positive sentinel lymph nodes and their associated basin does not appear to carry overall survival benefit compared to patients undergoing wide local excision alone.[33–35] Generally, patients with clinically negative nodes and primary melanomas with Breslow thickness greater than 1 mm are routinely offered SLNB. This reasoning derives from observed risk of sentinel lymph node metastases based on Breslow depth.

As a result of the low positivity rate in primary melanomas of less than 1 mm, SLNB is not routinely recommended for thin lesions.[36] Among thin melanomas, primary tumors of Breslow thickness less than or equal to 1 mm have a less than 5% nodal metastasis rate, and those less than 0.76 mm have a less than 2% nodal metastasis rate.[36–41] However, there are certain subgroups among these thin melanomas that may be at higher than expected risk based on factors other than the Breslow thickness. For example, tumors with a mitotic rate greater than zero have been associated with higher sentinel lymph node positivity rates (8.7% for ≤1 mm and 12.3% ≥ 0.76 mm).[39] For this special subgroup of thin melanomas, SLNB may be more seriously considered. In addition, lymphovascular invasion has also been implicated with a greater likelihood of sentinel lymph node positivity.[42] The utility of SLNB is a matter of debate in thick (≥ 4 mm) melanomas as well. Some believe that the high risk of occult disease at the time of presentation makes SLNB less useful because of an overall poor prognosis.[43] Others assert the utility of SLNB even in thick melanoma, citing statistically significant differences in 5 year overall survival rates in positive versus negative SLNB of melanomas greater than 4 mm.[44]

The 2010 AJCC guidelines recommend SLNB for greater than 4 mm melanomas without radiographic evidence of regional lymph node involvement. These guidelines recommend SLNB for patients with melanomas less than or equal to 1 mm if ulcerated or with one or more mitoses per millimeter squared.[45] A summary of the guidelines for SLNB recommendations can be found in Table 28-1.

In summary, melanoma is an increasingly common tumor that is usually best managed surgically. Wide local excision is the preferred initial management for primary tumors and is dictated by depth of invasion. Special body sites and tumor types may require modification of standard techniques, and Mohs micrographic surgery can be a useful technique for lentigo maligna when combined with rush permanent sections or immunohistochemistry to enhance the delineation of peripheral tumor margins. Although SLNB is useful for staging and prognosis, it confers no therapeutic survival benefit and should be offered only when clinically appropriate.

REFERENCES

1. Siegel R, Naishadham D, Jemal A. Cancer statistics. *CA Cancer J Clin.* 2012;62(1):10–29.
2. Bailey EC, Sober AJ, Tsao H, Mihm MC Jr, Johnson TM. Cutaneous melanoma. In: Goldsmith LA, Katz SI, Gilchrest BA, Paller AS, Leffell DJ, Dallas NA, eds. *Fitzpatrick's Dermatology in General Medicine.* 8th ed. New York, NY: McGraw-Hill; 2008.

3. Coit DG, Andtbacka R, Anker CJ, et al. Melanoma. *J Natl Compr Canc Netw*. 2012;10(3):366–400.
4. Bichakjian CK, Halpern AC, Johnson TM, et al. Guidelines of care for the management of primary cutaneous melanoma. American academy of dermatology. *J Am Acad Dermatol*. 2011;65(5):1032–1047.
5. Karimipour DJ, Schwartz JL, Wang TS, et al. Microstaging accuracy after subtotal incisional biopsy of cutaneous melanoma. *J Am Acad Dermatol*. 2005;52(5):798–802.
6. Ross MI. Excision of primary melanoma. In: Balch CM, Houghton AN, Sober AJ, Soong SJ, eds. *Cutaneous Melanoma*. 5th ed. St. Louis, MO: Quality Medical Publishing; 2009:251.
7. Veronesi U, Cascinelli N. Narrow excision (1-cm margin). A safe procedure for thin cutaneous melanoma. *Arch Surg*. 1991; 126(4):438–441.
8. Veronesi U, Cascinelli N, Adamus J, et al. Thin stage I primary cutaneous malignant melanoma. Comparison of excision with margins of 1 or 3 cm. *N Engl J Med. 1988*;318(18):1159–1162.
9. Balch CM, Urist MM, Karakousis CP, et al. Efficacy of 2-cm surgical margins for intermediate-thickness melanomas (1 to 4 mm). Results of a multi-institutional randomized surgical trial. *Ann Surg*. 1993;218(3):262–267; discussion 267–269.
10. Karakousis CP, Balch CM, Urist MM, Ross MM, Smith TJ, Bartolucci AA. Local recurrence in malignant melanoma: long-term results of the multiinstitutional randomized surgical trial. *Ann Surg Oncol*. 1996;3(5):446–452.
11. Balch CM, Soong SJ, Smith T, et al. Long-term results of a prospective surgical trial comparing 2 cm vs. 4 cm excision margins for 740 patients with 1–4 mm melanomas. *Ann Surg Oncol*. 2001;8(2):101–108.
12. Pasquali S, Haydu LE, Scolyer RA, et al. The importance of adequate primary tumor excision margins and sentinel node biopsy in achieving optimal locoregional control for patients with thick primary melanomas. *Ann Surg*. 2013;258(1):152–157.
13. Thomas JM, Newton-Bishop J, A'Hern R, et al. Excision margins in high-risk malignant melanoma. *N Engl J Med*. 2004;350(8):757–766.
14. Krown SE, Chapman PB. Defining adequate surgery for primary melanoma. *N Engl J Med*. 2004;350(8):823–825.
15. Khayat D, Rixe O, Martin G, et al. Surgical margins in cutaneous melanoma (2 cm versus 5 cm for lesions measuring less than 2.1-mm thick). *Cancer*. 2003;97(8):1941–1946.
16. Cohn-Cedermark G, Rutqvist LE, Andersson R, et al. Long term results of a randomized study by the Swedish melanoma study group on 2-cm versus 5-cm resection margins for patients with cutaneous melanoma with a tumor thickness of 0.8–2.0 mm. *Cancer*. 2000;89(7):1495–1501.
17. Johnson TM, Sondak VK. Melanoma margins: the importance and need for more evidence-based trials. *Arch Dermatol*. 2004;140(9):1148–1150.
18. Kunishige JH, Brodland DG, Zitelli JA. Surgical margins for melanoma in situ. *J Am Acad Dermatol*. 2012;66(3):438–444.
19. National Comprehensive Cancer Network. NCCN clinical practice guidelines in oncology (NCCN guidelines): melanoma; Version v4.2014.
20. Thompson JF, Kam PC. Isolated limb infusion for melanoma: a simple but effective alternative to isolated limb perfusion. *J Surg Oncol*. 2004;88(1):1–3.
21. Quinn MJ, Crotty KA, Thompson JF, Coates AS, O'Brien CJ, McCarthy WH. Desmoplastic and desmoplastic neurotropic melanoma: experience with 280 patients. *Cancer*. 1998;83(6): 1128–1135.
22. Cohen LM, MCall MW, Zax RH. Mohs micrograhic surgery for lentigo maligna and lentigo maligna melanoma. A follow-up study. *Dermatol Surg*. 1998;24:673–677.
23. Clayton BD, Leshin B, Hitchcock MG, Marks M, White WL. Utility of rush paraffin-embedded tangential sections in the management of cutaneous neoplasms. *Dermatol Surg*. 2000;26:671–678.
24. Bhardwaj SS, Tope WD, Lee PK. Mohs micrographic surgery for lentigo maligna and lentigo maligna melanoma using Mel-5 immunostaining: University of Minnesota experience. *Dermatol Surg*. 2006;32:690–696.
25. Garrison M, Nathanson L. Prognosis and staging in melanoma. *Semin Oncol*. 1996;23(6):725–733.
26. Slingluff CL Jr, Stidham KR, Ricci WM, Stanley WE, Seigler HF. Surgical management of regional lymph nodes in patients with melanoma. Experience with 4682 patients. *Ann Surg*. 1994; 219(2):120–123.
27. Morton DL, Wen DR, Wong JH, et al. Technical details of intraoperative lymphatic mapping for early stage melanoma. *Arch Surg*. 1992;127(4):392–399.
28. Morton DL, Cochran AJ, Thompson JF, et al. Sentinel node biopsy for early-stage melanoma: accuracy and morbidity in MSLT-I, an international multicenter trial. *Ann Surg*. 2005;242(3):302–311; discussion 311–313.
29. Stebbins WG, Garibyan L, Sober AJ. Sentinel lymph node biopsy and melanoma: 2010 update part I. *J Am Acad Dermatol*. 2010;62(5):723–734; quiz 735–736.
30. Balch CM, Buzaid AC, Soong SJ, et al. Final version of the American Joint Committee on Cancer staging system for cutaneous melanoma. *J Clin Oncol*. 2001;19(16):3635–3648.
31. Balch CM, Soong SJ, Gershenwald JE, et al. Prognostic factors analysis of 17600 melanoma patients: validation of the American Joint Committee on Cancer melanoma staging system. *J Clin Oncol*. 2001;19(16):3622–3634.
32. Reintgen M, Murray L, Akman K, et al. Evidence for a better nodal staging system for melanoma: the clinical relevance of metastatic disease confined to the sentinel lymph nodes. *J Surg Oncol*. 2013;20:668–674.
33. Nowecki ZI, Rutkowski P, Michej W. The survival benefit to patients with positive sentinel node melanoma after completion lymph node dissection may be limited to the subgroup with a primary lesion breslow thickness greater than 1.0 and less than or equal to 4 mm (pT2-pT3). *Ann Surg Oncol*. 2008;15(8):2223–2234.
34. van Akkooi AC, Bouwhuis MG, de Wilt JH, Kliffen M, Schmitz PI, Eggermont AM. Multivariable analysis comparing outcome after sentinel node biopsy or therapeutic lymph node dissection in patients with melanoma. *Br J Surg*. 2007;94(10):1293–1299.
35. Morton DL, Thompson JF, Cochran AJ, et al. Sentinel-node biopsy or nodal observation in melanoma. *N Engl J Med*. 2006;355(13):1307–1301.
36. Bleicher RJ, Essner R, Foshag LJ, Wanek LA, Morton DL. Role of sentinel lymphadenectomy in thin invasive cutaneous melanomas. *J Clin Oncol*. 2003;21(7):1326–1331.
37. Rousseau DL Jr, Ross MI, Johnson MM, et al. Revised American Joint Committee on Cancer staging criteria accurately predict sentinel lymph node positivity in clinically node-negative melanoma patients. *Ann Surg Oncol*. 2003;10(5):569–574.
38. Cascinelli N, Belli F, Santinami M, et al. Sentinel lymph node biopsy in cutaneous melanoma: the WHO melanoma program experience. *Ann Surg Oncol*. 2000;7(6):469–474.
39. Kesmodel SB, Karakousis GC, Botbyl JD, et al. Mitotic rate as a predictor of sentinel lymph node positivity in patients with thin melanomas. *Ann Surg Oncol*. 2005;12(6):449–458.
40. Wright BE, Scheri RP, Ye X, et al. Importance of sentinel lymph node biopsy in patients with thin melanoma. *Arch Surg*. 2008;143(9):892–899; discussion 899–900.
41. Wong SL, Brady MS, Busam KJ, Coit DG. Results of sentinel lymph node biopsy in patients with thin melanoma. *Ann Surg Oncol*. 2006;13(3):302–309.
42. Andtbacka RH, Gershenwald JE. Role of sentinel lymph node biopsy in patients with thin melanoma. *J Natl Compr Canc Netw*. 2009;7(3):308–317
43. Balch CM. The role of elective lymph node dissection in melanoma: rationale, results, and controversies. *J Clin Oncol*. 1988;6(1):163–172.
44. Gutzmer R, Satzger I, Thoms KM, et al. Sentinel lymph node status is the most important prognostic factor for thick (> or = 4 mm) melanomas. *J Dtsch Dermatol Ges*. 2008;6(3):198–203.
45. Balch CM, Gershenwald JE, Soong SJ, et al. Final version of 2009 AJCC melanoma staging and classification. *J Clin Oncol*. 2009;27(36):6199–6206.
46. Wong SL, Balch CM, Hurley P, et al. Sentinel lymph node biopsy for melanoma: American Society of Clinical Oncology and Society of Surgical Oncology joint clinical practice guideline. *J Clin Oncol*. 2012;30(23):2912–2918.

CHAPTER 29

Management of Advanced Nonmelanoma Skin Cancer

Catherine Lee Tran, Mark M. Tran, & Timothy S. Wang

INTRODUCTION

EPIDEMIOLOGY OF NONMELANOMA SKIN CANCER

Skin cancers are divided into two main groups: malignant melanoma (MM) and nonmelanoma skin cancer (NMSC). The term "NMSC" encompasses a wide variety of skin cancers including basal cell carcinomas (BCC), cutaneous squamous cell carcinomas (cSCC), dermatofibrosarcoma protuberans (DFSP), cutaneous lymphomas, adnexal tumors, and Merkel cell carcinoma (MCC), and only excludes malignancies involving melanocytes. BCC and cSCC comprise the vast majority of NMSC tumors (estimated between 75% and 80% and 20% and 25%, respectively)[1,2] and their incidence is approximately 18 to 20 times higher than that of MM.[3] This chapter will focus on the management of advanced BCC, cSCC, DFSP, and MCC.

The incidence of NMSC is highest in Australia and the lowest in parts of Africa.[4]

In the United States, the total number of NMSC cases is reported to be higher than lung, breast, prostate, and colon cancers combined.[5] Over one million new cases of NMSC are diagnosed each year in the United States alone, and this has continued to increase at a rate of approximately 3% to 8% since the 1960s.[3,6] NMSCs are also widely believed to be the most commonly diagnosed malignancy worldwide.[2,7]

BASAL CELL CARCINOMAS

BCC INCIDENCE AND RISK FACTORS. BCC is the most common type of cancer worldwide.[8] In the United States, the estimated annual incidence is estimated to be 0.1% to 0.5%.[9] It is especially common in light-skinned populations, with the estimated lifetime risk of developing BCC up to 30% in the United States white population.[10] The incidence is about 30% higher in men than in women,[11–13] and increases with age.[14] Interestingly, the incidence of BCC among Americans younger than 40 years of age, especially among women, seems to be increasing.[15]

Both environmental and genetic factors play a role in the development of BCC: these include ultraviolet (UV) radiation,[16–19] arsenic exposure,[20–22] history of radiation therapy (RT),[23–25] immunosuppression (from various causes including solid organ transplantation, HIV infection, or chronic steroid use secondary to autoimmune disorders),[26,27] fair skin,[28] light-colored eyes, red hair, northern European ancestry, older age, childhood freckling, history of blistering sunburns, history of tanning bed use,[29] smoking,[19,30] and genetic conditions, such as basal cell nevus syndrome (BCNS) and epidermolysis bullosa.[17,18,29,31–33] Of these, UV radiation is one of the most important causes of BCC. In addition to the total radiation dose, the timing and mode of exposure also seem to contribute to BCC development. Recent studies showed that acute, intense incremental UV exposure increases BCC risk more than similar doses of UV radiation delivered in a more chronic fashion over the same total period of time.[26,34] There have also been studies suggesting that childhood and adolescence are critical periods for establishing adult BCC risk, thus highlighting the importance of early photoprotective measures to prevent the development of BCCs.[16–19,33–35] Lifestyle factors such as smoking have also been suggested to contribute to the development of BCCs.[19,30]

Pathways involved in the growth, apoptosis, or differentiation of keratinocytes,[36–39] as well as genes that influence immune response such as CTLA1[40] also contribute to BCC development. Better understanding of these genetic abnormalities has led to a better understanding of BCC pathogenesis.

MOLECULAR PATHOGENESIS OF BCCs. Major advances in the understanding of the pathogenesis of BCCs have come from extensive studies of patients with BCNS and the subsequent discovery of mutations in the tumor suppressor gene, PTCH1. BCNS, also known as Gorlin's syndrome, is a rare, autosomal dominant syndrome, in which patients develop numerous BCCs starting in childhood, and are at risk of developing medulloblastomas and rhabdomyosarcomas.[41,42] BCNS is caused by loss-of-function mutations in the tumor suppressor gene, human PTCH1, on chromosome 9q22, which is the primary inhibitor of Hedgehog (Hh) signaling.[43,44] The Hh signaling pathway plays a critical role in embryonic growth and patterning, as well as in the maintenance of homeostasis postembryonically through effects on stem cells or progenitor cells in invertebrate and vertebrate organisms.[45] This signaling pathway is constitutively repressed under normal circumstances, and only activated by binding of Hh ligand, such as Sonic hedgehog (SHH), Indian hedgehog (IHH), and desert hedgehog (DHH), to the transmembrane receptor PTCH1.[46] When not bound by Hh ligand, PTCH1 receptor suppresses the activity of transmembrane protein Smoothened (SMO). When the PTCH receptor is bound by Hh ligand, the repression is released, thus permitting SMO to transmit downstream signals, leading to production of Gli family transcription factors (Fig. 29-1).[47–49] This receptor ligand association is reversible and has feedback

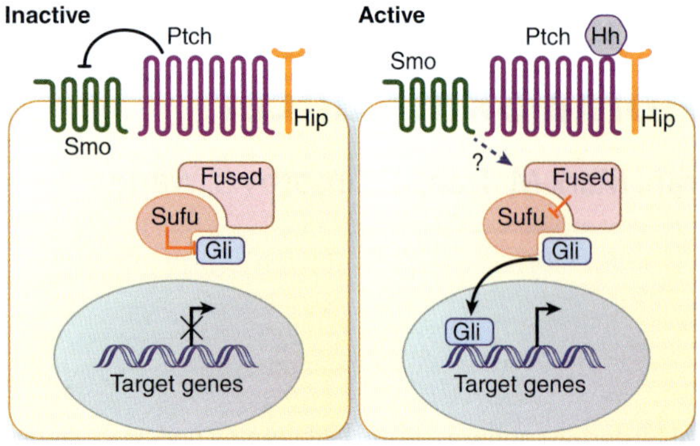

Figure 29-1 Molecular pathogenesis of basal cell carcinoma.

mechanisms to tightly control transcription and regulate downstream gene expression.[50] The possible regulation of Hh signaling by various molecular pathways, including Ras, nuclear factor-κB, and estrogen receptor-α, which thereby contributes to carcinogenesis, has also been postulated.[46]

This model demonstrates how either inactivating mutations in PTCH or activating mutations in SMO can result in constitutive signaling of Gli and downstream target genes. In patients with BCNS, the inactivating mutation of PTCH1 leads to constitutive overexpression of SHH signal, which has been implicated in the development of BCCs via activation of the transcription factors Gli.[51–56] Subsequent studies have demonstrated that approximately one-third of sporadic BCCs have acquired PTCH1 mutations.[57,58] Besides UV exposure targeting PTCH1,[59] the mechanisms involving SHH mutations in sporadic BCC are likely multifactorial, including activating mutations in the SMO gene, a reciprocal translocation between chromosomes 9q22.3 and 16p, and mutations in PTCH2.[60–63]

Studies of other genetic syndromes associated with multiple BCCs, such as Bazex–Dupré–Christol syndrome,[64] Rombo syndrome,[65] cartilage–hair hypoplasia syndrome,[66] and xeroderma pigmentosum,[67] have demonstrated other pathways, including DNA repair and telomere maintenance, that play an important role in BCC pathogenesis.[68] Recent studies have elucidated other molecular pathways that may contribute to its pathogenesis as well. The Wnt pathway is known to play a critical role in normal hair follicle development and cycling.[68] A mediator of Wnt signaling, β-catenin, was shown to be increased in both human and mouse BCCs.[69,70] Another study showed that active Wnt signaling is required for Hh-driven hamartomas by demonstrating that overexpression of the Wnt antagonist, Dkk1, in a mouse model, resulted in the inhibition of hamartomatous growth.[71]

Some pathways induce BCC formation by modulating Hh signaling. The epidermal growth factor receptor (EGFR)/MEK/ERK pathway was shown to modulate Gli-dependent transcription and induce oncogenic transformation of human keratinocytes.[68,72,73] Along with the PTCH pathway gene, the p53 tumor suppressor gene is another major target of UV radiation.[74] It plays a critical role in regulation of the cell cycle and apoptosis, and mutations in it were found to be present in about 56% of BCCs.[75] p53 can also influence BCC development via its influence on the Hh pathway, as shown in a study where complete loss of p53 resulted in upregulation of SMO in the interfollicular epidermis in mice.[76]

The important role of epithelial–stromal interaction in creating a favorable environment for tumor cell proliferation has also been demonstrated. Stromal cells isolated from human BCCs express increased levels of gremlin 1, which antagonizes the pro-differentiation factors, BMP2 and BMP4.[68,77]

TREATMENT OF BASAL CELL CARCINOMA.

Appropriate treatment of BCC is necessary due to the locally invasive and destructive nature of this tumor. The majority of BCCs represent only local disease and carry an excellent prognosis. The goal of treatment is complete tumor extirpation with maximal preservation of function and cosmesis. Currently, the widely accepted treatment modalities include: cryotherapy, electrodesiccation and curettage (ED&C), surgical excision, Mohs micrographic surgery (MMS), topical and intralesional agents (5-FU, imiquimod, resiquimod, ingenol mebulate, cyclooxygenase-2 inhibitors, cyclopamine), radiation therapy (RT), photodynamic therapy, and systemic chemotherapeutic agents (capecitabine, interferon, EGFR inhibitors, GDC-0449, LDE-225, vismodegib).[74,78] Several factors determine the recurrence potential of BCC, including size, location (Fig. 29-2), histopathologic subtype, perineural involvement, clinically indistinct borders, patient immune status, primary versus recurrent lesions, and history of radiation exposure to the affected area. These risk factors, as well as a thorough understanding of the different treatment modalities, including their associated risks, complications, cosmetic outcome, and recurrence rates, should be considered in order to make appropriate treatment choices.

Several studies have looked into various characteristics of BCC to determine the risk of tumor recurrence.[79–81] The National Comprehensive Cancer Network (NCCN) guidelines assess the risk factors for BCC recurrence, as well as proposed primary treatments for low-risk and high-risk BCCs (Table 29-1, Fig. 29-3).[82]

The majority of NMSC are low risk and can be successfully treated by ED&C, surgical excision, cryotherapy, photodynamic therapy, and topical agents. Patients with BCC who are not considered surgical candidates may be referred for radiotherapy, which has a 4 year locoregional control rate of 86% with a median time to recurrence of 40.5 months.[83] The use of radiotherapy may be limited in patients with tumors located near the eyes or on the eyelids,[84] which may be difficult to treat, and patients nearing their

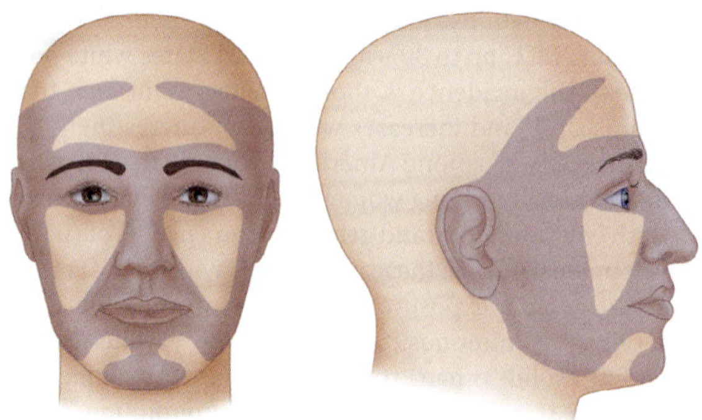

Figure 29-2 High-risk mask areas of face for basal and squamous cell carcinoma.

TABLE 29-1
Risk Factors for BCC Recurrence

Characteristic	Low Risk	High Risk
Primary vs. recurrent	Primary	Recurrent
Borders	Well defined	Poorly defined
Immunosuppression	No	Yes
Location: Eyelids, ears, nose, lips, genitals, hands, feet Cheeks, forehead, scalp, neck Trunk, extremities	Size <20 mm Size <10 mm Size <6 mm	Size ≥20 mm Size ≥10 mm Size ≥6 mm
Pathology	Nodular, superficial	Aggressive growth pattern
Perineural involvement	No	Yes
Site of previous radiation treatment	No	Yes

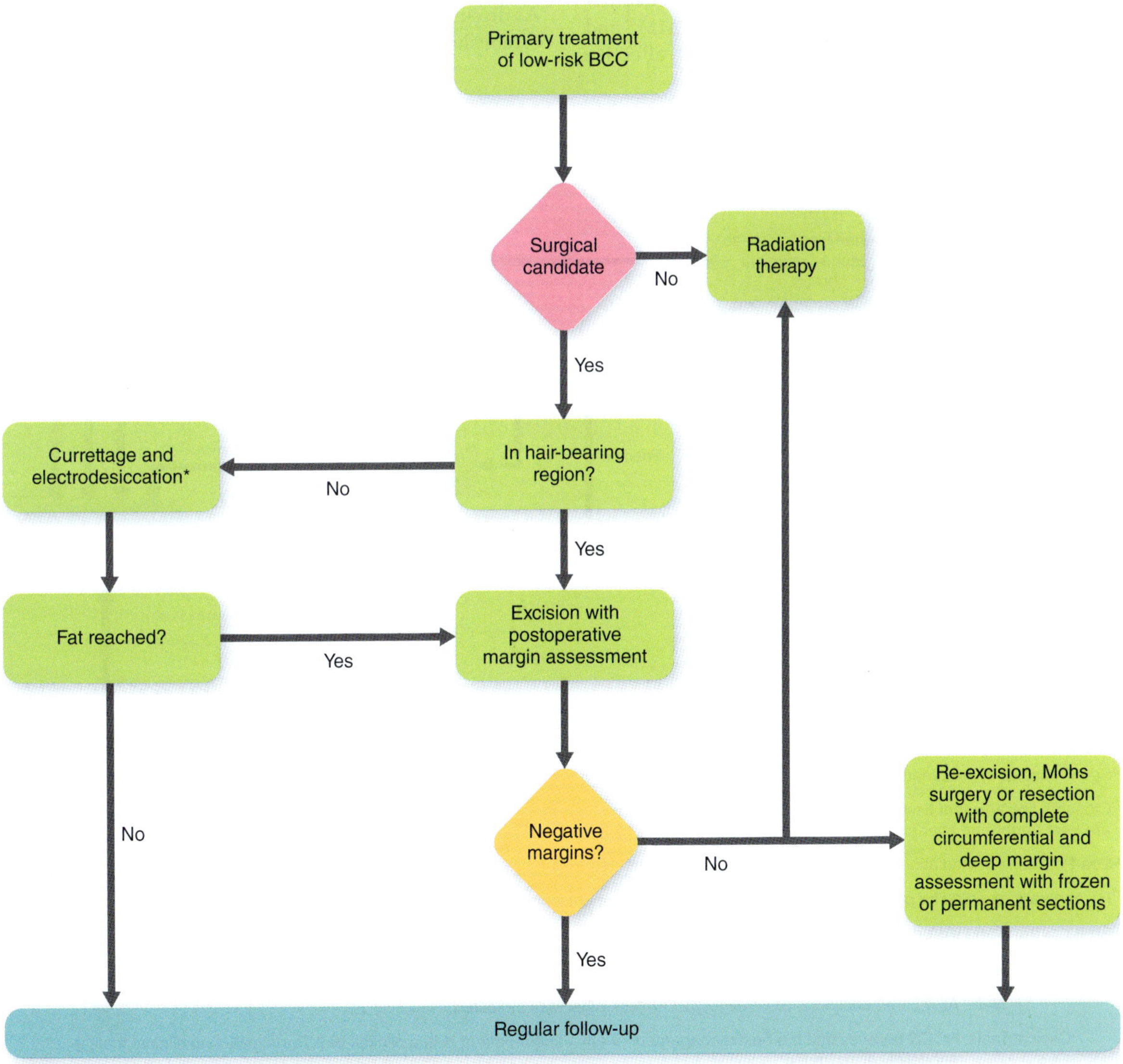

Figure 29-3 Treatment algorithm for basal cell carcinoma.

maximum safe lifetime dose of radiation.[85] Use of radiotherapy is contraindicated in Gorlin's syndrome[86] as well as in BCC that has recurred after prior radiotherapy.[84]

Certain BCCs are at higher risk for recurrence based on their size and location, as well as clinical and microscopic factors. Evidence-based treatment options for BCC are few because of the rarity of randomized, prospective studies comparing different treatment modalities and their recurrence rates. According to a large systematic review that included studies with at least 50 patients and 5 years' follow-up, totaling 9930 primary BCC cases, MMS had the lowest rate of recurrence, followed by surgical excision, cryosurgery, and ED&C.[87] The authors suggested that MMS be used for larger, morpheaform or recurrent BCCs located in danger zones (Fig. 29-4), and that surgical excision with 4 mm margins around the clinical borders of the tumor be used for well-circumscribed nodular or superficial BCCs <2 cm in diameter, as well as for re-excision of low-risk primary BCCs located on the trunk and extremities. They recommended that other treatment modalities be used in patients for whom surgery is contraindicated.[74,87] A Cochrane review analyzing randomized controlled trials examining BCC recurrence rates found that MMS and conventional surgical excision were the most effective treatments, followed by radiotherapy, cryotherapy, and photodynamic therapy.[88] ED&C can be a cost-effective and appropriate treatment choice for low-risk tumors if three important factors are kept in mind[74,82]:

1. This technique should not be used to treat lesions in hair-bearing sites because of the risk of tumor extending down hair follicles;
2. If the subcutaneous layer is reached during the ED&C procedure, surgical excision should be performed;
3. If curettage is performed based on the clinical appearance of tumor, a biopsy should be taken to confirm that there are no high-risk pathologic features. Further guidelines and treatment algorithms can be found on the NCCN website: http://www.nccn.org/.

Although surgical and other destructive treatments are considered the gold standard of therapy for localized BCC, advancements in understanding BCC pathogenesis have led to the development of targeted therapies for more advanced disease. These treatments are valuable for patients with unresectable tumors as well as metastases. As discussed earlier, the Hh signaling pathway is now well established as playing a critical role in BCC pathogenesis.

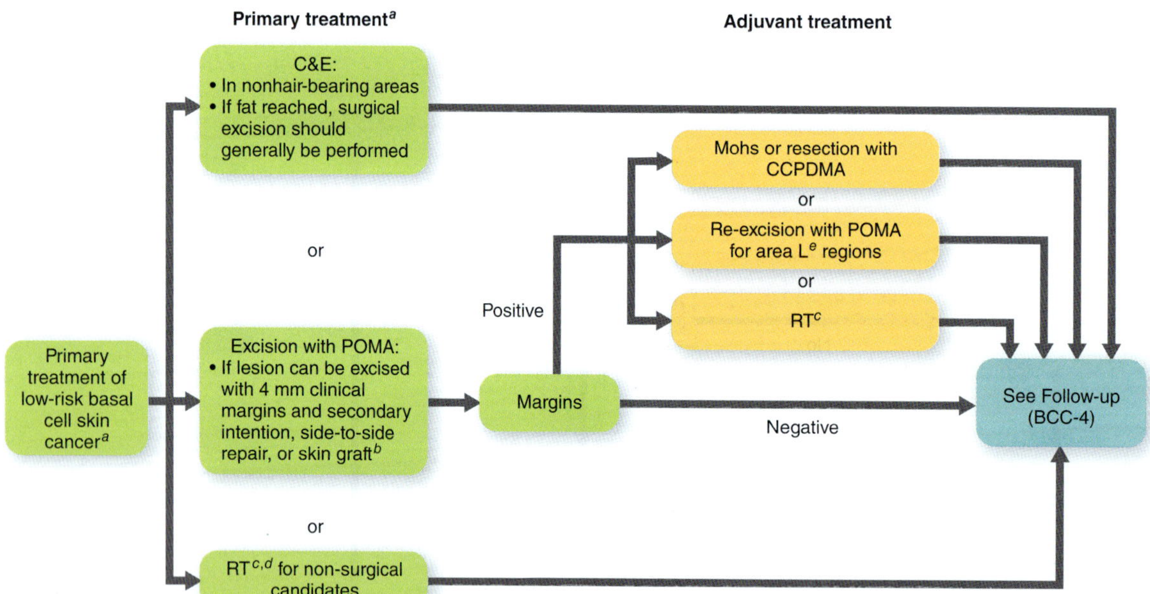

^a See Principles of Treatment for Basal Cell Skin Cancer (BCC-B).

^b Closures like adjacent tissue transfers, in which significant tissue rearrangement occurs, are best performed after clear margins are verified.

^c See Principles of Radiation Therapy for Basal Cell Skin Cancer (BCC-C).

^d RT generally reserved for patients over 60 y because of concerns about long term sequellae.

^e Area L = trunk and extremities (See BCC-A).

C&E = curettage and electrodesiccation

POMA = postoperative margin assessment

CCPDMA = complete circumferential peripheral and deep margin assessment with frozen or permanent sections

Note: All recommendations are category 2A unless otherwise indicated.

Clinical Trials: NCCN believes that the best management of any cancer patient is in a clinical trial. Participation in clinical trials is especially encouraged.

Figure 29-4 Treatment algorithm for high-risk basal cell carcinoma.

In 1998, it was observed that lambs developed cyclopia after maternal ingestion of corn lilies, which contain cyclopamine, a potent inhibitor of the Hh signaling pathway by direct binding to SMO.[89,90] Subsequent in vitro and in vivo studies demonstrated that the oral and topical administration of cyclopamine reduced BCC growth and development in mice and humans.[91,92] These observations led to the synthesis of a novel class of Hh antagonists derived from cyclopamine with improved pharmaceutical properties and in vitro potency.[93] Vismodegib (GDC-0449), a SMO inhibitor, showed promising results in a phase I trial of patients with locally advanced or metastatic BCC.[94,95]

In a phase II clinical trial of vismodegib, investigators observed such promising results among patients with locally advanced or metastatic BCC[96] and BCNS patients with multiple BCCs that the Data Safety Monitoring Board recommended ending the placebo arm of the study.[68] Vismodegib demonstrated a 30% response rate in patients with metastatic BCC (n = 33), and a 43% response rate in those with locally advanced BCC (n = 63); 21% showed complete responses (CRs).[97] More than 30% of patients reported adverse events including muscle spasms, alopecia, dysgeusia (taste disturbance), weight loss, and fatigue; seven deaths were noted. Acquired resistance during continuous vismodegib therapy has been reported in a case series in 21% of patients (n = 28) with advanced BCCs.[98] The novel use of vismodegib as a neoadjuvant to shrink a locally advanced BCC prior to resection has been reported recently in a patient with Gorlin's syndrome.[99]

Potential challenges in the use of Hh signaling pathway antagonists exist. Studies show that after dramatic reduction in tumor mass, a small population of residual tumor cells insensitive to Hh inhibition persist in both the mouse model[100] and in clinical trials of LDE225.[68,101] Another challenge is the development of resistance caused by mutations in SMO and amplification of downstream genes including Gli2 and cyclin D1.[102,103] Recently, an alternative SMO inhibitor, itraconazole, an FDA-approved antifungal agent, was found to inhibit Hh signaling pathway by binding SMO at a site different from that of cyclopamine, delaying BCC development in a mouse model.[104] Itraconazole is currently undergoing a phase II study to evaluate its potential as a BCC treatment option. Given the common adverse effects of systemic SMO inhibitors, including loss of taste, muscle spasms, hair loss, fatigue, and hyponatremia,[105–107] a topical formulation of SMO inhibitor LDE224 was developed, which produced a decrease in Hh gene expression in the majority of treated tumors without treatment-related side effects.[101] A number of inhibitors of the Hh signaling pathway with targets downstream of SMO, such as Gli transcription factors, or independent of SMO, are currently under investigation.[108–111]

SQUAMOUS CELL CARCINOMAS

INCIDENCE AND RISK FACTORS OF cSCC.

Cutaneous SCC (cSCC) is the second most common type of skin cancer in Caucasians after BCC, accounting for one-fifth of all cutaneous malignancies and 90% of all head and neck cancers.[1,112,113] In the United States, the incidence of SCC in men is 81 to 136 per 100,000 and 26 to 59 per 100,000 in women.[114] The risk factors for developing cSCCs include fair skin, male gender, older age (>65 years old), increased sun exposure, and immunosuppression such as solid organ transplantation.[115] For the last several decades, the incidence of cSCCs has been rising. This is likely attributable to several factors including an expanding older population; the incidence of cSCC is three times higher for those over the age of 75 compared to those between 50 to 55 years of age.[116] Additionally, there is a growing population of solid organ transplant recipients whose immunosuppression and longevity of transplant predispose these patients to numerous and high-risk cSCCs.[15,113,114,117,118]

While the majority of cSCCs are minimally invasive in their early stages, the potential for metastasis exists[115] with an approximately 2% to 3% overall rate of regional metastasis to lymph nodes of the head and neck, primarily to parotid lymph nodes.[119] When cSCCs do metastasize, they account for 20% of all skin cancer-related deaths.[120] Thus, with an increase in the geriatric population and longer life expectancy of immunosuppressed patients, the incidence of cSCC will likely continue to rise.

cSCC most frequently develops on sun-exposed areas of the skin.[2,119] Up to 75% of NMSCs occur in the head and neck region[121] with 68% of all cSCCs occurring on the head and neck.[122] Epidemiologic studies support the role of UV light in NMSC pathogenesis since increased rates are correlated with proximity to the equator[2,117,123] and are also seen in areas of ozone depletion, such as Australia, where the incidence of NMSC is approximately 1000 to 2000 per 100,000 per year.[1,2,4] Northern European countries have much lower rates of NMSC.[122]

The increased incidence of NMSCs following transplantation has been well documented.[124–128] One report documented a three- to five-fold increase in cancer risk in the posttransplant population compared to the general population[129] with the incidence of de novo malignancy in this population ranging between 6% and 18% in some studies.[127] Interestingly, the types and distributions of cancers that affect this population are quite different from those of the general population.[130] While the most common tumors in the general population are breast, prostate, colon, and lung cancers, the most common types of malignancies in transplant recipients are cSCC, BCC, and non-Hodgkin's lymphoma, with the most common sites of involvement being on the head and neck.[129–131] The cSCCs in immunocompromised patients are clinically aggressive; these patients tend to develop multiple lesions with a higher rate of recurrence and a higher rate of metastasis.[124] In particular, transplant patients have a 65 times greater risk of developing cSCCs compared to age-matched controls.[132]

CLINICAL AND HISTOLOGIC FEATURES OF HIGH-RISK SCC

Staging. The staging system most often used for NMSCs is the American Joint Commission on Cancer (AJCC) TNM system. The seventh edition of AJCC (Tables 29-2 and 29-3) includes the clinical and histologic features that should be taken into account to better ascertain the prognosis and natural history of cSCCs.

Pathogenesis. cSCC is thought to manifest as a spectrum of progressive changes, from actinic keratoses (AKs) to SCC in situ (SCCIS), invasive cSCC, and metastatic SCC.

According to the classic multistep model of carcinogenesis, mutations in tumor suppressor genes may cause development of precursor lesions with increased genetic instability, and additional mutations in oncogenes permit the emergence of invasive carcinoma.[133,134] In the case of cSCC, the mechanism leading to genomic instability is likely due to UVB-induced inactivation of p53,[135] as demonstrated in a study where p53 knockout mice developed increased numbers of AKs and cSCCs after UV-B exposure,[136] as well as a number of studies confirming the presence of p53 mutations in majority of cSCCs.[137–139] In addition to UV radiation induced signature mutations (CC→TT and C→T), aberrant activation of EGFR and Fyn, an Src-family tyrosine kinase, were shown to down-regulate p53 in a c-Jun-dependent manner.[140,141]

TABLE 29-3

Staging of Basal and Squamous Cell Skin Cancer by Prognostic and Histologic Groups

Prognostic Groups	Stage 0	Tis, N0, M0
	Stage I	T1, N0, M0
	Stage II	T2, N0, M0
	Stage III	T3 **OR**
		Tis-T3 with N1
	Stage IV	T4 **OR**
		Tis-T3 with N2 **OR**
		N3 **OR**
		M1
Histologic Grade	GX	can not be assessed
	G1	well differentiated
	G2	moderately differentiated
	G3	poorly differentiated
	G4	undifferentiated

TABLE 29-2

Staging of Basal and Squamous Cell Skin Cancer by Size/Presence of Lymph Node Involvement or Metastases

Primary Tumor (excludes eSCC of eyelid)		
Stage	*Definition*	*High-Risk Features*
Tx	Cannot be assessed	Depth >2 mm Clark level ≥4 On ear or non–hair-bearing lip Poorly or not differentiated
T0	No evidence of primary tumor	
Tis	Carcinoma in situ	
T1	≤2 cm and <2 high risk features	
T2	>2 cm OR has ≥2 high risk features	
T3	Invades maxilla, mandible, orbit, or temporal bones	
T4	Invades axial or appendicular skeleton or perineural skull base	
Regional Lymph Node Involvement		
Stage	*Definition*	
NX	Lymph nodes can not be assessed	
N0	No lymph node metastasis	
N1	Involves single lymph node ≤3 cm	
N2a	≥3 cm to ≤6 cm in single lymph node OR	
N2b	≤6 cm in multiple ipsilateral lymph nodes OR	
N2c	≤6 cm in bilateral or contralateral lymph nodes	
N3	Metastasis >6 cm in lymph node	
Distant Metastasis		
Stage	*Definition*	
M0	None	
M1	Present	

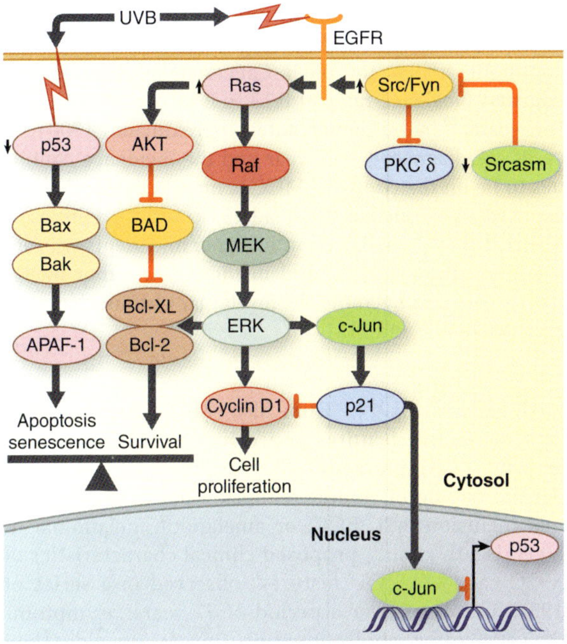

Figure 29-5 Key signaling pathways involved in the formation of cSCC. Mutations induced by UVB exposure can perturb multiple cellular pathways, thereby contributing or leading to the formation of cSCC. Thick arrows signify an increase or decrease in signaling in SCC. Red T-bars indicate inhibitory relationships.

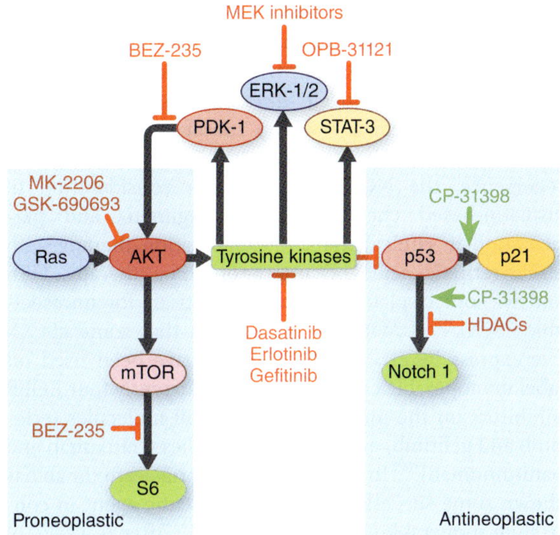

Figure 29-6 Potential pathways that may be targeted by small molecules to treat AKs and cSCCs. Key signaling pathways driving cutaneous neoplasia are shown. Small molecules that can permeate the epidermis and target these signaling deficits may have therapeutic potential. Arrows denote stimulatory relationships and T-bars denote inhibitory relationships. (Reproduced with permission from Ratushny V, Gober MD, Hick R, Ridky TW, Seykora JT. From keratinocyte to cancer: the pathogenesis and modeling of cutaneous squamous cell carcinoma. *J Clin Invest.* 2012;122:464–472.)

Recently, amplification and activating mutations of Ras oncogene, a family of GTP-binding proteins that activates the Raf/Mek/Erk1/Erk2 kinase pathway, have been found in SCCs and AKs.[142–145] The Ras family of proto-oncogenes promotes cellular growth and proliferation, and aberrant Ras activation can result in tumorigenic phenotypes.[145] Interestingly, one study showed that activation of oncogenic Ras alone was not sufficient to induce SCC, but that it was necessary to couple Ras overexpression with activation of the cell cycle progression mediator CDK4, or to modulate NF-κB activity to bypass Ras-mediated G1 arrest and induce epidermal tumorigenesis (Figs. 29-5 and 29-6).[134,146,147]

TREATMENT. The approach to treating cSCC depends on its risk classification according to the NCCN. The NCCN characterizes high-risk cSCC as having any of the following risk factors: large diameter (>2 cm or >1 cm on cheeks, forehead, scalp, or neck, or >6 mm on other areas of face, genitalia, hands, feet), depth >4 mm or beyond the papillary dermis, ill-defined margins, recurrence after definitive treatment, immunosuppression, prior radiation, chronic inflammation, rapid growth, neurological symptoms, perineural or vascular invasion, moderately or poorly differentiated histology, infiltrative or acantholytic pattern, or mucin production.[81] For non high-risk cSCC, the NCCN considers standard surgical excision adequate, in which the margin assessment is made from representative tissue sections. For high-risk cSCC, complete margin analysis is advised by the NCCN either by MMS or excision with complete circumferential peripheral and deep margin assessment (CCPDMA). Standard excision is permissible for tumors greater than 2 cm on the trunk and extremities with no other high-risk factors, which can be excised with a 1 cm clinical margin with a primary closure.[81] In MMS, the surgeon performs the complete margin assessment whereas the pathologist performs this assessment in CCPDMA. Lower recurrence rates have been reported with MMS in a systematic review comparing MMS to standard excision.[148] The cure rate of primary cSCC with MMS (97%) is reported to be higher than that of standard excision (92%); similarly, the cure rate of recurrent disease is reportedly higher following MMS (90%–94%) than after standard excision (77%).[148,149]

RT is another treatment option for cSCC but is reserved for tumors that that are difficult to treat surgically, particularly on the eyelids, lips, and ears.[150] While radiation can be used as a primary treatment option for cSCCs, it is important to note that reported cure rates are higher with surgical therapy, and that there are long-term cutaneous risks of radiation and as well as short-term scheduling challenges.[151] As monotherapy, radiation is generally reserved for patients in whom surgery would lead to unacceptable cosmetic or functional impairment, patients with inoperable tumors, or in whom the risks of surgery outweigh the benefits. With high-risk cSCC, local control rates with RT range from 80% to 85%.[152] When implemented in the right context, RT may match surgery in restoring oral function and cure rates for lower lip cSCC.[153] In cSCC with aggressive features, RT has been reportedly used as adjuvant therapy to surgery and chemotherapy with some degree of efficacy.[152,154,155]

Chemotherapy as a treatment modality for metastatic cSCC thus far remains inconsistently effective. Combinations of cisplatin with 5-flourouracil (5-FU), doxorubicin, or bleomycin have been reported to yield some degree of efficacy, with a subset achieving CRs in some cases.[155–160] For distant metastatic disease or regional recurrence, the NCCN recommends consideration of cisplatin-based chemotherapeutic regimens and participation in clinical trials.[158] Combination therapy with 13-*cis*-retinoic acid and interferon-alpha therapy, with and without cisplatin, are in clinical trials for unresectable cSCC.[159,161] With the recognition that some cSCCs overexpress EGFR, EGFR inhibitors have been used off label in inoperable cases.[162] There are currently four EGFR inhibitors on the market: two are small molecules (erlotinib and gefitinib) and two are antibodies (cetuximab and panitumumab).[163] In a phase II clinical trial, cetuximab has shown some success as a monotherapeutic agent in controlling inoperable or metastatic cSCC: after 6 weeks of treatment, 69% of enrolled patients were observed to have some degree of disease control.[164]

Combined radiotherapy and EGFR inhibition have also shown promising results compared to monotherapy alone. In an NEJM 2006 article, the authors demonstrated that, in patients with locally advanced head and neck SCC, radiotherapy with cetuximab achieved 49.0 months median survival compared to 29.3 months after radiotherapy alone.[153] A paper reviewing case reports and a phase II trial concluded that cetuximab combined with radiotherapy is superior to cetuximab alone; combination therapy showed a total response in 50% of advanced SCC cases.[165] As radiotherapy combined with EGFR inhibition has gained traction for advanced cSCC treatment, clinical trials are underway to elaborate the cutaneous side effects due to radiation versus cetuximab in a large national prospective study in Germany as of 2013.[166] In very high-risk SCC, characterized by lymphovascular or extracutaneous invasion, cetuximab appears to confer an advantage in controlling disease in combination with surgery and/or radiation in a recent retrospective study at an academic institution.[167]

Comparison studies of radiotherapy with adjunctive cisplatin-based chemotherapy versus adjunctive EGFR inhibition are sparse. One recent retrospective study of patients receiving these combination interventions shows the superiority of adjunctive cisplatin ($n = 18$) over adjunctive cetuximab ($n = 29$): 83% of patients achieved a 3 year disease-specific survival period in the cisplatin group compared with 18% in the cetuximab group.[156]

The advent of EGFR inhibitors marks an exciting period of discovery of new molecular targets for treatment of advanced cSCC. With novel molecules targeting alternative pathways, including PI3 K-AKT, ALK-1, NOTCH1, and Hh, new monotherapeutic or adjuvant agents promise new ways to control disease or at least overcome tumor resistance to EGFR inhibition.[168]

MERKEL CELL CARCINOMA

EPIDEMIOLOGY AND RISK FACTORS.

MCC is a rare, aggressive neuroendocrine carcinoma of the skin, with a high risk of recurrence and metastasis. Overall, MCC has a 1 year survival rate of approximately 80% and a 2 year survival rate of approximately 50%. It most commonly affects the older Caucasian population with adjusted incidence rates of 0.18 to 0.41 per 100,000 person-years.[169] In the United States, approximately 1500 new cases are diagnosed each year and the incidence continues to be on the rise.[162,170] MCC is more common in sun-exposed areas, such as the head, neck, and extremities.[171] The risk of MCC is significantly higher in patients who are immunosuppressed[172,173] and in those with other malignancies, including multiple myeloma, chronic lymphocytic leukemia, and MM.[174,175]

PRESENTATION.

Clinically, MCC lesions often lack distinctive features and can present as a rapidly growing, asymptomatic, flesh-colored to bluish-red dermal papule or nodule, clinically mimicking epidermal inclusion cyst, BCC, or amelanotic melanoma. In 2008, Heath et al.[176] proposed clinical characteristics of MCC called "AEIOU features" observed in a series of 195 MCC cases over a period of 27 years: asymptomatic; expanding rapidly; immune suppression, older than 50 years; and UV-exposed site on person of fair skin. Maintaining vigilance and a high index of suspicion for biopsy followed by histopathologic confirmation facilitates a timely diagnosis.

STAGING.

Once the diagnosis is established, the tumor is staged according to AJCC TNM criteria (Tables 29-4 and 29-5).[177] The staging system was first released in 2010; the criteria and stage groupings are based on the analysis of National Cancer Database data from more than 4000 MCC patients with at least 5 years' follow-up. Figure 29-7 shows the significant difference in survival rates found between patients presenting with local, regional, and distant metastatic disease.[178]

PATHOGENESIS.

Although the molecular pathogenesis of MCC has not yet been completely elucidated, multiple factors appear to contribute to the development of MCC, including immunosuppression, UV exposure and Merkel cell polyomavirus. The relative risk of MCC development increases significantly with immunosuppression, with a 13 fold increase in the HIV population[172] and a 10 fold increase in solid organ transplant patients.[173] There are multiple reports to support the possible important role of UV radiation exposure in the etiology of MCC. In one study of 195 cases of MCC, the lesions were observed to arise in sun-exposed areas 81% of the time.[176] In one population-based study of 425 cases of MCC from nine areas of the United States, the Surveillance, Epidemiology, and End Results (SEER) Program database demonstrated that regional incidence rates of both cancers increased with increasing sun exposure as measured by the UV-B solar index.[179] One prospective study of 1380 patients with psoriasis who were treated with oral psoralen and UV-A photochemotherapy (PUVA) showed an increased risk of MCC development in the PUVA treated group compared to controls.[180] In addition, a C-to-T mutation, a typical UV-B induced mutation, is found in MCC cell lines, further supporting

TABLE 29-4
Staging of Merkel Cell Carcinoma

Primary Tumor	
Stage	*Definition*
Tx	Cannot be assessed
T0	No evidence of primary tumor
Tis	Carcinoma in situ
T1	≤2 cm
T2	>2 cm and ≤5 cm
T3	>5 cm
T4	Invades musculoskeletal structures
Regional Lymph Node Involvement	
Stage	*Definition*
NX	Lymph nodes cannot be assessed
pNX	Lymph nodes cannot be assessed on pathology
cN0	Lymph nodes cannot be detected clinically
pN0	No lymph node metastasis detected on pathology
N1a	Micrometastasis (diagnosed after sentinel or elective lymphadenopathy)
N1b	Macrometastasis (clinically detectable and confirmed by biopsy or therapeutic lymphadenopathy)
N2	In-transit metastasis (distinct from and distal to primary lesion or between primary lesion and draining regional lymph node)
Distant Metastasis	
Stage	*Definition*
Mx	Cannot be assessed
M0	None
M1a	In skin, subcutaneous tissue or distant lymph nodes
M1b	In lungs
M1c	In other visceral site

the role of sun exposure as a factor contributing to MCC development.[181]

The observation of clonal integration of polyomavirus (MCPyV) in human MCC by Feng et al. in 2008 initiated great interest in the study of viral tumorigenesis.[182–184] MCPyV is a nonenveloped, double-stranded DNA virus with a reported prevalence in MCC lesions ranging from 77% to 86%.[182,185–187] Notably, it is not exclusively observed in MCC, but has also been detected in normal skin and cSCC.[188–192] Some studies also attempted to demonstrate the association of improved survival with the presence of MCPyV[187,193]; other studies were not able to show the prognostic relevance of MCPyV.[186,194] Although the emerging role of MCPyV provides promising insights into the etiology

TABLE 29-5
Prognostic Staging of Merkel Cell Carcinoma

Prognostic Groups	Stage 0	Tis, N0, M0
	Stage IA	T1, pN0, M0
	Stage IB	T1, cN0, M0
	Stage IIA	T2-T3, pN0, M0
	Stage IIB	T2-T3, cN0, M0
	Stage IIC	T4, N0, M0
	Stage IIIA	Tis-T4, N1a, M0
	Stage IIIB	Tix-T4, N1b/N2, M0
	Stage IV	M1
Histologic Grade	GX	Cannot be assessed
	G1	Well differentiated
	G2	Moderately differentiated
	G3	Poorly differentiated
	G4	Undifferentiated

of MCC, the exact molecular pathogenesis has yet to be elucidated fully.

TREATMENT. Currently, the main treatment modalities for MCC are surgical resection and radiotherapy, although much controversy exists regarding the specific role of each modality. The following are the updated NCCN consensus recommendations for the treatment of MCC.

Wide local excision (WLE) of the primary tumor with negative margins is the standard treatment for newly diagnosed MCC patients without evidence of metastasis. The current recommendation for surgical margins depends on the clinical size of the tumor: a 1 cm margin for <2 cm

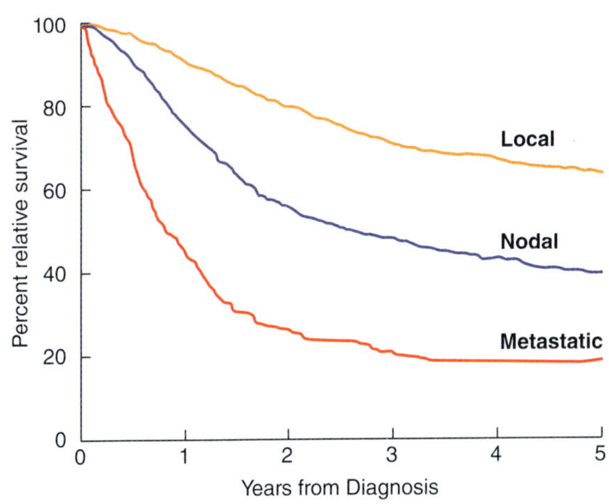

Local (n = 2356)	91%	80%	71%	67%	64%
Nodal (n =937)	75%	56%	48%	43%	39%
Metastatic (n = 277)	44%	26%	20%	18%	18%

Figure 29-7 Survival rates among patients presenting with local, regional, and distant metastatic Merkel cell carcinoma.

tumors and 2 cm margins for >2 cm tumors.[195] Almost one-third of clinically node-negative patients have microscopic nodal disease; therefore, for untreated primary tumors, sentinel lymph node (SLN) biopsy is recommended at the time of WLE, examined by both hematoxylin and eosin (H&E) and immunoperoxidase staining, including CK20.[177,178,196] If the SLNs are positive, completion lymph node dissection with subsequent radiotherapy of the basin is recommended.[178]

MCC has been shown to be a radiosensitive tumor, and radiotherapy is currently used as an adjuvant therapy to surgical excision in the majority of cases. In one study of 1254 MCC patients, surgery combined with local radiotherapy was shown to significantly decrease the incidence of local and regional recurrence compared with a control group treated with surgery alone.[197] Another study demonstrated improved survival in patients who underwent adjuvant RT.[198] In inoperable cases radiation monotherapy can provide an alternative therapeutic option.[199,200]

The role of chemotherapy in MCC treatment remains controversial. In general, MCC chemotherapy regimens are adapted from those used for small cell carcinoma of the lung. The most common agents include a combination of platinum-containing agents with etoposide, which are associated with significant morbidity and, rarely, mortality.[201] There have been no randomized trials evaluating the efficacy of chemotherapy. Even in patients with locally advanced or distant disease showing initial response to chemotherapy, chemotherapy thus far has not shown any survival benefit.[202] Chemotherapy is, therefore, used mostly as palliative treatment in disseminated disease rather than as primary or adjuvant therapy.

DERMATOFIBROSARCOMA PROTUBERANS

EPIDEMIOLOGY AND PRESENTATION.

DFSP is a rare, locally aggressive mesenchymal neoplasm with a generally low malignant potential. Its incidence ranges from 0.8 to 4.5 cases per million people per year,[203–205] accounting for 2% to 6% of all soft-tissue sarcomas diagnosed in the United States[206,207] It typically affects middle-aged individuals[208] with males more commonly affected than females (3:2 ratio),[209] and presents as an erythematous to violaceous dermal plaque or exophytic tumor with surrounding telangiectases.[210] The most commonly involved anatomic sites include the trunk (47%), followed by the lower extremity (20%), upper extremity (18%), and head and neck (14%).[211] The lesions show an initial indolent radial growth pattern with satellite peripheral nodules; if untreated, the lesion grows vertically, invading underlying structures including subcutaneous tissue, fascia, muscle, or bone with satellite nodules coalescing into a larger tumor to give it its "protuberant" appearance.[212] The diagnosis is made by histologic evaluation, often confirmed by immunohistochemistry, most notably by the presence of CD34, hyaluronate, and vimentin, and the absence of factor XIIIa and S100.[203,213]

PATHOGENESIS.

DFSP is characterized by a specific cytogenetic abnormality. In 1997 Simon et al.[214] identified the fusion gene COL1A1/PDGFB resulting from the rearrangement of upstream regions of the COL1A1 gene in 17q21 to 17q22 and exon 2 of PDGF in 22q13.1. This translocation results in the deregulation of platelet-derived growth factor-beta (PDGFB) expression, thus producing continuous autocrine activation of tyrosine kinase PDGF Receptor B (PDGFRB).[215–217] This mechanism is thought to be fundamental to the development of DFSP, as this fusion gene was observed to be present in nearly all cases of DFSP.[215,218] The fusion gene product COL1A1/PDGFB provides a useful molecular diagnostic test as well as a target for new molecular therapeutic options.

TREATMENT.

The standard of care in the treatment of patients with localized DFSP is complete resection with negative margins. The NCCN guidelines recommend some form of complete histologic surgical margin evaluation whenever possible, implementing different approaches including: MMS; modified MMS (MMS technique with an additional final margin taken for permanent section assessment); CCPDMA; and 2 to 4 cm margins to investing fascia of muscle or pericranium with clear pathologic margins, when clinically feasible.[219] Recent studies conducted in different parts of the world consistently show a significant decrease in the rate of recurrence (under 10%), compared to the recurrence rate of 20% to 60% reported in older studies.[206,211,220–224] Especially in anatomically challenging areas such as head and neck, MMS was shown to achieve a high cure rate, with the local recurrence rate averaging approximately 1.5%.[220,225–233]

The efficacy of RT as primary therapy for DFSP is still controversial given the scant data available.[234,235] Currently, RT is not indicated routinely and is mostly utilized in the adjuvant setting when negative margins cannot be achieved surgically.[210,219,234–238]

DFSP metastasis to the lymph nodes is extremely rare. Although the management strategy is controversial, lymphadenectomy is generally recommended for patients with lymph node spread.[239,240] In extremely rare cases of hematogenous metastases, the lungs are the most common site of involvement, followed by brain, bone, and other soft tissues. For isolated, resectable metastatic disease, resection is recommended.[241,242]

Systemic treatment is indicated for metastatic disease and surgically unresectable cases. As discussed previously, the majority of DFSP tumors have the characteristic fusion gene product, COL1A1/PDGFB, which is the molecular target of the small molecule tyrosine kinase inhibitors (TKI), such as imatinib, sunitinib, and sorafenib. Imatinib, a chemotherapeutic agent commonly used in the treatment of chronic myelogenous leukemia and gastrointestinal stromal tumors, inhibits the PDGFR and other receptor tyrosine kinases, such as c-kit. There have been multiple studies, including large retrospective series and multicenter prospective phase II trials, demonstrating that most patients with advanced DFSP with this specific translocation benefit from imatinib therapy.[217,243–251] Interestingly, one case report in a patient with locally advanced DFSP with a negative 17,22 translocation by RT-PCR showed a partial response to imatinib.[252] These promising results promoted interest in the use of imatinib in the neoadjuvant setting for large unresectable or recurrent tumors. Early studies have demonstrated potential benefits, including

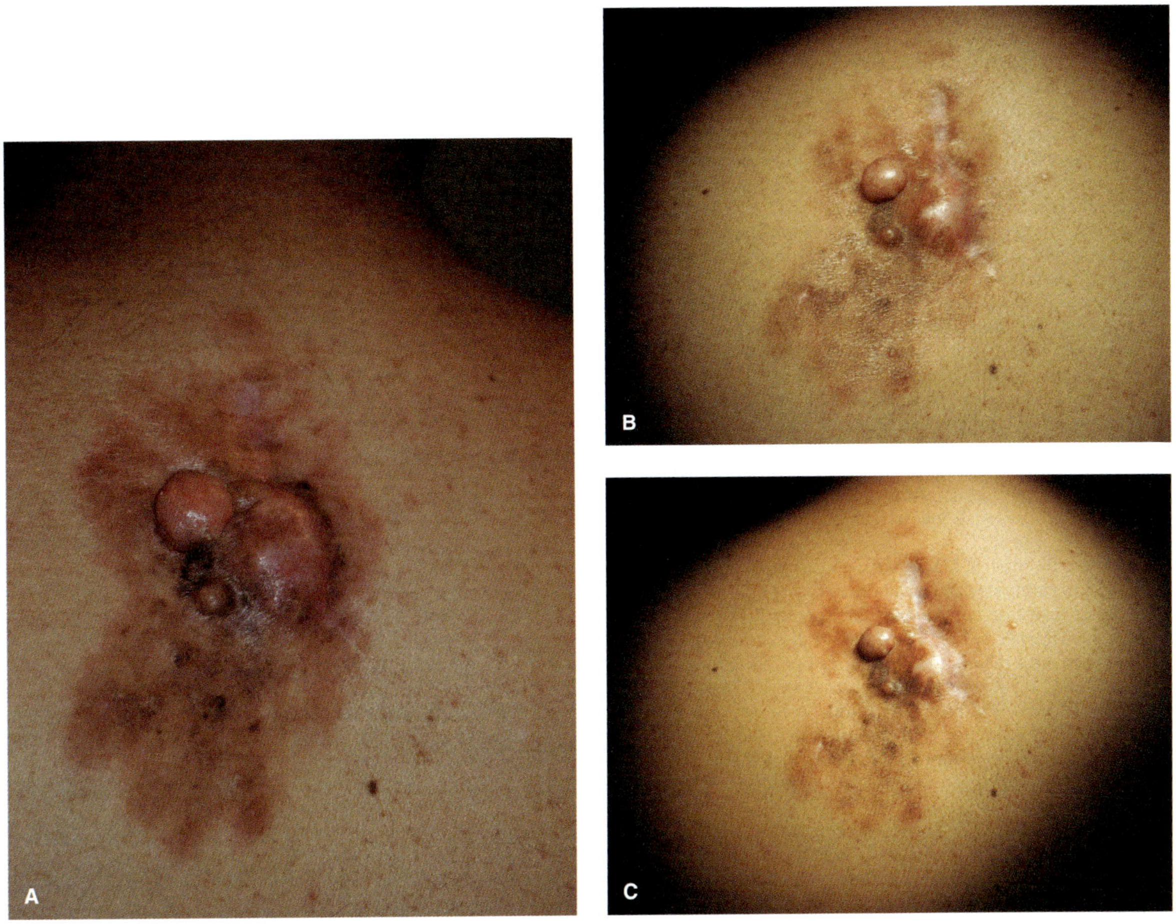

Figure 29-8 A. Patient with large recurrent DFSP of left upper back. The patient was started on imatinib to decrease the size of his lesion prior to Mohs surgery. **B.** The DFSP has shrunk considerably in thickness after 6 weeks of imatinib therapy. **C.** The lesion has shrunk still further after 9 weeks of imatinib, making it much easier to process the patient's specimen during Mohs micrographic surgery. (Used with permission of Désirée Ratner, MD.)

a decreased extent of excision and reconstruction and an improved rate of complete resection with negative margins.[212,248,249,253–257] The current NCCN guidelines recommend molecular analysis prior to initiation of imatinib. In the United States and Europe, imatinib treatment is indicated for adult patients with unresectable, recurrent and/or metastatic DFSP (Fig. 29-8).

The management of advanced NMSC appears to be entering a new phase of creative growth as new molecular targets are being discovered and translational research materializes into clinical applications.[258] The age of rationally designed molecular medicine not only instills hope but also raises concern for untoward effects that have yet to be elucidated. As new generations of drugs reach the clinic, we have reasons to be cautiously optimistic regarding the prognosis of those patients with advanced NMSC who were considered beyond hope just a generation ago.

REFERENCES

1. Buettner PG, Raasch BA. Incidence rates of skin cancer in Townsville, Australia. *Int J Cancer*. 1998;78:587–593.
2. Palme CE, MacKay SG, Kalnins I, Morgan GJ, Veness MJ. The need for a better prognostic staging system in patients with metastatic cutaneous squamous cell carcinoma of the head and neck. *Curr Opin Otolaryngol Head Neck Surg*. 2007;15:103–106.
3. Diepgen TL. The costs of skin disease. *Eur J Dermatol*. 2006;16:456–460.
4. Lomas A, Leonardi-Bee J, Bath-Hextall FA. Systematic review of worldwide incidence of nonmelanoma skin cancer. *Br J Dermatol*. 2012;166:1069–1080.
5. John Chen G, Yelverton CB, Polisetty SS, et al. Treatment patterns and cost of nonmelanoma skin cancer management. *Dermatol Surg*. 2006;32:1266–1271.
6. Jemal A, Siegel R, Ward E, Murray T, Xu J, Thun MJ. Cancer statistics. *CA Cancer J Clin*. 2007;57:43–66.
7. Talmi YP. Problems in the current TNM staging of nonmelanoma skin cancer of the head and neck. *Head Neck*. 2007;29:525–527.
8. WHO. Solar ultraviolet radiation: global burden of disease from solar ultraviolet radiation. WHO at http://www.who.int/uv/publications/solaradgbd/en/index.html. Accessed January 12, 2013.
9. Miller DL, Weinstock MA. Nonmelanoma skin cancer in the United States: incidence. *J Am Acad Dermatol*. 1994;30:774–778.
10. American cancer society cancer facts and figures 2010. at http://www.cancer.org/acs/groups/content/@epidemiologysurveilance/documents/document/acspc-026238.pdf. Accessed January 12, 2013.
11. Hannuksela-Svahn A, Pukkala E, Karvonen J. Basal cell skin carcinoma and other nonmelanoma skin cancers in

Finland from 1956 through 1995. *Arch Dermatol.* 1999;135: 781–786.
12. Green A, Battistutta D, Hart V, Leslie D, Weedon D. Skin cancer in a subtropical Australian population: incidence and lack of association with occupation. The Nambour Study Group. *Am J Epidemiol.* 1996;144:1034–1040.
13. Chuang TY, Popescu A, Su WP, Chute CG. Basal cell carcinoma. A population-based incidence study in Rochester, Minnesota. *J Am Acad Dermatol.* 1990;22:413–417.
14. Scotto J, Fears TR, Fraumeni JF Jr. Incidence of nonmelanoma skin cancer in the United States in collaboration with Fred Hutchinson. Cancer Research Center. 1983.
15. Christenson LJ, Borrowman TA, Vachon CM. Incidence of basal cell and squamous cell carcinomas in a population younger than 40 years. *JAMA.* 2005;294:681–690.
16. Vitasa BC, Taylor HR, Strickland PT, et al. Association of nonmelanoma skin cancer and actinic keratosis with cumulative solar ultraviolet exposure in Maryland watermen. *Cancer.* 1990;65:2811–2817.
17. Van Dam RM, Huang Z, Rimm EB, et al. Risk factors for basal cell carcinoma of the skin in men: results from the health professionals follow-up study. *Am J Epidemiol.* 1999; 150:459–468.
18. Zanetti R, Rosso S, Martinez C, et al. Comparison of risk patterns in carcinoma and melanoma of the skin in men: a multicentre case-case-control study. *Br J Cancer.* 2006; 94:743–751.
19. Boyd AS, Shyr Y, King LE Jr. Basal cell carcinoma in young women: an evaluation of the association of tanning bed use and smoking. *J Am Acad Dermatol.* 2002;46:706–709.
20. Karagas MR, Tosteson TD, Blum J, Morris JS, Baron JA, Klaue B. Design of an epidemiologic study of drinking water arsenic exposure and skin and bladder cancer risk in a U.S. population. *Environ Health Perspect.* 1998;106(suppl 4):1047–1050.
21. Tao SS, Bolger PM. Dietary arsenic intakes in the United States: FDA total diet study, September 1991-December 1996. *Food Addit Contam.* 1999;16:465–472.
22. Boonchai W, Green A, Ng J, Dicker A, Chenevix-Trench G. Basal cell carcinoma in chronic arsenicism occurring in Queensland, Australia, after ingestion of an asthma medication. *J Am Acad Dermatol.* 2000;43:664–669.
23. Ron E, Modan B, Preston D, Alfandary E, Stovall M, Boice JD Jr. Radiation-induced skin carcinomas of the head and neck. *Radiat Res.* 1991;125:318–325.
24. Lichter MD, Karagas MR, Mott LA, Spencer SK, Stukel TA, Greenberg ER. Therapeutic ionizing radiation and the incidence of basal cell carcinoma and squamous cell carcinoma. The New Hampshire Skin Cancer Study Group. *Arch Dermatol.* 2000;136:1007–1011.
25. Karagas MR, McDonald JA, Greenberg ER, et al. Risk of basal cell and squamous cell skin cancers after ionizing radiation therapy. For The Skin Cancer Prevention Study Group. *J Natl Cancer Inst.* 1996;88:1848–1853.
26. Ramsay HM, Fryer AA, Hawley CM, Smith AG, Nicol DL, Harden PN. Factors associated with nonmelanoma skin cancer following renal transplantation in Queensland, Australia. *J Am Acad Dermatol.* 2003;49:397–406.
27. Euvrard S, Kanitakis J, Claudy A. Skin cancers after organ transplantation. *N Engl J Med.* 2003;348:1681–1691.
28. Gudbjartsson DF, Sulem P, Stacey SN, et al. ASIP and TYR pigmentation variants associate with cutaneous melanoma and basal cell carcinoma. *Nat Genet.* 2008;40:886–891.
29. Ferrucci LM, Cartmel B, Molinaro AM, Leffell DJ, Bale AE, Mayne ST. Indoor tanning and risk of early-onset basal cell carcinoma. *J Am Acad Dermatol.* 2012;67(4):552–562. doi:10.1016/j.jaad.2011.11.940
30. Milán T, Verkasalo PK, Kaprio J, Koskenvuo M. Lifestyle differences in twin pairs discordant for basal cell carcinoma of the skin. *Br J Dermatol.* 2003;149:115–123.
31. Fine JD, Johnson LB, Weiner M, Li KP, Suchindran C. Epidermolysis bullosa and the risk of life-threatening cancers: the National EB Registry experience, 1986–2006. *J Am Acad Dermatol.* 2009;60:203–211.
32. Vitasa BC, Taylor HR, Strickland PT, et al. Association of nonmelanoma skin cancer and actinic keratosis with cumulative solar ultraviolet exposure in Maryland watermen. *Cancer.* 1990;65:2811–2817.
33. Boyd AS, Shyr Y, King LE Jr. Basal cell carcinoma in young women: an evaluation of the association of tanning bed use and smoking. *J Am Acad Dermatol.* 2002;46:706–709.
34. Kricker A, Armstrong BK, English DR, Heenan PJ. Does intermittent sun exposure cause basal cell carcinoma? a case-control study in Western Australia. *Int J Cancer.* 1995; 60:489–494.
35. Gallagher RP, Hill GB, Bajdik CD, et al. Sunlight exposure, pigmentary factors, and risk of nonmelanocytic skin cancer. I. Basal cell carcinoma. *Arch Dermatol.* 1995;131:157–163.
36. Stacey SN, Gudbjartsson DF, Sulem P, et al. Common variants on 1p36 and 1q42 are associated with cutaneous basal cell carcinoma but not with melanoma or pigmentation traits. *Nat Genet.* 2008;40:1313–1318.
37. Rafnar T, Sulem P, Stacey SN, et al. Sequence variants at the TERT-CLPTM1 L locus associate with many cancer types. *Nat Genet.* 2009;41:221–227.
38. Stacey SN, Sulem P, Masson G, et al. New common variants affecting susceptibility to basal cell carcinoma. *Nat Genet.* 2009;41:909–914.
39. Stacey SN, Sulem P, Jonasdottir A, et al. A germline variant in the TP53 polyadenylation signal confers cancer susceptibility. *Nat Genet.* 2011;43:1098–1103.
40. Welsh MM, Applebaum KM, Spencer SK, Perry AE, Karagas MR, Nelson HH. CTLA4 variants, UV-induced tolerance, and risk of non-melanoma skin cancer. *Cancer Res.* 2009;69:6158–6163.
41. Howell JB, Caro MR. The basal-cell nevus: its relationship to multiple cutaneous cancers and associated anomalies of development. *AMA Arch Derm.* 1959;79:67–77; discussion 77–80.
42. Gorlin RJ, Goltz RW. Multiple nevoid basal-cell epithelioma, jaw cysts and bifid rib. A syndrome. *N Engl J Med.* 1960; 262:908–912.
43. Hahn H, Wicking C, Zaphiropoulous PG, et al. Mutations of the human homolog of drosophila patched in the nevoid basal cell carcinoma syndrome. *Cell.* 1996;85:841–851.
44. Johnson RL, Rothman AL, Xie J, et al. Human homolog of patched, a candidate gene for the basal cell nevus syndrome. *Science.* 1996;272:1668–1671.
45. Li C, Chi S, Xie J. Hedgehog signaling in skin cancers. *Cell Signal.* 2011;23:1235–1243.
46. Kudchadkar R, Lewis K, Gonzalez R. Advances in the treatment of Basal cell carcinoma: hedgehog inhibitors. *Semin Oncol.* 2012;39:139–144.
47. Lum L, Beachy PA. The hedgehog response network: sensors, switches, and routers. *Science.* 2004;304:1755–1759.
48. Rohatgi R, Scott MP. Patching the gaps in Hedgehog signalling. *Nature Cell Biol.* 2007;9:1005–1009.
49. Varjosalo M, Taipale J. Hedgehog signaling. *J Cell Sci.* 2007; 120:3–6.
50. Bonifas JM, Pennypacker S, Chuang PT, et al. Activation of expression of hedgehog target genes in basal cell carcinomas. *J Invest Dermatol.* 2001;116:739–742.
51. Booth DR. The hedgehog signalling pathway and its role in basal cell carcinoma. *Cancer Metastasis Rev.* 1999;18:261–284.
52. Dahmane N. Activation of the transcription factor Gli1 and the Sonic hedgehog signalling pathway in skin tumours. *Nature.* 1997;389:876–881.
53. Eichberger T. FOXE1, a new transcriptional target of GLI2 is expressed in human epidermis and basal cell carcinoma. *J Invest Dermatol.* 2004;122:1180–1187.
54. Green J. Basal cell carcinoma development is associated with induction of the expression of the transcription factor Gli-1. *Br J Dermatol.* 1998;139:911–915.
55. Wicking C, Smyth I, Bale A. The hedgehog signalling pathway in tumorigenesis and development. *Oncogene.* 1999;18: 7844–7851.
56. Duman Scheel M, Weng L, Xin S, Du W. Hedgehog regulates cell growth and proliferation by inducing Cyclin D and Cyclin E. *Nature.* 2002;417:299–304.
57. Gailani MR. The role of the human homologue of Drosophila patched in sporadic basal cell carcinomas. *Nature Genet.* 1996;14:78–81.

58. Wolter M. Mutations in the human homologue of the Drosophila segment polarity gene patched (PTCH) in sporadic basal cell carcinomas of the skin and primitive neuroectodermal tumors of the central nervous system. *Cancer Res.* 1997;57:2581–2585.
59. Zhang H. Role of PTCH and p53 genes in early-onset basal cell carcinoma. *Amer J Pathol.* 2001;158:381–385.
60. Xie J. Activating Smoothened mutations in sporadic basal-cell carcinoma. *Nature.* 1998;391:90–92.
61. Jin Y. The reciprocal translocation t(9;16)(q22;p13) is a primary chromosome abnormality in basal cell carcinomas. *Cancer Res.* 1997;57:404–406.
62. Smyth I. Isolation and characterization of human patched 2 (PTCH2), a putative tumour suppressor gene inbasal cell carcinoma and medulloblastoma on chromosome 1p32. *Hum Mol Genet.* 1999;8:291–297.
63. Motoyama J. Ptch2, a second mouse Patched gene is co-expressed with Sonic hedgehog. *Nature Genet.* 1998; 18:104–106.
64. Vabres P, De Prost Y. Bazex-Dupré-Christol syndrome: a possible diagnosis for basal cell carcinomas, coarse sparse hair, and milia. *Am J Med Genet.* 1993;45:786.
65. Michaëlsson G, Olsson E, Westermark P. The Rombo syndrome: a familial disorder with vermiculate atrophoderma, milia, hypotrichosis, trichoepitheliomas, basal cell carcinomas and peripheral vasodilation with cyanosis. *Acta Derm Venereol.* 1981;61:497–503.
66. Mäkitie O, Pukkala E, Teppo L, Kaitila I. Increased incidence of cancer in patients with cartilage-hair hypoplasia. *J Pediatr.* 1999;134:315–318.
67. Kraemer KH, Patronas NJ, Schiffmann R, Brooks BP, Tamura D, DiGiovanna JJ. Xeroderma pigmentosum, trichothiodystrophy and Cockayne syndrome: a complex genotype-phenotype relationship. *Neuroscience.* 2007;145:1388–1396.
68. Kasper M, Jaks V, Hohl D, Toftgård R. Basal cell carcinoma - molecular biology and potential new therapies. *J Clin Invest.* 2012;122:455–463.
69. Adolphe C, Hetherington R, Ellis T, Wainwright B. Patched1 functions as a gatekeeper by promoting cell cycle progression. *Cancer Res.* 2006;66:2081–2088.
70. El-Bahrawy M, El-Masry N, Alison M, Poulsom R, Fallowfield M. Expression of beta-catenin in basal cell carcinoma. *Br J Dermatol.* 2003;148:964–970.
71. Yang SH, Andl T, Grachtchouk V, et al. Pathological responses to oncogenic Hedgehog signaling in skin are dependent on canonical Wnt/beta3-catenin signaling. *Nat Genet.* 2008;40:1130–1135.
72. Kasper M, Schnidar H, Neill GW, et al. Selective modulation of Hedgehog/GLI target gene expression by epidermal growth factor signaling in human keratinocytes. *Mol Cell Biol.* 2006;26:6283–6298.
73. Schnidar H, Eberl M, Klingler S, et al. Epidermal growth factor receptor signaling synergizes with Hedgehog/GLI in oncogenic transformation via activation of the MEK/ERK/JUN pathway. *Cancer Res.* 2009;69:1284–1292.
74. Kwasniak LA, Garcia-Zuazaga J. Basal cell carcinoma: evidence-based medicine and review of treatment modalities. *Int J Dermatol.* 2011;50:645–658.
75. Soehnge H, Ouhtit A, Ananthaswamy ON. Mechanisms of induction of skin cancer by UV radiation. *Front Biosci.* 1997;2:538–551.
76. Wang GY, Wang J, Mancianti M-L, Epstein EH Jr. Basal cell carcinomas arise from hair follicle stem cells in Ptch1(+/−) mice. *Cancer Cell.* 2011;19:114–124.
77. Sneddon JB, Zhen HH, Montgomery K, et al. Bone morphogenetic protein antagonist gremlin 1 is widely expressed by cancer-associated stromal cells and can promote tumor cell proliferation. *Proc Natl Acad Sci U.S.A.* 2006;103:14842–14847.
78. Epstein EH. Basal cell carcinomas: attack of the hedgehog. *Nat Rev Cancer.* 2008;8:743–754.
79. Batra RS, Kelley LC. Predictors of extensive subclinical spread in nonmelanoma skin cancer treated with Mohs micrographic surgery. *Arch Dermatol.* 2002;138:1043–1051.
80. Walling HW, Fosko SW, Geraminejad PA, Whitaker DC, Arpey CJ. Aggressive basal cell carcinoma: presentation, pathogenesis, and management. *Cancer Metastasis Rev.* 2004;23:389–402.
81. Miller SJ, Alam M, Andersen J, et al. Basal cell and squamous cell skin cancers. *J Natl Compr Canc Netw.* 2010;8:836–864.
82. NCCN Practice Guidelines in Oncology—v.1.2010: Basal cell and squamous cell skin cancers.at http://www.nccn.org
83. Kwan W, Wilson D, Moravan V. Radiotherapy for locally advanced basal cell and squamous cell carcinomas of the skin. *Int J Radiat Oncol Biol Phy.* 2004;60:406–411.
84. Telfer NR, Colver GB, Morton CA. Guidelines for the management of basal cell carcinoma. *Br J Dermatol.* 2008; 159:35–48.
85. Mills WA. Regulatory consideration in radiation protection. *Health Phys.* 1985;48:701–704.
86. Loncaster J, Swindell R, Slevin F, Sheridan L, Allan D, Allan E. Efficacy of photodynamic therapy as a treatment for Gorlin syndrome-related basal cell carcinomas. *Clinl Oncol.* 2009;21:502–508.
87. Thissen MR, Neumann MH, Schouten LJ. A systematic review of treatment modalities for primary basal cell carcinomas. *Arch Dermatol.* 1999;135:1177–1183.
88. Bath-Hextall FJ, Perkins W, Bong J, Williams HC. Interventions for basal cell carcinoma of the skin. *Cochrane Database Syst Rev.* John Wiley & Sons, Ltd; 2007. At http://onlinelibrary.wiley.com/doi/10.1002/14651858.CD003412.pub2/abstract
89. Binns W, James LF, Shupe JL, Everett GA. Congenital cyclopian-type malformation in lambs induced by maternal ingestion of a range plant, veratrum californicum. *Am J Vet Res.* 1963;24:1164–1175.
90. Chen JK, Taipale J, Cooper MK, Beachy PA. Inhibition of Hedgehog signaling by direct binding of cyclopamine to Smoothened. *Genes Dev.* 2002;16:2743–2748.
91. Athar M, Li C, Tang X, et al. Inhibition of smoothened signaling prevents ultraviolet B-induced basal cell carcinomas through regulation of Fas expression and apoptosis. *Cancer Res.* 2004;64:7545–7552.
92. Tabs S, Avci O. Induction of the differentiation and apoptosis of tumor cells in vivo with efficiency and selectivity. *Eur J Dermatol.* 2004;14:96–102.
93. Tremblay MR, Nevalainen M, Nair SJ, et al. Semisynthetic cyclopamine analogues as potent and orally bioavailable hedgehog pathway antagonists. *J Med Chem.* 2008;51:6646–6649.
94. Von Hoff DD, LoRusso PM, Rudin CM, et al. Inhibition of the hedgehog pathway in advanced basal-cell carcinoma. *N Engl J Med.* 2009;361:1164–1172.
95. LoRusso PM, Rudin CM, Reddy JC, et al. Phase I trial of hedgehog pathway inhibitor vismodegib (GDC-0449) in patients with refractory, locally advanced or metastatic solid tumors. *Clin Cancer Res.* 2011;17:2502–2511.
96. Sekulic A, Migden MR, Oro AE, et al. CO14. A pivotal study evaluating efficacy and safety of the hedgehog pathway inhibitor (HPI) vismodegib (GDC-0449) in patients with locally advanced (la) or metastatic (m) basal cell carcinoma (BCC). *Melanoma Res.* 2011;21:e9.
97. Sekulic A. Migden MR, Oro AE, et al. Efficacy and safety of vismodegib in advanced basal-cell carcinoma. *N Engl J Med.* 2012;366:2171–2179.
98. Chang AL, Oro AE. Initial assessment of tumor regrowth after vismodegib in advanced Basal cell carcinoma. *Arch Dermatol.* 2012;148:1324–1325.
99. Chang AL, Atwood SX, Tartar DM, Oro AE. Surgical excision after neoadjuvant therapy with vismodegib for a locally advanced basal cell carcinoma and resistant basal carcinomas in Gorlin syndrome. *JAMA Dermatol.* 2013;149:639–641.
100. Hutchin ME, Kariapper MS, Grachtchouk M, et al. Sustained Hedgehog signaling is required for basal cell carcinoma proliferation and survival: conditional skin tumorigenesis recapitulates the hair growth cycle. *Genes Dev.* 2005;19: 214–223.
101. Skvara H, Kalthoff F, Meingassner JG, et al. Topical treatment of Basal cell carcinomas in nevoid Basal cell carcinoma syndrome with a smoothened inhibitor. *J Invest Dermatol.* 2011;131:1735–1744.

102. Buonamici S, Williams J, Morrissey M, et al. Interfering with resistance to smoothened antagonists by inhibition of the PI3 K pathway in medulloblastoma. *Sci Transl Med.* 2010;2:51ra70.
103. Dijkgraaf GJ, Alicke B, Weinmann L, et al. Small molecule inhibition of GDC-0449 refractory smoothened mutants and downstream mechanisms of drug resistance. *Cancer Res.* 2011;71:435–444.
104. Kim J, Tang JY, Gong R, et al. Itraconazole, a commonly used antifungal that inhibits Hedgehog pathway activity and cancer growth. *Cancer Cell.* 2010;17:388–399.
105. Tang JY, Mackay-Wiggan JM, Aszterbaum M, et al. Inhibiting the hedgehog pathway in patients with the basal-cell nevus syndrome. *N Engl J Med.* 2012;366:2180–2188.
106. Hall JM, Bell ML, Finger TE. Disruption of sonic hedgehog signaling alters growth and patterning of lingual taste papillae. *Dev Biol.* 2003;255:263–277.
107. St-Jacques B, Dassule HR, Karavanova I, et al. Sonic hedgehog signaling is essential for hair development. *Curr Biol.* 1998;8:1058–1068.
108. Lauth M, Bergström A, Shimokawa T, Toftgård R. Inhibition of GLI-mediated transcription and tumor cell growth by small-molecule antagonists. *Proc Natl Acad Sci U.S.A.* 2007;104:8455–8460.
109. Hyman JM, Firestone AJ, Heine VM, et al. Small-molecule inhibitors reveal multiple strategies for Hedgehog pathway blockade. *Proc Natl Acad Sci U.S.A.* 2009;106:14132–14137.
110. Beauchamp EM, Ringer L, Bulut G, et al. Arsenic trioxide inhibits human cancer cell growth and tumor development in mice by blocking Hedgehog/GLI pathway. *J Clin Invest.* 2011;121:148–160.
111. Kim J, Lee JJ, Kim J, Gardner D, Beachy PA. Arsenic antagonizes the Hedgehog pathway by preventing ciliary accumulation and reducing stability of the Gli2 transcriptional effector. *Proc Natl Acad Sci U.S.A.* 2010;107:13432–13437.
112. Salehi Z, Mashayekhi F, Shahosseini F. Significance of eIF4E expression in skin squamous cell carcinoma. *Cell Biol Int.* 2007;31:1400–1404.
113. Johnson TM, Rowe DE, Nelson BR, Swanson NA. Squamous cell carcinoma of the skin (excluding lip and oral mucosa). *J Am Acad Dermatol.* 1992;26:467–484.
114. Weinberg AS, Ogle CA, Shim EK. Metastatic cutaneous squamous cell carcinoma: an update. *Dermatol Surg.* 2007;33:885–899.
115. Alam M, Ratner D. Cutaneous squamous cell carcinoma. *N Engl J Med.* 2001;344:975–983.
116. Holme SA, Malinovszky K, Roberts DL. Changing trends in non-melanoma skin cancer in South Wales, 1988–98. *Br J Dermatol.* 2000;143:1224–1229.
117. Veness MJ. Defining patients with high-risk cutaneous squamous cell carcinoma. *Australas J Dermatol.* 2006;47:28–33.
118. Hampton T. Skin cancer's ranks rise: immunosuppression to blame. *JAMA.* 2005;294:1476–1480
119. Venessa M. Advanced non melanoma skin cancers of the head and neck: an overview on management. *Cancer Forum.* 2006;30:195–201.
120. Rowe DE, Carroll RJ, Day CL Jr. Prognostic factors for local recurrence, metastasis, and survival rates in squamous cell carcinoma of the skin, ear, and lip. Implications for treatment modality selection. *J Am Acad Dermatol.* 1992;26:976–990.
121. Moore BA, Weber RS, Prieto V, et al. Lymph node metastases from cutaneous squamous cell carcinoma of the head and neck. *Laryngoscope.* 2005;115:1561–1567.
122. Urbach F. Geographic distribution of skin cancer. *J Surg Oncol.* 1971;3:219–234.
123. Staples M, Marks R, Giles G. Trends in the incidence of nonmelanocytic skin cancer (NMSC) treated in Australia 1985–1995: are primary prevention programs starting to have an effect? *Int J Cancer.* 1998;78:144–148.
124. Euvrard S, Kanitakis J, Pouteil-Noble C, et al. Comparative epidemiologic study of premalignant and malignant epithelial cutaneous lesions developing after kidney and heart transplantation. *J Am Acad Dermatol.* 1995;33:222–229.
125. Hartevelt MM, Bavinck JN, Kootte AM, Vermeer BJ, Vandenbroucke JP. Incidence of skin cancer after renal transplantation in The Netherlands. *Transplantation.* 1990;49:506–509.
126. Lanza RP, Cooper DK, Cassidy MJ, Barnard CN. Malignant neoplasms occurring after cardiac transplantation. *JAMA.* 1983;249:1746–1748.
127. Penn I. Tumors after renal and cardiac transplantation. *Hematol Oncol Clin North Am.* 1993;7:431–445.
128. Bernstein D, Baum D, Berry G, et al. Neoplastic disorders after pediatric heart transplantation. *Circulation.* 1993;88:II230–237.
129. Pollard JD, Hanasono MM, Mikulec AA, Le QT, Terris DJ. Head and neck cancer in cardiothoracic transplant recipients. *Laryngoscope.* 2000;110:1257–1261.
130. Gourin CG, Terris DJ. Head and neck cancer in transplant recipients. *Curr Opin Otolaryngol Head Neck Surg.* 2004;12:122–126.
131. Penn I. Cancers in renal transplant recipients. *Adv Ren Replace Ther.* 2000;7:147–156.
132. Jensen P Hansen S, Møller B, et al. Skin cancer in kidney and heart transplant recipients and different long-term immunosuppressive therapy regimens. *J Am Acad Dermatol.* 1999;40:177–186.
133. Fearon ER, Vogelstein B. A genetic model for colorectal tumorigenesis. *Cell.* 1990;61:759–767.
134. Ratushny V, Gober MD, Hick R, Ridky TW, Seykora JT. From keratinocyte to cancer: the pathogenesis and modeling of cutaneous squamous cell carcinoma. *J Clin Invest.* 2012;122:464–472.
135. Brash DE, Rudolph JA, Simon JA, et al. A role for sunlight in skin cancer: UV-induced p53 mutations in squamous cell carcinoma. *Proc Natl Acad Sci U.S.A.* 1991;88:10124–10128.
136. Jiang W, Ananthaswamy HN, Muller HK, Kripke ML. p53 protects against skin cancer induction by UV-B radiation. *Oncogene.* 1999;18:4247–4253.
137. Kubo Y, Urano Y, Yoshimoto K, et al. p53 gene mutations in human skin cancers and precancerous lesions: comparison with immunohistochemical analysis. *J Invest Dermatol.* 1994;102:440–444.
138. Ziegler A, Jonason AS, Leffell DJ, et al. Sunburn and p53 in the onset of skin cancer. *Nature.* 1994;372:773–776.
139. Nelson MA, Einspahr JG, Alberts DS, et al. Analysis of the p53 gene in human precancerous actinic keratosis lesions and squamous cell cancers. *Cancer Lett.* 1994;85:23–29.
140. Kolev V, Mandinova A, Guinea-Viniegra J, et al. EGFR signalling as a negative regulator of Notch1 gene transcription and function in proliferating keratinocytes and cancer. *Nat Cell Biol.* 2008;10:902–911.
141. Zhao L, Li W, Marshall C, et al. Srcasm inhibits Fyn-induced cutaneous carcinogenesis with modulation of Notch1 and p53. *Cancer Res.* 2009;69:9439–9447.
142. Pierceall WE, Goldberg LH, Tainsky MA, Mukhopadhyay T, Ananthaswamy HN. Ras gene mutation and amplification in human nonmelanoma skin cancers. *Mol Carcinog.* 1991;4:196–202.
143. Spencer JM, Kahn SM, Jiang W, DeLeo VA, Weinstein IB. Activated ras genes occur in human actinic keratoses, premalignant precursors to squamous cell carcinomas. *Arch Dermatol.* 1995;131:796–800.
144. Boukamp P. Non-melanoma skin cancer: what drives tumor development and progression? *Carcinogenesis.* 2005;26:1657–1667.
145. Khavari PA. Modelling cancer in human skin tissue. *Nat Rev Cancer.* 2006;6:270–280.
146. Ridky TW, Chow JM, Wong DJ, Khavari PA. Invasive three-dimensional organotypic neoplasia from multiple normal human epithelia. *Nat Med.* 2010;16:1450–1455.
147. Dajee M, Lazarov M, Zhang JY, et al. NF-kappaB blockade and oncogenic Ras trigger invasive human epidermal neoplasia. *Nature.* 2003;421:639–643.
148. Rowe DE, Carroll RJ, Day CL Jr. Prognostic factors for local recurrence, metastasis, and survival rates in squamous cell carcinoma of the skin, ear, and lip. Implications for

treatment modality selection. *J Am Acad Dermatol.* 1992; 26:976–990.
149. Leibovitch I, Huilgol SC, Selva D, Hill D, Richards S, Paver R. Cutaneous squamous cell carcinoma treated with Mohs micrographic surgery in Australia I. Experience over 10 years. *J Am Acad Dermatol.* 2005;53:253–260.
150. Jambusaria-Pahlajani A., Hess SD, Katz KA, Berg D, Schmults CD. Uncertainty in the perioperative management of high-risk cutaneous squamous cell carcinoma among Mohs surgeons. *Arch Dermatol.* 2010;146:1225–1231.
151. Sandulache VC, Ow TJ, Daram SP, et al. Residual nodal disease in patients with advanced-stage oropharyngeal squamous cell carcinoma treated with definitive radiation therapy and posttreatment neck dissection: Association with locoregional recurrence, distant metastasis, and decreased survival. *Head Neck.* 35;2012:1454–1460.doi:10.1002/hed. 23173
152. Veness M, Richards S. Role of modern radiotherapy in treating skin cancer. *Australas J Dermatol.* 2003;44:159–166; quiz 167–168.
153. Bonner JA, Harari PM, Giralt J, et al. Radiotherapy plus cetuximab for squamous-cell carcinoma of the head and neck. *N Engl J Med.* 2006;354:567–578.
154. Loeffler JS, Larson DA, Clark JR, Weichselbaum RR, Norris CM Jr, Ervin TJ. Treatment of perineural metastasis from squamous carcinoma of the skin with aggressive combination chemotherapy and irradiation. *J Surg Oncol.* 1985;29:181–183.
155. Fujisawa Y, Umebayashi Y, Ichikawa E, Kawachi Y, Otsuka F. Chemoradiation using low-dose cisplatin and 5-fluorouracil in locally advanced squamous cell carcinoma of the skin: a report of two cases. *J Am Acad Dermatol.* 2006;55: S81–S85.
156. Ley J, Mehan P, Wildes TM, et al. Cisplatin versus cetuximab given concurrently with definitive radiation therapy for locally advanced head and neck squamous cell carcinoma. *Oncology.* 2013;85:290–296.
157. DeConti RC. Chemotherapy of squamous cell carcinoma of the skin. *Semin Oncol.* 2012;39:145–149.
158. Sadek H, Azli N, Wendling JL, et al. Treatment of advanced squamous cell carcinoma of the skin with cisplatin, 5-fluorouracil, and bleomycin. *Cancer.* 1990;66:1692–1696.
159. Shin DM, Glisson BS, Khuri FR, et al. Phase II and biologic study of interferon alfa, retinoic acid, and cisplatin in advanced squamous skin cancer. *J Clin Oncol.* 2002;20:364–370.
160. Guthrie TH Jr, McElveen LJ, Porubsky ES, Harmon JD. Cisplatin and doxorubicin. An effective chemotherapy combination in the treatment of advanced basal cell and squamous carcinoma of the skin. *Cancer.* 1985;55:1629–1632.
161. Brewster AM, Lee JJ, Clayman GL, et al. Randomized trial of adjuvant 13-cis-retinoic acid and interferon alfa for patients with aggressive skin squamous cell carcinoma. *J Clin Oncol.* 2007;25:1974–1978.
162. Lemos B, Nghiem P. Merkel cell carcinoma: More deaths but still no pathway to blame. *J Invest Dermatol.* 2007;127: 2100–2103.
163. Alter M, Satzger I, Mattern A, Kapp A, Gutzmer R. Treatment of advanced cutaneous squamous cell carcinomas with epidermal growth factor receptor inhibitors. *Dermatology.* 2013;227:289–294.doi:10.1159/000355181
164. Maubec E, Petrow P, Scheer-Senyarich I, et al. Phase II study of cetuximab as first-line single-drug therapy in patients with unresectable squamous cell carcinoma of the skin. *J Clin Oncol.* 2011;29:3419–3426.
165. Wollina U. Cetuximab in non-melanoma skin cancer. *Expert Opin Biol Ther.* 2012;12:949–956.
166. Habl G, Potthoff K, Haefner MF, et al. Differentiation of irradiation and cetuximab induced skin reactions in patients with locally advanced head and neck cancer undergoing radioimmunotherapy: the HICARE protocol (head and neck cancer: immunochemo and radiotherapy with erbitux) - a multicenter phase IV trial. *BMC Cancer.* 2013;13:345.
167. O'Bryan KW, Sherman WH, Niedt GW, Taback B, Manolidis S, Ratner D. An evolving paradigm for the work-up and management of very high risk cutaneous squamous cell carcinomas. *J Am Acad Dermatol.* 2013;69(4):595–602.
168. Psyrri A, Seiwert TY, Jimeno A. Molecular pathways in head and neck cancer. *Am Soc Clin Oncol Educ Book.* 2013;246–255.doi:10.1200/EdBook_AM.2013.33.246
169. Albores Saavedra J. Merkel cell carcinoma demographics, morphology, and survival based on 3870 cases: a population based study. *J Cutaneous Pathol.* 2010;37:20–27.
170. Hodgson NC. Merkel cell carcinoma: Changing incidence trends. *J Surg Oncol.* 2005;89:1–4.
171. Hitchcock CL, Bland KI, Laney RG 3rd, Franzini D, Harris B, Copeland EM 3rd. Neuroendocrine (Merkel cell) carcinoma of the skin. Its natural history, diagnosis, and treatment. *Ann Surg.* 1988;207:201–207.
172. Engels EA, Frisch M, Goedert JJ, Biggar RJ, Miller RW. Merkel cell carcinoma and HIV infection. *Lancet.* 2002;359:497–498.
173. Busam KJ, Jungbluth AA, Rekthman N, et al. Merkel cell polyomavirus expression in merkel cell carcinomas and its absence in combined tumors and pulmonary neuroendocrine carcinomas. *Am J Surg Pathol.* 2009;33:1378–1385.
174. Howard RA. Merkel cell carcinoma and multiple primary cancers. *Cancer Epidemiol Biomarkers Prev.* 2006;15:1545–1549.
175. Kaae J. Merkel cell carcinoma: incidence, mortality, and risk of other cancers. *J Natl Cancer Inst.* 2010;102:793–801.
176. Heath M, Jaimes N, Lemos B, et al. Clinical characteristics of Merkel cell carcinoma at diagnosis in 195 patients: the AEIOU features. *J Amer Acad Dermatol.* 2008;58:375–381.
177. Lemos BD, Storer BE, Iyer JG, et al. Pathologic nodal evaluation improves prognostic accuracy in Merkel cell carcinoma: analysis of 5823 cases as the basis of the first consensus staging system. *J Am Acad Dermatol.* 2010;63: 751–761.
178. Wang TS, Byrne PJ, Jacobs LK, Taube JM. Merkel cell carcinoma: update and review. *Semin Cutan Med Surg.* 2011;30:48–56.
179. Miller RW, Rabkin CS. Merkel cell carcinoma and melanoma: etiological similarities and differences. *Cancer Epidemiol Biomarkers Prev.* 1999;8:153–158.
180. Lunder EJ, Stern RS. Merkel-cell carcinomas in patients treated with methoxsalen and ultraviolet A radiation. *N Engl J Med.* 1998;339:1247–1248.
181. Van Gele M. Mutation analysis of P73 and TP53 in Merkel cell carcinoma. *Br J Cancer.* 2000;82:823–826.
182. Feng H, Shuda M, Chang Y, Moore PS. Clonal integration of a polyomavirus in human Merkel cell carcinoma. *Science.* 2008;319:1096–1100.
183. Sastre-Garau X, Peter M, Avril MF, et al. Merkel cell carcinoma of the skin: pathological and molecular evidence for a causative role of MCV in oncogenesis. *J Pathol.* 2009; 218:48–56.
184. Shuda M, Feng H, Kwun HJ, et al. T antigen mutations are a human tumor-specific signature for Merkel cell polyomavirus. *Proc Natl Acad Sci U S A.* 2008;105:16272–16277.
185. Kassem A, Schöpflin A, Diaz C, et al. Frequent detection of Merkel cell polyomavirus in human Merkel cell carcinomas and identification of a unique deletion in the VP1 gene. *Cancer Res.* 2008;68:5009–5013.
186. Schrama D, Peitsch WK, Zapatka M, et al. Merkel cell polyomavirus status is not associated with clinical course of Merkel cell carcinoma. *J Invest Dermatol.* 2011;131:1631–1638.
187. Sihto H, Kukko H, Koljonen V, Sankila R, Böhling T, Joensuu H. Clinical factors associated with Merkel cell polyomavirus infection in Merkel cell carcinoma. *J Natl Cancer Inst.* 2009;101:938–945.
188. Kassem A, Technau K, Kurz AK, et al. Merkel cell polyomavirus sequences are frequently detected in nonmelanoma skin cancer of immunosuppressed patients. *Int J Cancer.* 2009;125:356–361.
189. Rollison DE, Giuliano AR, Messina JL, et al. Case-control study of Merkel cell polyomavirus infection and cutaneous squamous cell carcinoma. *Cancer Epidemiol Biomarkers Prev.* 2012;21:74–81.
190. Murakami M, Imajoh M, Ikawa T, et al. Presence of Merkel cell polyomavirus in Japanese cutaneous squamous cell carcinoma. *J Clin Virol.* 2011;50:37–41.

191. Dworkin AM, Tseng SY, Allain DC, Iwenofu OH, Peters SB, Toland AE. Merkel cell polyomavirus in cutaneous squamous cell carcinoma of immunocompetent individuals. *J Invest Dermatol.* 2009;129:2868–2874.
192. Foulongne V, Dereure O, Kluger N, Molès JP, Guillot B, Segondy M. Merkel cell polyomavirus DNA detection in lesional and nonlesional skin from patients with Merkel cell carcinoma or other skin diseases. *Br J Dermatol.* 2010;162:59–63.
193. Bhatia K, Goedert JJ, Modali R, Preiss L, Ayers LW. Merkel cell carcinoma subgroups by Merkel cell polyomavirus DNA relative abundance and oncogene expression. *Int J Cancer.* 2010;126:2240–2246.
194. Handschel J, Müller D, Depprich RA, et al. The new polyomavirus (MCPyV) does not affect the clinical course in MCCs. *Int J Oral Maxillofac Surg.* 2010;39:1086–1090.
195. Miller SJ, Alam M, Andersen J, et al. Merkel Cell Carcinoma. *J Natl Compr Canc Netw.* 2009;7:322–332.
196. Gupta SG, Wang LC, Peñas PF, Gellenthin M, Lee SJ, Nghiem P. Sentinel lymph node biopsy for evaluation and treatment of patients with Merkel cell carcinoma: the Dana-Farber experience and meta-analysis of the literature. *Arch Dermatol.* 2006;142:685–690.
197. Lewis KG, Weinstock MA, Weaver AL, Otley CC. Adjuvant local irradiation for Merkel cell carcinoma. *Arch Dermatol.* 2006;142:693–700.
198. Mojica P, Smith D, Ellenhorn JD. Adjuvant radiation therapy is associated with improved survival in merkel cell carcinoma of the skin. *J Clin Oncol.* 2007;25:1043–1047.
199. Veness M, Foote M, Gebski V, Poulsen M. The role of radiotherapy alone in patients with merkel cell carcinoma: reporting the Australian experience of 43 patients. *Int J Radiat Oncol Biol Phys.* 2010;78:703–709.
200. Pape E, Rezvoy N, Penel N, et al. Radiotherapy alone for Merkel cell carcinoma: a comparative and retrospective study of 25 patients. *J Am Acad Dermatol.* 2011;65:983–990.
201. Garneski KM, Nghiem P. Merkel cell carcinoma adjuvant therapy: Current data support radiation but not chemotherapy. *J Am Acad Dermatol.* 2007;57:166–169.
202. Voog E, Biron P, Martin J-P, Blay J-Y. Chemotherapy for patients with locally advanced or metastatic Merkel cell carcinoma. *Cancer.* 1999;85:2589–2595.
203. Gloster HM Jr. Dermatofibrosarcoma protuberans. *J Am Acad Dermatol.* 1996;35:355–374; quiz 375–376.
204. Criscione VD, Weinstock MA. Descriptive epidemiology of dermatofibrosarcoma protuberans in the United States, 1973 to 2002. *J Am Acad Dermatol.* 2007;56:968–973.
205. Rouhani P, Fletcher CD, Devesa SS, Toro JR. Cutaneous soft tissue sarcoma incidence patterns in the U.S.: an analysis of 12,114 cases. *Cancer.* 2008;113:616–627.
206. Chang CK, Jacobs IA, Salti GI. Outcomes of surgery for dermatofibrosarcoma protuberans. *Eur J Surg Oncol.* 2004; 30:341–345.
207. Kransdorf MJ. Malignant soft-tissue tumors in a large referral population: distribution of diagnoses by age, sex, and location. *AJR Am J Roentgenol.* 1995;164:129–134.
208. Laskin WB. Dermatofibrosarcoma protuberans. *CA Cancer J Clin.* 1992;42:116–125.
209. Rutgers EJ, Kroon BB, Albus-Lutter CE, Gortzak E. Dermatofibrosarcoma protuberans: treatment and prognosis. *Eur J Surg Oncol.* 1992;18:241–248.
210. Lindner N, Scarborough M, Powell G. Revision surgery in dermatofibrosarcoma protuberans of the trunk and extremities. *Eur J Surg Oncol.* 1999;25:392–397.
211. Fiore M, Miceli R, Mussi C, et al. Dermatofibrosarcoma protuberans treated at a single institution: a surgical disease with a high cure rate. *J Clin Oncol.* 2005;23:7669–7675.
212. Malhotra B, Schuetze SM. Dermatofibrosarcoma protruberans treatment with platelet-derived growth factor receptor inhibitor. *Curr Opin Oncol.* 2012;24:419–424.
213. Haycox CL, Odland PB, Olbricht SM, Piepkorn M. Immunohistochemical characterization of dermatofibrosarcoma protuberans with practical applications for diagnosis and treatment. *J Am Acad Dermatol.* 1997;37:438–444.
214. Simon MP, Pedeutour F, Sirvent N, et al. Deregulation of the platelet-derived growth factor B-chain gene via fusion with collagen gene COL1A1 in dermatofibrosarcoma protuberans and giant-cell fibroblastoma. *Nat Genet.* 1997;15:95–98.
215. Sjöblom T, Shimizu A, O'Brien KP, et al. Growth inhibition of dermatofibrosarcoma protuberans tumors by the platelet-derived growth factor receptor antagonist STI571 through induction of apoptosis. *Cancer Res.* 2001;61:5778–5783.
216. McArthur GA. Dermatofibrosarcoma protuberans: a surgical disease with a molecular savior. *Curr Opin Oncol.* 2006;18:341–346.
217. Kiuru-Kuhlefelt S, El-Rifai W, Fanburg-Smith J, et al. Concomitant DNA copy number amplification at 17q and 22q in dermatofibrosarcoma protuberans. *Cytogenet Cell Genet.* 2001;92:192–195.
218. Patel KU, Szabo SS, Hernandez VS, et al. Dermatofibrosarcoma protuberans COL1A1-PDGFB fusion is identified in virtually all dermatofibrosarcoma protuberans cases when investigated by newly developed multiplex reverse transcription polymerase chain reaction and fluorescence in situ hybridization assays. *Hum Pathol.* 2008;39:184–193.
219. National Comprehensive Cancer Network (NCCN) guidelines. At www.nccn.org
220. DuBay D, Cimmino V, Lowe L, Johnson TM, Sondak VK. Low recurrence rate after surgery for dermatofibrosarcoma protuberans: a multidisciplinary approach from a single institution. *Cancer.* 2004;100:1008–1016.
221. Farma JM, Ammori JB, Zager JS, et al. Dermatofibrosarcoma protuberans: how wide should we resect? *Ann Surg Oncol.* 2010;17:2112–2118.
222. Cai H, Wang Y, Wu J, Shi Y. Dermatofibrosarcoma protuberans: clinical diagnoses and treatment results of 260 cases in China. *J Surg Oncol.* 2012;105:142–148.
223. Mentzel T, Beham A, Katenkamp D, Dei Tos AP, Fletcher CD. Fibrosarcomatous ('high-grade') dermatofibrosarcoma protuberans: clinicopathologic and immunohistochemical study of a series of 41 cases with emphasis on prognostic significance. *Am J Surg Pathol.* 1998;22:576–587.
224. Fields RC, Hameed M, Qin LX, et al. Dermatofibrosarcoma protuberans (DFSP): predictors of recurrence and the use of systemic therapy. *Ann Surg Oncol.* 2011;18:328–336.
225. Gloster HM Jr, Harris KR, Roenigk RK. A comparison between Mohs micrographic surgery and wide surgical excision for the treatment of dermatofibrosarcoma protuberans. *J Am Acad Dermatol.* 1996;35:82–87.
226. Snow SN, Gordon EM, Larson PO, Bagheri MM, Bentz ML, Sable DB. Dermatofibrosarcoma protuberans: a report on 29 patients treated by Mohs micrographic surgery with long-term follow-up and review of the literature. *Cancer.* 2004;101:28–38.
227. Wacker J, Khan-Durani B, Hartschuh W. Modified Mohs micrographic surgery in the therapy of dermatofibrosarcoma protuberans: analysis of 22 patients. *Ann Surg Oncol.* 2004;11:438–444.
228. Nouri K, Lodha R, Jimenez G, Robins P. Mohs micrographic surgery for dermatofibrosarcoma protuberans: university of Miami and NYU experience. *Dermatol Surg.* 2002;28:1060–1064; discussion 1064.
229. Robinson JK. Dermatofibrosarcoma protuberans resected by Mohs' surgery (chemosurgery). A 5-year prospective study. *J Am Acad Dermatol.* 1985;12:1093–1098.
230. Ratner D, Thomas CO, Johnson TM, et al. Mohs micrographic surgery for the treatment of dermatofibrosarcoma protuberans. Results of a multiinstitutional series with an analysis of the extent of microscopic spread. *J Am Acad Dermatol.* 1997;37:600–613.
231. Haycox CL, Odland PB, Olbricht SM, Casey B. Dermatofibrosarcoma protuberans (DFSP): growth characteristics based on tumor modeling and a review of cases treated with Mohs micrographic surgery. *Ann Plast Surg.* 1997;38:246–251.
232. Nelson RA, Arlette JP. Mohs micrographic surgery and dermatofibrosarcoma protuberans: a multidisciplinary approach in 44 patients. *Ann Plast Surg.* 2008;60:667–672.
233. Lemm D, Mügge L-O, Mentzel T, Höffken K. Current treatment options in dermatofibrosarcoma protuberans. *J Cancer Res Clin Oncol.* 2009;135:653–665.

234. Suit H, Spiro I, Mankin HJ, Efird J, Rosenberg AE. Radiation in management of patients with dermatofibrosarcoma protuberans. *J Clin Oncol.* 1996;14:2365–2369.
235. Ballo MT, Zagars GK, Pisters P, Pollack A. The role of radiation therapy in the management of dermatofibrosarcoma protuberans. *Int J Radiat Oncol Biol Phys.* 1998;40:823–827.
236. Sun LM, Wang CJ, Huang CC, et al. Dermatofibrosarcoma protuberans: treatment results of 35 cases. *Radiother Oncol.* 2000;57:175–181.
237. Haas RL, Keus RB, Loftus BM, Rutgers EJ, van Coevorden F, Bartelink H. The role of radiotherapy in the local management of dermatofibrosarcoma protuberans. Soft Tissue Tumours Working Group. *Eur J Cancer.* 1997;33:1055–1060.
238. Dagan R, Morris CG, Zlotecki RA, Scarborough MT, Mendenhall WM. Radiotherapy in the treatment of dermatofibrosarcoma protuberans. *Am J Clin Oncol.* 2005;28:537–539.
239. Mavili ME, Gursu KG, Gokoz A. Dermatofibrosarcoma with lymph node involvement. *Ann Plast Surg.* 1994;32:438–440.
240. Lal P, Sharma R, Mohan H, Sekhon MS. Dermatofibrosarcoma protuberans metastasizing to lymph nodes: a case report and review of literature. *J Surg Oncol.* 1999;72:178–180.
241. Connelly JH, Evans HL. Dermatofibrosarcoma protuberans. A clinicopathologic review with emphasis on fibrosarcomatous areas. *Am J Surg Pathol.* 1992;16:921–925.
242. Westermann GW, Buerger H, Kappes U, Matzkies F, Kisters K. Dermatofibrosarcoma protuberans with lung metastasis in a patient with progressive systemic sclerosis. *South Med J.* 2002;95:363–365.
243. Maki RG, Awan RA, Dixon RH, Jhanwar S, Antonescu CR. Differential sensitivity to imatinib of 2 patients with metastatic sarcoma arising from dermatofibrosarcoma protuberans. *Int J Cancer.* 2002;100:623–626.
244. Rutkowski P, Van Glabbeke M, Rankin CJ, et al. Imatinib mesylate in advanced dermatofibrosarcoma protuberans: pooled analysis of two phase II clinical trials. *J Clin Oncol.* 2010;28:1772–1779.
245. Labropoulos SV, Fletcher JA, Oliveira AM, Papadopoulos S, Razis ED. Sustained complete remission of metastatic dermatofibrosarcoma protuberans with imatinib mesylate. *Anticancer Drugs.* 2005;16:461–466.
246. Abbott JJ, Erickson-Johnson M, Wang X, Nascimento AG, Oliveira AM. Gains of COL1A1-PDGFB genomic copies occur in fibrosarcomatous transformation of dermatofibrosarcoma protuberans. *Mod Pathol.* 2006;19:1512–1518.
247. Wang J, Morimitsu Y, Okamoto S, et al. COL1A1-PDGFB fusion transcripts in fibrosarcomatous areas of six dermatofibrosarcomas protuberans. *J Mol Diagn.* 2000;2:47–52.
248. Kerob D, Pedeutour F, Leboeuf C, et al. Value of cytogenetic analysis in the treatment of dermatofibrosarcoma protuberans. *J Clin Oncol.* 2008;26:1757–1759.
249. McArthur GA, Demetri GD, van Oosterom A, et al. Molecular and clinical analysis of locally advanced dermatofibrosarcoma protuberans treated with imatinib: Imatinib Target Exploration Consortium Study B2225. *J Clin Oncol.* 2005;23:866–873.
250. Mizutani K, Tamada Y, Hara K. et al. Imatinib mesylate inhibits the growth of metastatic lung lesions in a patient with dermatofibrosarcoma protuberans. *Br J Dermatol.* 2004;151:235–237.
251. Rubin BP, Schuetze SM, Eary JF, et al. Molecular targeting of platelet-derived growth factor B by imatinib mesylate in a patient with metastatic dermatofibrosarcoma protuberans. *J Clin Oncol.* 2002;20:3586–3591.
252. Lemm D, Muegge LO, Hoeffken K, et al. Remission with Imatinib mesylate treatment in a patient with initially unresectable dermatofibrosarcoma protuberans–a case report. *Oral Maxillofac Surg.* 2008;12:209–213.
253. Savoia P, Ortoncelli M, Quaglino P, Bernengo MG. Imatinib mesylate in the treatment of a large unresectable dermatofibrosarcoma protuberans: a case study. *Dermatol Surg.* 2006;32:1097–1102.
254. Wright TI, Petersen JE. Treatment of recurrent dermatofibrosarcoma protuberans with imatinib mesylate, followed by Mohs micrographic surgery. *Dermatol Surg.* 2007;33:741–744.
255. Price VE, Fletcher JA, Zielenska M, et al. Imatinib mesylate: an attractive alternative in young children with large, surgically challenging dermatofibrosarcoma protuberans. *Pediatr Blood Cancer.* 2005;44:511–515.
256. Han A, Chen EH, Niedt G, Sherman W, Ratner D. Neoadjuvant imatinib therapy for dermatofibrosarcoma protuberans. *Arch Dermatol.* 2009;145:792–796.
257. Kérob D, Porcher R, Vérola O, et al. Imatinib mesylate as a preoperative therapy in dermatofibrosarcoma: results of a multicenter phase II study on 25 patients. *Clin Cancer Res.* 2010;16:3288–3295.
258. Liu LS, Colegio OR. Molecularly targeted therapies for nonmelanoma skin cancers. *Int J Dermatol.* 2013;52:654–665.

CHAPTER 30

Skin Cancer in the Organ Transplant Patient

Sasha Jenkins, Maren Cotes, & Fiona Zwald

INTRODUCTION

Advances in the management of solid organ transplantation recipients (OTR) have led to improved overall survival. However, patients face many consequences of being on long-term immunosuppression, including an increased risk of developing premalignant and malignant skin cancers. This is likely to pose an increasing challenge to dermatologists, as the number of patients receiving a solid organ transplant continues to grow and the life expectancy of these patients continues to increase. Skin cancers are the most common malignancy posttransplantation, comprising almost 40% of posttransplant malignancies, and tend to behave more aggressively than in nontransplant patients.[1] The increased risk of skin cancer impacts patient morbidity and quality of life post transplantation, and management of such cases places a significant burden on diminishing health care resources.

EPIDEMIOLOGY

Nonmelanoma skin cancers (NMSC) are the most frequent cutaneous malignancies in OTRs, with squamous cell carcinomas (SCC) and basal cell carcinomas (BCC) representing about 90% to 95% of the total in multiple reported cohorts.[2,3] Although the incidence of both types of malignancies is increased, the rate of SCC is disproportionately higher. In the immunocompetent population, BCC is the more common type of NMSC. However, in the transplant population the ratio is reversed with the ratio of SCC to BCC of at least 4:1.[4,5] Although the risk of BCC is increased 10 to 16 fold, SCC occurs at a frequency 65 times that of the general population.[1,6] OTRs are also at increased risk for developing other premalignant and malignant cutaneous conditions, including actinic keratoses (AKs), Bowen's disease (SCC in situ), malignant melanoma (MM), Kaposi's sarcoma, Merkel cell carcinoma (MCC), atypical fibroxanthoma (AFX), lymphoma, and angiosarcoma.[7–10] However, the incidence of SCC predominates in this population.

The majority of transplant patients usually develop multiple SCCs. The time period between transplantation and development of a skin cancer varies from a few months to up to 20 years, depending on the length of time after transplantation, the level of sun exposure, skin type, and other risk factors predisposing to SCC (Table 30-1).[1] About 25% of OTRs will develop a second SCC within 13 months and 50% within 3.5 years of their first SCC.[11] The increased incidence of SCC in OTRs is such that the diagnosis of a first SCC has been shown to be predictive of the development of additional NMSC within 5 years.[12]

Transplant recipients have a five-fold increase in the risk of MM, which accounts for 6.2% of posttransplantation skin cancers in adults and 15% in children.[7,13] The mean time following transplantation to the development of melanoma is 5 years.[4] OTRs also tend to have lower survival rates than immunocompetent patients.[14]

The risk of skin cancers in the pediatric transplant population (<18 years old) is also increased compared to the general pediatric population. In a Dutch pediatric kidney transplant recipient population, the standardized risk for development of NMSC was found to be 222 fold higher than in the general pediatric population.[15] Skin cancers typically arise 12 to 15 years after transplantation, at an average age of 26 to 28 years.[15] SCCs are also more common than BCCs in pediatric OTRs. In one series, NMSC spread to lymph nodes was more common in pediatric transplant recipients compared to adults.[16] In this same series, lip SCC occurred more frequently in children than adults, and was associated with a higher rate of lymph node metastases.[16]

RISK FACTORS AND PATHOGENESIS

UV radiation exposure is the primary carcinogen promoting NMSC development in OTRs, which is easily appreciated considering that these lesions occur with greatest frequency on sun-exposed sites. Increased total sun burden prior to transplant (as measured by Fitzpatrick skin type, latitude of residence, and occupational and leisure sun exposure history) is correlated with an increased risk of skin cancer following transplantation.[5,17]

TABLE 30-1
Risk Factors for Development of Skin Cancers in Organ Transplant Recipients

- Fitzpatrick skin type I to III
- Increasing age at transplantation
- Duration and level of immunosuppression
- Type of organ transplant (heart/lung > kidney > liver)
- Previous transplant
- Squamous cell carcinoma before transplant
- History of lymphoma pre/posttransplant
- Pre-transplant end organ disease (e.g., rheumatoid arthritis, systemic lupus erythematosus, or autoimmune hepatitis)
- Liver transplant recipients with psoriasis on previous biologic therapy/psoralen plus ultraviolet A light phototherapy

Male gender and age greater than 50 years at the time of transplantation are associated with an early increase in NMSC number. Younger patients initially have a lower risk of developing a cutaneous neoplasm, but due to cumulative immunosuppression, their risk increases dramatically as they age.[18] OTRs with a history of NMSC are at high risk of developing a second skin malignancy and, therefore, require frequent skin screening examinations due to their elevated risk.[12,19]

Risk for the development of cutaneous malignancy is also related to the type, intensity, and duration of immunosuppression. Although individual immunosuppressive agents act via different mechanisms to potentiate the effects of photocarcinogenesis, studies have failed to demonstrate a consistent correlation between individual agents and overall risk of keratinocyte malignancy. Instead, it appears that the intensity and duration of immunosuppression is more closely associated with increased risk. Patients on triple therapy are more likely to develop skin cancer than those on dual or monotherapy.[20]

UV EXPOSURE AND MOLECULAR CHANGES

The role of UV radiation in the induction and promotion of cutaneous carcinogenesis is manifold; it is the major mutagen causing keratinocyte DNA damage and also leads to suppression of antigen presentation by Langerhans cells in the skin, thereby inducing tolerance to aberrant photodamaged cells. The combination of decreased immunosurveillance and immunosuppressive medications leads to down-regulation of the host response against cutaneous neoplasms in OTRs.[21]

The p53 tumor suppressor gene is the most commonly mutated gene in skin cancer and is particularly sensitive to UV-induced damage. p53 mutations are detected in up to 60% of NMSCs in OTRs, and the majority (78%) have UV-specific C to T transitions at dipyrimidine sites.[22] Normal-appearing skin adjacent to known cutaneous carcinoma in OTRs is found to have aberrant p53 patches with greater frequency than in matched, immunocompetent controls. These patches represent microscopic precursors of SCC and can serve as markers for increased SCC risk.[23]

HPV

The role of human papillomavirus (HPV) infection in cutaneous carcinogenesis is less well defined. Up to 90% of OTRs will develop HPV-induced verrucous lesions as a result of their immunosuppressed status. In addition, HPV DNA is detected in up to 75% of SCCs from OTRs versus 37% of SCCs from immunocompetent controls.[24] It is hypothesized that inactivation of cell cycle regulatory proteins p53 and pRb by viral oncogenes E6 and E7 may act synergistically with UV-induced DNA damage to promote keratinocyte tumorigenesis.[25] Additional study is needed to further elucidate the role of HPV infection in the promotion of NMSC in the transplant population.

IMMUNOSUPPRESSION

OTRs require lifelong immunosuppression to prevent potentially fatal organ rejection and to preserve graft organ function. This includes both initial and long-term maintenance immunosuppression. Induction therapy is an aggressive immunosuppressive regimen started before, at the time of, or immediately following transplantation in order to deplete or modify T-cell responses at the time of initial allograft antigen presentation. Therapy consists of treatment with either a lymphocyte-depleting agent (antithymocyte globulin, antilymphocyte globulin [OKT3], or muromonab CD3) or an IL-2 receptor antagonist (basiliximab and daclizumab), and is intended to reduce acute rejection rates and improve the efficacy of subsequent immunosuppression.[1] Increased rates of posttransplantation lymphoproliferative disorder and NMSC are seen after induction with lymphocyte-depleting antibodies.[26]

Maintenance immunosuppression is typically achieved with a combination of immunomodulatory agents; the goal of treatment is long-term prevention of graft rejection and ongoing preservation of graft function. In general, higher doses of immunosuppressive agents are used during the immediate posttransplant period, followed by dose reduction in stable patients to minimize toxicity.

Immunosuppressive agents can compound the effects of UV exposure in OTRs and accelerate cutaneous carcinogenesis independent of their role in depressing immune surveillance. Cyclosporine A has been shown to promote the formation of skin cancers via multiple mechanisms, including increased secretion of TGFβ, increased expression of vascular endothelial growth factor (VEGF), decreased p53-induced apoptosis, inhibition of nucleotide excision repair following photodamage, and tolerance of keratinocyte survival under conditions of increased genotoxic stress following UV radiation via inhibition of mitochondrial permeability transition pore opening.[27–32] Cyclosporine A has also been shown to induce ATF3 production through inhibition of the calcineurin/NFAT pathway, resulting in inhibition of p53-dependent cellular senescence and uncontrolled tumor growth.[33]

The active metabolite of azathioprine, 6-thioguanine, is incorporated into keratinocyte DNA, resulting in abnormal photosensitivity with decreased UV-A minimal erythema dose (MED-A) and accelerated photocarcinogenesis.[34,35] The use of azathioprine has also been shown to increase cellular susceptibility to mutagenesis via inhibition of postreplicative DNA mismatch repair.[36] It has also been demonstrated that azathioprine exposure can lead to BCCs on nonphotoexposed skin with unusual G:C to A:T transitions in the *PTCH* gene at nondipyrimidine sites.[37] Hofbauer et al.[38] recently demonstrated the photosensitizing effects of azathioprine in renal transplant patients, by replacing azathioprine with mycophenolate mofetil and measuring the MED following UV-A radiation. The mean MED response was much higher, demonstrating a marked reduction in photosensitivity in renal transplant patients in whom the conversion to mycophenolate mofetil occurred.

VORICONAZOLE

Other nonimmunosuppressive agents commonly used in the treatment of OTRs with potential to increase risk of posttransplant malignancy include voriconazole. Voriconazole, a second-generation triazole antifungal used for treatment and prophylaxis of invasive aspergillosis in lung transplant recipients, has been shown to increase the risk of NMSC; a potential mechanism may be via a phototoxic reaction in which the voriconazole N-oxide metabolite is excited by radiation in the UV-B range. Predisposition to cutaneous toxicity is seen in individuals with genetic polymorphisms of the cytochrome p450 enzyme CYP2C19.[39] There have been multiple reports documenting aggressive and multifocal SCCs in immunocompromised patients undergoing treatment with voriconazole, and it has recently been shown that a longer duration of treatment leads to increased numbers of NMSCs, supporting its role in accelerated keratinocyte carcinogenesis.[40–43] In a study of lung transplant recipients on voriconazole, Zwald et al. determined that length of time after transplantation, age, skin type I or II and months of exposure to voriconazole were found to be independent risk factors for the number of skin cancers after lung transplantation. Duration of voriconazole exposure was found to correlate with NMSC number. All patients exposed to voriconazole should be educated about their increased risk of skin cancer and should have regular dermatologic follow-up for skin cancer screening. Physicians caring for lung transplant recipients should consider alternatives to voriconazole in patients at risk.[43]

MANAGEMENT

PATIENT EDUCATION

Patient education regarding adequate sun protective measures and appropriate sunscreen application is the most important tool in managing and preventing skin cancer in solid OTRs. At the Emory Transplant Specialty Dermatology clinic, patient education in sun protection is integrated into the care of OTRs both pre- and post-transplantation. Education includes counseling on sun protection, appropriate sunscreen and sun-protective clothing use, and strong recommendations against the use of tanning salons. Sun-associated behavior modification posttransplant has been proven to reduce the risk of developing NMSC, even in patients with a history of prior SCC.[44] Vitamin D deficiency is a consequence of aggressive photoprotection, and OTRs should be screened and supplemented accordingly. The American Academy of Dermatology recommends daily supplementation with 1000 IU of D3 in adults who regularly and properly practice photoprotection.

PATIENT ACCESS TO SPECIALTY TRANSPLANT DERMATOLOGY CLINICS

Specialty transplant dermatology clinics offer more timely access to the care of OTRs, who represent a complex patient population with numerous and aggressive skin cancers. Comprehensive and effective multidisciplinary dermatologic care of these patients is a necessity. Regardless of clinic design, an organized and firmly established clinic model to allow proactive and ongoing care for these patients is important for education, prevention, and early intervention.[45] Ideally, all patients should be seen prior to transplantation for a total body skin examination to evaluate and treat preexisting lesions, and this examination should be repeated in the immediate posttransplant period. At the Emory Transplant Dermatology Clinic patients are stratified according to risk factors, such as prior history of skin cancer, cumulative lifetime sun exposure, duration of time posttransplant, skin type, and history of sunburns. Patients are scheduled for evaluation and follow-up based on their individual risk factors. All OTRs are, therefore, evaluated pre- and posttransplant as per protocol. This system enables those patients at high risk to be evaluated in a more timely fashion (Table 30-2).[46]

TABLE 30-2
Follow-Up Intervals for Total Body Skin Examination for Solid Organ Transplantation

Patient Risk Factor	Interval for Total Body Skin Examination (No. of Months)
No skin cancer/field disease	12
Field disease	3–6
One nonmelanoma skin cancer	3–6
Multiple nonmelanoma skin cancers	3
High-risk squamous cell carcinoma or melanoma	3
Metastatic squamous cell carcinoma or melanoma	1–3

Patients also receive information about performing self-skin examinations for suspicious lesions, and high-risk patients with a known history of skin cancer are taught how to perform a pertinent lymph node examination. The development of cutaneous malignancy negatively impacts patients' quality of life following transplantation, and intervention with regular skin examinations not only lessens morbidity associated with skin cancer but can improve overall quality of life in the posttransplant period.[47,48] In our practice we have established a system that authorizes designated transplant coordinators to overbook transplant patients with new or concerning lesions that may occur between regularly scheduled follow-up visits so that they may be evaluated in a more timely fashion. This arrangement is easily facilitated through the use of electronic medical records. All of the aforementioned recommendations allow for better utilization of diminishing clinical resources.

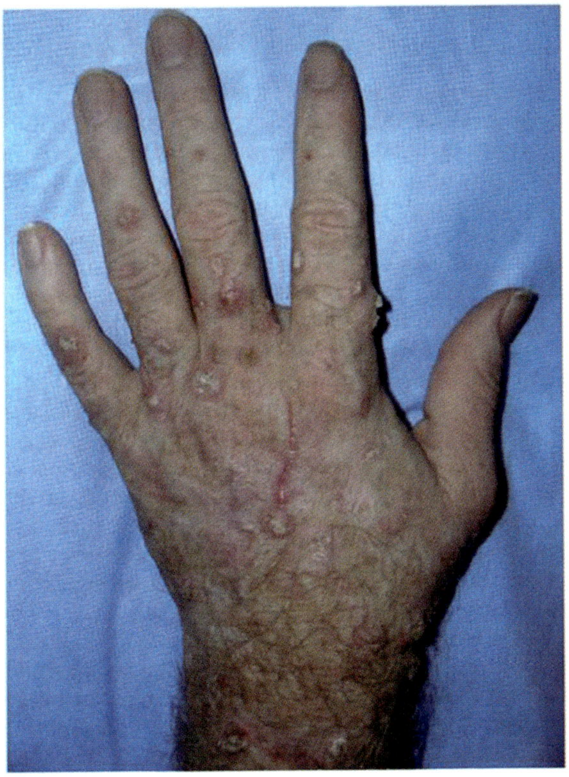

Figure 30-1 Field disease on the dorsum of the hand in a renal transplant recipient.

CONCEPT OF FIELD CANCERIZATION

Total body skin examination in OTRs can be challenging due to the presence of diffuse areas of photodamage with "field cancerization" in which it can be exceedingly difficult to determine which of the many keratotic lesions may be an actual skin cancer (Fig. 30-1). AKs and verrucae are associated with areas of actinic damage and represent clinical and subclinical lesions of epidermal dysplasia. Warts, AKs, and porokeratoses should be treated aggressively at first development, and if they are painful, have an atypical appearance, are enlarging, or do not respond to usual therapy, should be immediately biopsied for histological evaluation.

The use of curettage and other destructive modalities is useful in the treatment of individual lesions. The implementation of cyclical topical therapies has been added to traditional surgical approaches in the treatment of clinical and subclinical lesions in large, sun-exposed sites (field therapy), with good success in reducing overall burden of premalignant disease. Various modalities will be explored in greater detail below and may be employed in repeated rotation for the treatment of larger areas of field cancerization.[49]

TOPICAL THERAPIES

TOPICAL 5-FLUOROURACIL 5%.

Topical 5-fluorouracil (5-FU) is an antimetabolite that has been used for nearly 50 years in treating premalignant skin disease in the immunocompetent population and is commonly used for field treatment in OTRs. Its effect is mediated by disruption of RNA synthesis as well as via inhibition of thymidylate synthetase leading to decreased DNA synthesis.[50,51] Despite its widespread use, there are few randomized controlled trials examining the efficacy of 5-FU in OTRs. A single study performed in 2007 compared the use of methyl 5-aminolevulinate photodynamic therapy (MAL-PDT) with a typical 3 week course of twice daily application of 5-FU in transplant recipients and found that the 5-FU group experienced only an 11% rate of complete clearance of the treated fields, with a mean decrease in lesional area of 79%.[52] This is in marked contrast to prior studies of 5-FU in immunocompetent hosts, where rates of complete clearance of the treated field as high as 90% have been reported, likely secondary to the background immunosuppression seen in OTRs.[53]

5-FU can be used repeatedly in OTRs and no studies to date have reported adverse effects on graft function. Application under occlusion (chemowraps), applied weekly and left in place for 5 to 7 days, may increase efficacy and may be useful for treating larger areas of disease.[54] Table 30-3 provides an explanation of the chemowrap technique: in brief, topical 5-FU is applied under occlusion to affected areas on the forearms, dorsal hands, and/or lower extremities. The patient returns for weekly assessments by the dermatologist with care being taken to avoid the occurrence of superficial infection or skin ulceration. At the end of treatment, any lesions that remain should be biopsied to rule out invasive disease. Curettage of lesions prior to chemowrap application may shorten duration of therapy.

TABLE 30-3
Chemowrap Application

1. Wash affected area (either leg or arm) with soap and water.
2. Apply thick coat of 5-fluorouracil (should be white).
   - For the forearms, start on the dorsal hand and extend to below the elbow.
   - For the lower leg, start on the midfoot and extend to the upper calf.
   - For both areas, treat circumferentially, both affected and nonaffected skin.
3. For the lower leg, apply a Vaseline gauze on the anterior of ankle.
4. Apply a zinc-impregnated gauze, such as (Unna paste) with a 50% overlap over 5-FU.
5. Cover with Kerlix with minimal overlap.
6. Cover with 6 in coban or self-adhering wrap.
7. Patient removes wrap after 1 wk, washes area and returns to clinic for reapplication.
8. Continue as necessary, usually 4–12 wk.

IMIQUIMOD 5% CREAM.

Imiquimod is a member of the imidazoquinoline group, possesses antiviral and antitumor activities, and is approved by the FDA for treatment of condyloma acuminata, AKs, and superficial BCCs less than 2 cm on the neck, body, or extremities in immunocompetent adults. Its activity is thought to be mediated in part by interactions with Toll-like receptor (TLR) 7 and stimulation of both innate and adaptive immune responses.[55–57] A 2007 study examining the efficacy and safety of topical 5% imiquimod in OTRs demonstrated reduced cutaneous dysplasia with complete clearance rates of AKs as high as 62%. No adverse effects on graft organ function were noted during or following treatment with imiquimod on areas of 100 cm^2 three times per week over 16 weeks.[58] Combination with 5% 5-FU (imiquimod applied Monday, Wednesday, and Friday and 5-FU applied twice daily on off days) may enhance efficacy of each individual agent and has been used successfully to treat lower extremity SCC in situ in renal transplant recipients.[59]

INGENOL MEBUTATE. Ingenol mebutate is a recently approved topical medication for the treatment of AKs on the scalp, trunk, and extremities. It is derived from the milkweed plant, *Euphorbia peplus*, and is a hydrophobic macrocyclicditerpene ester. The proposed mechanism of action in immunocompetent hosts involves rapid lesion necrosis and specific neutrophil-mediated, antibody-dependent cellular cytotoxicity.[60] Clearance rates with ingenol mebutate in immunocompetent hosts are comparable to those achieved with topical imiquimod and 5-FU, with the major advantage being a short 2 or 3 day treatment course. Adverse effects are similar to those seen with other topical treatments for premalignant skin disease and include erythema, flaking, scaling, crusting, swelling, vesiculation, pustulation, erosions, or ulceration.[61] Ingenol mebutate has not yet been studied exclusively in OTRs or other immunosuppressed populations and it remains to be seen what role it will play in the care of such patients.

PHOTODYNAMIC THERAPY

Several recent studies have examined the efficacy of PDT in the treatment of field cancerization in OTRs. PDT employs a topical photosensitizer followed by exposure to a noncoherent light source; light is absorbed by the photosensitizing agent and subsequently generates reactive oxygen species. MAL is a methyl ester of aminolevulinic acid (ALA) and is converted into photo-activated porphyrin preferentially in cancer cells.[62] Three separate studies evaluating the efficacy of topical PDT with MAL for AKs in OTRs demonstrated complete clearance rates of 64% to 89% and a 71% to 76% decrease in number of AKs. These studies all followed similar protocols, which involved curettage of lesions prior to treatment, and use of noncoherent red light.[52,63,64] The most notable adverse effect associated with PDT is moderate to severe pain during treatment.

A small study followed 12 high-risk OTRs who received cyclic PDT using 20% 5-ALA and blue light every 4 to 8 week intervals over 2 years and monitored development of further SCC compared to pretreatment; the median reduction in invasive and in situ SCC at 12 and 24 months posttransplant was 79% and 95% respectively, showing promise for this treatment modality.[65]

PDT has previously been demonstrated as a successful therapy for BCCs in immunocompetent patients, and was recently shown to be effective for treating similar lesions in the transplant population: MAL-PDT was used to treat 18 transplant recipients with BCCs with only one recurrence at 26 months post treatment.[66]

ACITRETIN

Systemic retinoids, specifically acitretin, have demonstrated utility in suppressing AK and SCC development in OTRs.[67] This is the result of multiple downstream effects secondary to the binding of acitretin to the nuclear retinoid receptor, including promotion of cell maturation and differentiation as well as down-regulation of proto-oncogene expression.[68–70] Retinoids can be used both to prevent morbidity from multiple primary NMSCs as well as to decrease the risk of mortality from a single, high-risk tumor. Chemoprevention with acitretin should be considered in transplant recipients, particularly those developing multiple NMSCs annually (5–10 per year), those with extensive actinic damage and a history of multiple skin cancers, in those patients with a history of high-risk SCCs or metastatic SCC, and in patients with eruptive keratoacanthomas.[71] It is important to recognize that this is a long-term therapy; cessation of treatment results in prompt recurrence and rebound effect of premalignant/malignant skin disease that can be difficult to control.[72,73]

The side effect profile of acitretin therapy in OTRs is similar to that seen in the immunocompetent population and includes mucocutaneous xerosis, elevated serum lipids, and transaminitis. These effects appear to be dose related.[74] Initiation of therapy at low doses (10 mg every other day) and increasing at 10 mg increments at 2 to 4 week intervals to a goal dose of 20 to 25 mg daily can minimize side effects by preventing sudden onset of severe mucocutaneous symptoms. Baseline fasting lipids, comprehensive metabolic panel and complete blood count should be obtained and rechecked at 2 to 4 weeks and then at monthly intervals for the first 3 months of therapy. Acitretin is a teratogen and pregnancy category X and should never be used during pregnancy. The use of retinoids in women of childbearing age must be carefully weighed against these risks and regular pregnancy testing is critical. Other contraindications to use include severe lipid abnormalities refractory to standard therapies.

CAPECITABINE

Capecitabine is the first FDA-approved oral chemotherapeutic agent and was initially used in patients with metastatic breast cancer and later in patients with both metastatic and primary colon cancer. In 2006, Peramiquel et al.[75] reported inflammation and regression of AKs in patients receiving capecitabine and shortly thereafter the use of this medication was explored in patients at high risk for NMSC, including OTRs.

Capecitabine is a prodrug of 5-FU and the final step in its conversion is mediated in peripheral tissues by thymidine phosphorylase, which is expressed at greater levels in some carcinomas. Before starting therapy patients must be tested for activity of dihydropyrimidine dehydrogenase, an enzyme involved in uracil and thymine metabolism as deficiency can lead to toxicity following exposure.

Two retrospective reviews examined the use of low-dose oral capecitabine in OTRs with recurrent NMSC.[76,77] In these studies patients were treated in repeated 3 week cycles of 1 to 1.5 g/m^2 daily for 14 days, followed by 7 days of no treatment. A smaller study, which included only three patients, reported a dramatic decrease in the number of malignant skin lesions requiring excision in the 6 months following study onset compared to the 6 months immediately prior (only one lesion excised compared to a total of 35 excisions in the preceding 6 months). A study of 15 solid OTRs demonstrated a significant decrease in the incidence of SCCs in 80% of treated patients. In addition, 40% of patients had reduction in the rate of BCC occurrence, and 53.3% of patients had a decrease in number of AKs. No evidence of rebound after stopping therapy was reported. However, in this study 73% of patients eventually developed grade 3 or 4 toxicities, most commonly fatigue (40%), hand–foot syndrome (20%), and diarrhea (20%), and 33% of patients had discontinued treatment by 1 year. No cases of graft rejection were reported in either publication.

These early reports of capecitabine use in OTRs suggest that overall this is a relatively safe treatment, especially at low doses, but further prospective studies are needed to characterize its long-term safety and efficacy in the transplant population. Use of capecitabine in our institution is performed in close collaboration with medical oncology and the transplant team.

SURGICAL TREATMENT

MANAGEMENT OF BASAL CELL CARCINOMA

The management of BCC in OTRs is similar to management in immunocompetent patients. Although several small case series have reported successes with treatments such as PDT and 5% imiquimod cream in OTRs,[66,78] surgical treatment remains the standard of care. The AAD/ACMS/ASDSA/ASMS 2012 Appropriate Use Criteria for Mohs Micrographic Surgery (MMS) report deemed MMS the appropriate therapy for immunocompromised patients with BCCs of any size or histologic subtype on the face, neck, scalp, ears, genitalia, hands, feet, nail units, nipples/areolae, ankles, and pretibial surfaces. MMS was felt to be inappropriate for the same patient population with primary nodular BCCs ≤0.5 cm or primary superficial BCCs ≤1 cm on the trunk or extremities (excluding those areas mentioned previously).[79]

MANAGEMENT OF SQUAMOUS CELL CARCINOMA

LOW-RISK SCC. The treatment of low-risk SCC in OTRs is similar to that in immunocompetent individuals with use of standard excision with a minimum of 4 mm surgical margins recommended per the National Comprehensive Network (NCCN) guidelines. In addition, cyclical use of topical therapies, including 5-FU and imiquimod, or use of PDT is a necessity given the presence of field cancerization that can progress to SCC in situ and SCC. Addition of a systemic retinoid should be considered in patients at risk for developing multiple SCCs.

TABLE 30-4

High-risk Features of SCC in Organ Transplant Patients

- Large size (>2 cm)
- Multiple squamous cell carcinomas
- High-risk location (ear, lips, over parotid gland, scalp, or temple)
- In-transit metastatic lesion
- Recurrence
- Histology
  - Poorly differentiated
- Perineural invasion
  - Deep invasion

HIGH-RISK SCC. Features attributable to high-risk SCC include large size (>2 cm), location (ear, lips, scalp, temple, over parotid gland), histology of the lesion (poor differentiation, perineural invasion or deep invasion), especially if occurring in an immunocompromised patient (Table 30-4, Fig. 30-2).[73] Patients with high-risk SCC should be treated and monitored aggressively given their increased risk of developing metastases. In these patients, MMS is recommended to achieve rapid and complete tumor extirpation, especially for tumors located on the head and neck. Alternatively, high-risk SCC can be removed with a wider margin of at least 10 mm per NCCN guidelines. Preoperative CT/MRI or PET/CT may be required to evaluate for deep extension or nodal involvement in such lesions.

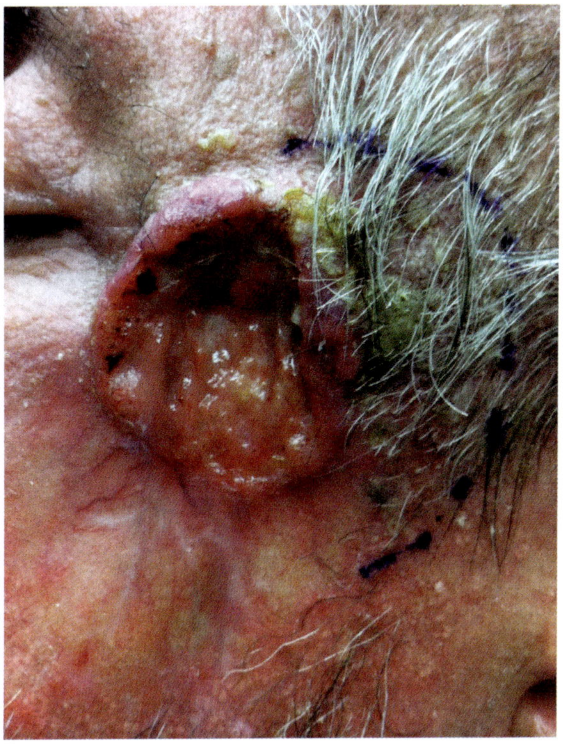

Figure 30-2 High-risk SCC on the left temple in a renal transplant patient.

TABLE 30-5
Indications for Radiation Therapy in Treatment of SCCs in Organ Transplant Recipients

- Nonsurgical candidates
- Adjuvant therapy for incomplete tumor resection
- Adjuvant therapy for lymph node involvement
- Adjuvant therapy for perineural tumor involvement

Adjuvant therapy with either node dissection and/or radiation therapy should also be considered, especially if perineural invasion is present, even in the absence of clinically palpable lymphadenopathy. Radiation therapy used as a primary treatment option leads to lower cure rates than surgical therapy, and should be reserved for patients where tumors are inoperable or when the risks of surgery outweigh the benefits. The use of radiation therapy in transplant patients is outlined in Table 30-5.[73]

Radiation therapy following tumor removal has better outcomes than surgery alone, according to nonrandomized case series data.[80] In patients with perineural invasion, adjuvant radiation therapy (ART) reduces the incidence of local recurrence.[81] Per NCCN guidelines, adjuvant radiation should be used at the primary tumor site if substantial perineural invasion is identified, defined as "involvement of more than just a few small sensory nerve branches or large nerve involvement," though in reality, its use is not always restricted to carcinomas involving large nerves.[82] Salvage radiation carries a higher risk of local, regional, and distant recurrence, but might be required in settings where there are positive margins following MMS or excision.[82,83]

Head and neck SCC with disease metastatic to the lymph nodes portends a poor prognosis. Treatment of these patients may require referral to ENT surgery for parotidectomy with or without neck dissection along with ART to improve local and regional control.[73,84] The addition of radiation therapy following lymphadenectomy can result in a 73% 5 year disease-free survival.[85] The NCCN recommends ART in all head and neck SCC nodal metastases, and it should be considered in cases of SCC on the trunk and extremities following lymphadenectomy.[82] Patients should be followed closely, with frequent PET-CT or MRI.

The role of chemotherapy in treatment of high-risk SCC remains unclear.[73] Metastatic SCC may be treated with cisplatin monotherapy or in combination with other systemic agents, such as methotrexate, 5-FU, bleomycin, and doxorubicin, all with limited efficacy data. Capecitabine, the oral 5-FU prodrug, has been used as monotherapy as well as in combination with subcutaneous interferon, with possible improved outcomes.[86,87] The use of capecitabine with cisplatin or paclitaxel in SCC of head and neck has shown favorable outcomes in phase II trials.[88,89] Therapy targeting epidermal growth factor receptors (EGFR), such as cetuximab, is being explored in treatment of SCC in clinical trials, but is being used off-label currently to treat SCC.[90] The NCCN guidelines recommend consideration of cisplatin-based therapy and clinical trial participation for metastatic disease or regional recurrence.[82]

In-transit metastases of high-risk SCC in OTRs present as rapidly enlarging subcutaneous nodules with no epidermal extension in close proximity to the primary or recurrent tumor (Fig. 30-3). Treatment of these lesions must be individualized, but usually requires wide surgical excision followed by wide-field ART.[73,91]

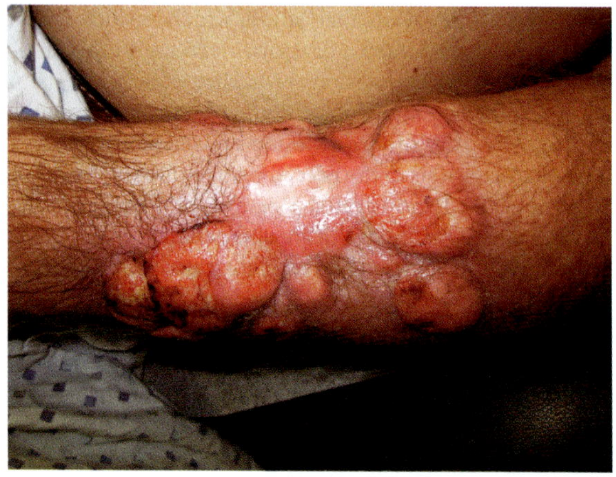

Figure 30-3 In-transit SCC in a lung transplant patient.

SENTINEL LYMPH NODE BIOPSY

Surgical staging of the primary nodal basin achieved by sentinel lymph node biopsy (SLNB) has been shown to be a prognostic factor in melanoma. There are emerging data indicating that SLNB may have a role in high-risk SCC. Lymph node involvement from high-risk SCC has an increased risk of recurrence and death.[92] SLNB may accurately detect subclinical lymph node metastasis in patients, potentially allowing for the earliest possible therapeutic lymphadenectomy if the SLNB is positive.[73,93] Prospective studies are needed to determine which risk factors predict nodal and distant metastases, and thus which patients warrant a SLNB. A recent study by Kwon et al. analyzed the results of SLNB in 128 patients with high-risk SCC without nodal involvement clinically. A positive SLNB was found in 14% of cases. Of the high-risk cases, SLNB had a negative predictive value of 97.8% and a false negative rate of 15%. Despite the high negative predictive value, long-term follow-up and close monitoring of these patients is recommended, as most of the data were derived from studies with a short follow-up period.[94]

MANAGEMENT OF OTHER MALIGNANCIES: MELANOMA

OTRs have a three- to five-fold increased risk for development of MM, with similar risk factors as those in the general population.[4] Three main clinical scenarios arise; namely, pre-transplant MM, donor-transmitted MM, and de novo MM occurring posttransplantation.[95] The management of pre-transplant MM and de novo MM occurring posttransplantation is the same as in immunocompetent individuals. MM in situ and thin melanoma (<1 mm) in the transplant population have recurrence and survival estimates similar to those in the general population. A minimum wait time of 2 years prior to transplantation is suggested for MM with a Breslow depth less than 1 mm and no clinical evidence of metastasis. More advanced MM may have a more aggressive course in transplant recipients. SLNB may be of additional prognostic benefit. Revision of immunosuppression in the management of de novo melanoma in collaboration with the transplant team should be considered. Larger prospective studies utilizing uniform staging criteria or, at minimum, Breslow depth, are required to assess true risk and outcome of MM in the immunosuppressed transplant population. Emphasis remains on patient education and regular screening to provide early detection of MM.[95]

MERKEL CELL CARCINOMA

OTRs are also at risk for development of MCC, with an estimated relative risk of 5 to 10 compared to the general population.[96] MCC tend to develop 7 to 8 years posttransplant, and often arise on the head and neck.[97] In OTRs, MCC behaves aggressively with rapid growth, ulceration, and a poor prognosis. Treatment of MCC is based on extent of disease, with local disease requiring wide local excision with 2.5 to 3 cm margins or MMS. SLNB with or without complete dissection, and ART, usually to the primary site and affected lymph node, is recommended.[97] Reduction of immunosuppression should also be considered.

ATYPICAL FIBROXANTHOMA AND UNDIFFERENTIATED PLEOMORPHIC SARCOMA

AFX and undifferentiated pleomorphic sarcoma (UPS) have a higher rate of local recurrence and metastasis in OTRs.[9] Treatment should be aggressive, with MMS or WLE (2 cm margins) followed by wide-field ART.[9] McCoppin et al. describe their experience in OTRs and outline the value of MMS in the treatment of AFX in immunocompromised patients. Progression to UPS and a possible role of immunosuppression are also discussed.[9]

THE ROLE OF REVISION OF IMMUNOSUPPRESSION

Patients who develop more than 5 to 10 high-risk SCCs per year or those with a high risk of metastasis from a cutaneous malignancy may benefit from a revision of immunosuppression. A 2006 consensus survey by the International Transplant Skin Cancer Collaborative (ITSCC) and the Skin Care in Organ Transplant Patients Europe (SCOPE) supports reduction/alteration of immunosuppression as an adjuvant management strategy for patients with substantial morbidity and mortality resulting from MM or NMSC. Multiple hypothetical scenarios were modeled by the consensus group with the conclusion that more aggressive revision of immunosuppression (weighed against the concomitant increased risk of allograft failure) was warranted in those patients with higher-risk skin malignancies.[71]

Multiple factors must be considered if contemplating a reduction in immunosuppression, including patient age, previous history of rejection, and type of allograft. Patient survival from melanoma or NMSC must be balanced with survival and quality of life related to their graft function. The patient's transplant physician should make all decisions regarding adjustment or reduction of immunosuppression, with dermatology acting in a consulting role.

There are several ways to achieve reduction in immunosuppression. The dosage of therapy may be lowered, or for patients on multidrug regimens, especially triple therapy, it may be possible to discontinue an agent without significantly impairing graft function. Another reasonable strategy is conversion from a calcineurin inhibitor and antimetabolite-based immunosuppressant regimen to one based on a mammalian target of rapamycin (mTOR) inhibitor (sirolimus or everolimus). Sirolimus is a potent, nonnephrotoxic immunosuppressant with both antitumor and antiangiogenic properties. Several studies have shown a significant decrease in the rate of de novo malignancies in those patients treated with an mTOR inhibitor as part of their immunosuppressive regimen, and it has been demonstrated to trigger regression of pre-existing NMSC in OTRs.[98–101] Two recent, multicenter, open label, controlled trials have been published examining the use of sirolimus in renal transplant recipients with a history of NMSC.[102,103] Patients were randomized either to continue calcineurin inhibitor therapy or convert to sirolimus. One study demonstrated that yearly NMSC rates were significantly lower within the sirolimus group (this reduction was seen in the rate of SCC development but not in that of BCCs), and that a lower proportion of patients receiving sirolimus developed new or recurrent NMSC or new SCCs compared with patients on other regimens. However, discontinuation rates secondary to adverse events were significantly higher with sirolimus.[102]

The second study investigated the rate of survival free of new NMSC at 2 years of treatment and did not demonstrate a significant difference in the number of new SCCs between sirolimus and calcineurin inhibitor in the intention to treat analysis; however, the length of disease-free survival was significantly increased in the sirolimus group. Rates of drug-related adverse events were high, and 23% of patients treated with sirolimus discontinued the drug prior to study completion. The authors did note that patients on progressive conversion protocols (>7 day transition from calcineurin inhibitors to sirolimus) had lower rates of discontinuation and serious adverse events than those on rapid protocols.[103]

Despite its promising anticarcinogenic properties, sirolimus is not appropriate therapy for patients within the first 6 months following transplant due to its deleterious effects on wound healing. Other reported adverse effects include hyperlipidemia, myelosuppression, proteinuria, edema, pneumonitis, thrombotic microangiopathy, and acneiform eruptions.

EMERGING THERAPIES

SCCs have an overexpression and amplification of EGFR. Cetuximab, a monoclonal antibody to the EGFR receptor, has been used in metastatic SCC of the head and neck. However, as mentioned earlier, the clinical use of this treatment in cutaneous SCC is currently being evaluated in phase I and II clinical trials. Cetuximab is fairly well tolerated, with the most common side effect being acneiform eruptions. The use of cetuximab in lung transplant patients should be cautioned, given that there are a few case reports in the literature of fatal alveolar hemorrhage.[104] A retrospective review comparing the treatment of high-risk SCC versus very-high-risk SCC (defined as perineural, parotid, cartilaginous, or bony invasion, in-transit metastasis, or regional or distant metastasis) in immunocompetent patients showed that patients with very-high-risk SCC treated with adjuvant cetuximab, or cetuximab and radiation, had a small benefit.[105] Another case series described eight patients, four with SCC and four with BCC, treated with cetuximab with a 62.5% complete remission. However, in the patients who achieved remission with cetuximab, there was a 63% relapse rate.[106] Future phase III trials need to be pursued to investigate further the role of chemotherapy in the treatment of SCC.

CONCLUSION

Treatment of skin cancer in OTRs can be challenging and requires a multidisciplinary approach. Education of these patients and frequent total body skin examinations are essential. Aggressive management with early biopsy, topical therapy, surgical excision, and use of adjuvant therapy is crucial to improving skin cancer related morbidity and mortality in these high-risk patients.

REFERENCES

1. Zwald FO, Brown M. Skin cancer in solid organ transplant recipients: advances in therapy and management: part I. Epidemiology of skin cancer in solid organ transplant recipients. *J Am Acad Dermatol.* 2011;65(2):253–261; quiz 62.
2. Jensen P, Moller B, Hansen S. Skin cancer in kidney and heart transplant recipients and different long-term immunosuppressive therapy regimens. *J Am Acad Dermatol.* 2000;42 (2 Pt 1):307.
3. Winkelhorst JT, Brokelman WJ, Tiggeler RG, Wobbes T. Incidence and clinical course of de-novo malignancies in renal allograft recipients. *Eur J Surg Oncol.* 2001;27(4):409–413.
4. Euvrard S, Kanitakis J, Claudy A. Skin cancers after organ transplantation. *N Engl J Med.* 2003;348(17):1681–1691.
5. Ulrich C, Schmook T, Sachse MM, Sterry W, Stockfleth E. Comparative epidemiology and pathogenic factors for nonmelanoma skin cancer in organ transplant patients. *Dermatol Surg.* 2004;30(4 Pt 2):622–627.
6. Lindelof B, Sigurgeirsson B, Gabel H, Stern RS. Incidence of skin cancer in 5356 patients following organ transplantation. *BrJ Dermatol.* 2000;143(3):513–519.
7. Penn I. Malignant melanoma in organ allograft recipients. *Transplantation.* 1996;61(2):274–278.
8. Koljonen V, Kukko H, Tukiainen E, et al. Incidence of Merkel cell carcinoma in renal transplant recipients. *Nephrol Dial Transplant.* 2009;24(10):3231–3235.
9. McCoppin HH, Christiansen D, Stasko T, et al. Clinical spectrum of atypical fibroxanthoma and undifferentiated pleomorphic sarcoma in solid organ transplant recipients: a collective experience. *Dermatol Surg.* 2012;38(2):230–239.
10. Ahmed I, Hamacher KL. Angiosarcoma in a chronically immunosuppressed renal transplant recipient: report of a case and review of the literature. *Am J Dermatopathol.* 2002;24 (4):330–335.
11. Otley CC, Stasko T. *Skin Disease in Organ Transplantation.* New York, NY: Cambridge University Press; 2008.
12. Euvrard S, Kanitakis J, Decullier E, et al. Subsequent skin cancers in kidney and heart transplant recipients after the first squamous cell carcinoma. *Transplantation.* 2006;81(8): 1093–1100.
13. Hollenbeak CS, Todd MM, Billingsley EM, Harper G, Dyer AM, Lengerich EJ. Increased incidence of melanoma in renal transplantation recipients. *Cancer.* 2005;104(9):1962–1967.
14. Brewer JD, Christenson LJ, Weaver AL, et al. Malignant melanoma in solid transplant recipients: collection of database cases and comparison with surveillance, epidemiology, and end results data for outcome analysis. *Arch Dermatol.* 2011;147(7):790–796.
15. Euvrard S, Kanitakis J, Cochat P, Claudy A. Skin cancers following pediatric organ transplantation. *Dermatol Surg.* 2004;30(4 Pt 2):616–621.
16. Penn I. De novo malignancy in pediatric organ transplant recipients. *J Pediatr Surg.* 1994;29(2):221–226; discussion 227–228.
17. Terhorst D, Drecoll U, Stockfleth E, Ulrich C. Organ transplant recipients and skin cancer: assessment of risk factors with focus on sun exposure. *Br J Dermatol.* 2009;161(Suppl 3):85–89.
18. Moloney FJ, Comber H, O'Lorcain P, O'Kelly P, Conlon PJ, Murphy GM. A population-based study of skin cancer incidence and prevalence in renal transplant recipients. *Br J Dermatol.* 2006;154(3):498–504.
19. Mackenzie KA, Wells JE, Lynn KL, et al. First and subsequent nonmelanoma skin cancers: incidence and predictors in a population of New Zealand renal transplant recipients. *Nephrol Dial Transplant.* 2010;25(1):300–306.
20. Campistol JM, Eris J, Oberbauer R, et al. Sirolimus therapy after early cyclosporine withdrawal reduces the risk for cancer in adult renal transplantation. *J Am Soc Nephrol.* 2006; 17(2):581–589.
21. Runger T. Ultraviolet light. In: Bolognia JL, Jorizzo JL, Shaffer JV. *Dermatology*: Elselvier; 2012:1455–1465.
22. Queille S, Luron L, Spatz A, et al. Analysis of skin cancer risk factors in immunosuppressed renal transplant patients shows high levels of UV-specific tandem CC to TT mutations of the p53 gene. *Carcinogenesis.* 2007;28(3):724–731.
23. de Graaf YG, Rebel H, Elghalbzouri A, et al. More epidermal p53 patches adjacent to skin carcinomas in renal transplant recipients than in immunocompetent patients: the role of azathioprine. *Exp Dermatol.* 2008;17(4):349–355.
24. Stockfleth E, Nindl I, Sterry W, Ulrich C, Schmook T, Meyer T. Human papillomaviruses in transplant-associated skin cancers. *Dermatol Surg.* 2004;30:604–609.
25. Dang C, Koehler A, Forschner T, et al. E6/E7 expression of human papillomavirus types in cutaneous squamous cell dysplasia and carcinoma in immunosuppressed organ transplant recipients. *Br J Dermatol.* 2006;155(1):129–136.
26. Gutierrez-Dalmau A, Campistol J. Immunosuppressive therapy and malignancy in organ transplant recipients; a systematic review. *Drugs.* 2007;67(8):1167–1198.
27. Norman KG, Canter JA, Shi M, Milne GL, Morrow JD, Sligh JE. Cyclosporine A suppresses keratinocyte cell death through MPTP inhibition in a model for skin cancer in organ transplant recipients. *Mitochondrion.* 2010;10(2):94–101.
28. Thoms KM, Kuschal C, Oetjen E, et al. Cyclosporin A, but not everolimus, inhibits DNA repair mediated by calcineurin: implications for tumorigenesis under immunosuppression. *Exp Dermatol.* 2011;20(3):232–236.
29. Prashar Y, Khanna A, Sehajpal P, Sharma VK, Suthanthiran M. Stimulation of transforming growth factor-beta 1 transcription by cyclosporine. *FEBS lett.* 1995;358(2):109–112.
30. Guba M, von Breitenbuch P, Steinbauer M, et al. Rapamycin inhibits primary and metastatic tumor growth by antiangiogenesis: involvement of vascular endothelial growth factor. *Nat Med.* 2002;8(2):128–135.
31. Shihab FS, Bennett WM, Isaac J, Yi H, Andoh TF. Nitric oxide modulates vascular endothelial growth factor and receptors in chronic cyclosporine nephrotoxicity. *Kidney Int.* 2003;63(2):522–533.
32. Rivera A, Maxwell SA. The p53-induced gene-6 (proline oxidase) mediates apoptosis through a calcineurin-dependent pathway. *J Biol Chem.* 2005;280(32):29346–29354.
33. Wu X, Nguyen BC, Dziunycz P, et al. Opposing roles for calcineurin and ATF3 in squamous skin cancer. *Nature.* 2010; 465(7296):368–372.

34. Perrett CM, Walker SL, O'Donovan P, et al. Azathioprine treatment photosensitizes human skin to ultraviolet A radiation. *Br J Dermatol.* 2008;159(1):198–204.
35. O'Donovan P, Perrett CM, Zhang X, et al. Azathioprine and UVA light generate mutagenic oxidative DNA damage. *Science.* 2005;309(5742):1871–1874.
36. Swann PF, Waters TR, Moulton DC, et al. Role of postreplicative DNA mismatch repair in the cytotoxic action of thioguanine. *Science.* 1996;273(5278):1109–1111.
37. Harwood CA, Attard NR, O'Donovan P, et al. PTCH mutations in basal cell carcinomas from azathioprine-treated organ transplant recipients. *Br J Cancer.* 2008;99(8):1276–1284.
38. Hofbauer GF, Attard NR, Harwood CA, et al. Reversal of UVA skin photosensitivity and DNA damage in kidney transplant recipients by replacing azathioprine. *Am J Transplant.* 2012;12(1):218–225.
39. Epaulard O, Leccia MT, Blanche S, et al. Phototoxicity and photocarcinogenesis associated with voriconazole. *Med Mal Infect.* 2011;41(12):639–645.
40. Brunel AS, Fraisse T, Lechiche C, Pinzani V, Mauboussin JM, Sotto A. Multifocal squamous cell carcinomas in an HIV-infected patient with a long-term voriconazole therapy. *AIDS.* 2008;22(7):905–906.
41. McCarthy KL, Playford EG, Looke DF, Whitby M. Severe photosensitivity causing multifocal squamous cell carcinomas secondary to prolonged voriconazole therapy. *Clin Infect Dis.* 2007;44(5):e55–e56.
42. Vanacker A, Fabre G, Van Dorpe J, Peetermans WE, Maes B. Aggressive cutaneous squamous cell carcinoma associated with prolonged voriconazole therapy in a renal transplant patient. *Am J Transplant.* 2008;8(4):877–880.
43. Zwald FO, Spratt M, Lemos BD, et al. Duration of voriconazole exposure: an independent risk factor for skin cancer after lung transplantation. *Dermatol Surg.* 2012;38(8):1369–1374.
44. Ulrich C, Jurgensen JS, Degen A, et al. Prevention of non-melanoma skin cancer in organ transplant patients by regular use of a sunscreen: a 24 months, prospective, case-control study. *Br J Dermatol.* 2009;161(Suppl 3):78–84.
45. Christenson LJ, Geusau A, Ferrandiz C, et al. Specialty clinics for the dermatologic care of solid-organ transplant recipients. *Dermatol Surg.* 2004;30(4 Pt 2):598–603.
46. Otley CC. Organization of a specialty clinic to optimize the care of organ transplant recipients at risk for skin cancer. *Dermatol Surg.* 2000;26(7):709–712.
47. O'Reilly F, Traywick C, Pennie ML, Foster JK, Chen SC. Baseline quality of life and anxiety in solid organ transplant recipients: a pilot study. *Dermatol Surg.* 2006;32(12):1480–1485.
48. Moloney FJ, Keane S, O'Kelly P, Conlon PJ, Murphy GM. The impact of skin disease following renal transplantation on quality of life. *Br J Dermatol.* 2005;153(3):574–578.
49. Ulrich C. Topical treatment of field cancerization. *Cancer Treat Res.* 2009;146:439–446.
50. Eaglsterin WH, Weinstien GD, Frost P. Fluorouracil: mechanims of action in human skin and actinic keratoses. I. Effect on DNA synthesis *in vivo. Arch Dermatol.* 1970;101:132–139.
51. Tsai E, Zackheim H, Kim Y. Topical and intralesional chemotherapeutic agents. In: Wolverton S, ed. *Comprehensive Dermatologic Drug Therapy.* 2nd ed. Philadelphia, PA: Elsevier; 2007:643–653.
52. Perrett CM, McGregor JM, Warwick J, et al. Treatment of post-transplant premalignant skin disease: a randomized intrapatient comparative study of 5-fluorouracil cream and topical photodynamic therapy. *Br J Dermatol.* 2007;156(2):320–328.
53. Pearlman DL. Weekly pulse dosing: effective and comfortable topical 5-fluorouracil treatment of multiple facial actinic keratoses. *J Am Acad Dermatol.* 1991;25(4):665–657.
54. Ritchie SA, Patel MJ, Miller SJ. Therapeutic options to decrease actinic keratosis and squamous cell carcinoma incidence and progression in solid organ transplant recipients: a practical approach. *Dermatol Surg.* 2012;38(10):1604–1621.
55. Sauder DN. Immunomodulatory and pharmacologic properties of imiquimod. *J Am Acad Dermatol.* 2000;43(1 Pt 2):S6–S11.
56. Ito T, Amakawa R, Kaisho T, et al. Interferon-alpha and interleukin-12 are induced differentially by Toll-like receptor 7 ligands in human blood dendritic cell subsets. *J Exp Med.* 2002;195(11):1507–1512.
57. Kovach BT, Stasko T. Use of topical immunomodulators in organ transplant recipients. *Dermatol Ther.* 2005;18(1):19–27.
58. Ulrich C, Busch JO, Meyer T, et al. Successful treatment of multiple actinic keratoses in organ transplant patients with topical 5% imiquimod: a report of six cases. *Br J Dermatol.* 2006;155(2):451–454.
59. Smith KJ, Germain M, Skelton H. Squamous cell carcinoma in situ (Bowen's disease) in renal transplant patients treated with 5% imiquimod and 5% 5-fluorouracil therapy. *Dermatol Surg.* 2001;27(6):561–564.
60. Rosen RH, Gupta AK, Tyring SK. Dual mechanism of action of ingenol mebutate gel for topical treatment of actinic keratoses: rapid lesion necrosis followed by lesion-specific immune response. *J Am Acad Dermatol.* 2012;66(3):486–493.
61. Lebwohl M, Swanson N, Lawrence AL, Melgaard A, Xu Z, Berman B. Ingenol mebutate gel for actinic keratosis. *N Engl J Med.* 2012;366:1010–1019.
62. Peng Q, Soler AM, Warloe T, Nesland JM, Giercksky KE. Selective distribution of porphyrins in skin thick basal cell carcinoma after topical application of methyl 5-aminolevulinate. *J Photochem Photobiol B.* 2001;62(3):140–145.
63. Dragieva G, Prinz BM, Hafner J, et al. A randomized controlled clinical trial of topical photodynamic therapy with methyl aminolaevulinate in the treatment of actinic keratoses in transplant recipients. *Br J Dermatol.* 2004;151(1):196–200.
64. Piaserico S, Belloni Fortina A, Rigotti P, et al. Topical photodynamic therapy of actinic keratosis in renal transplant recipients. *Transplant Proc.* 2007;39(6):1847–1850.
65. Willey A, Mehta S, Lee PK. Reduction in the incidence of squamous cell carcinoma in solid organ transplant recipients treated with cyclic photodynamic therapy. *Dermatol Surg.* 2010;36(5):652–658.
66. Guleng GE, Helsing P. Photodynamic therapy for basal cell carcinomas in organ-transplant recipients. *Clin Exp Dermatol.* 2012;37(4):367–369.
67. Chen K, Craig JC, Shumack S. Oral retinoids for the prevention of skin cancers in solid organ transplant recipients: a systematic review of randomized controlled trials. *Br J Dermatol.* 2005;152(3):518–523.
68. Schule R, Rangarajan P, Yang N, et al. Retinoic acid is a negative regulator of AP-1-responsive genes. *Proc Natl Acad Sci U S A.* 1991;88(14):6092–6096.
69. Hansen LA, Sigman CC, Andreola F, Ross SA, Kelloff GJ, De Luca LM. Retinoids in chemoprevention and differentiation therapy. *Carcinogenesis.* 2000;21(7):1271–1279.
70. Wright TI, Spencer JM, Flowers FP. Chemoprevention of nonmelanoma skin cancer. *J Am Acad Dermatol.* 2006;54(6):933–946; quiz 47–50.
71. Otley CC, Berg D, Ulrich C, et al. Reduction of immunosuppression for transplant-associated skin cancer: expert consensus survey. *Br J Dermatol.* 2006;154(3):395–400.
72. Kovach BT, Sams HH, Stasko T. Systemic strategies for chemoprevention of skin cancers in transplant recipients. *Clin Transplant.* 2005;19(6):726–734.
73. Zwald FO, Brown M. Skin cancer in solid organ transplant recipients: advances in therapy and management: part II. Management of skin cancer in solid organ transplant recipients. *J Am Acad Dermatol.* 2011;65(2):263–279; quiz 80.
74. Patton TJ, Zirwas MJ, Wolverton SE. Systemic retinoids. In: Wolverton SE, ed. *Comprehensive Dermatologic Drug Therapy.* 2nd ed. Philadelphia, PA: Elsevier; 2007:275–300.
75. Peramiquel L, Dalmau J, Puig L, Roé E, Fernández-Figueras MT, Alomar A. Inflammation of actinic keratoses and acral erythrodysesthesia during capecitabine treatment. *J Am Acad Dermatol.* 2006;55(5 Suppl):S119–S120.
76. Endrizzi BT, Lee PK. Management of carcinoma of the skin in solid organ transplant recipients with oral capecitabine. *Dermatol Surg.* 2009;35(10):1567–1572.
77. Jirakulaporn T, Endrizzi B, Lindgren B, Mathew J, Lee PK, Dudek AZ. Capecitabine for skin cancer prevention in solid organ transplant recipients. *Clin Transplant.* 2011;25(4):541–548.

78. Vidal D, Alomar A. Efficacy of imiquimod 5% cream for basal cell carcinoma in transplant patients. *Clin Exp Dermatol.* 2004;29(3):237–239.
79. Conolly SM, Baker DR, Coldiron BM, et al. AAD/ACMS/ASDSA/ASMS 2012 Appropriate use criteria for Mohs Micrographic Surgery. *J Am Acad Dermatol.* 2012;67(4):531–550.
80. Jambusaria-Pahlajani A, Hess SD, Katz KA, Berg D, Schmults CD. Uncertainty in the perioperative management of high-risk cutaneous squamous cell carcinoma among Mohs surgeons. *Arch Dermatol.* 2010;146(11):1225–1231.
81. Ross AS, Whalen FM, Elenitsas R, Xu X, Troxel AB, Schmults CD. Diameter of involved nerves predicts outcomes in cutaneous squamous cell carcinoma with perineural invasion: an investigator-blinded retrospective cohort study. *Dermatol Surg.* 2009;35(12):1859–1866.
82. Miller SJ, Alam M, Andersen J, et al. Basal cell and squamous cell skin cancers. *J Natl Compr Canc Netw.* 2010;8(8):836–864.
83. Kwan W, Wilson D, Moravan V. Radiotherapy for locally advanced basal cell and squamous cell carcinomas of the skin. *Int J Radiat Oncol Biol Phys.* 2004;60(2):406–411.
84. Stasko T, Brown MD, Carucci JA, et al. Guidelines for the management of squamous cell carcinoma in organ transplant recipients. *Dermatol Surg.* 2004;30(4 Pt 2):642–650.
85. Veness MJ, Morgan GJ, Palme CE, Gebski V. Surgery and adjuvant radiotherapy in patients with cutaneous head and neck squamous cell carcinoma metastatic to lymph nodes: combined treatment should be considered best practice. *Laryngoscope.* 2005;115(5):870–875.
86. Cartei G, Cartei F, Interlandi G, et al. Oral 5-fluorouracil in squamous cell carcinoma of the skin in the aged. *Am J Clin Oncol.* 2000;23(2):181–184.
87. Wollina U, Hansel G, Koch A, Köstler E. Oral capecitabine plus subcutaneous interferon alpha in advanced squamous cell carcinoma of the skin. *J Cancer Res Clin Oncol.* 2005;131(5):300–304.
88. Hitt R, Jimeno A, Rodriguez-Pinilla M, et al. Phase II trial of cisplatin and capecitabine in patients with squamous cell carcinoma of the head and neck, and correlative study of angiogenic factors. *Br J Cancer.* 2004;91(12):2005–2011.
89. Bentzen JD, Hansen HS. Phase II analysis of paclitaxel and capecitabine in the treatment of recurrent or disseminated squamous cell carcinoma of the head and neck region. *Head & neck.* 2007;29(1):47–51.
90. ClinicalTrials.gov. Phase III randomized study of adjuvant intensity-modulated radiotherapy with versus without cetuximab in patients with locally advanced resected squamous cell carcinoma of the head and neck. ClinicalTrials.gov identifier: NCT00956007. http://clinicaltrials.gov/show/NCT00956007. Accessed Aug. 6, 2014.
91. Carucci JA, Martinez JC, Zeitouni NC, et al. In-transit metastasis from primary cutaneous squamous cell carcinoma in organ transplant recipients and nonimmunosuppressed patients: clinical characteristics, management, and outcome in a series of 21 patients. *Dermatol Surg.* 2004;30(4 Pt 2):651–655.
92. Mullen JT, Feng L, Xing Y, et al. Invasive squamous cell carcinoma of the skin: defining a high-risk group. *Ann Surg Oncol.* 2006;13(7):902–909.
93. Ross AS, Schmults CD. Sentinel lymph node biopsy in cutaneous squamous cell carcinoma: a systematic review of the English literature. *Dermatol Surg.* 2006;32(11):1309–1321.
94. Kwon S, Dong ZM, Wu PC. Sentinel lymph node biopsy for high-risk cutaneous squamous cell carcinoma: clinical experience and review of literature. *World J Surg Oncol.* 2011; 9:80.
95. Zwald FO, Christenson LJ, Billingsley EM, et al. Melanoma in solid organ transplant recipients. *Am J Transplant.* 2010;10(5):1297–1304.
96. Nghiem P, Jamies N. Merkel cell carcinoma in organ transplant recipients. In: Otley CC, Stasko T, eds. *Skin Disease in Organ Transplantation.* New York, NY: Cambridge University Press; 2008:190–194.
97. Poulsen M. Merkel-cell carcinoma of the skin. *Lancet Oncol.* 2004;5(10):593–599.
98. Kauffman HM, Cherikh WS, Cheng Y, Hanto DW, Kahan BD. Maintenance immunosuppression with target-of-rapamycin inhibitors is associated with a reduced incidence of de novo malignancies. *Transplantation.* 2005;80(7):883–889.
99. Yakupoglu YK, Buell JF, Woodle S, Kahan BD. Individualization of immunosuppressive therapy. III. Sirolimus associated with a reduced incidence of malignancy. *Transplant Proc.* 2006; 38(2):358–361.
100. Fernandez A, Marcen R, Pascual J, et al. Conversion from calcineurin inhibitors to everolimus in kidney transplant recipients with malignant neoplasia. *Transplant Proc.* 2006;38(8): 2453–2455.
101. de Fijter JW. Use of proliferation signal inhibitors in non-melanoma skin cancer following renal transplantation. *Nephrol Dial Transplant.* 2007;22(Suppl 1):i23–i26.
102. Campbell SB, Walker R, Tai SS, Jiang Q, Russ GR. Randomized controlled trial of sirolimus for renal transplant recipients at high risk for nonmelanoma skin cancer. *Am J Transplant.* 2012;12(5):1146–1156.
103. Euvrard S, Morelon E, Rostaing L, et al. Sirolimus and secondary skin-cancer prevention in kidney transplantation. *N Engl J Med.* 2012;367(4):329–339.
104. Leard LE, Cho BK, Jones KD, et al. Fatal diffuse alveolar damage in two lung transplant patients treated with cetuximab. *J Heart Lung Transplant.* 2007;26(12):1340–1344.
105. O'Bryan K, Ratner D, eds. *Evolving Paradigm for the Workup and Management of Very High Risk Cutaneous Squamous Cell Carcinoma.* Chicago, IL: American College of Mohs Surgery; 2012.
106. Kalapurakal SJ, Malone J, Robbins KT, Buescher L, Godwin J, Rao K. Cetuximab in refractory skin cancer treatment. *J Cancer.* 2012;3:257–261.

SECTION 4

Aesthetic and Laser Procedures

CHAPTER 31

Cosmeceuticals and Topical Agents

Zoe Diana Draelos

INTRODUCTION

Topical agents are important in procedural dermatology. They can prevent infection, improve the skin barrier, minimize pain, create an environment for wound healing, decrease scarring, and enhance skin appearance. The most basic of topical agents important for skin health are cleansers designed to maintain a healthy biofilm key to the prevention of wound infection. A specialized subset of cleansers are hand sanitizers used by physicians and patients alike, as the most accessible source of pathogens for wound infection is the hands. Moisturizers are sometimes required due to the overly aggressive effects of cleansers and are useful in improving postprocedural skin appearance and creating an environment for barrier repair and healing. Many scar creams are specialized moisturizers with an important subset considered as FDA 510(k) cleared prescription products. Some contain interesting new ingredients, such as stem cell extracts and peptides, engineered to promote healing with market crossover into the anti-aging market. This chapter discusses these technologies and their relevance to procedural dermatology.

THE SKIN BIOFILM

The skin biofilm assumes great importance in procedural dermatology because it can become a source of organisms resulting in postprocedural complications. The biofilm covers every inch of the skin and is composed of sebum, eccrine and apocrine secretions, environmental dirt, cosmetics, skin care products, bacteria, yeast, and fungal organisms. It can be diminished, but not eliminated. Even after aggressive skin cleansing, the biofilm begins to reappear almost immediately. This begs the question as to whether the biofilm is an asset or hindrance to the success of dermatologic procedures. A healthy biofilm can be an asset to procedural dermatology because there is a limit to how many bacterial and fungal organisms can live in a square centimeter of skin. Colonization with nonpathogenic organisms, such as *Malassezia furfur* and *Staphylococcus epidermidis*, can limit the ability of pathogenic organisms, such as *Candida albicans* and methicillin-resistant *Staphylococcus aureus* (MRSA), to grow. On the other hand, it has been suggested that inadvertent injection of biofilm organisms into the skin with fillers has resulted in sterile granuloma formation. Nevertheless, the biofilm must be controlled to prevent postprocedural infections.

The main method of controlling the biofilm is through cleansing. Cleansing temporarily removes the biofilm, but recolonization occurs rapidly in a contaminated world. It is thought that the pH of healthy skin is 5, but this is really the pH of the biofilm. The slightly acidic biofilm pH limits the growth of organisms and must be maintained. For this reason, it is important to understand the role of skin cleansing in procedural dermatology.

SKIN CLEANSING

Skin cleansing is an important mechanism for procedural infection prevention, and represents a complex interaction between the skin surface, physical rubbing, and the chemistry of the cleanser. Even though cleansing is a routine skin hygiene event, it is technologically profound. The invention of soap ranks along with clean water and public sewers as one of the major advances providing improved health in the United States.

There are three types of traditional cleansers classified as soap: true soaps, syndets, and combars. True soaps, such as Ivory (Procter & Gamble) are composed of long-chain fatty acid alkali salts with a pH of 9 to 10. These true soaps can alkalinize the skin biofilm, which some researchers believe can contribute to irritation. If the biofilm is alkalinized, healthy skin will rapidly regain its slightly acidic pH, but this may not be the case in skin disease. True soaps do an excellent job of removing surface sebum, but can also remove the intercellular lipids.

The need to remove only surface sebum, leaving the skin barrier undamaged, led to the development of synthetic detergents, known as syndets. Syndets contain less than 10% soap. It is for this reason that they can be used frequently for daily bathing without causing eczematous disease in most individuals. Syndets also have a lower pH of 5.5 to 7, which is closer to natural neutral skin pH, resulting in less alkalinization of the skin. However, this point is somewhat controversial. There are people who design cleansers that believe a pH as close to neutral as possible is desirable, as it does not alter the pH of the skin. This is in contrast to the Japanese, who believe that skin cleansers should be formulated at a slightly acidic pH, because they feel that bacterial killing occurs better in an acidic environment. Others state that the cleanser pH does not matter, as healthy skin returns to its normal pH rapidly after cleansing. The controversy has yet to be resolved.

The most important cleansers from a dermatologic procedural standpoint are the combars. These are products that contain both soap and syndet cleansers, usually with an added topical antibacterial, such as triclosan (Dial, Dial Corporation; Irish Spring, Colgate-Palmolive). Triclosan is chemically known as 2,4,4'-trichloro-2'-hydroxydiphenyl ether. It is a chlorinated phenolic compound that is also used as a surgical scrub. Triclosan kills organisms by damaging the cell membrane, but has weak activity against gram-negative bacteria, such as *Pseudomonas*. Recent FDA concerns have been expressed regarding the widespread use of triclosan and its environmental impact, accompanied by concerns of possible growing bacterial resistance. Nevertheless, triclosan remains an important pre- and post-procedural cleanser to normalize the biofilm and prevent infection.

HAND SANITIZERS

Hand sanitizers represent a subset of cleansers with unique importance to procedural dermatology. Not only are hand sanitizers used by dermatologists to clean the hands prior to surgery in some cases, but patients can also use hand sanitizers to minimize infection following invasive procedures. In 2007, USA Today listed hand sanitizers as one of the 25 inventions, along with cell phones, that changed modern life during the past 25 years. Hand sanitizers fall into several categories on the basis of composition: alcohols, quaternary ammonium compounds, and triclosan, discussed previously under antibacterial cleansers.

The largest category of hand sanitizers is based on alcohols. Alcohols have been used for disinfection for over 100 years and are highly effective because they nonspecifically denature proteins. The most effective alcohol used in hand sanitizers is ethanol, which is generally recognized as safe and effective by the FDA. Ethanol has excellent killing properties against both gram-positive and gram-negative bacteria and fungal organisms, but is not effective against bacterial spores and has variable efficacy in killing enveloped viruses.

Quaternary ammonium compounds, such as benzalkonium chloride or benzethonium chloride, represent another category of hand sanitizers. While the ethanol-based hand sanitizers are flammable, the quaternary ammonium compounds are not and can be used around cautery and laser equipment. Quaternary ammonium compounds adsorb to the cytoplasmic membrane of microbes causing leakage of cytoplasmic contents. They are bacteriostatic against gram-positive bacteria and some gram-negative bacteria and are also fungistatic. They are not active against nonenveloped viruses. It is interesting to note that some species of *S. aureus* carry a gene that allows resistance to quaternary ammonium compounds. These organisms are more likely to be antibiotic resistant as well. Quarternary ammonium compound hand sanitizers may not be the best choice when MRSA is a concern.

The Center for Disease Control (CDC) considers hand sanitizers to be a mainstay in the prevention of worldwide disease transmission. Alcohol-based hand sanitizers have become an international standard for hand hygiene and are endorsed by the World Health Organization (WHO) as part of its Patient Safety Initiative.[1] However, hand sanitizers do not kill all organisms. For example, hand sanitizers are not effective against *Clostridium difficile*, which has become another antibiotic resistant organism. A study in health care workers demonstrated better skin condition with the use of hand sanitizers as opposed to frequent hand washing, attesting to their mildness when used repeatedly.[2]

MOISTURIZERS

Skin cleansing is important to normalize the biofilm and prevent infection postprocedurally, but maintenance of the skin barrier is equally important to prevent infection and promote healing. In viable epidermis, the nucleated cells possess tight gap and adherens junctions with desmosomes and cytoskeletal elements that contribute to the barrier. In the stratum corneum, the skin barrier is formed by protein rich intervening intercellular lipids that are synthesized in the keratinocytes during epidermal differentiation and extruded into the extracellular domains. These lipids are composed of ceramides, free fatty acids, and cholesterol, which covalently bind to the cornified envelope proteins. Changes in these intercellular lipids and alterations in epidermal differentiation lead to barrier defects and delayed postprocedural healing.

Moisturizers that are medically relevant increase skin hydration and improve skin tactile characteristics. They do so by leaving a skin film that creates an artificial barrier, thereby decreasing evaporation of water from the skin to the lower humidity atmosphere. Moisturizers do not moisturize the skin. In the strictest sense, the word "moisturizer" is a misnomer, as moisturizers do not add water to the skin. Any water in a moisturizer formulation is a vehicle that evaporates, possibly drying the skin further, without enhancing skin water content. This explains why frequent application of moisturizers will further damage xerotic skin due to repeated wetting and drying of the skin surface.

Moisturizers hydrate the skin by decreasing transepidermal water loss (TEWL) and attracting water to the dehydrated stratum corneum and epidermis. Substances that reduce TEWL are oily and occlusive (Table 31-1).

TABLE 31-1

Moisturizing Ingredients Minimizing Transepidermal Water Loss

Silicone: dimethicone, cyclomethicone
Vegetable oils: grape seed, borage, jojoba, sesame seed
Alcohols: cetyl alcohol, stearyl alcohol
Petroleum derivatives: petrolatum, mineral oil

Substances that attract water to the skin are known as humectants (Table 31-2). The best moisturizers delivering skin hydration will contain both occlusive and humectant ingredients. The sum of these skin effects results in an environment that is optimal for barrier repair and healing in a postprocedural setting.

EMOLLIENTS AND SCAR CREAMS

An interesting subset of moisturizers used postprocedure are emollients and scar creams. As the wounded skin heals, the edges of the corneocytes fold, creating an irregular skin surface. This irregular surface feels rough when stroked due to increased skin friction. Emollients, which are thin oily substances, deposit between the desquamating corneocytes and function like glue to stick the corneocyte back onto the skin surface, decreasing friction and creating soft, smooth skin. All of the substances listed in Table 31-1 can also be considered emollients and form the basis for many over-the-counter (OTC) scar creams. The friction reducing ability of the emollient ingredients also allows easier massage of the re-epithelialized skin, thereby increasing elasticity and possibly minimizing hypertrophic scarring. In addition to emollients, scar creams may contain topical antibiotics and botanical anti-inflammatories, such as onion extract.

POSTPROCEDURAL BARRIER PRODUCTS

A newer postprocedural moisturizer has been labeled as a barrier repair product. This class of creams differs from traditional nonprescription moisturizers because the FDA has approved them as a 510(k) device. The 510(k) device approval process was originally developed to ensure the safety of equipment with an on/off switch. Lasers, light devices, cardiac pacemakers, and insulin pumps represent equipment requiring this type of approval. Although creams are not traditionally thought of as "devices," they received approval because they induce a physical change in the skin. This physical change was documented as an increase in skin hydration resulting from a decrease in TEWL.

Much like the previously described moisturizers, barrier repair products place a water impervious film over the skin surface, which decreases TEWL. TEWL is elevated when the skin barrier is damaged, representing the physiologic signal for barrier repair initiated by ceramide synthesis. By decreasing TEWL, barrier creams hydrate the skin and create an environment optimal for healing. There are a variety of different formulations that presently have 510(k) approval and produce barrier repair by different mechanisms. These 510(k)-approved barrier creams are reviewed next based on their unique active ingredient.

TABLE 31-2

Humectant Moisturizing Ingredients

Glycerin
Sorbitol
Propylene glycol, ethylene glycol
Hyaluronic acid
Sodium PCA
Proteins (collagen, keratin), peptides, and amino acids
Vitamins (A, D, E)
Urea
Lactic acid

CERAMIDE

Ceramide synthesis is the first step in healing a postprocedure damaged skin barrier. Nine different ceramides have been identified and many have been synthetically duplicated for inclusion in moisturizer formulations. The ceramides are distinguished by their polar head group architecture, as well as by their hydrocarbon chain properties.[3] A ceramide-dominant, triple-lipid barrier repair formulation received 510(k) approval in April 2006 containing capric acid, cholesterol, conjugated linolenic acid and the TEWL reducing agents candelilla wax and petrolatum.[4] The unique aspect of this cream is that the ratio of the triple lipid combination mimics that of physiologic lipids. However, as of this writing, the product is temporarily unavailable due to patent issues (EpiCeram, Promius).[5]

HYALURONIC ACID

Another endogenous component of the skin necessary for the maintenance of hydration postprocedurally is hyaluronic acid, a glycosaminoglycan found in the dermis. Hyaluronic acid acts as a humectant and is a component of the extracellular matrix. It is believed to stimulate neutrophil migration, fibroblast proliferation, and neoangiogenesis. Ivanov evaluated the effect of a hyaluronic acid sodium salt in the healing of episiotomy and cesarean section surgical wounds and found a lower incidence of edema and decreased wound exudate.[6]

Two hyaluronic acid–containing products have received 510(k) approval (Bionect, Innocutis; Hylatopic, Onset Therapeutics). One contains 0.2% hyaluronic acid sodium salt, which functions as a humectant, in combination with other humectants, such as glycerol and a 70% sorbitol solution (Bionect). In addition to humectants, occlusive ingredients are required to keep the water attracted by the humectant from evaporating into the environment. These are oily substances, such as an emulsifying wax, that physically block TEWL. Most good moisturizers use ingredients with occlusive and humectant properties to increase skin hydration. The same hyaluronic acid sodium salt is combined in a foam formulation with glycerin as an added humectant accompanied by dimethicone and petrolatum as occlusives (Hylatopic, Onset Therapeutics). Both of these products are recommended by the manufacturer for postprocedural use following laser resurfacing.

LICORICE EXTRACT

Other 510(k) device barrier creams contain a variety of botanical extracts designed to reduce postprocedural inflammation. One currently marketed product contains glycyrrhetinic acid and Vitis vinifera extracts (Atopiclair, currently for sale). In addition, it contains allantoin, alpha-bisabolol, hyaluronic acid, and shea butter. Glycyrrhetinic acid is a licorice extract that was reported to be safe by the Cosmetic Ingredient Review, and has the ability to block gap junction intracellular communication and inflammation.[7]

In addition to the anti-inflammatory effect of glycyrrhetinic acid, the Vitis vinifera extract, derived from grapes, and the alpha-bisabolol, derived from chamomile, also serve as antioxidant, anti-inflammatory ingredients. Finally, allantoin, a heterocyclic organic compound, is a time tested anti-inflammatory as assessed by the Cosmetic Ingredient Review.[8] The combination of various botanical anti-inflammatories may be helpful in managing postprocedural erythema, although studies for this indication have not been published.

PETROLATUM

The oldest wound care product and the very first therapeutic moisturizer ever developed was petrolatum. Petrolatum is a semisolid mixture of hydrocarbons obtained through the dewaxing of heavy mineral oils. Pure cosmetic grade petrolatum is practically odorless and tasteless. Other hydrocarbon contaminants in lower quality petrolatum may account for a distinct chemical smell noted with some products. Petrolatum first appeared in the US Pharmacopoeia in 1880 and has been a widely used ingredient in skin care products and topical pharmaceuticals ever since. It is interesting to note that petrolatum has never been duplicated synthetically. Some barrier repair creams contain petrolatum as their primary ingredient (Eletone, Ferndale). Petrolatum remains the gold standard for barrier repair ingredients because it is the substance closest to the natural intercellular lipids and it can intercalate into the intercellular spaces.[9] It may be that the beneficial effect of topical antibiotics in postprocedural wound care is not related to the bacitracin or neomycin, but rather to the petrolatum vehicle.

DIMETHICONE AND SILICONE GEL SHEETING

A newer alternative to petrolatum as a barrier repair ingredient is dimethicone, one of a family of silicone oils. These oils are less greasy than petrolatum and possess better aesthetic properties but are not as efficacious as petrolatum in reducing TEWL. Silicone originates from silica, which is found in sand, quartz, and granite. It derives its properties from the alternating silica and oxygen bonds, known as siloxane bonds, which are exceedingly strong. These strong bonds account for the tremendous thermal and oxidizing stability of silicone. Silicone is resistant to decomposition from ultraviolet radiation, acids, alkalis, ozone, and electrical discharges. The silicone used in topical preparations is an odorless, colorless, nontoxic liquid, which is excellent at reducing friction and can be used to massage a wound to minimize hypertrophic scar formation. To date there is no report of toxicity from the use of topical silicone.[10] A combination of cyclomethicone, a cyclic higher viscosity silicone, and dimethicone are used in barrier creams that are resistant to water removal (Tetrix, Valeant).[11,12]

Silicone is also used to promote healing and minimize scarring in the form of gel sheeting. The gel sheets are affixed to the re-epithelialized wound. Exactly how the gel works has never been proven, but it can reduce TEWL thus creating an environment conducive to wound healing.

PARAFFIN WAX

Another time-tested occlusive agent to decrease TEWL is paraffin wax. Liquid paraffin combined with paraffin wax is the basis for another barrier cream designed to be used in the management of superficial wounds, dermal ulcers, donor sites, burns, and radiation dermatitis (Biafine, OrthoNeutrogena). The wax provides an artificial barrier that remains in place until healing can occur. In addition, it was demonstrated that the formulation was chemotactic for macrophages and increased the IL-1/IL-6 ratio in epidermal wounds in normal human volunteers.[13] This wax-based formulation also improved healing following the treatment of actinic keratoses.[14]

TOPICAL STEM CELLS AND HEALING

Another topical trend in postprocedural healing is the use of stem cell technology. Although there is little scientific dermatologic data to support the use of such products, their tremendous penetration into the boutique cosmeceutical marketplace makes them a worthwhile topic for discussion. Stem cells are pluripotent cells that can differentiate into many different structures. The ability of stem cells to differentiate and remain differentiated is the key to survival of complex multiorgan life, such as humans. Once differentiated, liver cells must remain liver cells, kidney cells must remain kidney cells, and skin cells must remain skin cells. This is accomplished through epigenetic changes that repress selected gene sequences that should no longer be transcribed. If these gene sequences are mistakenly available for transcription, cancer may occur. There is nevertheless tremendous interest in stem cells as a source of materials for replenishing the aging body and also for promoting wound healing.

STEM CELL EXTRACTS

The majority of stem cells used in cosmeceuticals are derived from plants rather than animals. This eliminates the possibility of disease transmission and also keeps with current industry standards of avoiding animal cruelty; however, it also raises the issue as to whether plant stem cells can truly have an effect on human physiology. In actuality, the stem cells are not used in the skin healing products, but rather substances that are present in the stem cell extract. The stem cells are used as bioreactors to produce highly pure and refined raw materials to include in cosmeceutical formulations.

Some of the more popular stem cell extracts are derived from berries, such as raspberries, blueberries, and strawberries, because they contain high levels of anthocyanins, representing a new category of highly potent antioxidants with anti-inflammatory activity. The anti-inflammatory properties are felt to be beneficial in wound healing preparations.

Stem cells used for extract preparation can be obtained from berries, leaves, stems, twigs, or roots, but leaf stem cells are most commonly cultivated because they are the site of photosynthesis and require excellent oxidative stress protection yielding high quantities of antioxidants. The stem cells are cultured under controlled laboratory conditions to obtain the purest extracts possible, which are free from environmental contaminants including heavy metals, pesticides, and fungal toxins. When plant materials are concentrated, so are the contaminants. Stem cell derived materials also have greater consistency of contents. The plant materials are cultured under optimal conditions to yield a more standard composition than those grown outdoors, which may vary based on factors such as weather, soil condition, or fertilizer application. Consistency is the key to obtaining a reliable extract for reproducible results.

STEM CELL CULTIVATION

Many dermatologists mistakenly think that the entire stem cell is placed in the skin care product, but this is not the case. The stem cell is used to obtain the extract that is then placed into formulation. It is not possible to maintain live stem cells in cosmeceutical emulsions. Osmotic conditions, lack of suitable growth media, and preservatives make this impossible.

Stem cells are obtained from the plant leaves after they have been sterilized in 70% ethanol for 15 minutes and 1% bleach for an additional 15 minutes followed by washing three times with sterile water. The original plant material for culture must come from outdoors, but all contaminants must be removed for successful culture. The leaves are then cut into thin 0.5 cm pieces and placed on an agar culture plate containing plant growth hormones, such as kinetin, an active agent advertised in dermatology to promote healing and decrease the appearance of aging. Plant callus is then formed, and can be collected. The callus is then cultured to form single cells, which are recultured in a liquid medium. The cells are then filtered for removal from the media and homogenized. The mixture is centrifuged to remove the soluble components and lyophilized to obtain a powder that represents the cosmeceutical ingredient, which is added to the wound healing product. An example of the constituents of a raspberry extract obtained in this manner, containing numerous antioxidants, is listed in Table 31-3.[15]

TABLE 31-3
Raspberry Extract Constituents

Phenolic acids
Ferulic acid
Caffeic acid
Protocatechuic acid
Gallic acid
Coumaric acids
Ellagic acid pentose derivatives
Ellagitannins
Flavonoids
Quercetin
Quercetin rhamnoside
Quercetin glucoside
Methyl-derivative of quercetin
Kaempferol glucoside
Anthocyanins
Pelargonidin
Pelargonidin glucoside
Resveratrol glucoside

Stem cell technology is the first step in standardizing botanical cosmetic ingredients and achieving dose consistency and purity. However, stem cell technology does not mean that plant cells can somehow interact with human cells to promote wound healing or induce slowing of aging. Stem cells are simply chemical factories to yield high-quality ingredients that might be beneficial in creating an environment for wound healing. This technology is in its infancy and certainly will be an area to follow for future developments.

PEPTIDES AND WOUND HEALING

Peptides are the cellular messengers of the body that allow the modulation of receptors, activate enzyme release, and regulate the production of proteins. Peptides are present in many of the new generation cosmeceuticals, but were originally developed for wound healing purposes. They are considered safe when topically applied, as peptides are ingested on a regular basis when consuming meat. Allergic reactions to topical peptide formulations have not been reported to date. This discussion examines peptides and their role in postprocedural skin care.

Peptides are formed from amino acids that are selected by the protein chemist to achieve a specific functional goal. The peptide families that have been identified thus far are listed in Table 31-4. The first peptides introduced into the wound healing marketplace were carrier peptides, which were then adapted to the anti-aging skin care market. From the

TABLE 31-4 Peptide Families
Carrier peptides
Signal peptides
Neurotransmitter peptides
Enzyme-modulating peptides

carrier peptides, the next development was signal peptides designed to mimic a natural body structure and turn on or off production of an endogenous protein. Neurotransmitter peptides were then developed that interrupted acetylcholine release. Finally, enzyme-modulating peptides that directly or indirectly inhibit enzyme functioning were produced.

CARRIER PEPTIDES

The first commercialized peptides were carrier peptides. These peptides were designed to hook to another ingredient and facilitate transportation of the agent to the active site. The first carrier peptide was designed to deliver copper, a trace element necessary for wound healing. From a wound healing application, a peptide known as GHK-Cu was commercialized into a line of skin care products to minimize the appearance of fine lines and wrinkles (Neutrogena, J&J). GHK-Cu is composed of glycine, histidyl and lysine hooked to copper and was found to induce dermal keratinocyte proliferation. GHK was originally isolated from human plasma and then synthetically engineered.

SIGNAL PEPTIDES

The largest peptide family currently used in marketed cosmeceuticals is the signal peptides. Signal peptides stimulate collagen, elastin, fibronectin, proteoglycan, and glycosaminoglycan production, creating the appearance of younger looking skin. The most popular signal peptide is palmitoyl pentapeptide, commercially known as Matrixyl (Olay Regenerist, P&G). Palmitoyl pentapeptide, abbreviated Pal-KTTKS, is composed of the amino acids threonine, lysine, and serine. It is a procollagen I fragment demonstrated to stimulate the production of collagen I, III, and IV in vitro. It is used in a low concentration of four parts per million, as it theoretically acts as a "signal," by way of which one molecule has a cascading effect. The idea is to present the body with procollagen fragments that will down-regulate the production of collagenase, thereby increasing dermal collagen.

NEUROTRANSMITTER PEPTIDES

Neurotransmitter peptides function by inhibiting the release of acetylcholine at the neuromuscular junction. They are similar to botulinum toxin in that both selectively modulate synaptosome-associated protein of 25,000 Daltons, more commonly known as SNAP-25. Botulinum toxin A proteolytically degrades SNAP-25 while acetyl hexapeptide-3, a neurotransmitter peptide, mimics the N-terminal end of the SNAP-25 protein that inhibits the SNARE (soluble N-ethyl-maleimide-sensitive factor attachment protein receptor) complex formation. Acetyl hexapeptide-3 is commercially known as Argireline (Centerchem). It supposedly functions topically to relax muscles, much like a weak short-lived botulinum toxin, by inhibiting vesicle docking through prevention of the SNARE complex formation. This muscle relaxation reduces the appearance of facial wrinkles.

ENZYME-MODULATING PEPTIDES

Enzyme-modulating peptides directly or indirectly inhibit the function of a key enzyme in some metabolic processes. Many of these peptides are extracted from botanical sources rather than engineered through protein chemistry. Soy proteins, already used in cosmeceuticals for the reduction of postinflammatory hyperpigmentation, possess another peptide that inhibits the formation of proteases. Rice proteins possess a peptide that inhibits matrix metalloproteinase (MMP) activity. These naturally occurring peptides are presently used in a number of marketed cosmeceuticals.

It is important to recognize that peptide chemistry is still in its infancy. Peptides hold the promise to modulate skin healing and functioning, but good studies remain elusive. The dermatologist should closely watch this family of cosmeceutical ingredients, as their true potential has not yet been fully realized.

CONCLUSION

There are a variety of topical products worthy of discussion relevant to procedural dermatology. These include cleansers and hand sanitizers that can restore a healthy biofilm following skin injury from filler injectables, chemical peeling, laser resurfacing, or cancer removal with reconstruction. After cleansing of the skin, a moisturizer is usually applied. The moisturizer can improve the appearance of the skin by smoothing scale in the area of the procedure, but also can create an environment for optimal healing. Specialized scar and barrier repair creams are a subset of moisturizers using many of the same ingredients, but also incorporating new technologies. Two of the most interesting relevant technologies are stem cell extracts and peptides. Over time, new topical agents with enhanced formulations will be developed, which will be likely to have increasing relevance and utility for the procedural dermatologist.

REFERENCES

1. Harbarth S, Pittet D, Grady L, et al. Interventional study to evaluate the impact of an alcohol-based hand gel in improving hand hygiene compliance. *Pediatr Infect Dis J.* 2002; 21:489–495.
2. Boyce JM, Kelliler S, Vallande N. Skin irritation and dryness associated with two hand hygiene regimens. *Infect Control Hosp Epidemiol.* 2000;21:442–448.
3. Garidel P, Fölting B, Schaller I, Kerth A. The microstructure of the stratum corneum lipid barrier: mid-infrared spectroscopic studies of hydrated ceramide: palmitic acid: cholesterol model systems. *Biophys Chem.* 2010;150(1–3): 144–156.

4. Madaan A. Epiceram for the treatment of atopic dermatitis. *Drugs Today (Barc).* 2008;44(10):751–755.
5. Sugarman JL, Parish LC. Efficacy of a lipid-based barrier repair formulation in moderate-to-severe pediatric atopic dermatitis. *J Drugs Dermatol.* 2009;8(12):1106–1111.
6. Ivanov C, Michova M, Russeva R, Batashki I. Clinical application of bionect (Hyaluronic acid sodium salt) in wound care by cesarean section and episiotomy. *Akush Ginekol (Sofiia).* 2007;46(Suppl 4):20–26.
7. Eberlein B, Eicke C, Reinhardt HW, Ring J. Adjuvant treatment of atopic eczema: assessment of an emollient containing N-palmitoylethanolamine (ATOPA Study). *J Eur Acad Dermatol Venereol.* 2008;22(1):73–82.
8. Becker LC, Bergfeld WF, Belsito DV, et al. Final report of the safety assessment of allantoin and its related complexes. *Int J Toxicol.* 2010;29(Suppl 3):84S–97S.
9. Morrison DS. Petrolatum: a useful classic. *Cosmet Toilet.* 1996;111:59–69.
10. Ruiz MA, Hernandez A, Llacer JM, Gallardo V. Silicone chemistry. *Cosmet Toilet.* 1998;113:57–62.
11. Slade HB, Fowler J, Draelos ZD, Reece BT, Cargill DI. Clinical efficacy evaluation of a novel barrier protection cream. *Cutis.* 2008;82(Suppl 4):21–28.
12. Slade HB, Fowler J, Reece BT, Cargill DI. Clinical safety evaluation of a novel barrier protection cream. *Cutis.* 2008; 82(Suppl 4):16–20.
13. Coulomb B, Friteau L, Dubertret L. Biafine applied on human epidermal wounds is chemotactic for macrophages and increases the IL-1/IL-6 ratio. *Skin Pharmacol.* 1997;10 (5–6):281–287.
14. Cohen JL, Jorizzo JL, Kircik LH. Use of a topical emulsion for wound healing. *J Support Oncol.* 2007;5(10 Suppl 5):1–9.
15. Barbulova A, Tito A, Carola A, et al. Raspberry stem cell extract to protect skin from inflammation and oxidative stress. *Cosmet Toilet.* 2010;125(7):38–47.

CHAPTER 32

Chemical Peels

Christopher B. Harmon & Tarek M. Fakhouri

INTRODUCTION

Maintaining a youthful appearance through the rehabilitation of photoaged skin is a topic of growing interest among the general population. To meet this need, rejuvenation techniques such as chemical peeling, dermabrasion, and laser resurfacing have been developed. Of these, chemical peeling has the longest record of safety and efficacy while being an easily accessible modality to the clinician. Chemical peeling is also low in cost and has a relatively quick recovery time.[1]

MECHANISM OF ACTION

Chemical peeling is the result of application of a chemical agent to the facial skin to create an injury to a specific depth, thereby inducing rejuvenation via wound repair. The degree of tissue penetration and ensuing injury by the peeling agent is dependent on several factors including skin preparation, anatomic site, duration of peeling, and the strength of the compound.[1] The depth of the injury is used to classify chemical peels into several categories. Superficial chemical peels cause epidermal injury. Medium-depth chemical peels cause injury to the level of the upper dermis. Deep chemical peels cause injury that extends to the level of the mid-dermis.

HISTORY OF USE

Chemical peeling has been practiced since ancient times. Cleopatra was known to use an alpha hydroxyacid (AHA) (lactic acid) from sour milk to smoothen her skin. Of historical interest to dermatology, Unna first described the use of trichloroacetic acid (TCA), salicylic acid, resorcinol, and phenol in 1882. Mackee, in 1903, treated facial scars with phenol and began publishing his results in 1952. In the 1940s, Eller and Wolff summarized the peeling formulas available at that time and used phenol, resorcinol, salicylic acid, and carbon dioxide (CO_2).[2] In the 1960s, Brown, Baker, and Gordon described a modified phenol solution with Septisol, croton oil, and water while Ayres began experimenting with TCA.[3–6] The work of Stegman in the 1980s characterized the histologic depth of many chemical cauterants and heralded a controlled scientific approach to chemical peeling.[7] Van Scott's work on AHAs in the 1970s and 1980s laid the foundation for the most popular superficial peeling agent, glycolic acid (GA).[8]

PEEL CLASSIFICATION

Peels are classified based on the achievable depth of penetration, which determines the clinical effect of the agent. Superficial peels (0.06 mm depth) lead to exfoliation and regeneration of the entire epidermis while very superficial peels only affect the stratum corneum. Medium-depth peels (0.45 mm depth) will destroy the epidermis and induce inflammation within the papillary dermis. Deep peels (0.6 mm depth) will induce inflammation into the reticular dermis and induce new collagen production.[7]

PROPER PATIENT SELECTION

As with any procedure, patient selection is key to optimizing outcomes and special attention should be paid to features of the patient's history and physical examination in attempt to identify factors that may contribute to intraoperative or postoperative problems. As a general rule, the deeper the peel the more care must be exercised in patient selection. Although patients of all skin types are often able to tolerate superficial peels, medium and deep peels carry more risk. Patients with Fitzpatrick skin types III to VI have higher risk of postoperative dyschromia than patients of lighter skin types (Table 32-1).[1,9]

Enquiry should be made regarding prior recent resurfacing procedures, face-lift surgery, and isotretinoin therapy within the past 6 months as these factors may increase the risk of complications.[10] A history of hypertrophic or keloidal scar formation is a relative contraindication to medium-depth peels and a contraindication to deep peels. A history of prior radiation treatment or photodynamic therapy must also be carefully considered as they may impact the skin's ability to repopulate the epidermis if significant numbers of pilosebaceous units have been obliterated.[11]

TABLE 32-1
The Fitzpatrick Classification of Skin Types

Skin Type	Color	Reaction to Sun
I	Very white, freckled	Always burns
II	White	Usually burns
III	White to olive	Sometimes burns
IV	Brown	Rarely burns
V	Dark brown	Very rarely burns
VI	Black	Never burns

TABLE 32-2
Photoaging Groups According to the Glogau Classification

Mild (28–35 yrs)	Moderate (35–50 yrs)	Advanced (50–65 yrs)	Severe (60–75 yrs)
Little wrinkling or scarring	Early wrinkling; mild scarring	Persistent wrinkling or moderate acne scarring	Severe wrinkling, photoaging, gravitational and dynamic forces affecting skin
No keratoses	Sallow color with early actinic keratoses	Discoloration with telangiectasias and actinic keratoses	Actinic keratoses ± skin cancer
Little or no makeup	Little makeup	Wears makeup always	Wears makeup with poor coverage

Patients with dermatologic disorders such as atopic dermatitis, rosacea, seborrheic dermatitis, and psoriasis may be at increased risk of postoperative complications including disease exacerbation, prolonged erythema, contact hypersensitivity, and delayed healing. Individuals with rosacea and vasomotor instability may develop an exaggerated inflammatory response to the peeling agent with prolonged postoperative erythema. A history of "cold sores" can predispose to post-peel herpes simplex virus reactivation following medium or deep peeling. Similarly, cigarette smoking can delay healing of the treated area.

The Glogau system classifies the severity of photodamage, taking into account the degree of epidermal and dermal degenerative effects (Table 32-2).[12] These categories are devised to project which patients need therapeutic intervention. Patients with mild photoaging are best treated with superficial chemical peeling in combination with a medical or cosmeceutical agent. Patients with moderate or advanced photoaging achieve maximal benefit from medium-depth chemical peeling whereas individuals with severe photoaging need deep peeling or resurfacing plus cosmetic surgical intervention to improve gravitational changes.

SUPERFICIAL PEELS

The most common peeling agents for superficial peels are AHA (e.g., GA), beta hydroxyacids (BHA) (e.g., salicylic acid), Jessner's solution (JS) (resorcinol 14 g, salicylic acid 14 g, lactic acid 14 mL, and ethanol 100 mL), CO_2 slush, and TCA. Very light superficial peels injure only the stratum corneum, causing exfoliation without necrosis. Agents used for very light peels include low concentrations of GA (10%–40%), TCA (10%–20%), JS, and salicylic acid. Light superficial peels injure the entire epidermis and are performed using GA 70%, TCA (25%–35%), or solid CO_2 slush.[1,13]

Sample Consent Form

CONSENT FOR CHEMICAL PEEL

I, ______________ request and authorize Dr. ______________ to perform a chemical peel of the skin in order to improve the following condition(s): ____
______________________________________.

I know that the practice of medicine and surgery is not an exact science; therefore, reputable practitioners cannot properly guarantee the quality of the results or freedom from complications. I acknowledge that the nature and effects of this procedure, risks involved, as well as alternative methods of treatment, have been explained to me to my satisfaction.

By signing this consent, I acknowledge that I understand the following facts about chemical peeling:

1. There is no guarantee that the results will be satisfactory to me.
2. There is some discomfort associated with these procedures. I may be given pain medicines prior to the procedure.
3. Multiple procedures may be necessary to achieve the desired results, especially with "light" chemical peels consisting only of JS or TCA.
4. There is a risk of complications such as, but not limited to, any of the following: edema (swelling), hyperpigmentation (increased pigmentation) that might be blotchy, hypopigmentation (decreased pigmentation) that might be blotchy, persistent erythema (redness) in some areas after the procedure, infection, allergic reaction, scarring (this is a very rare complication).
5. Exposure to sun may increase the possibility of swelling and redness.
6. Photographs of the affected areas, before, during, and after treatment, shall be held for your medical records; unless, in the judgment of the doctor, medical research or science will benefit from their use.
7. I understand that this procedure may be considered cosmetic even though it is the recommended procedure for my condition. I agree to pay for this procedure and will be fully responsible for these charges in the event that my insurance does not cover this surgery.
8. The estimated cost of this procedure is $______________.

Patient:______________________________ Date:____________

Witness:______________________________ Date:____________

INDICATIONS FOR SUPERFICIAL PEELS.

Superficial chemical peels can be used for comedonal acne, postinflammatory erythema or pigmentation, epidermal melasma, and mild photoaging (Glogau I and II).[14] Multiple peeling sessions are necessary to obtain maximal result and are usually performed on a weekly or biweekly frequency.[1] Results are enhanced by daily use of a retinoid and, when used for pigmentary lesions, daily kojic acid or hydroquinone may improve efficacy.[15] Prior to initiation of a treatment course for photoaging, the patient and physician must understand the limitations of that course. The improvement will be subtle and the effect of multiple superficial peels will never equal the effect of a medium-depth or deep peel. Superficial peels only affect the epidermis and are unable to effect improvement in dermal processes, such as deep rhytides.

SUPERFICIAL PEEL PROTOCOLS.

GA is an AHA that is naturally present in sugar cane. GA can be obtained in unbuffered concentrations of 50% to 70%. Following degreasing with acetone, GA 70% is applied to the skin evenly with a gauze pad or cotton swab. GA 70% will induce epidermolysis in 3 to 7 minutes depending upon the patient. The acid must be neutralized by rinsing with water or 5% sodium bicarbonate once appropriate peeling has occurred, typically 2 to 4 minutes after application. Mild erythema with scaling may occur for an hour post procedure.[16]

TCA 10% to 35% can be used for very light to light superficial peels. TCA should be formulated using a weight-in-volume method. For example, a 25% TCA solution is made by adding 30 g of TCA to enough water to make a 100 mL solution. Adding 25 g of TCA to 100 mL would produce a weaker concentration and is inappropriate. Following degreasing with acetone, hexachlorophene, or chlorhexidine gluconate, TCA is applied with a gauze pad or cotton-tipped applicator. As with all peels, the TCA is applied to cosmetic units individually, beginning with the thickest and most sebaceous skin and progressing to the thinnest and most delicate skin of the eyelids. The TCA is applied uniformly and a fan or ice pack may be used to alleviate the discomfort of areas that have come to a complete frost. Immediate erythema of the treated site is followed by a frost that usually persists for less than an hour.[17] Exfoliation without vesiculation begins on postoperative day 2 and lasts from 3 to 5 days.

JS is used for very light or in combination with TCA for medium-depth peels. JS must be kept in a dark bottle, otherwise it will become an irritating solution that can discolor the fingernails. JS is applied similarly to TCA with wrung-out or wet gauze sponge application. Dilution is not performed and neutralization is unnecessary. Additional coats will increase the strength of the peel and the patient's response to the number of coats should be monitored. The number of coats is typically increased based on patient tolerability. JS has the advantage of being a single solution that does not require dilution or timing of the duration of application.[18,19]

MEDIUM-DEPTH PEELS

Due to its low cost, ease of application, and efficacy, the benchmark standard for medium-depth chemical peels was 50% TCA. When used alone, this agent produced acceptable results in ameliorating fine wrinkles and actinic damage.[20] However, in strengths of 50% or higher, TCA can result in increased risk of scarring and has since fallen out of favor as a single agent chemical peel as a result. More recently, combinations of 35% TCA with other chemical and physical agents have been found to be equally effective in producing this level of controlled damage with a much lower risk of scarring.[19,21,22]

Brody[21] pioneered the use of solid CO_2 applied with acetone to the skin before the application of 35% TCA. Freezing the skin surface prior to application of TCA breaks up the epidermal barrier and allows for more even penetration, and the penetration using this combination is deeper than with 35% TCA alone. Monheit[19] demonstrated similar results with the use of JS prior to application of 35% TCA. JS destroys the epidermal barrier, allowing for deeper and more even penetration of the 35% TCA. Coleman and Futrell[22] demonstrated similar efficacy and safety using the combination of 70% GA prior to the application of 35% TCA. Tse et al.[23] compared the GA/TCA 35% and JS/TCA 35% medium-depth peels in the treatment of fine wrinkling, actinic keratoses (AKs), and lentigines. Although both methods produced similar clinical responses and had similar healing times, patients treated with GA/TCA 35% experienced more pain than those treated with JS/TCA 35%. The JS/TCA 35% peel produced a more intense inflammatory response, and clinically post-peel erythema was more prolonged. Although all three medium-depth peel combinations have proven to be as effective as the use of 50% TCA with a greater safety margin, the JS/TCA 35% combination enjoys widespread use and will be discussed later.

INDICATIONS FOR MEDIUM-DEPTH PEELS.

Medium-depth chemical peels may be used to treat mild-to-moderate photoaging including pigmentary changes, lentigines, AKs, acne scarring, unwanted epidermal growths, dyschromias, and rhytides (Fig. 32-1).[24] Although most often performed for photoaging, the efficacy of medium-depth chemical peels in the treatment of AKs is well substantiated.

Lawrence et al.[25] compared the efficacy and safety of the JS/TCA 35% medium-depth peel to that of 5% fluorouracil (5-FU) in the treatment of severe facial actinic damage. Both treatments reduced the number of AKs by 75% and produced equivalent reductions in keratinocyte atypia, hyperkeratosis, parakeratosis, and inflammation. The majority of patients preferred the peel to 5-FU because of the single application and less morbidity. Witheiler et al.[26] compared the long-term efficacy and safety of JS/TCA to 5-FU in the treatment of widespread facial AKs. Both treatments resulted in an 80% decrease in AKs, and the reduction in clinically apparent lesions was stable for 1 year after treatment. However, the investigators noted a sharp increase in the mean number of AKs between 12 and 32 months after both treatments, and these findings indicate the importance of 12 to 18 month follow-up visits. In both studies, a single treatment of JS/TCA 35% was compared to 3 weeks of 5-FU cream applied b.i.d.

CONTRAINDICATIONS.

There are no absolute contraindications for medium-depth chemical peeling. However, the risk/benefit ratio of a medium-depth chemical

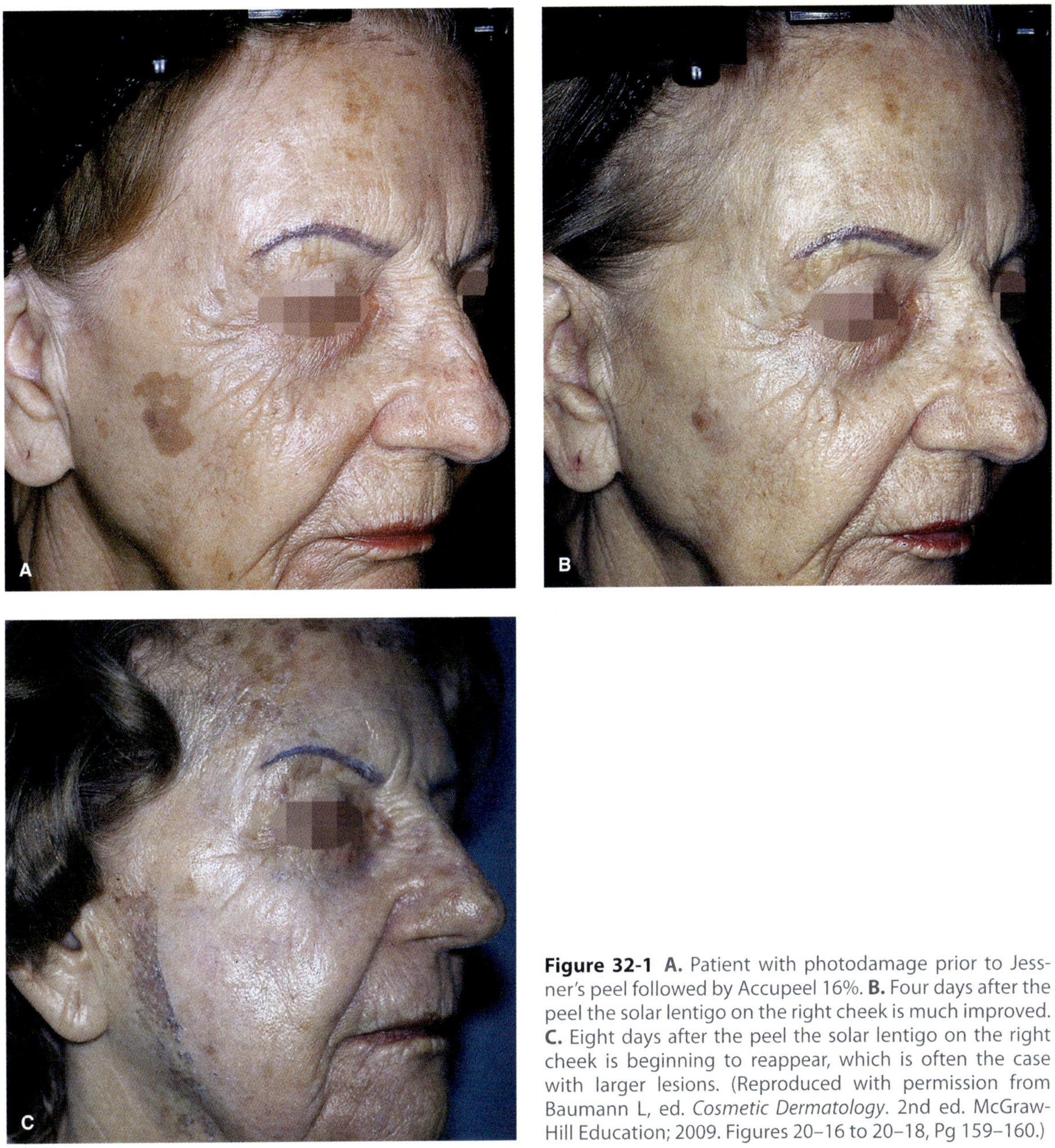

Figure 32-1 A. Patient with photodamage prior to Jessner's peel followed by Accupeel 16%. **B.** Four days after the peel the solar lentigo on the right cheek is much improved. **C.** Eight days after the peel the solar lentigo on the right cheek is beginning to reappear, which is often the case with larger lesions. (Reproduced with permission from Baumann L, ed. *Cosmetic Dermatology*. 2nd ed. McGraw-Hill Education; 2009. Figures 20–16 to 20–18, Pg 159–160.)

peel may be unfavorable in patients with dermatologic disorders that koebnerize, a history of radiation or photo dynamic therapy for acne, recent isotretinoin use, a history of hypertrophic scarring, or a darker skin phenotype.

PREPROCEDURE EDUCATION AND PREPARATION. Patients should be aware that the procedure requires application of a peeling agent to the skin that will cause moderate pain, stinging, and burning. Methods to alleviate this pain include: local anesthesia, pre- and intraoperative pain medications, and a fan blowing cool air on the treatment site. Normal postoperative expectations include oozing of clear fluid, mild-to-moderate edema, erythema, and skin peeling. Patients must be informed of the possible complications including allergic reactions, scarring, postoperative infection, and pigmentary dyschromia. The consent form should be signed (see **Sample Consent Form**), and the patient is then given a prescription for valcyclovir 500 to 1000 mg b.i.d. to t.i.d. for 14 days with instructions to begin taking this medication 1 day prior to the procedure. Patients should also be instructed to purchase a jar of a petrolatum-based emollient for use after the procedure.

Skin preparation prior to medium-depth peeling is important to avoid post-peel complications and increase efficacy following the peel. Adjunctive agents should be started 6 weeks prior to peeling, the most important of which is a topical retinoid. Tretinoin 0.025% to 0.1% is used for its ability to decrease stratum corneum thickness, increase the rate of epidermal turnover, and decrease corneocyte adhesion.[20] Exfoliants such as AHAs can be used to stimulate epidermal growth by disrupting the stratum corneum. Finally, broad-spectrum sunscreens and hydroquinone 4% to 8% are useful in patients with dyschromias and those at risk for postprocedure inflammatory dyspigmentation.

MEDIUM-DEPTH JS/TCA 35% PEEL PROTOCOL

TRAY SET UP AND STORAGE OF MATERIALS. The set up tray should include Septisol Soap, 4 oz.; acetone, 8 oz.; JS solution, 4 oz.; and TCA 35%, 1 oz.[19,27] All of these chemicals are available from Delasco Dermatologic Lab & Supply, Inc (Delasco, Council Bluffs, IA; tel. 800–831–6273). Additional items include a midsized electric fan, 1 L prechilled normal saline, 2 × 2 gauze pads, 4 × 4 gauze pads, and cotton-tipped swabs. Chemical components of the set up tray are stored at room temperature and have a shelf life of up to 2 years. Staff should review the chemical expiration dates to ensure quality.

PROCEDURE PREPARATION AND ANESTHESIA. Prophylactic valcyclovir 500 to 1000 mg b.i.d. to t.i.d. should have been initiated 1 day prior to the procedure and should be continued for a total of 14 days. Documentation is reviewed including the consent form and the operative site (Table 32-3). Preoperative photographs are taken and archived. Medium-depth chemical peels are usually performed with mild preoperative sedation in combination with a nonsteroidal anti-inflammatory drug (NSAID). Choices include 50 mg of i.m. or p.o. meperidine, 5 mg of p.o. diazepam, 5 mg of i.v. midazolam, 25 mg of p.o. vistaril, and p.o. aspirin 325 mg. Aspirin can be continued 24 hours postoperatively if tolerated as its anti-inflammatory effect is especially helpful in reducing swelling and relieving pain.[24] If given before surgery, that may be all that the patient requires during the postoperative phase.

INTRAOPERATIVE SAFETY CONCERNS. The major safety concern regarding the medium-depth chemical peel is eye injury from the peeling agent or prep materials. The physician should wear protective eyewear, damp swabs containing JS or TCA should never be carried over the patient's eyes, and care must be taken when applying the peeling agent to the eyelids and periorbital regions. The patient should be instructed to keep their eyes closed at all times during the procedure. We apply the peeling agent to the eyelids with a damp cotton-tipped swab. In addition to these precautions, it is prudent to have appropriate eye lavage gear available.

PROCEDURE TECHNIQUE. The patient should be positioned with the head elevated at 30 degrees and the eyelids closed. To remove oil and debris, facial skin is scrubbed thoroughly with Septisol soap, 4 × 4 gauze pads and water, then rinsed with water and dried. This process may be repeated depending on the amount of oil and debris present. The intent is to debride the skin of stratum corneum and excessive scale.

Next, the skin surface is degreased by scrubbing with 2 × 2 gauze pads dampened with acetone. The cleansed skin should be palpated to check for the presence of oil, and if any is felt, degreasing should be repeated. Three applications for females and up to five applications for males may be required. Thorough degreasing is necessary to ensure even penetration of the peel and uniform results. The fan is switched on, pointed toward the patient's face, and left in this position for the duration of the procedure.

After degreasing, a single coat of JS is applied to the area using cotton-tipped swabs or 2 × 2 gauze pads. The forehead is treated first, followed by the cheeks, then the nose and chin, and finally the eyelids. This process may be repeated to ensure complete and even coverage. Proper application of the JS results in a faint frost that is superimposed on a background of erythema (level I frosting).

TABLE 32-3
Procedure checklist

☐ Prophylactic antiviral medication
☐ Informed consent signed
☐ Photos taken
☐ Preoperative medications given
☐ Liquid nitrogen treatment to keratoses if needed
☐ Apply septisol
☐ Apply acetone
☐ Turn on fan
☐ Apply JS
☐ Apply TCA
☐ Apply cool saline compresses
☐ Postoperative instructions given
☐ Procedure note documented in chart

Sample Postoperative Instructions

POST CHEMICAL PEEL INSTRUCTIONS (MEDIUM-DEPTH)

POSTOPERATIVE CARE

1. Starting tomorrow morning
   a. Soak the treated area for 15 minutes, four times a day using a solution of one tablespoon white vinegar in one pint of cool water on a washcloth. Any scabs present should be gently soaked off if possible. DO NOT PICK TO REMOVE DEAD SKIN OR SCABS.
   b. After soaking, pat the skin dry with a towel and apply a layer of Eucerin® cream over the entire face. Reapply whenever the skin feels dry.
2. Sleep on your back with your head elevated on a few pillows for the first few days if the face is swollen.
3. Avoid strenuous exercise for 2 weeks to avoid irritating the skin.
4. Do not expose the skin to the sun for 2 weeks. After complete healing, it will be able to tolerate sunscreens. We recommend Shade UVA Guard.
5. Most chemical peels today are supplemented by the use of creams such as retinoic acid (Retin-A), which cause a constant turnover of the top layers of skin, further improving its integrity. Your physician will instruct you when to resume the appropriate strength of Retin-A.

**Do not use AHA or Retin-A products until directed by physician

POSTOPERATIVE EXPECTATIONS

1. Mild/moderate redness is expected for 7 days after the procedure and will fade gradually over a 4 to 6 week period
2. Oozing of clear fluid from the surgical site may occur for 3 to 7 days
3. Mild-to-moderate swelling is normal and may last 3 to 7 days

---

Sample Chemical Peel Operative Note

CHEMEXFOLIATION OPERATIVE NOTE

Name:____________________

Date:____________________

Diagnosis:____________________

Procedure: 1. Local destruction of ____________________ lesions.

2. Chemexfoliation of the ____________________ using ____________________

____

Surgeon:____________________

Assistant:____________________

Description of the procedure: The individual lesions and areas for chemical removal were outlined and scrubbed with septisol and acetone to degrease and remove stratum corneum. A regional block using the ____________________ nerve with ____________________ anesthetic was performed. ____________________

Solution was painted over the area until frosting was evident. Individual lesions were destroyed with ____________________, and the regional area(s) of the ____________________ were painted carefully with cotton tips until frosted. After____________________, the areas were covered with saline saturated 4 × 4 gauze. The patient tolerated the procedure well.

Physician:____________________

Signature:____________________

The frosting from JS is much lighter than that produced by TCA and produces a feeling of heat.

After the JS has completely dried, TCA 35% is applied with one to four cotton-tipped swabs or 2 × 2 gauze until a light frost appears. The amount of TCA delivered to the skin surface is dependent on the degree of saturation of the swabs or gauze. More saturated gauze or swabs are applied with broad strokes over the forehead and cheeks. Two moist swabs or a less saturated gauze pad are used to treat the lips and chin, and one semidry swab is used to carry the TCA within 2 to 3 mm of the lid margin.

Application of TCA to the eyelids can be challenging due to the profuse tearing that accompanies coating of the sensitive eyelid skin. Placing a dry cotton swab at the medial and lateral canthi can soak up excess tears. By applying a slight amount of horizontal tension with the dry swabs, the eyelid skin can be delicately stretched, making it easier to evenly coat the area. Application of TCA to the eyelids is best done by rolling the swab in the direction opposite to that of application.

As with the application of JS, the forehead is treated first, followed by the cheeks, then the nose, chin, and finally the eyelids. The white frost from application of the

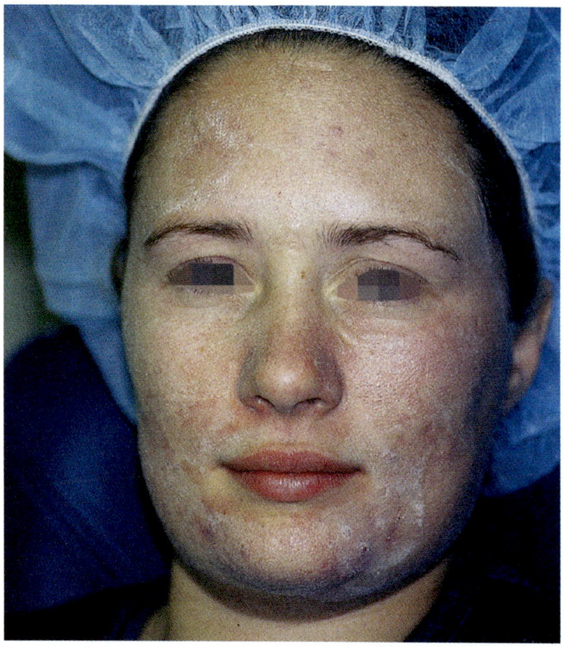

Figure 32-2 The white frost appears 2 minutes after application of a salicylic acid peel. (Reproduced with permission from Baumann L, ed. *Cosmetic Dermatology*. 2nd ed. McGraw-Hill Education; 2009. Fig 20–7, Pg 151.)

TCA appears on the treated area within 30 seconds to 2 minutes. Before re-treating the area, at least 3 to 4 minutes should elapse to ensure that frosting has reached its peak. Additional applications of TCA to previously treated areas will increase the depth of penetration and the risk of complications. For this reason, TCA should be carefully reapplied to unfrosted areas. Feathering of the solution into the hairline and around the rim of the jaw and brow conceals the demarcation line between treated and untreated areas. After the application of TCA is completed, cool saline compresses are applied to the entire face to dilute the solution, and these should remain in place for at least 10 to 20 minutes with the fan running.

Achieving level II to level III frosting will ensure desired efficacy. Most medium-depth peels use a level II frosting, which is defined as white-coated frosting with erythema showing through (Fig. 32-2). The zygomatic arch, bony prominences of the jaw line, and chin should only receive up to a level II frosting as risk of scarring is high in these areas. Level III frosting, defined as solid enamel frosting with faint background erythema, should be reserved for areas of heavy actinic damage or thick skin.

POSTPROCEDURE CARE. The patient should be instructed to soak the treated area with 0.25% acetic acid (one tablespoon white vinegar in one pint of warm water) using a clean washcloth up to four times per day. After soaking, the area should be gently patted dry and a thin layer of emollient applied. After 24 hours, the patient can shower and clean gently with a mild nondetergent cleanser. Some oozing of clear fluid from the treated area as well as mild-to-moderate swelling are normal in postoperative findings that may last 3 to 7 days. Patients should be advised that the peeled skin will look and feel tight and that excessive manipulation such as rubbing or picking can lead to scarring. A low-potency topical steroid may be used in patients who complain of pruritus. Patients should be informed that pre-existing pigmented lesions will darken considerably and appear grayish-brown.

Patients will experience a variable degree of erythema and edema. Edema peaks at 48 hours and may persist for several days. The patient should be instructed to sleep on his or her back with head elevated for the first few days if the face is swollen. Patients should also avoid strenuous exercise and not expose the treated skin to the sun for 4 to 6 weeks. The erythema intensifies as desquamation becomes complete within 4 to 5 days after the procedure. After 7 days the bright red color has faded to pink and has the appearance of a sunburn. Frequent brief follow-up visits are important to ensure normal healing. We schedule visits on postoperative days 1, 3, and 10. After re-epithelialization is complete, 7 to 10 days postprocedure, sunscreen, cosmetics, and retinoids may be restarted as tolerated. Patients should be advised that a post-peel regimen of sunscreen, retinoid, and an exfoliating agent, such as AHA, is necessary to maintain the benefits gained. Medium-depth chemical peels should not be repeated for a period of 6 months.

DEEP CHEMICAL PEELING

Patients with Glogau group III to IV photodamage may require deep chemical peeling or laser resurfacing to correct the dermal damage. Due to its unpredictability and risk of scarring, TCA ≥45% is no longer used for deep chemical peeling. The Baker–Gordon peel, described in 1961, produces reliable results and is the most commonly used formula for deep chemical peeling.[28] The Baker–Gordon peel formula must be freshly prepared and stirred vigorously prior to application.[29] The two main variations of deep chemical peeling with the Baker–Gordon formula are occluded (with zinc oxide tape) and unoccluded.

The tape, placed directly after the phenol is applied to each cosmetic unit, increases the penetration of the Baker's phenol solution and is helpful for very deep rhytides. The taped Baker–Gordon phenol peel creates damage to the midreticular dermis and carries a significant risk of scarring and overpenetration.[24] The unoccluded technique as modified by McCollough requires more skin cleansing and application of a greater amount of solution to achieve deep penetration.[30] However, it does not produce as deep a peel as the occluded method.

INDICATIONS FOR DEEP CHEMICAL PEELING. Deep chemical peeling is indicated for patients with severe photoaging (Glogau groups III and IV).

CONTRAINDICATIONS TO DEEP CHEMICAL PEELING. Phenol is toxic to the kidneys and liver, and may induce cardiac arrhythmias. It is, therefore, contraindicated in patients with a history of arrhythmia, who are on pro-arrhythmic medications, or who have hepatic or renal disease. Deep chemical peeling should not be performed within 6 months of using isotretinoin or having a medium or deep chemical peel.

In addition, deep chemical peeling carries the risk of persistent erythema and pigmentary disturbance. This can be particularly problematic for male patients and those with Fitzpatrick skin types III to VI. Other relative contraindications to deep peeling include patients with a koebnerizing condition, a history of radiation or photodynamic therapy for acne, and a history of abnormal wound healing.

PREPROCEDURE EDUCATION AND PREPARATION. As with medium-depth chemical peeling, patients who are undergoing deep chemical peeling should be aware that the procedure requires application of a peeling agent to the skin that will cause pain, stinging, and burning. This pain is managed by preoperative sedation. Patients should be fully informed of the risks to the heart, liver, and kidneys and a thorough preoperative evaluation must be performed. A baseline electrocardiogram and baseline labs (liver function tests, blood urea nitrogen, creatinine, complete blood count, and electrolytes) should be obtained and verified as normal. The patient's medications should be reviewed to ensure that an arrhythmogenic medication is not present.

Normal postoperative expectations include oozing of clear fluid, moderate-to-severe edema, erythema, and skin peeling. Close follow-up during epithelialization is required and the patient must also be aware that it is normal for postprocedure erythema to last up to 90 days. Patients must be informed of the possible complications including allergic reaction, scarring, postoperative infection, persistent erythema (<90 days), and pigmentary dyschromia. The consent form should be signed (see **Sample Consent Form**), and the patient is then given a prescription for valcyclovir 500 to 1000 mg b.i.d. to t.i.d. for 14 days with instructions to begin taking this medication 1 day prior to the procedure. Patients should also be instructed to purchase a jar of a petrolatum-based emollient for use after the procedure.

BAKER–GORDON PEEL PROTOCOL

TRAY SET UP AND STORAGE OF MATERIALS

The Baker–Gordon peel formula must be prepared fresh, and consists of 3 mL SUP liquid phenol 88%, 2 mL tap water, 8 drops of Septisol, and 3 drops of croton oil.[5,24,28,30–32] Additional items include cotton-tipped applicators, waterproof zinc oxide tape cut into short strips (if performed with occlusion), and ice packs.

PROCEDURE PREPARATION AND ANESTHESIA. Prior to administration of sedation and analgesics, the surgeon outlines the limits of the operative field with a surgical pen with the patient in a sitting position. On the day of the procedure the patient should be NPO and skip breakfast. Documentation is reviewed including the consent form and operative site (Table 32-3). Preoperative photographs are taken. The patient is then placed on cardiac monitoring equipment, including a pulse oximeter and automated blood pressure cuff, and an infusion of lactated Ringer's solution is begun. Administration of 500 mL of lactated Ringer's before the procedure and 1 L during and after the peel facilitates excretion of the phenol by the kidneys and decreases the risk of arrhythmia. Intravenous (IV) midazolam is titrated slowly at 1 mg per dose up to a maximum of 5 mg. IV fentanyl citrate is given in 50 ug doses to a maximum of 2 ug/kg over 90 to 120 minutes. These medications should be administered and monitored by an anesthesiologist or anesthetist.

INTRAOPERATIVE SAFETY CONCERNS. Phenol is systemically absorbed and is toxic to the liver, kidneys, and heart.[33] Intraoperative arrhythmia is the most feared complication. Patients should be monitored closely and the peel must proceed slowly (10–15 minutes between cosmetic units). Slow application of the phenol in conjunction with pre, intra, and postoperative IV hydration prevents serum phenol from rising to toxic levels, thereby minimizing risk of renal toxicity and arrhythmia. As with medium-depth peels, deep-peeling agents should never be carried over the eyes or introduced into the eye. Should this occur, flushing with mineral oil is necessary as water can increase the strength of the phenol. If the phenol is accidentally spilled on staff or the patient, propylene glycol or glycerol can be used to decontaminate the area.

PROCEDURE TECHNIQUE. Following adequate sedation and monitoring the face is cleansed and degreased with hexachlorophene (Septisol) with special attention to sebaceous areas. If performing an occluded peel, the facial hair is shaved to avoid discomfort during tape removal.

The phenol formula is then carefully applied with a cotton-tipped applicator to cosmetic units in this sequence: forehead, perioral area, right cheek, left cheek, nose, and periorbital area. After treatment of a cosmetic unit frosting occurs rapidly and, if performing a deep peel with occlusion, the tape should be placed just after the phenol has been applied. Tape is applied in at least two layers over all treated areas except the periorbital area and earlobes. Microfoam tape is often used on the perioral area as it is elastic. Waiting 15 minutes before treating the next cosmetic unit is necessary to allow the body to clear any systemically absorbed phenol and prevent toxicity. The peel may be extended just over the mandibular rim in order to blend the treated and untreated areas. The periorbital area must be treated conservatively to avoid overpenetration and scarring.

The peeling agent creates an immediate burning sensation for 15 to 20 seconds that subsides and then returns after 20 minutes, persisting for up to 8 hours. Ice packs and opioid analgesics are usually adequate for pain control. A short course of systemic steroids may be employed to lessen the inflammatory response. For unoccluded peels, petrolatum is applied and a biosynthetic dressing is placed.

POSTPROCEDURE CARE. Patients should return on postoperative day 1 for encouragement and evaluation. The tape mask is easily removed at 48 hours due to the action of the wound exudate on the adhesive. Removal of the tape mask may be performed at 24 hours if the patient is very uncomfortable. Postoperative edema can be substantial and cause the eyelids to swell shut. This can be alleviated by sleeping, with the aid of hypnotics, in a sitting or elevated position.

Wet to dry soaks with 0.25% acetic acid should be performed three to five times daily. The acetic acid has antibacterial activity against gram-negative organisms and *Pseudomonas* and is mildly debridant. Following soaks, the patient should apply bland emollients. Occlusive salves prevent crusting and speed re-epithelialization. Milia may develop during re-epithelialization and may be manually extracted if they do not resolve spontaneously. Strict photoprotection is necessary until re-epithelialization occurs at 8 to 12 days. Pruritus may be managed with moisturizers, low-potency topical steroids, ice packs, and NSAIDs. As with medium-depth peels, resumption of a skin care regimen that includes sunscreen and a retinoid is necessary to maintain the results. Peak results can be seen 3 to 4 months postoperatively and repeat peeling should not be performed for at least 6 months postoperatively.

CHEMICAL PEEL COMPLICATIONS

Many of the complications seen with chemical peeling can be recognized early, and the surgeon should be well acquainted with the normal postoperative appearance and the normal time frame required for healing.[33] Complications may arise intraoperatively or postoperatively. Intraoperative errors include incorrect peel pharmacology and solution misplacement. As described earlier, all solutions must be fresh and at the proper concentration. Application should be deliberate and systematic, and care must be taken to avoid spills or introduction of the solutions into the eye. Saline and sodium bicarbonate should be present to dilute TCA or neutralize GA. Mineral oil should be present for Baker–Gordon phenol peels. Postoperative complications include infection, persistent erythema, scarring, pigment alteration, and, in the case of phenol, systemic toxicity.

Frequent postoperative visits are necessary to recognize the early onset of bacterial infection. Infection may present as delayed wound healing, ulcerations, or a buildup of necrotic material with excessive scabbing, crusting, purulent drainage, and odor. The use of 0.25% acetic acid soaks to debride crust and remove residual necrotic debris as well as the removal of the ointment with each soak may deter bacterial growth. Infection should be treated empirically with coverage for both *Staphylococcus* and *Pseudomonas* until cultures and susceptibility testing are available to guide therapy. Early recognition and institution of appropriate antibiotics will prevent the spread of infection and minimize scarring.

Herpes simplex virus reactivation most commonly occurs on perioral skin and often manifests itself 7 to 10 days after the procedure. Unusual and unexpected pain occurring 3 or 4 days postoperatively may herald the onset of viral infection. The risk of scarring is high and all patients must be treated prophylactic antiviral medications. A 14 day course of valcyclovir 500 to 1000 mg b.i.d. to t.i.d. should be initiated 1 day prior to the procedure for prophylaxis. If herpetic lesions appear, treatment should be at a dose of 1000 mg t.i.d. If caught early, herpetic infections usually do not scar.

Persistent erythema is a rare syndrome in which the skin remains erythematous and/or pruritic beyond the 15 to 30 days that is normally expected for a medium-depth chemical peel or 60 to 90 days expected for a deep peel. In addition to infectious etiologies, this condition can result from allergic or irritant contact dermatitis, exacerbation of prior skin disease, or a genetic susceptibility to erythema. Persistent erythema is indicative of poor wound healing and the presence of excessive angiogenic factors, which can induce scarring. After ruling out infectious agents, the erythema can be treated with topical, systemic, or intralesional steroids if focal thickening is present.[24] Biosynthetic membranes (e.g., Vigilon, C.R. Bard, Inc., Covington, GA) can provide a protective barrier and speed resolution of this process. If thickening or scarring becomes evident, other measures that may be helpful include the daily use of silicone sheeting and the 585 nm pulsed dye laser.[34,35] With prompt intervention, scarring may be averted.

Medium and deep peels carry the risk of scarring. A history of prior peel, dermabrasion, or isotretinoin use within 6 months may be risk factors for scarring. A personal or family history of hypertrophic scarring carries increased risk. Postrhytidectomy full-thickness skin sloughing may occur from peels performed earlier than 3 months post procedure.[33] Patients who have had a blepharoplasty within 6 months are at risk of lower lid ectropion after deep peeling.[33] Scars may be treated with topical or intralesional steroids, silicon gel sheeting, pulsed dye laser, or simple massage.

Patients with Fitzpatrick skin types I to III ordinarily have few problems with pigmentation after peeling. Type IV skin can be peeled but may leave an obvious demarcation between peeled and unpeeled skin. Type VI skin will hyperpigment after peeling and may not return to normal for up to 2 years. In addition, type VI skin may heal with a visibly lighter skin tone. Type V skin can be unpredictable and often hyperpigments.[36] Oral contraceptives, estrogens, photosensitizing drugs, sunlight, and pregnancy within 6 months of a peel may exacerbate post-peel hyperpigmentation. Combination therapy with a topical retinoid, hydroquinone 4% to 6%, and a low-potency topical steroid can alleviate post-peel hyperpigmentation.[37]

Deep peeling with phenol carries the risk of cardiac arrhythmia, nephrotoxicity, and hepatotoxicity. Cardiac arrhthymias are associated with treating 50% or more of the face within 60 minutes. Anxiety and exercise increase ectopic beats while sedation and relaxation can decrease ectopic beats. In patients who were deliberately peeled rapidly (30 minutes) tachycardia was noted first followed by premature ventricular contractions, bigeminy, paroxysmal atrial tachycardia, and ventricular tachycardia. Severe cases can progress to atrial fibrillation. Diuresis allows metabolism and excretion of phenol and reduces arrhythmias. If an arrhythmia occurs the peel should be stopped until a normal sinus rhythm is sustained for 15 minutes. The procedure may then be resumed with extension of the peel intervals by an additional 15 minutes.[38–40]

REFERENCES

1. Monheit GD, Chastain MA. Chemical peels. *Facial Plast Surg Clin North Am*. 2001;9:239–255, viii.
2. Eller JJ, Wolff S. Skin peeling and scarification. *JAMA*. 1941; 116: 934–938.
3. Ayres S 3rd. Dermal changes following application of chemical cauterants to aging skin. Superficial chemosurgery. *Arch Dermatol*. 1960;82:578–585.
4. Ayres S 3rd. Superficial chemosurgery in treating aging skin. *Arch Dermatol*. 1962;85:385–393.

5. Brown AM, Kaplan LM, Brown ME. Phenol-induced histological skin changes: hazards, technique, and uses. *Br J Plast Surg.* 1960;13:158–169.
6. Baker TJ. Chemical face peeling and rhytidectomy. A combined approach for facial rejuvenation. *Plast Reconstr Surg Transplant Bull.* 1962;29:199–207.
7. Stegman SJ. A comparative histologic study of the effects of three peeling agents and dermabrasion on normal and sun-damaged skin. *Aesthetic Plast Surg.* 1982;6:123–135.
8. Van Scott EJ, Yu RJ. Control of keratinization with alpha-hydroxy acids and related compounds. I. Topical treatment of ichthyotic disorders. *Arch Dermatol.* 1974;110:586–590.
9. Fitzpatrick TB. The validity and practicality of sun-reactive skin types I through VI. *Arch Dermatol.* 1988;124:869–871.
10. Rubenstein R, Roenigk HH Jr, Stegman SJ, Hanke CW. Atypical keloids after dermabrasion of patients taking isotretinoin. *J Am Acad Dermatol.* 1986;15:280–285.
11. Wolfe SA. Chemical face peeling following therapeutic irradiation. *Plast Reconstr Surg.* 1982;69:859–862.
12. Glogau RG, Matarasso SL. Chemical face peeling: patient and peeling agent selection. *Facial Plast Surg.* 1995;11:1–8.
13. Clark CP 3rd. Office-based skin care and superficial peels: the scientific rationale. *Plast Reconstr Surg.* 1999;104: 854–864; discussion 65–66.
14. Bergfeld W, Tung R, Vidimos A, Vellanki L, Remzi B, Stanton-Hicks U. Improving the cosmetic appearance of photoaged skin with glycolic acid. *J Am Acad Dermatol.* 1997; 36:1011–1013.
15. Garcia A, Fulton JE Jr. The combination of glycolic acid and hydroquinone or kojic acid for the treatment of melasma and related conditions. *Dermatol Surg.* 1996;22:443–447.
16. Van Scott EJ, Yu RJ. Hyperkeratinization, corneocyte cohesion, and alpha hydroxy acids. *J Am Acad Dermatol.* 1984; 11:867–879.
17. Resnik SS. Chemical peeling with trichloroacetic acid. *J Dermatol Surg Oncol.* 1984;10:549–550.
18. Stagnone JJ. Chemabrasion, a combined technique of chemical-peeling and dermabrasion. *J Dermatol Surg Oncol.* 1977; 3:217–219.
19. Monheit GD. The Jessner's + TCA peel: a medium-depth chemical peel. *J Dermatol Surg Oncol.* 1989;15:945–950.
20. Monheit GD. Medium-depth chemical peels. *Dermatol Clin.* 2001;19:413–425, vii.
21. Brody HJ. Variations and comparisons in medium-depth chemical peeling. *J Dermatol Surg Oncol.* 1989;15:953–963.
22. Coleman WP 3rd, Futrell JM. The glycolic acid trichloroacetic acid peel. *J Dermatol Surg Oncol.* 1994;20:76–80.
23. Tse Y, Ostad A, Lee HS, et al. A clinical and histologic evaluation of two medium-depth peels. Glycolic acid versus Jessner's trichloroacetic acid. *Dermatol Surg.* 1996;22:781–786.
24. Monheit GD. Chemical peels. *Skin Therapy Lett.* 2004;9:6–11.
25. Lawrence N, Cox SE, Cockerell CJ, Freeman RG, Cruz PD Jr. A comparison of the efficacy and safety of Jessner's solution and 35% trichloroacetic acid vs 5% fluorouracil in the treatment of widespread facial actinic keratoses. *Arch Dermatol.* 1995;131:176–181.
26. Witheiler DD, Lawrence N, Cox SE, Cruz C, Cockerell CJ, Freemen RG. Long-term efficacy and safety of Jessner's solution and 35% trichloroacetic acid vs 5% fluorouracil in the treatment of widespread facial actinic keratoses. *Dermatol Surg.* 1997;23:191–196.
27. Monheit GD. The Jessner's-trichloroacetic acid peel. An enhanced medium-depth chemical peel. *Dermatol Clin.* 1995;13:277–283.
28. Baker TJ, Gordon HL. Chemical face peeling. In: *Surgical rejuvenation of the face.* St. Louis, MO: Mosby; 1986.
29. Hetter GP. An examination of the phenol-croton oil peel: part I. Dissecting the formula. *Plast Reconstr Surg.* 2000;105: 227–239; discussion 49–51.
30. Beeson WH, McCollough EG. Chemical face peeling without taping. *J Dermatol Surg Oncol.* 1985;11:985–990.
31. Alt TH. Occluded Baker-Gordon chemical peel: review and update. *J Dermatol Surg Oncol.* 1989;15:980–993.
32. Maloney BP, McCollough EG. Deep-depth chemical peeling. *Facial Plast Surg.* 1995;11:30–38.
33. Brody HJ. Complications of chemical resurfacing. *Dermatol Clin.* 2001;19:427–438, vii-viii.
34. Alster T. Laser scar revision: comparison study of 585-nm pulsed dye laser with and without intralesional corticosteroids. *Dermatol Surg.* 2003;29:25–29.
35. Alster T, Zaulyanov L. Laser scar revision: a review. *Dermatol Surg.* 2007;33:131–140.
36. Spira M, Gerow FJ, Hardy SB. Complications of chemical face peeling. *Plast Reconstr Surg.* 1974;54:397–403.
37. Kligman AM, Willis I. A new formula for depigmenting human skin. *Arch Dermatol.* 1975;111:40–48.
38. Truppman ES, Ellenby JD. Major electrocardiographic changes during chemical face peeling. *Plast Reconstr Surg.* 1979;63:44–48.
39. Price NM. EKG changes in relationship to the chemical peel. *J Dermatol Surg Oncol.* 1990;16:37–42.
40. Gross BG. Cardiac arrhythmia during phenol face peeling. *Plast Reconstr Surg.* 1984;73:590–594.

CHAPTER 33

Photodynamic Therapy for Nonmelanoma Skin Cancer and Precursor Lesions

Katrine Togsverd-Bo & Merete Haedersdal

INTRODUCTION

Photodynamic therapy (PDT) is increasingly used in both USA and Europe for the treatment of actinic keratosis (AK) and selected cases of nonmelanoma skin cancer (NMSC). Being a minimally invasive therapy, PDT is especially suitable for the treatment of multiple lesions, field cancerization and lesions located in areas where optimal cosmetic outcome is essential.[1,2] The principle of PDT involves the combination of a photosensitizer, oxygen, and light to produce selective cytotoxic damage of dysplastic cells. In dermatology, PDT is used with a topically applied photosensitizer, which allows for specific lesion targeting.

Topical PDT was introduced in 1990 when Kennedy and Pottiers applied 5-aminolevulinic acid (ALA), a precursor of the endogenous photosensitizer, protoporphyrin IX (PpIX), directly on skin tumors.[3,4] The use of a topically applied photosensitizer was a major advantage compared to the previously used photosensitizers, which required intravenous administration and produced long-lasting phototoxicity.[5] Since the introduction of PDT with ALA or its methylated ester, methyl aminolevulinate (MAL), intensive research has established PDT in dermatology and the concept of PDT is now substantially documented for the treatment of NMSC and precursor lesions. PDT is performed with both ALA and MAL for AK lesions and besides, MAL-PDT is approved in Europe for the treatment of Bowen's disease (BD, squamous cell carcinoma [SCC] in situ), and superficial and small nodular basal cell carcinomas (BCC).[1,2] Furthermore, PDT is administered as off-label treatment for photoaged skin, acne, and selected skin conditions of inflammatory, infectious, and neoplastic origin.

MECHANISMS OF PHOTODYNAMIC THERAPY

The mechanism of PDT involves the simultaneous presence of a photosensitizer, oxygen, and light. A photosensitizer is a molecule that absorbs light of appropriate wavelengths to initiate a photochemical reaction.[6] When a photosensitizer absorbs light, an electron is transferred to a higher energy orbital and the photosensitizer enters the excited singlet state (Fig. 33-1).[7] The excited singlet state is very unstable and thus, the photosensitizer emits excess energy as either fluorescence and/or heat, or undergoes intersystem crossing to form a more stable excited triplet state (Fig. 33-1).[7] From the triplet state, PpIX can either (i) decay to the ground state, (ii) react directly with the substrate to form free radicals (type I reaction), or (iii) react directly with tissue oxygen to form singlet oxygen ($^1O_2$) (type II reaction).[8]

The main mechanism of action in PDT is the type II reaction, in which the excited PpIX reacts with molecular oxygen to form $^1O_2$.[7,9] $^1O_2$ is highly unstable and reacts with nearby molecules, including PpIX itself, causing cellular damage and ultimately cell death.[10] During type I and II reactions, PpIX itself is degraded by a process known as photobleaching, which is useful for dosimetry of the PDT response.[11]

The biologic PDT response involves direct cell death due to reaction with $^1O_2$, indirect tissue damage due to vasculature damage and shutdown, as well as inflammation and immune activation.[6,12] Direct cell death is mainly mediated through apoptosis but also involves necrosis and autophagous processes.[10,12] These processes are accompanied by microvascular damage, which is considered an important contributor to tumor destruction.[13] In

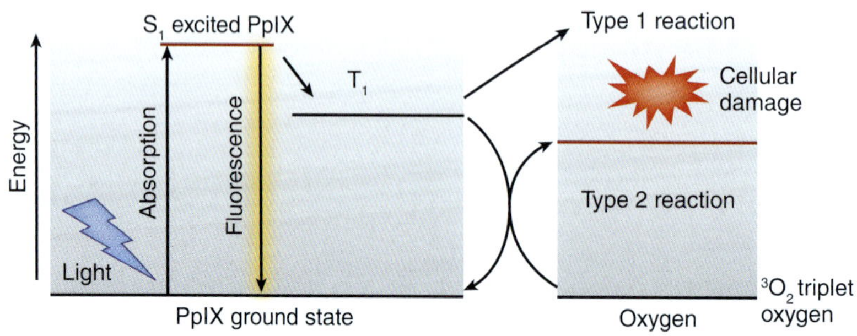

Figure 33-1 The photodynamic process.

addition, PDT raises an inflammatory response, including recruitment of antigen-presenting cells that may stimulate the host immune response.[14] The immune response is believed to play an important role in the long-term efficacy of PDT in tumor treatment.[12,15]

PHOTOSENSITIZING AGENTS

Topical PDT in dermatology is currently licensed with two PpIX prodrugs, ALA and its methylated ester, MAL. Both are endogenously converted to PpIX by the heme biosynthetic pathway and relatively selectively concentrated in dysplastic tissue, which is possibly due to facilitated penetration and increased PpIX metabolism in dysplastic tissue.[5,16,17] When ALA or MAL is exogenously applied, the normal feedback mechanism is bypassed and PpIX accumulates intracellularly in phototoxic concentrations.[4]

ALA is a small, hydrophilic molecule (molecular weight, MW, 168 Da) and a zwitterion (both positively and negatively charged groups) at physiological pH.[18] These characteristics make ALA unstable in aqueous formulations and impair its penetration through lipophilic environments such as the stratum corneum.[19] To improve the bioavailability of PpIX in dysplastic lesions, the more lipophilic and stable MAL was introduced. MAL is slightly larger than ALA (MW 182 Da) but penetrates and accumulates more readily in lipophilic structures.[20,21] MAL is selective with regard to PpIX accumulation in diseased skin and produces a higher lesion/normal tissue concentration ratio than ALA.[22,23] Recently, a nanoemulsion of ALA has been developed in order to improve ALA stability and increase its skin surface penetration, thereby enhancing PpIX tissue distribution.[24]

LIGHT SOURCES FOR PDT

Ideally, light sources used for PDT must have emission spectra that match the PpIX absorption spectrum as well as considerable skin penetration to photoactivate accumulated PpIX within the target lesions.[6] Light penetration is influenced by absorption of skin chromophores and by scattering of photons. Absorption and scattering effects are more pronounced for shorter than longer visible wavelengths and thus, the penetration of light is deeper for longer than shorter visible wavelengths.[25] PpIX has a maximum absorption band in the blue light spectrum (Soret band, 405–415 nm) and substantially weaker absorption in the green (506–540 nm), yellow (572–582 nm), and red (628–635 nm) wave bands (Fig. 33-2). Although PpIX absorption is substantially higher at 405 nm, blue light penetrates poorly into the dermis, whereas red light has a deep skin penetration and may drive PDT reactions down to 4 mm.[26] Correspondingly, clinical studies have found red light to be superior for PDT treatment of BD and BCC.[2,27,28]

Clinically and experimentally, a wide range of light sources have been used for PDT. These include noncoherent light sources with narrowband light-emitting diodes (LED); broadband light sources such as fluorescent lamps, metal halide and xenon arc lamps; as well as daylight and coherent laser light. Furthermore, pulsed light sources such as intense pulsed light (IPL) and long-pulsed dye lasers

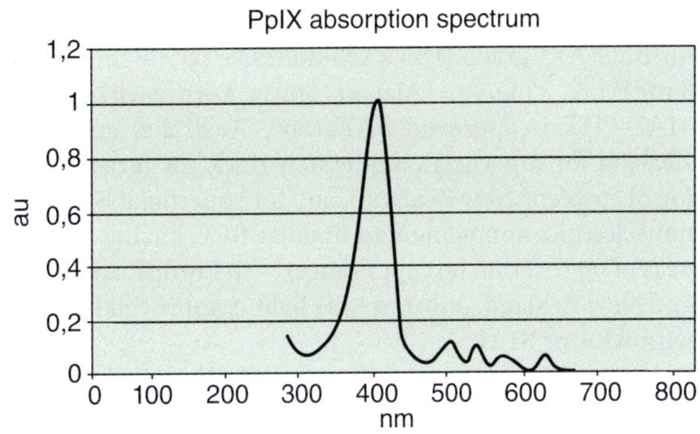

Figure 33-2 The PpIX absorption spectrum in arbitrary units (au). PpIX has absorption peaks around 405 to 430 nm (Soret band), 506 to 540 nm, 572 to 582 nm, and 628 to 635 nm.

(LPDLs) are widely used in PDT for the treatment of especially photodamaged skin, but also for acne and AK.[29–34]

Noncoherent light sources in the visible light spectrum are now widely used for PDT as they are inexpensive, require little maintenance and may cover wide illumination areas. A number of continuous, noncoherent light sources with emission spectra in the visible spectrum are available.[35] That is, blue light is available as a blue fluorescent lamp at 400 to 450 nm with emission peak at 417 nm (BLU-U, DUSA Pharmaceuticals, USA). Red light is provided as narrowband LED light at 630 ± 3 nm (Aktilite, Galderma, France) or 633 ± 4 nm (Omnilux, Phototherapeutics, UK) and as broadband light sources at 560 to 710 nm (i.e., Waldmann, Waldmann Medizintechnic, Germany; PhotoDyn, Hydrosun Medizintechnik; Paterson lamp, Paterson Institute, UK). Compared to the broadband light sources, narrowband LED light produces higher complete response rates and may also induce a more pronounced PDT response in the deeper skin layers.[26,36] However, pain intensities during illumination are also significantly higher in narrowband compared to broadband red light.[36] Narrowband as well as broadband continuous light sources have shown to produce higher degrees of PpIX photobleaching than pulsed light sources, including in deeper tissue layers, possibly due to oxygen depletion during delivery of light.[37,38]

INDICATIONS AND LICENSES

In the USA, PDT is approved for the treatment of superficial and moderately thick (Olsen grade I and II), nonhyperkeratotic, nonhyperpigmented AK of the face and scalp using ALA combined with blue light exposure and MAL combined with red LED exposure.[39] In USA and South America, ALA is currently marked as Levulan Kerastick 20% hydroalcoholic (Dusa Pharmaceuticals, Wilmington, MA, USA) and MAL is licensed as Metvixia cream (Galderma International, Paris, France) containing 16.8% MAL as hydrochloride. In Canada, Metvix 16.8% is approved for thin or nonhyperkeratotic and nonpigmented AK on the face and scalp and for primary superficial BCC outside the central zone of the face. In Europe, ALA was recently approved for grade I and II AK of the face and scalp as a nanoemulsion gel with 7.8% ALA (Ameluz,

Biofrontera Bioscience GmbH, Leverkusen, Germany) and for mild AK (grade I) as a self-adhesive patch containing 8 mg ALA, 2 mg/cm^2 (Alacare, Spirig, Bern, Switzerland). MAL-PDT is approved in Europe, Australia, and New Zealand for superficial, moderately thick AK (grade I–II), for BD (except New Zealand), and for superficial BCC and nonsclerotic, nonpigmented nodular BCC having a thickness of up to 2 mm (except France).[1,2] In Europe, Australia, and New Zealand, only red LED light is approved for PDT with ALA or MAL.

ALA-PDT with Levulan Kerastick is licensed for application at 14 to 18 hours followed by blue light illumination with a fluorescent lamp (BLU-U, Dusa Pharmaceuticals, Wilmington, MA, USA) at 400 to 450 nm in a dose of 10 J/cm^2, 10 mW/cm^2 irradiance, corresponding to an illumination time of 1,000 seconds.[40] PDT with ALA nanoemulsion, ALA patch and MAL is licensed using red narrowband LED light at 630 ± 3 nm (Aktilite CL 128, Galderma International, France), or 633 ± 4 nm (Omnilux, Phototherapeutics, UK) at 37 J/cm^2 and 68 mW/cm^2 irradiance, which corresponds to an illumination time of approximately 9 minutes. ALA nanoemulsion and MAL cream require an incubation time of 3 hours while ALA patch must incubate on the skin lesion for 4 hours before illumination. If narrowband light sources are not tolerated due to intense pain during illumination, broadband light sources at 570 to 650 nm, such as the Waldmann 1200 (Waldmann Medizintechnic, Germany) in a dose of 170 J/cm^2 may be used; however clearance rates are reported to be slightly lower (61%–72% vs. 68%–85% of AK lesions).[36]

ACTINIC KERATOSES

AKs are the most common premalignant lesion and characteristically, the lesions often appear in chronically sun-damaged skin as a sign of field cancerization. AK may develop into SCCs, which have metastatic potential, especially in immunosuppressed patients.

Since the introduction of ALA-PDT in 1990, a large body of evidence has established PDT with both ALA and MAL as an effective treatment of AK and field-cancerized skin with superior cosmetic outcomes compared to conventional destructive therapies (Fig. 33-3).[2] Studies have reported lesion response rates from 71% to 96% at 1 to 3 months after PDT of the face and scalp while lower clearance rates of 44% to 70% are reported for AKs located on the trunk or extremities.

In clinical studies, ALA-PDT has been applied in a variety of different protocols, whereas MAL-PDT in most studies is used according to the approved protocols.

The effect of ALA-PDT, applied according to the licensed protocol (ALA 14–18 hours, 417 ± 5 nm, 10 J/cm^2, 10 mW/cm^2), was compared to placebo in a multicenter, randomized controlled trial involving a total of 243 patients with multiple AK.[40] At 8 weeks follow-up, the AK response rate was 83% after one treatment, and retreatment of remaining lesions increased the response rate to 91% after 3 months (31% and 25% after placebo treatment). Similar clearance rates were found in smaller clinical studies following one or two treatments of ALA-PDT although ALA incubation varied from 1 to 6 hours and illumination

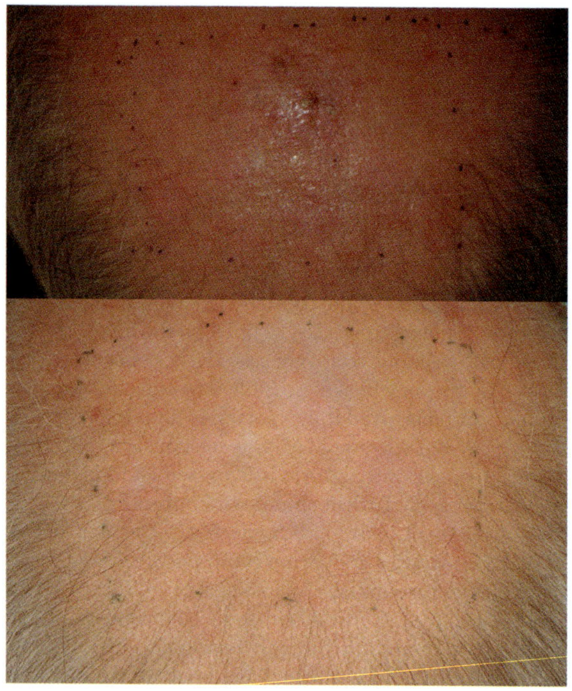

Figure 33-3 Field-cancerized skin with actinic keratoses before (top) and 3 months after MAL-PDT treatment (bottom).

was provided by broadband light sources and pulsed light sources such as IPL and LPDL.[1,30,41,42]

In clinical studies, MAL-PDT (MAL 3 hours, 570–650 nm, 75 J/cm^2, 50–250 mW/cm^2) has established efficacy rates of 89% to 93% at 3 months after two treatments given at 1 to 2 week intervals.[43–45] In a multicenter randomized study of thin and moderately thick AK, a narrowband red LED (630 ± 3 nm, 37 J/cm^2, 50 mW/cm^2) was used to compare two MAL-PDT treatments at 7 day intervals versus a single treatment that was repeated at 3 months if required.[46] The study found a single treatment to be as effective as two treatments, clearing 92% and 87% of lesions, respectively. This led to a revision of the EU license for MAL-PDT, recommending an initial single treatment, repeated at 3 months if required.

The efficacy of PDT depends, similar to topical treatments for AK, on the thickness of the lesion. Using a single PDT treatment, studies have reported response rates of 75% to 93% for thin lesions; 64% to 83% for moderately thick lesions and 39% to 52% for thick lesions.[5,6,16–18] Hence, two PDT treatments at 1 to 2 week intervals are recommended for thick lesions.

PDT has previously been compared to other treatments for AK, mainly cryotherapy but also 5-fluorouracil (5-FU) and imiquimod.[46,48,50–51] Studies comparing PDT and cryotherapy found similar response rates from one or two treatments of PDT compared to cryotherapy, while cosmetic outcomes were superior for PDT with 80% to 90% excellent results for PDT vs. 51% for cryotherapy.[45,47] PDT has shown equivalent efficacy compared to 5-FU with lesion clearances of 79% and 80% respectively at 1 month and 73% and 70% at 6 months. In smaller studies comparing PDT and imiquimod, data have been somewhat ambiguous, since comparisons have shown both PDT and imiquimod to be superior for AK treatment.[48,59]

BOWEN'S DISEASE

PDT is an effective treatment for BD, clearing on average 80% to 93% of lesions.[27,47,50] Immediate response rates at 3 months range from 88% to 100%, and responses at 12 months range from 80% to 95%, which is significantly better than cryotherapy (67%) and similar to 5-FU treatment (83%).[47] At 2 years follow-up, 68% of lesions remained clear after PDT, 60% after cryotherapy and 59% after 5-FU, with cosmetically superior results of PDT compared to cryotherapy and 5-FU.[4]

While PDT is effective for BD, significantly lower response rates are found for invasive SCC.[51] In view of the metastatic potential of SCC, PDT cannot be recommended for treatment of invasive SCC.

BASAL CELL CARCINOMA

BCCs are the most common cancers in the USA, Australia, and Europe, and worldwide the incidence is increasing. In Europe, Australia, and New Zealand, MAL-PDT is approved for primary, superficial BCC and low-risk nodular BCC. High risk tumors are not suitable for treatment with PDT. High risk tumors include those with (i) size greater than 2 cm diameter; (ii) location in the central facial region (H-zone, especially around eyes, nose, lips, and ears); (iii) clinically poorly defined tumor margins; (iv) pigmented BCC; (v) aggressive histologic subtype and perivascular or perineural invasion; (vi) recurrent tumors; and (vi) tumors in immunosuppressed patients.[52]

Superficial BCCs are reported to respond well to PDT with clearance rates of approximately 85% at 12 months after two treatments. At 5 years' follow-up, recurrences have been reported in 25% of cases, which is similar to cryotherapy (26%), but with PDT resulting in significantly better cosmetic outcomes than cryotherapy (excellent results in 60% of PDT patients vs. 16% of cryotherapy patients).[53]

In studies on nodular BCC, two MAL-PDT treatments at 1 to 2 week intervals achieved complete remission of low-risk tumors in 82% to 91% of cases within 1 year posttreatment. In these low-risk tumors, complete remission was sustained in 78% to 86% of lesions at 3 to 5 years' follow-up, whereas PDT treatment of high-risk BCC showed recurrence rates of 38% at 3 years' follow-up.[1]

Long-term complete response of MAL-PDT for primary, low-risk BCC has been compared to surgical excision in a randomized controlled trial.[54] Treatment response at 3 months showed 98% to 99% of surgically excised lesions cleared after surgical excision, versus 92% of PDT-treated lesions, declining to 96% and 83% at 12 months' follow-up.[5] At 5 years posttreatment, surgical excision resulted in higher sustained response rates of 96% compared to 76% of lesions after PDT, whereas cosmetic outcomes favored PDT, with good or excellent outcomes in 87% of cases after PDT compared to 54% after surgery (Fig. 33-4).

In summary, there is increasing evidence that MAL-PDT is becoming established as an effective treatment modality for primary, superficial BCC and as a reasonable treatment for primary, low-risk nodular BCC.[1,2,55] PDT may be considered for nodular BCC in cases where surgical excision is relatively contraindicated or when other factors, such as patient preference, comorbidities and/or cosmetic considerations result in a willingness to accept higher risk of recurrence. A recent European PDT guideline advises a minimum of 1 year follow-up for patients receiving PDT for nodular BCC.[1]

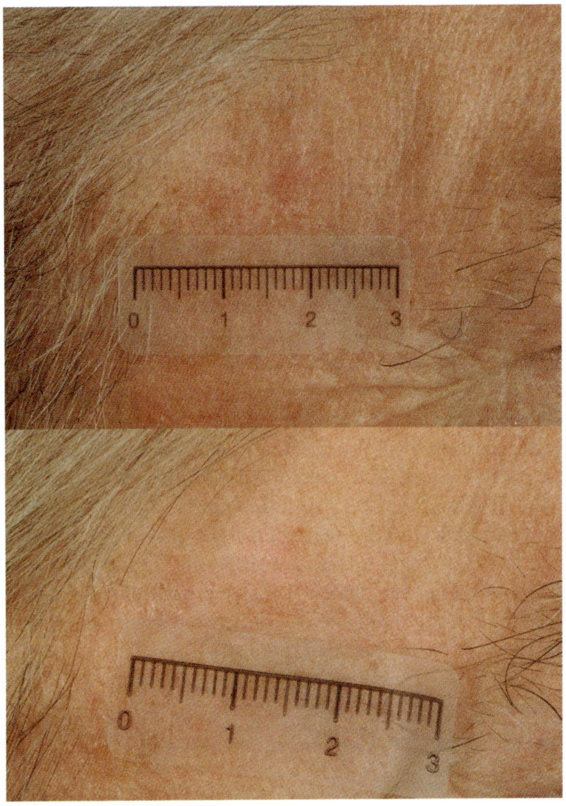

Figure 33-4 Basal cell carcinoma before (top) and 6 months after two MAL-PDT treatment at 7 day interval (bottom).

FIELD CANCERIZATION AND SKIN CANCER PREVENTION

Field cancerization is characterized by multifocal areas of clinical and subclinical premalignant and malignant lesions that primarily appear in chronically sun-damaged skin.[56,57] Field-directed PDT is an attractive treatment modality for field cancerization, as it may be used for multiple lesions and large skin areas with excellent cosmetic results. The preventative potential of field-directed PDT for facial AKs in immunocompetent patients demonstrated a significant delay in development of new AKs up to 6 months compared to control sites, highlighting its potential as a preventive measure.[58] Recent studies have shown that PDT reduces the histological features of actinic damage and expression of early oncogenic markers such as p53 mutations in field-cancerized skin.[59,60] These findings support the preventative effect of PDT in skin carcinogenesis.

Patients receiving long-term immunosuppressive therapy such as organ transplant recipients (OTRs) are at particularly high risk of developing dysplastic field changes and multiple carcinomas. These patients require multiple sessions of field-directed therapies, frequent screening for malignancies and long-term follow-up of treated tumors.[61] As in immunocompetent patients, field-directed PDT in OTR also prevents the development of new AK.[58,62,63] In renal OTR, one MAL-PDT session significantly delayed the development of new AKs in an intrapatient randomized study (9.6 vs. 6.8 months for control sites).[63] In a multicenter study, repeated sessions of MAL-PDT were initially more effective than lesion-targeted cryotherapy for prevention of new AKs (65 vs. 103 AKs in control areas at 6 months).[62] However, the superiority was lost by 27 months, suggesting that continued treatments are required to maintain a sustained, protective effect. Repeated PDT cycles (6–8 treatments per year) showed a reduced incidence of new SCC in transplant recipients,[64] whereas a single PDT treatment did not protect against SCC development at 2 year follow-up.[65]

In summary, field-directed PDT is evolving as a suitable therapeutic option for the prevention of AKs in OTR and immunocompetent patients having multiple dysplastic lesions. For these patients, field-directed treatment is preferred over lesion-targeted therapy.

OFF-LABEL USE

PDT is reported as off-label treatment for photoaged skin, selected inflammatory and infectious diseases and neoplastic diseases other than NMSC.

PDT is increasingly used for photoaged skin, often in combination with filtered pulsed light sources and lasers.[66] Multiple studies have demonstrated improvement of fine wrinkles, mottled hyperpigmentation, tactile roughness and sallowness by addition of ALA or MAL compared to light alone.[67–70] These results are supported by immunohistochemical analyses that revealed both upregulation of collagen production and increased epidermal proliferation.[60] To minimize phototoxic reactions after treatment, most studies have used short incubation periods (0.5–1 hour) with ALA or MAL but several protocols are currently being used for photodynamic photorejuvenation.

During the past decade, PDT has been extensively studied as a treatment modality for inflammatory acne, although without current existing consensus on optimal protocols for photosensizers, incubation time, light source, or dosimetry.[71] However, the literature suggests that sebaceous glands are reduced after longer incubation periods (3 hours) with a photosensitizing agent followed by red light exposure rather than short incubation (10–30 minutes) and blue light exposure.[71] The mechanism of action seems to involve an antibacterial effect upon *Proprionibacterium acnes,* selective destruction of sebaceous glands and possible immunologic changes in the acne lesions.[71,72] PDT with different protocols and light sources has demonstrated a 38% to 88% reduction in inflammatory lesions at 12 weeks after 2 to 3 PDT treatments, whereas no consistent reduction in noninflammatory lesions was seen.[23,32,71] However, PDT treatment of acne has been associated with intense posttreatment inflammatory skin reactions, which at the moment does not bolster support of PDT as a first-line therapy for acne. Case series and individual reports have described the potential of PDT to treat a variety of other inflammatory diseases such as localized scleroderma, necrobiosis lipoidica diabeticorum and perioral dermatitis, but PDT appears to have a limited role in treating psoriasis.[73]

In the treatment of infectious diseases, ALA- and MAL-PDT have shown to be a potential option for refractory viral warts, with clearance rates of 56% to 75% following two to six treatments.[1,74] In genital warts, clearance rates of 66% to 89% have been reported following one to four ALA-PDT treatments.[1] In case reports of early stage, localized cutaneous T-cell lymphoma, ALA- and MAL-PDT successfully cleared plaque lesions, whereas solid tumors responded less effectively.[75] Intraepithelial neoplasia of the vulva also responded to PDT with complete histological clearance of vulvar intraepithelial neoplasia (VIN) grade II to III in 57% to 73% of lesions at 1 year posttreatment.[70,76] However, studies have reported high recurrence rates of up to 50%, which calls for optimization of the protocols used.[70]

TREATMENT PROCEDURES

Topical PDT is a three-step process that involves lesion preparation, incubation with ALA or MAL, and light exposure. An example of the most commonly used equipment is displayed in Figure 33-5.

LESION PREPARATION

Careful preparation of the treated lesion is essential to optimize treatment outcome.[77] Preparation depends on the type of lesion and is performed in the clinic immediately prior to treatment. Lesion marking may be useful in the treatment of BD and BCC, since a margin of 5 mm of normal skin surrounding the tumor should be treated along with the lesion.[78,79]

When treating AKs, all scale and crust should be removed and the stratum corneum disrupted to facilitate sufficient depth of penetration of ALA and MAL. Gentle

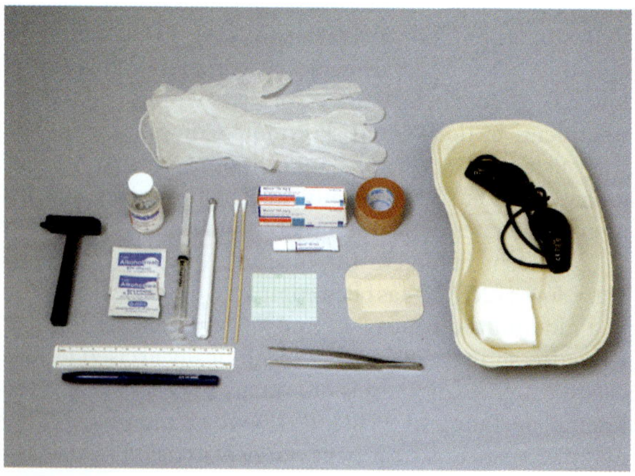

Figure 33-5 Equipment used for PDT treatment: disposable razor, ruler and pen, disposable gloves, disinfection swabs, local anaesthesia, needle and syringe, curette, swabs for application of MAL cream, MAL cream, adhesive dressing, nontransparent tape and bandage, cotton buds, and protective glasses for illumination. Forceps may be used in tumor debulking when treating BCC.

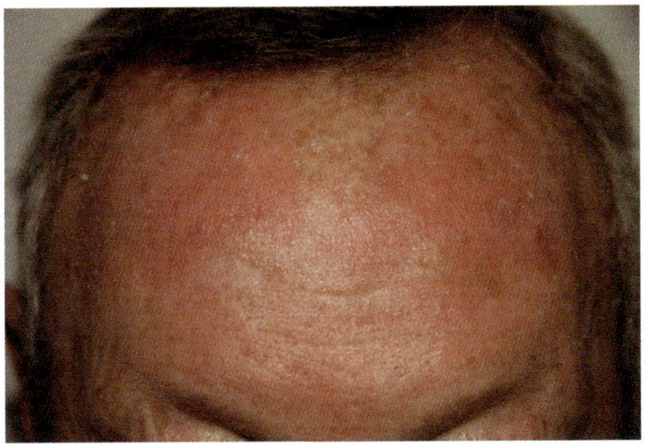

Figure 33-6 Field-cancerized skin immediately after curettage of the entire treatment area. No bleeding or oozing of the skin is present.

curettage or scraping with the edge of a scalpel blade is carefully performed to avoid bleeding. In field-directed PDT, curettage of the entire treatment area must be performed evenly (Fig. 33-6).

The preparation of BCC requires a deeper scraping with careful removal of overlying epidermal keratin and debulking of the exposed tumor material. Local anesthesia of the lesion may be required. The intention is to remove the central core of the tumor without performing a full curettage of the lesion (Fig. 33-7). Tumor debulking is usually performed immediately before PDT, but may be undertaken a few days prior to treatment.[79,80] Any bleeding or oozing of the lesion must cease before application of MAL in order to ensure cream penetration into the lesion. Bleeding may be stopped by compression, whereas hemostasis with diathermy, trichloroacetic acid, iron, or aluminum chloride may affect the outcome of PDT due to coagulation of blood in the treatment area.[79,80]

APPLICATION OF PHOTOSENSITIZER

Following lesion preparation, ALA or MAL is applied directly to the lesion site and the surrounding 5 mm of normal skin. Incubation of the photosensitizing agent should take place at room temperature as cold skin temperatures may reduce the rate of PpIX formation.[17] High ambient temperature may on the other hand cause excessive sweating and thus dilute the drug concentration.[79]

The application technique and incubation time depends on the photosensitizing agent and formulation used.

ALA FORMULATED IN A LIQUID SOLUTION

- Mix the ALA powder and alcohol solution of the aminolevulinic acid stick immediately (<2 hours) before AK application.
- Apply the prepared solution to uniformly wet the surface of the AK. Repeat when the initial application has dried.
- Incubate for 14 to 18 hours without occlusion, avoiding bathing or washing of the lesion.

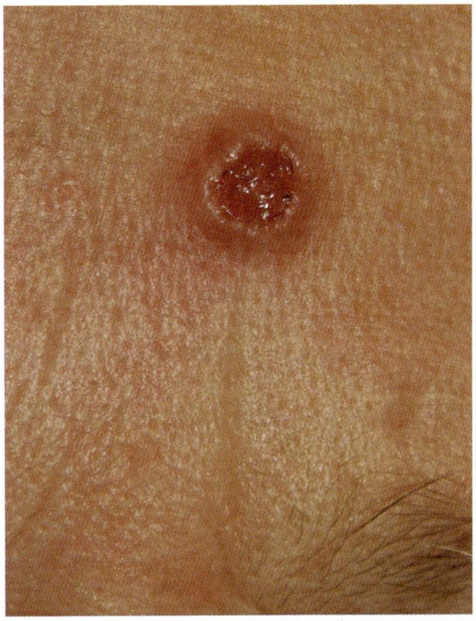

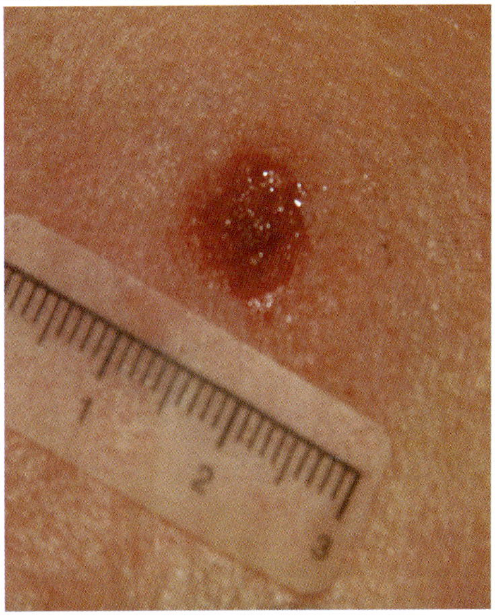

Figure 33-7 Lesion preparation of nodular basal cell carcinoma before (above) and after tumor debulking (below).

- Following incubation, the treatment area should be gently rinsed with water and dried before illumination.

ALA PATCH

- Apply the patch and incubate for 4 hours.
- Following incubation, remove the patch and rinse the treatment area with water.

ALA NANOEMULSION

- Following lesion preparation, lesions must be wiped with an ethanol or isopropyl alcoholol-soaked cotton pad to degrease the skin. The gel is then applied in a 1 mm thick layer to the entire lesional area avoiding application close to eyes, nostrils, mouth, and ears.

- Allow the gel to dry for approximately 10 minutes before the treatment area is covered with occlusive light-impermeable dressing. Incubate for 3 hours.
- Following incubation, the occlusive dressing is removed and the treatment area cleaned with saline and gauze.

MAL CREAM

- Apply MAL cream in a 1 mm thick layer to the entire lesion to be treated.
- Treatment area must be covered with occlusive light-impermeable dressing and incubated for 3 hours.
- Following incubation, the occlusive dressing is removed and the treatment area cleaned with saline and gauze.

ILLUMINATION

Illumination with blue or red light is performed according to the following:

- Adjust and fix the distance from lamp to patient according to manufacturer's instructions.
- During illumination, patient and medical personnel should wear suitable protective glasses, whereas untreated surrounding skin needs no protection (Fig. 33-8). It is advisable that illumination be performed under the surveillance of a health care professional in order to pause or interrupt illumination if needed.
- After illumination, it is recommended that treated skin be protected from ambient light for 24 to 48 hours to avoid additional local photosensitivity reactions.

REACTIONS AND ADVERSE EFFECTS

Although generally well-tolerated, PDT treatment is associated with pain and phototoxic reactions such as localized inflammation, erythema, edema, crusting, and scaling of the treated skin. Less frequently, whealing urticaria, contact dermatitis, infection, and hyperpigmentation may occur.[81]

ACUTE AND SHORT-TERM REACTIONS

Frequently observed reactions include pain during illumination and posttreatment inflammatory skin reactions. **Pain** during illumination can be a significant adverse effect, which may deter some patients from receiving continued treatments. Patients describe pain as a burning, stinging sensation that peaks within the first few minutes of illumination and continues throughout the entire illumination period. Pain intensities vary widely between patients but the majority of patients report moderate-to-severe intensities (66% of patients).[82] Factors associated with severe pain intensities include high amounts of accumulated PpIX at illumination, anatomical regions such as scalp and face, large treatment areas, red narrowband LED light source and illumination with high irradiances.[82–84] Pain issues are most typically managed by the use of cold water spray and pauses during illumination, which provide slight-to-moderate reductions of pain intensities.[81] For more effective pain reduction, local anesthesia and facial nerve blocks of forehead and scalp may be used (pain intensities reduced from 6.4 to 1.0 on visual analogue scale).[85] Continuous activation of PpIX with daylight irradiation is significantly less painful and at the same time as effective as conventional PDT with LED.[86] Thus, daylight-mediated PDT may be an alternative treatment modality for pain management.

Following PDT, **inflammatory skin reactions** such as erythema and edema occur in more than 60% of patients.[78] Reactions are usually of mild-to-moderate intensities and typically last for 1 to 4 days. In severely photodamaged skin with high amounts of accumulated PpIX, inflammatory skin reactions may be intense, including development of crusts and sterile pustules (Fig. 33-9) whereas erosions and bleeding are less frequently observed. These reactions usually resolve within 2 to 3 weeks but posttreatment erythema may persist for 1 to 2 months.[78]

Skin cultures to exclude infections may be indicated, although uncommonly required (<1% of cases).[78] During healing, scaling and itching of the skin is common and application of a bland emollient may reduce discomfort.

Whealing urticaria is an uncommon reaction, considered due to exaggerated histamine release as part of an immediate, short-lived urticarial response during

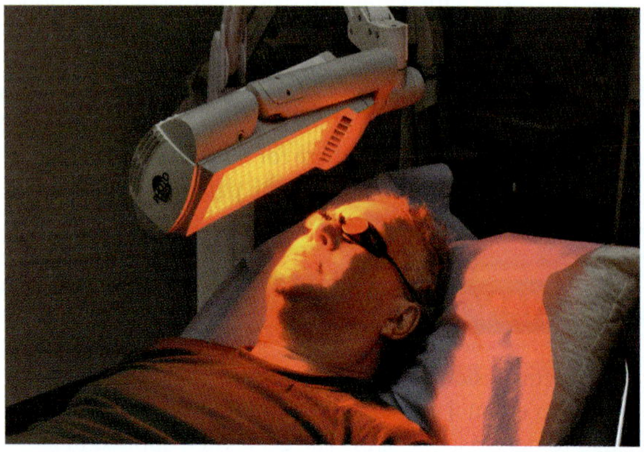

Figure 33-8 Illumination with narrowband red LED light (630 nm, Aktilite CL 128, Galderma International, France).

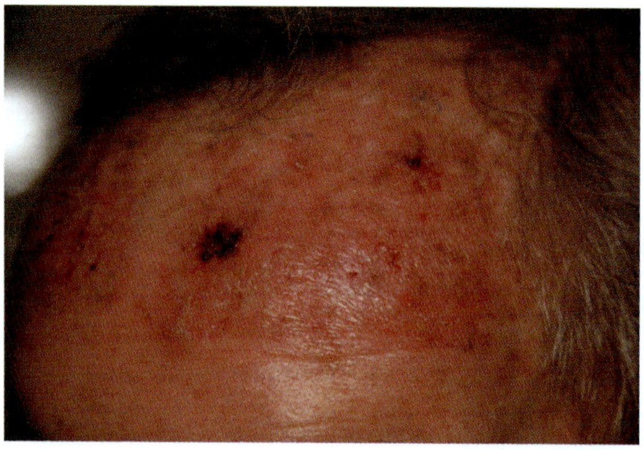

Figure 33-9 Moderate-to-severe inflammatory skin reactions with erythema, swelling, pustules, and crusts 3 days following field-directed PDT of AKs on the forehead.

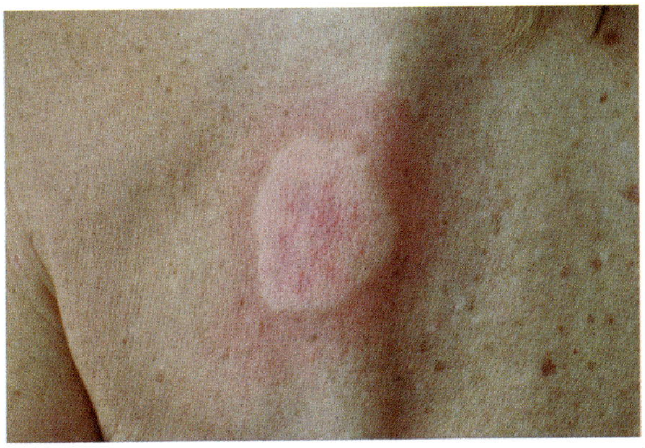

Figure 33-10 Whealing urticaria immediately after PDT illumination due to histamine release.

illumination (Fig. 33-10).[87] Urticaria occurs in approximately 1% of treated patients[78] but has been reported to occur in 3.8% of patients who received more than 7 PDT treatments.[87] As the reaction is mediated through H_1-receptors, prophylactic treatment with antihistamines reduces itch and whealing and permits illumination to be continued.

Contact dermatitis may occur from MAL-PDT and is most frequently observed in patients exposed to repeated PDT treatments.[78] MAL sensitization may be considered in patients with prolonged dermatitis after PDT treatment. The diagnosis is confirmed by patch test with MAL cream *as is*. The risk of sensitization to MAL is estimated in 0.5% of patients but may occur in up to 3% in patients having five or more PDT treatments.[88] If sensitization to MAL is induced, MAL-PDT should be stopped and future treatments may instead be performed using ALA as the photosensitizing agent.

LONG-TERM REACTIONS

Long-term adverse reactions after PDT include pigmentary changes such as hyper- and hypopigmentation as well as atrophic scarring. Transient hyperpigmentation has been described in 5% to 6% of cases following PDT and usually resolves within 3 to 6 months.[54,78,81] The increase in pigmentation is considered due to increased activity of melanocytes activated by PDT and may be prevented through adequate sun protection.[89] In contrast, hypopigmentation due to phototoxic damage of melanocytes is relatively uncommon following PDT.[78] Atrophic or hypertrophic scarring is an infrequent adverse effect after PDT and is mainly observed following skin infections.[78] However, atrophy may occur due to of local tumor destruction and removal of tumor tissue as part of the debulking procedure. Thus, PDT in itself carries a low risk of scarring and, therefore, may be considered as a reasonable treatment when cosmesis constitutes a major concern.

NEW PERSPECTIVES

The main limitations of PDT include pain during illumination and the resources required for patients and health care personnel. Furthermore, reduced clearance rates and high recurrence rates of thick AKs and nodular BCC compared to thin lesions is a further disadvantage, particularly when those recurrence rates are compared to those of surgical excision. In order to improve PDT in these areas, research within recent years has focused on (i) daylight-mediated PDT as a simplified, pain-reducing treatment modality and (ii) fractional laser-assisted PDT, which increases ALA and MAL skin penetration, for intensified treatment procedures.

DAYLIGHT-MEDIATED PDT

Daylight-mediated PDT is based on continuous photoactivation of small amounts of PpIX during daylight exposure rather than photobleaching large amounts of accumulated PpIX by lamp illumination. The concept was developed by Professor Hans Christian Wulf, Copenhagen, Denmark, and the current body of evidence includes five landmark studies on AK carried out by Dr. Stine R. Wiegell from 2006 to 2012.[90–95] In daylight-mediated PDT, sunscreen is applied before lesion preparation, which is followed by application of MAL cream without occlusion. Patients are subsequently exposed to home-based ambient daylight for 2 hours, which provides an effective light dose and makes it unnecessary for patients to return to the clinic for light exposure (Fig. 33-11).[91]

Daylight comprises ultraviolet radiation as well as visible light and infrared light in a range from 280 to 1000,000 nm, which covers PpIX absorption of blue and red visible wavelengths.[91] Daylight PDT studies have been performed in Scandinavia and the PpIX effective

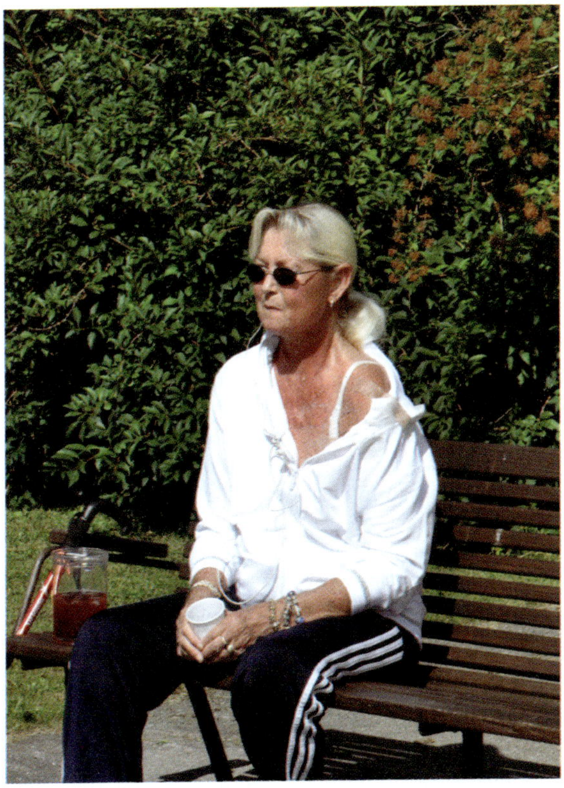

Figure 33-11 Daylight-PDT treatment of AK on the chest performed in the hospital garden.

light dose depends on latitude, weather conditions, and time of year. In a recent study, measurements on effective PpIX light dose found that daylight PDT may be performed until the middle of November in Turin and all year round in Israel.[91]

The existing body of evidence on the efficacy of daylight-PDT for multiple AKs on the face and scalp consists of five randomized clinical trials. In the first study, 30 patients were treated in a split-site fashion with daylight-mediated PDT versus conventional PDT with red LED light given in a hospital setting.[95] The study found that daylight-mediated PDT was as effective as conventional PDT (79% and 71% reduction of AK lesions at 3 month follow-up) and significantly less painful (mean maximal pain score of 2.0 vs. 6.7 on 10 point scale).[5] In the second study, patients were treated in a home-based setting with 8% and 16% MAL application and subsequent daylight exposure (77% cure of AKs at 3 months for 16% MAL and 80% for 8% MAL).[94] Recently, two multicenter studies including a large patient population (n = 120 patients with 2,768 thin, moderately and thick AKs of the face and scalp) substantiated daylight-PDT as a promising concept, especially for patients with large field-cancerized areas that can easily be exposed to sunlight.[92,93]

FRACTIONAL LASER-ASSISTED PDT

Ablative fractional resurfacing (AFR) creates microscopic vertical holes of ablated tissue that are surrounded by a thin layer of coagulated tissue.[96] In an in vivo porcine study these vertical channels facilitated the biodistribution of topically applied MAL into deep skin layers and promoted an intensified PDT response in the deep dermal compartment.[97,98] At the mid-dermal level corresponding to 1 mm skin depth, MAL-induced PpIX fluorescence intensities were approximately 50 times higher in hair follicle epithelium and dermal fluorescence intensities approximately 15 times higher as compared with non-AFR treated samples when AFR pretreatment was performed. In a recent randomized study, the efficacy and safety of AFR-assisted PDT was compared to conventional PDT for AK treatment in field-cancerized skin (Fig. 33-12).[99] The study showed AFR pretreatment to be significantly more effective in the treatment of especially thick AKs compared to conventional PDT, with 87.5% vs. 58.8% of moderately and thick AKs cleared at 3 months after treatment.[101] AFR-pretreatment increased the accumulated amount of PpIX prior to illumination and facilitated an intensified PDT response in terms of enhanced efficacy as well as phototoxic reactions post-treatment. Initial clinical attempts have been made to investigate the feasibility of fractional laser-assisted PDT for nodular BCC[100] and this treatment modality is currently under examination in an IRB-approved clinical trial for difficult-to-treat BCCs of the face.

Daylight-PDT as well as fractional laser-assisted PDT techniques are not FDA approved and thus far constitute research-based off-label indications. The use of these as routine treatments must await additional data from clinical trials.

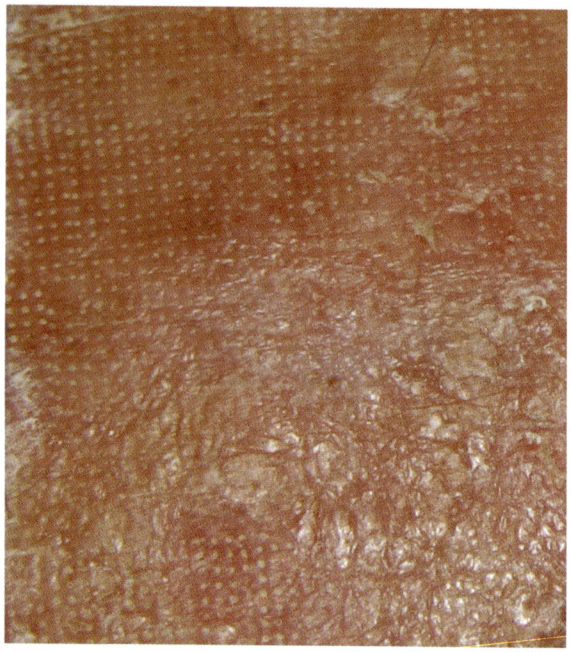

Figure 33-12 Ablative fractional laser pattern before MAL application for intensified PDT procedure in field-cancerized skin of the scalp.

REFERENCES

1. Morton CA, Szeimies RM, Sidoroff A, Braathen LR. European guidelines for topical photodynamic therapy part 1: treatment delivery and current indications - actinic keratoses, Bowen's disease, basal cell carcinoma. *J Eur Acad Dermatol Venereol.* 2012;27(5):536–544.
2. Braathen LR, Szeimies RM, Basset-Seguin N, et al. Guidelines on the use of photodynamic therapy for nonmelanoma skin cancer: an international consensus. International Society for Photodynamic Therapy in Dermatology, 2005. *J Am Acad Dermatol.* 2007;56(1):125–143.
3. Kennedy JC, Pottier RH. Endogenous protoporphyrin IX, a clinically useful photosensitizer for photodynamic therapy. *J Photochem Photobiol B.* 1992;14(4):275–292.
4. Kennedy JC, Pottier RH, Pross DC. Photodynamic therapy with endogenous protoporphyrin IX: basic principles and present clinical experience. *J Photochem Photobiol B.* 1990;6(1–2):143–148.
5. Kennedy JC, Marcus SL, Pottier RH. Photodynamic therapy (PDT) and photodiagnosis (PD) using endogenous photosensitization induced by 5-aminolevulinic acid (ALA): mechanisms and clinical results. *J Clin Laser Med Surg.* 1996;14(5): 289–304.
6. Henderson BW, Dougherty TJ. How does photodynamic therapy work? *Photochem Photobiol.* 1992;55(1):145–157.
7. Redmond RM. Photophysics and photochemistry in photodynamic therapy. In: Hamblin MR, Mroz P, ed. *Advances in Photodynamic Therapy. Basic, Translational, and Clinical.* 1st ed. Boston, MA: Artech House; 2008:41–58.
8. Moan J, Juzeniene A. The role of oxygen in photodynamic therapy. In: Hamblin MR, Mroz P, ed. *Advances in Photodynamic Therapy. Basic, Translational, and Clinical.* 1st ed. Boston, MA: Artech House; 2008:135–149.
9. Moan J, Sommer S. Oxygen dependence of the photosensitizing effect of hematoporphyrin derivative in NHIK 3025 cells. *Cancer Res.* 1985;45(4):1608–1610.
10. Buytaert E, Dewaele M, Agostinis P. Molecular effectors of multiple cell death pathways initiated by photodynamic therapy. *Biochim Biophys Acta.* 2007;1776(1):86–107.

11. Nowis D, Golab J. Photodynamic therapy and oxidative stress. In: Hamblin MR, Mróz P, ed. *Advances in Photodynamic Therapy Basic, Translational and Clinical.* 1st ed. Norwood, MA: Artech House; 2008:151–178.
12. Garg AD, Nowis D, Golab J, Agostinis P. Photodynamic therapy: illuminating the road from cell death towards anti-tumour immunity. *Apoptosis.* 2010;15(9):1050–1071.
13. Agostinis P, Berg K, Cengel KA, et al. Photodynamic therapy of cancer: an update. *CA Cancer J Clin.* 2011;61(4):250–281.
14. Mroz P, Szokalska A, Wu MX, Hamblin MR. Photodynamic therapy of tumors can lead to development of systemic antigen-specific immune response. *PLoS One.* 2010;5(12):e15194.
15. Korbelik M. PDT and Inflammation. In: Hamblin MR, Mróz P, ed. *Advances in Photodynamic Therapy Basic, Translational, and Clinical.* 1st ed. Norwood, MA: Artech House;2008: 255–266.
16. Peng Q, Warloe T, Moan J,et al. Distribution of 5-aminolevulinic acid-induced porphyrins in noduloulcerative basal cell carcinoma. *Photochem Photobiol.* 1995;62(5):906–913.
17. Juzeniene A, Juzenas P, Kaalhus O, Iani V, Moan J. Temperature effect on accumulation of protoporphyrin IX after topical application of 5-aminolevulinic acid and its methylester and hexylester derivatives in normal mouse skin. *Photochem Photobiol.* 2002;76(4):452–456.
18. Fotinos N, Campo MA, Popowycz F, Gurny R, Lange N. 5-Aminolevulinic acid derivatives in photomedicine: characteristics, application and perspectives. *Photochem Photobiol.* 2006;82(4):994–1015.
19. van den Akker JT, Iani V, Star WM, Sterenborg HJ, Moan J. Topical application of 5-aminolevulinic acid hexyl ester and 5-aminolevulinic acid to normal nude mouse skin: differences in protoporphyrin IX fluorescence kinetics and the role of the stratum corneum. *Photochem Photobiol.* 2000;72(5):681–689.
20. Uehlinger P, Zellweger M, Wagnieres G, Juillerat-Jeanneret L, van den Bergh H, Lange N. 5-Aminolevulinic acid and its derivatives: physical chemical properties and protoporphyrin IX formation in cultured cells. *J Photochem Photobiol B.* 2000;54(1):72–80.
21. Peng Q, Moan J, Warloe T, et al. Build-up of esterified aminolevulinic-acid-derivative-induced porphyrin fluorescence in normal mouse skin. *J Photochem Photobiol B.* 1996;34(1):95–96.
22. Fritsch C, Homey B, Stahl W, Lehmann P, Ruzicka T, Sies H. Preferential relative porphyrin enrichment in solar keratoses upon topical application of delta-aminolevulinic acid methylester. *Photochem Photobiol.* 1998;68(2):218–221.
23. Wiegell SR, Wulf HC. Photodynamic therapy of acne vulgaris using 5-aminolevulinic acid versus methyl aminolevulinate. *J Am Acad Dermatol.* 2006;54(4):647–651.
24. Szeimies RM, Radny P, Sebastian M, et al. Photodynamic therapy with BF-200 ALA for the treatment of actinic keratosis: results of a prospective, randomized, double-blind, placebo-controlled phase III study. *Br J Dermatol.* 2010;163(2):386–394.
25. Anderson RR. Laser-Tissue Interactions. In: Almound G, ed.*Cutaneous Laser Surgery. The art and science of selective photothermolysis.* 2nd ed. St. Louis, Missouri: Mosby; 1999:1–18.
26. Juzeniene A, Juzenas P, Ma LW, Iani V, Moan J. Effectiveness of different light sources for 5-aminolevulinic acid photodynamic therapy. *Lasers Med Sci.* 2004;19(3):139–149.
27. Morton CA, Whitehurst C, Moore JV, MacKie RM. Comparison of red and green light in the treatment of Bowen's disease by photodynamic therapy. *Br J Dermatol.* 2000;143(4): 767–772.
28. Valentine RM, Wood K, Brown CT, Ibbotson SH, Moseley H. Monte Carlo simulations for optimal light delivery in photodynamic therapy of non-melanoma skin cancer. *Phys Med Biol.* 2012;57(20):6327–6345.
29. Alexiades-Armenakas M. Laser-mediated photodynamic therapy. *Clin Dermatol.* 2006;24(1):16–25.
30. Alexiades-Armenakas MR, Geronemus RG. Laser-mediated photodynamic therapy of actinic keratoses. *Arch Dermatol.* 2003;139(10):1313–1320.
31. Brancaleon L, Moseley H. Laser and non-laser light sources for photodynamic therapy. *Lasers Med Sci.* 2002;17(3):173–186.
32. Haedersdal M, Togsverd-Bo K, Wiegell SR, Wulf HC. Long-pulsed dye laser versus long-pulsed dye laser-assisted photodynamic therapy for acne vulgaris: A randomized controlled trial. *J Am Acad Dermatol.* 2008;58(3):387–394.
33. Alexiades-Armenakas M. Intense pulsed light-mediated photodynamic therapy. *J Drugs Dermatol.* 2005;4(5):657–658.
34. Babilas P, Knobler R, Hummel S, et al. Variable pulsed light is less painful than light-emitting diodes for topical photodynamic therapy of actinic keratosis: a prospective randomized controlled trial. *Br J Dermatol.* 2007;157(1):111–117.
35. Moseley H, Ibbotson S, Woods J, et al. Clinical and research applications of photodynamic therapy in dermatology: experience of the Scottish PDT Centre. *Lasers Surg Med.* 2006; 38(5):403–416.
36. Dirschka T, Radny P, Dominicus R, et al. Photodynamic therapy with BF-200 ALA for the treatment of actinic keratosis: results of a multicentre, randomized, observer-blind phase III study in comparison with a registered methyl-5-aminolaevulinate cream and placebo. *Br J Dermatol.* 2012;166(1): 137–146.
37. Togsverd-Bo K, Idorn LW, Philipsen PA, Wulf HC, Haedersdal M. Protoporphyrin IX formation and photobleaching in different layers of normal human skin: methyl- and hexylaminolevulinate and different light sources. *Exp Dermatol.* 2012; 21(10):745–750.
38. Strasswimmer J, Grande DJ. Do pulsed lasers produce an effective photodynamic therapy response? *Lasers Surg Med.* 2006;38(1):22–25.
39. Olsen EA, Abernethy ML, Kulp-Shorten C, et al. A double-blind, vehicle-controlled study evaluating masoprocol cream in the treatment of actinic keratoses on the head and neck. *J Am Acad Dermatol.* 1991;24(5 pt 1):738–743.
40. Piacquadio DJ, Chen DM, Farber HF, et al. Photodynamic therapy with aminolevulinic acid topical solution and visible blue light in the treatment of multiple actinic keratoses of the face and scalp: investigator-blinded, phase 3, multicenter trials. *Arch Dermatol.* 2004;140(1):41–46.
41. Apalla Z, Sotiriou E, Panagiotidou D, Lefaki I, Goussi C, Ioannides D. The impact of different fluence rates on pain and clinical outcome in patients with actinic keratoses treated with photodynamic therapy. *Photodermatol Photoimmunol Photomed.* 2011;27(4):181–185.
42. Morton CA, Brown SB, Collins S, et al. Guidelines for topical photodynamic therapy: report of a workshop of the British Photodermatology Group. *Br J Dermatol.* 2002;146(4): 552–567.
43. Freeman M, Vinciullo C, Francis D, et al. A comparison of photodynamic therapy using topical methyl aminolevulinate (Metvix) with single cycle cryotherapy in patients with actinic keratosis: a prospective, randomized study. *J Dermatolog Treat.* 2003;14(2):99–106.
44. Pariser D, Loss R, Jarratt M, et al. Topical methyl-aminolevulinate photodynamic therapy using red light-emitting diode light for treatment of multiple actinic keratoses: a randomized, double-blind, placebo-controlled study. *J Am Acad Dermatol.* 2008;59(4):569–576.
45. Szeimies RM, Karrer S, Radakovic-Fijan S, et al. Photodynamic therapy using topical methyl 5-aminolevulinate compared with cryotherapy for actinic keratosis: a prospective, randomized study. *J Am Acad Dermatol.* 2002;47(2):258–262.
46. Tarstedt M, Rosdahl I, Berne B, Svanberg K, Wennberg AM. A randomized multicenter study to compare two treatment regimens of topical methyl aminolevulinate (Metvix)-PDT in actinic keratosis of the face and scalp. *Acta Derm Venereol.* 2005;85(5):424–428.
47. Morton C, Horn M, Leman J, et al. Comparison of topical methyl aminolevulinate photodynamic therapy with cryotherapy or Fluorouracil for treatment of squamous cell carcinoma in situ: results of a multicenter randomized trial. *Arch Dermatol.* 2006;142(6):729–735.
48. Hadley J, Tristani-Firouzi P, Hull C, Florell S, Cotter M, Hadley M. Results of an investigator-initiated single-blind

split-face comparison of photodynamic therapy and 5% imiquimod cream for the treatment of actinic keratoses. *Dermatol Surg.* 2012;38(5):722–727.

49. Serra-Guillen C, Nagore E, Hueso L, et al. A randomized pilot comparative study of topical methyl aminolevulinate photodynamic therapy versus imiquimod 5% versus sequential application of both therapies in immunocompetent patients with actinic keratosis: clinical and histologic outcomes. *J Am Acad Dermatol.* 2012;66(4):e131–e137.
50. Morton CA, Whitehurst C, Moseley H, McColl JH, Moore JV, MacKie RM. Comparison of photodynamic therapy with cryotherapy in the treatment of Bowen's disease. *Br J Dermatol.* 1996;135(5):766–771.
51. Calzavara-Pinton PG, Venturini M, Sala R, et al. Methylaminolaevulinate-based photodynamic therapy of Bowen's disease and squamous cell carcinoma. *Br J Dermatol.* 2008;159(1):137–144.
52. Madan V, Lear JT, Szeimies RM. Non-melanoma skin cancer. *Lancet.* 2010;375(9715):673–685.
53. Basset-Seguin N, Ibbotson SH, Emtestam L, et al. Topical methyl aminolaevulinate photodynamic therapy versus cryotherapy for superficial basal cell carcinoma: a 5 year randomized trial. *Eur J Dermatol.* 2008;18(5):547–553.
54. Rhodes LE, de Rie MA, Leifsdottir R, et al. Five-year follow-up of a randomized, prospective trial of topical methyl aminolevulinate photodynamic therapy vs surgery for nodular basal cell carcinoma. *Arch Dermatol.* 2007;143(9):1131–1136.
55. Telfer NR, Colver GB, Morton CA. Guidelines for the management of basal cell carcinoma. *Br J Dermatol.* 2008; 159(1):35–48.
56. Slaughter DP, Southwick HW, Smejkal W. Field cancerization in oral stratified squamous epithelium; clinical implications of multicentric origin. *Cancer.* 1953;6(5):963–968.
57. Young AR. Cumulative effects of ultraviolet radiation on the skin: cancer and photoaging. *Semin Dermatol.* 1990;9(1): 25–31.
58. Apalla Z, Sotiriou E, Chovarda E, Lefaki I, Devliotou-Panagiotidou D, Ioannides D. Skin cancer: preventive photodynamic therapy in patients with face and scalp cancerization. A randomized placebo-controlled study. *Br J Dermatol.* 2010;162(1):171–175.
59. Bagazgoitia L, Cuevas SJ, Juarranz A, Jaen P. Photodynamic therapy reduces the histological features of actinic damage and the expression of early oncogenic markers. *Br J Dermatol.* 2011;165(1):144–151.
60. Szeimies RM, Torezan L, Niwa A, et al. Clinical, histopathological and immunohistochemical assessment of human skin field cancerization before and after photodynamic therapy. *Br J Dermatol.* 2012;167(1):150–159.
61. Zwald FO, Brown M. Skin cancer in solid organ transplant recipients: advances in therapy and management: part II. Management of skin cancer in solid organ transplant recipients. *J Am Acad Dermatol.* 2011;65(2):263–279.
62. Wennberg AM, Stenquist B, Stockfleth E, et al. Photodynamic therapy with methyl aminolevulinate for prevention of new skin lesions in transplant recipients: a randomized study. *Transplantation.* 2008;86(3):423–429.
63. Wulf HC, Pavel S, Stender I, Bakker-Wensveen CA. Topical photodynamic therapy for prevention of new skin lesions in renal transplant recipients. *Acta Derm Venereol.* 2006;86(1):25–28.
64. Willey A, Mehta S, Lee PK. Reduction in the incidence of squamous cell carcinoma in solid organ transplant recipients treated with cyclic photodynamic therapy. *Dermatol Surg.* 2010;36(5):652–658.
65. de Graaf YG, Kennedy C, Wolterbeek R, Collen AF, Willemze R, Bouwes Bavinck JN. Photodynamic therapy does not prevent cutaneous squamous-cell carcinoma in organ-transplant recipients: results of a randomized-controlled trial. *J Invest Dermatol.* 2006;126(3):569–574.
66. Kohl E, Karrer S. Photodynamic therapy for photorejuvenation and non-oncologic indications: overview and update. *G Ital Dermatol Venereol.* 2011;146(6):473–485.
67. Kohl E, Torezan LA, Landthaler M, Szeimies RM. Aesthetic effects of topical photodynamic therapy. *J Eur Acad Dermatol Venereol.* 2010;24(11):1261–1269.
68. Dover JS, Bhatia AC, Stewart B, Arndt KA. Topical 5-aminolevulinic acid combined with intense pulsed light in the treatment of photoaging. *Arch Dermatol.* 2005;141(10): 1247–1252.
69. Gold MH, Bradshaw VL, Boring MM, Bridges TM, Biron JA. Split-face comparison of photodynamic therapy with 5-aminolevulinic acid and intense pulsed light versus intense pulsed light alone for photodamage. *Dermatol Surg.* 2006; 32(6):795–801.
70. Hillemanns P, Wang X, Staehle S, Michels W, Dannecker C. Evaluation of different treatment modalities for vulvar intraepithelial neoplasia (VIN): CO(2) laser vaporization, photodynamic therapy, excision and vulvectomy. *Gynecol Oncol.* 2006;100(2):271–275.
71. Sakamoto FH, Torezan L, Anderson RR. Photodynamic therapy for acne vulgaris: a critical review from basics to clinical practice: part II. Understanding parameters for acne treatment with photodynamic therapy. *J Am Acad Dermatol.* 2010;63(2):195–211.
72. Sakamoto FH, Lopes JD, Anderson RR. Photodynamic therapy for acne vulgaris: a critical review from basics to clinical practice: part I. Acne vulgaris: when and why consider photodynamic therapy? *J Am Acad Dermatol.* 2010;63(2):183–193.
73. Morton CA, Szeimies RM, Sidoroff A, Braathen LR. European guidelines for topical photodynamic therapy part 2: emerging indications - field cancerization, photorejuvenation and inflammatory/infective dermatoses. *J Eur Acad Dermatol Venereol.* 2012;27(6):672–679.
74. Stender IM, Na R, Fogh H, Gluud C, Wulf HC. Photodynamic therapy with 5-aminolaevulinic acid or placebo for recalcitrant foot and hand warts: randomised double-blind trial. *Lancet.* 2000;355(9208):963–966.
75. Edstrom DW, Porwit A, Ros AM. Photodynamic therapy with topical 5-aminolevulinic acid for mycosis fungoides: clinical and histological response. *Acta Derm Venereol.* 2001;81(3):184–188.
76. Fehr MK, Hornung R, Schwarz VA, Simeon R, Haller U, Wyss P. Photodynamic therapy of vulvar intraepithelial neoplasia III using topically applied 5-aminolevulinic acid. *Gynecol Oncol.* 2001;80(1):62–66.
77. Peng Q, Soler AM, Warloe T, Nesland JM, Giercksky KE. Selective distribution of porphyrins in skin thick basal cell carcinoma after topical application of methyl 5-aminolevulinate. *J Photochem Photobiol B.* 2001;62(3):140–145.
78. FDA. Metvixia Label information. 20-11-2012. Ref Type: Pamphlet.
79. Christensen E, Warloe T, Kroon S, et al. Guidelines for practical use of MAL-PDT in non-melanoma skin cancer. *J Eur Acad Dermatol Venereol.* 2010;24(5):505–512.
80. Morton CA. Methyl aminolevulinate (Metvix) photodynamic therapy - practical pearls. *J Dermatolog Treat.* 2003; 14(suppl 3):23–26.
81. Ibbotson SH. Adverse effects of topical photodynamic therapy. *Photodermatol Photoimmunol Photomed.* 2011;27(3):116–130.
82. Halldin CB, Gillstedt M, Paoli J, Wennberg AM, Gonzalez H. Predictors of pain associated with photodynamic therapy: a retrospective study of 658 treatments. *Acta Derm Venereol.* 2011;91(5):545–551.
83. Wiegell SR, Skiveren J, Philipsen PA, Wulf HC. Pain during photodynamic therapy is associated with protoporphyrin IX fluorescence and fluence rate. *Br J Dermatol.* 2008; 158(4):727–733.
84. Valentine RM, Ibbotson SH, Brown CT, Wood K, Moseley H. A quantitative comparison of 5-aminolaevulinic acid- and methyl aminolevulinate-induced fluorescence, photobleaching and pain during photodynamic therapy. *Photochem Photobiol.* 2011;87(1):242–249.
85. Halldin CB, Paoli J, Sandberg C, Gonzalez H, Wennberg AM. Nerve blocks enable adequate pain relief during topical photodynamic therapy of field cancerization on the forehead and scalp. *Br J Dermatol.* 2009;160(4):795–800.

86. Wiegell SR, Wulf HC, Szeimies RM, et al. Daylight photodynamic therapy for actinic keratosis: an international consensus: International Society for Photodynamic Therapy in Dermatology. *J Eur Acad Dermatol Venereol.* 2012;26(6):673–679.
87. Kaae J, Philipsen PA, Haedersdal M, Wulf HC. Immediate whealing urticaria in red light exposed areas during photodynamic therapy. *Acta Derm Venereol.* 2008;88(5):480–483.
88. Korshoj S, Solvsten H, Erlandsen M, Sommerlund M. Frequency of sensitization to methyl aminolaevulinate after photodynamic therapy. *Contact Dermatitis.* 2009;60(6):320–324.
89. Karrer S, Bosserhoff AK, Weiderer P, Landthaler M, Szeimies RM. Influence of 5-aminolevulinic acid and red light on collagen metabolism of human dermal fibroblasts. *J Invest Dermatol.* 2003;120(2):325–331.
90. Wiegell SR, Heydenreich J, Fabricius S, Wulf HC. Continuous ultra-low-intensity artificial daylight is not as effective as red LED light in photodynamic therapy of multiple actinic keratoses. *Photodermatol Photoimmunol Photomed.* 2011;27(6):280–285.
91. Wiegell SR, Wulf HC, Szeimies RM, et al. Daylight photodynamic therapy for actinic keratosis: an international consensus: International Society for Photodynamic Therapy in Dermatology. *J Eur Acad Dermatol Venereol.* 2012;26(6):673–679.
92. Wiegell SR, Fabricius S, Gniadecka M, et al. Daylight-mediated photodynamic therapy of moderate to thick actinic keratoses of the face and scalp: a randomized multicentre study. *Br J Dermatol.* 2012;166(6):1327–1332.
93. Wiegell SR, Fabricius S, Stender IM, et al. A randomized, multicentre study of directed daylight exposure times of 1(1/2) vs. 2(1/2) h in daylight-mediated photodynamic therapy with methyl aminolaevulinate in patients with multiple thin actinic keratoses of the face and scalp. *Br J Dermatol.* 2011;164(5):1083–1090.
94. Wiegell SR, Haedersdal M, Eriksen P, Wulf HC. Photodynamic therapy of actinic keratoses with 8% and 16% methyl aminolaevulinate and home-based daylight exposure: a double-blinded randomized clinical trial. *Br J Dermatol.* 2009;160(6):1308–1314.
95. Wiegell SR, Haedersdal M, Philipsen PA, Eriksen P, Enk CD, Wulf HC. Continuous activation of PpIX by daylight is as effective as and less painful than conventional photodynamic therapy for actinic keratoses; a randomized, controlled, single-blinded study. *Br J Dermatol.* 2008;158(4):740–746.
96. Manstein D, Herron GS, Sink RK, Tanner H, Anderson RR. Fractional photothermolysis: a new concept for cutaneous remodeling using microscopic patterns of thermal injury. *Lasers Surg Med.* 2004;34(5):426–438.
97. Haedersdal M, Katsnelson J, Sakamoto FH, et al. Enhanced uptake and photoactivation of topical methyl aminolevulinate after fractional CO_2 laser pretreatment. *Lasers Surg Med.* 2011;43(8):804–813.
98. Haedersdal M, Sakamoto FH, Farinelli WA, Doukas AG, Tam J, Anderson RR. Fractional CO(2) laser-assisted drug delivery. *Lasers Surg Med.* 2010;42(2):113–122.
99. Togsverd-Bo K, Haak CS, Thaysen-Petersen D, Wulf HC, Anderson RR, Haedesdal M. Intensified photodynamic therapy of actinic keratoses with fractional CO(2) laser: a randomized clinical trial. *Br J Dermatol.* 2012;166(6):1262–1269.
100. Haedersdal M, Togsverd-Bo K, Paasch U. Case reports on the potential of fractional laser-assisted photodynamic therapy for basal cell carcinomas. *Lasers Med Sci.* 2012;27(5):1091–1093.

CHAPTER 34

Noninvasive Skin Tightening Technology

Andrew A. Nelson

Loose, sagging skin is an unfortunate but often inevitable part of the aging process. These changes are particularly troublesome on facial and neck skin where they result in deep, static rhytides. Traditionally, surgical procedures incorporating skin removal and suspension sutures were utilized to remove the excess skin and reposition the remaining skin to recreate a younger facial structure and appearance. Most commonly these procedures consist of a facelift or necklift, which are often performed together to achieve better results. Due to the increasing epidemic of obesity, and the changes in skin tone and tightness following weight loss, demand for skin tightening of nonfacial skin has also increased dramatically in recent years. Although invasive surgical procedures remain the gold standard for large-scale skin tightening and removal, many patients are concerned about the downtime, healing, and cost associated with these procedures. As a result, patients are increasingly turning to noninvasive procedures to tighten their loose skin and minimize the aging process, and cosmetic skin tightening has become a rapidly enlarging field.

There are now multiple noninvasive treatment options to achieve skin tightening. The most commonly utilized technologies include laser, radiofrequency (RF), and ultrasound. These noninvasive treatment options are most appropriate for those patients with mild-to-moderate skin laxity. Patients with significant skin laxity, such as severe jowl formation, are typically better candidates for surgical lifting procedures. Although there are significant differences between these new, noninvasive technologies, in general, their goal is to tighten existing skin via controlled dermal heating to stimulate collagen remodeling and neocollagenesis. There are advantages and disadvantages to each technology, and as a result, no single technology is best for all patients. Furthermore, it is often difficult to predict who will benefit most from one procedure or another. Thus, it is important to be familiar with all of these technologies to be able to offer each patient the treatment that best achieves their cosmetic goals.

It is important to remember that many of the treatments we discuss in this chapter may not be specifically FDA cleared for skin tightening; instead, they may be approved for other uses, such as deep dermal heating or cellulite improvement. Many of the treatments we discuss in this chapter may, therefore, represent off-label indications for these devices. In addition, we will not focus on noninvasive fat contouring technologies in this chapter; these technologies are discussed elsewhere in this book.

BASIC SCIENCE OF COLLAGEN

Aging results in damage to collagen, which manifests itself as fragmentation of the collagen fibers and solar elastosis. This occurs as a result of extrinsic damage such as sun exposure and smoking, as well as intrinsic effects including genetics. Tissue tightening technologies focus on dermal heating to tighten existing, damaged collagen and stimulate neocollagenesis. It is, therefore, important to have an understanding of the basic science of collagen.

Collagen is a triple helical structure, held together by interstrand hydrogen bonds. As collagen is heated, these bonds are broken down, allowing the lattice to unwind. When the lattice unwinds, the coils shorten and contract. The hydrogen bonds then reform in this more compact, tightened configuration. Typically, this is seen histologically as collagen fibers with greater diameters and shorter lengths.[1] Controlled heating also stimulates the formation of new collagen (neocollagenesis), further contributing to the tissue tightening effect. Collagen denaturation is dependent on time and temperature[2]; higher temperatures are associated with shorter treatment times, but may result in increased patient discomfort and a higher risk of thermal burns. Lower temperatures require longer exposure times, but may be safer. Although the overall goal of the technologies are similar, the exact mechanism of action through which each technology achieves controlled heating of collagen differs, and treatment exposure times vary as well.[3]

EPIDERMAL COOLING

Noninvasive skin tightening technologies attempt focused heating of dermal collagen to remodel existing collagen and stimulate neocollagenesis. Although the technologies have advanced techniques to focus the heat, there remains some nonspecific bulk heating of surrounding tissues. This can be a significant challenge, as nonspecific epidermal heating can result in thermal burns, dyspigmentation, and potential scarring. As a result, many of these technologies incorporate epidermal cooling devices to reduce these risks. There are several different types of epidermal cooling devices, including dynamic (spray) cooling and contact cooling (Pelletier). When selecting a noninvasive skin tightening device, providers must have a good understanding of the proper functioning of that device's cooling mechanisms to offer safe, effective skin tightening for their patients.

PATIENT SELECTION

Patient selection and education are critical for proper implementation of noninvasive skin tightening devices. In general, noninvasive skin tightening devices work best in patients with mild-to-moderate skin laxity, requiring either facial or non-facial skin tightening. Patients with significant excess skin, manifesting as severe jowls, nasolabial folds, deep rhytides, or excess body skin are not ideal candidates. These patients may achieve some skin tightening with noninvasive technologies, but are likely better treated with an invasive surgical procedure to achieve more clinically significant skin tightening.

Patients should also be educated about the likely outcomes of noninvasive skin tightening. It is essential that patients have realistic expectations. It is important to note that improvement may be unpredictable. If a patient expects a noninvasive skin tightening procedure to produce an outcome similar to that of a surgical facelift or abdominoplasty, that patient will inevitably be disappointed. These patients should either not be treated, or the physician should ensure that they are educated to be more realistic in their expectations. Patients should also be educated that with certain technologies a series of treatments over an extended time period will likely be necessary to achieve a better outcome.

Patients with mild-to-moderate skin laxity and realistic treatment expectations will achieve the greatest benefit from noninvasive skin tightening. By selecting the proper patients and educating them appropriately, physicians can help these patients to achieve their treatment goals.

LASER DEVICES

Laser (Light Amplification by Stimulated Emission of Radiation) devices were among the first technologies to be FDA cleared for skin tightening. Lasers produce monochromatic, high intensity, coherent light. The effect of lasers on tissue is generally predicted by the theory of selective photothermolysis. According to selective photothermolysis, there are four main chromophores in the skin: water, melanin, oxyhemoglobin, and deoxyhemoglobin.[4] The central tenet of selective photothermolysis is that by utilizing a laser with a wavelength selectively absorbed by the target chromophore, with sufficient energy to heat the target, and an appropriate pulse duration to contain the energy within the target, the target can be specifically heated while minimizing the unintended spread of energy to surrounding tissue. In order to heat collagen and effectively remodel it, it is necessary to target water within the dermis as the chromophore. There are multiple wavelengths of light that can target water, and, therefore, several wavelengths that should theoretically stimulate collagen remodeling and neocollagenesis.

Initially, fully ablative lasers such as the carbon dioxide (CO_2) and erbium:yttrium-aluminum-garnet (Er:YAG) were studied for tissue tightening. Although these ablative lasers were very effective in reducing rhytides and surface changes, the results on skin tightening were more modest and may have been related to wound contraction rather than collagen remodeling.[5,6] In addition, the several weeks of healing time associated with traditional ablative resurfacing made it a less desirable option for patients. In an effort to reduce the downtime associated with fully ablative lasers, fractionated nonablative and ablative technologies were developed. These fractionated technologies treat only a portion of the epidermal surface, known as microthermal zones. By only treating a portion of the skin surface, typically 5% to 25%, it is possible to reduce the downtime and healing associated with ablative laser resurfacing. Fractionated ablative lasers can be used to effectively treat rhytides, surface irregularities, melasma, and multiple other indications; however, their effect on skin tightening remains modest.[7] Fractionated ablative lasers are more fully discussed elsewhere in this book, and will not be discussed further in this section.

Nonablative infrared lasers (750 nm through 1 mm wavelength) have become widely utilized for noninvasive skin tightening. These lasers target water in the dermis as their major chromophore. There are several reasons for utilizing infrared wavelengths for skin tightening. First, the depth of laser penetration is directly related to its wavelength; the longer the wavelength of light, the deeper its penetration. Second, longer wavelengths are less well absorbed by melanin; this means that these infrared wavelengths are not absorbed by epidermal melanin, reducing the risk of thermal burns of the epidermis. Third, with less absorption of light by epidermal melanin, the infrared lasers generate a higher effective fluence of energy at the level of the dermal collagen – the target of tissue tightening. Finally, these infrared lasers do not produce ablation (removal) of the epidermis, thereby significantly reducing downtime and healing.

The original infrared devices for skin tightening were lasers with wavelengths in the mid-infrared range. One of the early devices utilized a 1320 nm Nd:YAG laser to target dermal water (CoolTouch, CoolTouch Corporation, Roseville, CA). In a clinical study, however, this device resulted in minimal or mild reduction in wrinkles.[8] Similarly, a 1450 nm diode laser was developed for acne scarring and dermal remodeling (SmoothBeam, Syneron Inc., Irvine, CA). Again, in a clinical study, mild-to-moderate improvement in facial rhytides was observed following a series of treatments, along with a possibly increased expression of collagen.[9,10] These devices produced modest improvements in skin tone, texture, and in some cases, skin tightening. More recently, broadband infrared devices have been developed in an attempt to increase clinical efficacy. A broadband infrared lamp, emitting wavelengths from 1100 to 1800 nm, has been developed that produces dermal heating from 1 to 2 mm in depth (Titan, Cutera, Brisbane, CA). By incorporating effective pre and post cooling, a prolonged multisecond heating cycle can be utilized. With these improvements, the broadband infrared device may achieve effective noninvasive skin tightening.

Erbium glass-based lasers have also been developed to target dermal collagen. Fraxel re:store (Solta Medical Inc., Hayward, CA) utilizes a 1550 nm erbium-doped fiber to target dermal water; this device utilizes nonablative fractional photothermolysis to deliver the laser energy through thermally confined microthermal zones. There is another device utilizing a flashlamp system with a specific codoped Yb-Er:phosphate glass material to generate a 1540 nm wavelength (Lux1540 handpiece, Palomar

Medical Technologies Inc., Burlington, MA). This device also utilizes a fractionated delivery system to target the dermis. These erbium glass systems can be used to treat fine lines, wrinkles, acne scars, and a myriad of other indications. They may also have a modest effect on skin tightening through dermal heating.

CLINICAL OUTCOMES

Infrared lasers for skin tightening (1100–1800 nm) are best used in patients seeking mild-to-moderate improvement in fine lines and skin tone as well as skin tightening. Patients seeking more significant improvements are better candidates for surgical interventions. Often, the degree of improvement is difficult to predict prior to treatment.

In a clinical trial of a broadband infrared device (Titan, Cutera, Brisbane, CA), the greatest skin tightening was noted over the malar region, the neck, and the body of the mandible; however, the average tightening in these areas was 10%, 10%, and 12%, respectively.[11] In another clinical study of skin laxity in Asian skin, 23% of patients reported mild skin tightening, 15% reported moderate improvement, and 54% reported significant improvement 3 months following a series of treatments.[12] This again emphasizes that while skin tightening can be achieved with broadband infrared devices, these improvements are mild to moderate in most cases, and there can be a great deal of variability in patient outcomes.

Erbium glass systems (Fraxel re:store, Solta Medical, Hayward, CA) can also be used to achieve mild-to-moderate skin tightening (Fig. 34-1). In a study of Asian patients with acne scarring, facial images of patients were analyzed with computer software to indicate that, in addition to scar remodeling, skin tightening was achieved following a series of noninvasive erbium glass laser treatments.[13] Erbium-doped fiber lasers can also be used to improve photodamage, dyspigmentation, and rhytides. In a study of 50 patients, significant improvement in photodamaged facial and non-facial skin (Fig. 34-2) was achieved, including a reduction in rhytides.[14] However, other authors have noted that while superficial rhytides may improve with nonablative fractional erbium-doped fiber lasers, moderate and deeper rhytides do not improve as significantly as with previous ablative laser treatment options.[15] As a result, many physicians consider these nonablative fractional laser treatment options to be better options for superficial dyspigmentation, photodamage, and superficial rhytides. Although mild skin tightening may also be observed following nonablative fractional erbium glass laser treatments, significant skin tightening is less likely to be achieved. Thus, these technologies may be a good option for patients seeking mild-to-moderate skin tightening with the simultaneous treatment of photodamage.

PATIENT EDUCATION AND ADVERSE EVENTS

Treatment protocols and algorithms have evolved over the years since these devices were developed. Initially, many of the devices utilized a single pass, single treatment protocol with high energy levels. Unfortunately, the highest energy levels may increase the risk of discomfort, thermal burns, and scarring. More recent treatment algorithms utilize lower energy, multiple pass treatments. Many of the devices now require a series of two to four separate treatments in order to achieve efficacy.

Side effects of infrared devices include mild erythema and edema immediately following the treatment, which are typically transient. Although new protocols have reduced the risk of serious adverse effects, there is still the potential for thermal burns and scars, particularly if the cooling system on the technology is not functioning properly during the treatment.

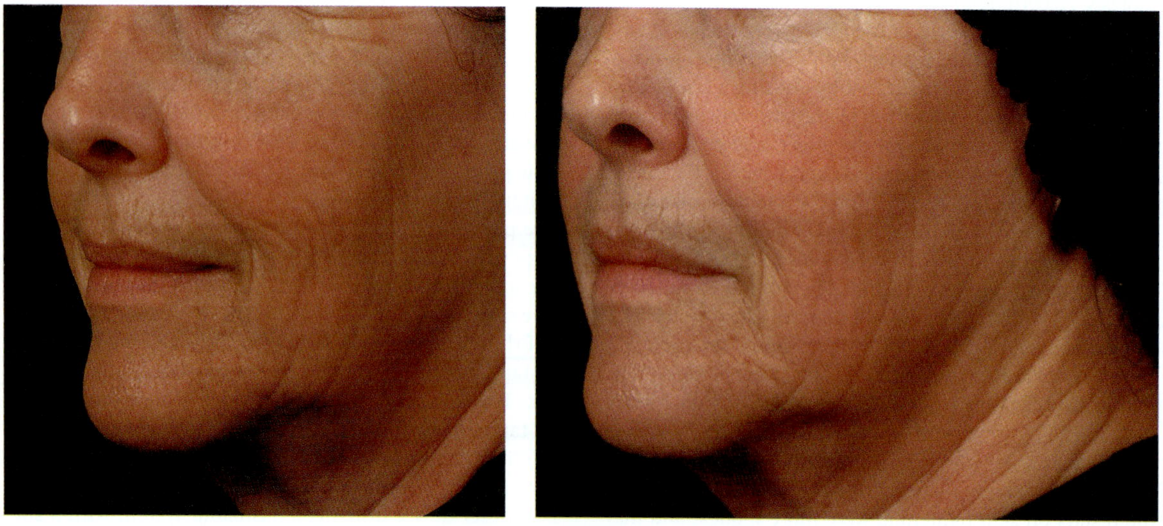

Figure 34-1 Clinical results showing skin tightening and a reduction in rhytides following two treatments with a 1550 nm noninvasive device. (Reproduced from Beasley KL, Weiss RA. Nonablative fractional lasers. In: Goldman MP, Fitzpatrick RE, Ross EV, Kilmer SL, Weiss RA, eds. *Lasers and Energy Devices for the Skin*. 2nd ed. Boca Raton, FL: CRC Press; 2013, with permission.)

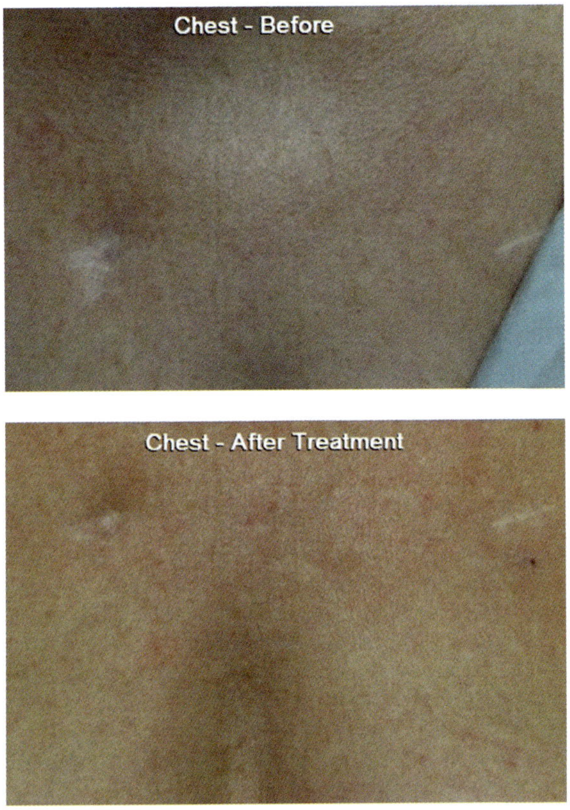

Figure 34-2 Clinical improvement of photodamaged chest following two treatments with a 1550 nm noninvasive device. (Reproduced from Beasley KL, Weiss RA. Nonablative fractional lasers. In: Goldman MP, Fitzpatrick RE, Ross EV, Kilmer SL, Weiss RA, eds. *Lasers and Energy Devices for the Skin*. 2nd ed. Boca Raton, FL: CRC Press; 2013, with permission.)

RADIOFREQUENCY

Radiofrequency (RF) devices are chromophore independent, focused heating sources. These devices utilize oscillating current, which is passed through the tissue target. The alternating flow of electricity causes increased molecular vibration and friction, which in turn generates heat.[16] Different RF devices utilize differing frequencies, but most devices for tissue tightening incorporate frequencies in the MHz range. The frequency of an RF device has an effect on tissue penetration, with lower frequency devices typically offering a greater depth of penetration and heating. As RF heating does not depend on a specific molecule absorbing the energy, it does not follow the principle of selective photothermolysis and is, therefore, chromophore independent. This property is beneficial in that RF is safe to use in all skin types, even skin types V and VI.

There are many different RF devices currently on the market, and there are likely to be many more added in coming years. Rather than focusing specifically on each device, we will group the devices into a few categories. First, RF devices can be divided based upon their polarity: monopolar, bipolar, and multipolar. Monopolar devices utilize a single positive pole incorporated into the handpiece and a ground (return) electrode placed somewhere on the patient's body. In this configuration, the current passes from the handpiece through the patient's body and exits through the return electrode. Monopolar devices in theory allow for greater depth of penetration than bipolar and multipolar devices, but may have an increased risk of unintended spread of the current throughout the body. Bipolar RF devices, in contrast, utilize a handpiece that incorporates both the positive and negative poles to create a closed electrical circuit with a fixed distance between the positive and negative electrodes. The distance between the two electrodes helps to determine the ultimate depth of penetration of the RF energy, which is typically considered to be a depth of penetration equal to one-half of the distance between the electrodes. Bipolar RF devices may not allow energy to penetrate as deeply as monopolar devices, but may be safer due to the closed controlled electrical circuit. Relatively new devices known as multipolar RF have also been developed. These multipolar devices are best considered as a type of sequential bipolar device. They utilize multiple bipolar electrodes, set at a variety of distances apart. When the device discharges RF energy from these multiple bipolar electrode pairs, it effectively heats the dermis at differing levels. These new multipolar devices may potentially offer greater efficacy due to the multiple treatment depths that can be achieved with a single treatment.

In addition to the polarity of an RF device, the technologies can be divided based upon the manner in which the energy is delivered. RF energy can be delivered via a static, stamping motion with in which the RF handpiece is held in a single position while energy is delivered, and then the handpiece is moved before the next RF pulse is delivered. RF can also be delivered in a moving, dynamic pattern where the handpiece is constantly rotated or moved across the skin surface while the energy is delivered. Dynamic devices may allow for larger areas to be treated more efficiently, while static devices may allow for the treatment of smaller more targeted areas. Finally, RF energy can be fractionated, similar to fractional lasers. As a result of all of these differences, it is important for physicians to carefully research each individual technology prior to incorporating these devices into their practice.

There are many different RF devices available that typically fall into one of three categories determined by the polarity of the device (Table 34-1). Further subdivisions and variations of each of these categories also exist. In addition to pure RF devices, RF can be combined with other technologies such as lasers or intense pulsed light. A full description of each of these numerous combination devices is beyond the scope of this review.

CLINICAL OUTCOMES

As a result of so many different RF technologies being available, a comprehensive review of all clinical trials is not possible in this chapter. Rather, we will focus on a few specific trials and RF technologies. Initial studies of a static, monopolar RF device (Thermage, Solta Medical, Hayward, CA) revealed mild-to-moderate improvements in periorbital wrinkling, cheek and neck skin laxity, nasolabial folds, marionette lines, and jowls (Fig. 34-3).[17–19]

TABLE 34-1
Radiofrequency Devices for Skin Tightening, Divided According to Method of RF Energy Delivery

Monopolar RF Devices	Bipolar Devices	Multipolar Devices
TruSculpt (Cutera, Brisbane, CA)	Accent (has both unipolar and bipolar handpieces) (Alma Lasers, Buffalo Grove, IL)	Venus Freeze (combines multipolar RF with magnetic pulsed fields) (Venus Concept, Toronto, ON, Canada)
Thermage Comfort Pulse Technology (Solta Medical, Hayward, CA)	ePrime (Syneron Inc., Irvine, CA)	Apollo (tripolar RF) (Pollogen LTD, Jerusalem, Israel)
Exilis (BTL Industries, Framingham, MA)	VelaShape (Syneron Inc., Irvine, CA)	EndyMed Pro (EndyMed Medical Ltd, Caesarea, Israel)
Pelleve (Ellman International, Hicksville, NY)	eMatrix (Syneron Inc., Irvine, CA)	Reaction (Viora, Jersey City, NJ)
	Forma (InMode Inc., Yokenam, Israel)	

A novel dynamic moving monopolar RF device (Pelleve, Ellman International, Oceanside, NY) has also been shown to improve patients' overall skin laxity, texture, wrinkles, and overall appearance by 30% to 50%, 1 year following a series of treatments.[20] Similarly, another dynamic monopolar device with incorporated Pelletier cooling (Exilis, BTL Industries, Framingham, MA) has been observed to improve skin texture and skin tightening both for facial and non-facial indications (Fig. 34-4).

Bipolar and multipolar RF devices have also been reported to result in improved patient appearance with increased skin tightening. A bipolar, multifrequency, suction-assisted RF device (Reaction, Viora Inc., Jersey City, NJ) resulted in improved thigh skin laxity appearance in 57% of patient-assessed outcomes and 78% of investigator-assessed subjects.[21] In addition, a novel bipolar RF device (Forma, InMode Inc., Yokenam, Israel) with built-in sensors including epidermal thermal, impedance, and contact sensors has been observed to achieve effective skin tightening following a series of treatments (Fig. 34-5). The built-in feedback sensors allow for prolonged, controlled dermal heating while limiting the risk of overheating or burning the treatment area. A multipolar RF device (EndyMed PRO, EndyMed Medical, Caesarea, Israel) has also been shown to result in skin tightening and improve the appearance of cellulite.[22]

Although many of these devices appear to help patients achieve mild-to-moderate improvement in skin tightening following a series of noninvasive RF treatments, many studies do not adequately quantify the degree of improvement. Furthermore, head-to-head comparison studies between these different RF devices are lacking. It is, therefore, difficult to state with any certainty which device, if any, is superior.

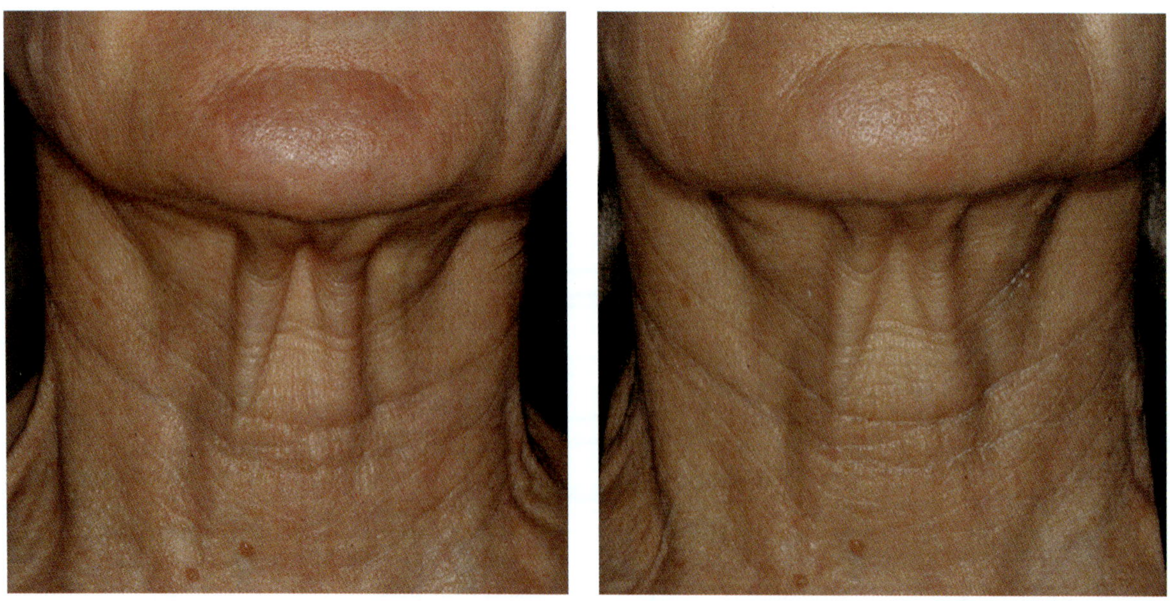

Figure 34-3 Clinical improvement with tightening of neck skin and improved band appearance 4 months following a series of monopolar RF treatments. (Photo used with permission of Dr. Suzanne Kilmer, Laser & Skin Surgery Center of Northern California, Sacramento, CA.)

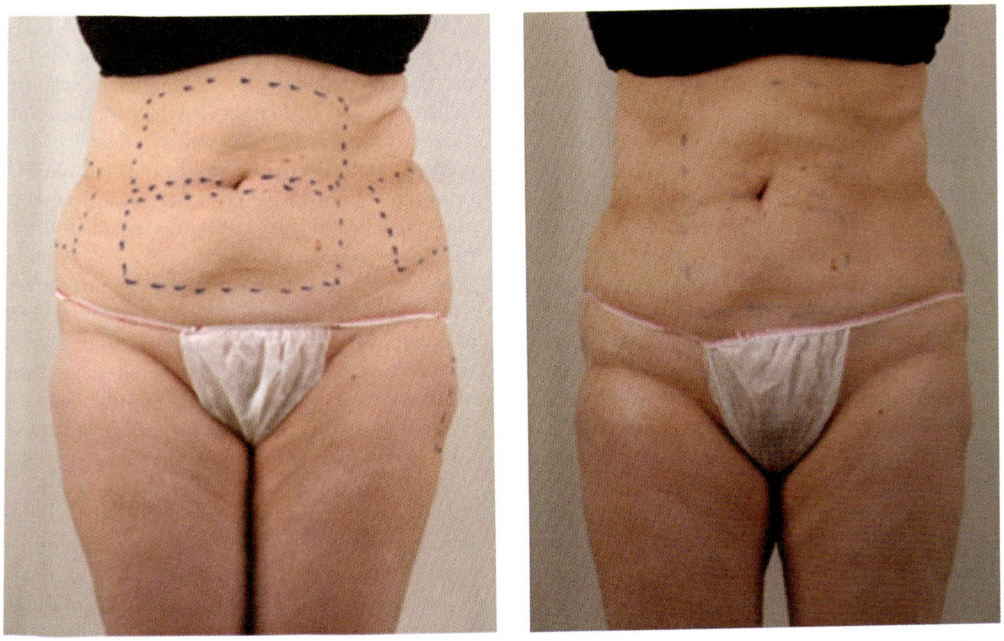

Figure 34-4 Clinical improvement showing skin tightening of the abdomen following series of three dynamic monopolar RF treatments. (Reproduced from Garibyan L, Jalian HR, Avram MM,Weiss RA. Body contouring: Noninvasive fat reduction. In: Goldman MP, Fitzpatrick RE, Ross EV, Kilmer SL, Weiss RA, eds. *Lasers and Energy Devices for the Skin*. 2nd ed. Boca Raton, FL: CRC Press; 2013, with permission.)

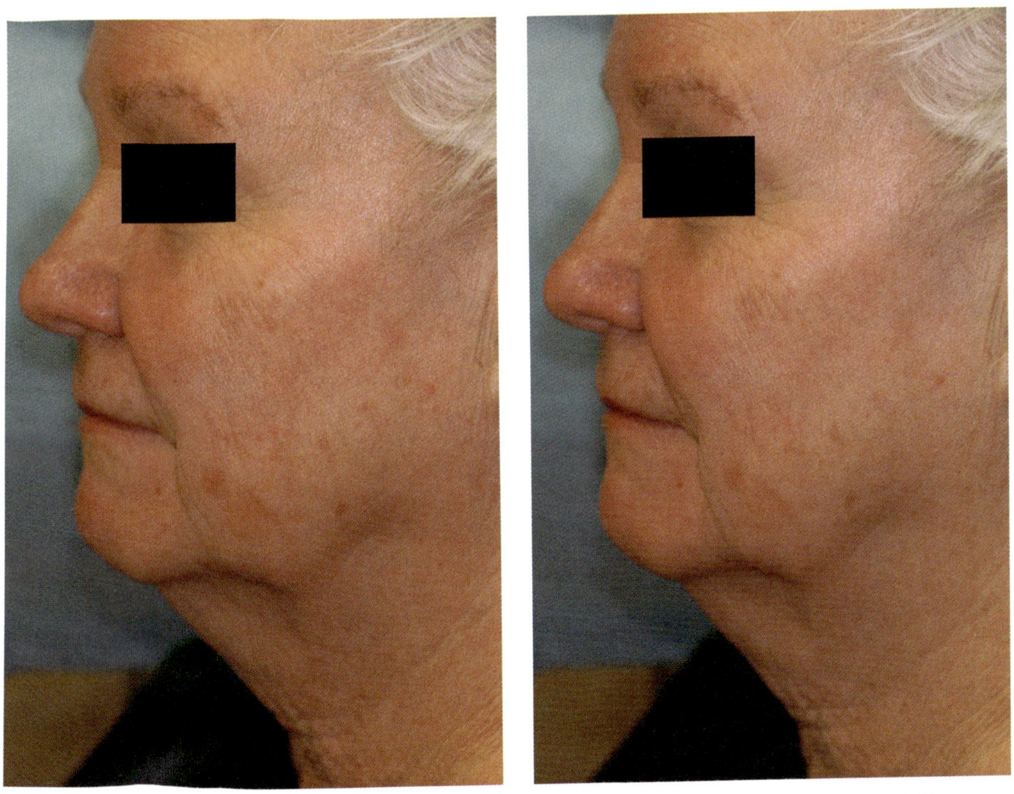

Figure 34-5 Clinical improvement in skin tightening, skin texture and rhytide reduction following a series of four nonablative bipolar radiofrequency treatments. (Photo used with permission of Dr. Andrew Nelson, Nelson Dermatology, Saint Petersburg, FL.)

PATIENT EDUCATION AND ADVERSE EVENTS

Patients should be educated regarding the extent of improvement to be seen with RF skin tightening. In most cases, mild-to-moderate improvement in rhytides along with some skin tightening will be observed. Most RF devices typically require a series of 4 to 6 weekly treatments for greatest efficacy; patients must be able to commit to a series of treatments. It is important to note that improvement, if any, may be modest. Patients with significant, deep rhytides are likely better candidates for a surgical procedure. Following RF skin tightening, the skin typically appears erythematous and slightly edematous; this may last a few hours. The skin typically feels warm to touch immediately after treatment, and patients may occasionally note that the treated area feels hot. With many RF devices, patients can return to their normal activities the day after treatment.

Reports of thermal burns and scars with RF devices, particularly first generation monopolar devices, exist. These complications have been reported with newer devices as well.[23] As a result RF devices have begun incorporating temperature and skin impedance monitoring, allowing for real time feedback and control of dermal heating. These modifications make the treatment more comfortable while also limiting the risk of burns, scars, and electrical arcing. There is concern regarding possible RF interference with implanted cardiac pacemakers and defibrillators, known as electromagnetic interference (EMI); theoretically, bipolar and multipolar RF devices may carry a lower risk as they have a closed electrical circuit. Although in general, current RF devices are safe and efficacious treatment options for skin tightening in patients of all skin types, RF devices are probably not the ideal noninvasive skin tightening technology for patients with implanted cardiac devices.

ULTRASOUND DEVICES

Ultrasound devices utilize mechanical compression waves above the range of hearing to have their effect on tissue. As the acoustic waves pass through the tissue, they cause vibration of the molecules. This vibration leads to friction between molecules, which in turn, generates heat in the tissue target. Most patients are familiar with diagnostic ultrasound devices, which utilize low energy, nonfocused energy; these devices allow for imaging of the tissue without directing energy at any one area long enough to generate sufficient heating. More recently, focused ultrasound devices have been developed, which specifically focus convergent ultrasound waves at a specific target. High-intensity focused ultrasound (HIFU) devices were initially used for medical treatments of deep structures, such as ultrasound lithotripsy of kidney stones or ultrasound ablation of solid organ cancers. Such depth of treatment is not seen in other dermatologic technologies. HIFU has also been adapted to allow for treatment of subcutaneous fat (Liposonix, Solta Medical Inc., Hayward, CA), a technology which is discussed in more detail in the chapter on body contouring in this book.

Recently, microfocused ultrasound (MIFU) technology has been developed, which allows for the targeting of dermis, subcutaneous tissues and fascia, resulting in skin tightening. The Ulthera device (Ulthera Inc., Mesa, AZ) is currently the only FDA-cleared MIFU device for skin tightening. In contrast to previous technologies, MIFU has been reported not only to heat collagen in the dermis, but also to effectively heat deeper structures including the superficial muscular aponeurotic system (SMAS), which connects muscles of facial expression to the dermis of the face. The SMAS is often tightened during surgical facelifts in order to provide longer-lasting results. Theoretically, heating and remodeling the SMAS with a noninvasive device should result in a longer-lasting, more clinically apparent result. However, to date, there are no definitive data to support this conclusion and further studies are required.

MIFU utilizes short pulse durations, with high frequency transducers, to produce focused beams of ultrasound energy, resulting in small areas of coagulative necrosis known as thermal injury zones (TIZs). The depth of the TIZ is a function of the frequency of the ultrasound energy. Higher frequencies penetrate less deeply and, therefore, result in a more superficial TIZ. Lower frequencies penetrate more deeply, resulting in a deeper TIZ. MIFU devices utilize an initial low-energy imaging mode in order to visualize the intended target as well as determine the depth of the target. The device then uses one of several transducers to treat the intended target. The frequencies of the handpiece are fixed at 7 MHz (3 and 4.5 mm focal depth), 4 MHz (4.5 mm focal depth), and 19 MHz (1.5 mm focal depth). The transducers deliver energy in straight-line patterns, with the TIZs separated from each other by 0.5 to 5 mm of untreated skin. The device utilizes short pulse durations with low energy to limit the size of the TIZ, effectively controlling the zone of heating and limiting damage to surrounding tissue. As the energy is directed to the deep dermis and SMAS, rather than epidermis, superficial cooling may not be necessary. Also, due to the fractionated nature of the treatment with normal untreated skin between TIZs, recovery may be faster.

CLINICAL OUTCOMES

Initial studies, including those performed for FDA clearance for MIFU, analyzed the effect of this technology on eyebrow position. In a study of 36 patients, 86% were observed to have clinically significant brow lift 90 days after a single treatment with the 7 MHz, 4.5 mm transducer; the mean eyebrow lift was 1.7 mm.[24] Notably, edema and erythema were common, with an average pain score of 7/10 on a visual analog scale. MIFU has also been studied for its effect on skin tightening on the lower face and jowls. In a study of 10 patients with multiple passes (initial pass with 4 MHz, 4.5 mm transducer, followed by the 7 MHz, 3 mm transducer), 25% of patients were noted to have significant improvement in jowls as well as lower face tightening, 50% of patients were observed to have moderate improvement, and 25% were noted to have mild improvement.[25] MIFU has also been noted to result in mild-to-moderate skin tightening of the décolletage following a single treatment (Fig. 34-6).[26] MIFU can also be used for non-facial applications including in areas such as

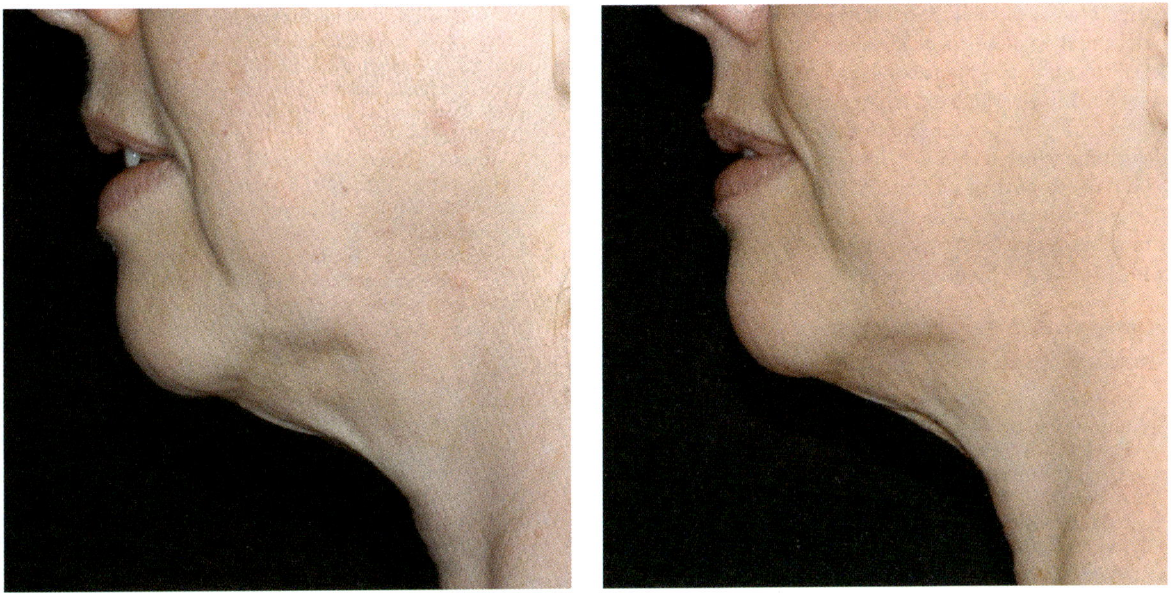

Figure 34-6 Clinical improvement with reduction of jowls and tightening of neck skin 3 months following a single microfocused ultrasound (MIFU) treatment. (Photo used with permission of Dr. Suzanne Kilmer, Laser & Skin Surgery Center of Northern California, Sacramento, CA.)

the arms, knees, and medial thighs, to produce skin tightening and lifting.[27]

If multiple transducers are to be utilized, the patient's deeper tissue zones are usually treated first, followed by treatment of more superficial tissue levels. In areas with relatively thin skin, the more superficial transducers should be utilized. It is thought that by layering multiple different levels of treatment, greater clinical efficacy can be achieved. However, as the technology is relatively new, exact treatment protocols and parameters continue to evolve.

As noted earlier, in clinical studies, patients have reported relatively high pain scores during the procedure. As a result, topical anesthesia alone is not sufficient for many patients to tolerate the procedure, particularly with the lower frequency, more deeply penetrating handpieces. Multiple pain reduction techniques have been reported in the literature to diminish the discomfort of MIFU devices, including nerve blocks and local anesthesia, nonsteroidal anti-inflammatory agents, oral anxiolytics, oral/intramuscular/intravenous narcotics, and conscious sedation. Their use depends upon the office facility and the physician's comfort level with these techniques. More recently, less aggressive treatment regimens have been employed that generate less pain.

PATIENT EDUCATION AND ADVERSE EVENTS

Patients should be advised that MIFU is most effective in patients with mild-to-moderate skin laxity. More severe cases should be referred for excisional procedures.

Following MIFU treatment, patients typically notice erythema and edema, which may last several days. Skin tenderness in the treatment area may last for several weeks following the procedure. More significant side effects including nodule formation and motor nerve paresthesias have also been reported; these appear to be temporary, but can last 2 to 6 weeks. Motor nerve paresthesias seem to occur more commonly in "danger areas" where the motor nerves are relatively superficial; the nerves at greatest risk appear to be the temporal branch of CNV (trigeminal nerve) and the marginal mandibular branch of CNVII.[27]

CONCLUSIONS

Noninvasive skin tightening is a rapidly expanding area of cosmetic rejuvenation, particularly as patients are increasingly eschewing invasive surgical procedures. Patients can safely and effectively achieve collagen tightening, remodeling, and contraction with noninvasive treatments. These procedures typically result in mild-to-moderate skin tightening, although at times improvement can be difficult to discern. Many patients with severe volume loss, jowling, and substantial excess skin may not be ideal candidates for these noninvasive procedures. It is, therefore, extremely important to educate patients with severe lax skin and volume loss that a traditional facelift, abdominoplasty or other surgical intervention may be a better option. As a result, patient selection is a critical component in achieving satisfaction following noninvasive skin tightening. Ideal candidates are typically patients with mild-to-moderate skin laxity, no significant facial volume loss, and realistic outcome expectations.

In recent years, multiple new skin tightening technologies have evolved, initially consisting of infrared lasers and more recently including RF devices and focused ultrasound technologies. All of these technologies similarly target collagen for focused heating, remodeling of existing collagen and stimulation of neocollagenesis. As a result, multiple different options and devices are available to help patients achieve their skin rejuvenation goals. Unfortunately, to date, head-to-head studies comparing these different technologies are lacking; as a result, it is difficult to state objectively which technology or device, if any, is most efficacious. It is therefore up to the individual provider to determine which technology best fits their practice as well as the needs of their patients. With proper patient selection and education as to realistic expectations, patients can achieve satisfactory skin tightening and rejuvenation with any of these noninvasive technologies.

REFERENCES

1. Zelickson BD, Kist D, Bernstein E, et al. Histological and ultrastructural evaluation of the effects of a radiofrequency-based nonablative dermal remodeling device: a pilot study. *Arch Dermatol.* 2004;140(2):204–209.
2. Akeson WH. Application of the Arrhenius equation to rat tail tendon collagen. *Nature.* 1963;199:185–186.
3. Dierickx CC. The role of deep heating for noninvasive skin rejuvenation. *Lasers Surg Med.* 2006;38(9):799–807.
4. Anderson RR, Parrish JA. Selective photothermolysis: precise microsurgery by selective absorption of pulsed radiation. *Science.* 1983;220(4596):524–527.
5. Koch RJ, Cheng ET. Quantification of skin elasticity changes associated with pulsed carbon dioxide laser skin resurfacing. *Arch Facial Plast Surg.* 1999;1(4):272–275.
6. Fitzpatrick RE, Rostan EF, Marchell N. Collagen tightening induced by carbon dioxide laser versus erbium: YAG laser. *Lasers Surg Med.* 2000;27(5):395–403.
7. Hunzeker CM, Weiss ET, Geronemus RG. Fractionated CO2 laser resurfacing: our experience with more than 2000 treatments. *Aesthet Surg J.* 2009;29(4):317–322.
8. Chan HH, Lam LK, Wong DS, Kono T, Trendell-Smith N. Use of 1320 nm Nd:YAG laser for wrinkle reduction and the treatment of atrophic acne scarring in Asians. *Lasers Surg Med.* 2004;34(2):98–103.
9. Tanzi EL, Williams CM, Alster TS. Treatment of facial rhytides with a nonablative 1450-nm diode laser: a controlled clinical and histologic study. *Dermatol Surg.* 2003;29(2):124–128.
10. Nouri K, Zhang YP, Singer L, et al. Effect of the 1450 nm diode non-ablative laser on collagen expression in an artificial skin model. *Lasers Surg Med.* 2005;37(1):97–102.
11. Carniol PJ, Dzopa N, Fernandes N, Fernandes N, Carniol ET, Renzi AS. Facial skin tightening with an 1100–1800 nm infrared device. *J Cosmet Laser Ther.* 2008;10(2):67–71.
12. Chan HH, Yu CS, Shek S, Yeung CK, Kono T, Wei WI. A prospective, split face, single-blinded study looking at the use of an infrared device with contact cooling in the treatment of skin laxity in Asians. *Lasers Surg Med.* 2008;40(2):146–152.
13. Dainichi T, Kawaguchi A, Ueda S, et al. Skin tightening effect using fractional laser treatment: I. A randomized half-side pilot study on faces of patients with acne. *Dermatol Surg.* 2010;36(1):66–70.
14. Wanner M, Tanzi EL, Alster TS. Fractional photothermolysis: treatment of facial and nonfacial cutaneous photodamage with a 1550-nm erbium-doped fiber laser. *Dermatol Surg.* 2007;33(1):23–28.
15. Geronemus RG. Fractional photothermolysis: current and future applications. *Lasers Surg Med.* 2006;38(3):169–176.
16. Weiss RA. Noninvasive radio frequency for skin tightening and body contouring. *Semin Cutan Med Surg.* 2013;32(1):9–17.
17. Fritz M, Counters JT, Zelickson BD. Radiofrequency treatment for middle and lower face laxity. *Arch Facial Plast Surg.* 2004;6(6):370–373.
18. Alster TS, Tanzi E. Improvement of neck and cheek laxity with a nonablative radiofrequency device: a lifting experience. *Dermatol Surg.* 2004;30(4 Pt 1):503–507.
19. Fitzpatrick R, Geronemus R, Goldberg D, Kaminer M, Kilmer S, Ruiz-Esparza J. Multicenter study of noninvasive radiofrequency for periorbital tissue tightening. *Lasers Surg Med.* 2003;33(4):232–242.
20. Taub AF, Tucker RD, Palange A. Facial tightening with an advanced 4-MHz monopolar radiofrequency device. *J Drugs Dermatol.* 2012;11(11):1288–1294.
21. Kassim AT, Goldberg DJ. Assessment of the safety and efficacy of a bipolar multi-frequency radiofrequency device in the treatment of skin laxity. *J Cosmet Laser Ther.* 2013;15(2):114–117.
22. Elman M, Harth Y. Novel multi-source phase-controlled radiofrequency technology for non-ablative and micro-ablative treatment of wrinkles, lax skin and acne scars. *Laser Ther.* 2011;20(2):139–144.
23. Mayoral FA, Vega JM. Multiple facial burns with the new thermage CPT system. *J Drugs Dermatol.* 2011;10(11):1320–1321.
24. Alam M, White LE, Martin N, Witherspoon J, Yoo S, West DP. Ultrasound tightening of facial and neck skin: a rater-blinded prospective cohort study. *J Am Acad Dermatol.* 2010;62(2):262–269.
25. Lee HS, Jang WS, Cha YJ, et al. Multiple pass ultrasound tightening of skin laxity of the lower face and neck. *Dermatol Surg.* 2012;38(1):20–27.
26. Fabi SG, Massaki A, Eimpunth S, Eimpunth S, Pogoda J, Goldman MP. Evaluation of microfocused ultrasound with visualization for lifting, tightening, and wrinkle reduction of the décolletage. *J Am Acad Dermatol.* 2013;69(6):965–971.
27. Alster TS, Tanzi EL. Noninvasive lifting of arm, thigh, and knee skin with transcutaneous intense focused ultrasound. *Dermatol Surg.* 2012;38(5):754–759.

CHAPTER 35

Ablative and Fractional Ablative Resurfacing

Arisa E. Ortiz, Mitchel P. Goldman, & Richard E. Fitzpatrick

INTRODUCTION

Laser resurfacing began in the 1980s with fully ablative (confluent) skin resurfacing to address cosmetic concerns of aging skin. Chronologic aging contributes to deteriorating skin texture and tone. This process is exacerbated by years of ultraviolet light exposure leading to photodamage in the form of lentigines, rhytides, texture irregularity, and telangiectasia. Traditional resurfacing was first performed with a 10,600 nm carbon dioxide (CO_2) laser and later evolved with the 2940 nm erbium-doped yttrium aluminum garnet (Er:YAG) laser either as a short pulse after CO_2 laser or alone as a long-pulsed Er:YAG laser.

CO_2 laser resurfacing is based on the theory of selective photothermolysis.[1,2] Briefly, selective photothermolysis allows for the selective targeting of a chromophore by choosing a specific wavelength and appropriate pulse duration for that chromophore. The 10,600 nm wavelength specifically targets water as the primary chromophore to completely ablate the epidermis and the superficial dermis. A fluence of 5 J/cm^2 has been determined to be necessary to vaporize epidermal cells. The delivered energy must be within the thermal reaction time of the target, which is less than 1 ms for epidermal cells. The re-epithelialized skin has a more youthful appearance with improved texture and tone. For decades, fully ablative CO_2 lasers were considered the gold standard in skin resurfacing for rhytides, photodamage, and scars.[3–5] The results seen with traditional resurfacing are predictable and successful, but coincide with a risk of scarring, dyspigmentation, and prolonged downtime dependent on the extent of nonspecific thermally damaged tissue remaining after tissue vaporization. As a result, alternative approaches to circumvent the side-effect profile of traditional CO_2 and Er:YAG lasers were developed.

The nonablative laser-resurfacing devices that appeared on the market were initially met with great enthusiasm, but quickly fell out of favor due to marginal clinical improvement.[6,7] Nonablative technology was significantly advanced in 2004 with the introduction of fractional photothermolysis.[8] In fractional photothermolysis, the laser beam is pixilated, delivering the energy to only a specific fraction of the epidermal and dermal architecture. The undamaged intervening areas of skin allow for more rapid healing and an improved side-effect profile. The first laser to employ this technology was a 1550 nm erbium-doped fiber laser. Although fractional nonablative devices showed more improvement than traditional nonablative devices, the results were still less impressive compared to ablative resurfacing and required a series of treatments.[9] This led to the development of fractional ablative devices. Fractional ablative resurfacing produces significantly better clinical results than those seen with nonablative technologies and approaches but does not achieve the results seen with fully ablative resurfacing. Significant clinical improvement, along with decreased downtime and an enhanced safety profile, has advanced the adoption of fractional ablative lasers. This chapter will review the indications, patient selection, perioperative management and anesthesia, and complications for traditional ablative and fractional ablative lasers.

ABLATIVE LASERS

TECHNOLOGY

Traditional ablative resurfacing began in the 1980s with the 10,600 nm CO_2 laser. The 10,600 nm wavelength is in the far-infrared electromagnetic spectrum. The specific chromophore at this wavelength is water. Therefore, CO_2 lasers are able to ablate the skin without regard for the presence of melanin or hemoglobin. In order to achieve successful ablation of the skin, without the risk of scarring, the extent of nonspecific thermal damage should be limited to about 100 to 150 μm. This may be achieved with a CO_2 laser fluence above the vaporization threshold of the skin (5 J/cm^2) and a pulse duration shorter than the thermal relaxation time of the skin (1 ms).[10–12] Fluences below the vaporization threshold will only achieve coagulation and longer pulse durations result in an increased risk of scarring.

The advent of short-pulsed high-power CO_2 lasers and lower energy rapidly scanning continuous-wave CO_2 lasers significantly reduced the risks seen with the previous generation of continuous-wave CO_2 laser devices. The short-pulsed, high-power CO_2 laser can deliver 500 mJ in 600 μs to 1 ms, resulting in 5 J/cm^2.[13] This fluence can be achieved with either a 3 mm spot or a computerized pattern generator that rapidly and precisely places several 2.25 mm spots in different patterns. Rapidly scanning continuous-wave CO_2 lasers use optomechanical flash scanners connected to conventional continuous-wave CO_2 lasers to focus small-diameter beams that distribute the energy into a train of pulses with a dwell time less than 1 ms, mimicking a truly pulsed laser. Few systems employ this technology currently, as more technical expertise is required than with shuttered pulse lasers, which raises safety concerns.

Further progression in ablative technology led to the 2940 nm Er:YAG laser. The 2940 nm wavelength is better absorbed by water due to its closer approximation to water's peak absorption at 2935 nm. This allows for more precise ablation compared to the CO_2 laser. At the same time, the increased absorption by water limits its depth of penetration to only 1 to 3 μm per J/cm^2 and results

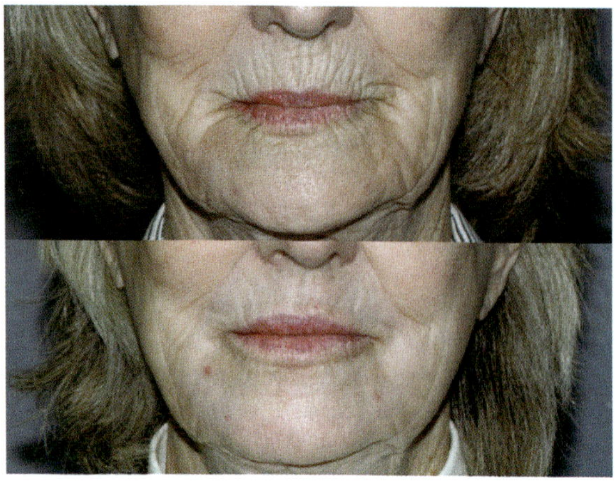

Figure 35-1 A patient with deep static perioral rhytides at baseline (*top*). Dramatic improvement of perioral lines after CO_2 laser resurfacing (*bottom*). (Photographs used with permission of Richard E. Fitzpatrick, MD.)

in more bleeding from decreased thermal coagulation of blood vessels when pulses less than 500 ms are used.

Comparative studies between CO_2 lasers and short-pulsed (500 ms) Er:YAG lasers tend to favor the CO_2 laser for skin resurfacing. However, the results are often very similar when the Er:YAG is pulsed in the 6 to 10 ms range as these lasers can then produce an area of nonspecific thermal damage similar to that achieved with CO_2 ablation.[14,15]

INDICATIONS

The primary indication for ablative laser resurfacing is photoaging. This includes static rhytides, texture irregularity, telangiectasia, and lentigines. Other indications include scarring, actinic cheilitis, actinic keratoses, seborrheic keratoses, benign epidermal lesions (verrucae, sebaceous hyperplasia, epidermal nevi, and the like) and rhinophyma.

With the introduction of fractional ablation, confluent full-surface ablation has fallen out of favor due to its prolonged downtime and high-risk safety profile. However, there is still a role for traditional ablation when treating deep static periorbital and perioral rhytides (Fig. 35-1), as well as benign epidermal lesions and rhinophyma (Fig. 35-2), which are particularly difficult to improve with fractional devices. Precancerous lesions and superficial skin cancers are also more effectively treated with confluent ablation, as fractional ablation theoretically should only treat a fraction of the lesion.

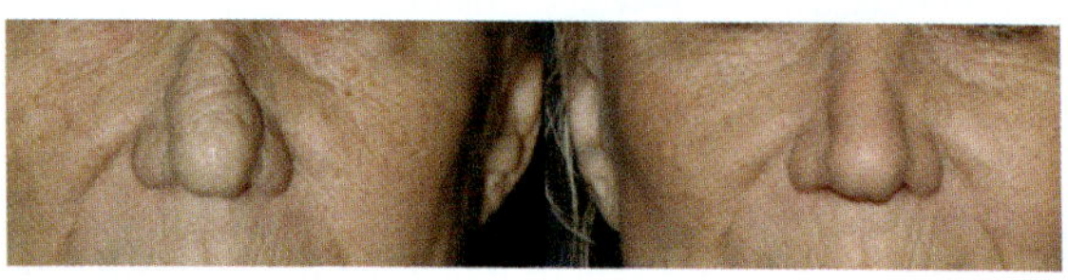

Figure 35-2 A patient with moderate rhinophyma at baseline (left). Result after traditional resurfacing (right). (Photographs used with permission of Richard E. Fitzpatrick, MD.)

PATIENT SELECTION

It is essential to thoroughly evaluate patients prior to initiation of treatment. Ideal patients have realistic expectations of cosmetic outcomes and a clear understanding of the amount of downtime required. Patients must also understand the side effects associated with traditional confluent full-surface ablation. Patients with Fitzpatrick skin types I through III have the highest incidence of hypopigmentation following full-surface and even fractional ablation because they have the least active and least dense concentrations of melanocytes. Although skin types IV through VI may develop relative hypopigmentation, they are at a much greater risk of significant postinflammatory hyperpigmentation (PIH). Traditional ablation is not advised in darker-skinned patients unless the physician is extremely well versed in lasers and wound healing.

A complete medical history is very important for the selection of appropriate patients. Patients with a history of keloids should be treated with caution, as laser resurfacing may trigger keloid formation. Recent or concurrent isotretinoin use during laser procedures is a relative contraindication, as scarring has been reported from laser procedures, dermabrasion, and chemical peeling in association with isotretinoin.[16,17] Although collagen synthesis and wound healing has been shown to be unaffected by isotretinoin,[18] it is still prudent to avoid elective laser procedures after recent isotretinoin use. The exact washout time for isotretinoin has not been determined, but 6 months seems to be sufficient. Likewise, patients with dermatologic diseases that koebnerize, such as vitiligo or psoriasis, should be discouraged from elective procedures that may worsen their condition.

Areas with few adnexal structures, such as the neck, chest, and hands, should not be treated because of their greater risk of scarring. Areas that have been previously irradiated have the same risk of scarring due to the loss of adnexal structures.

PERIOPERATIVE MANAGEMENT AND ANESTHESIA

This section will briefly describe the appropriate management of patients undergoing traditional ablation. A more exhaustive discussion will follow in the fractional ablative section, since there is great overlap between the two techniques.

Prophylaxis with antiviral agents and antibiotics is generally recommended to prevent herpes simplex outbreaks and secondary bacterial infections.[19] Antifungal and antiyeast medications may also be prescribed, but are not the standard of care.[20]

Several options exist for anesthesia, including a combination of topical agents, local infiltration, nerve blocks, and systemic tranquilizing and analgesic agents. The CO_2 lasers tend to be more painful than the short-pulsed Er:YAG lasers, whereas long-pulsed Er:YAG lasers are associated with similar pain levels. This is thought to be from greater tissue heating of type C pain fibers.

Postoperative management of edema may include the use of a short course of oral or intramuscular corticosteroids, but we recommend against this practice in general as it may increase the risk of postoperative infection or suppression of neocollagenesis. The care of exudate and skin sloughing includes saline, deionized water, or diluted white vinegar soaks, cool compresses, head elevation, and the use of petrolatum ointment. Erythema may persist for several months. Therefore, the need for sun avoidance and protection should be emphasized to reduce the risk of PIH.[21,22]

COMPLICATIONS

The most notable complications of confluent laser ablation are scarring and delayed-onset hypopigmentation. Delayed-onset hypopigmentation presents 6 to 12 months after the procedure. It is estimated that over 50% of patients have this complication.[23] However, we rarely see this complication when using conservative settings and limiting nonspecific thermal damage. Hypopigmentation tends to occur from deeper ablation, while superficial ablation generally results in hyperpigmentation. Scarring generally occurs from too much thermal necrosis/nonspecific thermal damage, excessively deep ablation, or wound infection that extends the depth of injury beyond that which was intended. Some areas are particularly prone to scarring, most notably areas of very thin skin such as the eyelids, neck, and chest. The neck is particularly at risk and should not be treated with confluent full-surface resurfacing, as even a single pass produced a 10% incidence of scarring in a small pilot study.[24] Other complications including infection, acneiform eruptions, and eczematous dermatitis are generally self-limited and resolve with proper care.

FRACTIONAL ABLATIVE LASERS

TECHNOLOGY

Fractional ablative technology has revolutionized the field of laser resurfacing due to its significantly improved safety profile, reduced healing time, and effective results. Fractional devices deliver columns of thermal injury, termed microthermal zones (MTZs) (includes areas of ablation and coagulation), while the surrounding skin remains untreated. Unaffected follicular units and their stem cells, as well as fibroblasts, aid in the healing process. This leads to a decreased healing time and a lower incidence of adverse outcomes.

The most significant variables that determine clinical efficacy and wound healing include the percentage of surface area treated (density), the diameter of the MTZs, and the depth of ablation. No studies to date have examined the effect of the ratio of ablation to coagulation within the MTZs. For example, the volume of injury might be similar, but if the volumes contain different ratios of ablation to coagulation, wound healing and cosmetic outcomes may be affected. Greater proportions of ablation seem to improve cosmetic outcome, while greater proportions of coagulation prolong healing time if excessive, but may be important in achieving tightening of treated skin. The optimal ratio of ablation:coagulation has yet to be elucidated. It is important to note that some manufacturers include surrounding coagulative necrosis in the density calculation, whereas other manufacturers only account for the zone of ablation.

Maximum ablation depths have been reported to extend over 1.5 mm into the dermis at higher energies (70 mJ).[25–27] Re-epithelialization occurs within 2 days, but collagen remodeling persists 3 months post procedure consistent with the presence of heat shock protein (HSP) 47 found on histology.[25] Initially, neocollagenesis is confined to the healing columns of ablation, and then becomes generalized throughout the dermis approximately 1 month post procedure.

There are currently three commercially available wavelengths that employ fractional ablative technology: 2790 nm erbium-doped:ytrrium-scandium-gallium-garnet laser (Er:YSGG); 2940 nm Er:YAG; and 10,600 nm CO_2 laser. By adjusting laser parameters, the different wavelengths may be able to produce essentially comparable results. Several fractional ablative devices are available with various treatment hand pieces, depth of ablation and coagulation, spot size, and shape (Table 35-1). Hand pieces can either deliver energy via a rolling or stamping mechanism.

INDICATIONS

The applications for fractionated devices are increasing rapidly. Although initial studies were directed toward reversal of photoaging, fractionated lasers are currently being used in many capacities.

Fractional deep dermal ablation has been shown to improve dyspigmentation, telangiectasia, and rhytides.[28] Specifically, fractional ablative resurfacing can significantly improve lentigines, seborrheic keratoses, actinic keratoses, telangiectasia, rhytides, textural irregularity, and skin laxity to some degree (Figs. 35-3 and 35-4). Although fractional lasers can achieve results that approach those of traditional resurfacing, they are not able to sustain the same level of improvement in wrinkle reduction. With time, the improvement in rhytides seen with fractional resurfacing seems to retrogress.[29] The same appears to be true with reduction of dyschromia. However, it has been shown to be safe to combine multiple lasers in the same treatment session with fractional ablative lasers resulting in more significant and longer lasting improvement. Our approach is to treat vascular lesions first with a vascular specific laser, such as the 595 nm pulsed dye laser or an Intense Pulsed Light device. Next, discrete brown spots (lentigines, seborrheic keratoses) are treated with a Q-switched (QS) laser (alexandrite or ruby) and/or an Intense Pulsed Light device insuring 100% coverage of the epidermal surface. Then, the pulsed CO_2 laser is used to treat upper and lower lip lines, followed by precise sculpting with a pulsed Er:YAG laser. Finally, the entire face, and at times the neck and chest, are treated with fractional CO_2. Alternatively, the Intense Pulsed Light device is utilized to treat the neck and chest. This treatment sequence is not provided to suggest that everyone can treat their patients as aggressively, but rather to demonstrate the compatibility of sequential multilaser treatments with fractional laser delivery. In fact, the greatest advantage of fractional lasers is their lower risk of complications such as infection and delayed long-term hypopigmentation combined with faster healing times.[30] There is also a decreased risk of scarring, especially away from the face. Prior to fractional technology, confluent resurfacing of the neck

TABLE 35-1
Currently Available Ablative Resurfacing devices.

Manufacturer/ Device	Type/Wavelength	Energy Output	Pulse Duration	Comments
Alma Lasers Harmony^{XL} platform Pixel 2940	Fractional Er:YAG Pixel/2940 nm	200–2500 mJ/P		Three tip options: 7 × 7 mm, 9 × 9 mm, 1 × 7 mm
Alma Lasers Harmony^{XL} platform Pixel CO_2	Fractional CO_2/10,600 nm	70 W	50–1000 μs	Three tip options: 7 × 7 mm, 9 × 9 mm, 1 × 7 mm
Alma Lasers Harmony^{XL} platform Pixel omnifit	Handpiece for CO_2 platforms/10,600 nm	30–100 W	N/A	Fits Coherent, Lumenis, and Sharplan CO_2 lasers
Cutera Xeo pearl fractional	Fractional Er:YSGG/2,790 nm	60–320 mJ/ microspot	600 μs	Deep ablation >1 mm. Real time calibration
Cynosure Smart skin	Fractional CO_2/10,600 nm	30 W	1–20 ms	Variable scanning patterns. Adjustable power, depth of ablation, dwell time, spot pitch, and scan shapes
DEKA SmartXide DOT	Fractional CO_2 scanner/10,600 nm	150 W/250 W	200–2000 μs	Adjustable ablation and dwell time Variable scanning modes
Ellman Elluminé fractionalCO_2 laser system	CO_2 fractional with scanner and flexible fiber/10,600 nm	Up to 105 mJ	2–7 ms	Adjustable scan density and pulse duration
Focus Medical NaturaLase CO_2	Fractional CO_2/10,600 nm	50 W	Up to 10 ms	Pending FDA approval
Hironic Co. MIXEL	Fractional CO_2/10,600 nm	60 mJ	Up to 5,000 μs	Adjustable scan size and beam size
ILOODA Co. Fraxis	Fractional CO_2/10,600 nm	Up to 30 W	0.1–5 ms	Fast scanning mode
LASERING MiXto SX	Fractional CO_2/10,600 nm	0.5–30 W	2.5–16 ms	Variable spot sizes with focusing handpieces
Lumenis UltraPulse active FX	Fractional CO_2/10,600 nm	1–225 mJ	<1 ms	CoolScan handpiece
Lumenis UltraPulse deep FX	Fractional CO_2/10,600 nm	2.5–50 mJ	<2 ms	120 μm spot size scanning handpiece with penetration depth up to 2 mm
Lumenis UltraPulse total FX	Fractional CO_2/10,600 nm	1–225 mJ	<2 ms	Combination of active/deep Fx
Lumenis Ultrapulse SCAAR FX	Fractional CO_2/10,600 nm	2.5–150 mJ	<2 ms	Increased depth of ablation to treat thicker scars
Lumenis AcuPulse multimode	Fractional CO_2/10,600 nm	1–170 mJ	<2 ms	
Lutronic eCO_2	Fractional CO_2/10,600 nm	Up to 240 mJ	Variable	Multiple tip sizes and shapes. Handpiece available for continuous wave
Palomar Starlux 500 platform Lux 2940 fractional	Fractional 2,940 nm	2–5.5 mJ/ 0.1 mm	0.25–5 ms	IPL platform with multiple handpieces for different applications
Sandstone Medical Technologies Matrix LS-40 with Ultrafine-FS fractional scanner	Fractional scanner (adapts to most CO_2 lasers CO_2)/10,600 nm	N/A	N/A	Fractional scanner with 150 mm focusing handpiece
Sandstone Medical Technologies Cortex resurfacing work station	CO_2 and Er:YAG/10,600 and 2,940 nm	Up to 40 W	Adjustable to 100 ms	Fractional CO_2 combined with Er:YAG and fractionated Erbium

TABLE 35-1 (*Continued*)

Manufacturer/ Device	Type/wavelength	Energy Output	Pulse Duration	Comments
Sciton Joule/ProFractional	Er:YAG/2,940 nm	Up to 400 J/cm^2	Variable	20- × 20 mm scanner with 250 μm spot size
Solta Medical Fraxel DUAL	1927 Thulium fiber laser/1927 nm	Up to 20 mJ/ MTZ	N/A	Intelligent Optical Tracking System (IOTS), adjusts to hand speed to provide uniform delivery of laser energy
Solta Medical Fraxel Re:Pair	Fractional CO_2 laser/10,600 nm	5–70 mJ/MTZ	N/A	Integrated smoke evacuation system. Also with IOTS
Syneron and Candela CO_2 RE	Fractional CO_2/ 10,600 nm	60 W	30–60 mJ 60–90 mJ 50–80 mJ 60–70 mJ 1–10 mJ	Multiple patterns allow for simultaneous superficial/deep treatment

and chest with CO_2 and Er:YAG lasers was a forbidden territory, with the exception of very conservative, superficial treatment.[31]

Another key indication for ablative fractional resurfacing is the treatment of scars. Interestingly, fractional resurfacing has exhibited the ability to improve both atrophic and hypertrophic scars.[26] Anecdotally, scarring seems to respond to lower density (<35%) and higher depth (>500 μm) treatment settings. No study to date has confirmed this belief.

Acne scarring, in particular, presents a treatment challenge to the laser surgeon and causes great psychological distress in the patient. Small box-car scars and rolling scars tend to respond well to ablative fractional lasers. In general, rolling scars will predictably respond well if the scar flattens and disappears with stretching of the scar between the fingers. Ice-pick scars, or scars that do not respond well to laser treatment alone, may require additional interventions such as subcision, punch excisions, fillers, or the trichloroacetic acid (TCA) chemical reconstruction of skin scars (CROSS) technique. The first study on fractional CO_2 laser resurfacing of acne scars showed clinical improvement of scarring in 23 out of 25 patients after 3 months.[32] Subjects received one to three treatments 1 month apart with treatment energies ranging from 20 to 100 mJ and total densities of 600 to 1600 MTZ/cm^2. No serious complications were noted. Patients had the added benefit of improvement in their overall appearance, including dyspigmentation and rhytides. Even patients with darker skin types can be safely treated for scarring with fractional ablative lasers given the decreased risk of PIH compared to confluent ablation (Fig. 35-5).

Surgical and traumatic scars have also shown promising results with ablative fractional technology (Fig. 35-6). Not only is there cosmetic improvement, but fractional ablative lasers have also produced functional improvement in pliability and increased range of motion.[33] The improvement in range of motion is almost instantaneous in certain cases. The mechanism by which this may occur is unclear,

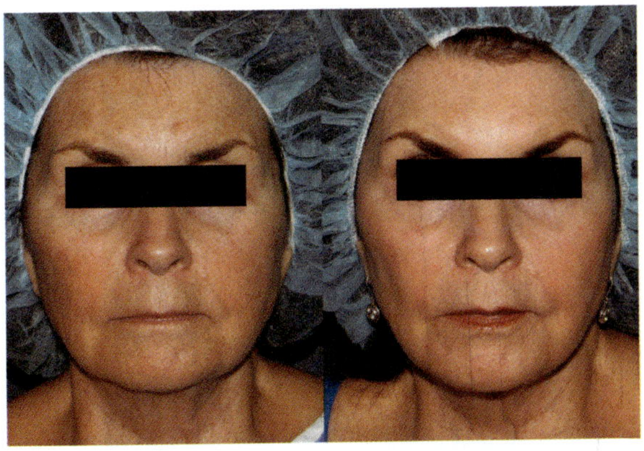

Figure 35-3 Seventy-three-year-old female with severe photodamage, static rhytides, and facial laxity prior to treatment (*left*). Four months after one fractional CO_2 laser treatment. Note improvement in lentigines, fine lines and jowl laxity (*right*). (Photographs used with permission of Mitchel P. Goldman, MD.)

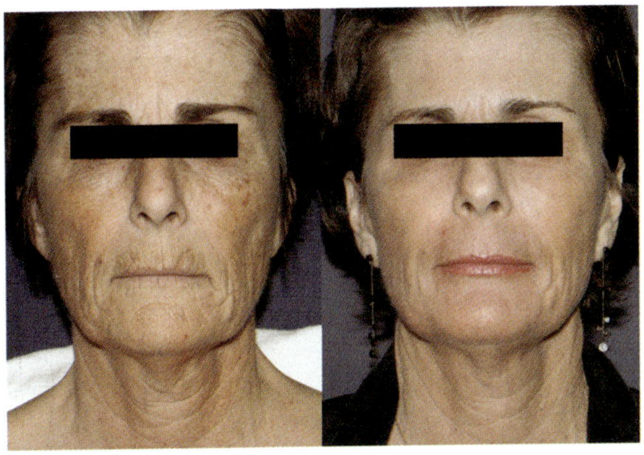

Figure 35-4 A female patient with severe dyspigmentation and static rhytides at baseline (*left*). Note almost complete resolution of lentigines and significant improvement in rhytides, particularly in the perioral region, after fractional CO_2 laser treatment (*right*). (Photographs used with permission of Richard E. Fitzpatrick, MD.)

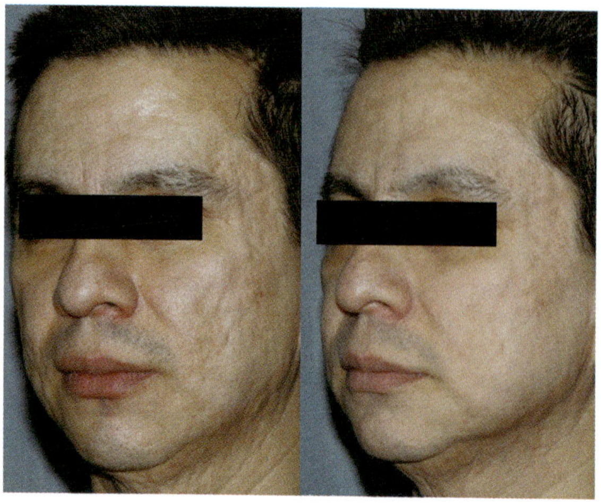

Figure 35-5 A male patient with skin type IV with severe atrophic acne scarring prior to treatment (*left*). Significant improvement in acne scars with no evidence of postinflammatory hyperpigmentation (*right*). (Photographs used with permission of Richard E. Fitzpatrick, MD.)

but appears to be due to the physical removal of a fraction of the scar tissue. Over time, the abnormal scar tissue is replaced by type III nascent collagen, which may also play a role in long-term improvement of function and cosmesis.

A newer indication for fractional ablation is tattoo removal. Traditionally, tattoo removal has been accomplished using QS and/or picosecond lasers. The addition of ablative fractional lasers after treatment with QS lasers may enhance tattoo removal by physically ablating some of the pigment while also allowing transepidermal extrusion of pigment through ablated channels. In the case of an allergic reaction to tattoo pigment, use of an ablative CO_2 laser may be considered instead of QS and/or picosecond lasers to prevent any systemic effects from release of tattoo ink into the blood stream.[34] This technique may prove to be an alternative paradigm for tattoo inks that are difficult to treat with currently available QS and picosecond lasers.

When used in conjunction with QS and picosecond lasers, the fractional ablative lasers provide another mechanism of pigment removal and are much less likely to cause hypopigmentation, as they are not targeting melanin and encourage melanocyte migration with wound healing. Another advantage is that the fractional ablative laser will treat any scarring associated with the QS laser.

There are numerous other promising applications for fractional ablative lasers, such as treatment of syringomas,[35] striae,[36] rhinophyma,[37] actinic cheilitis, regressed infantile hemangiomas, and repigmentation of delayed-onset hypopigmentation following confluent ablation.[26] Repigmentation may occur via the renewed stimulation of melanocytes, but this has yet to be investigated. The use of fractional ablative lasers for the treatment of premalignant and malignant lesions is limited by design as less than 100% of the skin surface is treated. A more promising approach to skin cancer therapy is the use of fractional ablative devices for enhanced drug delivery of medications such as methyl 5-aminolevulinate (MAL) or 5-aminolevulinate (ALA) for photodynamic therapy.[38] Drug delivery via fractional ablation is an exciting new arena because essentially any drug can be applied. The only potential limitations would be solubility and the molecular size of the drug.

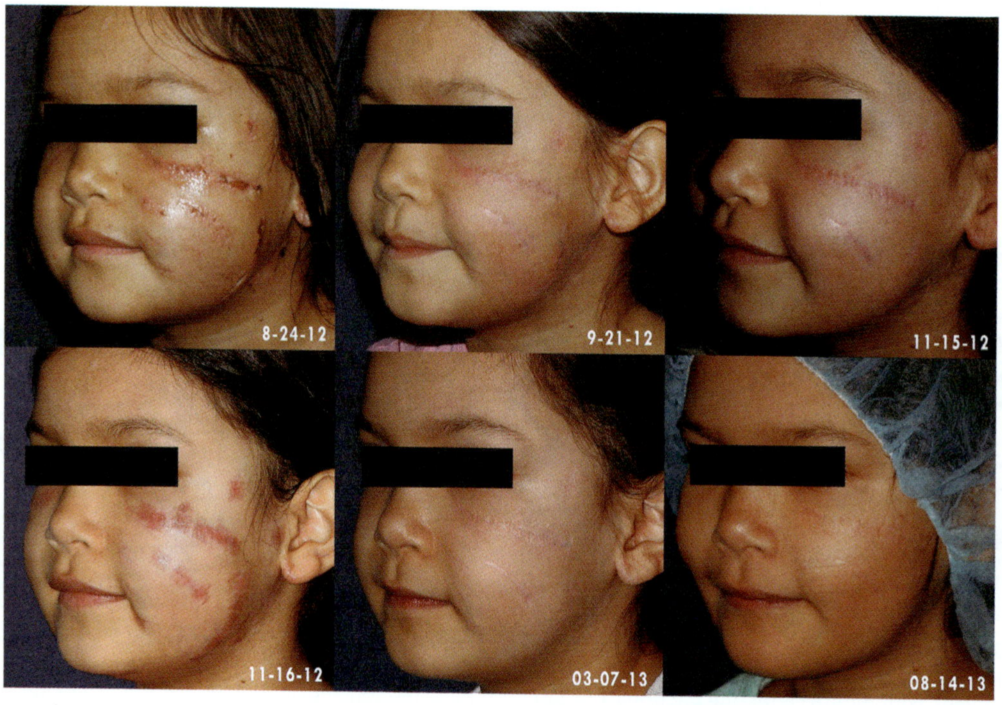

Figure 35-6 A 7 year-old female with traumatic facial scars prior to laser treatment (top left). Progression of improvement after two treatments with fractional CO_2 laser. Significant improvement of scarring 1 year after initial accident (bottom right). (Photographs used with permission of Mitchel P. Goldman, MD.)

PATIENT SELECTION

Appropriate patient selection is key to a successful resurfacing procedure. Evaluation of patients considering fractional ablative procedures is very similar to those seeking fully ablative procedures. However, there is greater flexibility in skin types, ages, and body sites that may be treated with fractional ablative lasers. Unlike traditional ablation, any skin phototype may be treated with fractional ablative lasers. Nevertheless, skin type V to VI should be treated with caution at low-density settings to decrease the risk of pigmentary complications.

PERIOPERATIVE MANAGEMENT AND ANESTHESIA

Standard prophylaxis with antivirals and antibacterials prior to treatment with fractional lasers has not been shown to prevent complications.[30] However, in certain high-risk patients, antiviral and antibiotic prophylaxis may be considered. An antiherpetic agent, such as valcyclovir, is initiated on the day of procedure and continued for about a week. Prophylactic antibiotics are usually penicillins, macrolides, or tetracyclines, such as minocycline, and are administered during the same time frame as the antivirals. We use minocycline because it almost always covers *Staphylococcus* species, as well as normal flora – which are the two most common groups of bacteria isolated from slow-healing wounds. Antifungals, such as fluconazole, may be given for prevention of secondary candidal or fungal infections. However, this is more dependent on the patient's history and is not the standard of care.

Pain is managed with a topical anesthetic agent, such as lidocaine or prilocaine cream, applied 1 hour prior to the procedure. This is not likely to be effective as a single agent unless conservative, minimally aggressive treatment parameters are chosen. Additional pain control can be achieved with supraorbital, infraorbital, nasalis, and mental nerve blocks immediately prior to the procedure. Local infiltration may be necessary in the preauricular area, as well as in other areas not covered by nerve blocks, which tend to be very painful even with the aforementioned techniques. Intramuscular nonsteroidal anti-inflammatory medications or oral antianxiolytics may also be used. Intravenous sedation may help to provide an easier experience for both the laser surgeon and the patient. It is imperative for patients receiving systemic medications that alter mental function to be properly monitored and to have a method of transport prearranged. During the procedure,

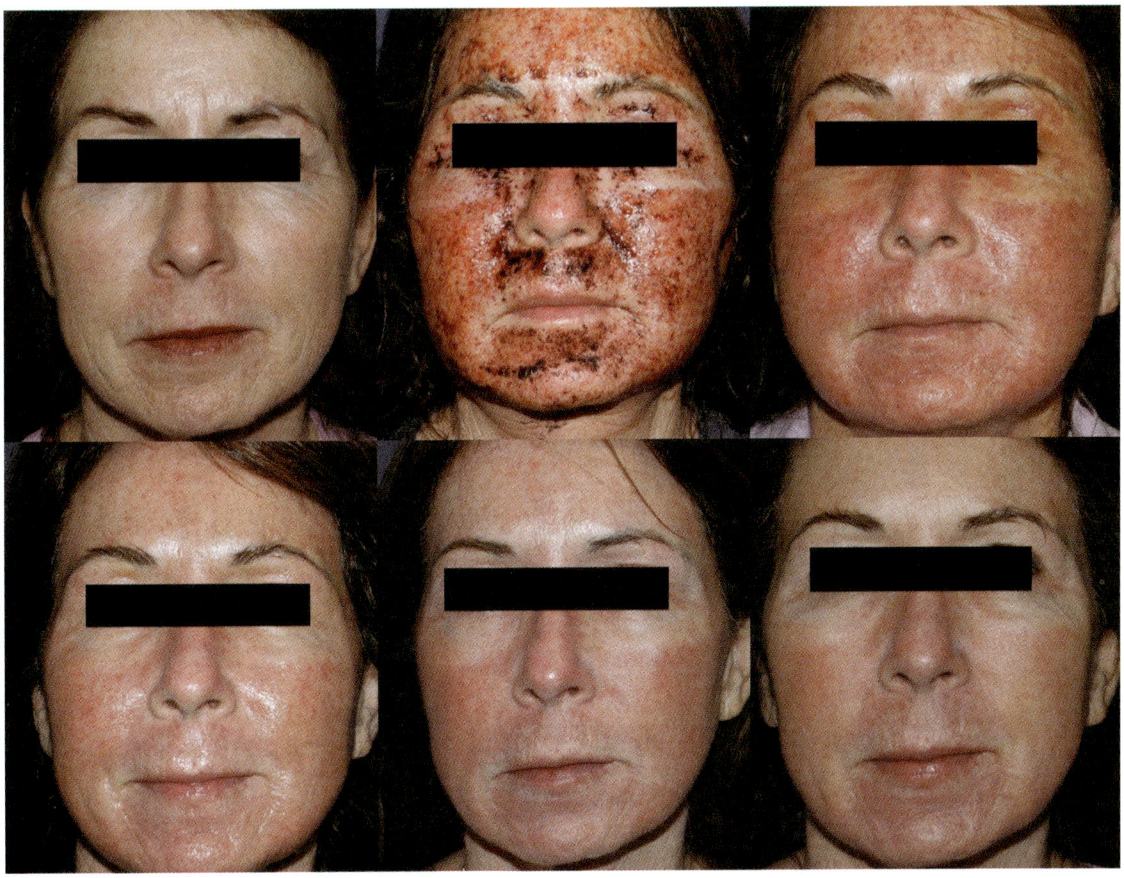

Figure 35-7 Typical progression of healing seen in a patient after fractional CO_2 laser resurfacing. The patient at baseline (*top left*), 1 day after procedure (*top middle*), 4 days after procedure (*top right*), 8 days after procedure (*bottom left*), 3 weeks after procedure (bottom middle), and 4 weeks after procedure (*bottom right*). Note that crusting has resolved by day 4 and that erythema can easily be covered with makeup by 1 week. (Photographs used with permission of Mitchel P. Goldman, MD.)

cold-air cooling can maximize comfort. Postoperative pain is generally minor, reminiscent of a mild sunburn. Thus, any increase in pain after the procedure should prompt an immediate in-office evaluation to rule out infection.

Postoperatively, patients should apply diluted vinegar soaks every few hours followed by application of petrolatum ointment for oozing and crusting, which may last up to 3 days (Fig. 35-7). Sun avoidance and protection is imperative to minimize the risk of PIH.

COMPLICATIONS

The primary advantage of fractional ablative resurfacing over full ablation is an improved safety profile. Most significant is its lower risk of scarring and delayed-onset hypopigmentation. This lower risk of scarring also extends to non-facial areas, such as the neck, chest, back, and extremities, which previously could not be treated with fully ablative lasers, although there have been a few cases of scarring and ectropion reported in the literature.[39–41] Scarring from fractional ablative lasers is almost always a result of improper technique or excessive energy and density settings (Fig. 35-8). It is important to minimize bulk heating by allowing the skin sufficient time to cool between passes. This is especially important when treating smaller anatomic areas. Ironically, the same laser that created the scar may later be used to treat the scar when proper settings are employed.

Infections with cutaneous herpes simplex virus (HSV) are rare, and generally present within the first week after treatment. It is imperative that the person performing the procedure be able to recognize and properly treat HSV infection in order to avoid delayed wound healing and scarring. Patients with active HSV infections on the day of procedure should not be treated to prevent dissemination. Postoperative bacterial infections with *Staphylococcus, Pseudomonas, and Klebsiella* have been reported.[42] Any increase in pain, erythema, erosions or crusting is usually a sign of infection.

Patients with darker skin types should be counseled that they are at high risk for PIH (Fig. 35-9). These patients may benefit from posttreatment with hydroquinone or other bleaching agents. Pretreatment with bleaching agents has not been found to be effective in preventing hyperpigmentation.[43] However, the use of a high-potency topical steroid in an ointment formulation with minimal preservatives and/or stabilizers twice daily for 2 days prior to treatment and 2 days post treatment may be beneficial in decreasing the incidence of PIH by shutting down the inflammatory cascade. Sun avoidance and protection are imperative for several weeks before and after treatment.[44]

Other minor complications may include acne exacerbation or milia formation. Occlusive ointments may play a significant role in the development of these lesions. These medications should, therefore, be discontinued and replaced with a lighter moisturizer after complete re-epithelialization has occurred, usually the third or fourth day after resurfacing. Others feel that thermal injury to the follicular openings and sebaceous gland ducts alters the maturation of the epidermis, resulting in blockage of the gland openings and subsequent milia formation as well as acne flares.

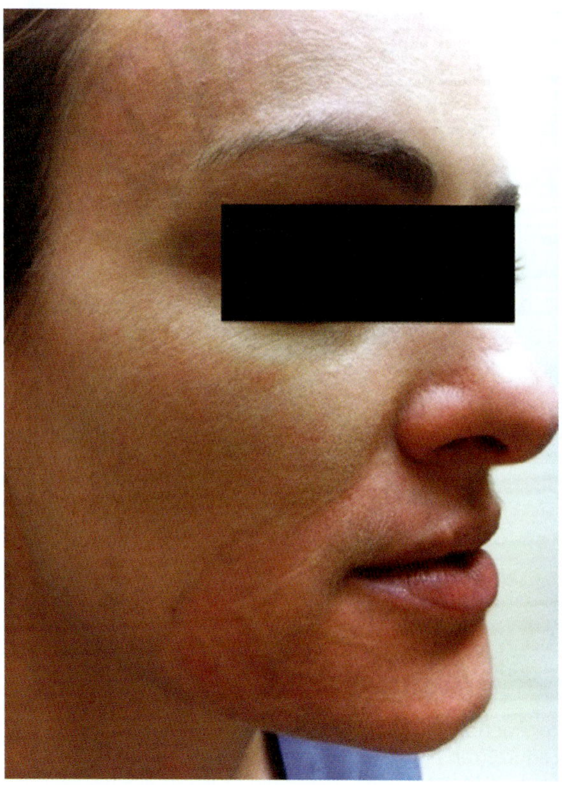

Figure 35-8 Scarring as a result of a fractional CO_2 laser treatment with excessive energy and density settings.

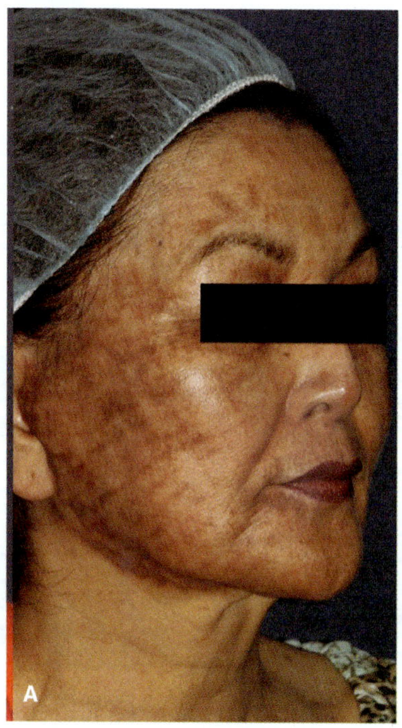

Figure 35-9 A. Postinflammatory hyperpigmentation in a patient with skin type IV after fractional CO_2 laser resurfacing.

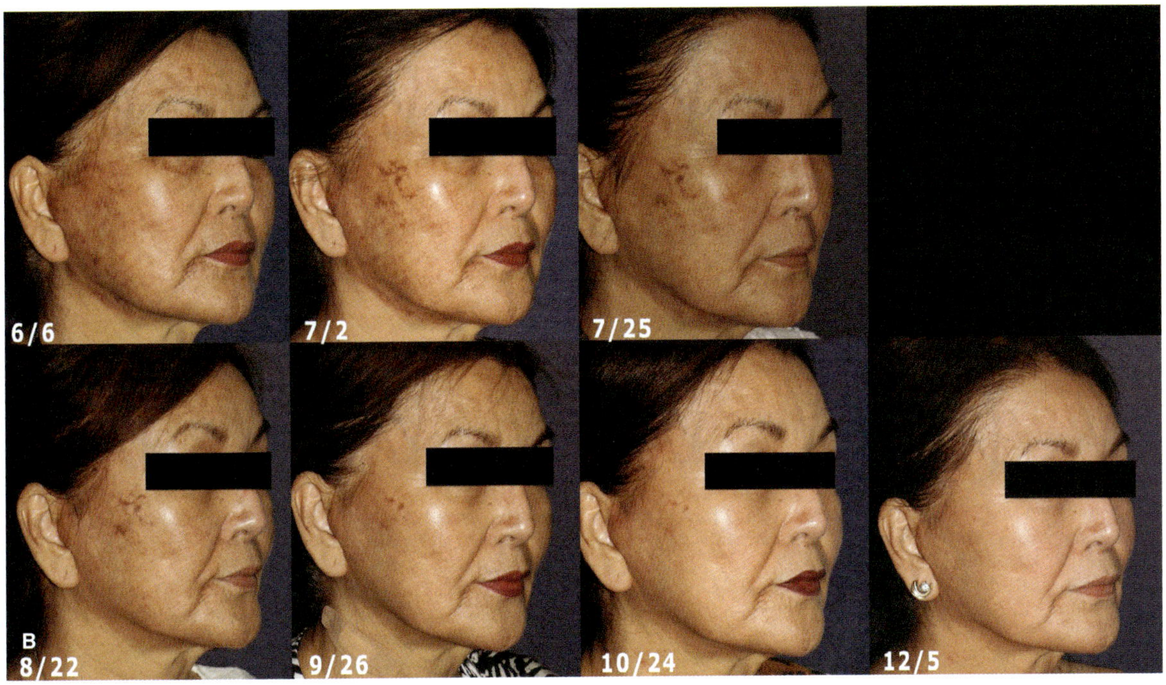

Figure 35-9 *(Continued)* **B.** Progressive improvement in hyperpigmentation after several courses of bleaching agents and intense pulsed light treatments.

CONCLUSION

The field of nonsurgical resurfacing has been transformed with the advent of fractional ablative technology. Despite results that fall short of the results of confluent ablation, fractional ablative technology has gained overwhelming favor over fully ablative procedures due to its more favorable side-effect profile, reduced recovery time, and overall efficacy. These qualities are inspiring the investigation of novel applications for fractional ablation of the skin and perhaps other organs as well.

REFERENCES

1. Anderson RR, Parrish JA. Selective photothermolysis: precise microsurgery by selective absorption of pulsed radiation. *Science*. 1983;220:524–527.
2. Altshuler GB, Anderson RR, Manstein D, Zenzie HH, Smirnov MZ. Extended theory of selective photothermolysis. *Lasers Surg Med*. 2001;29:416–432.
3. Waldorf HA, Kauvar AN, Geronemus RG. Skin resurfacing of fine to deep rhytides using a char-free carbon dioxide laser in 47 patients. *Dermatol Surg*. 1995;21:940–946.
4. Fitzpatrick RE, Goldman MP, Satur NM, Tope WD. Pulsed carbon dioxide laser resurfacing of photo-aged facial skin. *Arch Dermatol*. 1996;132:395–402.
5. Alster TS, West TB. Resurfacing of atrophic facial acne scars with a high-energy, pulsed carbon dioxide laser. *Dermatol Surg*. 1996;22:151–154; discussion 54–55.
6. Paithankar DY, Clifford JM, Saleh BA, Ross EV, Hardaway CA, Barnette D. Subsurface skin renewal by treatment with a 1450-nm laser in combination with dynamic cooling. *J Biomed Opt*. 2003;8:545–551.
7. Goldberg DJ. Non-ablative subsurface remodeling: clinical and histologic evaluation of a 1320-nm Nd:YAG laser. *J Cutan Laser Ther*. 1999;1:153–157.
8. Manstein D, Herron GS, Sink RK, Tanner H, Anderson RR. Fractional photothermolysis: a new concept for cutaneous remodeling using microscopic patterns of thermal injury. *Lasers Surg Med*. 2004;34:426–438.
9. Fisher GJ, Varani J, Voorhees JJ. Looking older: fibroblast collapse and therapeutic implications. *Arch Dermatol*. 2008;144:666–672.
10. Kauvar AN, Waldorf HA, Geronemus RG. A histopathological comparison of "char-free" carbon dioxide lasers. *Dermatol Surg*. 1996;22:343–348.
11. Walsh JT Jr, Flotte TJ, Anderson RR, Deutsch TF. Pulsed CO_2 laser tissue ablation: effect of tissue type and pulse duration on thermal damage. *Lasers Surg Med*. 1988;8:108–118.
12. Green HA, Domankevitz Y, Nishioka NS. Pulsed carbon dioxide laser ablation of burned skin: in vitro and in vivo analysis. *Lasers Surg Med*. 1990;10:476–484.
13. Yang CC, Chai CY. Animal study of skin resurfacing using the ultrapulse carbon dioxide laser. *Ann Plast Surg*. 1995;35:154–158.
14. Goldman MP, Manuskiatti W. Combined laser resurfacing with the 950-microsec pulsed CO_2 + Er:YAG lasers. *Dermatol Surg*. 1999;25:160–163.
15. Rostan EF, Fitzpatrick RE, Goldman MP. Laser resurfacing with a long pulse erbium:YAG laser compared to the 950 ms pulsed CO(2) laser. *Lasers Surg Med*. 2001;29:136–141.
16. Rubenstein R, Roenigk HH Jr, Stegman SJ, Hanke CW. Atypical keloids after dermabrasion of patients taking isotretinoin. *J Am Acad Dermatol*. 1986;15:280–285.
17. Bernestein LJ, Geronemus RG. Keloid formation with the 585-nm pulsed dye laser during isotretinoin treatment. *Arch Dermatol*. 1997;133:111–112.
18. Moy RL, Moy LS, Bennett RG, Zitelli JA, Uitto J. Systemic isotretinoin: effects on dermal wound healing in a rabbit ear model in vivo. *J Dermatol Surg Oncol*. 1990;16:1142–1146.
19. Manuskiatti W, Fitzpatrick RE, Goldman MP, Krejci-Papa N. Prophylactic antibiotics in patients undergoing laser resurfacing of the skin. *J Am Acad Dermatol*. 1999;40:77–84.
20. Conn H, Nanda VS. Prophylactic fluconazole promotes reepithelialization in full-face carbon dioxide laser skin resurfacing. *Lasers Surg Med*. 2000;26:201–207.
21. Goldman MP, Roberts TL 3rd, Skover G, Lettieri JT, Fitzpatrick RE. Optimizing wound healing in the face after laser abrasion. *J Am Acad Dermatol*. 2002;46:399–407.
22. Fitzpatrick RE, Williams B, Goldman MP. Preoperative anesthesia and postoperative considerations in laser resurfacing. *Semin Cutan Med Surg*. 1996;15:170–176.

23. Dijkema SJ, van der Lei B. Long-term results of upper lips treated for rhytides with carbon dioxide laser. *Plast Reconstr Surg.* 2005;115:1731–1735.
24. Fitzpatrick RE, Goldman MP, Sriprachya-Anunt S. Resurfacing of photodamaged skin on the neck with an UltraPulse((R)) carbon dioxide laser. *Lasers Surg Med.* 2001;28:145–149.
25. Hantash BM, Bedi VP, Kapadia B, et al. In vivo histological evaluation of a novel ablative fractional resurfacing device. *Lasers Surg Med.* 2007;39:96–107.
26. Hunzeker CM, Weiss ET, Geronemus RG. Fractionated CO_2 laser resurfacing: our experience with more than 2000 treatments. *Aesthet Surg J.* 2009;29:317–322.
27. Hantash BM, Bedi VP, Chan KF, Zachary CB. Ex vivo histological characterization of a novel ablative fractional resurfacing device. *Lasers Surg Med.* 2007;39:87–95.
28. Rahman Z, MacFalls H, Jiang K, et al. Fractional deep dermal ablation induces tissue tightening. *Lasers Surg Med.* 2009;41:78–86.
29. Ortiz AE, Tremaine AM, Zachary CB. Long-term efficacy of a fractional resurfacing device. *Lasers Surg Med.* 2010;42 :168–170.
30. Campbell TM, Goldman MP. Adverse events of fractionated carbon dioxide laser: review of 373 treatments. *Dermatol Surg.* 2010;36:1645–1650.
31. Fitzpatrick RE. CO_2 laser resurfacing. *Dermatol Clin.* 2001;19: 443–451, viii.
32. Walgrave SE, Ortiz AE, MacFalls HT, et al. Evaluation of a novel fractional resurfacing device for treatment of acne scarring. *Lasers Surg Med.* 2009;41:122–127.
33. Waibel J, Beer K. Ablative fractional laser resurfacing for the treatment of a third-degree burn. *J Drugs Dermatol.* 2009; 8:294–297.
34. Ibrahimi OA, Syed Z, Sakamoto FH, Avram MM, Anderson RR. Treatment of tattoo allergy with ablative fractional resurfacing: a novel paradigm for tattoo removal. *J Am Acad Dermatol.* 2011;64:1111–1114.
35. Cho SB, Kim HJ, Noh S, Lee SJ, Kim YK, Lee JH. Treatment of syringoma using an ablative 10,600-nm carbon dioxide fractional laser: a prospective analysis of 35 patients. *Dermatol Surg.* 2011;37:433–438.
36. Lee SE, Kim JH, Lee SJ, et al. Treatment of striae distensae using an ablative 10600-nm carbon dioxide fractional laser: a retrospective review of 27 participants. *Dermatol Surg.* 2010;36:1683–1690.
37. Serowka KL, Saedi N, Dover JS, Zachary CB. Fractionated ablative carbon dioxide laser for the treatment of rhinophyma. *Lasers Surg Med.* 2014;46(1):8–12.
38. Haedersdal M, Sakamoto FH, Farinelli WA, Doukas AG, Tam J, Anderson RR. Fractional CO(2) laser-assisted drug delivery. *Lasers Surg Med.* 2010;42:113–122.
39. Fife DJ, Fitzpatrick RE, Zachary CB. Complications of fractional CO_2 laser resurfacing: four cases. *Lasers Surg Med.* 2009;41:179–184.
40. Ross RB, Spencer J. Scarring and persistent erythema after fractionated ablative CO_2 laser resurfacing. *J Drugs Dermatol.* 2008;7:1072–1073.
41. Avram MM, Tope WD, Yu T, Szachowicz E, Nelson JS. Hypertrophic scarring of the neck following ablative fractional carbon dioxide laser resurfacing. *Lasers Surg Med.* 2009;41:185–188.
42. Ortiz AE, Tingey C, Yu YE, Ross EV. Topical steroids implicated in postoperative infection following ablative laser resurfacing. *Lasers Surg Med.* 2012;44:1–3.
43. Sriprachya-anunt S, Marchell NL, Fitzpatrick RE, Goldman MP, Rostan EF. Facial resurfacing in patients with Fitzpatrick skin type IV. *Lasers Surg Med.* 2002;30:86–92.
44. Chan HH, Manstein D, Yu CS, Shek S, Kono T, Wei WI. The prevalence and risk factors of post-inflammatory hyperpigmentation after fractional resurfacing in Asians. *Lasers Surg Med.* 2007;39:381–385.

CHAPTER 36

Nonablative Dermal Remodeling

Yoon-Soo Cindy Bae & David J. Goldberg

Although promising in their potential, ablative approaches to rejuvenating photodamaged skin, including both CO_2 and Er:YAG laser technology, are sometimes accompanied by untoward side effects and complications. The most common of these is postoperative erythema, experienced by virtually all patients treated with ablative resurfacing. Other potential risks induced by these dermal wounding lasers consist of delayed healing, postoperative pigmentary changes, and scarring, which may be seen not only in patients with lower Fitzpatrick skin types, but also in patients with higher Fitzpatrick skin types. These risks, in addition to a prolonged recovery period after treatment, have prompted the development of nonablative and more recently, fractionated resurfacing technologies.

The clinical improvement noted after ablative laser therapy results from dermal wounding, which stimulates new collagen formation and deposition in a parallel configuration. Techniques that induce a dermal wound without epidermal ablation should, therefore, theoretically produce cosmetic improvement of dermal photodamage and scarring. This idea led to the development of newer rejuvenating laser systems known as nonablative dermal remodeling systems, which can be classified into three main groups: mid-infrared lasers, visible lasers, and intense pulsed light (IPL) sources. These groups operate on the principles of selective photothermolysis, as they target either a discrete chromophore or dermal water. Despite having different targets, these lasers, whether directed at dermal microvasculature, pigment or tissue water, produce similar histologic changes due to thermal injury. These changes in dermal collagen account for the clinical improvement observed after treatment with these modalities. The recent study and development of radiofrequency (RF) devices and fractional laser delivery systems has expanded the approach to using nonablative treatments for dermal remodeling. This chapter will review what is currently known about these treatment modalities.

INFRARED LASERS

The water absorption coefficient is relatively low in the infrared portion of the electromagnetic spectrum (>700 nm), which allows for deeper laser tissue penetration. Mid-infrared lasers typically used for photorejuvenation include the 1320 nm neodymium:yttrium–aluminum–garnet (Nd:YAG) laser, the 1450 nm diode laser, and the 1540 nm ytterbium–erbium:phosphate glass, also known as the erbium:glass (Er:glass) laser. Light produced by all three lasers is absorbed by water, with the 1320 nm wavelength absorbed least. As a result, optical penetration depth by this laser is the greatest of the three devices, with effective heating to the depth of 400 μm compared to a depth of approximately 300 μm achieved by the 1450 nm diode laser.[1] In addition, the 1320 nm wavelength is associated with significant scattering, resulting in deposition of energy outside the laser beam and subsequent effective dermal heating. Although low throughout the mid-infrared spectrum, laser light absorption by epidermal melanin is approximately 1.6 times lower at 1540 nm compared to 1320 nm.[2] It has, therefore, been suggested that the former wavelength may be safer to use in darkly pigmented individuals.

In one of the first studies evaluating a nonablative approach to dermal remodeling, a 1064 nm Q-switched Nd:YAG laser was used in an attempt to improve rhytides.[3] Eleven subjects (Fitzpatrick skin types I, II) with Class I to II perioral or periorbital rhytides were treated using a Q-switched Nd:YAG laser at 5.5 J/cm^2 and a 3 mm spot size. The authors sought a nonspecific clinical endpoint of pinpoint bleeding. Subjects were treated only once and were evaluated 7, 30, 60, and 90 days after treatment for improvement of rhytides, healing, pigmentary changes, and erythema. Three patients (two perioral/one periorbital) were thought to have improvement, with results comparable to those following treatment with ablative resurfacing. Six patients (three perioral/three periorbital), were noted to have clinical improvement, but their results were not comparable to those achieved with ablative laser systems (Figs. 36-1 and 36-2). No clinical improvement was seen in two patients (one perioral/one periorbital) and no pigmentary change or scarring was seen in any of the treated subjects. At 1 month, 3 of 11 subjects showed persistent erythema at the treated sites, which eventually resolved at 3 months.

Of note, Q-switched Nd:YAG laser energy is not well absorbed by tissue water and results in relatively deep penetration into the skin; it is nonselectively placed within the dermis. The previous study was, therefore, modified by potentiating the Q-switched Nd:YAG laser using a topical carbon-assisted solution (Fig. 36-3).[4] This modification was thought to localize the cellular damage to the tissue immediately adjacent to the carbon, thereby minimally affecting the nontargeted tissue and requiring less than 10% of the typical energy output from CO_2 laser treatment.

With this new approach, 242 solar anatomic sites on 61 human subjects underwent three 1064 nm Q-switched Nd:YAG laser treatments. Parameters of treatment included a fluence of 2.5 J/cm^2, pulse duration of 6 to 20 nanoseconds, and a spot size of 7 mm. The treatment sites were evaluated at baseline, 4, 8, 14, 20, and 32 weeks for skin texture, skin elasticity, and rhytide reduction. All sites were treated at a baseline visit, and later at 4 and 8 weeks. At

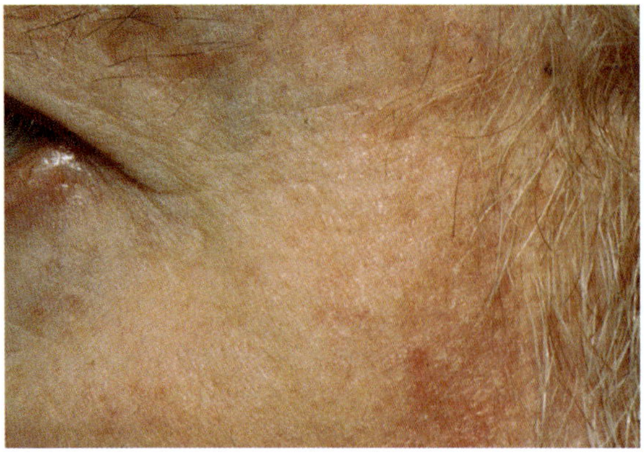

Figure 36-1 Periorbital rhytides before treatment with a Q-switched Nd:YAG Laser.

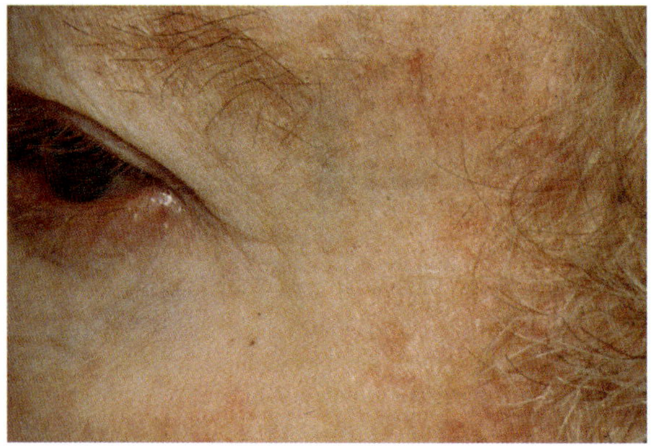

Figure 36-2 Improvement in rhytides after treatment with a Q-switched Nd:YAG Laser.

8 months, the investigators reported improvement in skin texture and skin elasticity, as well as reduction in wrinkles compared to baseline (Figs. 36-4 and 36-5). The majority of adverse events were limited to mild and brief erythema.

As a result of these earlier investigations, the first specifically nonablative laser to be marketed solely to the physician community was a 1320 nm Nd:YAG infrared laser. Nelson et al.[5] performed a study using one or more passes of the 1320 nm Nd:YAG laser on photoaged skin. The waveform consisted of three 200 usec laser pulses at a 100 Hz repetition rate. Laser energy was delivered through a 5 mm spot with fluences up to 10 J/cm^2. A dynamic cryogen cooling technique was applied immediately prior to laser treatment to produce selective subsurface skin heating without epidermal damage. Immediately after treatment, mild edema and erythema appeared in the treated skin. These side effects resolved within 2 days and at 2 months after treatment facial rhytides were noted to have improved. No persistent erythema or pigmentary changes were appreciated (Figs. 36-6 and 36-7).

The efficacy of the 1320 nm Nd:YAG laser has been compared to that of the 1450 nm diode laser, an infrared laser with lower peak powers, necessitating longer pulse durations to achieve optimal fluences.[6] A study of 20 patients (Fitzpatrick skin types I to V) with mild-to-moderate atrophic facial acne scars randomly received three successive monthly treatments with a long-pulsed 1320 nm Nd:YAG laser on one facial half and a long-pulsed 1450 nm diode laser on the contralateral facial half. Using digital photography and three-dimensional in vivo microtopography measurements, patients were evaluated at each treatment visit and at 1, 3, 6, and 12 months postoperatively. Histologic evaluations of cutaneous biopsies obtained before treatment, immediately after the first treatment, and at 1, 3, 6, and 12 months after the third treatment were performed. In the majority of patients studied, mild-to-moderate clinical improvement was observed after the series of three treatments. Patient satisfaction scores and in vivo microtopography measurements paralleled the photographic and histopathologic changes seen. Side effects of treatment were limited to mild transient erythema, edema, and hyperpigmentation. No scarring or adverse textural changes resulted from the use of either laser system. The authors concluded that the 1450 nm diode laser showed greater clinical scar response at the parameters studied (Figs. 36-8 and 36-9).[7]

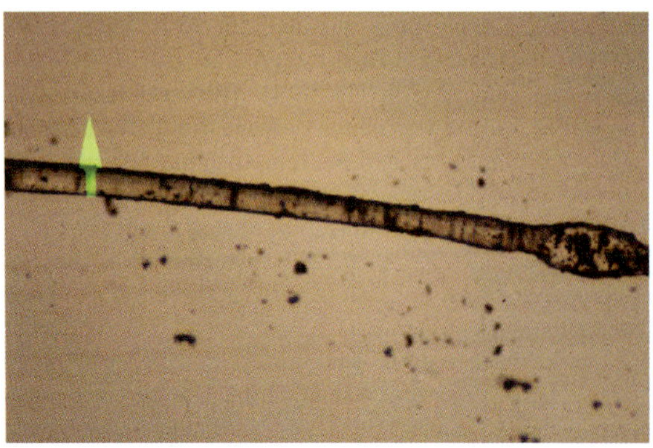

Figure 36-3 Topical carbon surrounding hair follicle used in carbon-assisted, low fluence Q-switched Nd:YAG Laser.

Dahan et al.[8] investigated the use of an Erbium glass 1540 nm laser in 20 patients to increase dermal thickness and firmness. Skin thickness and mechanical properties were measured before the first treatment, 1 month after the third treatment, 1 month after the fifth treatment, and 3 months after the fifth treatment. All patients reported an improvement in both skin tone and texture. Using ultrasound imaging, dermal thickness of the neck and forehead increased and a dramatic increase in firmness of the forehead skin was observed. No immediate or late adverse effects were noted throughout the treatment regimen. This study demonstrated that irradiation with a 1540 nm Er:glass laser emitted in a pulsed mode and coupled with an efficient contact cooling system increases dermal thickness and firmness, leading to clinical improvement in neck lines and forehead rhytides.

To address the potential postprocedural pigmentary changes after various laser treatments in patients with higher Fitzpatrick skin types, Badawi et al.[9] published a retrospective study analyzing nonablative scar treatments in dark skin types using a submillisecond Nd:YAG 1064 nm laser. The theory behind using microsecond pulse durations stems from the concept that this type of laser heating more selectively targets the microvasculature in the papillary dermis and melanocytes within the epidermis, without actually damaging larger dermal vessels or the epidermis.

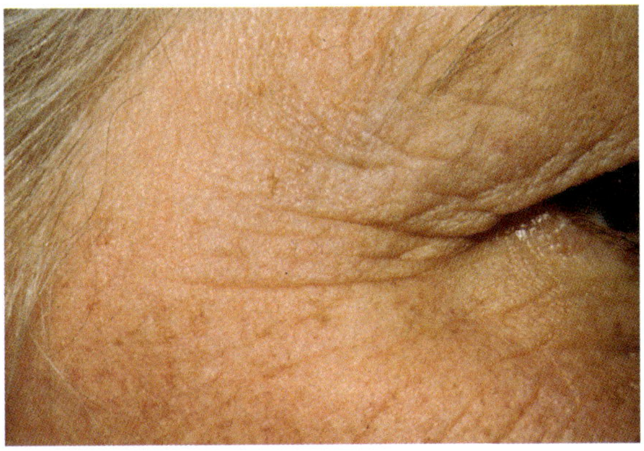

Figure 36-4 Periorbital rhytides before treatment with a carbon-assisted, low fluence Q-switched Nd:YAG Laser.

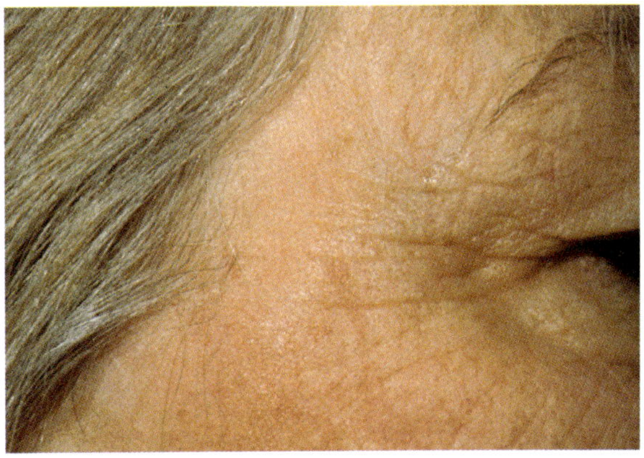

Figure 36-5 Improvement in rhytides after treatment with a carbon-assisted, low fluence Q-switched Nd:YAG laser.

In addition, bulk heating, using a 5 mm spot size and pulsing at 5 to 10 Hz, allows delivery of large amounts of energy in short pulses faster than the body can extract the heat. In nonselective heat conduction, no structures are specifically targeted, thereby permitting patients with higher Fitzpatrick skin types to be safely treated.[9]

In their retrospective review, 22 patients with Fitzpatrick skin types III to VI were enrolled and treated for an average of six sessions at an average of 24.5 day intervals. To optimize laser results and allow greater light penetration into the papillary dermis, the skin was treated with microdermabrasion throughout the submillisecond 1064 nm Nd:YAG laser treatment series (3 days minimum for microdermabrasion to laser treatment). The authors did not administer prophylaxis against postinflammatory hyperpigmentation. Assessment of pre and post procedure photographs by two blinded dermatologists and one plastic surgeon indicated improvements in scarring, texture, and postinflammatory hyperpigmentation. No transient or permanent hyper- or hypopigmentation was observed.[9] The authors recognized the need for prospective trials and possible split face trials to confirm treatment efficacy.[9]

PULSED DYE LASER

Dermal remodeling has also been demonstrated using another nonablative approach targeting hemoglobin, known as the pulsed dye laser (PDL). Histopathologic examination of 585 nm PDL-treated scars revealed improvement in dermal collagen. There was also an increase in the number of regional mast cells in the treated scars. As mast cells elaborate a variety of cytokines, their presence following irradiation and accompanying tissue revascularization may provide an explanation for therapeutic improvement following PDL treatment. Using this concept, Zelickson et al.[10] evaluated the use of PDL in the treatment of rhytides. The authors reported clinical improvement in 75% to 90% of mild-to-moderate rhytides and 40% of moderate-to-severe rhytides; however, the study results were tempered by cosmetically unacceptable purpura, which are commonly seen following PDL treatment (Figs. 36-10 and 36-11).

Although in the case of vascular lesions, the development of purpura is associated with effective treatment, Tanghetti et al.[11] questioned the efficacy of low dose or subpurpuric fluences using a PDL to treat photodamage (textural changes, rhytides). Prior studies demonstrated that multipass, subpurpuric treatments increase the depth of total tissue effect while reducing the risk of purpura.[12] Tanghetti et al. sought to investigate treatment methods and parameters to address the most effective approach, splitting 20 of their patients into two groups: one group receiving a series of four single-pass treatments at 2 week intervals and the other receiving a series of four double-pass treatments at similar intervals. Within each patient,

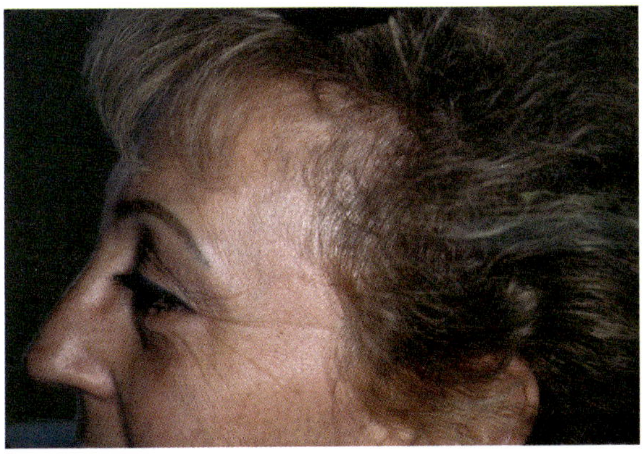

Figure 36-6 Patient before treatment with a 1320 nm Nd:YAG laser.

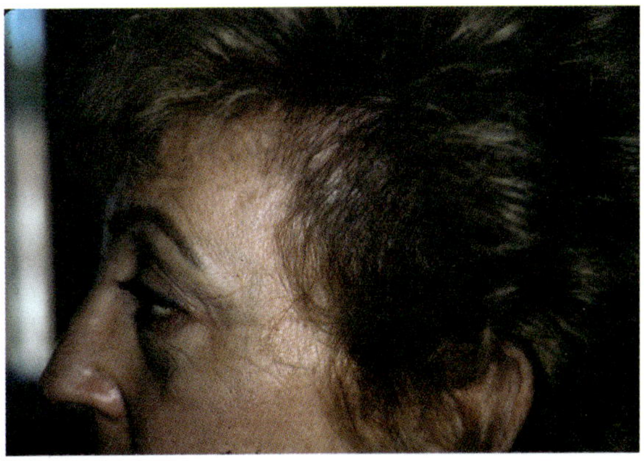

Figure 36-7 Patient 6 months after 1320 nm Nd:YAG laser treatment.

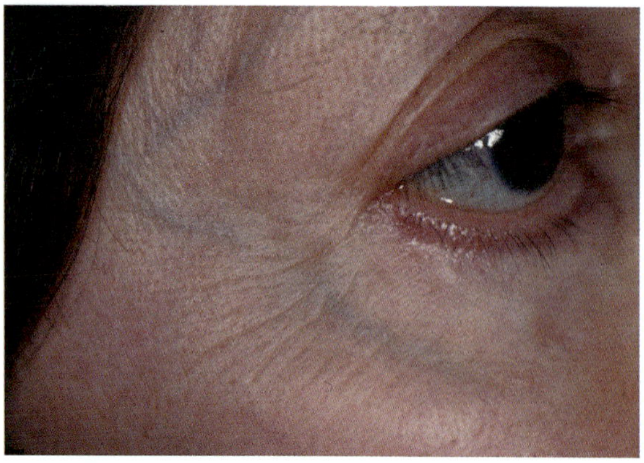

Figure 36-8 Periorbital rhytides before treatment with a 1450 nm diode laser.

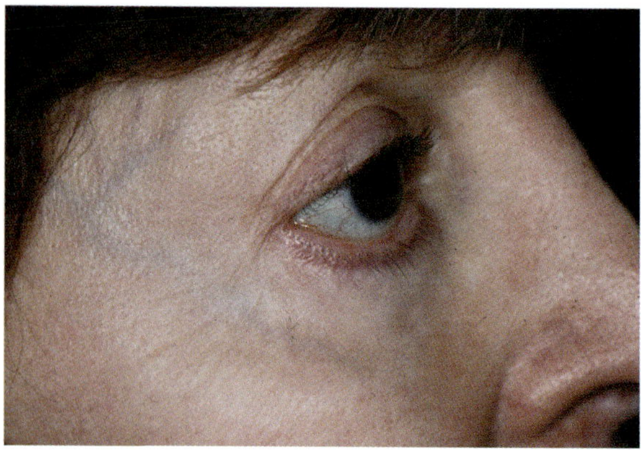

Figure 36-9 Improvement in rhytides after treatment with a 1450 nm diode laser.

one-half of the face was randomized to receive treatment with either the 585 or 595 nm wavelength. All treatments were provided using a pulse duration of 0.5 ms with a 10 mm handpiece. Treatment fluences were maintained just below the individual's subpurpuric threshold for each respective wavelength and ranged from 3 to 4 J/cm^2.

The Fitzpatrick skin type of each patient was not noted; however, the authors reported no adverse events from the study. Blinded observers rated an average overall improvement of 1.2 (scale of 1–4, four being exceptional improvement) in patients' facial rhytides and reported no difference between the 585 and 595 nm groups or even between the single or double pass groups when comparing photographs before treatment and 6 months after the last treatment. Of note, the authors mention that the majority of observed improvement was related to a reduction in superficial dyspigmentation. This study appears to support the use of subpurpuric fluences to achieve improvement of photodamage, although additional studies may be needed to confirm these findings.

INTENSE PULSED LIGHT

IPL, which targets both melanin and hemoglobin, has histologically revealed neocollagenesis after treatment of rhytides.[13] Compared to PDL, use of IPL has not demonstrated treatment related purpura. Goldberg et al. enrolled 30 subjects (Fitzpatrick skin types I, II) with Class I to II periorbital, perioral, and forehead rhytides and administered one to four IPL treatments. Noncoherent IPL was delivered to the skin using a 645 nm cutoff filter, which led to emission of light with wavelengths between 645 nm and 1100 nm. Light was delivered through a bracketed cooling device, in triple 7 ms pulses, with a 50 ms interpulse delay between the pulses. Delivered fluences were between 40 and 50 J/cm^2. The authors evaluated the degree of improvement 6 months after the last treatment using the following descriptive categories: (1) no improvement; (2) some improvement; (3) substantial improvement; and (4) total improvement.

Six months after the final treatment, five subjects were noted to have no improvement. Similarly, no subjects were noted to have total improvement. Some improvement was observed in 16 subjects, while nine subjects showed substantial improvement. All participants were evaluated for pigmentary changes, posttreatment blistering, erythema, and scarring. Blistering immediately after treatment occurred in three of the 30 subjects. All 30 subjects had posttreatment erythema. Six months after treatment, no pigmentary changes, erythema, or scarring were noted. The authors concluded that IPL could improve some rhytides (Figs. 36-12 and 36-13); however, the changes appeared to be more subtle than those seen after ablative resurfacing.[14]

The principle behind tightening of the skin with IPL rests on the theory that heating collagen fibers with

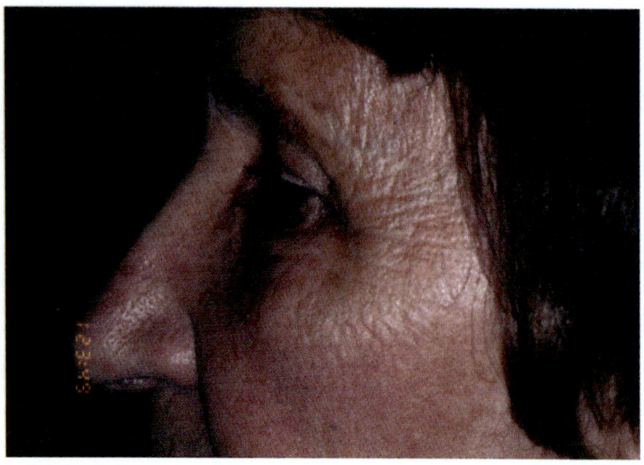

Figure 36-10 Periorbital rhytides before treatment with a pulsed dye laser.

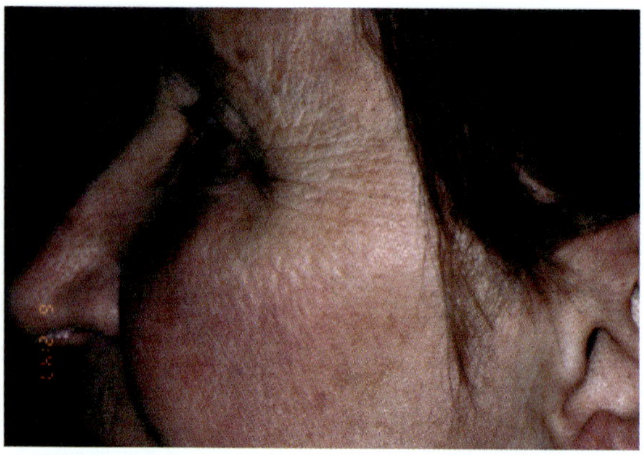

Figure 36-11 Improvement in rhytides after treatment with a pulsed dye laser.

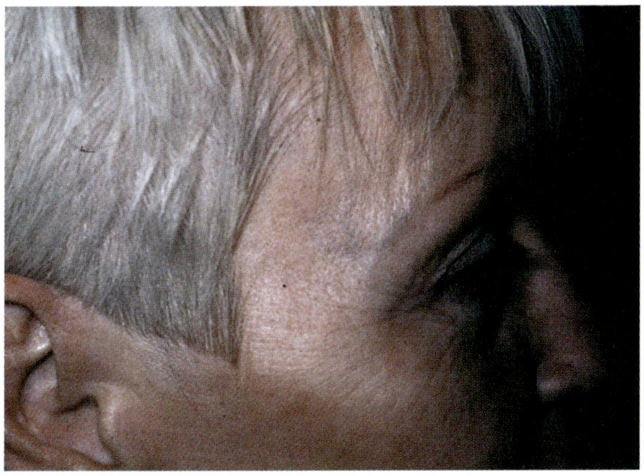

Figure 36-12 Periorbital rhytides before treatment with an Intense Pulsed Light source.

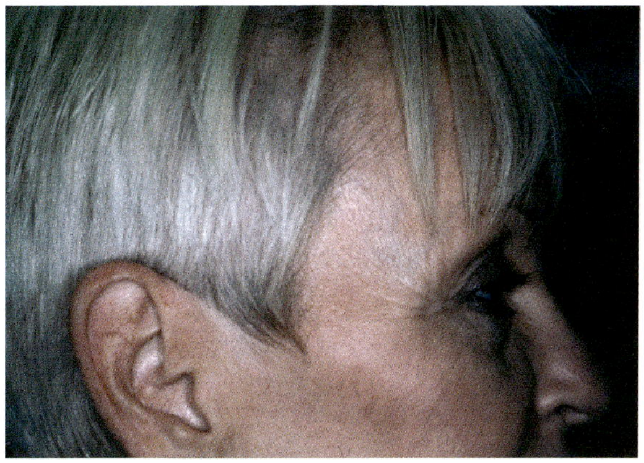

Figure 36-13 Improvement in rhytides after treatment with an Intense Pulsed Light source.

high-intensity light energy leads to their contracture. This may account for the textural changes described in skin treated with IPL, which has been reported as a secondary observation in several studies.[15] Furthermore, thermal stimulation of dermal fibroblasts by the higher wavelengths within the IPL spectrum has been shown to result in increased synthesis of extracellular matrix proteins, leading to at least partial replacement of the lost dermal volume seen due to the intrinsic and extrinsic aging process. Specifically, wavelengths in the 1200 nm spectrum are absorbed by water in the dermis, triggering a cytokine reaction, which in turn, stimulates the formation of new collagen I, III, and elastin.[16] Histological evaluation of the effects of five subsequent IPL treatments with 570 to 645 nm wavelengths showed epidermal thickening of 100 to 300 um, new rete ridge formation, a decrease in proportion of degenerated elastic fibers, and new dermal collagen formation.[17] In addition to new collagen formation, improvement in age-related vascular and pigmented lesions has also been described following IPL, as these wavelengths target both hemoglobin and melanin, although this limits its use among patients with higher Fitzpatrick skin types.[14,18]

Studies comparing the efficacy of PDL to that of IPL are limited although both modalities have been used for skin rejuvenation. Kono et al. compared IPL to long-pulsed pulsed dye laser (LPDL) in rejuvenating facial skin. Ten patients with Fitzpatrick skin types III to IV were enrolled; half of each patient's face was treated with IPL (six treatment sessions) and the other half with LPDL for three treatment sessions. The LPDL was used to treat facial rhytides with fluences between 10 and 12 J/cm^2 and a pulse duration of 20 ms, using a pulse stacking technique. The parameters for use of IPL for wrinkles included fluences between 27 and 40 J/cm^2 and a pulse duration of 20 ms. Overall, the investigators found no significant difference between IPL and LPDL in wrinkle reduction although the degree of improvement ranged from 26% to 100% with both modalities. No scarring or pigmentary changes were seen with either device. The authors pointed out that LPDL was significantly more effective than IPL in treating lentigines.[19] Thus, both modalities demonstrate promise in treating photodamaged facial skin.

RADIOFREQUENCY

In order to increase penetration depth so as to stimulate collagen contracture and produce skin tightening, RF devices have been developed. This technology uniformly delivers a volumetric heating effect into the deep dermis, which is potentiated by the tissue's resistance to current flow. Jacobson et al.[20] treated 24 patients with redundant nasolabial folds, marionette lines, and jowls with one to three RF passes using 106 to 144 J with the Thermacool system (Thermage; Hayward, CA). Seventeen of 24 patients demonstrated visible improvement 1 to 3 months after treatment. For patients who received more than a single treatment, it appeared that subsequent sessions further improved facial skin laxity. Similarly, patients who received more than one pass with the device appeared to benefit more than those who were treated with a single pass. Patients not only described a sensation of tightening in the treated areas but also noted visually observable improvement. Using a three-dimensional imaging system, a significant decrease in rhytide depth was demonstrated in two patients. However, subsequent studies failed to demonstrate statistically significant improvement.[21]

To broaden the application of nonablative RF devices, Ruiz-Esparza treated nine patients with laxity and rhytides of the lower eyelids (Fitzpatrick skin types not noted). A single treatment using a single pass on two patients, two passes in five patients, and three passes in two patients was performed and these patients were followed-up for 1 year. The authors noted improvement, with marked eyelid skin contraction and correspondingly high patient satisfaction. The author specifically treated anchoring points, or areas distal to the target area, to prevent complications including scarring, ectropion, and pigmentary changes seen with ablative laser resurfacing, blepharoplasty, or even chemical peels. The author therefore recommended use of RF devices to noninvasively contract the lax skin of the forehead to produce an eyebrow lift, as well as tightening the skin on the cheeks, neck, and other areas to produce visible lifting.[22] Overall, the patients enrolled in these studies did not experience any downtime or complications,[23] further supporting the application of RF technology to facial rhytides.

Continued improvement in RF devices has led to a novel electrosurgical technology that uses substantially lower energy. This resurfacing device uses a bipolar multielectrode-tipped stylet and an electrically conductive medium, usually isotonic sodium chloride solution.[24] Multielectrode RF resurfacing is a low-heat process compared with traditional electrosurgery; hence, the term *coblation* (*cold* + *ablation*) has been coined. Using a conductive medium, the device applies low-energy RF, which causes a vapor layer of ionized particles, or plasma field, to form around the electrodes.[24] These ionized particles possess sufficient energy to dissociate organic molecular bonds within the tissue. Investigations using this device on ex vivo human skin demonstrated no apparent epidermal ablation, but an increasing amount of residual thermal damage with increased pass number.[25] After three passes at 86, 108, and 139 V, the mean thickness of the layer of thermal damage was 97, 80, and 80 μm, respectively.[25] The similarity of this pattern of tissue damage to that associated with short-pulsed CO_2 laser resurfacing indicated that this RF device should be effective in cutaneous resurfacing, with rapid postoperative wound healing.

To apply this innovation to the treatment of rhytides, Grekin et al. prospectively enrolled 95 patients (Fitzpatrick skin types I to III) with periorbital (75 treatment sites) and perioral (50 sites) photodamage. The participants were treated with two to three passes at 125 or 139 V. Wrinkle and cosmetic improvement were evaluated by an independent panel of five evaluators. All evaluators discerned a positive mean improvement in wrinkling, both in periorbital and perioral anatomic sites, using photographs taken at baseline and 6 months after treatment, with greater improvement seen in patients with more severe wrinkling at baseline. An increased number of passes and higher voltage settings had a positive impact on wrinkle improvement. Transient postinflammatory hyperpigmentation occurred in 26% of periorbital and 4% of perioral sites. Hypertrophic scarring occurred in 3.8% of treatment sites, with all but one scar resolving by 6 months. Overall, healing was rapid, pain was minimal, and erythema largely resolved within 2 months. The authors concluded that treatment with the bipolar RF device led to less severe postoperative morbidity than usually occurs with ablative approaches.[26]

FRACTIONAL PHOTOTHERMOLYSIS

In 2003 the innovative concept of fractional photothermolysis (FP) was reported[27] and was followed in 2004 with development of an original prototype FP device.[28] With this modality, small columns of thermal injury known as "microthermal zones" (MTZs) were produced by light energy delivered in a pixilated fashion to the skin. This fractional emission of light differed from traditional ablative resurfacing, in which a uniform patch of epidermal and dermal injury was delivered using a flat, nonfractionated beam. With these initial prototype devices, the deep epidermis and dermis became necrotic in the individual MTZs, without being vaporized, and the stratum corneum remained histologically intact. Resurfacing with these initial fractional devices was termed "nonablative" and could be delivered using wavelengths only moderately absorbed by water (1410 nm, 1440 nm, 1540 nm, 1550 nm).[29] Because FP produces microscopic zones of thermal injury, the surrounding islands of normal tissue serve as a reservoir for re-epithelialization.[30] Histological studies demonstrated full epidermal healing occurring within the first 24 hours after the procedure.[30] This rapid barrier restoration lowered the risk of infection, erythema, changes in pigmentation, and other complications frequently associated with ablative resurfacing procedures.[29] Although results were far superior to those seen with nonfractionated nonablative technologies, multiple treatments, typically in the range of five to seven, were needed.

The efficacy of fractional nonablative photothermolysis in the treatment of photodamaged facial skin was first demonstrated in 2005.[31] In this study 12 subjects with facial rhytides were treated with a first generation laser using fluences of 6 to 20 J at 1 to 4 week intervals with densities of 2000 to 3000 MTZ/cm^2. Each participant received an average of four to five treatments and was assessed for improvement in texture, dyschromia, and wrinkles on the face, neck, and the chest. Significant improvement was seen in all clinical parameters, and was supported by histological evidence of new collagen formation. Side effects were minimal and limited to posttreatment erythema and mild edema that resolved within a few days.

In a subsequent study, the long-term efficacy of fractional nonablative photothermolysis in treating both facial and nonfacial photodamage, rhytides, and dyspigmentation was demonstrated.[32] Fifty patients (Fitzpatrick skin types I–III) underwent a series of three consecutive treatments (2000 MTZ/cm^2 at 8 mJ for facial areas; 1500–2000 MTZ/cm^2 at 8 mJ for nonfacial areas, Fraxel 750 SR) spaced 3 to 4 weeks apart. Two blinded physicians assessed clinical improvement with a three-point quartile grading scale. The investigators reported a mean improvement of 2.23, 2.10, and 1.96 at 3, 6, and 9 months after treatment, respectively. Similar results were observed for nonfacial areas, with a mean improvement of 1.85, 1.81, and 1.70 at 3, 6, and 9 months after treatment, respectively. An overall improvement of 51% to 75% was found in 73% (facial arm) and 55% (nonfacial arm) of patients 9 months after treatment. Adverse effects were limited and short-lived. The authors concluded that FP was a safe and effective treatment for facial and nonfacial photodamage, rhytides, and dyspigmentation with a favorable recovery and side-effect profile.

Investigations comparing fractional ablative versus fractional nonablative laser systems have been performed retrospectively.[33] Alajlan et al. reviewed patients with acne scars and Fitzpatrick skin types III to V. A total of 82 patients were recruited for the study, 45 of whom received an average of five sessions with the nonablative fractional laser (1550 nm) and 37 patients treated on average two times with the ablative fractional CO_2 laser. The average fluence, density, and time after treatment for the nonablative and ablative groups were 2.87 kJ and 125 mJ/cm^2, 17% and 30%, and 1 month and 2 months, respectively. The authors noted that both treatment modalities were effective in treating acne scars in ethnic skin with good patient satisfaction rates and a high safety profile. One of the side effects reported was postinflammatory hyperpigmentation; the severity and rate of occurrence decreased after initiating use of a topical bleaching formulation with hydroquinone 4% to 6% in combination with retinoic acid, glycolic acid, or Kojic acid for 6 to 8 weeks, beginning 1 week after treatment with the laser. One interesting finding mentioned in the study was improvement in pore size after treatment with the nonablative fractional laser. The investigators concluded that there was significantly less downtime in patients treated with the nonablative fractional laser and that patient satisfaction was comparable for the two approaches (71% for nonablative fractional laser and 65% for ablative CO_2 fractional laser). Although the analysis suggested comparability of the two systems, the authors acknowledged that prospective trials are needed to more rigorously evaluate the differences in efficacy between the ablative and nonablative fractional lasers. In addition, it was noted that patients with more severe cases of acne scarring were chosen for treatment with the ablative CO_2 fractional laser.[33]

In 2009, Hruza et al.[34] introduced the fractional RF device, the first nonlaser, nonlight based device capable of inducing fractional skin ablation, coagulation, and necrosis for skin rejuvenation. Brightman applied the term "sublative rejuvenation" to this technology, as it produces limited epidermal disruption with coagulative effects concentrated in the mid to deep dermis. Compared to lasers, RF energy produces higher volumetric heating through tissue impedance, which allows the diffusion of heat to deeper tissues.[35] This technology holds the greatest promise for the fractional resurfacing of patients with darker skin types.[36] Since the epidermis is mostly spared, fractional RF lowers the risk of scarring and postinflammatory hyperpigmentation in susceptible patients.

A recently introduced fractional RF device is the Matrix RF (Syneron Medical Ltd.). Matrix RF is the first bipolar RF-based aesthetic device capable of delivering ablative tunable RF energy to the skin in a nonhomogeneous fractional manner using an array of multielectrode pins. Hruza et al.[34] delivered fractional RF treatment using different tips at varying energies and coverage rates to the abdomen in individuals scheduled for abdominoplasty. Another group of subjects received three facial treatments scheduled at 3 to 4 week intervals. Histological findings immediately after treatment revealed well-demarcated zones of ablation, coagulation, necrosis, and subnecrosis up to a depth of 450 μm. Higher energy levels generated deeper tissue effects. Subjects undergoing facial treatment had minimal pain and no permanent side effects or significant downtime. Investigators' assessments of improvement in facial skin texture correlated with subjects' evaluations and were greater than 40% in approximately half of subjects. Eighty percent of the subjects were satisfied with the results.

Man and Goldberg aimed to evaluate the safety and efficacy of bipolar fractionated RF devices in improving skin texture, fine lines, and wrinkles in patients with Fitzpatrick skin types V and VI. Fifteen subjects each received three treatments to the full face with a fractionated bipolar RF device (Syneron Inc., Irvine, USA) 30 days apart. Patients were evaluated by the study investigator and a blinded investigator at each treatment and 90 days after the last treatment for treatment safety and efficacy. The authors reported a statistically significant improvement in wrinkles, texture, and fine lines in most subjects. Adverse events, specifically postinflammatory hyperpigmentation and hypopigmentation, were not seen in any of the patients, suggesting that the use of fractionated RF devices is a safe and effective method of skin rejuvenation for skin types V and VI (Figs. 36-14 and 36-15).[37]

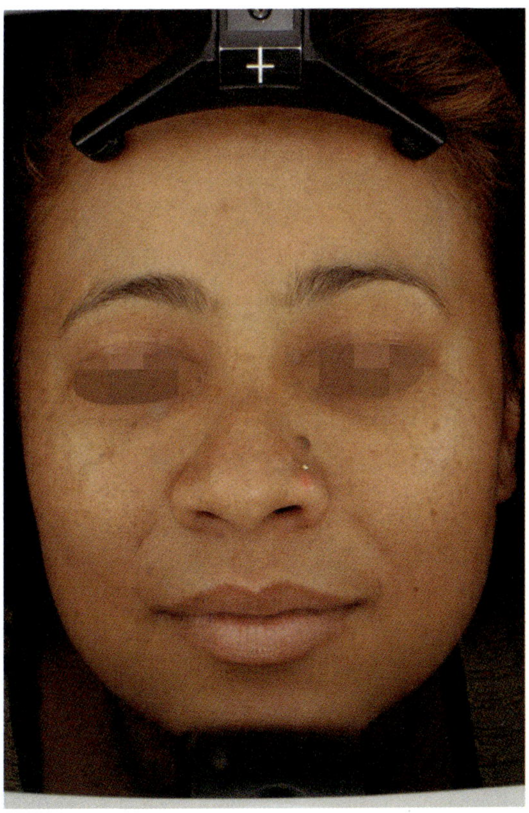

Figure 36-14 Before treatment of fine lines with a fractionated bipolar radiofrequency device.

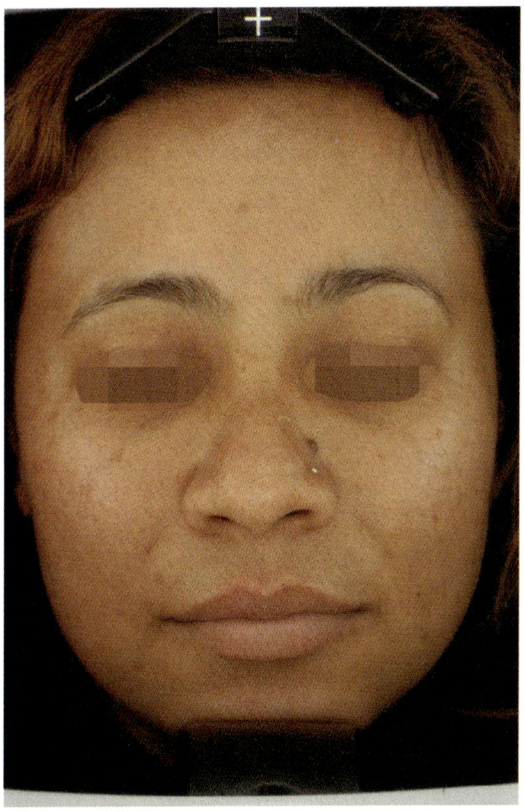

Figure 36-15 Improvement in fine lines after treatment with fractionated bipolar radiofrequency device--note lack of pigmentary changes after treatment.

Nonablative approaches, including nonablative fractionated systems, represent the newest approach to improving photodamaged skin. The degree of collagen remodeling and the decrease in epidermal pigmentary changes are not expected to be as great as those caused by other more destructive, ablative approaches or specific pigmented lesion lasers. However, with the advent of fractionated nonablative laser systems, dermal remodeling comparable to that achieved using ablative lasers has been achieved after multiple treatments. In addition, the advantages of nonablative therapies over ablative laser resurfacing are numerous. Patients do not develop open wounds, which reduces their risks of infection, dyspigmentation, and scarring in addition to minimizing downtime.[38] One of the other significant advances in nonablative FP is the ability to treat nonfacial areas, including the neck, chest, back, and extremities, which are prone to developing hypertrophic scarring if treated with traditional ablative or even fractionated ablative resurfacing.[39–41] With continued experience using fractionated RF technology, it is possible that the risk of treating patients with darker skin types for fear of postprocedure pigmentary changes may diminish significantly.[36,37] In the future, standardized treatment regimens controlling for differences in density and spot size could revolutionize the field of laser therapy for the treatment of superficial photodamage as well as deeper wrinkling in patients encompassing the full range of Fitzpatrick skin types.

REFERENCES

1. Hardaway CA, Ross EV, Barnette DJ, Paithankar DY. Nonablative cutaneous remodeling with a 1.45 micron mid-infrared diode laser: phase I. *J Cosmet Laser Ther*. 2002;4:3–8.
2. Mordon S, Capon A, Creusy C, et al. In vivo experimental evaluation of skin remodeling by using an Er:glass laser with contact cooling. *Laser Surg Med*. 2000;27:1–9.
3. Goldberg DJ, Whitworth J. Laser skin resurfacing with the Q switched Nd:YAG laser. *Dermatol Surg*. 1997;23:903–907.
4. Goldberg DJ, Metzler C. Skin resurfacing utilizing a low fluence Nd:YAG laser cut laser ther. 1999;1:23–27.
5. Nelson JS, Millner TE, Dave D, et al. Clinical Study of non ablative laser treatment of facial rhytides. *Lasers Surg Med*. 1998;17(suppl 9):150.
6. Sadick NS, Makino Y. Selective electro-thermolysis in aesthetic medicine: a review. *Laser Surg Med*. 2004;34:91–97.
7. Tanzi EL, Alster TS. Comparison of a 1450-nm diode laser and a 1320-nm Nd:YAG laser in the treatment of atrophic facial scars: a prospective clinical and histologic study. *Dermatol Surg*. 2004;30(2 Pt 1):152–157.
8. Dahan S, Lagarde JM, Turlier V, Courrech L, Mordon S. Treatment of neck lines and forehead rhytids with a nonablative 1540-nm Er:glass laser: a controlled clinical study combined with the measurement of the thickness and the mechanical properties of the skin. *Dermatol Surg*. 2004;30: 872–879.
9. Badawi A, Tome MA, Atteya A, Sami N, Morsy IA. Retrospective analysis of non ablative scar treatment in dark skin types using the sub millisecond Nd:YAG 1064 nm laser. *Lasers Surg Med*. 2011;43:130–136.
10. Zelickson BD, Kilmer SL, Bernstein E, et.al. Pulsed dye laser for sun damaged skin. *Lasers Surg Med*. 1999;25:229–236.
11. Tanghetti EA, Sherr EA, Alvarado SL. Multipass treatment of photodamage using the pulse dye laser. *Dermatol Surg*. 2003;29(7):686–690; discussion 690–691.
12. Bjerring P, Clement M, Heickendorff L, Egevist H, Kiernan M. Selective non-ablative wrinkle reduction by laser. *J Cutan Laser Ther*. 2000;2(1):9–15.
13. Goldberg DJ. New collagen formation after dermal remodeling with an intense pulsed light source. *J Cut Las Ther*. 2000; 2(2):59–61.
14. Goldberg DJ. Histologic changes after treatment with an intense pulsed light. *J Cut Las Ther*. 2000;2:53–56.
15. Weiss RA, Weiss MA, Beasley KL. Rejuvenation of photoaged skin: 5 years results with intense pulsed light of the face, neck and chest. *Dermatol Surg*. 2002;28(12):1115–1119.
16. Wong WR, Shyu WL, Tsai JW, Hsu KH, Pang JH. Intense pulsed light effects on the expression of extracellular matrix proteins and transforming growth factor beta-1 in skin dermal fibroblasts cultured within contracted collagen lattices. *Dermatol Surg*. 2009;35(5):816–825
17. Hernandez-Perez E, Ibiett EV. Gross and microscopic findings in patients submitted to nonablative full-face resurfacing using intense pulsed light: a preliminary study. *Dermatol Surg*. 2002;28(8):651–655.
18. Bitter PJ. Noninvasive rejuvenation of photoaged skin using serial, full-face intense pulsed light treatments. *Dermatol Surg*. 2000;26:835–843.
19. Kono T, Groff WF, Sakurai H, et al. Comparison study of intense pulsed light versus a long-pulse pulsed dye laser in the treatment of facial skin rejuvenation. *Ann Plast Surg*. 2007;59(5):479–483.
20. Jacobson LG, Alexiades-Armenakas MR, Bernstein L, Geronemus RG. Treatment of nasolabial folds and jowls with a non-invasive radiofrequency device. *Arch Dermatol*. 2003;139:1313–1320.
21. Hsu TS, Kaminer MS. The use of nonablative radiofrequency technology to tighten the lower face and neck. *Semin Cutan Med Surg*. 2003;22:115–123.
22. Ruiz-Esparza J, Gomez JB. Non-ablative radiofrequency tissue tightening of facial skin: the medical face lift: a report of 25 patients. *Lasers Surg Med Suppl*. 2003;15:36.
23. Ruiz-Esparza J. Noninvasive lower eyelid blepharoplasty: a new technique using nonablative radiofrequency on periorbital skin. *Dermatol Surg*. 2004;30(2 Pt 1):125–129.
24. Olhoffer IH, Leffell DJ. What's new in electrosurgery? Coblation: a new method for facial resurfacing. *Aesthet Dermatol Cosmet Surg*. 1999; 1:31–33.
25. Tope WD. Multi-electrode radio frequency resurfacing of ex vivo human skin. *Dermatol Surg*. 1999;25;348–352.
26. Grekin RC, Tope WD, Yarborough JM Jr, et al. Electrosurgical facial resurfacing: a prospective multicenter study of efficacy and safety. *Arch Dermatol*. 2000;136(11):1309–1316.
27. Huzaira M, Anderson RR, Sink K, Manstein D. Intradermal focusing of near-infrared optical pulses: a new approach for non-ablative laser therapy. *Lasers Surg Med*. 2003; 32(Suppl 15): 17–38.
28. Manstein D, Herron GS, Sink RK, Tanner H, Anderson RR. Fractional photothermolysis: a new concept for cutaneous remodeling using microscopic patterns of thermal injury. *Lasers Surg Med*. 2004:34(5):426–438.
29. Bogdan Allemann I, Kaufman J. Fractional photothermolysis–an update. *Lasers Med Sci*. 2010;25(1):137–144.
30. Laubach HJ, Tannous Z, Anderson RR, Manstein D. Skin responses to fractional photothermolysis. *Lasers Surg Med*. 2006;38:142–149.
31. Rokhsar CK, Fitzpatrick RE. The treatment of photodamage and facial rhytides with fractional photothermolysis. *Lasers in Surgery and Medicine*. 2005;Suppl 17:32.
32. Wanner M, Tanzi EL, Alster TS. Fractional photothermolysis: treatment of facial and nonfacial cutaneous photodamage with a 1550-nm erbium-doped fiber laser. *Dermatol Surg*. 2007;33(1):23–28.
33. Alajlan A, Alsuwaidan S. Acne scars in ethnic skin treated with both non-ablative fractional 1550 nm and ablative fractional CO_2 lasers: comparative retrospective analysis with recommended guidelines. *Lasers Surg Med*. 2001;43:787–791.
34. Hruza G, Taub AF, Collier SL, Mulholland SR. Skin rejuvenation and wrinkle reduction using a fractional radiofrequency system. *J Drugs Dermatol*. 2009;8(3):259–265.
35. Brightman L, Goldman MP, Taub AF. Sublative rejuvenation: experience with a new fractional radiofrequency system for skin rejuvenation and repair. *J Drugs Dermatol*. 2009;8(11 Suppl):s9–13.

36. Taub AF, Garretson CB. Treatment of acne scars of skin types II to V by sublative fractional bipolar radiofrequency and bipolar radiofrequency combined with diode laser. *J Clin Aesthet Dermatol*. 2011;4(10):18–27.
37. Man J, Goldberg DJ. Safety and efficacy of fractional bipolar radiofrequency treatment in Fitzpatrick skin types V-VI. *J Cosmet Laser Ther*. 2012;14(4):179–83.
38. Ciocon DH, Rokhsar CK. "Laser treatment of pigmentation associated with photoaging". In: Carniol PJ, Sadick NS, eds. *Clinical Procedures in Laser Skin Rejuvenation*. Boca Raton, FL: Informa Press; 2007.
39. Ciocon DH, Rokhsar CK. Fractional resurfacing of difficult to treat anatomical locations. In: Mckenna J, Clements S, eds. *US Dermatology Review*. London: Touch Briefings; 2007.
40. Avram MM, Tope WD, Yu T, Szachowicz E, Nelson JS. Hypertrophic scarring of the neck following ablative fractional carbon dioxide laser resurfacing. *Lasers Surg Med*. 2009;41(3):185–188.
41. Fife D, Fitzpatrick RE, Zachary CB. Complications of fractional CO_2 laser resurfacing: four cases. *Lasers Surg Med*. 2009;41:179–184.

CHAPTER 37

Fillers

Jason Emer & Heidi A. Waldorf

INTRODUCTION

Much has been written about selection of filling agents and anatomic considerations for soft-tissue augmentation. An increased understanding of the volumetric changes that occur with aging and their effect on our perception of beauty has changed the way we use fillers over the last decade. Rather than filling individual wrinkles, modern soft-tissue augmentation focuses on replenishing lost fat pads, providing increased structural support and volume, and constructing facial contours. Injections may be done by bolus to lift or by fanning along vectors. In recent years, the availability of new tools has introduced still more possibilities for variation in the injection procedure. Although manufacturers may claim improved cosmetic results and fewer complications, is it the product being injected, the tool used to inject, the injection technique, the injector or a combination that is responsible? Herein, we describe injection techniques with and without the use of blunt-tipped microcannulas for facial contouring, and we outline when and where their use can provide a less traumatic, reliable, and versatile technical option for the treatment of facial aging.

OVERVIEW

Blunt-tipped microcannulas are sterile, disposable (single use) surgical steel injection tips available in a range of gauges and lengths (Fig. 37-1). They may be used in places or situations in which there is a significant risk of the cutting bevels of the hypodermic needle causing tissue trauma and vessel injury with resultant complications. Most short-term adverse effects, such as pain, erythema, edema, and ecchymosis, are considered to be expected injection-related complications and are more from the injection technique rather than the filler itself.[1,2] Although there are reports of serious complications such as skin necrosis, blindness, or stroke, complications of soft-tissue filling generally can be avoided with proper technique and patient and material selection.[3–5]

Blunt-tipped cannulas have a long-standing history of use in the injection of autologous fat (fat transfer) for volume restoration and have only become popular for dermal fillers over the past few years following their introduction in Europe.[6,7] The large size and flexibility of these cannulas makes them suitable for use with dermal fillers in the subcutaneous and supraperiosteal planes, although smaller sizes (larger gauges) are available and may be useful for intradermal injections, which require greater precision in their placement.[8,9] The proposed benefits, as compared to sharp needle injection, include the reduction in postinjection bleeding and ecchymosis (atraumatic injection), a decrease in the number of injection entry points, decreased risk of inadvertent intravascular injection, and less patient discomfort during injection (Table 37-1).[10] Additively, this equates to a reduced risk of adverse events. Other potential benefits include the increased ability for large volume or panfacial volume restoration from a single entry point, increased precision and safety in higher risk areas (i.e., glabella, nasal dorsum, temple, orbital rim, and neck), and better control of product placement in a single level plane. This limits downtime and increases patient satisfaction. Studies also suggest the potential for collagenesis

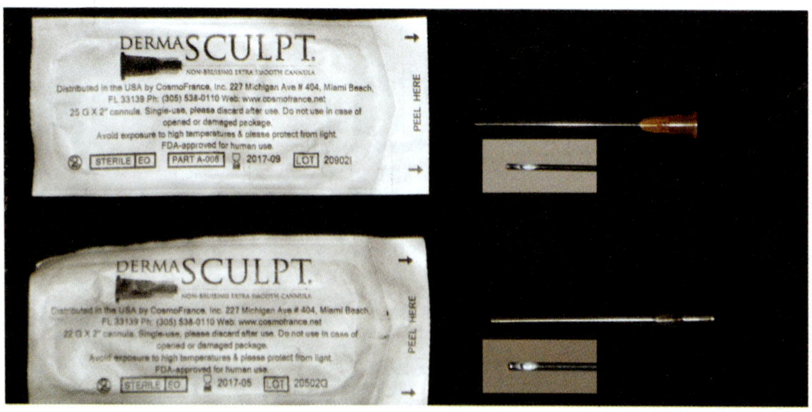

Figure 37-1 Microcannula examples. There are many types of microcannulas, but all have blunt ends and distal port sites in common (see insets). This company (DermaSculpt, CosmoFrance, Inc.) makes hubs of various colors to correlate with the microcannula gauge. Various lengths are available, but the most commonly used in dermatology range from 1 to 2.75 in.

TABLE 37-1

Advantages and Disadvantages of Microcannulas Versus Sharp Needles

	Advantages	Disadvantages
Needle	Quick Supplied with product Inexpensive	Sharp Increased puncture sites Risk of neurovascular injury in danger zones Increased risk of bruising and swelling
Microcannula	Blunt-tipped	Time consuming
	Increased safety in neurovascular danger zones	Requires sharp needle for initial puncture (entry site)
	Fewer puncture sites	Difficult to use in thick/sebaceous skin or in areas of previous trauma, surgery, or scarring
	Decreased risk of bruising and swelling	More expensive
	Subcision effect may promote neocollagenesis	Requires increased technical skill for use

from multiple back-and-forth subdermal passes of the microcannula (fanning injection technique), even without the addition of fillers, via the mechanical stimulation of fibroblasts.[11,12] Increased treatment times (depending on experience level) and added cost/procedural steps may hinder naive injectors. Some fear overstatement of the safety profile of these cannulas and report that smaller gauge (30 gauge) blunt-tipped cannulas, especially if inflexible, can puncture vessels, nerves, and the orbital septum.[13] Large-bore blunt cannulas have been reported to cause middle cerebral artery infarction and vision loss, at least in the fat transfer literature, more so with high-pressure bolus injections.[14,15] Nonetheless, choosing the smallest bore flexible cannula (preferably 22 gauge or larger), using constant movement (avoiding static injections), avoiding high injection pressures by depositing small aliquots of product, injecting into multiple planes so as to avoid wide tunnels, evenly distributing product and preventing pooling, as well as understanding surgical anatomy, can promote good aesthetic outcomes.

A study of 26 patients injected with a hyaluronic acid filler (HA; Restylane, Q-Med, Sweden) using reinforced, rigid microcannulas (Pix'L, Esthetique, Ltd., Limassol, Cyprus) into the periorbital and eyebrow region demonstrated high rates of patient satisfaction (85% reported satisfied or very satisfied) with fewer complications, including irregularities, inflammatory reactions, and ecchymosis (three cases of bruising, four cases of lymphatic stasis) as compared to published results.[16] Patients were evaluated immediately after injection, 10 to 25 days afterward, and 3 months post treatment. It was noted that product was evenly distributed throughout the treatment areas and produced excellent aesthetic improvement with a low rate of hematoma or posttreatment edema.

Furthermore, a recent double-blind, randomized, controlled clinical trial comparing the use of a proprietary 21 gauge, 30 mm metallic blunt-tipped cannula to a standard sharp needle (30 gauge, 13 mm) for nasolabial fold augmentation (n = 25) reported fewer side effects, such as pain, edema, redness, and hematoma, with the new tool as compared to the standard needle.[17] On evaluation 3 days after injection, there was a bilateral decrease in the Modified Fitzpatrick Wrinkle Scale (MFWS) indicating clinical improvement in both of the nasolabial folds.

Most recently, a study of 96 patients aged 30 to 76 years old desiring either facial, décolleté, or hand augmentation were treated with an HA filler (Restylane or Perlane; Juvederm, Allergan, Irvine, CA; Hydrelle, Ankia Therapeutics, Inc., Bedford, MA) either with a microcannula (DermaSculpt, CosmoFrance, Inc., Miami Beach, FL; 18, 22, 25, 27, or 30 gauge; 25, 38, 50, 70 mm) with a blunt-tip and side port or hypodermic sharp needle (27 gauge, 0.5 or 1.5 in). Overall clinical improvement was equivalent with both implantation devices but pain, bruising, and ecchymosis were reduced with the use of the blunt-tipped microcannulas, leading to faster recovery times in these patients.[18]

It should also be noted that while the approval of blunt-tipped microcannulas enables them to be used for fluid injection or aspiration, use with soft-tissue fillers is considered off-label by the United States Food and Drug Administration (USFDA). This caveat should be noted to the patient and included in the informed consent prior to injection. Each filler product is specifically approved for use with the sharp needle(s) that are packaged with it. Four brands of blunt-tipped microcannulas are currently approved by the USFDA as 510(k) Hypodermic Single Lumen Needle devices: DermaSculpt, TSK (distributed by Merz Aesthetics, Inc., San Mateo, CA), Magic Needle (Needle Concept, France), and SoftFil (SoftFil-USA, Kerylos Corporation, Los Angeles, CA).

INJECTION PATTERN AND INJECTION TECHNIQUES

GENERAL APPROACHES

Appropriate injection technique can help ensure successful outcome and limit the risk of contour irregularities or excessively superficial placement with subsequent patient dissatisfaction. Serious complications from administration are rare, but can occur, including vascular occlusion or embolism with resulting skin necrosis, blindness, or stroke. Many injection patterns are recognized such as fanning, serial puncture, cross-hatching, and linear threading; the choice of pattern is based on the location to be injected and the product utilized (Fig. 37-2).[19]

Recently, two novel techniques have been defined that offer alternative means of delivering the product.[20,21] The tower technique involves injecting filler in a vertical manner (at a 90 degree angle to the base of the injection site) and while withdrawing the syringe, small deposits of filler are placed between the tissue planes to help build

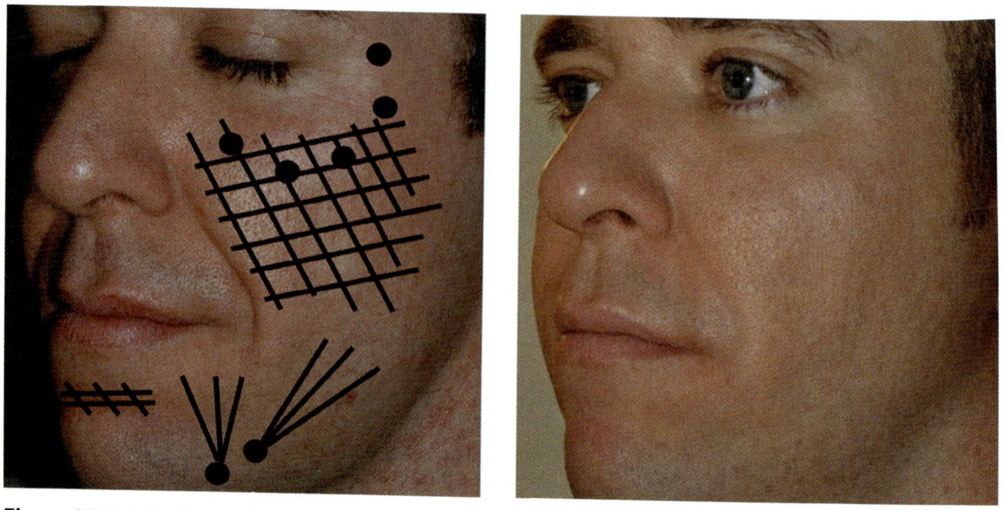

Figure 37-2 Injection technique with sharp needle. Before (*left*) and after (*right*) 3.0 cc of calcium hydroxylapatite (Radiesse) mixed with 0.3 cc of 2% lidocaine with 1:100,000 epinephrine to the midface (cross-hatching and supraperiosteal depot) as well as the marionette and mandibular angle (supraperiosteal depot and fanning). 0.8 cc of a hyaluronic acid gel filler (Juvederm Ultra) mixed with 0.1 cc of 2% lidocaine with 1:100,000 epinephrine was used (linear threading) on the lower cutaneous lip/chin for contouring and lifting. Notice, the nasolabial fold itself was not treated, but a clear improvement is noted.

"towers" or "columns" in the tissue. This limits lateralization of filler and helps for lifting (vertical extension) as it provides self-support. This technique has been recommended in areas where no base is present, such as the nasolabial folds, marionette lines, the upper and lower lip, and cheeks. The vertical supraperiosteal depot technique uses a single, small depot of soft-tissue filler material placed on the bone or periosteum. The orbital rim, zygomatic bone, mandible, bridge of the nose, and the entire forehead can utilize this technique. Finally, the "fern" or "bridging" technique involves a combination of linear threading and serial puncture. The needle is inserted perpendicular to the fold and advanced a few millimeters away from the fold. This procedure is repeated along the extent of the fold in multiple passes alternating between the left and right sides of the fold. A scaffold of material lifts and supports the wrinkle. The "fern" technique is particularly beneficial along the length of the nasolabial fold or marionette lines.

The proper use of these patterns can help the injector more uniformly treat the desired areas with fewer side effects. Glogau et al. found in a prospective, blinded, controlled study of 283 patients randomized to midface volume correction of the nasolabial folds and oral commissures with HA filling agents (Restylane or Perlane) that local adverse events following injection were related to investigator technique and not to differences in the intrinsic properties of the filler or needle size.[22] The elements found to be associated with an increased risk of adverse events included injection techniques that increased the likelihood of dissection in the subepidermal plane such as fan-like projection, rapid injection, rapid flow rates, and higher volumes. Interestingly, injection techniques that increased epidermal damage or subcutaneous contact such as serial puncture or deep depot injections had no effect on adverse events. Thus, proper technique is essential to successful outcomes.

Unlike needles, cannulas have blunt-tips/ends and flexible or rigid bodies that offer increased safety by decreasing the chance for trauma to the surrounding soft tissue, nerves, or vessels. This correlates with less pain, bruising, and swelling post procedure. Decreased risk of ecchymosis is a major advantage especially in areas such as the nasojugal fold, upper eyelid, prejowl sulcus, and perioral regions in which bruising is commonplace (Fig. 37-3). Injectors may be able to perform the fan-like injection technique without the increased risk of side effects from fanning with hypodermic needles. The degree of flexibility (vs. rigidity) of the microcannulas can impact their clinical behavior. Longer (38 mm or more) and smaller gauge (27 or more) microcannulas tend to be more flexible, while shorter (25 mm or less) and larger gauge (23 or less) are more rigid. Physical characteristics can affect clinical outcome, and will influence the passage of filler through tissue as well as injection patterns.

ATLAS GUIDE TO INJECTION WITH MICROCANNULA

The approach to using cannulas is to properly clean the skin with alcohol and/or chlorhexidine, evaluate the skin areas to be treated, and decide on an entry point (Fig. 37-4A,B). Cannula injection is not completely atraumatic, and the initial entry point requires anesthesia and puncture with a needle larger than the cannula (typically 21 or 23 gauge) to penetrate the skin just beyond the bevel before cannula insertion (Fig. 37-4C,D). If bruising does occur during the use of microcannulas, it is typically at the insertion site of the pilot needle or in areas of increased tissue resistance (i.e., dense beard area, fibrosis from previous surgery, or acne scarring) or fragile vessels. A recent consensus statement reported the use of a 23 gauge sharp needle for 25 gauge microcannula and a

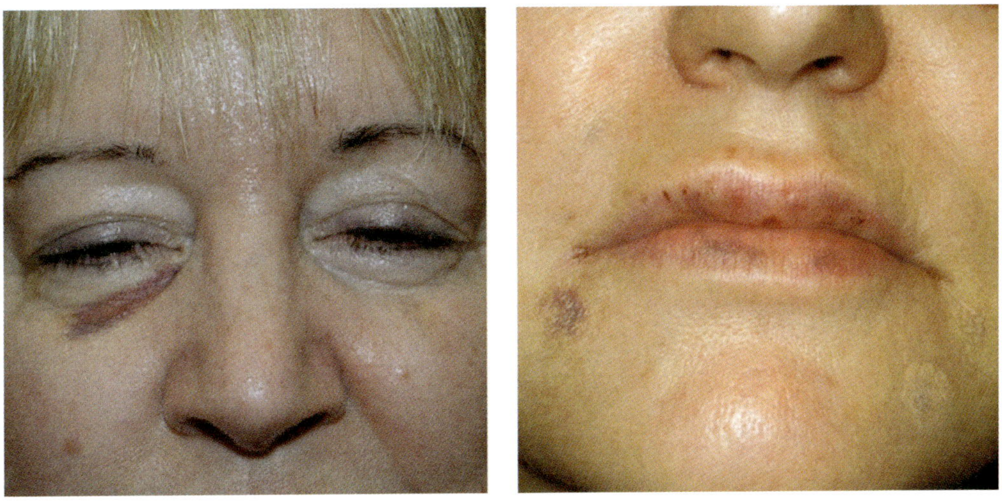

Figure 37-3 Ecchymosis of the tear trough (*left*) and lips (*right*) after injection of hyaluronic acid gel filler (Juvederm Ultra) using sharp needle (31 gauge) injection. Of note, both patients were taking aspirin.

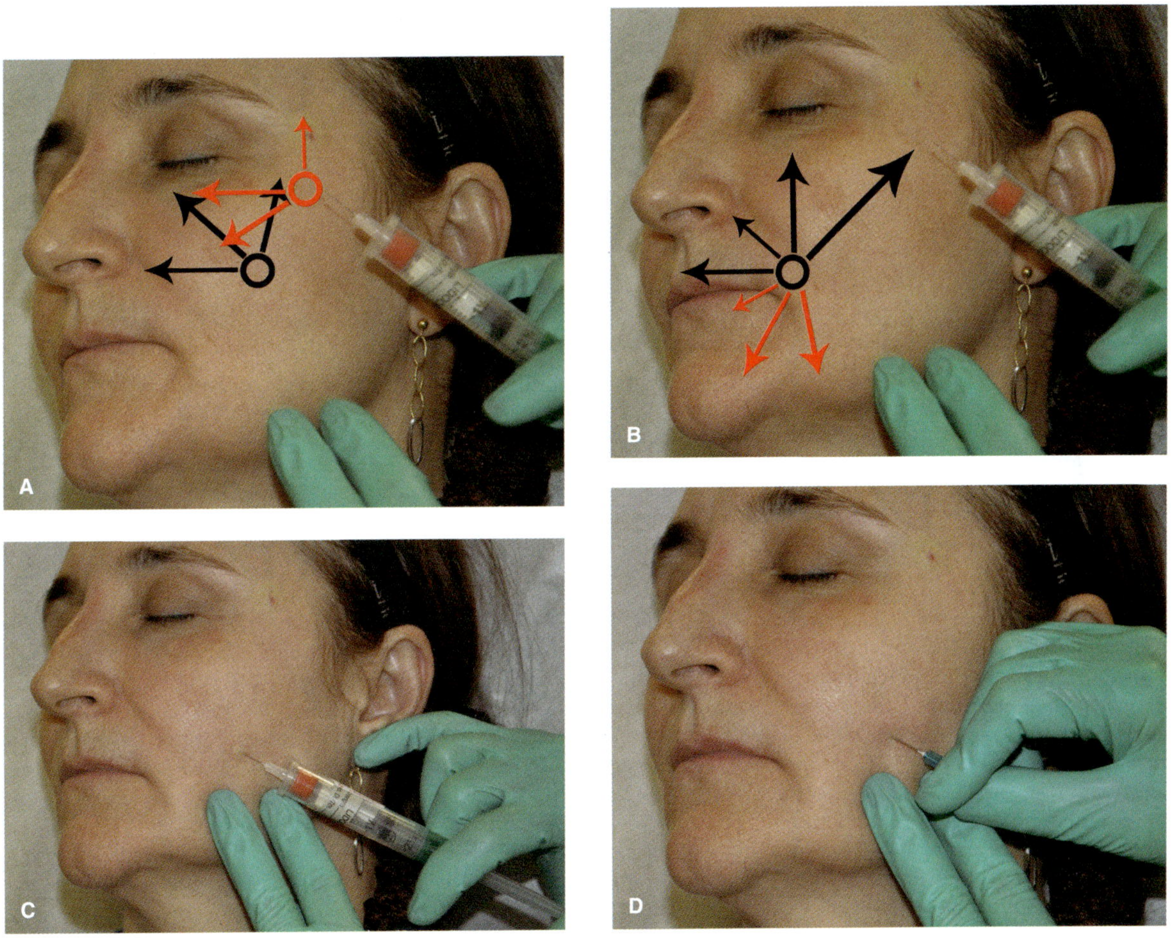

Figure 37-4 A, B. Using the midface (cheek/tear trough) as an example, a multitude of entry points can be used for microcannula insertion. Recontouring and volumization can be achieved from any of these sites. Optimal entry sites (*black arrows*) allow for a large area of treatment. Alternative sites (*red arrows*) allow for customized contouring and volumizing with the ability to treat nearby areas such as the temple or eyebrow for midface entry sites and nasolabial folds, cutaneous lip, and marionette lines/prejowl for upper cutaneous lip/lip corner entry sites. **C.** Anesthetic (2% lidocaine with 1:100,000 epinephrine) is injected intradermally into the area chosen as an entry site. **D.** Sharp needle (23 gauge) is punctured through the upper skin into the subcutaneous tissue to create a portal of entry for the microcannula. Care should be taken to limit superficial vessel injury and obtain the correct plane for insertion. (*continued*)

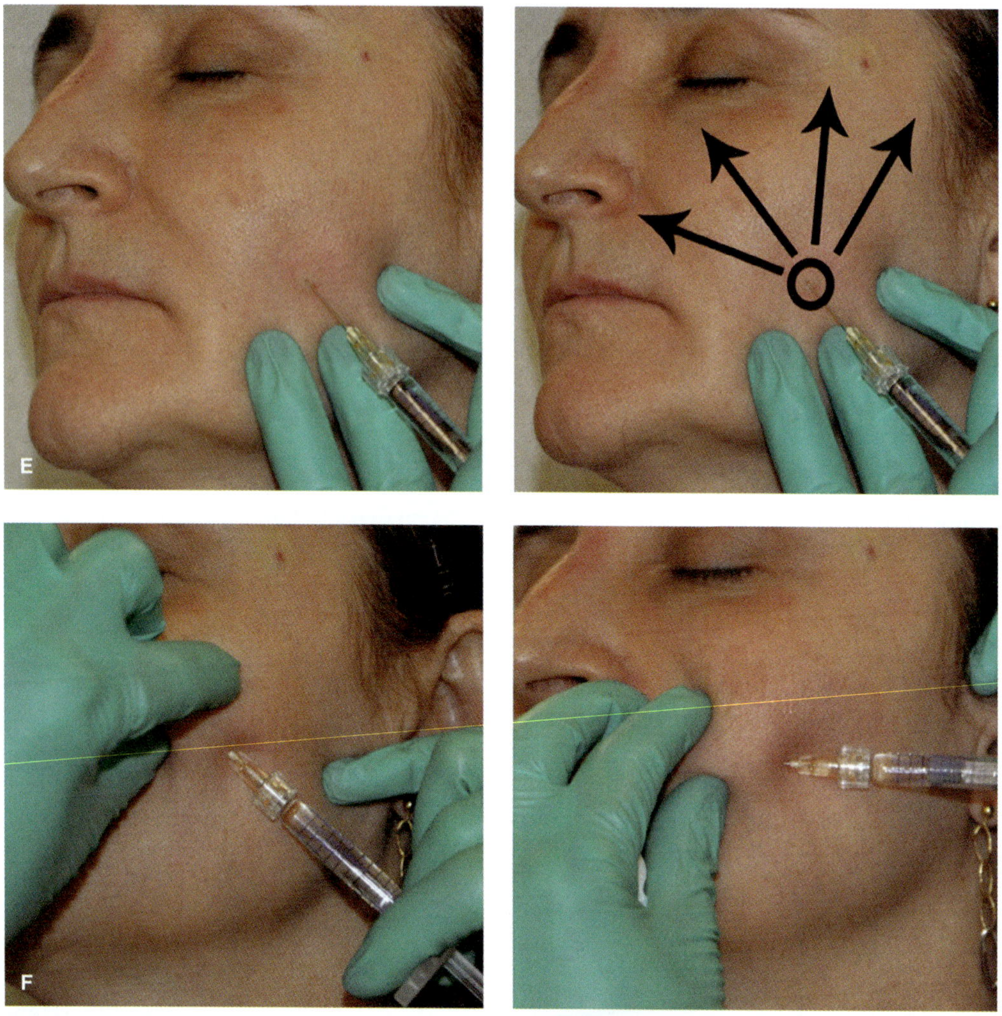

Figure 37-4 *(Continued)* **E.** The cannula is inserted into the subcutaneous layer (*left*) and multiple, retrograde linear threads are injected at vectors chosen to revolumize and recontour (*right*) the midface. Note one entry point allows for quick treatment of a large cosmetic area, with little, if any, pain. **F.** Pinching of the skin ensures proper placement of the microcannula in the correct plane, helps limit the risk of neurovascular injury, and allows for easier placement of filler while threading in vectors. It is important to retract the microcannula and redirect when switching vectors so an appropriate new tunnel can be created without overlapping filler planes.

26 gauge sharp needle for 27 gauge microcannula entry.[10] As the pilot needle is close in size to the microcannula, some injectors prefer to "pinch" the skin around the needle with the noninjecting/nondominant hand and have an assistant pull out the needle while their focus stays on the puncture site. The authors find that the use of a larger gauge pilot needle (21 or 23 gauge for 25 or 27 gauge microcannula entry) and using lidocaine with epinephrine to anesthetize and blanch the entry site so as to more easily see the resultant opening, allows the injector to remove the pilot needle without the help of an assistant, thereby reducing the risk of needle stick. If it is difficult to locate the entry site after the initial puncture, rubbing of the area with the sterile, gloved fingers can produce slight bleeding. The blunt-tipped, flexible microcannula is then maneuvered through the newly created entrance and positioned into the planned area of volume enhancement (Fig. 37-4E). Lifting the skin to guide the cannula through the plane and direction desired is helpful (Fig. 37-4F). The cannulas have a Luer-Lock tip and plastic hub to accommodate the most commonly used filler syringes from various companies (Fig. 37-1).

A major advantage of microcannulas is that with a single or double puncture site an entire lip, nasolabial fold, cheek, forehead, hand, mandible, or décolleté can be injected. A disadvantage is that anesthesia is typically required at the desired insertion sites (Table 37-1). Some have reported the use of topical anesthesia with a lidocaine-based mixture locally or with a polyvinyl gel composed of tetracaine 5% and lidocaine 5% (Anesthetic Peel-Off Mask, compounded by ApothéCure, Dallas, TX) over an entire area. Some time (about 30–60 minutes) later the cream/mask is removed and the area is cleansed, leaving it ready for injection. Injectable lidocaine with or without epinephrine (~0.05–0.1 cc/site) can be injected over the anticipated area for quicker treatment times. Niamtu reported the use of intraoral injections of lidocaine with epinephrine for augmentation of the lips, perioral, and nasolabial fold areas.[23] Nerve blocks can be used in an anxious patient or those with a low pain tolerance, but are likely unnecessary and can distort the anatomical site prior to injection, leading to unwanted clinical results such as improper product placement or overtreatment. The authors have found that utilizing injectable anesthetic for the insertion site and filling agents containing or mixed with anesthetic eliminates the need for additional topical or injectable anesthetic.

PEARLS OF INJECTION TECHNIQUES

The nasolabial folds, glabella, philtral columns, fine perioral and periocular rhytides, lips, forehead lines, and oral commissures do well with serial puncture or linear threading techniques. With serial puncture, multiple small depot injections are made along a wrinkle or crease, which allows for accurate material placement. The skin of the treatment area must be held taut between the thumb and forefinger as the needle tip is guided horizontally until it just barely penetrates the epidermis. Care must be taken to ensure that each injection is of equal volume and sequential so the overall picture is that of a smooth, continuous line that lifts or fills out the fold. Steady, continuous pressure on the syringe plunger produces a flow of material into the dermis. Molding and massaging can help to ensure that gaps are filled in and soften minor irregularities post treatment. Of note, HAs should be injected into the mid-to-deep dermis as to avoid the Tyndall effect (blue discoloration due to superficial placement) and superficial lumps and bumps.

Belotero (Merz Aesthetics, Inc., Franksville, WI), recently approved by the USFDA as a 1 mL prefilled glass syringe containing 22.5 mg/mL of crosslinked HA to be injected with 30 gauge, 0.5 in needles, can be implanted into the upper dermis with a lower risk of the aforementioned side effects due to its unique structure and ability to integrate into the dermis. Poly-L-lactic acid (PLLA; Sculptra, Sanofi-Aventis, Bridgewater, NJ) and calcium hydroxylapatite (CaHA; Merz Aesthetics, Inc., Franksville, WI) should be injected in the deep dermal, subcutaneous, or periosteal planes and superficial placement should be avoided.

Linear threading works well for the lips (along the "white roll"), nasolabial folds, lateral zygoma, angle of the mandible, and preauricular areas. The correct technique involves inserting the full length of the needle into the middle of the wrinkle or area to be enhanced and creating a tunnel that will be filled with the product by either an anterograde (while needle is advanced) or retrograde injection (while needle is withdrawn). Both techniques are acceptable and give excellent cosmetic results. Some may feel that the anterograde method is safer as it allows the material being injected to "push away" small cutaneous vessels and nerves and may decrease complications, most notably bruising and swelling. However, in areas that are highly vascular such as the glabella or lip, a retrograde method may be a better choice as it decreases the likelihood of an intra-arterial injection. The potential spaces in the vermillion border ("white roll") and philtral columns allow easy product flow and placement with antegrade injection.

For very large areas such as the cheek, midface, and marionette lines, the cross-hatching or fanning technique can be very effective. Cross-hatching works by creating a series of linear threads evenly spaced in a progressive grid, similar to a scaffold that works to ensure a large space is supported and filled. Several levels may be needed to help fill and lift the area of treatment, especially in the midface where there is no osseous backing of facial support. Fanning is similar to linear threading except that the needle is not completely withdrawn and is advanced in a different location (clockwise or counterclockwise) allowing for the same injection site to be used to fill a particular area. This limits the number of skin punctures needed and may decrease the risk of surface bruising and swelling.[24,25] However, the process of fanning the needle horizontally through the skin increases the chance of encountering small vessels and, therefore, carries a risk of deeper bruising if using a hypodermic sharp needle, and a lower risk if using blunt-tipped microcannulas. Alternatively, use of the depot method, where larger volumes of low viscosity product are injected and then massaged or molded to facial contours, limits both surface and deeper needle movement. Microcannulas should not be used for serial puncture or microaliquot injection techniques (including depot injections); this should be reserved for use with sharp needles.

AREA- AND PRODUCT-SPECIFIC CONSIDERATIONS

Physicians currently working with blunt-tipped microcannulas believe that there is a great benefit to using them, and that they achieve more pronounced volume restoration with fewer entry points. Longer microcannulas allow treatment of large areas and easy refinement in facial contours as compared to longer needles, which need more precision during injection and have increased tissue resistance in the subdermal plane, as compared to cannulas tracking in the subcutis (Table 37-2).

TABLE 37-2
Practical Pearls for the Use of Microcannulas

Select the smallest number of entry points to limit injection-related side effects
Use sharp needle of larger gauge than chosen microcannula size (e.g., 21 gauge needle for use of a 22 gauge microcannula)
Longer lengths (50 mm or more) for large placement areas
Short lengths (38 mm or less) for fine-tuning procedures or smaller treatment areas
Large gauges (18–25) for high-viscosity fillers and larger fill areas
Small gauges (27–30) for low-viscosity fillers and superficial placement
Placement of product should be in the deep subdermal, subcutaneous, or periosteal planes; avoid intradermal injection
Use a broad, multidirectional, fanning technique for even distribution of filler in large areas
Not for superficial injection of fine rhytides or for supraperiosteal depot injections of product
Optimal in neurovascular danger zones to lessen risk of injury

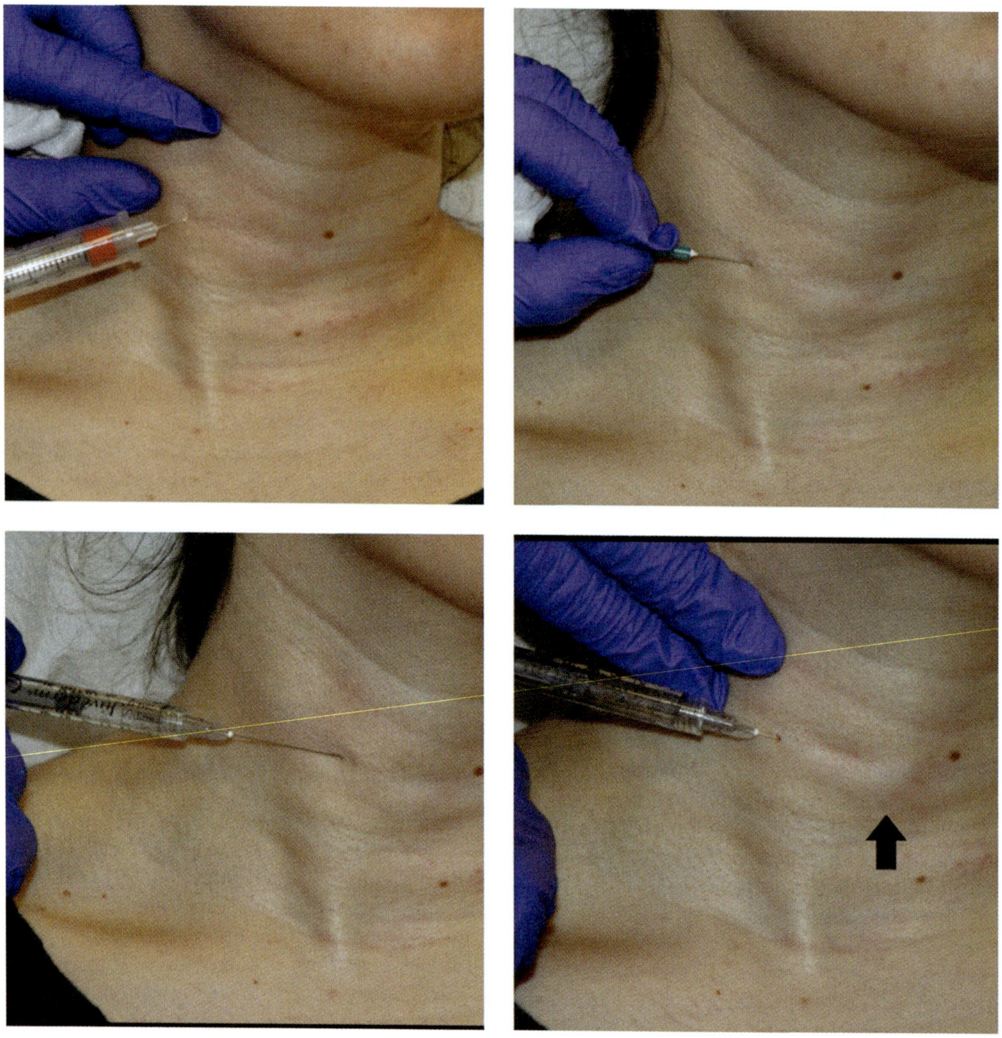

Figure 37-5 Microcannula injection for neck lines. Two percent lidocaine with 1:100,000 epinephrine is injected at a chosen entry site (*top left*) and sharp needle (23 gauge) is used to create portal of entry (*top right*). Microcannula (27 gauge, 50 mm) is inserted into the appropriate subcutaneous plane (*bottom left*) and hyaluronic acid filler (Juvederm Ultra) diluted 1:1 with 2% lidocaine is implanted in retrograde linear threads along the wrinkle crease. Note the tip of the cannula (*black arrow*) upon full insertion (*bottom right*). Longer cannulas lengths (50 mm or higher) are useful in areas such as the neck where large surface areas are required to be treated.

A recent consensus panel on the use of blunt-tipped microcannulas suggested the greatest utility from using 27 gauge, 1.25 in long sharp needles when injecting CaHA into the midface and the 22 gauge, 70 mm (2.75 in) blunt-tipped microcannulas or the 25 gauge, 1.5 in long sharp needle for the use of PLLA. One of the panel members has been utilizing a 22 gauge blunt-tipped microcannulas with a length of 50 mm (2 in) or longer for all facial areas. Nonetheless, as described previously, the specific characteristics and design of the cannula as well as the product chosen are both needed to determine the best injection technique.

For large areas of volume loss such as the cheeks, nasolabial folds, temples, mandible, chest, and neck (décolleté), longer cannulas (38 mm or more) will be required (Figs. 37-5 and 37-6). Larger gauges should be used with CaHA, PLLA, or more viscous HAs (such as Perlane, Juvederm Ultra Plus, Juvederm Voluma, unless thinned out). In the chest and neck (décolleté), temples or lips, a semirigid or fully rigid cannula may make injection easier, but has a higher risk of puncturing nearby vessels or nerves. For hand augmentation, very long, flexible cannulas (70 mm) are needed to cover the area using only a few entry points. Depending on the filler type, large-gauge (CaHA) or low-gauge (HAs) can be chosen.

In the periocular area including the tear trough and lateral eyebrow, many sizes and lengths of cannulas can be used depending on the area to be treated. The lips and perioral area (some argue) should never be injected with CaHa or PLLA as there is a high risk of nodule or lump/bump formation due to the high rate of muscle movement and the potential for granuloma formation and clumping with these products. A small gauge (27 or 25) and long length (38 or 50 mm) cannula is needed to cover the entire area through one entry site.

Overall, blunt-tipped microcannulas appear to be superior to sharp needles for the injection of fillers with regard to safety, but they do not replace them. In fact, needles are still necessary for fine-tuning asymmetries, areas of

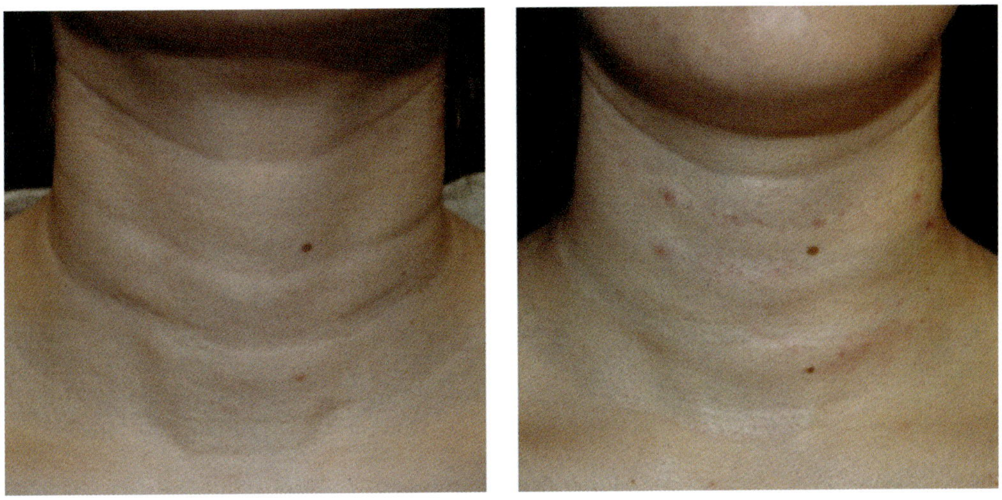

Figure 37-6 Before (*left*) and after (*right*) hyaluronic acid filler (Juvederm Ultra) injection with microcannula (27 gauge, 50 mm) for unwanted neck lines. Significant improvement is noted with minimal bruising, swelling, or erythema. Pinpoint bruising can be noted at areas of local injection of anesthesia and needle puncture entry sites.

under-treatment, the lip tubercles or philtral columns, for superficial placement including very small perioral or periocular lines, crepe skin on the lateral midface/preauricular, in the upper cheek/lower eyelid/tear trough, or for depot injections, especially periosteal injections on the mandible, zygoma, temporal fossa, or lateral orbital rim.

Microcannulas can be a first-line option for deep filler injection to areas of diffuse volume loss, but combining them with sharp needles to address superficial changes and focal volume loss can give an optimal balance of safety and efficacy with volume restoration plus contouring and shaping. Microcannulas are the authors' tool of choice for the upper face including the tear troughs, midcheek, temples, eyebrow, and forehead, as well as whenever the plunger on a syringe cannot be pulled back before injection. Thus, when using PLLA, a liquid solution, microcannulas are not necessary because intravascular injection is more easily avoided (Fig. 37-7). On the other hand, the plunger on a syringe of CaHA cannot be pulled backward, so use of fanning technique with a cannula provides an alternative to supraperiosteal bolus injection to reduce complications.

MICROCANNULA INJECTION TECHNIQUES BY LOCATION

TEMPLES. Temporal lifting is of the greatest benefit to individuals with signs of aging around the eyes and forehead. This procedure lifts the eyebrows, reduces crow's feet lines, contours the outer area of the eye, softens the hooding of the outer eyelid, and rids the person of a skeletonized appearance.[26] Those with temporal recession often report a perceived increase in age, disease status (HIV), or drug use (amphetamines). Some simply have had a recent profound weight loss and feel less youthful and upset over their sunken appearance. Thus, rejuvenation in this area can have a great effect both on a person's self-perception and the way in which others perceive them.[27]

Depending on the degree of temporal recession and the length of cannula chosen, as few as one to two entry points may be all that are required for rejuvenation in this location. Although all filling agents have been used, traditionally CaHA and/or PLLA are the primary products chosen as they provide a substantial amount of volumization with the need for less product and have longer-lasting results as compared to HAs. However, the introduction of a new HA (Juvederm Voluma) in the United States with better lifting

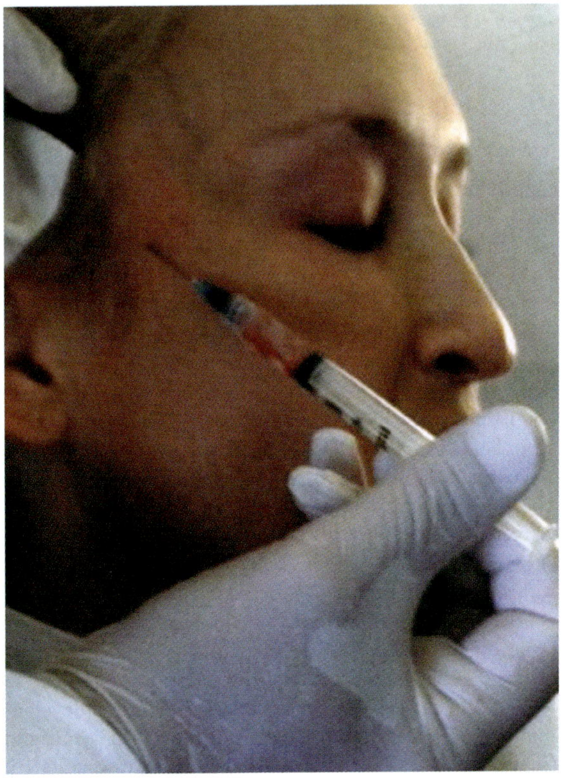

Figure 37-7 Aspiration prior to injection is much easier with poly-L-lactic acid as its consistency is fluid. Blood aspirate indicates an intravascular location of the needle and signals the practitioner to stop the procedure, remove the needle, and hold pressure over the area.

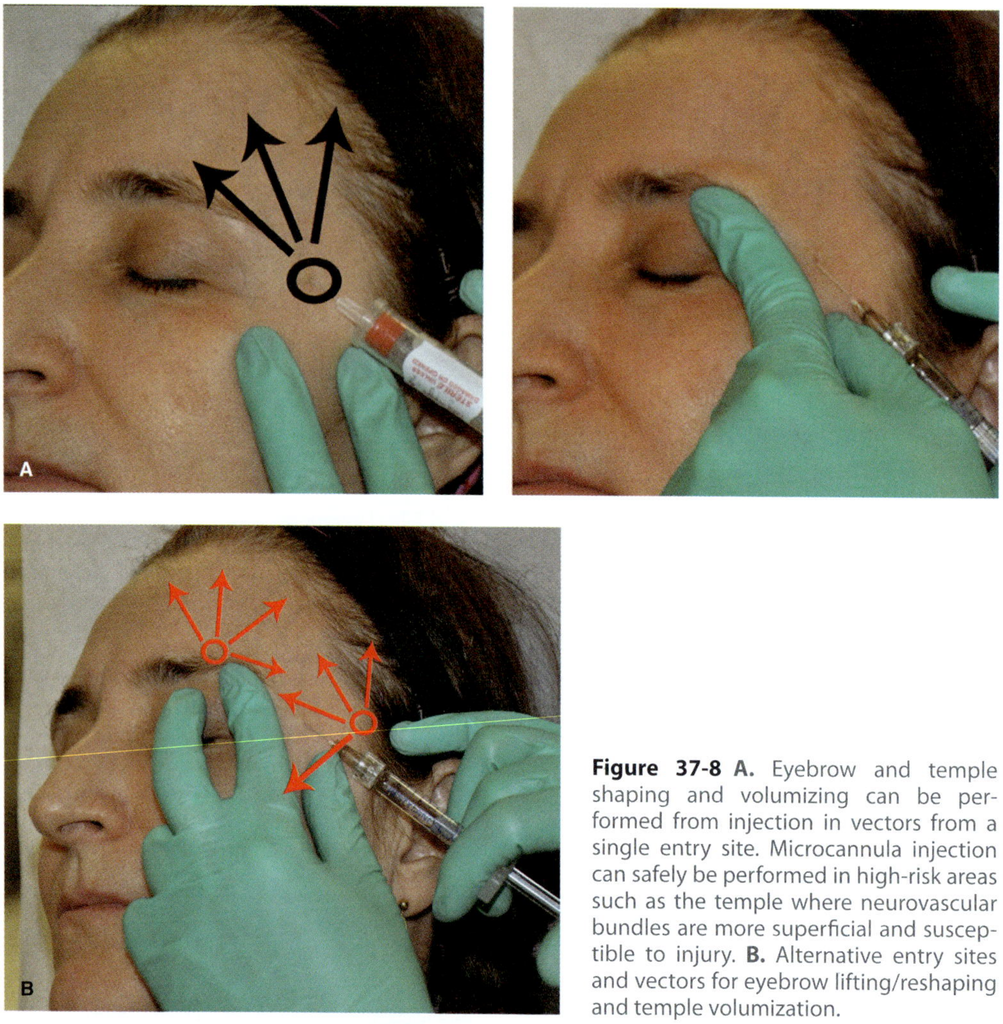

Figure 37-8 A. Eyebrow and temple shaping and volumizing can be performed from injection in vectors from a single entry site. Microcannula injection can safely be performed in high-risk areas such as the temple where neurovascular bundles are more superficial and susceptible to injury. **B.** Alternative entry sites and vectors for eyebrow lifting/reshaping and temple volumization.

capacity may change these recommendations. All fillers in this location have proven clinically effective and safe.[28–31]

With any gauge (ranging from 30 gauge for thinner HAs, to 27 gauge for CaHA, and 25 gauge for PLLA), 1 to 1.5 in sharp needle, vertically oriented depot injections are placed in a periosteal location along the temporal fossa (sphenoid and temporal bones) until adequate augmentation is seen. Some will use a single entry point midway between the lateral canthus and the tragus just superior to the zygomatic arch. Palpation of the temporal artery just anterior to the tragus/helix above the temporomandibular joint (TMJ) will prevent unanticipated puncturing of the artery or nearby vein. This area is high risk as it houses the temporal nerve and vessels, so care should be taken to avoid medial and superior injections that put the needle in a compromising zone. For this reason, blunt-tipped microcannulas may be preferred in this location to facilitate safer injections, especially in the more superficial planes. Deeper planes contain no anatomical structures that could influence the development of complications. Microcannula (flexible or semirigid) sizes ranging from 22 to 25 gauge, 38 to 70 mm in length are preferred for vectoring or fanning techniques. Serial puncture or large-volume depot injections should be done only with sharp needles along the periosteum. Entry points for the blunt-tipped microcannula include superior and lateral to the lateral canthus along the orbital rim, along the zygomatic arch midway between the hair line/helical rim and the lateral canthus/orbital rim, and along the superior hairline in a vector directly posterior to the lateral third of the eyebrow (Fig. 37-8A,B).

PERIORBITAL AND TEAR TROUGH.

Rejuvenation of the periorbital area gives significant patient satisfaction and optimal outcomes when performed properly.[32,33] Traditional injection with a sharp needle often requires multiple injection points; due to the increased vascularity in this area, significant bruising and bleeding can occur. Prolonged swelling ("festooning"), visible papules/product if injected superficially, and a Tyndall effect can also be seen if intradermal injections are not done fastidiously.[34,35] HA fillers are most commonly used, as PLLA and CaHA have been avoided due to their potential for causing asymmetry and nodule formation, although their use can be performed by an experienced injector with proper dilution.[36] A recent report demonstrated successful treatment of unwanted, improperly injected superficial CaHA with saline injections and erbium laser in the inferior periorbital area/eyelid.[37] With more commonly used deeper injection techniques (subcutaneous into fat pads and supraperiosteal), side effects are limited and large volume restoration and contouring can be performed.[38] Of importance, visual loss/change due to orbital infarction following filler injection has been documented in the literature, so meticulous injection technique and a thorough knowledge of anatomy are required to minimize the risk of catastrophic complications.[39–42]

For use of cannulas in the tear trough, some prefer a smaller diameter (27 or 30 gauge) and short (25 or 38 mm) length in the deep (subcutaneous or supraperiosteal) planes from an entry along the deformity or on the midcheek. However, the authors prefer approaching from the lateral cheek with a 25 or 27 gauge, 38 to 50 mm (1.5–2 in) cannula to reduce the risk of intravascular injection and reduce needle sticks near the lower lid, where there is a higher chance of subsequent ecchymosis or lymphedema (Fig. 37-4A). On the upper eyelid and below the eyebrow, better control can be obtained with shorter or semirigid cannulas. Longer (38 or 50 mm) and larger (25 or 22 gauge) cannulas can be used in multiple facial areas and if used in this area a single entry point placed in the superolateral midface (along the zygoma, lateral and inferior to the lateral canthus) gives access to both the lower eyelid and the lower forehead above the eyebrow, as well as access to the midface and tear trough.[10,18] In a recent case report, a single entry point inferior to the lateral canthus along the patient's tear trough deformity with subsequent insertion of a 27 gauge, 42 mm blunt, rigid microcannula demonstrated excellent clinical results without any patient discomfort or immediate bruising or swelling after 0.7 mL of an HA filler (into tear trough) was placed.[43] The single entry point has the benefits of limiting pain, bruising, and swelling, but also provides access to multiple facial sites at one time, thereby simplifying the injection technique. It is best to inject with a linear technique in a retrograde (while withdrawing) fashion. It is also recommended that the patient be injected in a seated rather than reclining position in order to achieve accurate filler placement and avoid overcorrection.

MIDDLE FACE – NASOLABIAL FOLDS AND CHEEKS.

Midface rejuvenation has undergone dramatic changes in recent years in both injection techniques and perception.[44] This has led to a paradigm shift in our therapeutic approach. Rather than using fillers to simply fill a line, with increased understanding of facial aging and changes that occur with the subcutaneous fat pads and craniofacial skeleton, we now account for the three-dimensional shape of the face, allowing for the use of fillers as lifting and sculpting agents. Tissue repositioning and contouring can be achieved by replacing atrophic and drooping fat pads with injection along the periosteum at areas of recession.

With the use of cannulas, large areas can be filled, lifted, and recontoured through few entrance points with almost no downtime. Vectoring the filler, along with injection directly into the fat pads, can lift the superficial skin drapery and provide a more natural, youthful appearance.

Possible entry points for the midface include just superior and lateral to the oral commissure on the upper cutaneous lip, giving easy access to the nasolabial folds, medial cheeks and marionette lines; in the central cheek midway between a line drawn posteriorly from the oral commissure and the superior helical rim (an alternative would be a lower entry point midway between a line drawn from the oral commissure and the tragus) providing full access to the medial and lateral cheeks including the zygomatic arch (Fig. 37-4A,B). Depending on the cannula length, as few as one or two entrance points can be used for complete midfacial treatment.

The midface requires longer cannulas (50 mm or more) to cover the large areas of volume loss. The 22 or 25 gauge sizes can be used for the most commonly used filler products (HA, CaHA, PLLA). Once the larger areas of loss have been refilled and contoured, focal areas of loss and the superficial drapery, reflecting a loss of elasticity from aging, can be addressed with sharp needle depot or small aliquot serial puncture techniques. HA filler superficially injected with a short needle (32 gauge, 4 mm mesotherapy needle) in a microdroplet injection technique (0.02 ml injections, to whole cheek, about 25 injections) was recently reported to target improvement in skin elasticity and provide excellent changes in appearance.[45] A fan-like injection technique with linear threads perpendicular to the direction of the smile lines in a superficial (subdermal) plane was used with the flexible blunt microcannula. The overall picture was that of a smoother skin surface and the disappearance of smile lines. For this technique, 27 to 30 gauge microcannulas, 38 mm or more in length, can be used. Long-term improvement from this technique comes from the pharmacologic characteristics of the filler product itself, as well as the mechanical stimulation (microtrauma) of the cannula through the plane of injection, promoting collagenesis. An advantage of utilizing a cannula for the midface is the ability to treat the pyriform aperture, an often neglected but important area to improve, from the same entry point and without using a sharp needle (Fig. 37-9).

LIPS AND LOWER FACE.

Flexible or rigid blunt-tipped microcannulas can be extremely useful in this area, as bruising and swelling are common complications from sharp needle injection. Niamtu[8] was the first to report the use of a rigid, blunt 0.9 mm (20 gauge), 5 cm fat injection microcannula to inject the entire lip and nasolabial fold with one entry point for each location (Fig. 37-10). An 18-gauge needle was used to make a puncture site at the site of injection (lateral vermillion border/oral commissure and along the inferior aspect of the nasolabial fold) and the microcannula was then inserted the entire length of the lip or fold and the filler injected in a retrograde, linear threading fashion. He concluded that there was less edema and bruising and a faster patient recovery as compared to using hypodermic needles.

The belly of the lip is an ideal location for use with microcannulas and the amount of filler can be tapered easily as the cannula is retracted to give more product placement in the middle of the lip and less as it is withdrawn laterally (Fig. 37-11). This gives a natural appearance rather than a "sausage"-type lip, which has no contour or shape. The vermillion is more difficult for cannula insertion although small gauge (27 or less) microcannulas can be used. Length will vary depending on the area to be treated, but longer lengths (50 mm or more) should rarely be needed. The vermillion border, Cupid's bow, philtral columns, and very fine perioral lines may require sharp needles for more precision when injecting.

The oral commissures can easily be treated with an entrance point directly lateral to the commissure, superolateral or inferolateral to the commissure, or a point superior to the prejowl sulcus. Areas where the microcannula should not be introduced include at the insertion of the

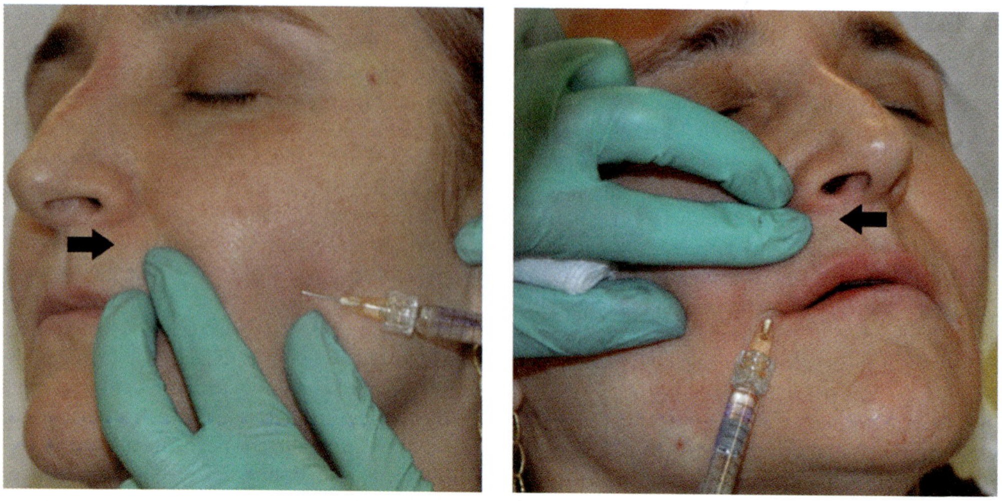

Figure 37-9 Cannula entry site options to reach the pyriform aperture (*black arrows*). The pyriform aperture is a heart- or pear-shaped opening in the skull that enlarges with age, influencing the shape and height of the nasal cartilaginous structures and upper cutaneous lip. Adding support to this area with soft-tissue filler can have a significant cosmetic influence on the shape of the upper cutaneous lip and nasal tip.

depressor anguli oris (DAO) muscle and platysma muscle on the mandibular angle. Various gauge diameters (22, 25, or 27), 38 mm or more in length, will be best for all filler types. It is best to proceed with caution when using CaHA or PLLA in the perioral areas as high movement due to the orbicularis oris muscle can increase the risk for nodule and granuloma formation. The lips should never be directly injected with CaHA or PLLA, even if significantly diluted.

The entire lower face including the mandibular angle/prejowl sulcus, chin, and lower cutaneous lip can all be accessed through an entrance point just superior and medial to the insertion of the DAO onto the mandible (Figs. 37-12 and 37-13). An additional site along the jawline just inferior to the ear lobule (similar sites used in neck liposuction) can access the entire preauricular area and mandibular angle. Longer microcannula lengths will be needed to access the entire length of the jaw (50 or 70 mm). Depot injections along the periosteum should still be performed with sharp needles; CaHA or PLLA are excellent products here. For the jawline itself, the senior author does prefer the use of a 25 or 27 gauge, 5/8 to 1 in needle to provide a sharp margin, especially in those who have had prior surgeries.

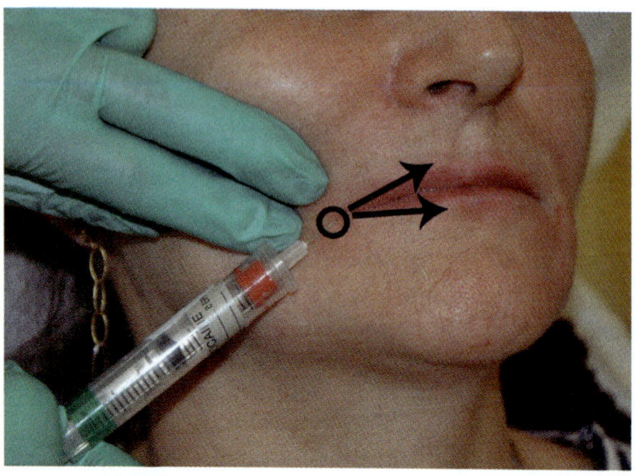

Figure 37-10 Anesthesia of microcannula entry site. Lip enhancement with microcannula is through one entry site at the lateral commissure. Opposing vectors can be used to contour and revolumize.

HANDS. Prominent signs of aging can be seen in a person's hands including increased vascularity, tendons, bony prominences, sun spots, and wrinkling of the skin (skin turgor), all a consequence of a complex interaction between genetics and environmental exposure (dermatoheliosis). Many have reported success with the use of fillers (mainly HA, CaHA, fat) in this area but proper technique is needed for adequate results.[46–49] A single entrance point on the dorsum of the hand at the wrist or in the finger web between the middle (third) and ring (fourth) fingers may be all that is needed. Alternatively, two entrance points can be made with the first between the index (second) and middle (third) fingers and the second between the ring (fourth) and little/pinky finger (fifth). Entering from the wrist and injecting proximal to distal provides easier access to the full surface of the hand but positioning the patient may be more difficult. Preferred microcannulas are 22 or 25 gauge and 38 mm. Fulton reported the use of an 18 gauge, 70 mm microcannula on the dorsum of the hand with excellent results 6 months after implantation of 2 mL of an HA filler.[18] Thus, the filler length and size should be customized to the individual and the product chosen.

If CaHA is used, and many consider this the filler of choice in this area due to its opacity, diluting 1:1 with 1% or 2% lidocaine lowers the viscosity of the filler and facilitates its spread through the tissue after implantation. The technique is not any different in this area than in others, but due to thin skin and increased vascularity it is imperative to choose an entry site that is not directly over a vein to prevent intravascular injection or increased bleeding/bruising from the procedure. The entry point is pinched and a needle (larger than the microcannula size

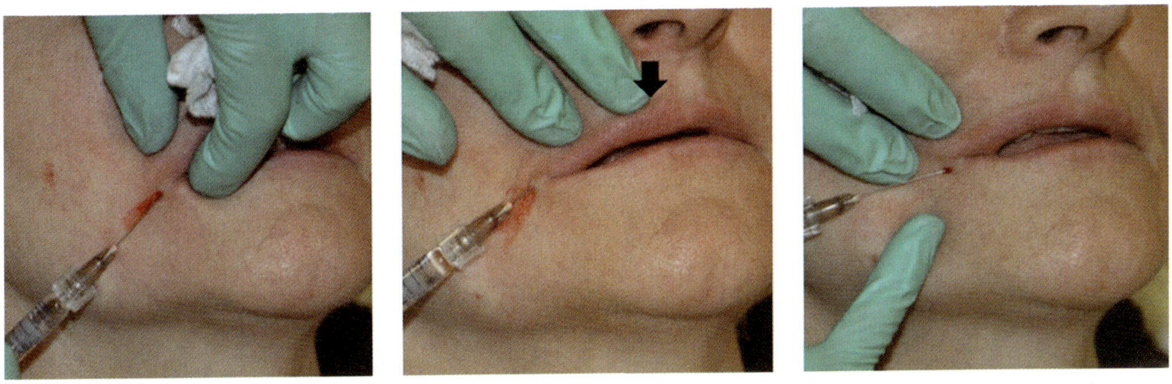

Figure 37-11 Microcannula (22 gauge, 50 mm) insertion into the lip is painless and easy due to blunt dissection (left). Upon full insertion, the tip of the cannula (*black arrow*, middle) can be noted at the medial portion of upper lip belly. Significant eversion and lip fullness are noted (right) after filler material (Restylane) is injected as the cannula is retracted.

chosen) is inserted to create a port site for the cannula. Without letting go, the needle is removed and the cannula inserted in a distal to proximal direction. The fanning injection technique should be utilized when using microcannulas for optimal results. More filler may be required in this area for adequate revolumization as compared to facial sites, especially if using an HA filler. Some like to have the patient clench their fist while injecting, as this can potentially help to prevent injecting distal to the metacarpophalangeal (MCP) joints or proximal to the wrist bones, which should both be avoided. However, this may obscure the skin laxity and compress veins, giving a false impression of adequate filling. After the injection is complete, massaging with a petrolatum or glycerin-based product and ice/cold packs should be used to ensure even placement of the product and decrease pain, bruising, or swelling post procedure.

DÉCOLLETÉ. Use of microcannulas in the décolleté region is a significant advantage as it can cover a wide area in a short period of time with little or no discomfort or bruising. Both the skin wrinkles (crinkling of skin) and prominent vascularity seen with aging can be treated with filler injections in this area. The use of the fanning injection technique with a 25 gauge, 38 mm or larger, flexible or semirigid microcannulas can be used in the vertical lines of this area. HA fillers are generally the products of choice in this area. CaHA is being used at dilutions of 2:1 or greater (mixed with 1% lidocaine plus 0.9% saline) in a similar manner to the technique in the hands with good results. Although highly diluted PLLA is used, there is a risk of leaving visible nodules in this thin-skinned area.

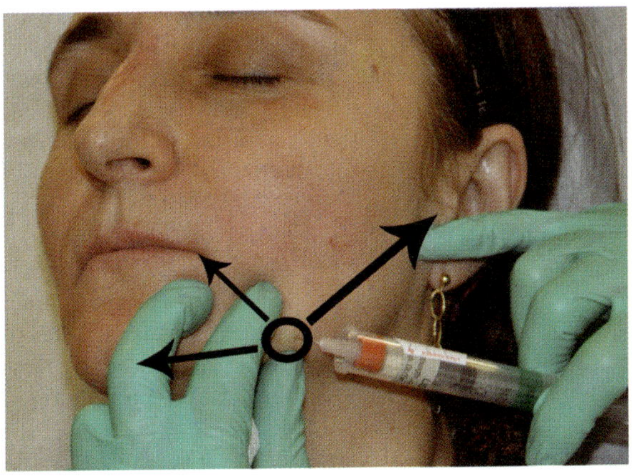

Figure 37-12 Vectors for lower face microcannula injection, author's preference. Multiple locations can be chosen to access an area consisting of the lower cutaneous lip/chin, marionette lines, prejowl/jawline, and preauricular region.

HIGH-RISK CONSIDERATIONS – NEUROVASCULAR

As stated previously, the clinical benefits of using blunt-tipped microcannulas include the near elimination of traumatic injection and risk to vital neurovascular structures. Certain anatomical regions are more sensitive to injury, either due to the nature of the skin at that location (decreased thickness) or the structures that lie beneath (vessels or nerves). The major anatomic vessels of concern when performing soft-tissue augmentation of the face include: (1) supratrochlear artery, (2) superior and inferior labial arteries, (3) angular artery, and (4) the parotid duct.[50] With the use of microcannulas of 27 gauge or larger, the chance of intravascular injection is nearly impossible, and vital structures will be pushed aside as the cannula transverses through the tissues. A 30 gauge cannula, especially if rigid, may still have the potential to cause injury and should be passed through tissue slowly with product extruded at low forces. The longer length of cannulas as compared to sharp needles (typically 13 mm/0.5 in to 19 mm/0.75 in) intrinsically decreases extrusion forces when injecting fillers in this manner.

With the recent popularity of filling temple concavities as well as correcting nasal contour irregularities, the superficial temporal artery as well as the dorsal nasal artery are areas of concern and caution. The periocular area and tear trough, temple and lateral brow, and angle of the mandible, may be more difficult to treat and challenging to a novice injector. Strict adherence to proper technique can help limit serious side effects in these locations, but minor side effects may be unavoidable and should be explained completely prior to treatment.

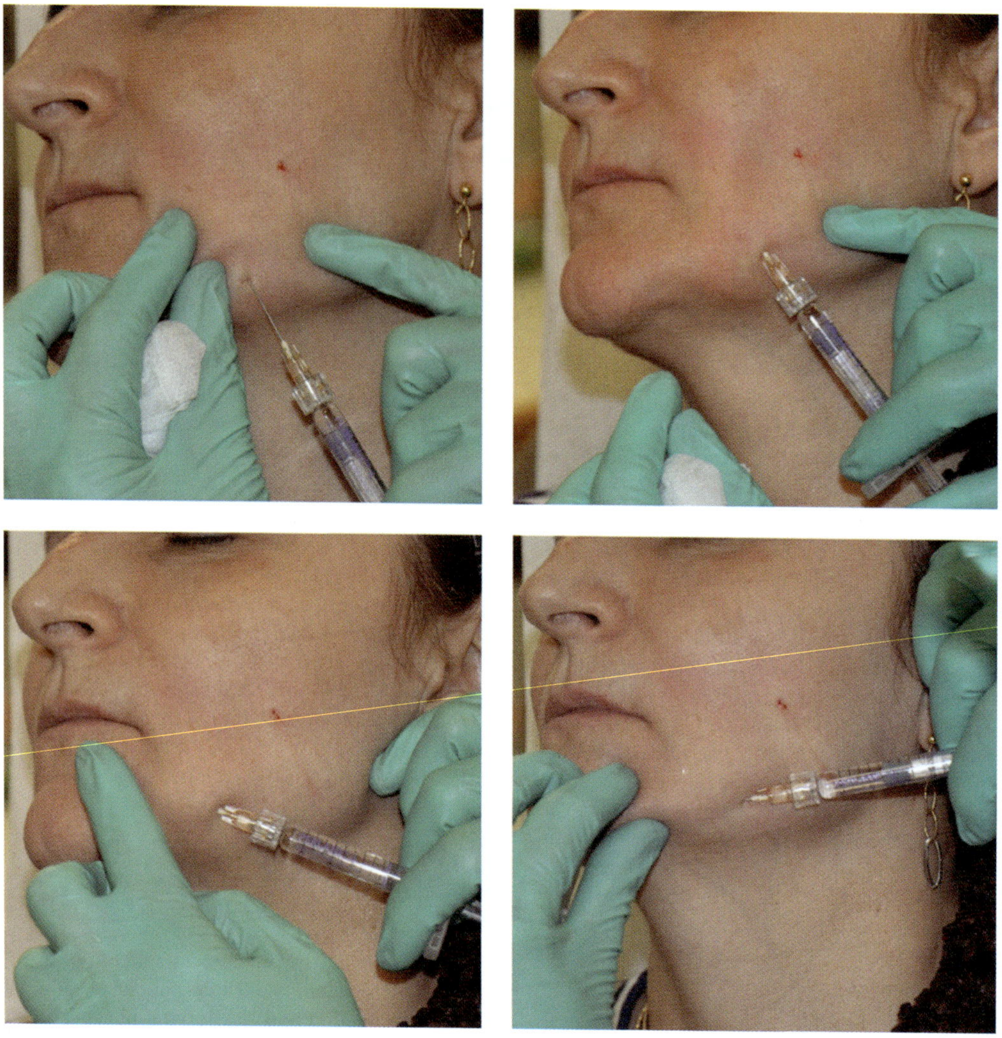

Figure 37-13 Microcannula (25 gauge, 38 mm) injection of the lower face involves reorienting in multiple vectors while in the subcutaneous plane. Pinching the skin helps to ensure accurate placement of product and depth of the microcannula.

For example, the periorbital area is surrounded by several major vessels and nerves that can be injured during careless injection or simple bad luck, and this type of injury could potentially result in visual impairment or blindness.[40,50,51] Injections above the bony border of the orbit can result in septal damage and possibly injury to the globe that may be irreversible.

The supratrochlear artery is at particularly high risk of injury from injection in the glabellar region and/or superior medial bony orbit. The superficial temporal artery is most vulnerable in the preauricular, lateral zygoma, and temporal locations. Vessel damage here can potentially lead to the devastating complication of unilateral scalp necrosis.

The superior and inferior labial arteries are at risk of injury with augmentation of the perioral area and lips, as these arteries supply the upper lip including some of the nasal ala and the lower lip and superior part of the chin, respectively. The angular artery (continuation of the facial artery) provides blood to the medial cheek, nasal ala, nasal sidewall, and dorsum of the nose. Care should be exercised when injecting near the alar groove, as excessive compression with large volumes of filler or frank injection directly into the vessel at this point can lead to nasal ala, nasal tip, nasolabial fold, and upper lip necrosis.[52,53]

Clinicians should take every precaution to avoid vascular compromise. If possible, aspirating prior to injection in anatomic danger zones can be helpful but proves quite difficult with viscous fillers and may only be more reliable in circumstances such as using PLLA. Intravascular injection may lead to immediate blanching followed by ischemia and necrosis (Fig. 37-14). When using local anesthesia either separately or mixed into a filling agent, it is important to know whether the anesthetic contains epinephrine so that the cause of blanching can be determined quickly. This is one reason that most clinicians prefer to use lidocaine without epinephrine during tissue augmentation, although the junior author believes the addition of epinephrine helps limit bruising.

Other structures can also be at risk. Like the artery, the superficial temporal nerve is vulnerable in the preauricular, lateral zygoma, and temporal locations. The temporal branch of the facial nerve is at risk over the lateral brow and the zygomatic branch of the facial nerve is at risk over the zygoma. Injury to the nerves in this location can lead

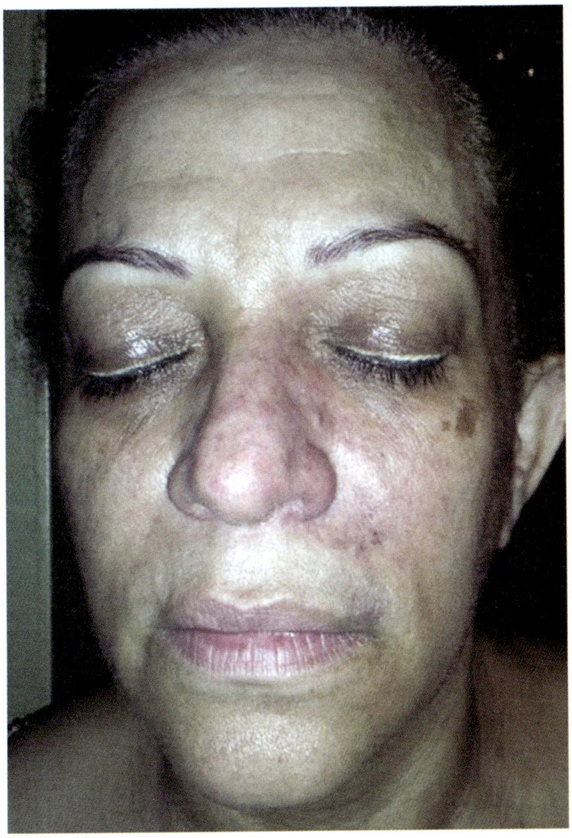

Figure 37-14 Impending necrosis. A dusky, reticulated patch is noted on the midface quickly after sharp needle injection of a hyaluronic acid gel (Juvederm Ultra) by the supraperiosteal injection technique. No long-term sequelae resulted, but the patient required treatment with hyaluronidase, nitroglycerin paste, aspirin, and warm compresses.

to the inability to move the eyebrow or close the upper eyelid on that side completely. Injections near the angle of the mandible put the marginal mandibular branch of the facial nerve at risk and injury to this nerve causes denervation of the depressors of the lip/mouth, leading to chronic drooling or the inability to chew/eat correctly. Finally, the parotid duct (Stensen's duct) enters the mouth at the level of the second molar and is vulnerable to trauma during midface and cheek augmentation, especially in patients with a more significant degree of aging, extreme weight loss, and HIV lipoatrophy. Decreased subcutaneous volume makes the duct more susceptible to injury.

To avoid complications when using microcannulas, in general a 27 gauge or larger diameter cannula should be used in place of a 30 gauge sharp needle and a 25 gauge microcannula or larger diameter cannula should be used in place of a 27 gauge sharp needle. Decreased extrusion forces facilitate increased and even flow of filler product, decreasing the potential for an inappropriately large filler bolus leading to asymmetries, vascular compression, or overtreatment.

CONCLUSION

Blunt-tipped microcannulas are a significant advantage in our armamentarium of options for soft-tissue filler injections. With any cosmetic procedure, the results are dependent upon the knowledge and skill of the practitioner and the safety and efficacy of the employed technique. Techniques for the use of blunt-tipped, flexible microcannulas have been described here, although more controlled studies with the use of microcannulas of various types are needed to determine proper guidelines for use as compared to traditional sharp hypodermic needles. For most patients a combination of blunt-tipped microcannulas and sharp needles will be needed for optimal volumization and contouring as well as precise treatment of fine rhytides and focal areas of volume loss. The proposed benefits, including decreased pain, bruising and swelling, as well as the ability to treat large areas with few puncture sites, are very attractive. Ultimately, however, evidence-based approaches are needed to determine the optimal locations and uses for these relatively new injection tools.

REFERENCES

1. Lafaille P, Benedetto A. Fillers: contraindications, side effects and precautions. *J Cutan Aesthet Surg.* 2010;3(1):16–19.
2. Andre P, Lowe NJ, Parc A, Clerici TH, Zimmermann U. Adverse reactions to dermal fillers: a review of European experiences. *J Cosmet Laser Ther.* 2005;7(3–4):171–176.
3. Sclafani AP, Fagien S. Treatment of injectable soft tissue filler complications. *Dermatol Surg.* 2009;35:1672–1680.
4. Levy LL, Emer JJ. Complications of minimally invasive cosmetic procedures: prevention and management. *J Cutan Aesthet Surg.* 2012;5(2):121–132.
5. Bailey SH, Cohen JL, Kenkel JM. Etiology, prevention, and treatment of dermal filler complications. *Aesthet Surg J.* 2011;31(1):110–121.
6. Coleman SR. Facial augmentation with structural fat grafting. *Clin Plast Surg.* 2006;33(4):567–577.
7. Zeichner JA, Cohen JL. Use of blunt tipped cannulas for soft tissue fillers. *J Drugs Dermatol.* 2012;11(1):70–72.
8. Niamtu J 3rd. Filler injection with micro-cannula instead of needles. *Dermatol Surg.* 2009;35(12):2005–2008.
9. Hertzog B, Andre P. The flexible needle, a safe and easy new technique to inject the face. *J Cosmet Dermatol.* 2010;9(3):251–252.
10. Sundaram H, Weinkle S, Pozner J, Dewandre L. Blunt-tipped microcannulas for the injection of soft tissue fillers: a consensus panel assessment and recommendations. *J Drugs Dermatol.* 2012;11(8):s33–s39.
11. Fisher GJ, Varani J, Voorhees JJ. Looking older: fibroblast collapse and therapeutic implications. *Arch Dermatol.* 2008;144(5):666–672.
12. Harris AK, Stopak D, Wild P. Fibroblast traction as a mechanism for collagen morphogenesis. *Nature.* 1981;290(5803):249–251.
13. Donofrio LM. Blunt-tipped microcannulas–a personal perspective. *J Drugs Dermatol.* 2012;11(8):s41–s42.
14. Feinendegen DL, Baumgartner RW, Schroth G, Mattle HP, Tschopp H. Middle cerebral artery occlusion AND ocular fat embolism after autologous fat injection in the face. *J Neurol.* 1998;245(1):53–54.
15. Feinendegen DL, Baumgartner RW, Vuadens P, et al. Autologous fat injection for soft tissue augmentation in the face: a safe procedure? *Aesthetic Plast Surg.* 1998;22(3):163–167.
16. Berros P. Periorbital contour abnormalities: hollow eye ring management with hyalurostructure. *Orbit.* 2010;29(2):119–125.
17. Hexsel D, Soirefmann M, Porto MD, Siega C, Schilling-Souza J, Brum C. Double-blind, randomized, controlled clinical trial to compare safety and efficacy of a metallic cannula with that of a standard needle for soft tissue augmentation of the nasolabial folds. *Dermatol Surg.* 2012;38(2):207–214.
18. Fulton J, Caperton C, Weinkle S, Dewandre L. Filler injections with the blunt-tip microcannula. *J Drugs Dermatol.* 2012;11(9):1098–1103.
19. Vleggaar D, Forte R. Cosmetic injectable devices: a review of the injection techniques. *J Drugs Dermatol.* 2006;5(10):951–956.

20. Van Eijk T, Braun M. A novel method to inject hyaluronic acid: the Fern Pattern Technique. *J Drugs Dermatol.* 2007;6(8):805–808.
21. Sattler G. The tower technique and vertical supraperiosteal depot technique: novel vertical injection techniques for volume-efficient subcutaneous tissue support and volumetric augmentation. *J Drugs Dermatol.* 2012;11(8):s45–s47.
22. Glogau RG, Kane MA. Effect of injection techniques on the rate of local adverse events in patients implanted with nonanimal hyaluronic acid gel dermal fillers. *Dermatol Surg.* 2008;34:S105–S109.
23. Niamtu J 3rd. Simple technique for lip and nasolabial fold anesthesia for injectable fillers. *Dermatol Surg.* 2005;31(10):1330–1332.
24. Rohrich RJ, Ghavami A, Crosby MA. The role of hyaluronic acid fillers (Restylane) in facial cosmetic surgery: review and technical considerations. *Plast Reconstr Surg.* 2007;120:41S–54S.
25. Carruthers JD, Carruthers A. Facial sculpting and tissue augmentation. *Dermatol Surg.* 2005;31:1604–1612.
26. Raspaldo H. Temporal rejuvenation with fillers: global faceculpture approach. *Dermatol Surg.* 2012;38(2):261–265.
27. Taub AF, Sarnoff D, Gold M, Jacob C. Effect of multisyringe hyaluronic acid facial rejuvenation on perceived age. *Dermatol Surg.* 2010;36(3):322–328.
28. Ross JJ, Malhotra R. Orbitofacial rejuvenation of temple hollowing with Perlane injectable filler. *Aesthet Surg J.* 2010; 30(3):428–433.
29. Moradi A, Shirazi A, Perez V. A guide to temporal fossa augmentation with small gel particle hyaluronic acid dermal filler. *J Drugs Dermatol.* 2011;10(6):673–676.
30. Lambros V. A technique for filling the temples with highly diluted hyaluronic acid: the "dilution solution". *Aesthet Surg J.* 2011;31(1):89–94.
31. Fitzgerald R, Vleggaar D. Facial volume restoration of the aging face with poly-l-lactic acid. *Dermatol Ther.* 2011;24(1):2–27.
32. Succi IB, da Silva RT, Orofino-Costa R. Rejuvenation of periorbital area: treatment with an injectable nonanimal noncrosslinked glycerol added hyaluronic acid preparation. *Dermatol Surg.* 2012;38(2):192–198.
33. Rzany B, Cartier H, Kestermont P, et al. Correction of tear troughs and periorbital lines with a range of customized hyaluronic acid fillers. *J Drugs Dermatol.* 2012;11:s27–s34.
34. Dayan SH, Arkins JP, Somenek M. Restylane persisting in lower eyelids for 5 years. *J Cosmet Dermatol.* 2012;11(3):237–238.
35. Nettar K, Maas C. Facial filler and neurotoxin complications. *Facial Plast Surg.* 2012;28(3):288–293.
36. Stewart DB, Morganroth GS, Mooney MA, Cohen J, Levin PS, Gladstone HB. Management of visible granulomas following periorbital injection of poly-L-lactic Acid. *Ophthal Plast Reconstr Surg.* 23(4):298–301.
37. Vrcek IM, Malouf P, Gilliland GD. A novel solution for superficially placed calcium hydroxylapatite (Radiesse) in the inferior eyelid. *Orbit.* 2012;31(6):431–432.
38. Vagefi MR, McMullan TF, Burroughs JR, White GL Jr, McCann JD, Anderson RL. Calcium hydroxylapatite for orbital volume augmentation. *Arch Facial Plast Surg.* 9(6): 439–442.
39. Roberts SA, Arthurs BP. Severe visual loss and orbital infarction following periorbital aesthetic poly-(L)-lactic acid (PLLA) injection. *Ophthal Plast Reconstr Surg.* 2012;28(3):e68–e70.
40. Sung MS, Kim HG, Woo KI, Kim YD. Ocular ischemia and ischemic oculomotor nerve palsy after vascular embolization of injectable calcium hydroxylapatite filler. *Ophthal Plast Reconstr Surg.* 2010;26(4):289–291.
41. Lazzeri D, Agostini T, Figus M, Nardi M, Pantaloni M, Lazzeri S. Blindness following cosmetic injections of the face. *Plast Reconstr Surg.* 2012;129(4):995–1012.
42. Kim YJ, Kim SS, Song WK, Lee SY, Yoon JS. Ocular ischemia with hypotony after injection of hyaluronic acid gel. *Ophthal Plast Reconstr Surg.* 2011;27(6):e152–e155.
43. Trevidic P. The Use of blunt-tipped cannulas for tear trough correction. *J Drugs Dermatol.* 2012;11:S38–S40.
44. Greco TM, Antunes MB, Yellin SA. Injectable fillers for volume replacement in the aging face. *Facial Plast Surg.* 28(1):8–20.
45. Landau M. Hyaluronic acid "skinboosters" and use of blunt injection microcannulas. *J Drugs Dermatol.* 2012;11(3): 41–43.
46. Park TH, Yeo KK, Seo SW, et al. Clinical experience with complications of hand rejuvenation. *J Plast Reconstr Aesthet Surg.* 2012;65(12):1627–1631.
47. Sadick NS, Anderson D, Werschler WP. Addressing volume loss in hand rejuvenation: a report of clinical experience. *J Cosmet Laser Ther.* 2008;10:237–241.
48. Brandt FS, Cazzaniga A, Strangman N, Coleman J, Axford-Gatley R. Long-term effectiveness and safety of small gel particle hyaluronic acid for hand rejuvenation. *Dermatol Surg.* 2012;38:1128–1135.
49. Butterwick KJ. Rejuvenation of the aging hand. *Dermatol Clin.* 2005;23:515–527.
50. Cohen JL, Brown MR. Anatomic considerations for soft tissue augmentation of the face. *J Drugs Dermatol.* 2009;8(1): 13–16.
51. Silva MT, Curi AL. Blindness and total ophthalmoplegia after aesthetic polymethylmethacrylate injection: case report. *Arq Neuropsiquiatr.* 2004;62(3B):873–874.
52. Grunebaum LD, Bogdan Allemann I, Dayan S, Mandy S, Baumann L. The risk of alar necrosis associated with dermal filler injection. *Dermatol Surg.* 2009;35:1635–1640.
53. Kassir R, Kolluru A, Kassir M. Extensive necrosis after injection of hyaluronic acid filler: case report and review of the literature. *J Cosmet Dermatol.* 2011;10(3):224–231.

CHAPTER 38

Injectables

Karen L. Connolly, David M. Ozog, & Joel L. Cohen

INTRODUCTION

Botulinum toxin (BoNT) has long been recognized as a potent neurotoxin, which causes symmetric flaccid paralysis upon ingestion of food contaminated with bacterial spores. *Clostridium botulinum*, a spore-forming, gram-positive, anaerobic bacterium, produces the toxin along with its associated proteins.[1]

The use of BoNT in medicine dates back to the 1970s, with its initial use in ophthalmology to treat strabismus via its paralyzing effects on the extraocular muscles. The first cosmetic use of BoNT in facial aesthetics occurred in the late 1980s.[2] Use of BoNT for facial rejuvenation now ranks as the number one cosmetic treatment in the United States.[3] The only current FDA-approved cosmetic indication for botulinum toxin type A (BoNT-A) in the United States is treatment of moderate-to-severe glabellar lines in adults, with three different BoNT-A agents: Ona- (Botox®. Allergan. Irvine, CA. USA), Abo- (Dysport®. Ipsen.), and Inco- (Xeomin®. Merz. Germany). However, the BoNT-A agents are commonly used off-label for other aesthetic purposes on the face, neck, and sometimes the upper chest.

In the United States, AbobotulinumtoxinA, IncobotulinumtoxinA, and OnabotulinumtoxinA are also approved by the FDA for the treatment of cervical dystonia. OnabotulinumtoxinA is approved for the treatment of blepharospasm, strabismus, and severe primary axillary hyperhidrosis that is inadequately managed by topical agents. IncobotulinumtoxinA is also approved for treatment of blepharospasm.

AVAILABLE TOXINS

Currently, seven serotypes of BoNTs exist (A–G), all resulting in temporary muscle paralysis. Only serotypes A and B are currently commercially available.[1] For the three preparations of BoNT-A licensed in the United States for cosmetic use, OnabotulinumtoxinA, AbobotulinumtoxinA, and IncobotulinumtoxinA, there is no standard equivalency ratio. Several clinical studies have attempted to determine a ratio specifically for OnabotulinumtoxinA and AbobotulinumtoxinA. A single unit of OnabotulinumtoxinA is approximately equivalent to 2 to 4 units of AbobotulinumtoxinA but this estimation varies between studies, physicians, countries, and by indication.[4–6] Although there are current investigations underway comparing the potency of IncobotulinumtoxinA and OnabotulinumtoxinA, a recent study suggests close to a 1:1 ratio between the products (Table 38-1).[7]

AbobotulinumtoxinA is supplied in a lyophilized form along with human serum albumin and lactose. OnabotulinumtoxinA is supplied in a vacuum-dried form containing human albumin. IncobotulinumtoxinA is supplied in a lyophilized form with human albumin and sucrose.

MECHANISM OF ACTION

Following injection of BoNT-A, the product diffuses over the target muscles and is absorbed into presynaptic motor nerve terminals. In order to enter the nerve, the toxin molecule initially binds to SV2, a synaptic vesicle protein that anchors the heavy chain of the toxin complex through receptor-mediated endocytosis. The toxin complex then enters the nerve, and once it is intra-neural, the heavy chain and light chain separate. The light chain then travels to the nerve terminus where it cleaves synaptosomal-associated protein (SNAP-25), a protein responsible for exocytosis and release of acetylcholine in synaptic vesicles.[8,9] The mechanism of action of botulinum toxin type B (BoNT-B) differs slightly from its type A counterpart; this serotype cleaves vesicle-associated membrane protein (VAMP, also called synaptobrevin) instead of SNAP-25, but the result is similar in that it blocks the exocytic release of Ach from the nerve terminus.[10] The effects of BoNT-A at doses used for cosmetic treatment begin within 2 to 5 days, peak at about 4 weeks, and start to wane by 2 to 3 months. They typically resolve completely by 6 months.[8]

PREPARATION OF THE NEUROMODULATOR FOR USE

Each of the three BoNT-A neuromodulator agents must be reconstituted for use. Reconstitution with unpreserved 0.9% sodium chloride is recommended in each of the three products' manufacturers' package inserts. However, recent literature has suggested that there is no change in OnabotulinumtoxinA's efficacy using saline preserved with benzyl alcohol, although decreased pain with injection has been noted.[11] There are also a few small studies analyzing reconstitution with an anesthetic.[12] Preserved saline has by far become the most common diluent for reconstitution in clinical practice.[13] The recommended manufacturers' reconstitution volumes for Dysport, Xeomin, and Botox for treatment of glabellar lines are detailed

TABLE 38-1
Botulinum Toxin Products Under Development in the United States

	BOTOX	BOTOX Cosmetic/ Vistabel®/ Vistabex®	Dysport/ Reloxin®	Dysport Cosmetic	Myobloc®/ NeuroBloc®	NT-201/ XEOMIN	PurTox®
Company	Allergan Inc.	Allergan Inc.	Ipsen Inc./Medicis Inc.	Ipsen Inc./Medicis Inc.	Solstice Neurosciences Inc.	Merz Pharmaceuticals	Mentor Corporation
Type	Type A-Hall strain	Type A-Hall strain	Type A	Type A	Type B	Type A-Hall strain	Type A-Hall strain
Approvals	In over 75 countries worldwide, including US and Canada	In over 16 countries, including United States, Canada, Italy, France	In over 65 countries; not approved in US or Canada	Germany, other European countries	Some European countries, US, Canada	Germany, other European countries, Mexico, Argentina	None
Active substance (molecular weight)	Botulinum toxin type A complex (900 kD)	Botulinum toxin type A complex (900 kD)	Botulinum toxin type A complex (900kD)[a]	Botulinum toxin type A complex (900kD)[a]	Botulinum toxin type B complex (700 kD)	Botulinum toxin type A, free from complexing proteins (150 kD)	Botulinum toxin type A, free from complexing proteins (150 kD)
Indications	Blepharospasm; cervical dystonia; glabellar lines; hyperhidrosis	Glabellar lines	Blepharospasm; cervical dystonia	Glabellar lines	Cervical dystonia	Blepharospasm; cervical dystonia; glabellar lines	Phase 3 for glabellar lines; Phase 1 for spasmodic torticollis/ cervical dystonia
Mode of action	SNAP-25	SNAP-25	SNAP-25	SNAP-25	VAMP	SNAP-25	SNAP-25
Pharmaceutical form	Powder dissolved in solution for injection	Powder dissolved in solution for injection	Powder dissolved in solution for injection	Powder dissolved in solution for injection	Solution	Powder dissolved in solution for injection	[b]
Units/vial	100	50	500	300 or 500	2500; 5000; 10,000	50 or 100	[b]
Volume	10 mL maximum	1.25 mL or 2.5 mL recommended	2.5 mL recommended	5 mL maximum	0.5 mL; 1 mL; 2 mL	8 mL maximum	[b]
Re-constitution	0.9% NaCl solution	0.9% NaCl solution	0.9% NaCl solution	0.9% NaCl solution	Prepared solution, dilutable	0.9% NaCl solution	0.9% NaCl solution
Storage	2°–8°C or <–5°C	2°–8°C or <–5°C	2°–8°C	2°–8°C	2–8°C do not freeze	Up to 25°C	[b]

Summary of botulinum toxin products approved or under development for cosmetic indications.
[a]The formulation contains complexes of variable size between 500 and 900 kD.[2]
[b]Data unavailable or unconfirmed.
SNAP-25 (synaptosomal associated protein with the molecular mass of 25 kD), an intracellular protein that is essential for synaptic vesicle transmission; it has been identified as the molecular target of BTX-A.; **VAMP (synaptobrevin)**, a protein involved in synaptic vesicle movement that has been identified as the molecular target of BTX-B.
Source: Adapted with permission from Carruthers A, Carruthers J. Botulinum toxin products overview. *Skin Therapy Lett*. 2008;13(6):1–4.

TABLE 38-2
Botulinum Toxin Reconstitution Guidelines

Product	Units (Unit Vial)	Volume of 0.9% Sodium Chloride (mL)	Resulting Concentration
Dysport	300	2.5	10 Units per 0.08 mL
Dysport	300	1.5	10 Units per 0.05 mL
Botox cosmetic	100	2.5	4 Units per 0.1 mL
Botox cosmetic	50	1.25	4 Units per 0.1 mL
Xeomin	50	0.25–5	Varies with dilution
Xeomin	100	0.5–8	Varies with dilution

in Table 38-2. However, in clinical practice reconstitution volumes can vary based on location and indication. Lower volumes are often used in areas where diffusion needs to be minimized (such as perioral injections for orbicularis oris) while higher volumes are sometimes used to facilitate spread of the medication when there are larger target areas (such as for axillary hyperhidrosis).

The product insert for Botox recommends that once opened and reconstituted, the product should be stored at 2° to 8°C and used within 24 hours. The vial is single-use and it is not recommended that it be frozen once reconstituted. For Dysport, the product insert similarly recommends the vial be single-use, stored at 2° to 8°C, used within 4 to 6 hours and protected from light. It also states the product should not be frozen once reconstituted. In contrast, Xeomin may be stored in unopened vials at room temperature at 20° to 25°C, refrigerated at 2° to 8°C, or in a freezer at −20° to −10°C, for up to 36 months. Once reconstituted, the Xeomin product insert states that the product should be used within 24 hours.

Despite the manufacturer's recommendation that a vial be single-use, some studies suggest that a reconstituted BoNT-A vial can be used and re-accessed for up to 6 weeks when stored with refrigeration, without loss of efficacy or contamination.[14] The majority of providers use each vial for more than one patient and sometimes store BoNT-A for greater than 1 week,[11,13,15] while in a busy cosmetic practice a bottle is often not in use for longer than a day or two.

BoNT-A is typically administered using a 30-gauge 13 mm (1/2 in) needle, but different syringes and needles can be used. A 0.3 mL 30 gauge insulin syringe (product number 3,28,438, manufactured by B-D Inc, Franklin Lakes, NJ) to decrease injection pain has been advocated by Flynn et al.[16]

PATIENT SELECTION AND PREOPERATIVE CONSULTATION

Photodamage, loss of skin elasticity with aging, and repeated muscular contractions all contribute to wrinkling. When evaluating a patient for treatment using neuromodulators, one must evaluate the extent of wrinkling caused by photodamage and distinguish this from wrinkling caused by repetitive movement of facial muscles. This will help predict the extent of improvement the patient may expect from treatment and factors into their overall aesthetic plan. The wrinkles caused by muscles of facial expression are arranged perpendicular to the vectors of muscle contraction. These can be temporary or persistent, and both forms can be improved with treatment using BoNT-A.[17] Analysis of facial movement, as well as recognition of any pre-existing asymmetry or ptosis, must be considered when deciding on the placement and dose of toxin to be used. Photographs are particularly important before and after the initial treatment session, as patients are often unaware of pre-existing baseline asymmetry and may later believe that this was caused by the neuromodulator treatment itself.

Realistic expectations regarding the degree of improvement expected and the eventual financial cost to the patient must be discussed in detail. Any off-label use of toxin should be clearly disclosed and ideally should be part of the consent form as well.

Contraindications for cosmetic use of BoNT-A include known hypersensitivity to any botulinum product, current infection at the proposed injection sites, and pre-existing neuromuscular junction disorders (myasthenia gravis, amyotrophic lateral sclerosis, and Lambert-Eaton Syndrome). Special precautions should be taken when treating patients with pre-existing swallowing or breathing difficulties, or who are taking high systemic doses of aminoglycosides or other medications interfering with neuromuscular release, which may potentiate the effect of BoNT-A. Interactions are also possible with certain medications, including chloroquine and hydroxychloroquine, which may antagonize the onset of BoNT-A activity. Cyclosporine can also potentially cause neuromuscular blockade.[9] Allergy to cow's milk protein is an additional contraindication to use of AbobotulinumtoxinA, which may contain trace amounts of this product.

AbobotulinumtoxinA, IncobotulinumtoxinA, and OnabotulinumtoxinA are Pregnancy Category C, and thus are not recommended for use during pregnancy. The excretion of BoNT-A or its metabolites in breast milk is possible, and their use is not recommended during lactation.

TECHNIQUES DIVIDED BY ANATOMIC LOCATION

GLABELLAR COMPLEX

The glabellar complex is the area most commonly treated with BoNT-A, and again is the only aesthetic area that is FDA-approved for injection of all three currently available BoNT-A products (Fig. 38-1). The corrugator and procerus muscles contract to produce a furrowed brow, which may give the impression of anger or sadness. These muscles are identified by asking the patient to frown or scowl. Three to five intramuscular injection points are typically used in this area (one in the belly of the procerus, and one to two injections along the corrugators). A single injection point

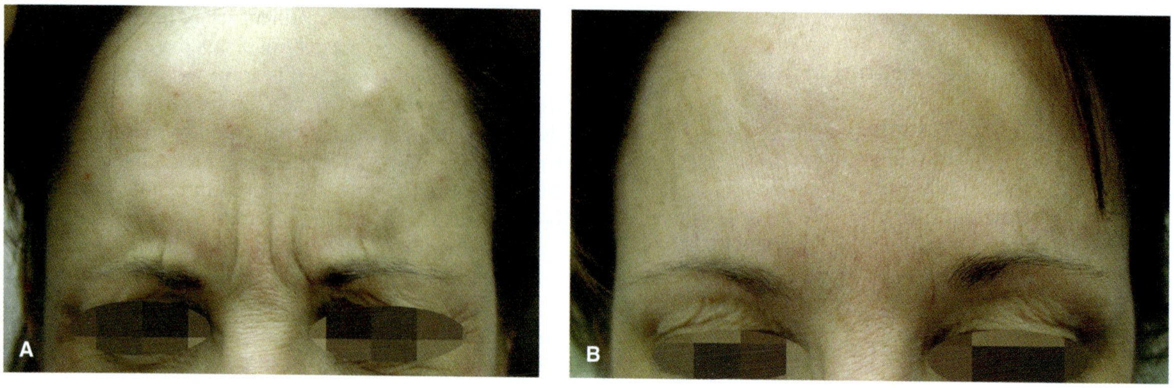

Figure 38-1 Glabellar lines (**A**) in a patient with maximal frown pretreatment and (**B**) attempting to frown after treatment (23 units Onabotulinumtoxin). (Photos used with permission of Joel L. Cohen, MD.)

in each corrugator may sometimes be preferred due to concern that the agent will spread to the adjacent frontalis muscle in some circumstances due to a patient's unique anatomy. When administering glabellar complex injections, grasping the muscles during contraction, and then asking the patient to relax, may allow for more precise targeting of the muscle belly. If possible, the needle should be placed intrafollicularly, as this has been shown to decrease pain on injection.[18] To minimize the risk of eyelid ptosis, some practitioners advocate that injections into the corrugators should be placed at least 1 cm superior to the supraorbital rim at the central area of the eyebrow. Palpating with a finger along the bony orbital rim can often identify this landmark.[3,19] However, it is important to tailor treatment to each patient, as too high an injection in patients with significant lateral brow-lid redundancy can result in brow ptosis if the lateral corrugator injection spreads to the adjacent frontalis muscle (Fig. 38-2) (Table 38-3).

Horizontal forehead lines or furrows are created by repeated contraction of the underlying frontalis muscle (Fig. 38-3). The significant variation in patient anatomy is reflected in the variety of techniques used to treat this location. In our opinion, successful treatment of this area is more challenging than treatment of either the glabellar complex or crow's feet. Some patients may decide later that they do not like either the physical appearance of a "treated forehead" or the "feeling" of the inability to raise their brow.

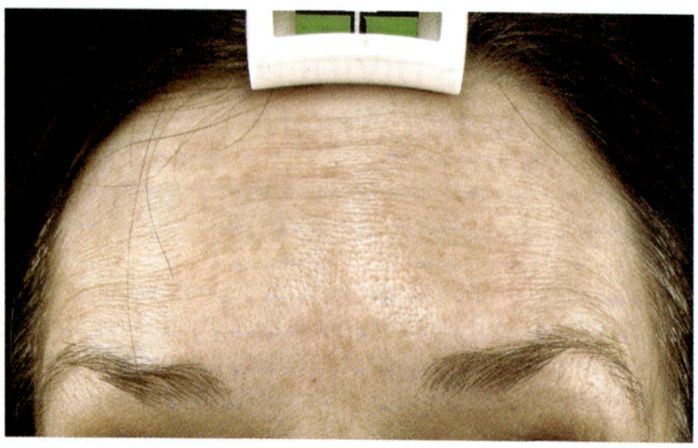

Figure 38-2 Medial brow depression from glabellar treatment with undesirable spread of BoNT-A to the medial frontalis muscle. The lateral brow shows an upward pull as frontalis fibers in that area persist, resulting in an artificial look. (Photo used with permission of Joel L. Cohen, MD.)

This is more common with older patients, probably due to downward repositioning of the brow after the neuromodulator agent relaxes the frontalis muscle. For this reason, injections have historically been located in the upper two-thirds of the forehead to allow for maintenance or elevation of brow position; in reality, however, this approach can lead to an odd or artificial appearance when the patient does elevate their brows, as only the most inferior portion of the frontalis is functioning in this case. For this reason, the authors recommend careful patient selection and clear-cut patient discussions. For many patients, we simply try to "soften" the overall musculature to make it less prominent and, therefore, less active in imprinting the skin with etched-in lines. Some patients want a total "knock-out" of all forehead movement and we try to deter them, but if they are young, lack significant dermatochalasis, and do not depend on their frontalis to raise their lateral brows, we may be more apt to perform this treatment (Fig. 38-4).

Brow ptosis is a complication that is usually avoidable with proper patient selection. Complete forehead paralysis should be discouraged in order to achieve a more natural aesthetic result, and lower starting doses are, therefore, preferable, although their duration of action may not be as great as those of higher doses. These points should be conveyed to the patient prior to their first treatment. Some patients will decide to try BoNT-A once to determine whether they like the look and feel of reduced or absent frontalis muscle activity. These patients should be seen the week after injection to determine whether additional toxin may be needed to balance any asymmetry in their appearance.

Multiple frontalis injection sites (sometimes eight or more) are typically placed using a superficial intramuscular injection technique. When injections are placed too medially, a quizzical eyebrow can result due to continued activity of the untreated lateral frontalis fibers. This can be corrected with additional BoNT-A injected into the lateral frontalis,[3,20] which can carry a risk of lateral brow droop, so it is essential to emphasize the need for lower dosages on the forehead, particularly for patients who have not yet had experience using this medication.

CROW'S FEET (OFF-LABEL INDICATION)

Wrinkles radiating outward from the lateral canthus while smiling are commonly known as crow's feet (Fig. 38-5). The

TABLE 38-3
Dosage Guidelines for Botulinum Toxin Injections

Number of Injection Points	Total Units Starting Dose		Anatomic Landmarks	Potential Complications
	Botox/Xeomin	Dysport		
Glabellar Complex				
3–5	20–30	50	Palpate the bony superior orbital rim and stay 1 cm above it	Ptosis, asymmetry of the brows
Horizontal Forehead Lines				
4–8	4–20	10–60	Upper two-thirds of the forehead	Eyebrow ptosis, quizzical eyebrow shape with injections placed too centrally
Crow's Feet				
1–5 per side	12–30 units	20–60	Stay 1–2 cm outside the external orbital rim. Avoid visible blood vessels by stretching underlying skin for better visualization.	Bruising, asymmetric smile with paralysis of zygomaticus major (injections too deep or inferior), ptosis (injections too deep)
Lateral Brow Lift and Eyebrow Shaping				
1 per side	12–16	20–40	Lateral eyebrow. Stay lateral to the orbital rim	Brow and eyelid ptosis can occur if injection is too close to the orbital rim
Bunny Lines				
1 per side	2–4	5–10	1 cm above the upper lateral nostril	Bruising, lip drooping if the levator labii alaeque nasi (LLAN) and levator labii superioris are targeted, or asymmetric smile due to knockout of LLAN and thus flattening of NLF as well
Nasal Droop				
Single injection at the base of the columella	3–5	8–12	Just superior to the angle of the columella and upper cutaneous lip	Upper lip ptosis (excess paralysis of depressor septi nasi). Pain.
Lower Eyelid Wrinkles				
1–2 per each under-eye	2–4	2–5	Mid-pupillary line, 2 mm below the lower eyelid margin	Eye dryness with higher doses
Chin Dimpling				
1 per side (2 total) or 1 midline injection	1–3	5–8	Bony jawline, close to the center	Injecting too high into the orbicularis oris can cause lower lip weakness and drooling. Injecting too laterally can cause slurred speech or asymmetrical smile if depressor labii inferioris injected.

(*Continued*)

TABLE 38-3 (*Continued*)
Dosage Guidelines for Botulinum Toxin Injections

Number of Injection Points	Total Units Starting Dose		Anatomic Landmarks	Potential Complications
	Botox/Xeomin	Dysport		
Perioral Wrinkles				
1–2 per upper lip side and 1 per lower lip side	6–10	10–20	Vermillion border (no more than 5 mm superior), philtrum (at least 1 mm lateral), mouth corners (at least 1.5 cm medial)	Overdosing: difficulty speaking, eating, drinking. Injection too close to the mouth corners: mouth asymmetry or drooping lip. Injection >5 mm superior to the vermillion border can cause lip ptosis, inversion, or eversion.
Downturned Oral Commissure				
1–2 per upper lip side and 1 per lower lip side	4–10	10–20	Vermillion border (no more than 5 mm superior), philtrum (at least 1 mm lateral), mouth corners (at least 1.5 cm medial)	Overdosing: difficulty speaking, eating, drinking. Injection too close to the mouth corners: mouth asymmetry or drooping lip. Injection >5 mm superior to the vermillion border can cause lip ptosis, inversion, or eversion.
Gummy Smile				
1 per side (2 total)	5	10	Lateral nasal ala	Asymmetric smile, excessive lengthening of the upper lip
Platysmal Bands				
Maximum of 10 points per side (20 total)	10–34	5–10 (maximum dose 100 total)	Injections start just below the jawline and continue to the mid-band	Dysphonia, dysphagia, neck weakness (excessive doses and too deep injection). Inefficacy (poor patient selection).
Masseter Hypertrophy				
1–3 points per side (up to 6 total)	40–60	60 for Caucasians, 120 for Asians	Jaw line for the superior-most injection. Continue to the mid-band.	Dysphonia, dysphagia, neck weakness (excessive doses and injecting too deep). Inefficacy (poor patient selection).
Primary Focal Hyperhidrosis				
1 per cm^2 30–40 total injection points per area	50–100 per axilla	150–300 per axilla	Minor's starch iodine test delineates affected area	Transient weakness of intrinsic hand muscles, intense pain with improper anesthesia of the palm or sole. Compensatory hyperhidrosis in untreated areas.

Note: Each table gives only a rough guideline for number of injection points and starting doses. Every patient's unique anatomy must be evaluated individually and treated accordingly.

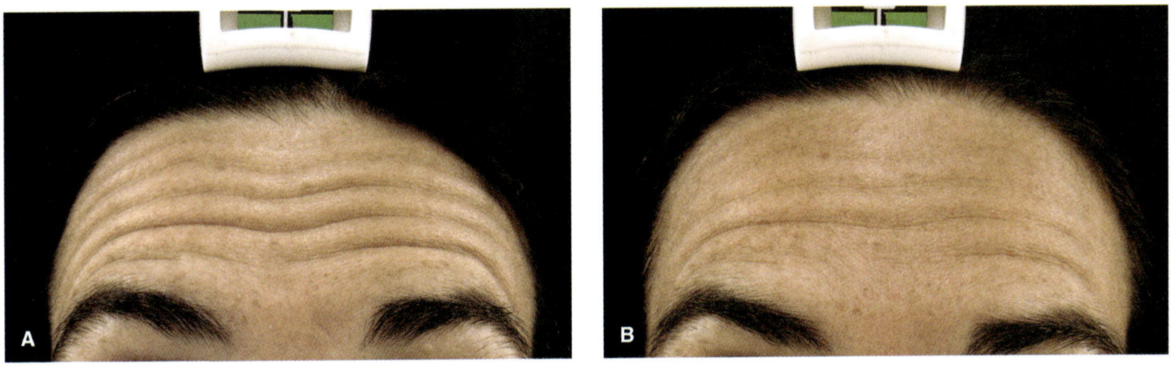

Figure 38-3 Horizontal forehead lines (**A**) at maximal eyebrow raise pre-treatment and (**B**) at maximal eyebrow raise posttreatment (7 units of IncoBotulinum toxin). Lower doses were used for a more "natural result," to simply lessen the muscular prominence of the frontalis. (Photos used with permission of Joel L. Cohen, MD.)

lateral fibers of the orbicularis oculi muscle are responsible for producing these lines. Significant patient variation exists in this area[21] and proper injection placement must be determined on an individual basis. Typically, three injection points are used, but anywhere from 1 to 5 injection points may be possible depending on individual patient characteristics. Injections are generally placed 1 to 2 cm lateral to the bony external orbital rim. The needle is typically pointed away from the orbit and injections are superficial, creating intradermal blebs. Superficial placement in this area minimizes bruising; stretching the skin can help the injector to visualize superficial veins so they can be avoided. Some individuals recruit fibers from the zygomaticus minor muscle in creating their crow's feet, which is important to note, as inadvertent paralysis of these fibers can result in an asymmetric smile. This is avoided by injecting superficially, as mentioned previously, as well as by making certain that the lowest injection point is not placed too far inferiorly.[3,20,21]

LATERAL BROW LIFT AND BROW SHAPING (OFF-LABEL INDICATION)

Drooping lateral eyebrows or brow-lid redundant skin can create a tired or unhappy expression. The "ideal" female eyebrow lies with the highest point of the arch above the lateral canthus. Contraction of the lateral orbicularis oculi

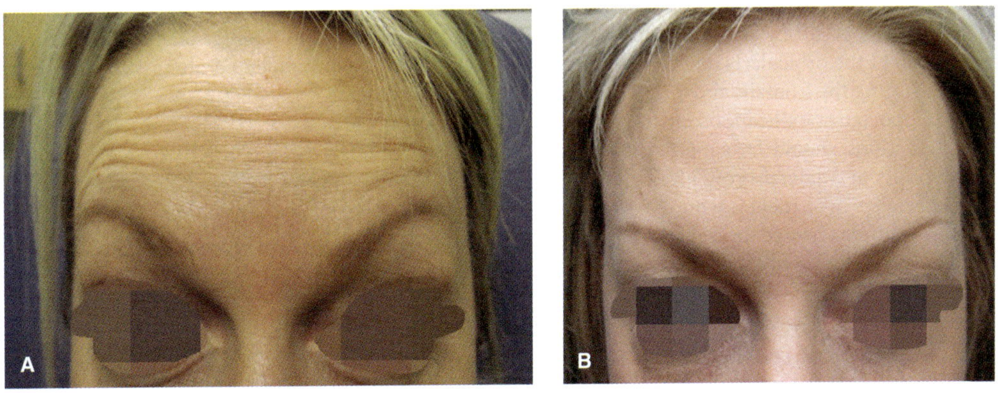

Figure 38-4 Horizontal forehead lines (**A**) in a subject before frontalis treatment upon lifting brows and (**B**) in a subject after treatment (32 units of Abobotulinumtoxin) upon attempting to lift brows. Patient desired a "frozen forehead" look despite being cautioned and advised againast it—as this is the way she has been treated with botulinum toxin at other facilities in the past. (Photos used with permission of Joel L. Cohen, MD.)

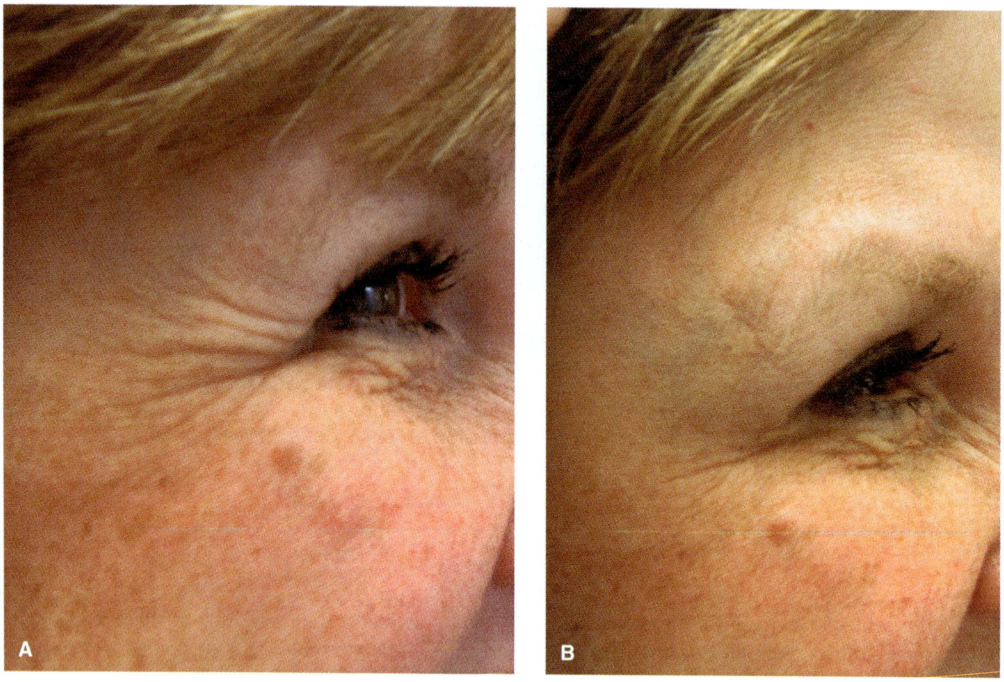

Figure 38-5 Crow's feet (**A**) in a subject pretreatment and (**B**) after treatment (Abobotulinumtoxin 30 units) at maximum smile. (Photos used with permission of Karen L. Connolly, MD.)

fibers depresses the lateral eyebrow, whereas the procerus and corrugators are responsible for depression of the central eyebrow. A lateral eyebrow lift can be achieved using toxin to block depression of the lateral eyebrow tail.[22,23] One lateral injection point is usually used per side specifically targeting the lateral orbicularis oculi at the eyebrow tail, or simply the point at which a squinting patient demonstrates maximal pull of the orbicularis oculi downward on the lateral brow. The injector must ensure that the injection point is at least 1 cm from any trailing lateral fibers of the inferior frontalis at the temporal fusion line; otherwise the attempt at lift by targeting only the superior lateral portion of the orbicularis oculi will be neutralized or offset by hitting the frontalis above it, which would drop the brow. Reported complications include eyelid and brow ptosis. Injections should be superficial and intramuscular.[3] Attempts at a lateral brow lift are not always successful, especially in patients who have excessive lid laxity; these patients would best be treated with a blepharoplasty .

BUNNY LINES (OFF-LABEL INDICATION)

"Bunny lines" radiate down the sides of the nose and occur due to contraction of the nasalis muscle on the proximal nasal sidewall (Fig. 38-6). These lines are often treated along with the glabellar complex to prevent recruitment; contraction of the procerus muscle itself can contribute to prominent "bunny lines" as well. One injection point per side is placed superficially to minimize bruising; this is usually placed high and medial on the proximal nasal sidewall into the belly of the musculature. Avoiding the laterally based levator labii alaeque nasi (LLAN) and levator labii superioris prevents lip ptosis, which can be a potential complication.[19,24] It is usually helpful to take a lateral approach to the nasalis muscle and to inject in a medial direction; this helps prevent unwanted diffusion to the laterally located lip elevators, which also contribute to the prominence of the nasolabial fold.[25] Not every patient's anatomy allows for a successful treatment result, and some patients, for unknown reasons, still maintain fairly prominent musculature of this area. As this area lies in the same horizontal plane as the crow's feet, this area is frequently injected along with the lateral canthal rhytids.

NASAL DROOP (OFF-LABEL INDICATION)

The depressor septi nasi muscles control the degree of nasal tip drooping. Treatment of this muscle group with toxin can potentially raise the nasal tip, increasing its distance from the upper lip and giving the nose a more youthful and fresher appearance; however, this treatment does not reliably create improvement. A single deep injection just superior to the angle of the columella and upper cutaneous lip is typically the point at which BoNT-A is placed. The injection can be painful, so icing the area beforehand will improve patient tolerance. Adverse effects include upper lip ptosis with excessive dosages.[19,26,27]

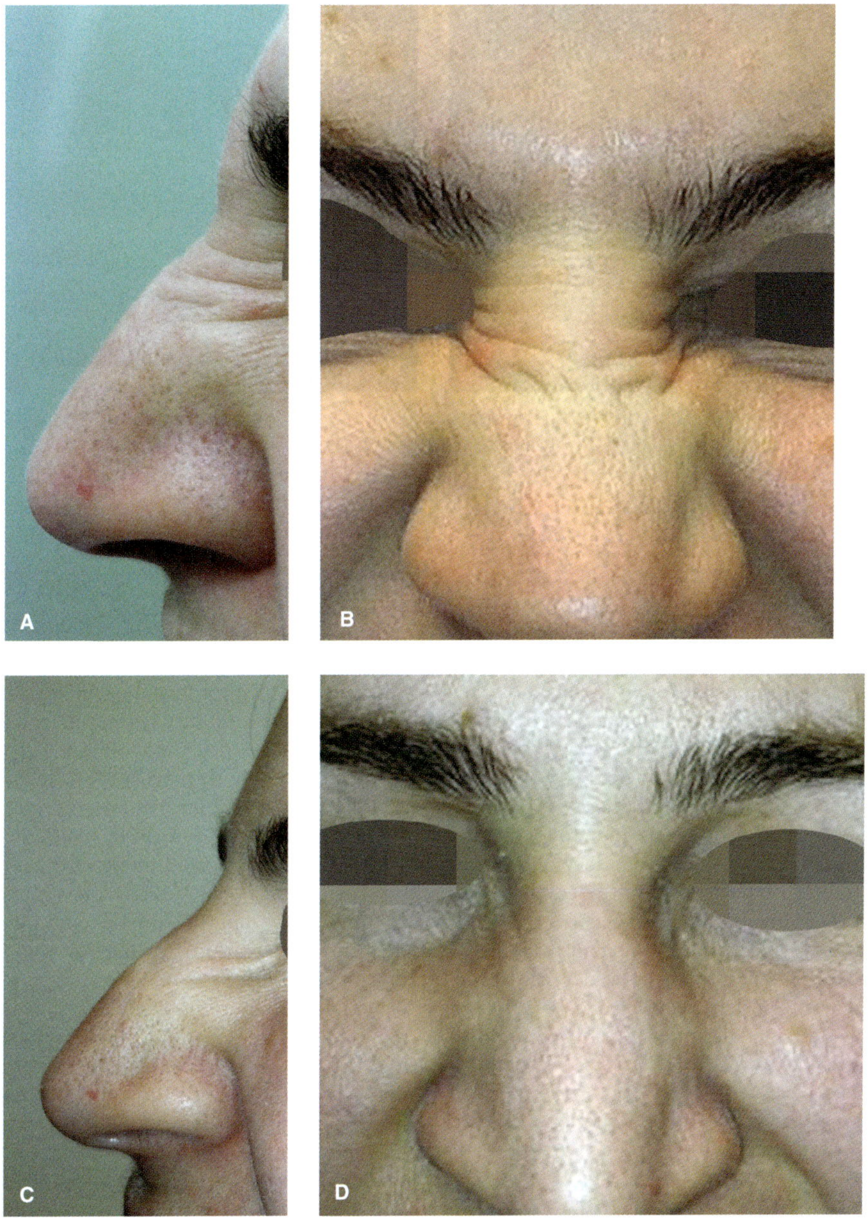

Figure 38-6 Patient (**A, B**) prior to treatment and (**C, D**) after treatment at maximum nose wrinkle. (Onabotulinumtoxin 16 units to glabellar complex and 4 units to bunny lines). (Photos used with permission of Karen L. Connolly, MD.)

LOWER EYELID WRINKLES (OFF-LABEL INDICATION)

Lower eyelid wrinkles can be caused by activity of the orbicularis oculi muscles and photodamage, and can also be hereditary, although a combination of all three causes is quite common. Wrinkling caused by hyperactivity of the inferior pre-tarsal orbicularis oculi can be treated using one injection point per side at the mid-pupillary line, approximately 2 mm below the lower lid margin. This technique is usually performed in conjunction with crow's feet injections, thereby producing more noticeable effects. These injections are superficial, should be done with the needle angled horizontally and away from the globe and should create a bleb in the skin. Patients must not have dry eyes or large eye bags, and must have a good snap test (demonstrating that the lower eyelids snap back into place immediately after pulling downward on the lower lid). This technique can also be used to achieve the effect of widening and rounding the eyes[19,28] especially if they have an almond shape. This procedure is best performed by experienced injectors.

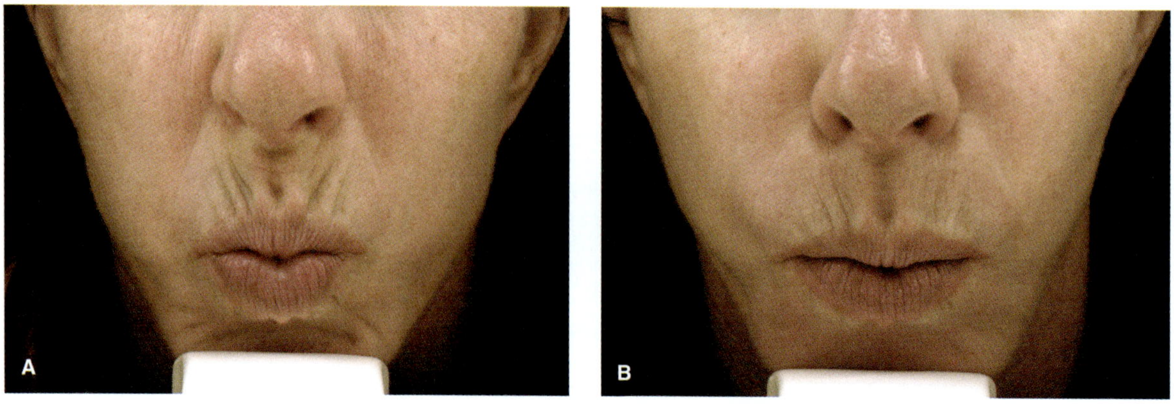

Figure 38-7 Perioral rhytides in (**A**) patient pretreatment upon contraction of the orbicularis oris and (**B**) posttreatment with BoNT-A (6 units OnaBotulinum toxin). (Photos used with permission of Joel L. Cohen, MD.)

CHIN DIMPLING (OFF-LABEL INDICATION)

The mentalis muscle is responsible for wrinkling and dimpling of the chin with animation, creating a peau d'orange appearance, as well as protrusion of the lower lip. Pushing the lower lip superiorly emphasizes this wrinkling. Treatment with BoNT can help smooth these depressions (sometimes called "golf ball chin") using one to two injection points at the jaw line. Injections are deep and intramuscular. Injecting too high must be avoided, as lower lip weakness and possibly drooling can occur if the orbicularis oris is targeted instead of the mentalis muscle.[3,19] Injections placed too laterally can affect the depressor labii inferioris (DLI), causing an asymmetric smile, so it is very important to inject the mentalis medially or even midline when targeting wrinkles in this area.

PERIORAL WRINKLES (OFF-LABEL INDICATION, ONLY FOR EXPERIENCED INJECTORS)

Vertical perioral wrinkles give an appearance of aging and are caused by movement of the orbicularis oris muscle, which closes the mouth and purses the lips (Fig. 38-7). Smoking, photoaging, playing a musical instrument, and whistling contribute to wrinkling in this area.[29] Two to six very superficial injection points along the upper lip and two along the lower lip are placed at the vermillion border. The medial points should be placed at least 1 mm lateral to the philtrum, and the lateral points at least 1.5 cm medial to the mouth corners. The high functional importance of this area must be considered and use of the lowest effective treatment dose is recommended. Potential adverse effects include upper lip ptosis with injections superior to the vermillion. Distortion of the Cupid's bow can be avoided by injecting lateral to the midline. Overtreatment with excessive doses can result in speech impairment, difficulty eating and drinking, and drooling. Injections in this area can also be quite painful.[3,19,29]

DOWNTURNED ORAL COMMISSURE (OFF-LABEL INDICATION)

Permanent downward angling of the lateral corners of the mouth conveys an unpleasant frowning appearance (Fig. 38-8). The depressor anguli oris (DAO) muscle is responsible for this expression, in opposition to the zygomaticus major and minor muscles, which elevate the corners of the lips to smile. Injection of BoNT-A into the DAO can allow a softening of the downward pull on the corners of the mouth by the zygomaticus muscles. A combination approach with toxin plus fillers can further improve marionette lines or melomental folds in this area (Fig. 38-8). One deep intramuscular injection is placed directly into the DAO, which is located along the mandibular line. Grasping the belly of the muscle during contraction helps to ensure proper placement.[3,19] It may also be helpful for the patient to contract the DAO (by displaying their lower teeth); the muscle can then be injected about 1 cm above the jawline. One should avoid the point on the posterior jawline at which the DAO and DLI come together as a V, and the needle should be aimed in a lateral direction to avoid unwanted diffusion to the adjacent DLI.

GUMMY SMILE (OFF-LABEL INDICATION, ONLY FOR EXPERIENCED INJECTORS)

Gummy smile is characterized by excessive gingival exposure and is mainly caused by excessive movement from the levator labii superioris alaeque nasi. Typically, greater than 2 to 3 mm of exposed gingiva is considered unaesthetic. When greater than 3 mm of exposed gingiva posterior to the canines is seen, the zygomaticus muscles are usually involved as well. Most commonly, a "gummy" smile is treated with one injection point on each side, at the site of convergence of the levator labii superioris alaeque nasi, zygomaticus minor, and levator labii superioris, just lateral to the nasal ala.[30–33]

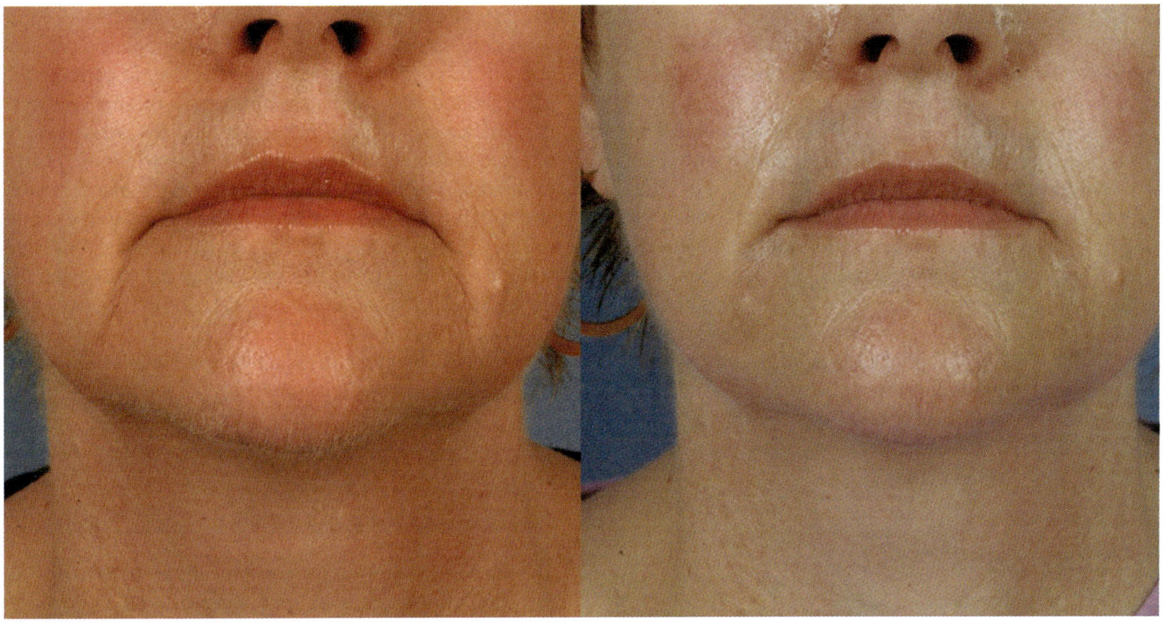

Figure 38-8 Downturned oral commissure treated by combining BoNT-A and a filler agent, in this case Restylane, to correct the appearance of a downturned smile. (Onabotulinumtoxin 3 units into each depressor anguli oris along with Restylane 0.35 cc into each oral commissure). (Photos used with permission of Joel L. Cohen, MD. Reprinted with permission from Cohen JL, Hirsch RJ. Challenge: correcting a downturned smile. *The Dermatologist*. 2006;14(2):52–53.)

PLATYSMAL BANDS (OFF-LABEL INDICATION)

The platysmal bands create prominent cord-like vertical bands as certain patients age, and can become prominent when speaking or smiling. Prominence of bands is best assessed with the patient pronouncing the letter "E." The ideal patient for treatment of these bands has retained elasticity of the neck skin and does not have excessive laxity or fat in this area. The patient should also have prominent platysmal banding *at rest*. The dose and number of injection points vary widely in the literature. The trend is toward lower toxin dosage in this area, which results in excellent clinical improvement while minimizing complications and reducing costs. Injections are placed by grasping the belly of the muscle along a band and starting at the jawline, moving down every 1.5 to 3 cm for each successive injection. Dosing is highly dependent on prominence of the patient's musculature. Our starting doses range from 12 to 34 units of Botox. Adverse effects, including dysphagia, neck weakness, and dysphonia are avoided by not exceeding maximum doses and using a horizontal superficial intramuscular injection technique, pulling the band away from the underlying strap muscles.[3,19] There is one report of a patient who received 60 units of Botox in the platysma and developed dysphagia, requiring a nasogastric tube for 6 weeks.[34]

The Nefertiti lift, as described by Levy, involves injection of BoNT-A along the inferior border of the mandible and the superior aspect of the most posterior platysmal band, resulting in a tighter appearance of the jawline. Fifteen to twenty units of Botox per side is the recommended starting dose.[35]

MASSETER HYPERTROPHY (OFF-LABEL INDICATION)

Hypertrophy of the masseter muscles can create a square shaped face and is common in Asian patients. In Caucasian patients, bruxism is associated with masseter hypertrophy, which can also be caused by regularly chewing bulky bubblegum or grinding ice. This hypertrophy can be treated using a deep three point injection technique per side, thereby weakening the masseter muscles, which can be palpated with the patient clenching the jaw. Injections are placed between a line connecting the earlobe and the corner of the mouth, and ending 1.5 cm above the mandibular angle. Alternatively, the area can be treated as a square with injections of the four corners and in the middle of the square. Potential adverse effects may occur with injections placed too close to the zygomaticus bone medially, which weaken the zygomaticus minor or major and cause a distorted smile, as well as weakened mastication if overdosing occurs. In Asian patients, higher doses are typically used than in Caucasian patients, who tend to have less hypertrophy. Clinical results are usually noted in 2 to 4 weeks,[19,36,37] but it often takes two treatment sessions about 3 months apart in our experience for more noticeable improvement to be documented by standardized photos.

PRIMARY FOCAL HYPERHIDROSIS

Primary idiopathic focal hyperhidrosis affects the axillae, palms, and soles and has a significant social impact on patients. The sympathetic nervous system innervates eccrine sweat glands and stimulates sweating via acetylcholine release. BoNT has emerged as an effective treatment for severe or refractory primary focal hyperhidrosis. Minor's starch iodine test can be helpful to delineate the initial treatment area, and is useful in cases requiring a "touch-up" to identify the exact area for additional treatment. The affected area is treated with a series of intradermal BoNT-A injections. Treatment of axillary hyperhidrosis is not all that painful and many times patients receive this treatment with only ice to the treatment area. On the palms and soles, most patients require at least ice, while others may try a topical anesthetic; less often nerve blocks of the palms or soles are performed due to significant pain with multiple injections in these sensitive areas.[38–42] Sometimes multiple modalities such as ice, a compressed air device, and a vibratory massage device can be useful to decrease pain through the Gates Principle of Afferent Overstimulation.[43,44]

AFTERCARE

Massage of the facial and neck treatment areas immediately after injection is not recommended by most experts, although it may be used when treating hyperhidrosis to avoid displacement or excessive movement of the product. Contraction of the injected area for approximately 2 hours after treatment is thought to increase product uptake.[3] Applying pressure and ice immediately after injection in areas prone to bleeding and ecchymoses (e.g., crow's feet) can be helpful.

COMPLICATIONS

COMMON ADVERSE EVENTS

The most common nonserious adverse events reported since licensure of OnabotulinumtoxinA are lack of effect (63%), injection site reaction (19%), ptosis (11%), muscle weakness (5%), and headache (5%).[45] The common injection site-related adverse events reported in package inserts for all three licensed BoNT-A products are similar and include localized pain, infection, inflammation, tenderness, swelling, erythema, bleeding, headache, respiratory infection, injection site pain, nasopharyngitis, nausea, blepharoptosis, and bruising.

Eyelid ptosis is uncommon with experienced injectors but can certainly occur with BoNT-A placement in the periorbital area including the glabellar complex. Alpha-adrenergic eye drops can be used in the treatment of BoNT-A–induced blepharoptosis through activation of Muller's muscle in the upper eyelid.[46]

SERIOUS ADVERSE EVENTS

Serious adverse events occur more commonly with the use of BoNTs for therapeutic as opposed to cosmetic use. A black box warning was added to the package inserts of Dysport, Botox, and Xeomin following postmarketing reports that BoNT products may spread distantly from the area of injection, causing systemic symptoms of botulism, although this seems to occur in therapeutic patients and not in cosmetic patients, as therapeutic patients are often treated with five to ten times the typical overall cosmetic dosages. Included in the warning are asthenia, generalized muscle weakness, diplopia, blurred vision, ptosis, dysphagia, dysphonia, dysarthria, urinary incontinence, and breathing difficulties. Death from breathing difficulties has also been reported. No serious adverse event from distant spread of toxin has been reported with cosmetic use of BoNT-A at the labeled dose. In the event of an overdose, an antitoxin is available from the CDC. However, it is only effective prior to onset of any clinically apparent BoNT effects.

IMMUNOGENICITY AND TREATMENT FAILURE

The immunogenicity of the complexing proteins in BoNT-A formulations has been a concern as well as development of neutralizing and nonneutralizing antibodies. However, the actual incidence of antibody conversion is very low, estimated at 0.28% for glabellar lines and 0.46% for axillary hyperhidrosis in patients treated with OnabotulinumtoxinA in a meta-analysis by Naumann et al.[47] Of the 2240 subjects, only three became nonresponsive to OnabotulinumtoxinA, indicating that the majority of antibodies formed did not affect the critical domain on the neurotoxin protein. A study by Lawrence and Moy[48] also failed to show neutralizing antibody production in 1554 patients treated with 50 units of AbobotulinumtoxinA at a variety of sites (although 0.32% of patients were seropositive for AbobotulinumtoxinA antibodies during the study). The package insert for IncobotulinumtoxinA reports a 1.1% rate of conversion to neutralizing antibodies in a group of 1080 subjects. However, the package insert goes on to assert that the majority of patients who developed neutralizing antibodies had been previously exposed to different botulinum neurotoxins. The longest effective interval between treatments is, therefore, generally recommended.[8]

MALE PATIENT POPULATION

Male patients are expressing increased interest in pursuing treatment with BoNT-A. In most areas men can be treated with the same techniques as in women but with higher doses, due to increased muscle mass. The glabella is a common area of treatment and the recommended starting dose of Botox is at least 25 units, and possibly as high as 35 to 40 units. Technique must be adjusted according to individual patient anatomy, as some male patients have a broader corrugator muscle, necessitating more lateral injection points.[49,50] Crow's feet are also common areas of treatment for male patients, requiring similar techniques with increased doses. It has been our experience that many men do better with lower doses in the forehead to simply soften the musculature, rather than attempting to completely paralyze the muscle.

CONCLUSION

As the use of non-invasive cosmetic procedures rises in prevalence, familiarity with the various injectable toxins will continue to hold importance for the cosmetic practitioner. The authors emphasize an individual approach to treatment with close evaluation of each patient's unique musculature and facial structure for optimal outcomes. With experience and detailed knowledge of facial anatomy, mastery of these techniques can be achieved.

REFERENCES

1. Aoki KR. Pharmacology and immunology of botulinum neurotoxins. *Int Ophthalmol Clin.* 2005;45(3):25–37.
2. Carruthers A. History of the clinical use of botulinum toxin A and B. *Clin Dermatol.* 2003;21(6):469–472.
3. Carruthers J, Fagien S, Matarasso SL; Botox Consensus Group. Consensus recommendations on the use of botulinum toxin type a in facial aesthetics. *Plast Reconstr Surg.* 2004;114(Suppl 6):1S–22S.
4. Karsai S, Raulin C. Current evidence on the unit equivalence of different botulinum neurotoxin A formulations and recommendations for clinical practice in dermatology. *Dermatol Surg.* 2009;35(1):1–8.
5. Wenzel R, Jones D, Borrego JA. Comparing two botulinum toxin type A formulations using manufacturers' product summaries. *J Clin Pharm Ther.* 2007;32(4):387–402.
6. Klein AW, Carruthers A, Fagien S, Lowe NJ. Comparisons among botulinum toxins: an evidence-based review. *Plast Reconstr Surg.* 2008;121(6):413e–422e.
7. Jandhyala R. Relative potency of incobotulinumtoxinA vs onabotulinumtoxinA a meta-analysis of key evidence. *J Drugs Dermatol.* 2012;11(6):731–736.
8. Sattler G. Current and future botulinum neurotoxin type A preparations in aesthetics: a literature review. *J Drugs Dermatol.* 2010;9(9):1065–1071.
9. Huang W, Foster JA, Rogachefsky AS. Pharmacology of botulinum toxin. *J Am Acad Dermatol.* 2000;43(2 Pt 1): 249–259.
10. Spencer JM. Botulinum toxin B: the new option in cosmetic injection. *J Drugs Dermatol.* 2002;1(1):17–22.
11. Alam M, Dover JS, Arndt KA. Pain associated with injection of botulinum A exotoxin reconstituted using isotonic sodium chloride with and without preservative: a double-blind, randomized controlled trial. *Arch Dermatol.* 2002;138(4):510–514.
12. Vadoud-Seyedi J, Simonart T. Treatment of axillary hyperhidrosis with botulinum toxin type A reconstituted in lidocaine or in normal saline: a randomized, side-by-side, double-blind study. *Br J Dermatol.* 2007;156(5):986–989.
13. Liu A, Carruthers A, Cohen JL, et al. Recommendations and current practices for the reconstitution and storage of botulinum toxin type A. *J Am Acad Dermatol.* 2012;67(3):373–378.
14. Trindade De Almeida AR, Secco LC, Carruthers A. Handling botulinum toxins: an updated literature review. *Dermatol Surg.* 2011;37(11):1553–1565.
15. Hexsel DM, De Almeida AT, Rutowitsch M, et al. Multicenter, double-blind study of the efficacy of injections with botulinum toxin type A reconstituted up to six consecutive weeks before application. *Dermatol Surg.* 2003;29(5):523–529; discussion 9.
16. Flynn TC, Carruthers A, Carruthers J. Surgical pearl: the use of the Ultra-Fine II short needle 0.3-cc insulin syringe for botulinum toxin injections. *J Am Acad Dermatol.* 2002;46(6):931–933.
17. Hillebrand GG, Liang Z, Yan X, et al. New wrinkles on wrinkling: an 8-year longitudinal study on the progression of expression lines into persistent wrinkles. *Br J Dermatol.* 2010;162(6):1233–1241.
18. Lewis T, Jacobsen G, Ozog D. Intrafollicular orifice injection technique for botulinum toxin type A. *Arch Dermatol.* 2008;144(12):1657–1658.
19. Ascher B, Talarico S, Cassuto D, et al. International consensus recommendations on the aesthetic usage of botulinum toxin type A (Speywood Unit)–Part II: Wrinkles on the middle and lower face, neck and chest. *J Eur Acad Dermatol Venereol.* 2010;24(11):1285–1295.
20. Ascher B, Talarico S, Cassuto D, et al. International consensus recommendations on the aesthetic usage of botulinum toxin type A (Speywood Unit)–Part I: upper facial wrinkles. *J Eur Acad Dermatol Venereol.* 2010;24(11):1278–1284.
21. Kane MA. Classification of crow's feet patterns among Caucasian women: the key to individualizing treatment. *Plast Reconstr Surg.* 2003;112(Suppl 5):33S–39S.
22. Ahn MS, Catten M, Maas CS. Temporal brow lift using botulinum toxin A. *Plast Reconstr Surg.* 2000;105(3):1129–1135; discussion 1136–1139.
23. Cohen JL, Dayan SH. Botulinum toxin type a in the treatment of dermatochalasis: an open-label, randomized, dose-comparison study. *J Drugs Dermatol.* 2006;5(7):596–601.
24. Carruthers J, Carruthers A. Botulinum toxin A in the mid and lower face and neck. *Dermatol Clin.* 2004;22(2):151–158.
25. Pessa JE, Brown F. Independent effect of various facial mimetic muscles on the nasolabial fold. *Aesthetic plast Surg.* 1992;16(2):167–171.
26. Dayan SH, Kempiners JJ. Treatment of the lower third of the nose and dynamic nasal tip ptosis with Botox. *Plast Reconstr Surg.* 2005;115(6):1784–1785.
27. Ghavami A, Janis JE, Guyuron B. Regarding the treatment of dynamic nasal tip ptosis with botulinum toxin A. *Plast Reconstr Surg.* 2006;118(1):263–264.
28. Flynn TC, Carruthers JA, Carruthers JA, Clark RE 2nd. Botulinum A toxin (BOTOX) in the lower eyelid: dose-finding study. *Dermatol Surg.* 2003;29(9):943–950; discussion 950–951.
29. Cohen JL, Dayan SH, Cox SE, Yalamanchili R, Tardie G. OnabotulinumtoxinA dose-ranging study for hyperdynamic perioral lines. *Dermatologic Surg.* 2012;38(9):1497–1505.
30. Mazzuco R, Hexsel D. Gummy smile and botulinum toxin: a new approach based on the gingival exposure area. *J Am Acad Dermatol.* 2010;63(6):1042–1051.
31. Mangano A. Current strategies in the treatment of gummy smile using botulinum toxin type A. *Plast Reconstr Surg.* 2012;129(6):1015e.
32. Hwang WS, Hur MS, Hu KS, et al. Surface anatomy of the lip elevator muscles for the treatment of gummy smile using botulinum toxin. *Angle Orthod.* 2009;79(1):70–77.
33. Sucupira E, Abramovitz A. A simplified method for smile enhancement: botulinum toxin injection for gummy smile. *Plast Reconstr Surg.* 2012;130(3):726–728.
34. Carruthers J, Carruthers A. Practical cosmetic Botox techniques. *J Cutan Med Surg.* 1999;3(Suppl 4):S49–S52.
35. Levy PM. The 'Nefertiti lift': a new technique for specific re-contouring of the jawline. *J Cosmet Laser Ther.* 2007; 9(4):249–252.
36. Choe SW, Cho WI, Lee CK, Seo SJ. Effects of botulinum toxin type A on contouring of the lower face. *Dermatol Surg.* 2005;31(5):502–507; discussion 507–508.
37. Kim NH, Chung JH, Park RH, Park JB. The use of botulinum toxin type A in aesthetic mandibular contouring. *Plast Reconstr Surg.* 2005;115(3):919–930.
38. Solish N, Bertucci V, Dansereau A, et al. A comprehensive approach to the recognition, diagnosis, and severity-based treatment of focal hyperhidrosis: recommendations of the Canadian Hyperhidrosis Advisory Committee. *Dermatol Surg.* 2007;33(8):908–923.
39. Vergilis-Kalner IJ. Same-patient prospective comparison of Botox versus Dysport for the treatment of primary axillary hyperhidrosis and review of literature. *J Drugs Dermatol.* 2011;10(9):1013–1015.
40. Naumann M, Lowe NJ, Kumar CR, Hamm H; Hyperhidrosis Clinical Investigators Group. Botulinum toxin type a is a safe and effective treatment for axillary hyperhidrosis over 16 months: a prospective study. *Arch Dermatol.* 2003;139(6):731–736.

41. Hornberger J, Grimes K, Naumann M, et al; Multi-Specialty Working Group on the Recognition, Diagnosis, and Treatment of Primary Focal Hyperhidrosis. Recognition, diagnosis, and treatment of primary focal hyperhidrosis. *J Am Acad Dermatol.* 2004;51(2):274–286.
42. Benohanian A. What stands in the way of treating palmar hyperhidrosis as effectively as axillary hyperhidrosis with botulinum toxin type A. *Dermatol Online J.* 2009;15(4):12.
43. Cohen JL, Cohen G, Solish N, Murray CA. Diagnosis, impact, and management of focal hyperhidrosis: treatment review including botulinum toxin therapy. *Facial Plast Surg Clin North Am.* 2007;15(1):17–30, v–vi.
44. Cohen JL, Solish N. Treatment of hyperhidrosis with botulinum toxin. *Facial Plast Surg Clin North Am.* 2003;11(4):493–502.
45. Cote TR, Mohan AK, Polder JA, Walton MK, Braun MM. Botulinum toxin type A injections: adverse events reported to the US Food and Drug Administration in therapeutic and cosmetic cases. *J Am Acad Dermatol.* 2005;53(3):407–415.
46. Karami M, Taheri A, Mansoori P. Treatment of botulinum toxin-induced eyelid ptosis with anticholinesterases. *Dermatol Surg.* 2007;33(11):1392–1394; discussion 1394–1395.
47. Naumann M, Carruthers A, Carruthers J, et al. Meta-analysis of neutralizing antibody conversion with onabotulinumtoxinA (BOTOX(R)) across multiple indications. *Mov Disord.* 2010;25(13):2211–2218.
48. Lawrence I, Moy R. An evaluation of neutralizing antibody induction during treatment of glabellar lines with a new US formulation of botulinum neurotoxin type A. *Aesthet Surg J.* 2009;29(Suppl 6):S66–S71.
49. Kane MA, Brandt F, Rohrich RJ, Narins RS, Monheit GD, Huber MB; Reloxin Investigational Group. Evaluation of variable-dose treatment with a new U.S. Botulinum Toxin Type A (Dysport) for correction of moderate to severe glabellar lines: results from a phase III, randomized, double-blind, placebo-controlled study. *Plast Reconstr Surg.* 2009;124(5):1619–1629.
50. Carruthers A, Carruthers J. Prospective, double-blind, randomized, parallel-group, dose-ranging study of botulinum toxin type A in men with glabellar rhytids. *Dermatol Surg.* 2005;31(10):1297–1303.

CHAPTER 39

Non-Invasive Fat Removal

H. Ray Jalian

INTRODUCTION

Fat fuels a 20 billion dollar industry in the United States. One hundred eight million Americans are on a diet every year.[1] The desire for weight loss and optimization of the human physique is hardly a new trend. As health care and sanitation have improved, the waist circumference of Americans has increased. With better availability of food has come an increased incidence of overweight people. The progression of this trend ushered in the era of weight loss regimens and schemes. This was apparent as early as the late nineteenth century in William Banting's "Letter on Corpulence, Addressed to the Public."[2] We are continuously inundated with a glut of "too good to be true" schemes, and the public's obsession with fat loss has never been greater.

In the 1920s, a primitive form of liposuction gained popularity in France but was largely abandoned after a French model suffered gangrene in her leg following the procedure in 1926. The late 1960s saw the re-emergence of liposuction, which evolved into suction assisted liposuction in the early 1980s, and shortly thereafter into tumescent liposuction, which enabled the procedure to be performed in the office setting. Currently, liposuction is the top cosmetic surgical procedure performed in the United States.[3] Despite its popularity, it is still an invasive surgical procedure and involves significant risks, including infection, anesthesia complications, and even death.[4,5] As a result, there is a significant desire for effective, safe non-invasive modalities for body contouring.

In the last 5 years, we have seen the introduction of several device-based treatments for body contouring and non-invasive fat reduction. Some of these technologies, such as cryolipolysis and lipid selective lasers, selectively target unique physical properties of adipocytes. Others, such as ultrasound and radiofrequency (RF), selectively heat adipose tissue or disrupt cell membranes to produce their effects. This chapter will serve as an overview of the various approaches to non-invasive body contouring.

CRYOLIPOLYSIS

Manstein et al. [6] introduced the concept of cryolipolysis, the use of controlled cooling to selectively damage adipocytes. The discovery of cold sensitivity of adipocytes is not a new observation, but rather was first described in the 1970s by Epstein. He described so-called "popsicle panniculitis" in three children who developed focal lipoatrophy of the cheek after prolonged exposure to a cold popsicle.[7] Indeed, numerous reports of cold induced lipoatrophy in various clinical situations support the cryo-sensitivity of adipocytes.[8–11] With these historical observations in mind, a series of pre-clinical experiments in swine demonstrated loss of superficial fat 3 months after a single application of cold without significant pigmentary alteration, textural changes, or scarring.[6,12]

The mechanism of action of cryolipolysis is hypothesized to be through apoptosis of adipocytes. Alternative mechanisms include cold and vacuum induced reperfusion injury and subsequent oxidative damage. Histology specimens from treatment areas demonstrate a delayed, mixed inflammatory lobular panniculitis, peaking at 2 to 4 weeks after treatment. As the inflammatory infiltrate subsides, variably sized adipocytes and widening of the fibrous septa are observed concurrent with the clinical reduction in fat.[6]

Numerous randomized clinical trials support the modest, but appreciable, clinical efficacy of cryolipolysis (Fig. 39-1). Initial clinical studies treated 32 subjects with focal adiposity of the "love handles" demonstrating decrease in adiposity by digital photography, blinded assessment and subject satisfaction. Ultrasonographic evaluation revealed an average 22% reduction in fat layer thickness in the treatment area.[13] Subsequent studies have demonstrated similar improvements by photographic as well as caliper measurements.[14,15] More recently, Garibyan et al. conducted a randomized trial evaluating the clinical efficacy of cryolipolysis using standardized three-dimensional photography. An average volumetric reduction of 50 cc was observed at the treatment site when compared to controls (personal communication, Lilit Garibyan, MD, PhD).

Currently, cryolipolysis is approved by the Food and Drug Administration (FDA) for the treatment of focal adiposity of the "love handles" and the abdomen. The current commercial device utilizes a variety of cup-shaped vacuum applicators with two cooling panels (CoolSculpting, Zeltiq Aesthetics, Inc, Pleasanton, CA). After application of a gel-saturated fabric, the vacuum draws the tissue inward to fill the applicator as well as facilitate cooling by causing relative vasoconstriction. There is a pre-determined cooling intensity factor (CIF), a value representing the rate of efflux of heat from the tissue, for a 60 minute cycle. Following treatment, the applicator is removed and the treatment area is manually massaged to homogenize the ice crystals.

Following initial clearance by the FDA in 2010, there have been over 700,000 treatment cycles of cryolipolysis performed. The majority of side effects are predictable and transient. Common and immediate side effects include erythema localized to the treatment site. Ecchymosis is not uncommon, particularly if the patient is on anticoagulants. Pain during the procedure is minimal, and decreases

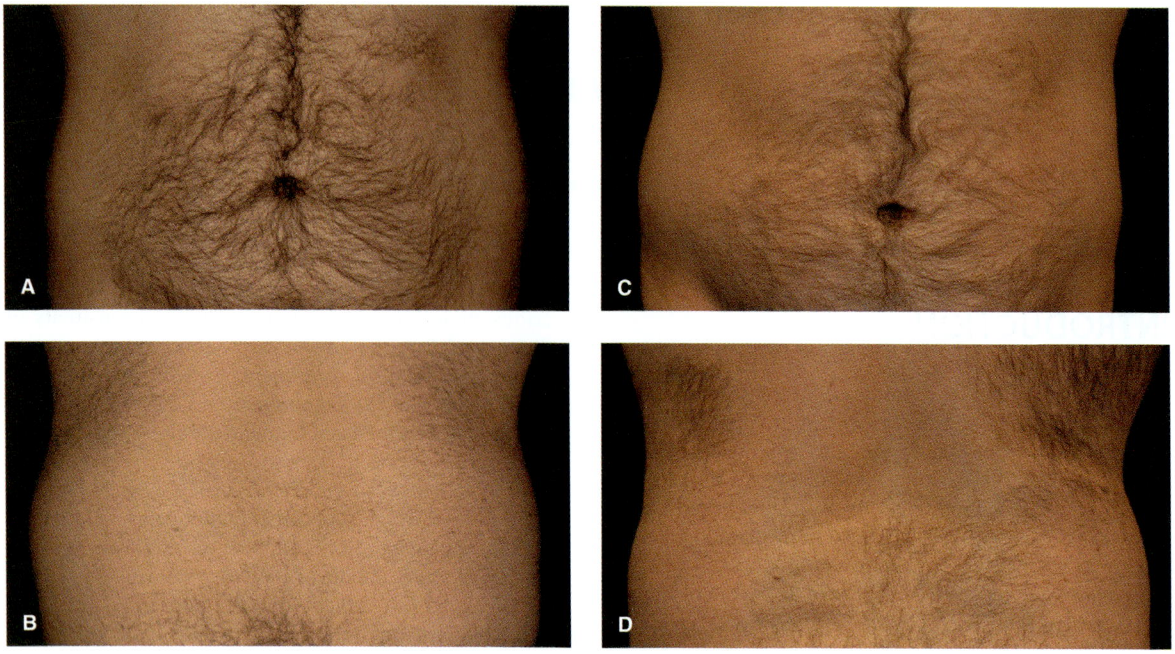

Figure 39-1 Cryolipolysis treatment of subject's left love handle. (**A**) Anterior and (**B**) posterior view prior to treatment. Three months following a single cycle to treatment area, there is a noticeable decrease in size of the love handle on the (**C**) anterior and (**D**) posterior view. Only treatment of left side was performed. Note no significant change in contralateral (untreated) site. (Photos used with permission of Lilit Garibyan, MD, PhD, Wellman Center for Photomedicine.)

further once the anesthetic effect of cooling takes effect. Alterations in cutaneous sensation were reported in the initial clinical trials, with up to 96% of subjects experiencing temporarily decreased sensation. This numbness largely resolves by 1 week posttreatment, though it can linger for up to 2 months.[16] No permanent cases of anesthesia have been reported. Posttreatment pain is limited, but rare cases of severe, intractable "shooting" and "jabbing" pain have been reported. The incidence is approximately one in 2000 and most commonly follows treatment with the larger applicator.[17] There is no significant increase in serum lipids or elevated liver function tests following cryolipolysis.[18] Cryolipolysis is relatively contraindicated in patients with cold sensitive dermatoses, including cryoglobulinemia, cold urticaria, Raynaud's syndrome, or paroxysmal cold induced hemoglobinuria.

With an increasing number of treatment cycles, rare side effects following cryolipolysis have emerged. Subcutaneous induration, described as generalized induration or discrete nodules (BB pellets to marbles) in the treatment area, was reported in a small subset of subjects. This side effect typically develops 2 weeks to 2 months post treatment, is transient in nature, and is often best appreciated by palpation. This phenomenon is self-limited and resolves in 3 to 6 months without any intervention.[19] Perhaps more concerning is the report of paradoxical adipose hyperplasia (PAH), which is delayed enlargement beyond baseline of the treatment site. The incidence of PAH is approximately one in 20,000 treated patients, although as new cases continue to emerge it may prove to be a more common phenomenon. Various anatomic locations have been reported including the flanks, abdomen, and upper back. No single, unifying characteristic has been identified among affected individuals at this time, although it seems to be more common in the male demographic. The onset of PAH is delayed several months following treatment. To date, no cases of PAH have resolved spontaneously and all have required either lipoplasty or abdominoplasty to correct the defect. The mechanism of action is largely unknown.[20]

ULTRASOUND

Ultrasound can non-invasively target adipocytes through nonthermal and thermal mechanisms. Ultrasound is a cyclic sound pressure wave with a frequency above the range of human hearing (>20 kHz). These waves pass through tissue, where they are scattered, reflected, or absorbed. Depending on the frequency of the incident ultrasound wave, various tissue interactions can occur. Low-intensity/low-frequency ultrasound results in nonthermal cavitation in the adipose tissue. In this case, the energy delivered has sufficient negative pressure to disrupt the molecular adhesion of the adipocytes, thus creating "holes" within the tissue. High-intensity focused ultrasound (HIFU) delivers energy of sufficient intensity to the adipose tissue to result in thermal ablation of adipocytes.

LOW-INTENSITY ULTRASOUND

Low-intensity, nonthermal ultrasound delivers concentrated energy to a precise depth in the subcutaneous tissue. This mechanical energy is used to disrupt fat cells without generating heat, thus sparing the neighboring structures such as skin, blood vessels, and nerves. This approach relies on the differential susceptibility of fat cells to mechanical stresses. A transducer utilizing an external guidance system directs a focused beam of energy into the tissue. Pulses of low intensity ultrasound waves alter adipocyte cellular membranes, generating cavitations within the tissue.[21,22]

Low-intensity ultrasound is approved by the FDA for circumference reduction of the waist, hips, and thighs. One of the initial studies to evaluate the efficacy of low-intensity ultrasound demonstrated a reduction in circumference measurements and fat thickness, as measured by ultrasonography, 1 month after three monthly treatments (UltraShape Ltd, Tel Aviv, Israel).[22] A larger study reported a mean reduction of approximately 2 cm in treatment area circumference and approximately 2.9 mm in fat thickness up to 12 weeks after a single treatment.[23] Side effects were minimal with subjects reporting mild pain, erythema, purpura, and rarely blister formation. No treatment related elevations in serum lipids were reported. Despite initial excitement, these results were not reproducible in a cohort of Asian subjects in a follow-up study.[24] Of note, none of the aforementioned studies had any histologic assessment of adipose tissue. Further studies are needed to determine the efficacy and the exact mechanism of fat loss.

HIGH-INTENSITY FOCUSED ULTRASOUND

HIFU has been used for nearly half a century for the non-invasive treatment of tumors of various organs,[25,26] but has only recently been evaluated as a method for the selective destruction of adipose tissue. High-energy ultrasonic waves are focused into the subcutaneous tissue, quickly raising the temperature above 56°C, resulting in coagulative necrosis of the adipocytes, and a subsequent reduction of the fat layer. Histology from pre-clinical and clinical studies demonstrates localized damage selective to the adipose tissue with sparing of the vasculature and nerve fibers within the treatment area. Gross examination of abdominoplasty specimens reveals well demarcated zones of necrosis limited to the treatment area. Microscopically, adipocyte necrosis is evident as demonstrated by disruption of cell membranes immediately after treatment. Two weeks following treatment, lipid-laden macrophages are present within the treatment zone. Resorption of lipids and healing are complete at approximately 14 weeks following a single treatment, corresponding to the observed clinical decrease at that time point. Examination of organs from distal organs in pre-clinical studies did not find any fat emboli.[27–29]

The second-generation HIFU device gained FDA clearance in 2011 (Solta Medical, Hayward, CA). Initial evidence for efficacy and safety in humans was based on two large case series of over 300 patients who had a single HIFU treatment to the anterior abdomen and flanks.[27,30] Waist circumference measurements taken 12 weeks post-treatment showed an average decrease of approximately 4.5 cm. Moreover, subject satisfaction was greater than 70% 3 months following treatment. A subsequent randomized control trial of 180 patients demonstrated a statistically significant decrease in waist circumference in the treatment group when compared to the sham treated control at 12 weeks following a single treatment.[31]

Side effects from HIFU occurred in approximately 10% of subjects and included prolonged tenderness, edema, ecchymoses, and hard lumps. All adverse events resolved within 1 to 3 months following treatment. The procedure is more painful than nonthermal ultrasound, and some study subjects did not tolerate the treatment. No increases in serum lipids or transaminases were noted.

RADIOFREQUENCY

RF has numerous applications in medicine, including RF cardiac ablation.[32] RF delivered at nonablative energy is used mainly to target dermal collagen in an attempt to tighten the skin. Quite simply, an RF current introduced into the tissue generates heat by transfer of energy from the electric field to charges in the tissue. RF can be delivered using monopolar, bipolar, and unipolar devices. In monopolar RF, a delivery electrode is placed over a target area and a return electrode is applied at a distant site. This allows a current to be generated that passes through the target tissue. In general, these monopolar devices have greater depth of penetration and are more painful. Delivery of energy can be static (e.g., short cycle in pulses) or dynamic (e.g., long cycles with a continuously moving handpiece). In bipolar RF devices both electrodes are incorporated into a single hand-piece. The depth of heating is determined by the distance between the electrodes. Unipolar RF systems function with one electrode and no grounding pad.

RF devices can non-invasively heat large volumes of tissue. By choosing the appropriate device and parameters of heat delivery, it is possible to selectively confine heat to the adipose tissue. Although the majority of studies using RF investigate efficacy for skin tightening and cellulite, more recently introduced devices are designed specifically for non-invasive body contouring. Large, peer-reviewed studies demonstrating the utility of these devices for this application are for the most part lacking. Nonetheless several devices have gained clearance by the FDA. These devices vary from static, pulsed monopolar devices (Thermacool TC, Solta Medical, Hayward, CA; Trusculpt, Cutera, Brisbane, CA) to dynamic monopolar devices (Exilis, BTL, Prague, Czech Republic). Further studies are needed to evaluate the efficacy of these devices.

The mechanism of action is largely unknown, although one study demonstrated thermal injury to adipocytes 9 days after treatment. Subsequent granulomatous inflammation coupled with foamy histiocytes was later observed within the adipose tissue. In the limited data available, there has been no associated increase in circulating serum lipids following treatment with an RF device.[33]

LOW-LEVEL LASER THERAPY

Low-level laser therapy (LLLT) is a relatively new area of photobiology based on the use of specific wavelengths of light to target cellular ultrastructure and alter cellular function. This technology is widely being applied to various applications in dermatology including treatment of androgenetic alopecia and wound healing.[34,35] The enthusiasm regarding the use of LLLT for targeting fat is based on the in vitro observation that transient pores can be induced in adipocytes after exposure to a 635 nm laser.[36] The formation of the pore is hypothesized to allow for the escape of lipid contents into the interstitial compartment with subsequent clearance from the body. Although initially utilized as a combination treatment with liposuction, LLLT alone is now used for fat reduction.

LLLT for non-invasive body contouring was FDA cleared in 2010. Many of the commercial devices contain multiple low-power laser diodes operating in the spectrum of red light (635 nm). Multiple treatment sessions are performed and often a nutritional supplement is concurrently administered throughout the treatment course. Although this approach appears to be quite safe, there are conflicting studies to support its efficacy.[37,38] In addition, unlike many of the technologies described previously, no histologic evidence of selective damage to adipocytes has been published following LLLT.

INFRARED LASERS

Selective photothermolysis involves the selection of a wavelength of light and pulse duration that sufficiently heat a specific target without damage to the surrounding tissue.[39] This confinement of heat allows for the targeting of individual chromophores without disruption of bystander tissue. Lipid-rich tissue has characteristic absorption within the infrared spectrum due to molecular vibrations of the carbon and hydrogen bonds. With this in mind, Anderson et al.[40] characterized the absorption spectrum of fat, and identified relative absorption peaks at 1210 nm and 1720 nm where the absorption of lipid is greater than that of water. A pilot human feasibility study investigated the use of a 1210 nm diode laser for the non-invasive destruction of fat. Punch biopsy specimens revealed damage to subcutaneous fat characterized by lipomembranous change.[41] Although microscopic samples demonstrated selective damage to the adipocytes, there are no large-scale clinical trials to support the use of this methodology for non-invasive fat reduction. Further studies and optimization of treatment parameters are needed to determine whether a 1210 nm wavelength laser may become a useful tool for the non-invasive selective destruction of fat.

CONCLUSION

Despite a historically tarnished track record, non-invasive fat reduction is now a reality. The last 5 years saw the introduction of various non-invasive fat technologies with novel approaches to target the adipose tissue. These devices, while not perfect, offer a predictable, safe approach to body contouring. As with any procedure, patient selection is key. It is important to set realistic expectations regarding clinical outcomes to avoid dissatisfaction. Interested patients should be informed that these technologies do not approach the degree of efficacy of liposuction. Ideal candidates are those that have focal adiposity that can be adequately targeted. Depending on the device chosen, multiple treatments may be necessary. Those that want dramatic results, have large amounts of fat, or desire global improvement are not ideal candidates. Moreover, those wishing to achieve noticeable weight loss or improvement in visceral fat will have negligible results.

The nascent nature of this field makes it difficult to compare the various technologies to determine whether one device is better than the other. Even with promising clinical results it is always important to approach these emerging technologies with a healthy dose of skepticism. Studies evaluating non-invasive body contouring are difficult to perform. Circumference measurements are inherently error-prone and susceptible to variation due to body positioning and variation in investigator methodologies. The same can be said regarding standardized photographs. Moreover some of these studies were not controlled for weight and thus can have variations based on weight changes. Finally, very few have looked at actual fat thickness by non-invasive means. Although some caliper measurements have been performed, these also are error-prone.[42] Longevity of results and long-term safety are still relatively unknown.

Despite the limitations and modest efficacy, non-invasive body contouring is now a reality and, just as the average waistline of Americans is growing, the demand for this technology is rising. As the technology continues to evolve, we are likely to see improved clinical efficacy, which perhaps will one day rival the dramatic effects of liposuction.

REFERENCES

1. 100 Million Dieters, $20 Billion: The Weight-Loss Industry by the Numbers. 2012. http://abcnews.go.com/Health/100-milliondieters-20-billion-weight-loss-industry/story?id = 16297197. Accessed November 20, 2013.
2. Banting W. *Letter on Corpulence, Addressed to the Public*. 2nd ed. London: Harrison and sons; 1863:22.
3. Statistics, Surveys & Trends. American Society of Aesthetic and Plastic Surgeons. 2012. http://www.surgery.org/media/news-releases/celebrating-15-years-of-trustworthy-plastic-surgery-statistics. Accessed August 7, 2014.
4. Grazer FM, de Jong RH. Fatal outcomes from liposuction: census survey of cosmetic surgeons. *Plast Reconstr Surg*. 2000;105(1):436–446; discussion 447–448.
5. Matarasso A, Swift RW, Rankin M. Abdominoplasty and abdominal contour surgery: a national plastic surgery survey. *Plast Reconstr Surg*. 2006;117(6):1797–1808.
6. Manstein D, Laubach H, Watanabe K, Farinelli W, Zurakowski D, Anderson RR. Selective cryolysis: a novel method of non-invasive fat removal. *Lasers Surg Med*. 2008;40(9):595–604.
7. Epstein EH Jr, Oren ME. Popsicle panniculitis. *N Engl J Med*. 1970;282(17):966–967.
8. Beacham BE, Cooper PH, Buchanan CS, Weary PE. Equestrian cold panniculitis in women. *Arch Dermatol*. 1980;116(9):1025–1027.
9. Collins HA, Stahlman M, Scott HW Jr. The occurrence of subcutaneous fat necrosis in an infant following induced hypothermia used as an adjuvant in cardiac surgery. *Ann Surg*. 1953;138(6):880–885.
10. Rotman H. Cold panniculitis in children. Adiponecrosis E frigore of Haxthausen. *Arch Dermatol*. 1966;94(6):720–721.
11. Solomon LM, Beerman H. Cold panniculitis. *Arch Dermatol*. 1963;88:897–900.
12. Zelickson B, Egbert BM, Preciado J, et al. Cryolipolysis for noninvasive fat cell destruction: initial results from a pig model. *Dermatol Surg*. 2009;35(10):1462–1470.
13. Kaminer M, Weiss R, Newman J. Visible cosmetic improvement with cryolipolysis: photographic evidence. In: *Annual Meeting of the American Society for Dermatologic Surgery*. 2009: Phoenix, AZ.

14. Dierickx CC, Mazer JM, Sand M, Koenig S, Arigon V. Safety, tolerance, and patient satisfaction with noninvasive cryolipolysis. *Dermatol Surg.* 2013;39(8):1209–1216.
15. Shek SY, Chan NP, Chan HH. Non-invasive cryolipolysis for body contouring in Chinese–a first commercial experience. *Lasers Surg Med.* 2012;44(2):125–130.
16. Coleman SR, Sachdeva K, Egbert BM, Preciado J, Allison J. Clinical efficacy of noninvasive cryolipolysis and its effects on peripheral nerves. *Aesthetic Plast Surg.* 2009;33(4):482–488.
17. Dover J, Saedi N, Kaminer M, et al. Side efects and risks associated with cryolipolysis. In: *Annual Meeting of the American Society for Laser Medicine and Surgery.* 2011. Grapevine, TX.
18. Klein KB, Zelickson B, Riopelle JG, et al. Non-invasive cryolipolysis for subcutaneous fat reduction does not affect serum lipid levels or liver function tests. *Lasers Surg Med.* 2009;41(10):785–790.
19. Jalian HR, Avram MM, Anderson RR. Rare side effects of cryolipolysis. In: *American Society for Laser Medicine and Surgery.* 2013: Boston, MA.
20. Jalian HR, Avram MM, Garibyan L, Mihm MC, Anderson RR. Paradoxical adipose hyperplasia following cryolipolysis. *JAMA Dermatology.* 2014;150(3):317–319.
21. Jewell ML, Solish NJ, Desilets CS. Noninvasive body sculpting technologies with an emphasis on high-intensity focused ultrasound. *Aesthetic Plast Surg.* 2011;35(5):901–912.
22. Moreno-Moraga J, Valero-Altés T, Riquelme AM, Isarria-Marcosy MI, de la Torre JR. Body contouring by non-invasive transdermal focused ultrasound. *Lasers Surg Med.* 2007;39(4):315–323.
23. Teitelbaum SA, Burns JL, Kubota J, et al. Noninvasive body contouring by focused ultrasound: safety and efficacy of the Contour I device in a multicenter, controlled, clinical study. *Plast Reconstr Surg.* 2007;120(3):779–789; discussion 790.
24. Shek S, Yeung CK, Kono T, Chan HH, et al. The use of focused ultrasound for non-invasive body contouring in Asians. *Lasers Surg Med.*, 2009;41(10):751–759.
25. Fruehauf JH, Back W, Eiermann A, et al. High-intensity focused ultrasound for the targeted destruction of uterine tissues: experiences from a pilot study using a mobile HIFU unit. *Arch Gynecol Obstet.* 2008;277(2):143–150.
26. Yoshizawa S, Ikeda T, Ito A, Ota R, Takagi S, Matsumoto Y. High intensity focused ultrasound lithotripsy with cavitating microbubbles. *Med Biol Eng Comput.* 2009;47(8):851–860.
27. Fatemi A. High-intensity focused ultrasound effectively reduces adipose tissue. *Semin Cutan Med Surg.* 2009;28(4):257–262.
28. Gadsden E, Aguilar MT, Smoller BR, Jewell ML. Evaluation of a novel high-intensity focused ultrasound device for ablating subcutaneous adipose tissue for noninvasive body contouring: safety studies in human volunteers. *Aesthet Surg J.* 2011;31(4):401–410.
29. Jewell ML, Desilets C, Smoller BR. Evaluation of a novel high-intensity focused ultrasound device: preclinical studies in a porcine model. *Aesthet Surg J.* 2011;31(4):429–434.
30. Fatemi A, Kane MA. High-intensity focused ultrasound effectively reduces waist circumference by ablating adipose tissue from the abdomen and flanks: a retrospective case series. *Aesthetic Plast Surg.* 2010;34(5):577–582.
31. Jewell ML, Baxter RA, Cox SE, et al. Randomized sham-controlled trial to evaluate the safety and effectiveness of a high-intensity focused ultrasound device for noninvasive body sculpting. *Plast Reconstr Surg.* 2011;128(1):253–262.
32. Alster TS, Lupton JR. Nonablative cutaneous remodeling using radiofrequency devices. *Clin Dermatol.* 2007;25(5):487–491.
33. Franco W, Kothare A, Ronan SJ, Grekin RC, McCalmont TH. Hyperthermic injury to adipocyte cells by selective heating of subcutaneous fat with a novel radiofrequency device: feasibility studies. *Lasers Surg Med.* 2010;42(5):361–370.
34. Avci P, Gupta A, Sadasivam M, et al. Low-level laser (light) therapy (LLLT) in skin: stimulating, healing, restoring. *Semin Cutan Med Surg.* 2013;32(1):41–52.
35. Avci P, Gupta GK, Clark J, Wikonkal N, Hamblin MR. Low-level laser (light) therapy (LLLT) for treatment of hair loss. *Lasers Surg Med.* 2014;46(2):144–151.
36. Neira R, Arroyave J, Ramirez H, et al. Fat liquefaction: effect of low-level laser energy on adipose tissue. *Plast Reconstr Surg.* 2002;110(3):912–922; discussion 923–925.
37. Elm CM, Wallander ID, Endrizzi B, Zelickson BD. Efficacy of a multiple diode laser system for body contouring. *Lasers Surg Med.* 2011;43(2):114–121.
38. Jackson RF, Dedo DD, Roche GC, Turok DI, Maloney RJ. Low-level laser therapy as a non-invasive approach for body contouring: a randomized, controlled study. *Lasers Surg Med.* 2009;41(10):799–809.
39. Anderson RR, Parrish JA. Selective photothermolysis: precise microsurgery by selective absorption of pulsed radiation. *Science.* 1983;220(4596):524–527.
40. Anderson RR, Farinelli W, Laubach H, et al. Selective photothermolysis of lipid-rich tissues: a free electron laser study. *Lasers Surg Med.* 2006;38(10):913–919.
41. Wanner M, Avram M, Gagnon D, et al. Effects of non-invasive, 1210-nm laser exposure on adipose tissue: results of a human pilot study. *Lasers Surg Med.* 2009;41(6):401–407.
42. Schmidt PK, Carter JE. Static and dynamic differences among five types of skinfold calipers. *Hum Biol.* 1990;62(3):369–388.

CHAPTER 40

Non-Invasive Body Contouring

Andrew A. Nelson & Mathew M. Avram

INTRODUCTION

Mankind has long been obsessed with achieving the so-called "perfect body"; in differing times and different circumstances, the ideal body has evolved. Currently, in our image-obsessed culture, many people possess a strong desire to lose weight to achieve their perfect body. Unfortunately, obesity is an epidemic in our culture and weight loss is a challenging goal for many. Although traditional dieting and exercise remain the best way to lose weight and maintain the weight loss, this may not work for all patients. Even patients who have achieved weight loss may continue to have small "problem areas." As a result, patients are increasingly turning to their physicians, desiring new technologies to help achieve body contouring and the ideal physique.

Historically, liposuction was the only means to achieve body contouring – other than diet and exercise. Although liposuction remains the gold standard, it is an invasive procedure with associated pain, bruising, downtime, and rarely, more serious side effects. Modern medicine has witnessed a dramatic movement toward minimal or no downtime procedures, as patients have become increasingly unwilling to tolerate prolonged healing or recovery times. While many topical agents have been reported to improve the appearance of cellulite, the improvements have typically been limited or modest in clinical experience.[1–4] The field of body contouring has rapidly evolved in the last several years with the introduction of numerous new technologies including lasers, RF devices, ultrasound devices, and cryolipolysis. Non-invasive fat removal procedures are now far more commonly performed than liposuction procedures. Non-invasive devices have been reported to have multiple beneficial effects including: improving the appearance of excess adipose tissue, reducing the overall volume of fat, reducing waist and thigh circumference, improving the appearance of cellulite, and skin tightening. Although these technologies are relatively new, and their potential utility must ultimately be determined by well-designed randomized scientific studies, the initial results and possibilities of some of these technologies are promising.

DETERMINING THE PATIENT'S STATUS AND TREATMENT GOALS

The first step in determining which therapeutic option is the best is to assess each patient individually and discuss their therapeutic goals. Depending on the patient's weight and individual body habitus, as well as their "problem areas" and goals, some devices may be a better option than others. As always, it is important to assess whether the patient has realistic goals as to the benefits of a procedure prior to any treatment.

The classic definition for obesity is based on a patient's body mass index (BMI = person's weight in kilograms divided by the square of their height in meters). This is a quick and easy calculation for patients and physicians. Obese patients are defined as those patients having a BMI>30. Typically, obese patients (BMI>30) are not good candidates for non-invasive body contouring and likely would benefit more from bariatric or other surgical interventions to help achieve meaningful weight loss. Thus, the simple BMI calculation may help to determine those patients who are not ideal candidates for non-invasive body contouring. Unfortunately, the BMI is also an oversimplification, as it does not necessarily take into account the patient's mixture of muscle and adipose tissue, or their overall body type. Many patients who present for non-invasive body sculpting may be in very good shape overall with a normal BMI, but feel plagued by only a few small problem areas, such as their thighs or flanks. For these patients, we, therefore, utilize measurements such as thigh circumference, waist circumference, skin fold thickness, visual assessment, and photographic comparisons pre- and post-procedure; these assessments more typically reflect the patient's ultimate clinical presentation and outcome.

It is also important to differentiate between fat and cellulite when assessing each patient.[5] Treatments for excess fat and cellulite are largely distinct. Excess fat and obesity are due to an overabundance of structurally normal adipocytes. In contrast, cellulite is best considered as a structural phenomenon of subcutaneous adipose tissue present in nearly all postpubertal females.[6,7] How then does normal fat become cellulite? This remains an area of ongoing research, but it is thought that cellulite may result from hormonal changes. Cellulite is rare in prepubertal females and males of any age, but is so common in postpubertal females that some researchers classify cellulite as a female secondary sexual characteristic. Estrogens are thought to stimulate lipogenesis while inhibiting lipolysis, thereby contributing to cellulite formation. Furthermore, it is believed that certain body areas have less effective lymphatic and vascular circulation, thereby contributing to the development of cellulite in these "high-risk areas." Ultrasound and magnetic resonance imaging (MRI) studies have documented the significant structural alterations between normal adipose tissue and abnormal cellulite structure.[8,9] In normal adipose tissue, the fibrous septae between the lobules of adipose tissue are arranged in an overlapping criss-cross pattern, creating greater tissue strength. Cellulite, on the other hand, has fibrous septae that are arranged parallel to each other, and perpendicular to the skin surface. This weaker structure allows for the focal herniation of adipose tissue, which ultimately contributes to the classic undulating, lumpy, "cottage cheese" appearance of cellulite. It remains unclear whether the presence of excess adipose tissue increases the risk of the development of cellulite. As a result of the differences between excess normal adipose tissue and structurally abnormal cellulite, we believe that excess fat and cellulite should be considered distinct entities and treated as such. Certain devices techniques that may be effective for treating cellulite may not treat excess adipose tissue, and vice versa.[10]

Once the patient has been evaluated and their treatment goals discussed, the patient and the treating physician can begin to effectively discuss the non-invasive body contouring options. Determining the best treatment option for each patient is dependent on clinical presentation, treatment goals, and most importantly, the patient's preferences.

NON-INVASIVE DEVICES

PHYSICAL TREATMENT OF FAT AND CELLULITE

Endermologie (LPG Systems, Valence, France) is an FDA-cleared device, which improves the appearance of cellulite through massage and kneading of the affected skin. The device combines positive and negative pressure created between two rollers to physically manipulate the patient's skin. The technique is thought to stimulate blood and lymphatic flow, thereby altering the architecture of the fat and improving the appearance of cellulite. It is less clear whether Endermologie has any effect on reducing unwanted excess adipose tissue. Modest clinical improvements in cellulite have been documented in clinical studies. A study by Gulec of 33 women who were treated with Endermologie for 15 sessions demonstrated a statistically significant improvement in the appearance of cellulite as assessed by a visual scale; however, few of the patients (5 of the 33) actually demonstrated clinical improvement.[11] A recent study by Collis et al.[12] compared twice-weekly treatment with Endermologie to a combination treatment of aminophylline cream and Endermologie; the authors concluded that Endermologie is not an effective treatment for cellulite, although 10 out of 35 patients with Endermologie-treated legs reported that their cellulite appearance improved clinically. In summary, Endermologie may result in modest improvements in the clinical appearance of fat and cellulite; however, it is likely that ongoing treatments would be necessary to maintain the improvement.

RADIOFREQUENCY DEVICES

Radiofrequency (RF) devices pass sinusoidal, alternating current through tissue, thereby causing ionic flow and ultimately heat from molecular friction. In essence, the tissue itself is the source of the heat, instead of the actual device. RF is, therefore, thought to create localized heat in the targeted tissue mass, while limiting the collateral spread of energy, neuromuscular reactions, or electrolysis. Adipocytes have high tissue resistance and relatively low heat transfer coefficients; as a result, adipose tissue can be readily heated by RF technologies and the heat will be relatively localized to the adipocytes. Recently, many RF devices have been advertised to improve the appearance of fat and cellulite.

The VelaSmooth and VelaShape (Syneron Medical Ltd, Irvine, CA) devices combine physical manipulation similar to Endermologie (massage and suction), with bipolar RF energy and broadband infrared light (700–2000 nm) to treat excess fat and cellulite. It has been proposed that these devices heat subcutaneous tissue and fat, resulting in increased blood flow and lipolysis in the treatment areas, thereby improving the appearance of fat and cellulite. In a randomized clinical study by Nootheti et al., patients were treated twice weekly for 6 weeks with either the VelaSmooth device or another laser device for cellulite (TriActive, Cynosure Inc, Westford, MA).[13] Seventy-five percent of patients were observed to have an improvement after comparing pre- and posttreatment photographs, but the results were modest. Patients were also observed to have a decrease in the upper and lower thigh circumference, as well as an improvement in the appearance of cellulite (Figs. 40-1 and 40-2). However, no statistically significant differences in the efficacies of the two devices were observed and no placebo group was included in the study. Bruising is a common side effect following treatment with the VelaSmooth device, likely related to the vacuum pressure and physical manipulation of the tissue rather than the RF technology itself.

Unipolar, volumetric RF devices with more diffuse, deep heating are also being studied for the treatment of fat and cellulite. Thirty patients were treated by Goldberg, et al. with a unipolar RF device (Accent, Alma Lasers US, Buffalo Grove, IL) every other week for a total of six treatment sessions; a decrease in mean leg circumference of 2.45 cm was observed, although the study was limited due to a lack of placebo or untreated controls.[14]

Recently, a novel RF device combining controlled RF heating and high-voltage ultrashort electrical pulses has been developed to treat adipose tissue (BodyFX, InMode Inc, Yokenam, Israel). The BodyFX system utilizes a vacuum system and traditional RF heating to warm the tissue and adipocytes to the range of 43 to 45 degrees Celsius. This heats the triglyceride droplet within the adipocyte and begins thermal adipocyte apoptosis. The BodyFX device then delivers high-voltage RF pulsing, which electroporates the cell membrane, basically poking a hole in the adipocyte membrane, leading to apoptosis of the adipocyte. These two mechanisms act synergistically to achieve greater levels of adipocyte apoptosis and greater clinical improvement. In initial studies, BodyFX has been shown to reduce circumferential measurements of treated areas, reduce the thickness of subcutaneous fat, induce direct adipocyte apoptosis, and simultaneously

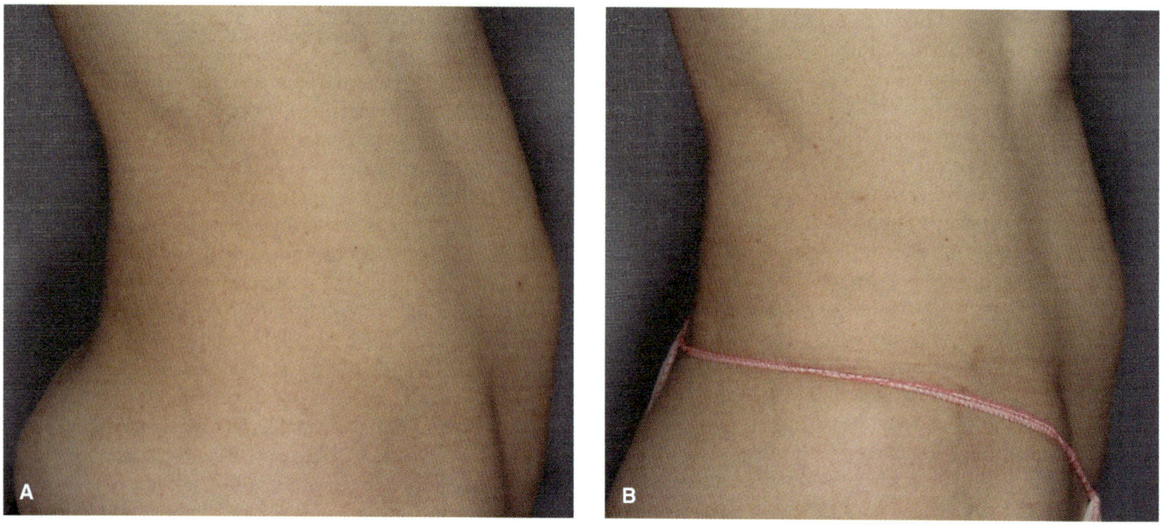

Figure 40-1 Clinical improvement in the appearance of the abdomen of a 60 year-old female before (**A**) and 3 months after (**B**) treatment with Velashape device. (Photos used with permission of Dr. Lori Brightman. Reprinted from, Wasserman DI, Avram M, Nelson AA. Approach to cellulite and fat. In: Kim J, Lask G, Nelson A, eds. *Comprehensive Aesthetic Rejuvenation: A Regional Approach.* 1st ed. New York, NY: Informa Healthcare; 2012:136–144.)

tighten skin through neocollagenesis in the treatment area (Fig. 40-3).[15] The BodyFX device represents another potential option for the treatment of excess fat, as it combines the added benefit of tightening the treatment area through traditional RF.

These RF technologies represent safe and efficacious therapeutic options for patients, although further clinical studies are necessary to establish their exact roles.

ULTRASOUND DEVICES

The diagnostic utility of ultrasound devices has long been established; more recently, focused ultrasound devices have been developed to treat adipocytes and the subcutis. The Liposonix device (Solta Medical, Hayward, CA) was recently FDA cleared for non-invasive waist circumference reduction.

A recent study by Jewell et al. of the Liposonix HIFU device (Solta Medical, Hayward, CA) reported improvement following a single treatment session.[16] One hundred and eighty patients were randomized to one of two different doses of HIFU or to a sham treatment. Twelve weeks following the single treatment, the patients treated with the higher HIFU dose had achieved a statistically significant improvement in waist circumference compared to the sham group (−2.44 cm vs. −1.43 cm). Patients were observed to have "improved" or "much improved"

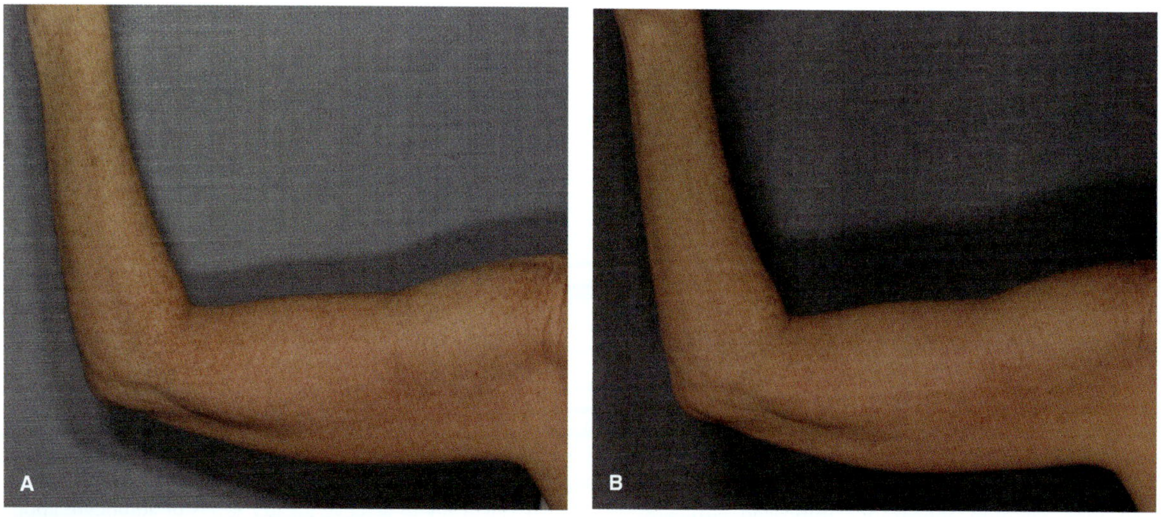

Figure 40-2 Clinical improvement in the appearance of the arms of a 55 year-old female before (**A**) and 6 months after (**B**) 5 treatments with the Velashape device (Radiofrequency level 3, infrared level 2, Vacuum level 1, treatment duration 7 minutes and 45 seconds). (Photos used with permission of Dr. Lori Brightman. Reprinted from, Wasserman DI, Avram M, Nelson AA. Approach to cellulite and fat. In: Kim J, Lask G, Nelson A, eds. *Comprehensive Aesthetic Rejuvenation: A Regional Approach.* 1st ed. New York, NY: Informa Healthcare;2012:136–144.)

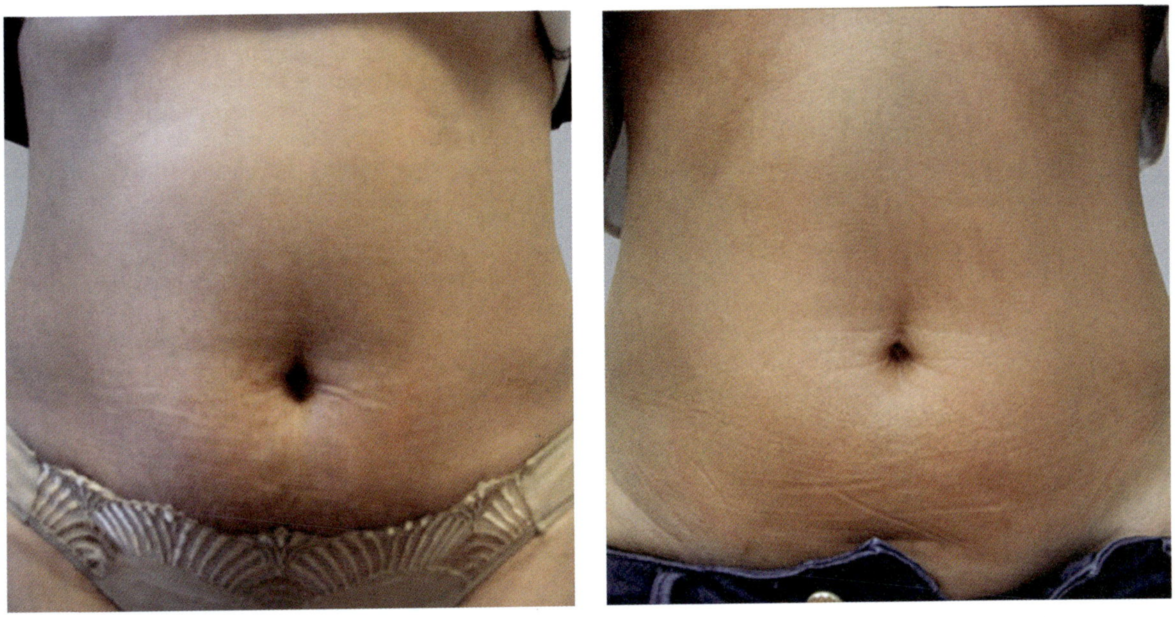

Figure 40-3 Clinical improvement showing a reduction of subcutaneous fat and tightening of skin in treatment area following a series of 6 BodyFX treatments. (Photo used with permission of InMode Inc., Yokenam, Israel.)

outcomes as assessed by physicians, and patients were satisfied with their treatments (Fig. 40-4). Common adverse events following the treatment included pain, bruising, and edema. However, no significant laboratory abnormalities were observed following treatment, including lipid profiles, markers of inflammation, coagulation, liver or renal function, hematologic assessments, or blood chemistry.

Another novel ultrasound technology, the UltraShape device (Syneron Inc., Irvine, CA) was recently FDA cleared for non-invasive reduction of abdominal circumference via mechanical (not thermal) fat cell destruction. A prospective, nonrandomized, controlled trial of 164 patients was conducted by Teitelbaum et al. to determine the efficacy of the device.[17] A total of 137 patients underwent one HIFU treatment to the abdomen, thighs, or flanks. Twelve weeks after the treatment, circumference reductions of the abdomen (mean reduction 2.3 cm), thighs (mean reduction 1.8 cm), and flanks (mean reduction 1.6 cm) were observed. The majority of the improvement in measured circumference was noted to occur within the first 2 weeks following treatment.

Ultrasound technologies represent a new and evolving area within the field of non-invasive fat treatment. Ultrasound technologies can also be incorporated into invasive liposuction procedures, known as ultrasound-assisted liposuction (UAL). Although this is an effective treatment method, it requires an invasive liposuction procedure. More recently, novel non-invasive HIFU technologies have been developed for improving the appearance of fat and cellulite. Although these devices require further

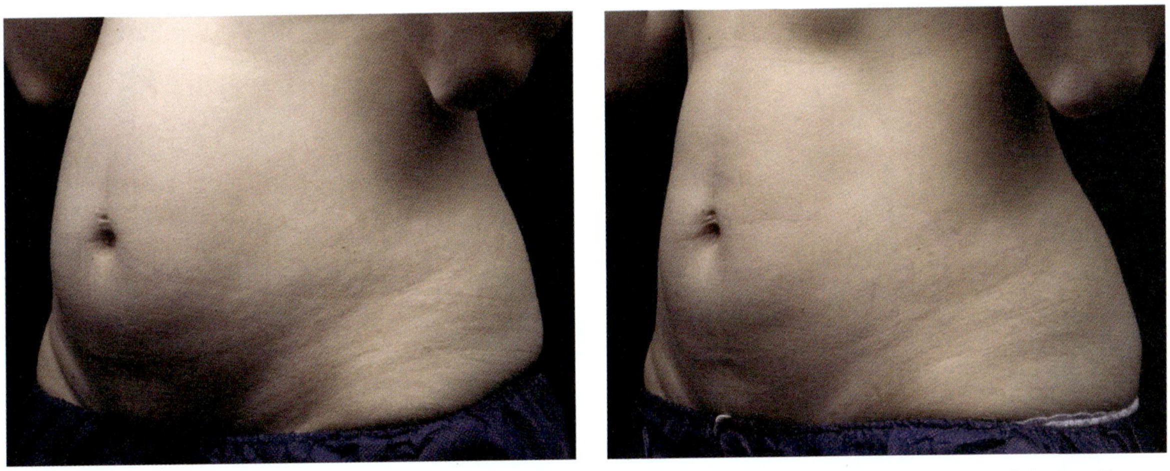

Figure 40-4 Clinical improvement following a single treatment with a high-intensity focused ultrasound device. (Reproduced with permission of Solta Medical, Inc.; courtesy of Solta Medical Aesthetic Center. Reprinted from Garibyan L, Jalian HR, Avram MM, Weiss RA. Body contouring: Non-invasive fat reduction. In: Goldman MP, Fitzpatrick RE, Ross EV, Kilmer SL, Weiss RA, eds. *Lasers and Energy Devices for the Skin*. 2nd ed. Boca Raton, FL: CRC Press; 2013.)

clinical study to determine their long-term efficacy and safety profile, they represent an exciting and promising opportunity within this field.

LASERS AND LIGHT SOURCES

Multiple novel light sources and laser technologies have been developed as therapeutic options for fat and cellulite. Historically, these laser devices were utilized as an adjunct with liposuction, known as laser-assisted liposuction (LAL). More recently, new non-invasive laser and light source devices have been marketed for the treatment of fat and cellulite. It is important to note that several devices which are marketed to improve fat and cellulite actually do not affect the adipocytes themselves, but rather, target the dermis in an attempt to stimulate collagen formation/remodeling. Devices with wavelengths in the near infrared region, as well as intense pulsed light (IPL) sources, fall into this category. At the time of this writing, few laser devices are FDA cleared for the direct treatment of fat and cellulite.

The TriActive device (Cynosure Inc, Bedford, MA) combines deep tissue massage and suction (similar to Endermologie), with contact cooling and a low-intensity diode laser (808 nm). The TriActive device is meant to improve the appearance of cellulite by increasing lymphatic drainage, improving blood flow, and tightening the skin in treated areas. Patients typically are treated with the device twice weekly, with progressive improvement following each treatment. In clinical studies, patients were noted to achieve objective reductions in hip and thigh circumference as well as subjective improvements in the appearance of cellulite, including a reduction in the appearance of skin dimpling, improvement in the overall contour of the limb, and improvement in overall skin texture (Fig. 40-5). TriActive

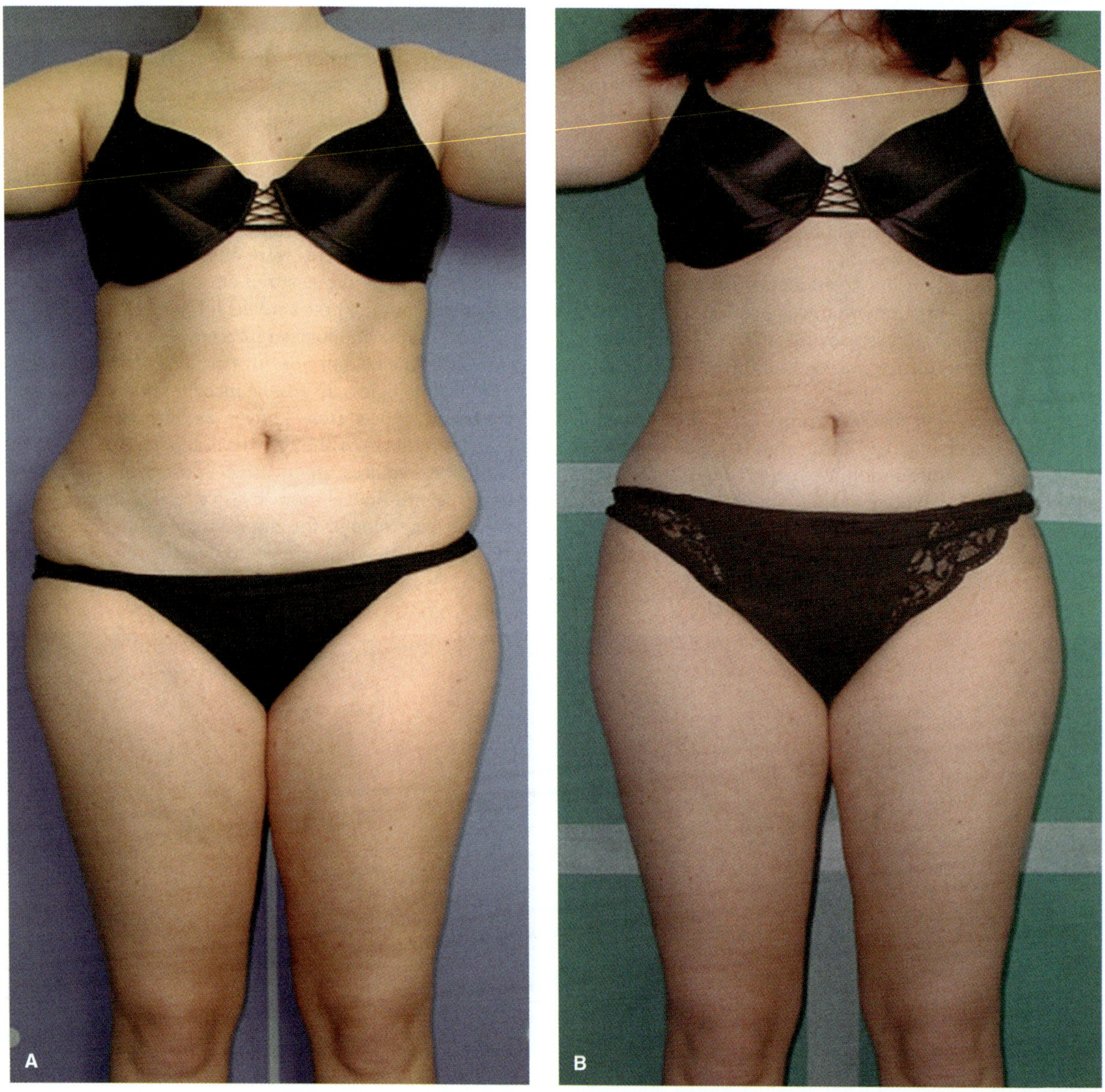

Figure 40-5 Clinical improvement in the appearance of abdominal cellulite and subcutaneous fat before (**A**) and after (**B**) 20 treatments with the Triactive device. (Photos used with permission of Dr. Andrea Pelosi. Reprinted from, Wasserman DI, Avram M, Nelson AA. Approach to cellulite and fat. In: Kim J, Lask G, Nelson A, eds. *Comprehensive Aesthetic Rejuvenation: A Regional Approach*. 1st ed. New York, NY: Informa Healthcare; 2012:136–144.)

treatments were generally well tolerated, although approximately 20% of patients developed mild bruising.

The SmoothShapes device (Eleme Medical, Merrimack, NH), combines two different wavelengths of laser with a physical massage system similar to Endermologie. The 915 nm diode wavelength is meant to liquefy fat, while the 650 nm wavelength is meant to improve fat membrane permeability, thereby allowing the adipocytes to be mobilized to the interstitium. A treatment session consists of multiple passes with the SmoothShapes device, and two to three treatment sessions are performed each week for best results. In clinical studies by Lach and Kulick, the SmoothShapes device results in reduction of the thickness of the subcutaneous fat pad, as assessed by MRI (Fig. 40-6).[18,19] The device was well tolerated with no significant associated adverse events.

The VelaSmooth and VelaShape (Syneron Medical Ltd, Irvine, CA) devices, as discussed previously, combine physical manipulation, bipolar RF energy, and broadband infrared light (700–2000 nm) to facilitate a multimodality approach to fat and cellulite treatment. The efficacy of these devices was previously discussed in the section regarding RF. In the future, more devices may approach fat and cellulite treatment through this multimodality approach in an effort to achieve greater efficacy.

Recently, a low-level laser device (Zerona, Erchnia Inc, McKinney, TX) was FDA cleared for the non-invasive reduction in circumference of hips, waist, and thighs. Zerona is a low-level diode laser (615 nm), which produces five independent beams. The center beam is fixed, while the four remaining beams can be individually adjusted allowing multiple body areas (abdomen, flank, thighs) to be treated simultaneously. The exact mechanism of action has not been elucidated, though it has been claimed that low-level laser therapy stimulates the fat cell to emulsify; the liquefied fat is then mobilized via a temporary pore in the cell membrane from inside the cell to the interstitium, where the fat is ultimately absorbed into the lymphatic system. Typically, Zerona treatments are performed every other day for a total of six treatments, with each treatment lasting approximately 40 minutes. There are other FDA-cleared low-level laser therapies. Further study will determine whether they constitute a significantly effective treatment option for excess adipose tissue.

CRYOLIPOLYSIS

CoolSculpting (Zeltiq Aesthetics, Pleasanton, CA) is a novel FDA-cleared device for non-invasive fat reduction. CoolSculpting utilizes cryolipolysis technology (controlled cold exposure) to selectively cool fat, thereby causing adipocyte apoptosis.[20] The treatment cycle lasts approximately 60 minutes, at the conclusion of which the skin is cool, firm, and erythematous. Following the treatment, the physician massages the area gently to break up any crystallized adipocytes. Over the next several weeks to months, the adipocytes undergo apoptosis, are mobilized and ultimately eliminated by the body. Typical treatment areas include the flank "love handles," the back "fat pads" and the abdomen "muffin top". In a recent clinical study, a significant reduction in the thickness of the fat in the treatment area was observed following a single CoolSculpting treatment (mean fat pad thickness reduction of 22.4%, as measured on ultrasound). Of the 32 patients in the study, all had achieved a significant visible contour improvement following a single treatment.[21,22] The best results were seen in patients with localized, discrete fat bulges. Treatments are typically well tolerated, although patients may develop bruising as well as transient altered sensation, numbness or even pain in the treatment area. Although the treatment and

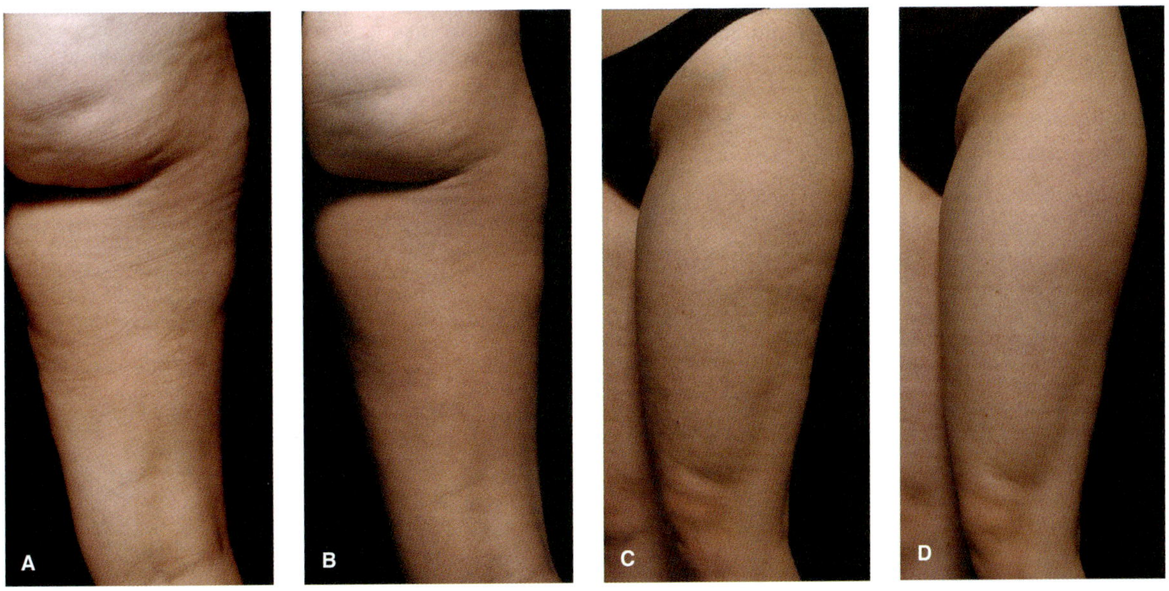

Figure 40-6 Clinical improvement in thigh circumference and texture before (**A, C**) and after (**B, D**) 8 treatments with the Smoothshapes device. (Photos used with permission of Dr. Khalil A. Khatri. Reprinted from, Wasserman DI, Avram M, Nelson AA. Approach to cellulite and fat. In: Kim J, Lask G, Nelson A, eds. *Comprehensive Aesthetic Rejuvenation: A Regional Approach*. 1st ed. New York, NY: Informa Healthcare; 2012:136–144.)

recovery from treatment are typically quite comfortable, significant pain can rarely be experienced in the area of treatment for 1 to 2 weeks.[23] CoolSculpting represents a safe, novel and efficacious, non-invasive treatment option for fat.

CONCLUSIONS

The last few years have witnessed profound changes in the field of body contouring with the development of safe, effective, non-invasive technologies. These non-invasive devices have been reported to have multiple beneficial effects including improving the appearance of excess adipose tissue, reducing the overall volume of fat, reducing waist and thigh circumference, improving the appearance of cellulite, and skin tightening. Although liposuction and surgical procedures remain the gold standard for patients seeking large volume fat removal, many patients prefer these novel non-invasive therapies as simple, no downtime alternatives to improve the appearance of limited fat and cellulite. For this reason, non-invasive treatments now far outnumber invasive procedures.

Physical manipulation devices, RF devices, ultrasound devices, lasers, and cryolipolysis have all been developed for the non-invasive treatment of fat and cellulite. Each technology has its own risks and benefits. Ultimately, rather than there being one single best technology for all patients, it is likely that different technologies will have specific patient types and situations for which they are best suited. As a result, it is important for physicians to assess each patient individually, discuss their current state and ultimate treatment goals, and choose a device accordingly. Ultimately, determining the best treatment option for each patient is dependent on clinical presentation, treatment goals, and most importantly, the patient's preferences. Some devices are better studied and more effective than others. Following these principles, it is possible for patients to undergo safe, effective, non-invasive treatments to treat unwanted fat and cellulite.

REFERENCES

1. Hamilton EC, Greenway FL, Bray GA. Regional fat loss from the thigh in women using 2% aminophylline. *Obes Res.* 1993;1: 95S.
2. Kligman AM, Pagnoni A, Stoudemayer T. Topical retinol improves cellulite. *J Dermatolog Treat.* 1999;10:119–125.
3. Pierard-Franchiemont C, Pierand GE, Henry F, Vroome V, Cauwenbergh G. A randomized, placebo controlled trial of topical retinal in the treatment of cellulite. *Am J Clin Dermatol.* 2000;1369–1374.
4. Rotunda AM, Avram MM, Avram AS. Cellulite: Is there a role for injectables? *J Cosmet Laser Ther.* 2005;7:147–154.
5. Avram MM. Cellulite: a review of its physiology and treatment. *J Cosmet Laser Ther.* 2004;6:181–185.
6. Nurnberger F, Muller G. So-called cellulite: an invented disease. *J Dermatol Surg Oncol.* 1978;4:221–229.
7. Rossi AB, Vergnanini AL. Cellulite: a review. *J Eur Acad Dermatol Venereol.* 2000;14:251–262.
8. Mirrashed F, Sharp JC, Krause V, Morgan J, Tomanek B. Pilot study of dermal and subcutaneous fat structures by MRI in individuals who differ in gender, BMI, and cellulite grading. *Skin Res Technol.* 2004;10:161–168.
9. Querleux B, Cornillon C, Jolivet O, Bittoun J. Anatomy and physiology of subcutaneous adipose tissue by in vivo magnetic resonance imaging and spectroscopy: relationships with sex and presence of cellulite. *Skin Res Technol.* 2002;8:118–124.
10. Hexsel DM, Mazzuco R. Subcision: a treatment for cellulite. *Int J Dermatol.* 2000;39:539–544.
11. Güleç AT. Treatment of cellulite with LPG endermologie. *Int J Dermatol.* 2009;48:265–270.
12. Collis N, Elliot LA, Sharpe C, Sharpe DT. Cellulite treatment: a myth or reality: a prospective randomized, controlled trial of two therapies, endermologie and aminophylline cream. *Plast Reconstr Surg.* 1999;104(4):1110–1114.
13. Nootheti PK, Magpantay A, Yosowitz G, Calderon S, Goldman MP. A single center, randomized, comparative, prospective clinical study to determine the efficacy of the Velasmooth system versus the Triactive system for the treatment of cellulite. *Lasers Surg Med.* 2006;38(10):908–912.
14. Goldberg DJ, Fazeli A, Berlin AL. Clinical, laboratory and MRI analysis of cellulite treatment with a unipolar radiofrequency device. *Dermatol Surg.* 2008;34(2):204–209.
15. Boisnic S, Divaris M, Nelson AA, Gharavi NM, Lask GP. A clinical and biological evaluation of a novel, noninvasive radiofrequency device for the long-term reduction of adipose tissue. *Lasers Surg Med.* 2014;46(2):94–103.
16. Jewell ML, Baxter RA, Cox SE, et al. Randomized sham-controlled trial to evaluate the safety and effectiveness of a high-intensity focused ultrasound device for noninvasive body sculpting. *Plast Reconstr Surg.* 2011;128(1):253–262.
17. Teitelbaum SA, Burns JL, Kubota J, et al. Noninvasive body contouring by focused ultrasound: safety and efficacy of the Contour I device in a multicenter, controlled, clinical study. *Plast Reconstr Surg.* 2007;120(3):779–789.
18. Kulick MI. Evaluation of a noninvasive, dual-wavelength laser-suction and massage device for the regional treatment of cellulite. *Plast Reconstr Surg.* 2010;125(6):1788–1796.
19. Lach R. Reduction of subcutaneous fat and improvement in cellulite appearance by dual-wavelength, low-level laser energy combined with vacuum and massage. *J Cosmet Laser Ther.* 2008;10(4):202–209.
20. Manstein D, Laubach H, Watanabe K, Farinelli W, Zurakowski D, Anderson RR. Selective cryolysis: a novel method of non-invasive fat removal. *Lasers Surg Med.* 2008;40(9): 595–604.
21. Dover J, Burns J, Coleman S, et al. A prospective clinical study of noninvasive cryolypolysis for subcutaneous fat layer reduction—Interim report of available subject data. Presented at the Annual Meeting of the American Society for Laser Medicine and Surgery. April 2009, National Harbor, MD.
22. Rosales-Berber IA, Diliz-Perez E. Controlled cooling of subcutaneous fat for body reshaping. Presented at the 15th World Congress of the International Confederation for Plastic, Reconstructive and Aesthetic Surgery. 2009, New Delhi, India.
23. Klein KB, Zelickson B, Riopelle JG, et al. Non-invasive cryolipolysis for subcutaneous fat reduction does not affect serum lipid levels or liver function tests. *Lasers Surg Med.* 2009;41(10): 785–790.

CHAPTER 41

Liposuction

Daniel P. Friedmann, Kimberly J. Butterwick, & Arisa E. Ortiz

INTRODUCTION

The popularity of liposuction has increased dramatically over the past two decades, with liposuction constituting 10% of all ambulatory cosmetic procedures performed in the United States between 1995 and 2010.[1] This interest, particularly among dermatologists and non-core cosmetic practitioners, has grown in large part due to Klein's introduction of the tumescent technique, allowing this procedure to be performed comfortably and less invasively under local anesthesia with minimal postoperative downtime, unparalleled patient safety, and improved aesthetic results.[2,3]

INDICATIONS

Diet- or exercise-resistant subcutaneous fat in virtually any area of the body can now be treated safely and effectively with tumescent liposuction, from excessively full jowls to thick ankles. Potential non-cosmetic indications for liposuction, such as breast reduction in women and the treatment of gynecomastia in men, are listed in Table 41-1.[4–11]

TABLE 41-1
Non-Cosmetic Indications for Tumescent Liposuction

Indications	Examples
Lipoma	▪ Solitary ▪ Angiolipoma ▪ Familial multiple lipomatosis ▪ Adiposis dolorosa (Dercum's disease)
Localized lipodystrophy	▪ Buffalo hump due to Cushing's syndrome ▪ Insulin-induced lipohypertrophy ▪ HAART-associated lipodystrophy
Endocrine	▪ Axillary hyperhidrosis or bromhidrosis ▪ Macromastia ▪ Gynecomastia or pseudogynecomastia
Reconstructive/Surgical	▪ Flap undermining or defatting ▪ Hematoma evacuation ▪ Post-surgical lymphedema

Adapted with permission from Coleman WP, Flynn TC. Liposuction. In: Bolgnia JL, Jorizzo JL, Rapini RP, eds. *Dermatology,* 2nd ed. Spain: Mosby; 2008:2346. Copyright Elsevier.

PATIENT SELECTION

CONSULTATION

Patients presenting for a liposuction consultation often have preconceived notions about the procedure, having heard both positive and negative reports from friends or via the internet. Although the advent of social media now connects individuals en masse, this may only potentiate the spread of biased and unreliable information.[12] Potential patients need to be properly informed and educated regarding tumescent liposuction, including the risks, benefits, alternatives, and a realistic appraisal of the postoperative course and expected results. The physician utilizes the consultation visit to determine whether the patient is mentally and physically healthy, has no contraindications to surgery, and has fatty deposits that are amenable to treatment. Once both the patient and the physician have adequate information, the decision to proceed can be made.

PATIENT SELECTION AND CONTRAINDICATIONS

The ideal patient is in excellent health, is not overweight, and has fatty deposits out of proportion to overall body shape, with otherwise normal skin tone and elasticity. These fatty deposit areas are primarily genetic in origin, gender specific, and resistant to diet and exercise. The ideal patient also has reasonable and realistic expectations. The ideal patient age range is 30 to 55 years old, as this group is generally mature enough to undergo this procedure and more likely to be free of underlying illnesses, with less risk of excessive skin laxity or other complicating factors.

Given that the majority of patients vary from this ideal in some manner, the consultation and preoperative examination enable the physician to screen and choose patients who are suitable for the procedure. The actual age of a prospective patient, for instance, is not as important as their overall mental and physical health. The authors have safely performed tumescent liposuction on patients from 18 to 85 years old. The extent of the procedure will also determine the ability of a particular patient to tolerate it. Patients with mild, controlled medical conditions such as diabetes or hypertension or elderly individuals in otherwise good health can, therefore, safely undergo a limited procedure under appropriate operative conditions.

It is important that the patient's weight be stable for several months prior to surgery. Patients with patterns of progressive or cyclical weight gain will most likely gain weight after surgery and have suboptimal results. Patients

TABLE 41-2
Medical Contraindications to Tumescent Liposuction

Contraindications
Morbid obesity
Pregnancy
Severe cardiovascular or renal disease
Severe coagulation disorder
Active hepatitis or chronic liver failure
Major immunosuppression
Active cancer
History of malignant hyperthermia

Republished with permission of Taylor & Francis Group LLC, from Butterwick KJ. Liposuction: consultation and preoperative considerations. In: Narins RS, ed. *Safe Liposuction and Fat Transfer.* New York, NY: Marcel Dekker, Inc; 2003:43. Permission conveyed through Copyright Clearance Center, Inc.

who have lost large amounts of fat in a short span will have very loose skin and are poor candidates for surgery. Although most patients are within 10 to 25 pounds of their ideal weight, some may be more than 20% heavier. Yet the majority of these patients have localized, disproportionate fatty deposits that would benefit from the procedure. Others may have a moderate degree of cellulite that will not improve with treatment along with significant underlying fatty deposits that may be dramatically recontoured. It is important to note that patients lose little weight with the procedure; however, the body-fat percentage is generally lower after liposuction and the basal metabolic rate (i.e., calories burned at rest) may increase.[13] The importance of weight maintenance postoperatively must be emphasized to patients to achieve optimal long-term results.

Prospective patients who are generally excluded from liposuction include those with medical contraindications (Table 41-2), excessively loose skin, unrealistic expectations – seeking perfection, immediate results, and/or substantial weight loss – and/or who are emotionally or psychologically unstable.[14,15] Certain personality traits and disorders, including perfectionism, eating disorders, and body dysmorphic disorder, have been suggested to correlate with dissatisfied cosmetic surgery patients.[16] Although excessively loose skin is typically a contraindication to treatment, older individuals who have poor skin tone but are more concerned about their shape in clothing than skin laxity may end up being happy patients.

PREOPERATIVE CONSIDERATIONS

If the initial consultation is successful and the patient has decided to undergo tumescent liposuction, a preoperative visit is scheduled with a trained nurse practitioner or registered nurse to prepare for the day of surgery. The recommended procedure is reviewed verbally, as are the detailed, written preoperative and postoperative instructions and the informed consent forms. In particular, patients need to be reminded that they cannot drive themselves home following the procedure and need to have someone monitor them for the first 24 hours. It is helpful to have a relative or close friend educated in postoperative care as well at the time of the visit. A detailed history and physical examination is also performed and preoperative laboratory studies, prescriptions, photographs, and informed consents are obtained.

MEDICAL/SURGICAL HISTORY

A detailed medical and surgical history is obtained to confirm that there are no contraindications to surgery. If there is a significant underlying medical condition, the patient's primary care physician is later contacted for medical clearance.

Ruling out patients with active liver disease is imperative as adequate hepatic function is essential for lidocaine metabolism.[17,18] Patients who are positive for hepatitis C or HIV but are otherwise healthy must nevertheless be approached with caution due to potentially compromised immune and liver function. HIV-positive patients may also exhibit unpredictable metabolism of lidocaine, independent of antiviral therapy.[19] Patients who have undergone chemotherapy may have an altered ability to metabolize lidocaine even with normal liver function tests, as reported in one case of lidocaine toxicity that occurred up to 2 years post treatment.[20] Immunocompromised patients are also poor candidates for liposuction due to their increased risk of infection and delayed wound healing.

Risk factors for thromboembolism should be identified. These include a prior history of thrombophlebitis, thrombophilia or thromboembolism, high-dose estrogen therapy, obesity, varicose veins, immobilization, and positive smoking history.[21] All allergies to medications, surgical materials, and postoperative dressings need to be noted.

A surgical history is helpful to screen for poor wound healing, a tendency for keloidal or hypertrophic scarring, infectious complications, and bleeding diatheses. Patients who have undergone recent abdominal surgery should wait 6 months or longer before undergoing liposuction in that area. Multiple abdominal surgeries may compromise results due to muscle laxity or adherent scarring. Multiple pregnancies may also signal weak abdominal musculature and the need for alternative procedures.

PHYSICAL EXAMINATION

NECK. When evaluating or photographing the head and neck, the ideal profile should be viewed with the head held in the Frankfurt horizontal plane, in which a horizontal line can be drawn through the highest point of the ear canal meatus and the lowest point of the orbital rim.[22] A 90° to 135° cervicomental angle, formed by the horizontal plane of the submentum and the vertical plane of the neck, and a defined inferior mandibular border are key anatomic features of a youthful neck that can become blunted with age and weight gain.[23] Grasping the submental fat and tucking it up under the chin to "remove" it from view can illustrate a postoperative result to patients. It is important to note that lax, photoaged neck skin may look more wrinkled postoperatively, and the patient should be advised appropriately.

POSTERIOR ARMS. The arms should be examined in the anatomic position as well as abducted perpendicularly from the body with thumbs up. Ideal patients have moderate amounts of excess fat localized to the posterior and lateral aspects of the arms with mild-to-minimal skin laxity. However, postoperative skin retraction can still produce excellent results in patients with large, hanging fat deposits and/or significant skin laxity as long as a sufficient amount of superficial fat remains to ensure skin smoothness.[24] The biceps area should be avoided in the majority of patients, given its thin overlying skin.

ABDOMEN, WAIST, AND FLANKS. The abdomen should be examined as a whole with the patient standing in anatomic position. Patients with prominent lower abdominal protrusion due to muscle diastasis, marked skin laxity, and/or visceral fat are likely poor candidates for liposuction.[25] Men with taut, protuberant abdomens due to visceral fat may still have ample subcutaneous tissue. Having the patient lie supine with back and hips slightly flexed may accentuate these deposits.[26] The presence or absence of a periumbilical or ventral hernia should always be documented as its presence may increase the risk of peritoneal perforation.

The male flanks lie just above the hips, extending between the iliac rim and the inferior costal margin, overlying the lateral oblique muscles (Fig. 41-1A). On the other hand, in female patients the anatomic area equivalent or slightly superior to the male flank is the waist. The female flanks lie infrascapularly, between the waist and the bra line (Fig. 41-1B).

HIPS, OUTER THIGHS, AND BUTTOCKS. The patient should be examined in a standing position. A gynecoid pattern of fat distribution predisposes women to commonly accumulate fat in all three of these areas. Fullness at the iliac crest of the hip and subtrochanteric area of the outer thigh, with an intervening lateral gluteofemoral depression, produce this "violin deformity"; downward and outward pressure from the buttock also augments lateral thigh protrusion.[27] Examination of the outer thighs should include an assessment for excess skin laxity, which can worsen postoperatively. Excess underlying musculature within the thigh and buttock may also limit results. Although areas of cellulite should be noted, patients must be informed that it may not improve with treatment.

MEDIAL THIGH AND KNEE. The thigh should be examined for overall shape with the patient standing. The ideal medial thigh has a slight proximal fullness, 2 to 8 cm posterior and inferior from the perineal–thigh crease, and tapers to a thin mid-thigh and knee. As the thin, inelastic skin of the medial thigh leads to notoriously poor postoperative skin retraction, preexisting wrinkling and sagging should be ruled out, as it may worsen postliposuction.[28,29]

Subcutaneous fat of the knee is primarily localized over the medial condyles of the tibia and femur and ideally ought to be relatively flat, with minimal associated fat in the patellar, infrapatellar, and lateral knee fat pads. The suprapatellar fat pad is a fibrofatty region that can become ptotic and wrinkled due to age, gravity, and the weight of the overlying anterior thigh.[30]

MEDICATIONS

A careful history of medication use is essential and includes prescription, over-the-counter, and herbal remedies. Particular attention is given to medications that affect clotting and should be avoided before or immediately following surgery. Medications or supplements containing aspirin, nonsteroidal anti-inflammatory agents, vitamin E, feverfew, or the four G's – ginkgo, ginseng, garlic, and ginger – are commonly discontinued 2 weeks prior to surgery to minimize intraoperative bleeding and bruising.[31] Long-term anticoagulation with warfarin or subcutaneous heparin is also a contraindication for surgery and should not be discontinued for elective procedures. To reduce cardiac stimulation, thyroid replacement therapy and pseudoephedrine are stopped 3 days, and appetite suppressants gradually discontinued 2 weeks, prior to surgery. Caffeine, alcohol, and tobacco products are also best avoided periprocedurally.

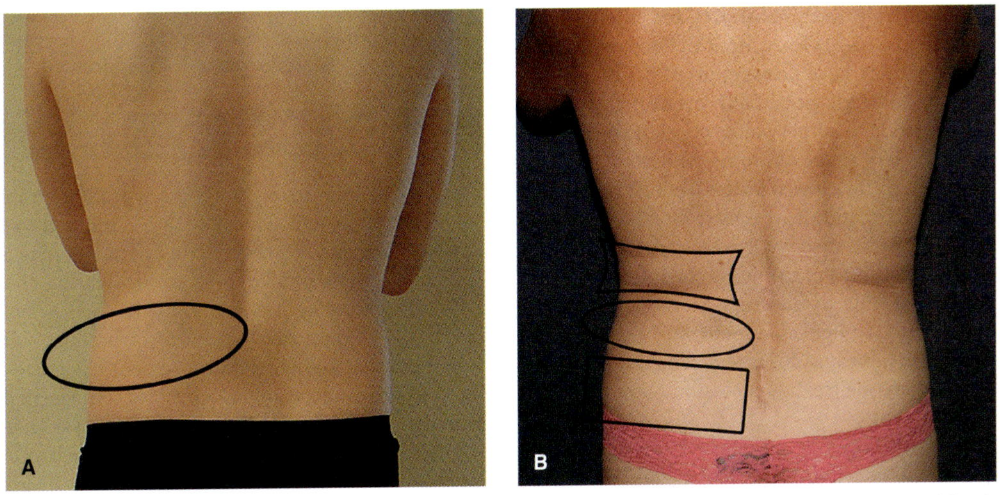

Figure 41-1 **A.** Male flanks marked by an ellipse. **B.** Female hip (*rectangle*), waist (*ellipse*), and flank (*polygon*). Note that the female waist is approximately equivalent to the male flank in anatomic position.

TABLE 41-3
Medications Potentially Affecting Lidocaine Metabolism

	CYP1A2 Inhibitors	CYP3A4 Inhibitors
Competitive Substrates	▪ Antidepressants (TCAs), Atypical Antipsychotics ▪ Propranolol, Verapamil ▪ Warfarin ▪ Some Chemotherapeutic and Hormonal Drugs (tamoxifen, estradiol)	▪ Antidepressants (TCAs and SSRIs), Atypical Antipsychotics, Benzodiazepines ▪ Propranolol, CCBs, Statins, Amiodarone ▪ Warfarin, Clopidogrel ▪ Chemotherapeutic & Hormonal Drugs ▪ Protease Inhibitors, Nevirapine ▪ Macrolide Antibiotics (not azithromycin) ▪ Azole Antifungals
Strong Inhibitors	▪ Fluoroquinolones (ciprofloxacin) ▪ Fluvoxamine ▪ CCBs (Verapamil) ▪ Herbs/Herbal Teas	▪ Protease Inhibitors (indinavir, ritonavir) ▪ Clarithromycin ▪ Chloramphenicol ▪ Itraconazole, Ketoconazole
Moderate Inhibitors		▪ Erythromycin, Fluconazole ▪ CCBs (diltiazem, verapamil)
Weak Inhibitors	▪ Caffeine ▪ Cimetidine	▪ Fluoxetine ▪ Cimetidine
Unspecified Inhibitors	▪ Amiodarone ▪ Interferon ▪ Isoniazid	▪ Amiodarone ▪ Ciprofloxacin ▪ Isoniazid ▪ Fluvoxamine

TCAs, tricyclic antidepressants; SSRIs, serotonin-specific receptor inhibitors; CCBs, calcium channel blockers.

Given that lidocaine is rapidly and almost exclusively eliminated by hepatic cytochrome P450 3A4 (CYP3A4) and 1A2 (CYP1A2), attention must be given to medications that inhibit or are competitively metabolized by these enzymatic pathways, as they may interfere with lidocaine metabolism and lead to elevations in lidocaine blood levels.[32,33] Although early in vitro studies implicated CYP3A4 as the main enzyme in lidocaine metabolism, recent clinical studies have confirmed that CYP1A2 is most likely principally responsible for the metabolic breakdown of lidocaine in subjects with normal liver function.[17] Antidepressants, antifungals, antivirals, and antibiotics are common culprits as substrates and inhibitors of both enzymes (Table 41-3). Toxic levels of lidocaine due to such drug interactions have been reported.[34] Patients are instructed to discontinue potentially problematic medications 2 weeks prior to surgery after checking with their prescribing physician. However, some patients may need to taper their medications over a longer period of time. For patients discontinuing antidepressants, lorazepam (1 mg PO qHS) may be prescribed for 1 week prior to surgery to mitigate any difficulties in tolerating the interruption in therapy. Patients unable to interrupt therapy with drugs that may interfere with lidocaine metabolism can still be treated, albeit with lidocaine doses reduced by at least 30% to 40%.[35] More than one treatment session may, therefore, be necessary.[36]

Preoperative prescriptions are started the day before surgery. Seven days of cefadroxil or cephalexin 500 mg PO b.i.d. (minocycline 100 mg PO q.d. if penicillin-allergic) are typically prescribed. Phytonadione (Vitamin K) 5 mg PO b.i.d. or arnica is also recommended for 10 days prior to surgery to minimize bruising.[37] For anxious patients, lorazepam 1 mg PO is prescribed for the night before and/or the morning of the procedure.

LABORATORY STUDIES

Preoperative laboratory studies for most liposuction procedures include a complete blood cell count with differential and platelet count, chemistry panel, prothrombin and partial thromboplastin times, serum pregnancy test, and serologies for hepatitis B and C and HIV.[38] An electrocardiogram is also ordered for patients over the age of 60. The surgeon reviews the results, preferably 2 weeks prior to surgery, and any abnormalities are addressed.

PHOTOGRAPHS

Digital, standardized preoperative photographs (with separate informed consent) are obtained, and every attempt is made to achieve consistent distance and background. The use of 45 degree strobe lighting ensures soft, natural-looking light and minimizes shadowing. Patients usually wear surgical underwear or bathing suits for the photographs. Baseline measurements may be obtained at this time, including weight, percentage of body fat, and circumferential measurements. Given that patients rarely have an accurate recollection of their preoperative anatomy, such as congenital irregularities or asymmetry, pretreatment photos are crucial. Postoperative photos are not taken until 3 to 6 months following treatment to document final results.

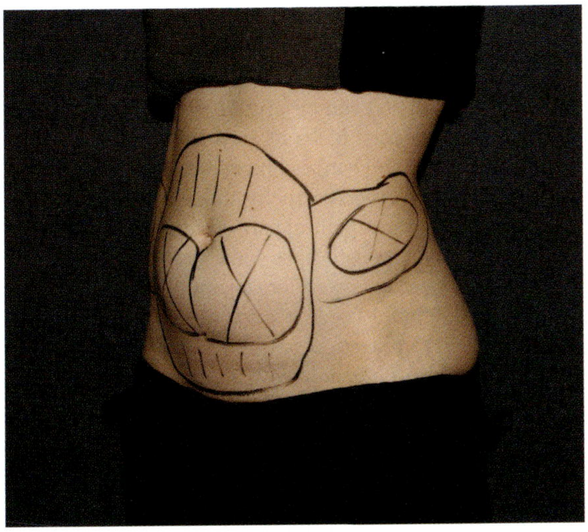

Figure 41-2 Preoperative topographical markings of the abdomen and anterior waist.

MARKING AND PREPARATION

Marking is performed immediately pre-procedure as a blueprint for surgery. A blue or black felt-tip permanent marker is used to topographically mark the area/s undergoing liposuction with the surgeon seated and the patient standing erect in anatomic position (Fig. 41-2). Bulges requiring more aggressive treatment, areas to be avoided, preexisting depressions, and side-to-side asymmetry can all be easily demarcated with this method. Once completed, the patient is transferred to the procedure room and the area/s to be treated is/are thoroughly cleansed with a chlorhexidine wash.

PERIOPERATIVE TECHNIQUES AND MANAGEMENT

TUMESCENT ANESTHESIA

BACKGROUND, PHARMACOKINETICS, AND SAFETY.

Tumescent liposuction is a technique based upon the direct infiltration of large volumes of dilute lidocaine with epinephrine in buffered physiologic saline, allowing for profound local anesthesia and hemostasis of skin and subcutaneous tissues without the need for general anesthesia.[39] Percutaneous infiltration of local anesthetic solution into subcutaneous tissue causes fluid spread and hydrodissection (known as bulk flow) throughout the interstitial connective tissue compartment that envelops adipocytes.[40] Although lidocaine is lipophilic and some portion of the infiltrated volume may be sequestered by fat cells directly, adipocyte swelling is not noted in tumesced areas.[41] The interstitial reservoir of lidocaine and its compressive effects on subcutaneous capillaries, combined with the vasoconstriction produced by epinephrine and the inherent relative avascularity of adipose tissue, slow the systemic absorption of lidocaine and lead to complete, prolonged anesthesia and hemostasis without third spacing.[42,43] Tumescence also hydraulically elevates subcutaneous tissue away from underlying structures, allowing for the safe treatment of areas such as the neck.[41]

Prior to tumescent anesthesia, liposuction was performed with either a "dry" or "wet" technique. Dry technique liposuction required general anesthesia and utilized no preoperative fluid infiltration, often leading to excessive bleeding and the need for intraoperative or postoperative intravenous (IV) fluids or blood transfusions. The prolonged recovery time and potential for disfiguring irregularities of the overlying skin also marred this procedure.[44] Wet and superwet techniques added the use of a vasoconstrictive solution of epinephrine. Although superwet liposuction is still widely used, it requires profound narcotic-induced anesthesia and has the potential for excessive bleeding and fluid overload secondary to intraoperative IV fluids.[45]

An unsubstantiated fear of lidocaine doses in excess of 7 mg/kg combined with a lack of understanding regarding lidocaine pharmacokinetics within subcutaneous tissues contributed to the popularity of such procedures and the shunning of tumescent technique liposuction by nondermatologic surgeons during its nascency.[44] Clinical studies have nevertheless confirmed that tumescent lidocaine dosages up to 45 mg/kg are exceedingly safe, with dosages up to 55 mg/kg likely being safe in the majority of patients, regardless of the speed of infiltration.[2,46,47] Lidocaine dosages in this range demonstrate peak plasma levels at 12 to 14 hours post-infiltration, well below the threshold for systemic toxicity (Fig. 41-3).[48] Despite overwhelming evidence to the contrary, the opinion that tumescent anesthesia is unsafe or unnecessary – or that tumescent anesthesia should be disregarded entirely – still endures outside of the dermatologic community.[49–51]

FORMULATION.

A guideline for lidocaine and epinephrine concentrations in tumescent anesthetic preparations, based on the authors' preferences and experience, is presented in Table 41-4. Nevertheless, more fibrous areas, such as the upper abdomen, breast, back, and periumbilical region, may require greater concentrations of lidocaine

TABLE 41-4
Tumescent Anesthetic Formulation

Ingredients	0.05%	0.1%
0.9% Normal saline	1 L	1 L
1% Lidocaine hydrochloride	500 mg (50 mL)	1000 mg (100 mL)
1:1000 Epinephrine (final concentration of 1:1,500,000)	0.65 mg (0.65 mL)	0.65 mg (0.65 mL)
8.4% Sodium bicarbonate	10 mEq (10 mL)	10 mEq (10 mL)
Optional: Triamcinolone acetonide	10 mg (1 mL)	10 mg (1 mL)

Note: Ingredients other than normal saline listed in mg or mEq (mL) needed to create 0.05% and 0.1% solution concentrations.

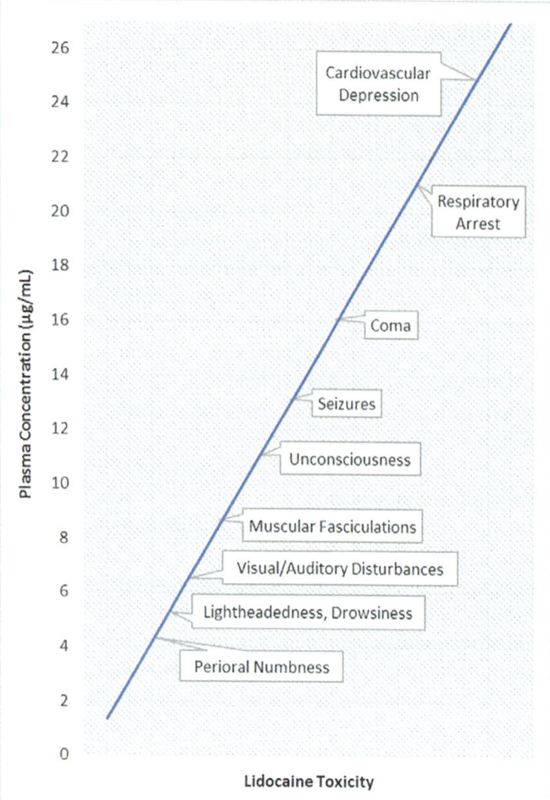

Figure 41-3 Plasma lidocaine levels and associated toxicity. The potential for lidocaine toxicity is clinically significant at plasma lidocaine concentrations >6 µg/mL. Adapted with permission from Butterwick KJ, Goldman MP, Sriprachya-Anunt S. Lidocaine levels during the first two hours of infiltration of dilute anesthetic solution for tumescent liposuction: rapid versus slow delivery. *Dermatol Surg.* 1999;25(9):681–685.

and epinephrine to achieve complete anesthesia and hemostasis.[52] Moreover, areas of greater skin laxity may require greater volumes of fluid, such as the upper inner thigh.[30] The appropriate volume of tumescent anesthetic is the minimal volume that will produce complete local anesthesia and hemostasis, albeit not necessarily complete tumescence (swelling or firmness) of tissue.[41]

A number of factors associated with tumescent solution can increase patient tolerance pre- and postprocedure. The addition of sodium bicarbonate (10 mEq/L) to anesthetic solution eliminates the burning and stinging associated with the acidic pH of commercially available lidocaine solutions.[44] Warming of anesthetic solution prior to infiltration dramatically increases tolerability with no significant hemodynamic effects.[53,54] Triamcinolone (10 mg/L), a highly lipophilic corticosteroid, may be added to decrease inflammation and tenderness postoperatively.

TECHNIQUE. A 25 G spinal needle is used to start infiltration in the deepest planes of a targeted subcutaneous compartment, followed by infusion of partially anesthetized, more superficial layers of fat. Infiltrating with a superficial-to-deep approach produces early induration of superficial layers, making infusion of deeper fat more technically difficult, and obscures the deep subcutaneous layers, impeding optimal tumescent anesthesia.[41] Once tissues are briefly – albeit sufficiently – anesthetized with a 25 G needle, a 20 G needle (or blunt-tipped larger cannula in non-fibrous areas) can be used. Pretreating infiltration sites with intradermal blebs of anesthetic solution (30 G needle, 5 mL syringe) can also increase patient comfort .If infiltration is performed correctly, these intradermal injections may be the most painful part of the entire procedure.

Most patients prefer to have some preprocedure anxiolytic and are typically given lorazepam 1 mg PO (with or without clonidine 0.1 mg PO) prior to the surgery. Patient comfort during infiltration is also directly related to the rate of tumescent infusion with variable-rate peristaltic pumps. Faster infiltration rates require premedication with IV analgesics (midazolam 1 to 3 mg, fentanyl 25 to 50 µg). Nevertheless, the convenience of rapid tumescent infiltration must be weighed against the inherent risks of intraoperative systemic narcotics and potentially uneven aesthetic results due to irregular tumescence.[41] Waiting 20 to 60 minutes after infiltration to allow for complete detumescence makes target fat easier to grasp and ensures maximal hemostasis, which enhances the comfort of the practitioner.

MICROCANNULAS AND LIPORASPIRATION

Profound vasoconstriction produced by tumescent anesthesia allows surgeons to use microcannulas with an inner diameter ≤2.2 mm. The decreased pain, greater ease of subcutaneous penetration, and more uniformly smooth results associated with microcannulas greatly outweigh any benefits that might arise from using larger cannulas.[55] However, small volumes of aspirate fat per stroke and the need for a greater number of cannula entry sites are relative disadvantages of microcannulas compared to their larger counterparts.

Microcannula entry sites may be either 2 mm incisions via an 11 blade or 1.0, 1.5, or 2 mm openings made via a biopsy punch. The latter (known as adits) may allow for less cannula-induced friction during treatment and better postoperative drainage than linear incisions.[56] Two-millimeter diameter adits are best placed in the inferior portion of a treated area to maximize drainage. The number of entry sites is dependent on a number of factors, typically increasing with larger and/or more fibrous areas and smaller microcannula diameters.[44] Entry sites should ideally be placed in natural skin folds, if possible, to minimize their postoperative appearance. Avoiding entry sites that are too small will also decrease cutaneous friction and trauma from microcannula movement.

Liposuction is typically started with smaller (16 or 14 G) microcannulas. As they produce less discomfort than larger (12 or 10 G) microcannulas, a surgeon utilizes them initially to ensure that target areas are properly anesthetized. The creation of small tunnels within the subcutaneous layer, especially in more fibrous areas, also increases the ease and efficiency of larger microcannulas.

When attached to an active, negative-pressure vacuum canister, a moving microcannula will rasp away small fragments of fat that are then immediately aspirated via suction, making lipoaspiration a more appropriate term than liposuction.[56] While the dominant hand moves the

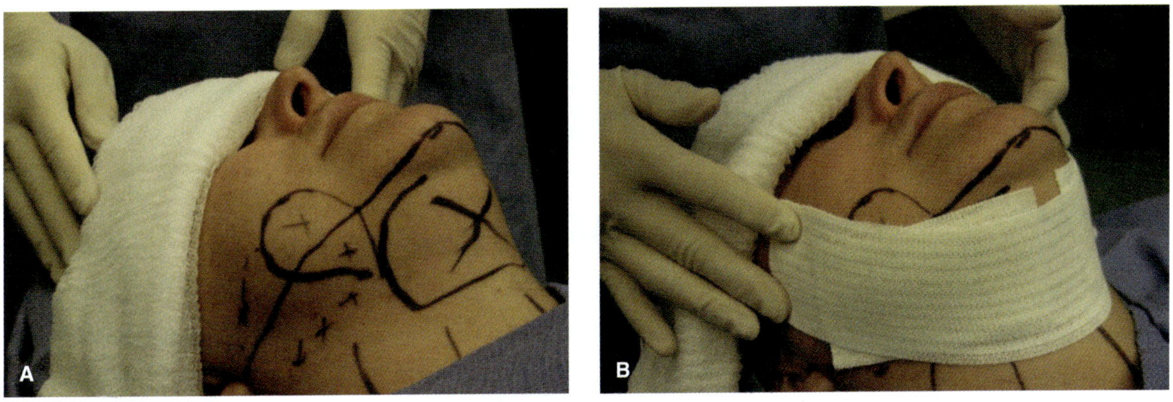

Figure 41-4 A. Operative position for tumescent liposuction of the neck. Three of the five entry sites are denoted with circles. The typical fanning pattern of treatment is shown with arrows. **B.** Foam tape applied with traction immediately post-treatment: two shorter pieces at the midline and a third, larger piece across the entire area help decrease central pooling. Tape is removed 24 to 48 hours post procedure.

microcannula in a fanning motion with long, smooth strokes, the non-dominant hand helps raise grasp and raise a subunit of skin and subcutaneous tissue. This allows for more efficient targeting of deep fat and enhances safety by elevating the tissues away from underlying structures. An even pinch test and topographic smoothness throughout the treatment area signify the end of treatment. Recent guidelines from the American Society for Dermatologic Surgery recommend removal of no more than 4 L of supranatant fat in a single session, whereas prior guidelines from the society and the American Academy of Dermatology advised limiting total aspirate volumes to 5 L.[14,57] A national survey published in 2004 reported single-session mean total aspirate and supranatant fat volumes of 1740 mL and 1160 mL, respectively.[57]

TECHNIQUE AND CONSIDERATIONS BY ANATOMIC LOCATION

The goal of tumescent liposuction is the three-dimensional contouring of subcutaneous adipose tissue at a given body site with optimal safety and enhanced cosmesis, although not necessarily a perfect result. The following are site-specific clinical techniques, pearls, and caveats for commonly treated areas.

NECK AND JOWLS. Once infiltration has been completed, patients may feel some anxiety due to the swelling and tautness of the area and must be reassured that this is normal and will loosen within minutes of starting the procedure. Typical volumes of infiltrated solution are 400 to 500 mL.

Standard neck liposuction utilizes five small entry sites: submental crease, two lateral submental, and two inferior to the angle of the mandible (Fig. 41-4A).[58] Although it may be tempting to perform the entire procedure through one site, crisscrossing and fanning via multiple sites leads to the most thorough and smooth result with a minimal risk of depression. The use of small microcannulas (16 G then 14 G) prevents superficial skin irregularities, and may maximize skin retraction by preserving subcutaneous connective tissue strands (Fig. 41-5). A thin, 3 to 5 mm layer of fat should also be left to prevent irregularities at the skin surface.[22]

Unlike other areas of the neck and lower face, the central to lateral submentum (submental crease to superior edge of the thyroid cartilage) can be treated aggressively. Jawline accentuation is achieved by directing the cannula 3 to 4 cm below the mandibular ramus. Deep fat near the ramus should be avoided to minimize the risk of marginal mandibular nerve injury. If necessary, treatment of the jowls and lower cheeks should be performed very conservatively with feathering (tunneling without suction) of the borders.[22]

POSTERIOR ARMS. Liposuction of 75% of the brachial circumference, sparing the thinner, more fibrous fat deposits of the anterior arm, leads to optimal outcomes in the majority of patients.[59] Suctioning is performed with the patient in a lateral decubitus position with their arm either at their side (for posterior/lateral compartment) or raised with their hand behind their head (for medial compartment). Long strokes with small microcannulas (14 or 16 G) directed relatively parallel to the long axis of the arm via incisions or 1.5 mm adits at the proximal or distal portions of the arm maximize cosmetic results (Fig. 41-6).[60] The authors have also found that treating the posterior and anterior axillary wings concurrently further increases patient satisfaction.

ABDOMEN AND FLANKS. The upper and lower abdomen are accessed via three suprapubic and two periumbilical crease entry sites. Two-millimeter adit sites in the suprapubic abdomen may provide the best postoperative drainage. Two additional incisions of the lateral abdomen at the level of the umbilicus allow access to the upper and lower abdomen for cross-tunneling, as well as the waist and flanks. Microcannula entry sites are also created over the spine for the latter. Incisions or adits above the level of the umbilicus and on the back should be limited in number due to potential post-inflammatory hyperpigmentation.

The relatively inelastic skin and fibrous fat of the upper abdomen mandates conservative treatment with a crisscrossing radial pattern of microcannula movement to

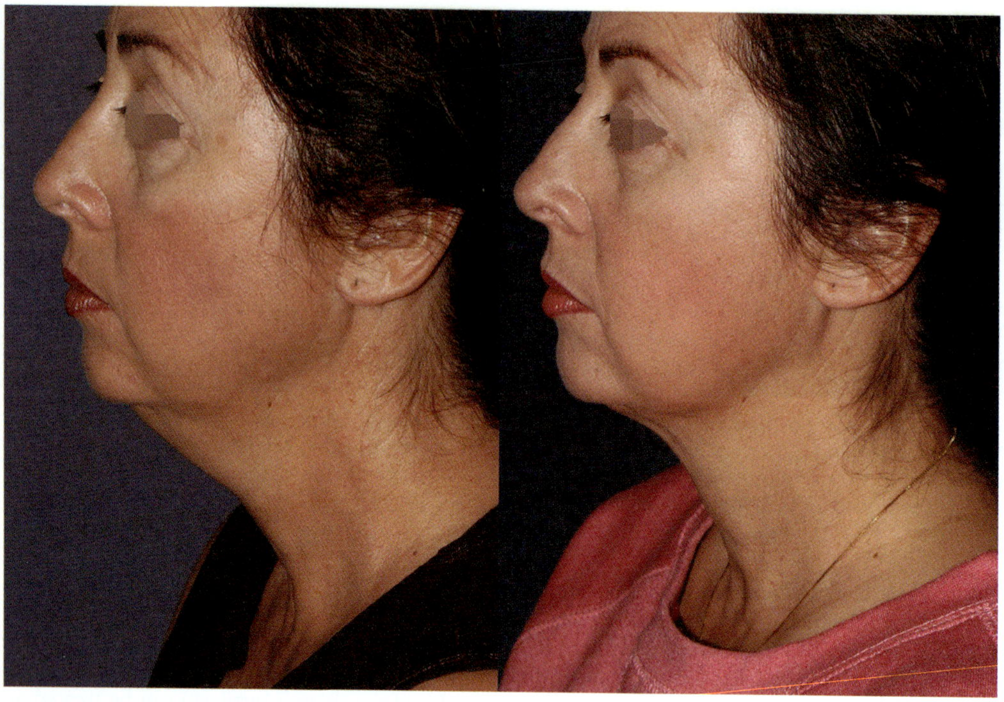

Figure 41-5 Tumescent liposuction of the neck. Preoperative (*left*) and 3 months postoperative (*right*). A total of 40 mL of fat removed in a single session.

ensure smooth results.[26] Forceful microcannula thrusts directed at the costal margin may lead to rib bruising or penetration of the diaphragm or pleural space. Attention should be given to the periumbilical area, to avoid leaving behind a "donut" of fat. Initial tunneling of highly fibrous subcutaneous tissue of the flanks (and waist in women) with a small microcannula (16 or 14 G) dramatically increases the ease of ensuing treatment with larger (12 or 10 G) microcannulas. Figures 41-7 and 41-8 demonstrate typical results in male and female patients.

HIPS, OUTER THIGHS, AND BUTTOCKS. With the patient in the lateral decubitus position, treatment of the hip is performed via three entry sites (superior, inferior, and posterior mid-lateral). Microcannula movement in this area is primarily in a vertical plane. The posterior incision site is also used to feather into the waist and anteriorly toward the abdomen.[27,61]

The ideal outer thigh position is in modified lateral decubitus with a midline wedge cushion, abducting and internally rotating the extremity to best approximate standing.

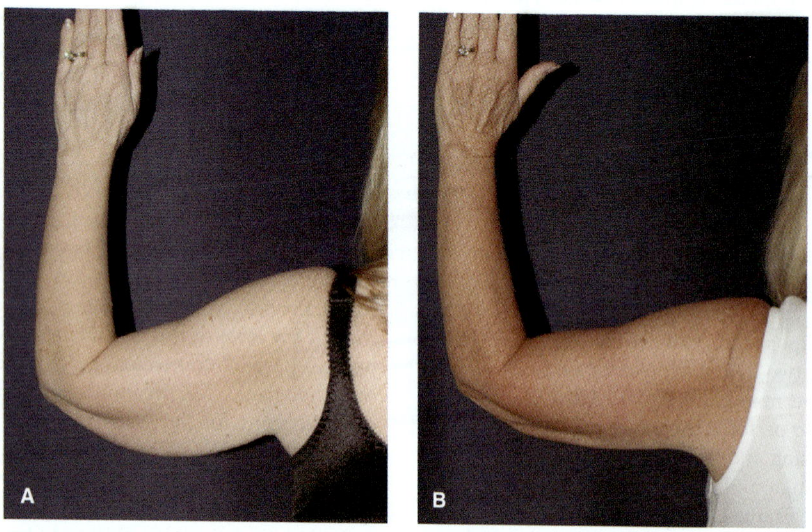

Figure 41-6 Tumescent liposuction of the posterior arm. Preoperative (**A**) and several months postoperative (**B**) with significant reduction in adiposity and associated laxity.

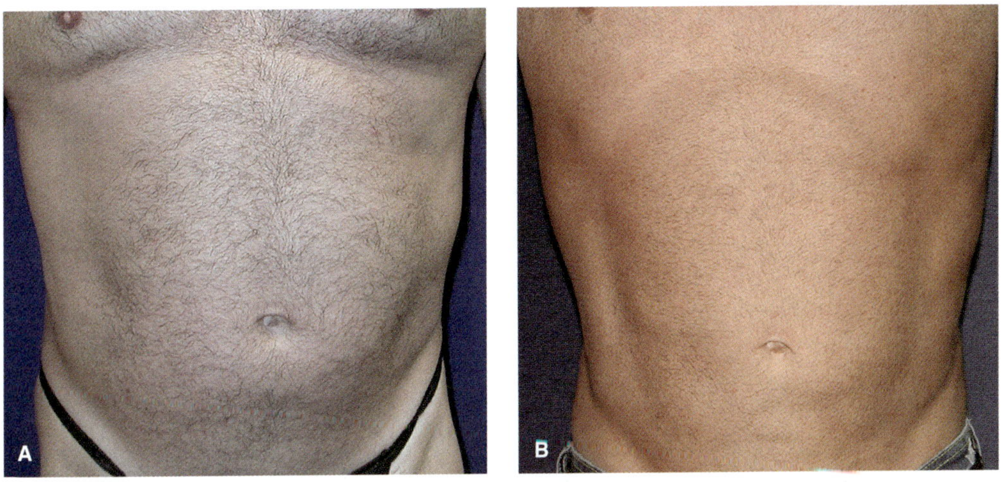

Figure 41-7 Tumescent liposuction of the male abdomen and flanks. Preoperative (**A**) and 6 months postoperative (**B**).

This position also limits oversuctioning by rotating away the greater trochanter. Entry sites are placed superiorly, inferiorly, and in the infragluteal crease. The latter can be used to blend the outer and posterior thigh together (Fig. 41-9). Circumferential treatment of thigh fat should never be performed in a single session due to the potential for compartment syndrome and persistent lymphedema.

Compared to the other two sites, the buttock is treated far less commonly. The area is treated with the patient prone and a pillow placed under the pelvis, with 1 to 3 microcannula entry sites placed infragluteally. The lateral gluteal (trochanteric) depression must be clearly marked preoperatively to avoid significantly suctioning this area. Buttock contraction emphasizes this area. Liposuction of the "banana fold," a convexity from the inferior gluteal crease to the posterior thigh that houses the ligament of Luschka, is best avoided or treated superficially only in a horizontal plane.[27,62] Injury to this infragluteal ligament may cause buttock drooping and herniation of fat into the posterior thigh.

MEDIAL THIGH AND KNEE. Liposuction of the proximal medial thigh, mid-thigh, and medial knee is first performed separately in each area then blended together. All three regions are performed in a lateral decubitus

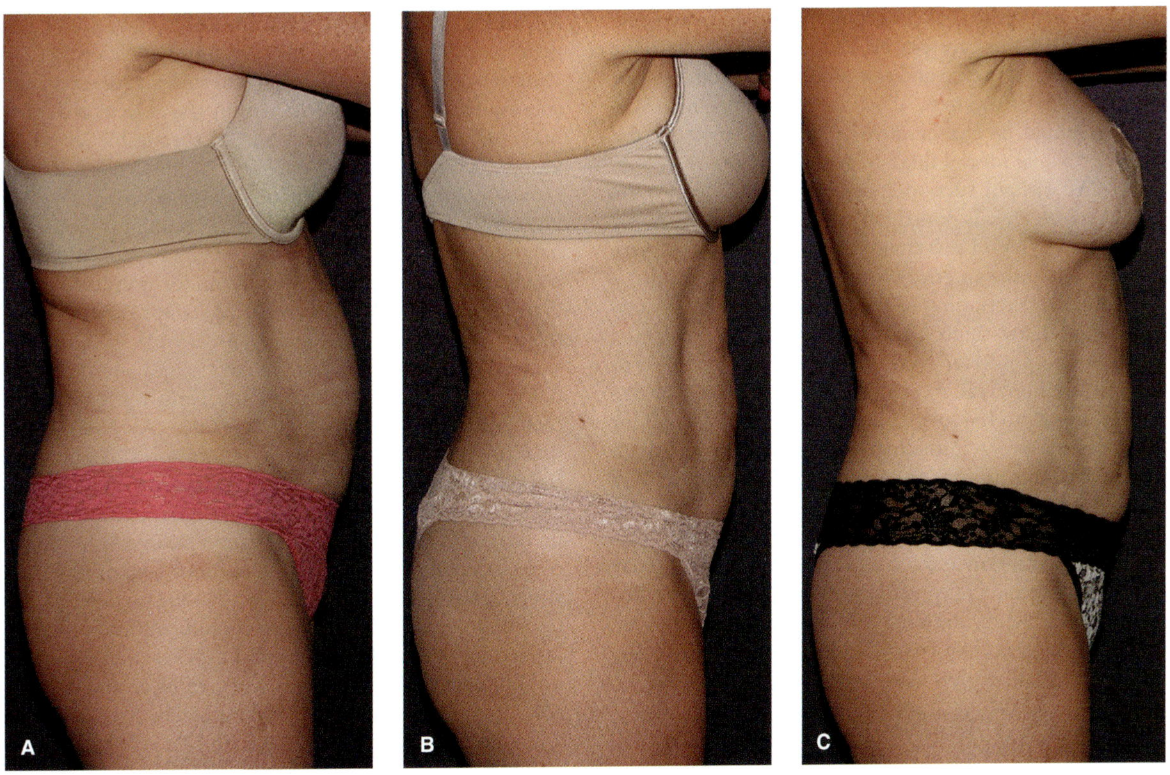

Figure 41-8 (**A**) Pre- and (**B**) 2 weeks and (**C**) 5 months following tumescent liposuction of the female abdomen, waist, and flanks.

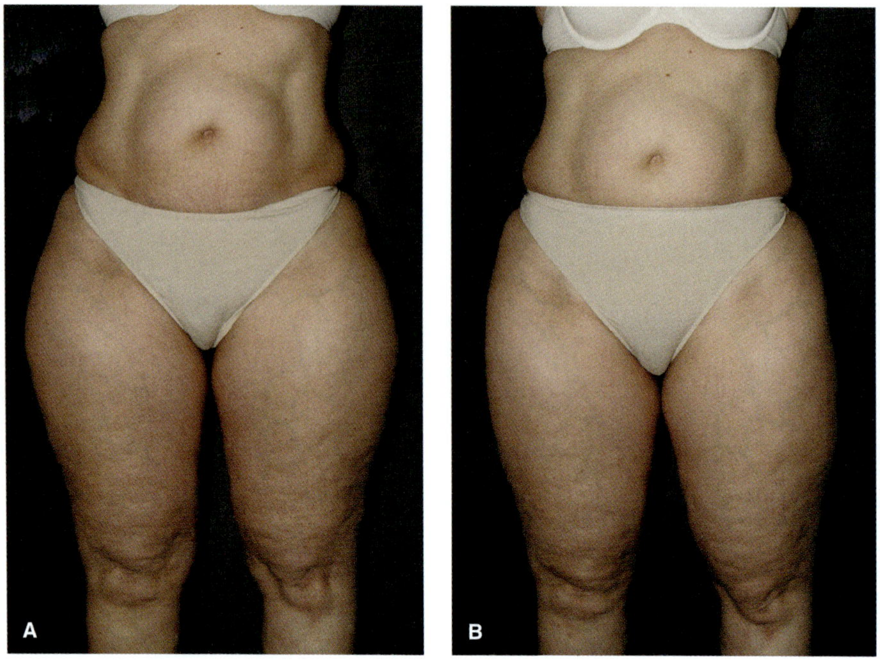

Figure 41-9 (**A**) Pre- and (**B**) several months following tumescent liposuction of the lateral thighs.

position with the contralateral extremity flexed high onto a foam cushion.

Proximal medial thigh fat is unique in its soft, nonfibrous nature, which makes the fat easily extracted and defects quick to develop. Placing an incision site at the distal aspect of the proximal medial thigh bulge or in the mid-thigh can result in depressions and should be avoided. Hidden entry sites are placed posteriorly, one near the mid-infragluteal crease and one placed 2 to 3 cm inferior and anterior to the first, allowing cross-tunneling. Suctioning should be conservative in the lowermost border of the proximal medial thigh to avoid excessive resection. Tunneling without suction is performed distally into the thicker, more fibrous mid-thigh fat. An incision site in the mid-anterior thigh 1 to 2 cm inferior to the inguinal crease can also target the anterior portion of the medial thigh.

Aggressive suctioning of the medial knee successfully tapers the distal thigh. Suction is primarily performed through one posterior incision site placed distal to (not within) the popliteal crease. A second incision site 2 to 3 cm superior to the medial popliteal crease is useful for conservative cross-tunneling, as well as for mid-thigh access. Fat pads inferior and medial to the patella are also treated aggressively. However, aggressive suctioning of the suprapatellar fat pad should be avoided, as inherently poor skin retraction and ptosis of the anterior thigh may cause sagging and creasing of the knee.[30] Tunneling without suction blends the knee to the mid-thigh and calf. The mid-thigh is then treated conservatively with long, smooth vertical strokes using preexisting entry sites.

LASER-ASSISTED LIPOSUCTION

The addition of Nd:YAG or diode laser lipolysis to standard liposuction techniques, known as laser-assisted liposuction (LAL), has been purported to improve aesthetic results and postoperative recovery compared to liposuction alone. Yet the prospective benefits achieved with LAL must be weighed against device costs and the risk of cutaneous thermal injury.

Although selective photothermal effects may play a role in LAL devices (ranging from 920 to 1440 nm), heat-generated sequelae most likely account for its potential clinical capabilities. Collagen thermocoagulation and subsequent neocollagenesis within the reticular dermis may enhance skin retraction.[63] Laser-induced blood vessel thrombosis and lymphatic channel closure may reduce postoperative ecchymosis and edema.[64] Greater fat emulsification from adipocyte cellular membrane degradation (adipolysis) may decrease the extent of mechanical damage produced by microcannulas (accelerating postoperative recovery) and improve the treatment of fibrous fat.[65–67]

Despite all of these possible advantages, studies comparing LAL to liposuction alone using the tumescent technique have shown mixed results. A randomized, double-blind study comparing 1064 nm LAL to liposuction alone in 220 split body areas demonstrated significantly less postoperative pain with LAL ($p < 0.0001$), but no differences in ecchymosis, edema, skin retraction, or overall cosmetic outcome.[68] A randomized, nonblinded study of posterior arms treated with 1064 nm LAL versus liposuction alone also found no significant differences in fat reduction or skin retraction.[69] Nevertheless, other nonblinded studies have shown greater – albeit modest – improvements in postoperative arm circumference and abdominal skin tightening with LAL.[70,71] More comparative studies are needed to solidify whether LAL has any true advantage over standard tumescent liposuction.[72]

ULTRASOUND- AND RADIOFREQUENCY-ASSISTED LIPOSUCTION

Ultrasound-assisted liposuction (UAL) utilizes internal pulsed or continuous ultrasound energy to produce adipocyte fragmentation and fat emulsification prior to suction.[73] A multicenter, randomized, subject-blinded study comparing superwet UAL to standard liposuction revealed only minor improvements in skin retraction and surgical hemostasis with UAL and no significant differences in satisfaction or postoperative induration, edema, or ecchymosis.[74] Subjects also reported greater postoperative pain, burning, numbness, and swelling with UAL.[75] The anecdotal nature of UAL benefits must be cautiously weighed against its lack of high-quality clinical data and ostensibly greater risk of burns, necrosis, and seromas.[76]

Radiofrequency-assisted liposuction (RFAL) has also been asserted to improve skin tightening and fat reduction. A suction cannula with an electrode tip delivers monopolar RF energy, while an external electrode reflects absorbed heat back into the dermis.[77] However, no studies have compared RFAL with standard liposuction techniques.[78,79]

POSTOPERATIVE CARE

Tumescent liposuction has an uncomplicated postoperative course with relatively low maintenance compared to non-tumescent liposuction under systemic anesthesia or other cosmetic surgical procedures.

IMMEDIATE POSTOPERATIVE PERIOD

Once tumescent liposuction is complete, the area is cleansed and absorbent pads or sanitary napkins are applied over the microcannula entrance sites to collect drainage, held in place with tape or tubular elastic netting. The treated area is then secured with a circumferential compression garment. Following tumescent liposuction of the neck, foam tape may be applied (Fig. 41-4B) to minimize bruising and pooling of fluid and free-floating adipocytes in the submental area. As tumesced areas remain at least partially anesthetized up to 18 to 24 hours post procedure, this prolonged anesthetic effect minimizes the need for potent oral analgesics.[50]

SHORT-TERM POSTOPERATIVE PERIOD

COMPRESSION. Compression garments serve a number of important functions during the postoperative period including decreasing edema and ecchymosis, mitigating discomfort, and accelerating patients' return to normal activities. Patients often maintain that the compression garment splints or supports the area that has been treated, making it less painful than when it is not in use. Open drainage and proper compression also virtually eliminate the risk of postoperative seromas.[80]

Hypertonic anesthetic solution remaining in subcutaneous tissue following tumescent liposuction (up to 80% of volume infiltrated) is unable to be resorbed due to widespread surgical disruption of lymphatic capillaries.[80] If left undrained, the hyperosmotic interstitial environment incites the diffusion of fluid out of the intravascular space, across the osmotic gradient, leading to longstanding lymphatic edema. Postoperative compression encourages drainage via open microcannula entry sites, minimizing post-liposuction edema.[81]

Bimodal compression, as advocated by dermatologist and tumescent liposuction pioneer Jeffrey Klein, involves two sequential degrees of compression in the postoperative period.[82] A high degree of uniform compression is used until 24 hours after drainage has ceased (i.e., a total of 2 to 4 days), at which time only a mild degree of compression (e.g., Spandex® garment) is needed.[83] Prolonged high-grade compression instead collapses lymphatic capillaries, blocking drainage of residual subcutaneous fluid and worsening edema postoperatively.[82] Mild continued compression offers patients physical comfort and maintains interstitial fluid hydrostatic pressures just high enough to slow transudate formation.[82] Nevertheless, once drainage has stopped, continued external compression is not essential and has no significant bearing on the ultimate cosmetic result.

Certain areas of the body have specific compression requirements, given their location or greater potential for adverse events. Patients undergoing liposuction of the submental area should be advised that focal areas of induration, representative of localized interstitial edema, always develop as an expected, temporary condition that resolve over a period of 4 to 8 weeks. A compressive chinstrap is worn 24 hours a day during the drainage phase, then may be used 2 to 4 hours a day for another 3 weeks.[22] Breasts have an increased risk of bleeding, ecchymosis, and hematoma formation in the immediate postoperative phase and require an exceptionally high degree of compression. Very high (first 12 to 18 hours), high (until 24 hours after drainage ceases), and mild compression can be achieved with a single, adjustable breast garment.[82] Circumferential thighs or calves and ankles have a greater risk for excessive or prolonged edema. The combination of a compression stocking (15 to 20 mm Hg), ankle-length support garment, and leg elevation during the first 3 days postoperatively will minimize edema formation. Twenty to thirty or 30 to 40 mm Hg stockings, depending on the amount of edema, are then used 24 hours a day for 1 week followed daily for 4 to 8 weeks.[30]

SURGICAL SITES. The vast majority of patients tolerate the postoperative period exceedingly well. Surgical site tenderness and mild edema are common short-term complaints. Over-the-counter oral analgesics or rarely a short course of low-dose narcotics are sufficient to control symptoms. Although nonthermal ultrasound, pulsed short-wave diathermy, and magnetic field therapy have all been studied post-liposuction, none lead to significant and reliable improvement in discomfort, edema, and bruising.[84–86] Ecchymosis, however, is generally mild, given the vasoconstrictive effects of tumescent anesthesia and post-treatment compression. If it develops, it is dependent in nature and migrates inferiorly; for example, purpura from tumescent liposuction of the neck tends to drift below the collar line.

Adit or incision sites should be left open for optimal drainage of residual anesthetic solution, preventing the occurrence of post-liposuction edema. Drainage usually ceases within 24 to 72 hours postoperatively with uniform, high-grade compression. As they are actively healing second intention wounds, erythema and mild ecchymosis surrounding the cutaneous openings are expected. Moist occlusive wound care without scab formation and proper sun protection will lead to a nearly imperceptible scar at 1 year post treatment. Although adit sites may lead to better postoperative drainage, the use of 2 mm incisions in darker skin types may minimize postinflammatory hyperpigmentation.

LONG-TERM POSTOPERATIVE PERIOD

Setting appropriate patient expectations prior to performing tumescent liposuction ensures that the majority of patients will be pleased with the subjective results. Pre- and postoperative digital photographs in a side-by-side format help illustrate the positive aesthetic changes and the importance of a healthy lifestyle. Weight should be measured at each follow-up visit, since it is not uncommon for unsatisfied patients to have gained weight in the postoperative period. Although liposuctioned areas will resist weight gain, fatty deposits may subsequently accumulate in other areas of the body, such as the breasts, abdomen, or viscera.[87–89] A survey performed by Rohrich et al.[90] found that 73% of patients who gained weight or 82% of those who did not gain weight post treatment were satisfied with results. However, only 29% of those who gained weight rated their appearance as good or excellent, compared to 79% of those who did not gain weight.

Touch-ups are performed no earlier than 6 months – and ideally beyond 1 year – following the original treatment session, allowing for maximum soft-tissue remodeling before evaluating final results. Obvious irregularities are often easily corrected by removing residual pockets of adipose tissue (Fig. 41-10). Incorrect endpoint assessment by the physician due to excess skin laxity or patient positioning, as well as patient hypersensitivity to parts or all of the procedure leading to incomplete fat removal, can all contribute to postoperative irregularity requiring touch-up treatment.[91] However, touch-ups for patient complaints that are not clinically appreciable by the physician or his/her staff should be avoided. Avoiding excessive fat resection further minimizes the incidence of patient dissatisfaction.

A retrospective review of 954 tumescent liposuction surgeries (1613 areas treated) by Butterwick et al.[91] reported a rate of 12.3% touch-up procedures (9% rate per area). The most common areas for touch-up, the neck and abdomen, were also the most common areas to be treated. The fibrous areas of the back, chest, and ankles, however, had the highest touch-up rate. Males and females had an equal incidence of touch-ups, with greater than 80% having the procedure 6 months or longer following their original surgery and 47% demonstrating a gain in weight during that time. More than one-third of those patients elected to have a second liposuction procedure, indicating overall satisfaction.

COMPLICATIONS

Large-scale studies have confirmed that liposuction performed solely with tumescent anesthesia using a clean surgical technique has remarkably few complications and no associated deaths (Table 41-5). The morbidity and

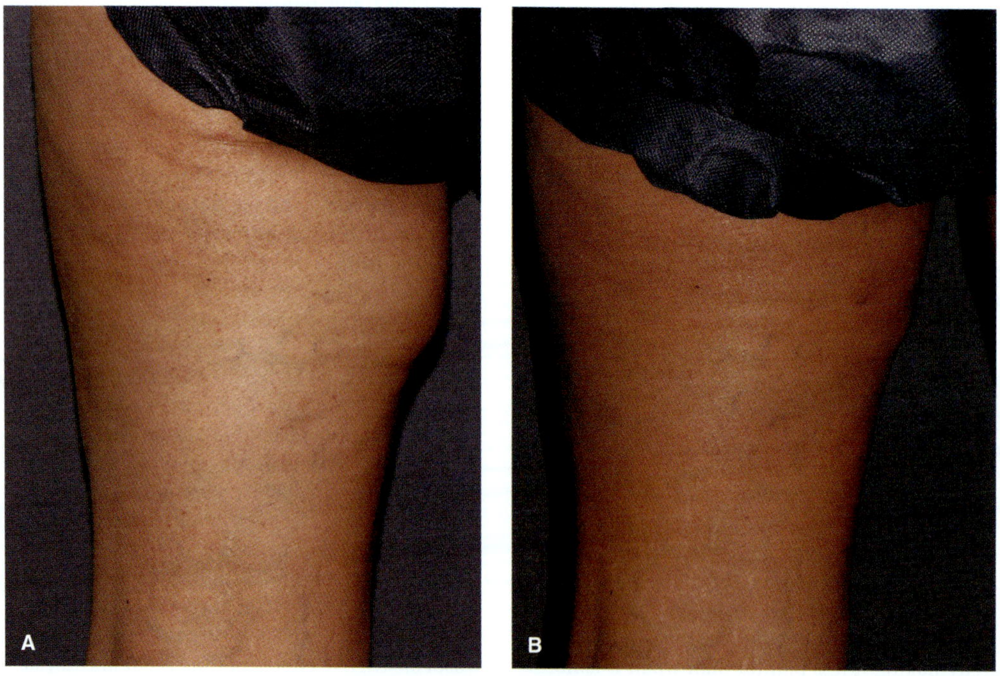

Figure 41-10 Residual adiposity of left proximal medial thigh from prior tumescent liposuction, before (**A**) and 2 months after (**B**) touch-up.

TABLE 41-5
Liposuction Safety Studies

Study	Anesthesia	Number of Cases	Fatality Rate (per 100,000)
Newman and Dolsky, 1984[92]	SA	5,458	0
Bernstein and Hanke, 1988[93]	29% SA, 71% local anesthesia[a]	9,478	0
Teimourian and Rogers, 1991[94]	SA	75,591	2.6
Dillerud, 1991[95]	57% SA 43% local anesthesia[a]	3,511	0
Hanke et al, 1995[96]	TLA	15,336	0
ASPRS Task Force on Liposuction, 1997[97]	SA	24,295	20.6
Jackson and Dolsky, 1999[98]	SA	200,000	2.4
Grazer and de Jong, 2000[99]	SA	496,245	19.1
Hughes, 2001[100]	SA	94,159	2.1
Housman et al, 2002[101]	91% TLA, negligible SA	66,570	0
Hanke et al, 2004[57]	TLA	668	0
Habbema, 2009[102]	TLA	3,240	0
Boeni, 2011[103]	TLA	4,380	0
Chia and Theodorou, 2012[104]	TLA	1,000	0

TLA, tumescent local anesthesia (including minimal conscious sedation); SA, systemic anesthesia (including general anesthesia or intravenous narcotics).
[a]The local anesthesia described here may also include a component of intravenous sedation with narcotics.

rare – albeit concerning – mortality seen with liposuction under general anesthesia is not simply a factor of the anesthesia itself, but is also directly related to the protracted or excessive procedures ("megaliposuction") or multiple concomitant procedures in a single session that it facilitates.[105] Although there have been numerous reports of mortality related to "tumescent liposuction," it is important to note that these cases did not represent true tumescent technique. All included the use of general or deep IV sedation and often additional, excessive intraoperative IV fluids or multiple concomitant procedures.[106–111] With true tumescent techniques as performed by dermatologic surgeons, it is not surprising that the incidence of intraoperative (visceral perforation, fluid overload) or postoperative (embolic) adverse events should be virtually eliminated since patients are alert and awake during the procedure and can resume normal activities almost immediately.

A national survey of tumescent liposuction by dermatologic surgeons revealed minimal morbidity and no life threatening complications, blood transfusions, or hospitalizations in 15,336 patients with 44,014 separate body areas.[96] The most frequent complications were scrotal or labial edema and ecchymosis (0.39%), mild localized infections (0.34%), cutaneous irregularities such as dimpling or retraction (0.26%), focal subcutaneous induration (0.20%), hematoma/seroma (0.17%), reactions to medications or tape (0.12%), and post-liposuction edema (0.10%). Cutaneous ulceration/necrosis, persistent postoperative pain or ecchymosis, and excessive postoperative somnolence or nausea all occurred rarely. Intraoperative tachycardia was extremely rare, given the highly dilute nature (1:1,000,000) of epinephrine.[80] A review of 10 year mandatory ambulatory surgery adverse event reports in Florida by Starling et al. also found no serious complications from tumescent liposuction; liposuction under general anesthesia, however, accounted for 32% of all cosmetic procedure-related deaths.[112]

The combination of excessive liposuction, iatrogenic hemodilution secondary to excessive intraoperative IV fluids, closure of microcannula insertion sites, and excessive external compression can also lead to a state of massive, progressive, osmotically mediated subcutaneous edema known as amplified liposuction edema (ALE).[81] Extreme cases of ALE can result in acute renal failure and fatal pulmonary and central nervous system edema.

CONCLUSION

Liposuction has evolved significantly in the past three decades. Once a procedure fraught with intraoperative and postoperative morbidity, the tumescent technique now allows liposuction to be performed purely as an outpatient procedure on awake patients with rare adverse events. Despite all of the new "bigger and better" technologies that have entered the marketplace to enhance the speed and results of treatment, the secret to successful liposuction remains unchanged: proper patient selection, patience, meticulous technique, an aesthetic eye, and excellent surgical staff.

REFERENCES

1. Ahn CS, Davis SA, Dabade TS, Williford PM, Feldman SR. Cosmetic procedures performed in the United States: a 16-year analysis. *Dermatol Surg.* 2013;39:1351–1359.
2. Klein JA. Tumescent technique for regional anesthesia permits lidocaine doses of 35 mg/kg for liposuction. *J Dermatol Surg Oncol.* 1990;16:248–263.
3. Tierney EP, Kouba DJ, Hanke CW. Safety of tumescent and laser-assisted liposuction: review of the literature. *J Drugs Dermatol.* 2011;10:1363–1369.
4. Jakubietz RG, Jakubietz DF, Gruenert JG, Schmidt K, Meffert RH, Jakubietz MG. Breast reduction by liposuction in females. *Aesthetic Plast Surg.* 2011;35:402–407.
5. Boni R. Tumescent power liposuction in the treatment of the enlarged male breast. *Dermatology (Basel).* 2006;213:140–143.
6. Choi CW, Kim BJ, Moon SE, Youn SW, Park KC, Huh CH. Treatment of lipomas assisted with tumescent liposuction. *J Eur Acad Dermatol Venereol.* 2007;21:243–246.
7. Chastain MA, Chastain JB, Coleman WP. HIV lipodystrophy: review of the syndrome and report of a case treated with liposuction. *Dermatol Surg.* 2001;27:497–500.
8. Lee D, Cho SH, Kim YC, Park JH, Lee SS, Park SW. Tumescent liposuction with dermal curettage for treatment of axillary osmidrosis and hyperhidrosis. *Dermatol Surg.* 2006;32:505–511.
9. Ooi A, Wong CH, Ong YS. Combined use of liposuction and arthroscopic shaver in lower-limb fasciocutaneous flap contouring. *J Plast Reconstr Aesthet Surg.* 2013;66:538–542.
10. Hansson E, Manjer J, Svensson H, Brorson H. Quality-of-life in patients with Dercum's disease–before and after liposuction. *J Plast Surg Hand Surg.* 2012;46:252–256.
11. Schmeller W, Hueppe M, Meier-Vollrath I. Tumescent liposuction in lipoedema yields good long-term results. *Br J Dermatol.* 2012;166:161–168.
12. Domanski MC, Cavale N. Self-reported "worth it" rating of aesthetic surgery in social media. *Aesthetic Plast Surg.* 2012;36:1292–1295.
13. Butterwick KJ, Goldman MP. Body fat analysis before and after liposuction as a means of objectively quantifying response to treatment. Presented at: American Society for Dermatologic Surgery Annual Meeting; 2000 November; Denver, CO.
14. Svedman KJ, Coldiron B, Coleman WP, et al. ASDS guidelines of care for tumescent liposuction. *Dermatol Surg.* 2006;32:709–716.
15. Javo IM, Sørlie T. Psychosocial characteristics of young Norwegian women interested in liposuction, breast augmentation, rhinoplasty, and abdominoplasty: a population-based study. *Plast Reconstr Surg.* 2010;125:1536–1543.
16. Javo IM, Pettersen G, Rosenvinge JH, et al. Predicting interest in liposuction among women with eating problems: a population-based study. *Body Image.* 2012;9:131–136.
17. Orlando R, Piccoli P, De Martin S, Padrini R, Floreani M, Palatini P. Cytochrome P450 1A2 is a major determinant of lidocaine metabolism in vivo: effects of liver function. *Clin Pharmacol Ther.* 2004;75:80–88.
18. Ben Said D, Ben Ali R, Ferchichi H, et al. Lidocaïne test for easier and less time consuming assessment of liver function in several hepatic injury models. *Hepatol Int.* 2011;5:941–948.
19. Luetkemeyer AF, Havlir DV, Currier JS. CROI 2013: complications of HIV disease, viral hepatitis, and antiretroviral therapy. *Top Antivir Med.* 2013;21:62–74.
20. Kelley L. Lidotoxic at low lidocaine levels. Presented at: World Congress on Liposuction; 2000; Detroit, MI.
21. Trussler AP, Tabbal GN. Patient safety in plastic surgery. *Plast Reconstr Surg.* 2012;130:470e–478e.
22. Butterwick KJ. Liposuction of the neck. In: Draelos ZD, ed. *Cosmetic Dermatology: Products and Procedures.* Singapore: Wiley-Blackwell; 2010:463–472.
23. Jacob CI, Berkes BJ, Kaminer MS. Liposuction and surgical recontouring of the neck: a retrospective analysis. *Dermatol Surg.* 2000;26:625–632.
24. Lillis PJ. Liposuction of the arms. *Dermatol Clin.* 1999;17:783–797.
25. Narins RS. Abdomen: hourglass abdomen, flanks, and modified abdominoplasty. In: Narins RS, ed. *Safe Liposuction and Fat Transfer.* New York, NY: Marcel Dekker, Inc; 2003:95–120.
26. Klein JA. Abdomen. In: Klein JA, ed. *Tumescent Technique: Tumescent Anesthesia and Microcannular Liposuction.* St. Louis, Mosby, Inc; 2000:297–324.
27. Cox SE. Violin: hips, outer thighs, and buttocks. In: Narins RS, ed. *Safe Liposuction and Fat Transfer.* New York, NY: Marcel Dekker, Inc; 2003:121–148.
28. Bernstein G. Liposuction of the thigh. *Dermatol Clin.* 1999;17:849–863.
29. Lillis PJ. Liposuction: how aggressive should it be? *Dermatol Surg.* 1996;22:973–976.
30. Butterwick KJ. Liposuction of the medial thigh, knee, calf, and ankle. In: Narins RS, ed. *Safe Liposuction and Fat Transfer.* New York, NY: Marcel Dekker, Inc; 2003:149–182.
31. Cupp MJ. Herbal remedies: adverse effects and drug interactions. *Am Fam Physician.* 1999;59:1239–1245.
32. Shiffman MA. Medications potentially causing lidocaine toxicity. *Am J Cosmet Surg.* 1998;15:227–228.
33. Klein JA. Cytochrome P450 3A4 and lidocaine metabolism. In: Klein JA, ed. *Tumescent Technique: Tumescent Anesthesia and Microcannular Liposuction.* St. Louis, MO: Mosby, Inc; 2000:131–141.
34. Klein JA, Kassarjdian N. Lidocaine toxicity with tumescent liposuction. A case report of probable drug interactions. *Dermatol Surg.* 1997;23:1169–1174.
35. Klein JA. Pharmacology of tumescent technique. In: Klein JA, ed. *Tumescent Technique: Tumescent Anesthesia and Microcannular Liposuction.* St. Louis, MO: Mosby, Inc; 2000:121–123.
36. Butterwick KJ. Liposuction: consultation and preoperative considerations. In: Narins RS, ed. *Safe Liposuction and Fat Transfer.* New York, NY: Marcel Dekker, Inc; 2003:41–68.
37. Rohrich R, Fodor PB, Petry JJ, et al. Preoperative and postoperative management of the body contour patient: a panel discussion. *Aesthet Surg J.* 1996;16:218–223.
38. Flynn TC, Narins RS. Preoperative evaluation of the liposuction patient. *Dermatol Clin.* 1999;17:729–734.
39. Klein JA. The tumescent technique for liposuction surgery. *Am J Cosm Surg.* 1987;4:263–267.
40. Klein JA. Pharmacokinetics of tumescent liposuction. In: Klein JA, ed. *Tumescent Technique: Tumescent Anesthesia and Microcannular Liposuction.* St. Louis, MO: Mosby, Inc; 2000:141–161.
41. Klein JA. Tumescent infiltration technique. In: Klein JA, ed. *Tumescent Technique: Tumescent Anesthesia and Microcannular Liposuction.* St. Louis, MO: Mosby, Inc; 2000:222–234.
42. Klein JA. Tumescent technique for local anesthesia improves safety in large-volume liposuction. *Plast Reconstr Surg.* 1993;92:1085–1098.
43. Samdal F, Amland PF, Bugge JF. Blood loss during liposuction using the tumescent technique. *Aesthetic Plast Surg.* 1994;18:157–160.
44. Klein JA. Tumescent technique chronicles. Local anesthesia, liposuction, and beyond. *Dermatol Surg.* 1995;21:449–457.
45. Klein JA. Superwet liposuction and pulmonary edema, In: Klein JA, ed. *Tumescent Technique: Tumescent Anesthesia and Microcannular Liposuction.* St. Louis, MO: Mosby, Inc; 2000:61–66.
46. Ostad A, Kageyama N, Moy RL. Tumescent anesthesia with a lidocaine dose of 55 mg/kg is safe for liposuction. *Dermatol Surg.* 1996;22:921–927.
47. Butterwick KJ, Goldman MP, Sriprachya-Anunt S. Lidocaine levels during the first two hours of infiltration of dilute anesthetic solution for tumescent liposuction: rapid versus slow delivery. *Dermatol Surg.* 1999;25:681–685.
48. Butterwick KJ, Goldman MP. Safety of lidocaine during tumescent anesthesia for liposuction. In: Hanke CW, Sattler G. *Liposuction.* Philadelphia, PA: Elsevier; 2005:33–37.
49. de Jong RH, Grazer FM. "Tumescent" liposuction alert: deaths from lidocaine cardiotoxicity. *Am J Forensic Med Pathol.* 1999;20:101.

50. Danilla S, Fontbona M, de Valdés VD, et al. Analgesic efficacy of lidocaine for suction-assisted lipectomy with tumescent technique under general anesthesia: a randomized, double-masked, controlled trial. *Plast Reconstr Surg.* 2013;132:327–332.
51. Matarasso A, Levine SM. Evidence-based medicine: liposuction. *Plast Reconstr Surg.* 2013;132:1697–1705.
52. Klein JA. Anesthetic formulation of tumescent solutions. *Dermatol Clin.* 1999;17:751–759.
53. Kaplan B, Moy RL. Comparison of room temperature and warmed local anesthetic solution for tumescent liposuction. A randomized double-blind study. *Dermatol Surg.* 1996; 22:707–709.
54. Robles-Cervantes JA, Martínez-Molina R, Cárdenas-Camarena L. Heating infiltration solutions used in tumescent liposuction: minimizing surgical risk. *Plast Reconstr Surg.* 2005;116:1077–1081.
55. Klein JA. Microcannulas. In: Klein JA, ed. *Tumescent Technique: Tumescent Anesthesia and Microcannular Liposuction.* St. Louis, MO: Mosby, Inc; 2000:235–247.
56. Klein JA. Surgical technique: microcannular tumescent liposuction. In: Klein JA, ed. *Tumescent Technique: Tumescent Anesthesia and Microcannular Liposuction.* St. Louis, MO: Mosby, Inc; 2000:248–270.
57. Hanke W, Cox SE, Kuznets N, Coleman WP 3rd. Tumescent liposuction report performance measurement initiative: national survey results. *Dermatol Surg.* 2004;30:967–977.
58. Langdon RC. Liposuction of neck and jowls: five-incision method combining machine-assisted and syringe aspiration. *Dermatol Surg.* 2000;26:388–391.
59. Klein JA. Arms. In: Klein JA, ed. *Tumescent Technique: Tumescent Anesthesia and Microcannular Liposuction.* St. Louis, MO: Mosby, Inc; 2000:427–439.
60. Donofrio LM. Liposuctions of the arms and back. In: Narins RS, ed. *Safe Liposuction and Fat Transfer.* New York, NY: Marcel Dekker, Inc; 2003:183–196.
61. Klein JA. Female hips and back and male flanks. In: Klein JA, ed. *Tumescent Technique: Tumescent Anesthesia and Microcannular Liposuction.* St. Louis, MO: Mosby, Inc; 2000:342–356.
62. Lack EB. Contouring the female buttocks: liposculpting the buttocks. *Dermatol Clin.* 1999;17:815–822.
63. Badin AZ, Moraes LM, Gondek L, Chiaratti MG, Canta L. Laser lipolysis: flaccidity under control. *Aesthetic Plast Surg.* 2002;26:335–339.
64. Badin AZ, Gondek LB, Garcia MJ, Valle LC, Flizikowski FB, de Noronha L. Analysis of laser lipolysis effects on human tissue samples obtained from liposuction. *Aesthetic Plast Surg.* 2005;29:281–286.
65. Goldman A, Gotkin RH. Laser-assisted liposuction. *Clin Plast Surg.* 2009;36:241–253.
66. Palm MD, Goldman MP. Laser lipolysis: current practices. *Sem Cutan Med Surg.* 2009;28:212–219.
67. Seckel BR, Doherty ST, Childs JJ, Smirnov MZ, Cohen RH, Altshuler GB. The role of laser tunnels in laser-assisted lipolysis. *Lasers Surg Med.* 2009;41:728–737.
68. Prado A, Andrades P, Danilla S, Leniz P, Castillo P, Gaete F. A prospective, randomized, double-blind, controlled clinical trial comparing laser-assisted lipoplasty with suction-assisted lipoplasty. *Plast Reconstr Surg.* 2006;118:1032–1045.
69. Woodhall KE, Saluja R, Khoury J, Goldman MP. A comparison of three separate clinical studies evaluating the safety and efficacy of laser-assisted lipolysis using 1,064, 1,320 nm, and a combined 1,064/1,320 nm multiplex device. *Lasers Surg Med.* 2009;41:774–778.
70. Goldman A, Wollina U, de Mundstock EC. Evaluation of tissue tightening by the subdermal Nd: YAG laser-assisted liposuction versus liposuction alone. *J Cutan Aesthet Surg.* 2011; 4:122–128.
71. DiBernardo BE, Reyes J. Evaluation of skin tightening after laser-assisted liposuction. *Aesthet Surg J.* 2009;29:400–407.
72. Fakhouri TM, El Tal AK, Abrou A, Mehregan DA, Barone F. Laser-assisted lipolysis: a review. *Dermatol Surg.* 2011; 38:155–169.
73. de Souza Pinto EB, Abdala PC, Maciel CM, dos Santos Fde P, de Souza RP. Liposuction and VASER. *Clin Plast Surg.* 2006;33:107–115.
74. Matarasso A. Discussion: a multicenter, prospective, randomized, single-blind, controlled clinical trial comparing VASER-assisted lipoplasty and suction-assisted lipoplasty. *Plast Reconstr Surg.* 2012;129:690e–691e.
75. Nagy MW, Vanek PF. A multicenter, prospective, randomized, single-blind, controlled clinical trial comparing VASER-assisted Lipoplasty and suction-assisted Lipoplasty. *Plast Reconstr Surg.* 2012;129:681e–689e.
76. Klein JA. Critique of ultrasonic liposuction. In: Klein JA, ed. *Tumescent Technique: Tumescent Anesthesia and Microcannular Liposuction.* St. Louis, MO: Mosby, Inc; 2000:271–280.
77. Mulholland RS. Nonexcisional, minimally invasive rejuvenation of the neck. *Clin Plast Surg.* 2014;41:11–31.
78. Theodorou SJ, Paresi RJ, Chia CT. Radiofrequency-assisted liposuction device for body contouring: 97 patients under local anesthesia. *Aesthetic Plast Surg.* 2012;36:767–779.
79. Duncan DI. Improving outcomes in upper arm liposuction: adding radiofrequency-assisted liposuction to induce skin contraction. *Aesthet Surg J.* 2012;32:84–95.
80. Klein JA. Post-tumescent liposuction care. Open drainage and bimodal compression. *Dermatol Clin.* 1999;17:881–889.
81. Klein JA. Postliposuction edema. In: Klein JA, ed. *Tumescent Technique: Tumescent Anesthesia and Microcannular Liposuction.* St. Louis, MO: Mosby, Inc; 2000:79–87.
82. Klein JA. Postliposuction care: open drainage and bimodal compression. In: Klein JA, ed. *Tumescent Technique: tumescent Anesthesia and Microcannular Liposuction.* St. Louis, MO: Mosby, Inc; 2000:281–293.
83. Fulton JE, Rahimi AD, Helton P. Modified tumescent liposuction. *Dermatol Surg.* 1999;25:755–766.
84. Butterwick KJ, Tse Y, Goldman MP. Effect of external ultrasound postliposuction: a side-to-side comparison study. *Dermatol Surg.* 2000;26:433–435.
85. Draper DO, Abergel RP, Castel JC, Schlaak C. Pulsed shortwave diathermy restricts swelling and bruising of liposuction patients. *Am J Cosm Surg.* 2000;17:17–20.
86. Man D, Man B, Plosker H. The influence of permanent magnetic field therapy on wound healing in suction lipectomy patients: a double-blind study. *Plast Reconstr Surg.* 1999;104:2261–2266.
87. Yun PL, Bruck M, Felsenfeld L, Katz BE. Breast enlargement observed after power liposuction: a retrospective review. *Dermatol Surg.* 2003;29:165–167.
88. Hernandez TL, Kittelson JM, Law CK, et al. Fat redistribution following suction lipectomy: defense of body fat and patterns of restoration. *Obesity (Silver Spring).* 2011;19:1388–1395.
89. Benatti F, Solis M, Artioli G, et al. Liposuction induces a compensatory increase of visceral fat which is effectively counteracted by physical activity: a randomized trial. *J Clin Endocrinol Metab.* 2012;97:2388–2395.
90. Rohrich RJ, Broughton G, Horton B, Lipschitz A, Kenkel JM, Brown SA. The key to long-term success in liposuction: a guide for plastic surgeons and patients. *Plast Reconstr Surg.* 2004;114:1945–1952.
91. Lawrence N, Butterwick KJ. Immediate and long-term postoperative care and touch-ups. In: Narins RS, ed. *Safe Liposuction and Fat Transfer.* New York, NY: Marcel Dekker, Inc; 2003:329–342.
92. Newman J, Dolsky RL. Evaluation of 5,458 cases of liposuction surgery. *Am J Cosmet Surg.* 1984;1:25–80.
93. Bernstein G, Hanke CW. Safety of liposuction: a review of 9478 cases performed by dermatologists. *J Dermatol Surg Oncol.* 1988;14:1112–1114.
94. Teimourian B, Rogers WB. A national survey of complications associated with suction lipectomy: a comparative study. *Plast Reconstr Surg.* 1989;84:628–631.
95. Dillerud E. Suction lipoplasty: a report on complications, undesired results, and patient satisfaction based on 3511 procedures. *Plast Reconstr Surg.* 1991;88:239–246.
96. Hanke CW, Bernstein G, Bullock S. Safety of tumescent liposuction in 15,336 patients. National survey results. *Dermatol Surg.* 1995;21:459–462.

97. Lipoplasty ATFO, Bruner JC. ASPRS Task Force on Lipoplasty, Bruner JG (Chair). 1997 Survey Summary Report. American Society of Plastic and Reconstructive Surgeons; 1998; Arlington Heights, IL.
98. Jackson RF, Dolsky RL. Liposuction and patient safety. *Am J Cosm Surg.* 1999;16:21–23.
99. Grazer FM, de Jong RH. Fatal outcomes from liposuction: census survey of cosmetic surgeons. *Plast Reconstr Surg.* 2000; 105:436–446.
100. Hughes CE. Reduction of lipoplasty risks and mortality: an ASAPS survey. *Aesthet Surg J.* 2001;21:120–127.
101. Housman TS, Lawrence N, Mellen BG, et al. The safety of liposuction: results of a national survey. *Dermatol Surg.* 2002; 28:971–978.
102. Habbema L. Safety of liposuction using exclusively tumescent local anesthesia in 3,240 consecutive cases. *Dermatol Surg.* 2009;35:1728–1735.
103. Boeni R. Safety of tumescent liposuction under local anesthesia in a series of 4,380 patients. *Dermatology.* 2011;222: 278–281.
104. Chia CT, Theodorou SJ. 1,000 consecutive cases of laser-assisted liposuction and suction-assisted lipectomy managed with local anesthesia. *Aesthetic Plast Surg.* 2012;36: 795–802.
105. Klein JA. Risks of systemic anesthesia. In: Klein JA, ed. *Tumescent Technique: Tumescent Anesthesia and Microcannular Liposuction.* St. Louis, MO: Mosby, Inc; 2000:32–42.
106. Platt MS, Kohler LJ, Ruiz R, Cohle SD, Ravichandran P. Deaths associated with liposuction: case reports and review of the literature. *J Forensic Sci.* 2002;47:205–207.
107. Uemura K, Kikuchi Y, Shintani-Ishida K, Nakajima M, Yoshida K. A fatal case of post-operative pulmonary thromboembolism with cosmetic liposuction. *J Clin Forensic Med.* 2006;13:41–43.
108. Gilliland MD, Coates N. Tumescent liposuction complicated by pulmonary edema. *Plast Reconstr Surg.* 1997;99:215–219.
109. Martínez MA, Ballesteros S, Segura LJ, García M. Reporting a fatality during tumescent liposuction. *Forensic Sci Int.* 2008;178:e11–e16.
110. Rao RB, Ely SF, Hoffman RS. Deaths related to liposuction. *N Engl J Med.* 1999;340:1471–1475.
111. Lehnhardt M, Homann HH, Daigeler A, Hauser J, Palka P, Steinau HU. Major and lethal complications of liposuction: a review of 72 cases in Germany between 1998 and 2002. *Plast Reconstr Surg.* 2008;121:396e–403e.
112. Starling J, Thosani MK, Coldiron BM. Determining the safety of office-based surgery: what 10 years of Florida data and 6 years of Alabama data reveal. *Dermatol Surg.* 2012;38(2):171–177.

CHAPTER 42

Hair Transplantation for Men and Women

Nicole E. Rogers & Marc R. Avram

INTRODUCTION

Between 40% and 50% of men and women suffer from male and female pattern hair loss. Over time, hair loss can have a profound impact on sense of self-image, self-awareness, and self-confidence. Hair provides an important frame to the face, and it also serves as a means of self-expression. Individuals may cut, color, and style their hair however they choose. The involuntary loss of this ability can be extremely distressing. When it affects young people in their teens and twenties, it can be especially devastating.

As hair restoration surgeons, we have the unique ability to help recreate our patients' sense of self-image and confidence. However the results of early hair transplantation were not always cosmetically acceptable. Hair transplantation for many still carries the stigma of oversized "pluggy" grafts and hairlines placed too low or unnaturally. It is imperative for novice surgeons to learn the conservative steps necessary for optimal, natural results. It is especially important to learn these steps so that we as practitioners of this profession do not repeat history.

Hair naturally grows in groupings of one to four hairs per follicular unit (FU) (Fig. 42-1). By separating the FUs from one another and allowing the hairs to remain as they do in nature, they can be relocated to areas of thinning with natural and undetectable results.

MEDICATIONS FOR HAIR LOSS

Presently, there are only two FDA-approved medications for hair loss that come in a variety of formulations (Fig. 42-2). Propecia® is a 1 mg finasteride pill that is taken once daily and is approved for use in men only. It works by blocking the enzyme 5-alpha reductase type II, which converts testosterone to dihydrotestosterone (DHT). DHT has been shown to have a miniaturizing effect on hair follicles and is believed to be one factor contributing to the development of male pattern hair loss. With ongoing use of finasteride, men can expect to have continued increases in both hair counts and hair thickness for up to 2 years before this effect reaches a plateau.[1,2]

Rogaine® (active ingredient minoxidil) is FDA approved for hair loss in both men (5% foam and solution) and women (2% solution). Recent evidence has shown that women can use the 5% once daily at bedtime with the same effects as seen using 2% twice daily.[3] Its exact mechanism of action is unknown but it is believed to work through a combination of local vasodilation, the opening of potassium channels, and possibly by down-regulating inflammation.[4] Even after surgery, minoxidil plays a potentially valuable role in speeding up the growth of transplanted follicles and stopping further loss.[5]

Low-level light therapy (LLLT) has also shown promise as a medical treatment for hair loss. Several devices exist on the market using 655 nm "red light" to shine directly on the hair follicle. The Hairmax Lasercomb received FDA 510(k) clearance as a medical device for the treatment of androgenetic alopecia in men in 2007. Additional clearance for females was obtained in 2011. Patients are instructed to use the device to comb through the scalp three times weekly for 15 minutes each time. So far the data is limited but promising and further independent studies will soon be available.[6]

HAIR LOSS CONSULTATION

During the consultation, it is important first to gain an understanding of how long the patient has been suffering

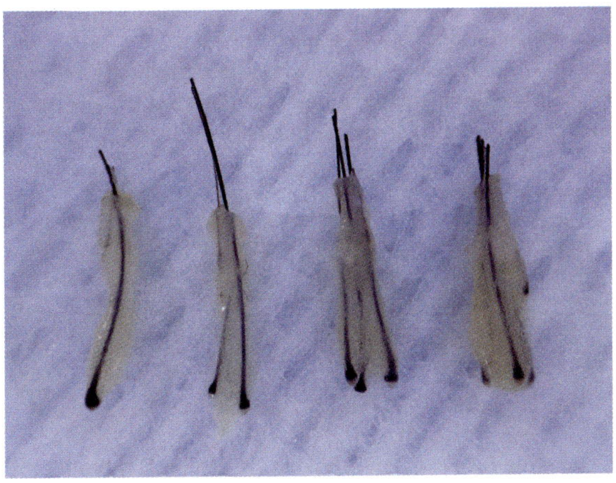

Figure 42-1 Hair follicles naturally grow in groupings of one, two, three, and four hairs.

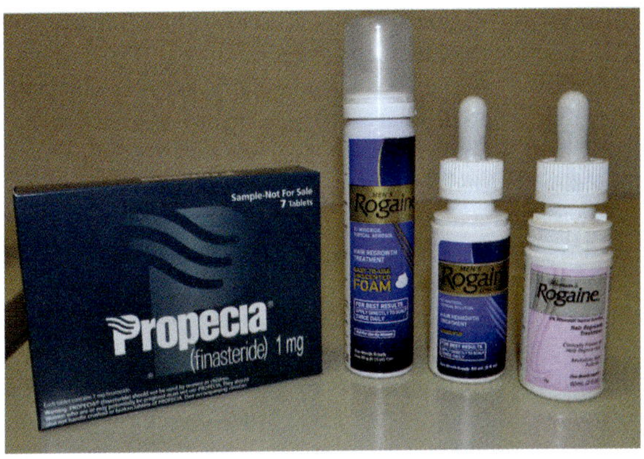

Figure 42-2 FDA-approved medications for hair loss include Propecia and Rogaine.

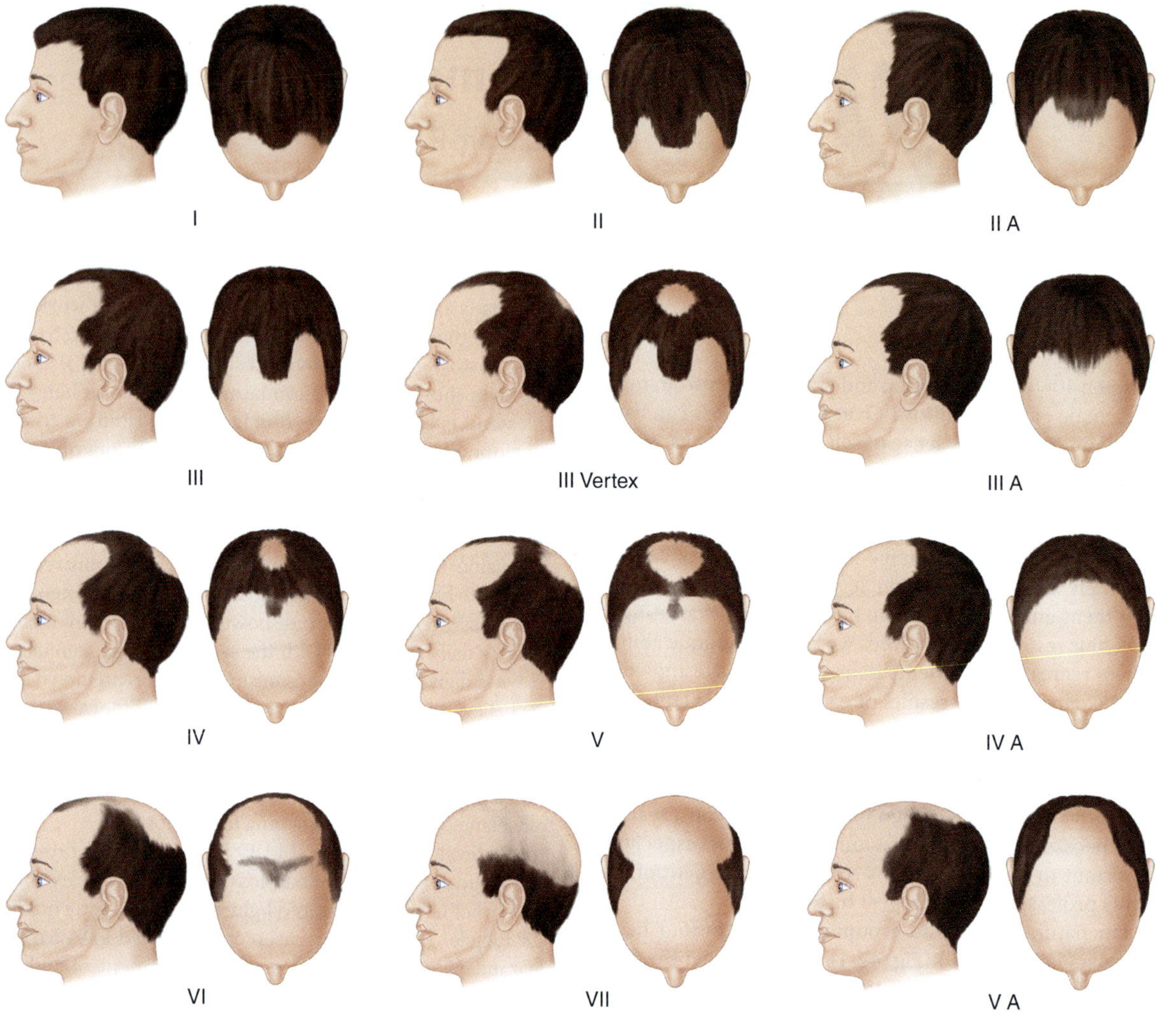

Figure 42-3 The Norwood system is used to classify male pattern hair loss.

from hair loss. If the time frame is as brief as 6 months, they may have a short-term condition called telogen effluvium, which can be due to childbirth, general anesthesia, major physiologic stress, changes in medications, thyroid disturbances, or other laboratory abnormalities. We encourage patients to bring any previous laboratory results with them or refer them to their internist or endocrinologist if further testing is necessary.

For the vast majority of patients seeking hair transplantation, their hair loss has been long-standing and they understand that there is a genetic component to their condition. They may have a brother, sister, parent, or uncle with severe hair loss. It is important to understand what treatments they have already tried (both prescription and over-the-counter supplements) and ask whether these have improved their hair loss. We encourage patients to continue their medications even if they proceed with hair transplantation because it will help to stabilize their ongoing loss.

Next, it is important to assess the age of the patient and their degree of hair loss. We discuss with patients the fact that androgenetic alopecia is an ongoing condition which can progress even after hair transplantation (hence the role of medications in preserving existing hairs). For men, we use the Norwood system to classify the existing distribution of hair loss (Fig. 42-3). In young patients, it can be difficult to predict how their hair loss will evolve over the succeeding 20 to 50 years. Family history can be helpful but not altogether predictive. Transplanting only the frontal 0.5 cm of the hairline or vertex in young men (early 20s) may leave them with unnatural-appearing results years later. In these cases, starting with medications for hair loss may be the best option.

For women, we use the Ludwig system to classify hair loss (Fig. 42-4). Female pattern hair loss does not usually result in a recession of the hairline but rather a loss of density in

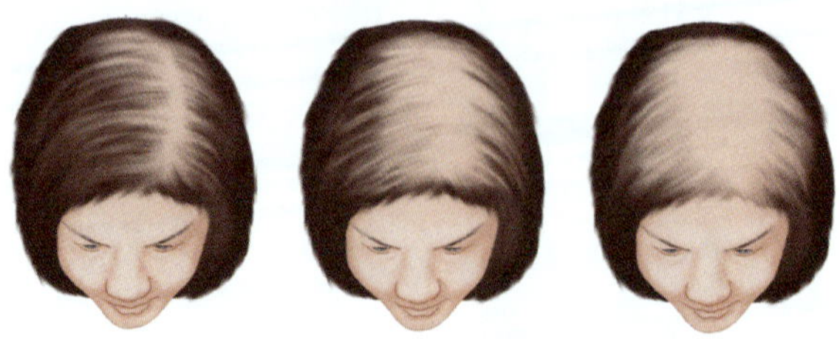

Figure 42-4 The Ludwig system is used to classify female pattern hair loss.

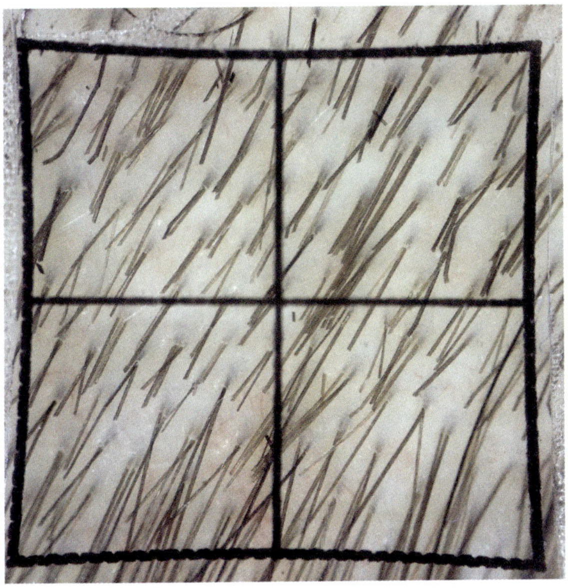

Figure 42-5 Magnified examination of the occipital scalp prior to hair surgery helps assess donor density.

the frontal one-half to two-thirds of the scalp. Women complain of a "see through" effect and feel self-conscious that others are looking at their scalp rather than their eyes. Generally, there are no risks to transplanting women but their results will be best if they have good donor hair density. If the hair on the occipital scalp is just as thin as it is elsewhere, surgery may not provide significant cosmetic benefit.

The physical examination involves assessing the existing distribution of the hair loss as well as the donor hair at the back of the scalp. It is important to examine the entire scalp to make sure that another condition is not causing the patient's hair loss. If there is ever any doubt as to the etiology of a patient's hair loss, a scalp biopsy should be performed. Thicker hairs will offer better coverage than hairs of fine, thin caliber. Dermoscopy can be helpful to assess whether patients have follicle miniaturization in the donor region as well. Generally, patients with good caliber and sufficient hair density (60–100 FUs/cm^2) make excellent candidates for hair transplantation (Fig. 42-5).

Realistic expectations are vital to the success of the procedure. Patients must understand how ongoing hair loss will impact the perceived density of a hair transplant over time (Net density = hair follicles transplanted – ongoing hair loss). Patients should understand before the procedure the areas in which their transplanted hair will appear natural 1 year *and* 10 years after the procedure. Transplanting on the frontal half of the scalp in both men and women will have the greatest cosmetic impact and is the cosmetically safest area in which to transplant for long-term results. Transplanting hairs to the vertex of the scalp will have the least cosmetic impact and has the greatest risk of developing an unnatural appearance over time, as existing hair is lost. Patients with body dysmorphic disorder (BDD) should be identified early because they may never be happy with surgical results. If a patient's goal is to achieve greater relative coverage of their scalp with a single procedure, and they understand that complete coverage may take two or more procedures, then a good outcome can be expected.

TABLE 42-1

List of Factors to Assess During Hair Transplant Consultation

Age of patient
Degree of hair loss
Duration of hair loss
Past treatments: Medications? Supplements?
Expectations: Reasonable? Any history of BDD?
General Health: Smoker? Cardiovascular risk factors?
Physical Examination: Caliber/color of donor hair

A complete list of factors to consider in the hair transplant consultation is shown in Table 42-1.

DAY OF SURGERY

Patients often arrive for their surgery slightly anxious and with some apprehension about what is about to take place. It is helpful to provide as much written material as possible about what to expect before the procedure and after it is complete. Patients are given ample time to review the packet and ask any final questions before signing the consent form. The surgical plan is reviewed, and baseline photographs can be taken and should document several different views of the patient if possible. After all consents are signed patients are given a mild sedative such as diazepam to relax. Their blood pressure is checked and if it is within normal limits the patient is escorted to the surgical suite to change into a gown. Patients are encouraged to wear a button down shirt so that at the end of the day they do not need to pull their shirt over their bandage.

The donor area is marked on the occipital scalp by pinning the hair up with a piece of tape and hairclips. If the hair is long enough (approximately 1–3 cm) it will cover the donor scar. The area is then trimmed using a razor and the patient is placed in a prone position. Specialized pillows are available to allow the patient to rest comfortably while prone. Some surgeons may offer headphones with music for distraction. We generally talk to our patients and keep an easy conversation going throughout the harvest and through the rest of the day.

ANESTHESIA AND DONOR HARVESTING

In the early days of hair transplantation, donor follicles were harvested from the occipital scalp using 4 to 6 mm punch trephines. When the hair was moved to areas of thinning, it continued to grow in oversized groupings of 10 to15 hairs. Since then, newer techniques have evolved, including both traditional strip excision and follicular unit extraction (FUE). These techniques offer more natural results and less noticeable scarring in the donor region.

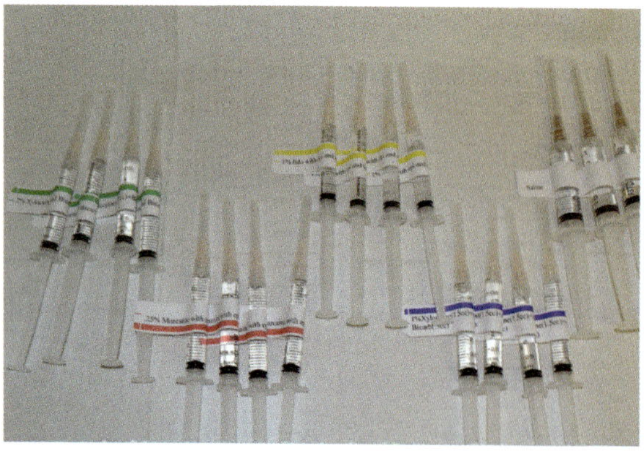

Figure 42-6 Local anesthesia using 0.5%, 1%, and 2% lidocaine as well as 0.25% bupivicane.

STRIP EXCISION

The gold standard for harvesting has traditionally been the strip excision, in which a long narrow strip is taken from the occipital scalp, below the top level of the ears. To avoid the creation of a wide scar, the strip should be no more than 1 to 1.5 cm wide. Some surgeons have had success with wider strips but caution should be used. Excess tension on the donor scalp can result in very wide scars, or worse, complete skin necrosis.

Various combinations of local anesthesia can be used to numb the donor area (Fig. 42-6), including 0.5%, 1%, and 2% lidocaine solutions with 1:1,00,000 epinephrine. We start with a buffered 2% lidocaine with epinephrine solution along the inferior aspect of the donor strip, where the occipital nerve originates. Bupivicane 0.25% is then added around the periphery of the donor strip to allow for longer-term anesthesia of the surrounding area after strip harvest (Fig. 42-7). Finally, saline is injected into the donor area to provide tumescence in the subcutis. This allows for firming of the skin and helps to elevate the follicles above any nerves and blood vessels below.

Next a single- or double-bladed scalpel with a #10 blade is used to remove the donor strip (Fig. 42-8). Care should be taken to angle the blade in the caudal direction so that it falls between existing hairs and does not transect any follicles. Some surgeons recommend just scoring the epidermis and using tension to dissect the dermis and subcutis.

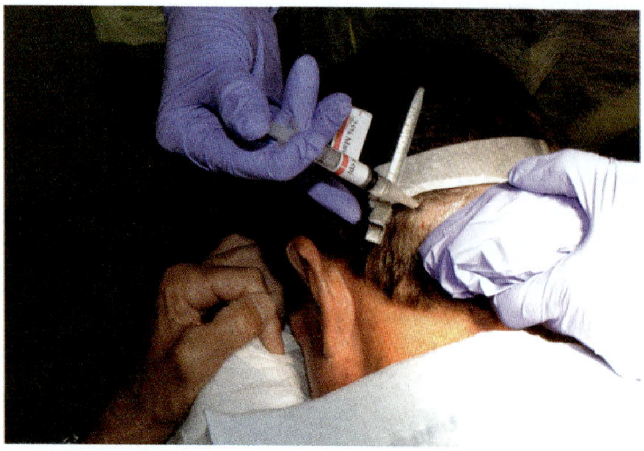

Figure 42-7 Injection of local anesthesia into the donor area prior to surgery.

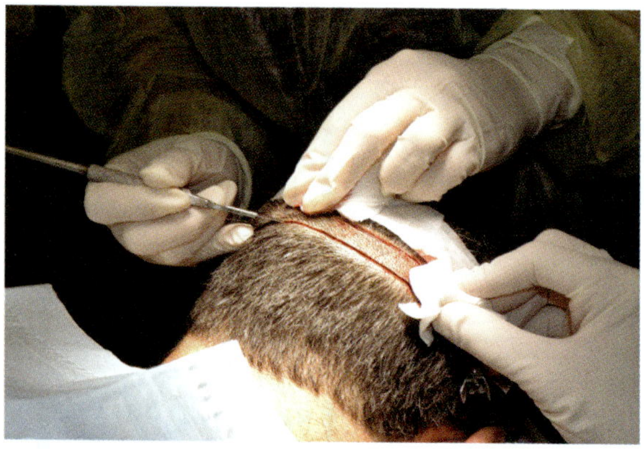

Figure 42-8 Harvesting of donor tissue from the occipital scalp.

Starting at one end, the strip should be lifted and gently separated from the underlying scalp tissue by working slowly across the scalp (Figs. 42-9 and 42-10). The edges should be tapered and when removed, the strip should be placed in saline until graft separation begins.

The donor site can be closed with either staples or sutures (Fig. 42-11). A variety of absorbable and nonabsorbable sutures can be used. The authors use both staples (MA) and running 3-0 or 4-0 polyglactin 910 sutures (NR). Undermining is generally not required and it is up to the surgeon whether to use local electrocautery for hemostasis. Staples and sutures must remain in place for 7 to 10 days, while dissolving sutures are a good option for out-of-town patients who cannot return for suture removal. Many advocate the use of a trichophytic closure technique to minimize the appearance of the scar. This is performed by removing a narrow, superficial ledge of epidermis from one or both wound edges so that when the hairs grow back, they will grow through the scar and help camouflage its appearance.

FOLLICULAR UNIT EXTRACTION (FUE)

In the last 5 years, there has been a trend toward "no scar" surgery, propelled both by patient desires and market forces. This form of donor harvest involves the removal of individual FUs one at a time using small (0.6–1 mm) manual or motorized punch devices. A larger donor area must

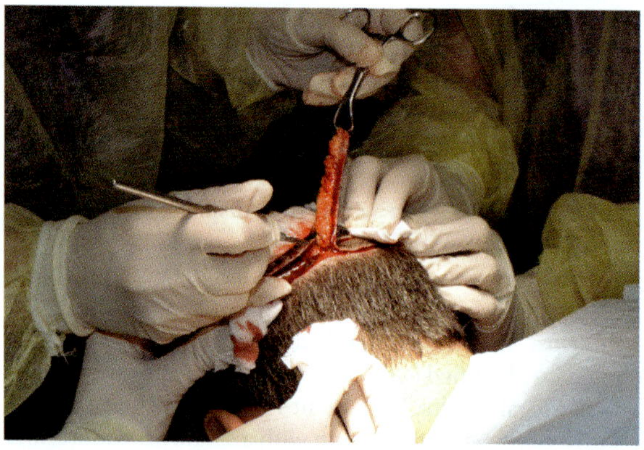

Figure 42-9 Removal of donor strip using sterile technique.

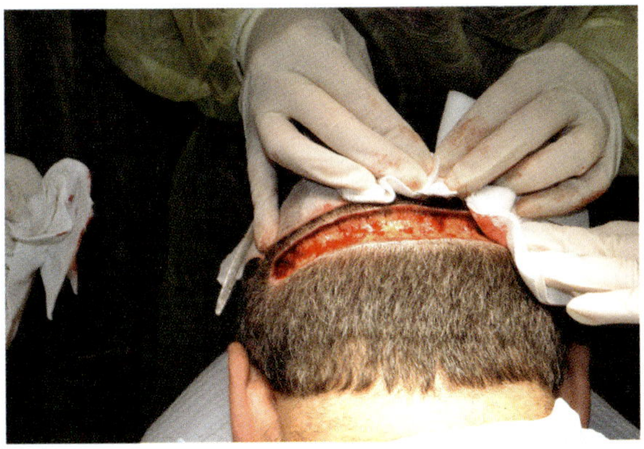

Figure 42-10 Subcutaneous fat remains after donor strip has been harvested.

be used and closely shaved to allow for harvesting of individual follicles. Most doctors use loupes or some form of magnification to correctly identify the angle of the follicle as it exits the scalp. Local anesthesia can be used and no closure is necessary for the pinpoint scars left behind. Patients simply keep the area clean and covered with a petrolatum based or antibiotic ointment while the sites are healing.

There are certain caveats to this technique. First, there can be considerably higher follicle transection rates seen with FUE, especially during the early phase of implementation. If the angle is not correct, or excess tension is placed on the follicle, it may be cut in half or lose its investing tissue. Either condition will deter subsequent growth. It is also considerably more time-consuming, as it provides just one-third to half the normal number of grafts within the same operative time. This can ultimately make this technique more expensive for the patients who choose it. Finally, patients may be left with reduced donor density in the event that they desire a traditional strip excision to be performed later. Time will tell how this technique compares with traditional strip excision.

ERGONOMICS AND PATIENT COMFORT

Local anesthesia is generally sufficient to achieve good hemostasis and maximal comfort for most patients. We

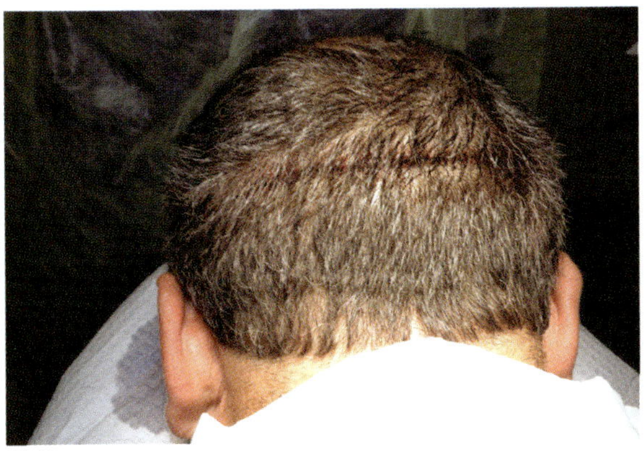

Figure 42-11 Donor scalp immediately following closure.

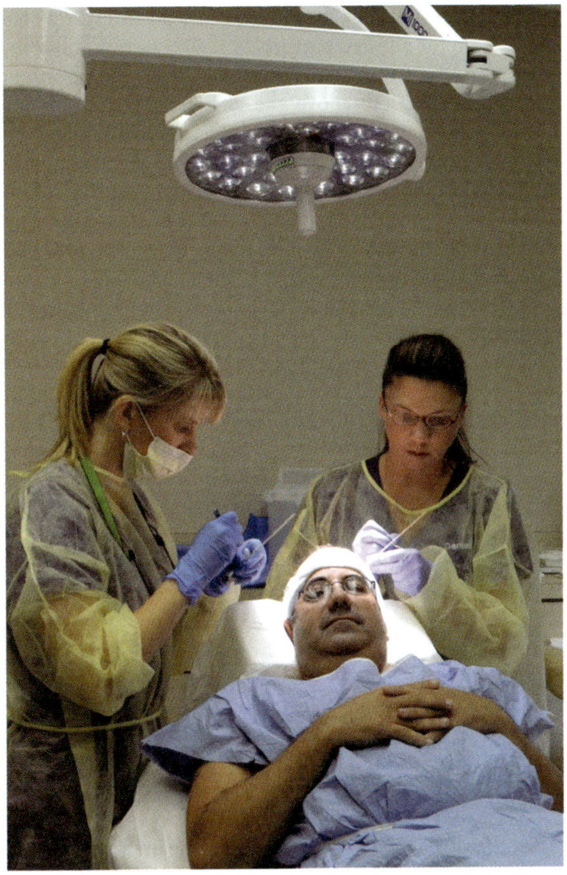

Figure 42-12 Patient is comfortably reclined during graft placement.

also provide oral diazepam but encourage those patients who take it not to drive after the procedure is over. In certain patients with above-average anxiety, it may be helpful to prescribe a stronger anxiolytic medication and allow them to take it before they come in (with consents signed beforehand) or to arrange for an anesthesiologist to be present for the procedure if the operating room is accredited for sedation and monitoring.

Patients are encouraged to let us know when they need to stretch or use the bathroom. Depending on the extent of the procedure it may be necessary to break for lunch in the middle of the day. A television is installed in the operating room and patients are invited to bring any movies or DVDs they would like to watch. Frequently they just enjoy talking and listening to music (Fig. 42-12). It is imperative to maintain a relaxed but professional atmosphere.

HAIRLINE DESIGN

The location and orientation of the hairline are both extremely important for the creation of natural results. The area that is transplanted must look cosmetically appropriate both in the present as well as 20 to 50 years after the procedure has been performed. For women, whose hairlines generally stay intact, this is less of an issue. However in men, hairlines that are placed too low, with FUs that are oriented radially or too perpendicular to the scalp (as in a picket fence) look unnatural and can lead to even worse self-esteem for affected patients.

In men, the frontal hairline should begin no less than approximately 9 cm above the glabella. Many surgeons create a 1 to 2 cm deep zone of reduced density along the frontal hairline, using hairs that are finer in caliber with only one hair per FU. Behind this hairline, larger FUs can be placed. It is imperative that the natural temporal recessions be preserved, since the appearance of a rounded hairline can be quite feminizing in a man. Under certain circumstances, men can benefit from hair restoration of the temples as well.

Many men request restoration of their balding vertex. The ability to fill in the vertex depends largely upon their age, degree of thinning, and amount of donor hair. Generally men in their 50s and 60s may be transplanted because their pattern of thinning is more well-established and less likely to advance rapidly. The vertex should not be transplanted in men aged 20 to 45 years whose future is less certain. If they have only a small hairless area, and it is transplanted but expands later, they will be left with a large, unnatural looking island of hair. As physicians we must educate patients about these possible scenarios and resist the temptation to give in to patients' (often misinformed) desires for hairline design.

GRAFT CREATION

After the donor strip is removed, it is cleaned and soaked in saline before being separated into individual FUs. To separate the units, the donor strip is first placed lengthwise on a hard surface such as a tongue depressor or a specifically designed plastic cutting board (Fig. 42-13). Individual strips are then slivered perpendicularly from the strip, each containing 10 to 25 FUs depending on the width of the strip (Fig. 42-14). As these strips are created, other members of the team begin separating each sliver into individual FUs of one to four hairs each, carefully preserving the conformation in which they naturally exist.

As the follicles are separated, they are placed in a petri dish with saline solution and a nonstick pad lining the bottom of the dish (Fig. 42-15). It is essential that the follicles stay moist during this step and throughout the procedure. If they dry out or become desiccated they will not survive the transplantation process. One must also be cautious not to place grafts that have become desiccated but, when placed back in saline, appear viable.

Much of what fueled the surge toward more natural results was the introduction of stereomicroscopic dissection of FU grafts. In 1994, Dr. B. L. Limmer published a landmark paper describing his technique of graft creation using microscopes with 10× magnification.[7] Since then, many surgeons have begun using magnification to assist in the separation and creation of FU grafts (Fig. 42-16). Others use eyewear such as loupes or drugstore glasses to magnify the hairs during dissection.

As the technicians create the grafts they record the numbers of grafts created. Some teams keep track of how many of each one-, two-, three-, and four-hair FU they create in order to know the total number of hairs transplanted in a single procedure. Others go by the total number of grafts regardless of how many of each size FU is created.

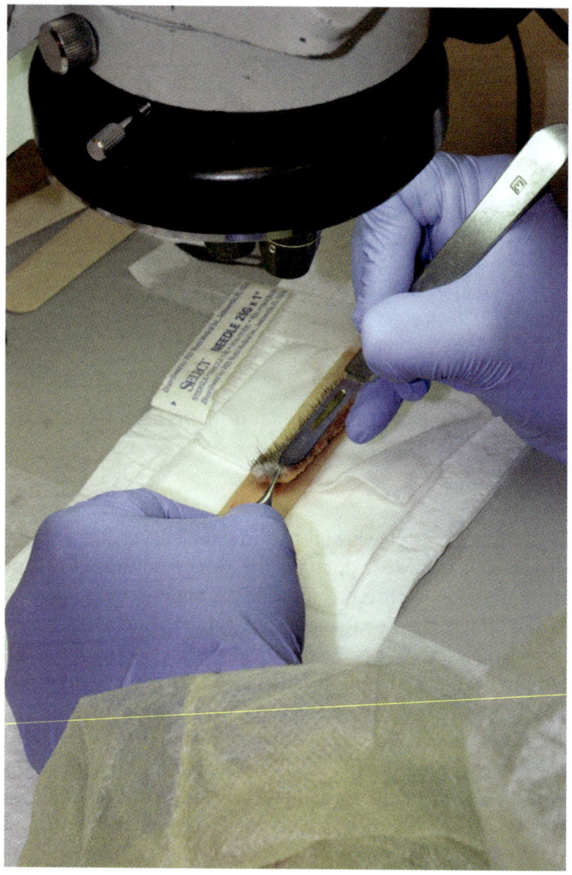

Figure 42-13 Strip is first slivered into thin slices of tissue 1 follicular unit wide.

RECIPIENT SITE CREATION

While the grafts are being created, the surgeon anesthetizes the area to be transplanted and creates recipient sites for the grafts. Often a 1% or 2% lidocaine ring block, injected carefully across the forehead, is sufficient to reduce the sensation of subsequent lidocaine injections posteriorly. Other doctors perform local nerve blocks by injecting the medial aspect of the eyebrows, from which

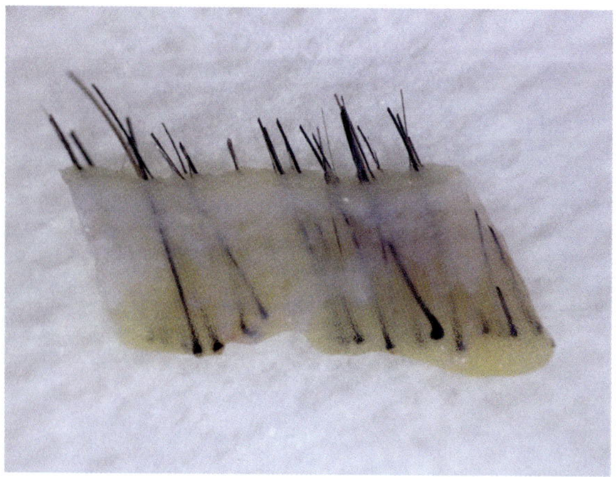

Figure 42-14 Single sliver in cross-section.

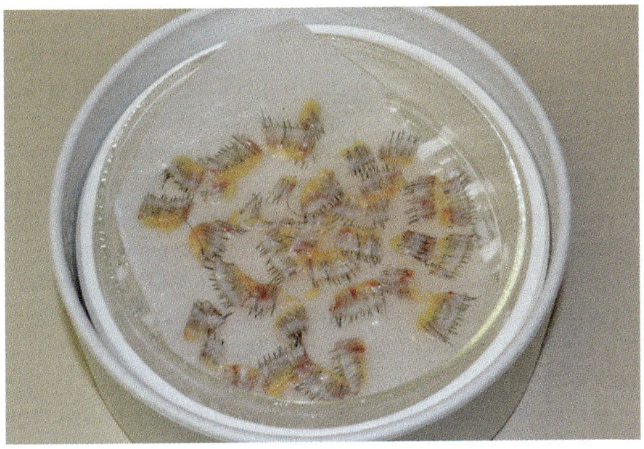

Figure 42-15 Slivers are kept chilled during graft dissection process.

the supraorbital and supratrochlear nerves exit their foramina. The skin should be numbed very superficially; often a 0.5% lidocaine concentration is sufficient. Regardless, the numbed area must be reinforced every 30 to 45 minutes to maintain anesthesia and to keep the patient comfortable. Layering with bupivicaine can also help reduce the frequency of injections needed.

Various tools are available for making recipient sites. Perhaps the most inexpensive and readily available tools are simple 18, 19, and 20 gauge needles. These correspond to

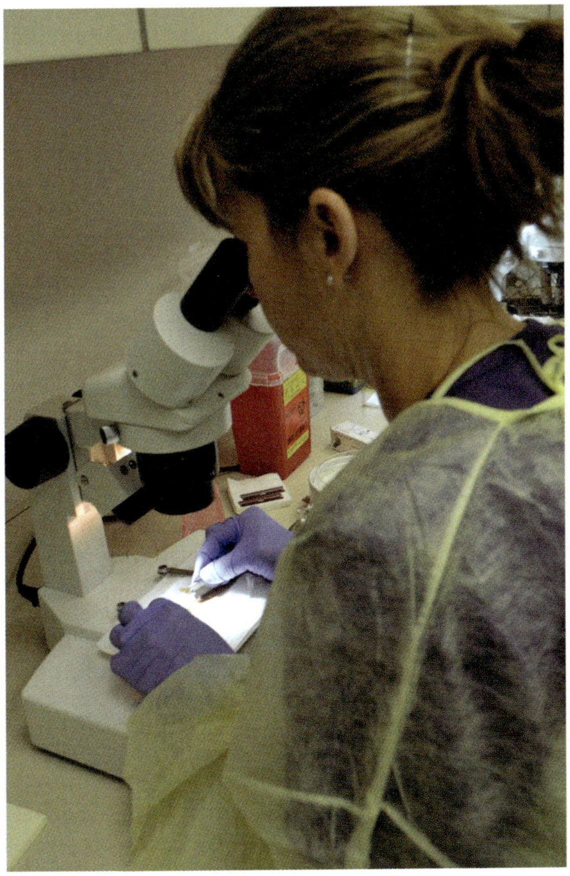

Figure 42-16 Microscopes can increase the ease and visibility of graft separation.

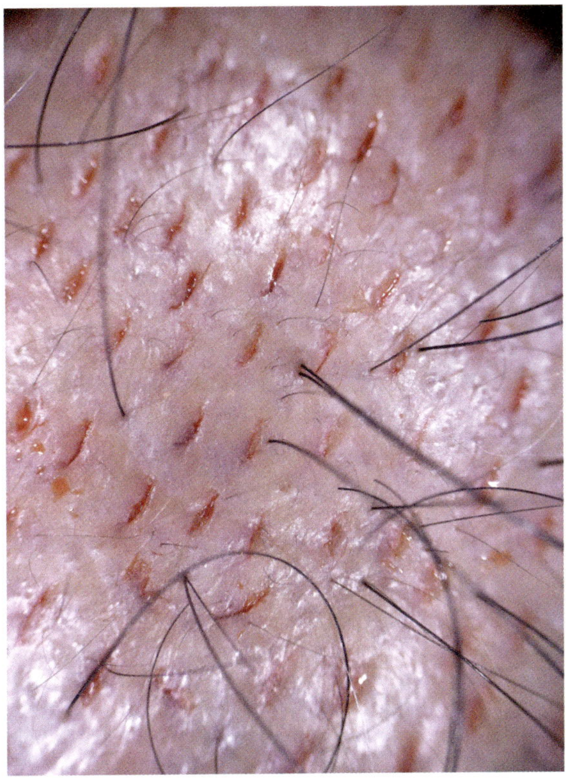

Figure 42-17 Microscopic examination of graft sites prior to graft placement.

widths of 1.25, 1.1, and 0.9 mm. Other commercially available tools are Minde blades and SP blades. The latter can be mounted on adjustable handles to control the depth of the blade as it enters the scalp. Other surgeons use chisel blades that are custom made or commercially available. Personal preference and ergonomics seem to be the most important factors in choosing what type of tool to use.

As the graft sites are created, the instrument handle should be angled forward, about 30 to 45 degrees up from the skin in front of the site. It is especially important that this be done along the frontal hairline where it is most visible. Some have argued that this angle cannot be too steep. The sites should be created in a random fashion, placing slits in and among the existing follicles (Fig. 42-17). Near the temporal recessions, the hair splits its direction of orientation. Medially, the hairs should therefore be angled centrally and toward the midline. Laterally they should be angled laterally and toward the chin. Again the narrower the angle is when the hairs emerge from the scalp, the more natural the results will appear (Fig. 42-18).

If sites are made on the vertex of the scalp, they should follow the direction of existing hairs, which may be a C-shaped whorl or a double S-shaped whorl. Again the hairs should be very acutely angled as they are transplanted. Otherwise, they will have an unnatural appearance if they exit too perpendicularly from the scalp.

As the graft sites are made, the total number is counted in order to know whether that number corresponds with the number of grafts created. Some bleeding can occur but is not usually more than can be handled with light pressure. The recipient area is repeatedly sprayed and cleaned with saline as the procedure progresses.

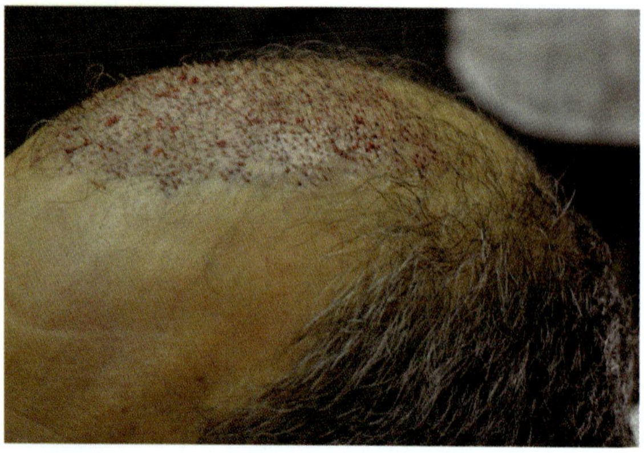

Figure 42-18 Patient immediately after placement of one to four hair follicular unit grafts.

GRAFT PLACEMENT

A number of different specialized forceps are used to place the grafts. They are narrow enough at the tips that they can be inserted slightly into the graft site, along with the graft, and then be released to leave the graft in place. Wooden cotton-tipped applicators are also used to hold the graft in place while it is again gently inserted the rest of the way into the graft site. Each graft should be picked up just above the base of the follicle with careful attention not to crush the bulb or the bulge area above it. A two-handed technique is usually necessary to "shimmy" the grafts in place, and patience is a virtue for those starting out.

Depending on the size and area being transplanted, it may be possible for one, two, or even three technicians to place the grafts at once. Patients with elevated blood pressures may have more "popping," a process which occurs when the hairs, once transplanted, come back out of their sites. Patience, good lighting and ergonomics are all essential to reduce eye strain and muscle fatigue. Technicians are also encouraged to take breaks as needed.

POSTOPERATIVE CARE

At the completion of surgery, long-acting bupivicaine can be injected again into the donor area to reinforce anesthesia during the evening hours. Antibiotic ointment is applied to the donor area, and Telfa dressings may or may not be applied to the frontal recipient areas. Conforming gauze bandages may be used to wrap the entire scalp to protect the donor area as well as the newly placed grafts. Patients are instructed to leave the bandage on overnight and remove it in the morning. If given a sedative, they are not allowed to drive home after the procedure.

That night, patients are encouraged to avoid exerting themselves. They may use the computer, read, or relax with a movie. Pain medication is prescribed. The day after surgery patients may gently pour warm water over their scalp, but they are instructed to wait 3 days before shampooing. They can return to full physical activities after 1 week. This includes running, biking, swimming, or weight-lifting.

A possible result of hair transplantation can be swelling of the forehead after surgery. This can occur as the anesthesia works its way down the face due to gravity. Two steps can be taken to prevent this. First, one can include an anti-inflammatory preparation such as triamcinolone in the local anesthetic solution. The second is to simply prescribe an oral anti-inflammatory medication such as prednisone to be taken for 3 to 5 days after surgery. Both techniques work well and many physicians use both with almost no patients reporting postoperative edema.

TABLE 42-2
Follicular Unit Extraction

Advantages	Disadvantages
No linear scar Potentially easier donor site healing	Potential for higher rate of transection of follicles during harvest More time-consuming Lower yield per harvest May need to shave large donor area

FUTURE TRENDS

Recently, robotic devices have been introduced for the purpose of hair transplantation. The ARTAS® system received FDA 510(k) clearance in April 2011 as an automated form of FUE. A computerized robot calculates the distance to the scalp and the angle of the exiting donor hairs. It then removes a 0.8 to 1.0 mm wide cylinder of tissue surrounding the hair as is done by the manual FUE technique described earlier. The advantages are less fatigue and eye strain for the physician, but these may be outweighed by the cost and space required. It is unclear whether robotic devices can offer lower transection rates than are seen with manual FUE. Further research and refinements to the device will help answer these questions.

The NeoGraft® device is another tool for FUE, although it does not have FDA device approval. Rather than using a robot, it implements a suction device to help remove the FUs once they are manually scored by the doctor. Physicians new to hair surgery should understand that the Neograft™ is a tool for (follicular unit) donor harvesting. Surgical skills are still required to design the hairline and artfully place the follicles back in the scalp. Again, time will tell whether the cost of this machine is balanced out by its benefit to the surgeon. Such products may be more helpful in marketing practices than in expediting or improving the surgical procedure.

Perhaps the most long-awaited advancement in hair transplantation is the ability to clone hairs. Presently we are limited by the amount of patient donor hair available. If one day we can take a small punch biopsy from the scalp and then replicate 1000 or 10,000 FUs from it, the field of hair transplantation will change dramatically. Far more patients will become candidates for the procedure and the donor harvest and graft creation process will no longer be necessary. Many private companies are attempting to develop this technique but it still appears to be years away.

CONCLUSION

Modern hair transplantation techniques offer results that are natural and undetectable. The separation of hairs into individual FUs was the lynchpin toward making this procedure cosmetically successful for patients in both the long and short run. Physician knowledge and experience is still essential in planning and executing an excellent hair transplant result. It will be exciting to see more tools and devices develop within this field. The most important innovations will be those that can increase hair follicle survival, reduce the amount of donor hair needed, and improve the patient's comfort and experience during the procedure.

REFERENCES

1. Price VH, Menefee E, Sanchez M, Ruane P, Kaufman KD. Changes in hair weight and hair count in men with androgenetic alopecia after treatment with finasteride, 1 mg daily. *J Am Acad Dermatol.* 2002;46:517–543.
2. Kaufman KD, Finasteride Male Pattern Hair Loss Study Group. Long-term (5-year) multinational experience with finasteride 1 mg in the treatment of men with androgenetic alopecia. *Eur J Dermatol.* 2002;12:38–49.
3. Peytavi UB, Hillmann K, Dietz E, Canfield D, Garcia Bartels N. A randomized, single-blind trial of 5% minoxidil foam once daily versus 2% minoxidil solution twice daily in the treatment of androgenetic alopecia in women. *J Am Acad Dermatol.* 2011;65:1126–1134.
4. Messenger AG, Rundegren J. Minoxidil: mechanisms of action on hair growth. *Br J Dermatol.* 2004;150:186–194.
5. Avram MR, Cole JP, Gandelman M, et al. The potential role of minoxidil in the hair transplantation setting. *J Derm Surg.* 2002;28:894–900.
6. Leavitt M, Charles G, Heyman E, Michaels D. HairMax Lasercomb laser phototherapy device in the treatment of male androgenetic alopecia: a randomized doubleblind, sham-device-controlled, multicentre trial. *Clin Drug Invest.* 2009;29:283–292.
7. Limmer BL. Elliptical donor stereoscopically assisted micrografting as an approach to further refinement in hair transplantation. *J Dermatol Surg Oncol.* 1994;20:789–793.

CHAPTER 43

Special Considerations for Hair Restoration Surgery

Marc R. Avram & Meena Singh

INTRODUCTION

Hair transplantation has been performed since the 1960s for the treatment of androgenetic alopecia. The technique of follicular unit transplantation (FUT) provides consistently natural appearing cosmetic outcomes for patients with this condition, and the majority of patients who seek consultation for hair restoration are seeking treatment for thinning hair as a result of female or male pattern hair loss. However, there is a subset of patients who require special consideration for hair restoration. In this chapter, we describe hair restoration surgery for scarring alopecia and corrective hair surgery.

The general public often perceives androgenetic alopecia as a normal variant of aging, but hair loss due to scarring alopecia is often more cosmetically disfiguring. Moreover, patients who seek corrective hair surgery typically do so because their previous surgery appears unnatural and they feel as though they *must* do something to correct their unnatural appearing, "pluggy" transplants. These patients need special consideration not only because they may be more troubled or devastated by the cosmetic appearance of the involved bald areas, but also because they will need special considerations regarding the techniques to be used for their corrective surgery to be successful.

HAIR RESTORATION SURGERY FOR CICATRICIAL (SCARRING) ALOPECIA

The term "cicatricial alopecia" will be used interchangeably with scarring alopecia in this section. Cicatricial or scarring denotes that the follicular epithelium has been replaced with fibrous connective tissue. Hair surgeons often use the term more broadly than dermatologists, with any cicatricial alopecia generally being defined as any form of inflammation or trauma that leads to a scarring process. This can, therefore, include scarring hair loss from cosmetic surgery, burns, or radiation. Cicatricial alopecia can be divided into primary and secondary cicatricial alopecias.[1] In primary cicatricial alopecia, the hair follicle is the target of the inflammation and disease activity.[2] In secondary cicatricial alopecia, the hair follicle just happens to be present in the area of disease activity, as in radiation dermatitis or burns. In this chapter, the various types of cicatricial alopecia will be discussed, as well as special considerations for transplanting patients with scarring alopecia.

INITIAL EVALUATION

Overall, hair transplantation into areas of scarring alopecia can be more challenging as the patient not only needs a suitable donor area, but the inflammatory stage of the scarring alopecia must also be inactive. It is, therefore, important that patients with scarring alopecias secondary to inflammatory scalp dermatoses be treated medically before considering surgery. Some patients respond to medical therapy within months, others over years. For some patients, reactivation of the inflammatory stage may occur post transplant and lead to loss of the transplanted hairs. Patients with primary scarring alopecia seeking hair transplant surgery should be aware of the impact that reactivation of inflammation would have on transplanted hair, as well as the need for regular follow-up with their dermatologist following surgery. In addition, scalp fibrosis and diminished blood supply may lead to decreased graft survival, as well as limited cosmetic improvement. For these reasons, when a patient seeks consultation for hair restoration, it is of utmost importance to have an accurate diagnosis for the cause of the alopecia and for patients to understand the challenges associated with transplanting hair in the setting of their scalp disease.

Importantly, patients may seek out consultation for what is believed to be androgenetic alopecia; however, they may in fact have a scarring alopecia that is mimicking androgenetic alopecia (Fig. 43-1). Because transplanting into scarring alopecia takes special consideration, it is critical that the surgeon not miss these diagnoses, as surgical outcomes may be suboptimal and lead to poor cosmetic results and patient dissatisfaction.

Making a proper diagnosis of cicatricial alopecia entails performing a detailed history and scalp examination.[3] (Tables 43-1 and 43-2). Helpful clues in diagnosing cicatricial alopecia include shiny atrophic skin with loss of follicular openings, as well as signs of inflammation, such as perifollicular erythema, hyperkeratosis, crust, dyschromia, pustules, and tufting or "doll hairs."[3] A hair pull test may also be performed. If oozing, bleeding, or crusting is present, tissue culture may be warranted. Additionally, a scalp biopsy is strongly recommended, if there is any doubt regarding the etiology of a patient's hair loss.[4]

HISTOPATHOLOGIC EXAMINATION

A biopsy can be useful not only to determine the diagnosis, but also to evaluate the potential for regrowth. If the alopecia is end-stage and has become permanent, histopathologic examination will reveal scar and perifollicular fibrosis with minimal lymphohistiocytic inflammation.[4] It

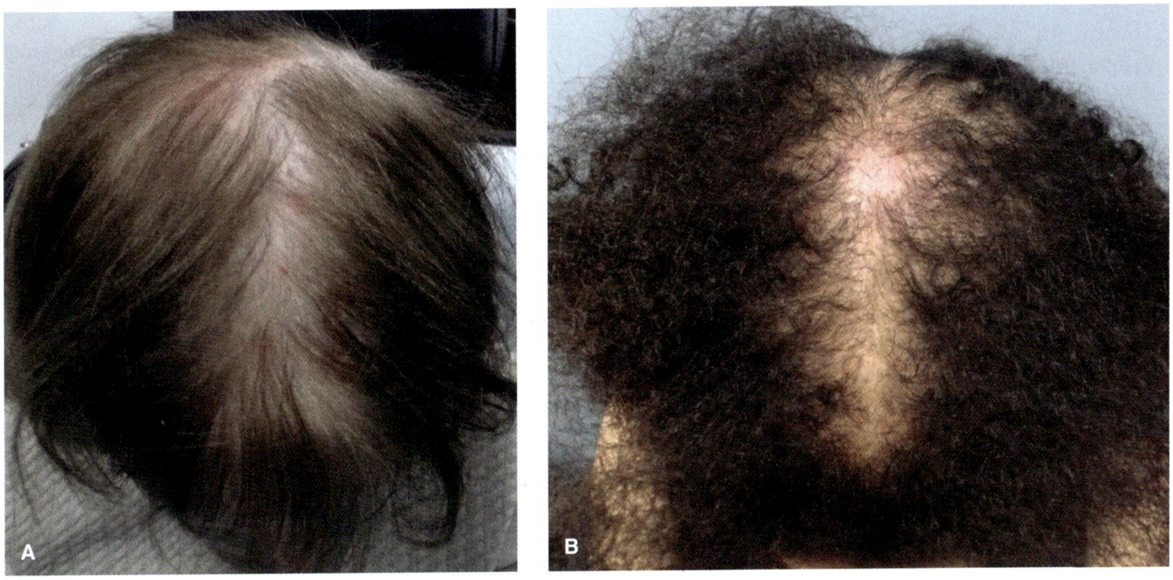

Figure 43-1 Hair transplant consults for female pattern hair loss. **A.** On close inspection, patient had perifollicular erythema, scale, and shiny, atrophic scalp skin. Biopsy was consistent with lichen planopilaris. **B.** Diffuse thinning with increased central part width and preservation of frontal hairline. Patient complained of tenderness of scalp and on closer inspection, there was a loss of follicular ostia and atrophic scalp skin, consistent with central centrifugal cicatricial alopecia (CCCA).

is also important to consider where to biopsy, how many biopsies to perform, and how the tissue is processed. The best diagnostic yield is produced when obtaining two biopsies for vertical and horizontal sectioning. If direct immunofluorescence (DIF) is warranted, the vertical section can be bisected using a no. 15 blade. One piece will be placed in formalin for Hematoxylin–Eosin (H&E) staining and the second piece will be placed in specialized media for DIF. DIF is typically performed when either lichen planopilaris (LPP) or lupus erythematosus (LE) is suspected.

PRIMARY CICATRICIAL (SCARRING) ALOPECIA

Primary cicatricial alopecias are areas of permanent, scarring hair loss due to an inflammatory disorder of the scalp. The etiology of this group of alopecias is largely unknown.

TABLE 43-1
Suggested Questions to Elicit History of Scarring Alopecia

Is the hair loss gradual or sudden?
Is the hair loss shedding or nonshedding?
Is there the presence of high fever or systemic disease?
Is there a recent stressor or medication exposure?
Is there the presence of harsh chemicals on hair such as relaxers or dyes?
Is there the presence of itching, burning, tenderness, or oozing?
Is there a history of traumatic hairstyling practices such as tight braids, weaves, or curlers?

The various inflammatory alopecias present with erythema, perifollicular papules, scale and pustules, and sometimes with bogginess. Ongoing inflammation leads to perifollicular fibrosis and eventual quiescence of the inflammation. Permanent loss of the hair follicle is thought to result from ongoing damage to the isthmus of the follicle, which destroys the stem cells and sebaceous glands.[5] These inflammatory alopecias at end-stage appear as scarring alopecias, presenting with shiny, atrophic patches of hair loss with loss of the follicular ostia.

CLASSIFICATION OF THE PRIMARY CICATRICIAL ALOPECIAS

The North American Hair Research Society proposed a working classification for primary cicatricial alopecias based on the type of perifollicular inflammation present: lymphocytic, neutrophilic, or mixed (Table 43-3).[6] We will discuss the more commonly seen types in brief that follows and focus more on the technical considerations for hair transplantation in these entities.

TABLE 43-2
On Scalp Examination, the Patient Should Be Evaluated for These Changes

Is the hair loss localized or diffuse?
Is there erythema, perifollicular papules, scales, or oozing?
Is there follicular plugging?
Is there cutaneous involvement?
Is there a loss of follicular ostia?
Are there doll hairs present?

TABLE 43-3
Proposed Classification for Primary Cicatricial Alopecias

Lymphocytic	Neutrophilic	Mixed
Chronic cutaneous lupus erythematosus	Folliculitis decalvans	Acne keloidalis
Lichen planopilaris	Dissecting cellulitis	Acne necrotica
Frontal fibrosing alopecia		Erosive pustular dermatosis
Pseudopelade of Brocq		
Central centrifugal cicatricial alopecia		
Alopecia mucinosa		

PREDOMINANTLY LYMPHOCYTIC PERIFOLLICULAR INFILTRATES

LUPUS ERYTHEMATOSUS

Chronic cutaneous LE can lead to discoid plaques on the scalp and scarring alopecia in its late stages. When active, it can present with atrophic, erythematous, hyper- or hypopigmented plaques with follicular plugging (Fig. 43-2). Lesions of LE seen in the external ear canal can be a clue to the diagnosis. Histopathologic examination demonstrates hyperkeratosis, follicular plugging, basement membrane thickening, vacuolar interface change at the dermoepidermal (DE) junction, pigment incontinence, dermal mucin deposition, and superficial and deep perifollicular and perivascular lymphocytic inflammation. DIF can demonstrate continuous granular deposition at the DE junction with IgG, IgM, IgA, and C3. Individuals with discoid LE who have systemic involvement should not be considered as candidates for hair transplantation.[7]

LICHEN PLANOPILARIS

LPP is another common cause of cicatricial alopecia. It is a common mimicker of androgenetic alopecia as its activity may be subclinical. LPP is more commonly seen in females and Caucasians with scattered patches of partial hair loss, perifollicular papules, erythema, and scale. It is commonly associated with pruritus, burning, and tenderness.[8]

Frontal fibrosing alopecia is thought to be a variant of LPP, typically occurring in postmenopausal women with a band of alopecia along the frontotemporal scalp, variably associated with perifollicular papules and eyebrow involvement (Fig. 43-3).[9] Graham–Little–Piccardi–Lassueur syndrome, another variant of LPP, demonstrates LPP on the scalp, keratosis pilaris on the extremities, and noncicatricial alopecia in the axilla and groin.[10] Histopathologic evaluation of LPP and its variants shows lichenoid interface dermatitis with dyskeratotic keratinocytes at the upper portions of the follicles. At

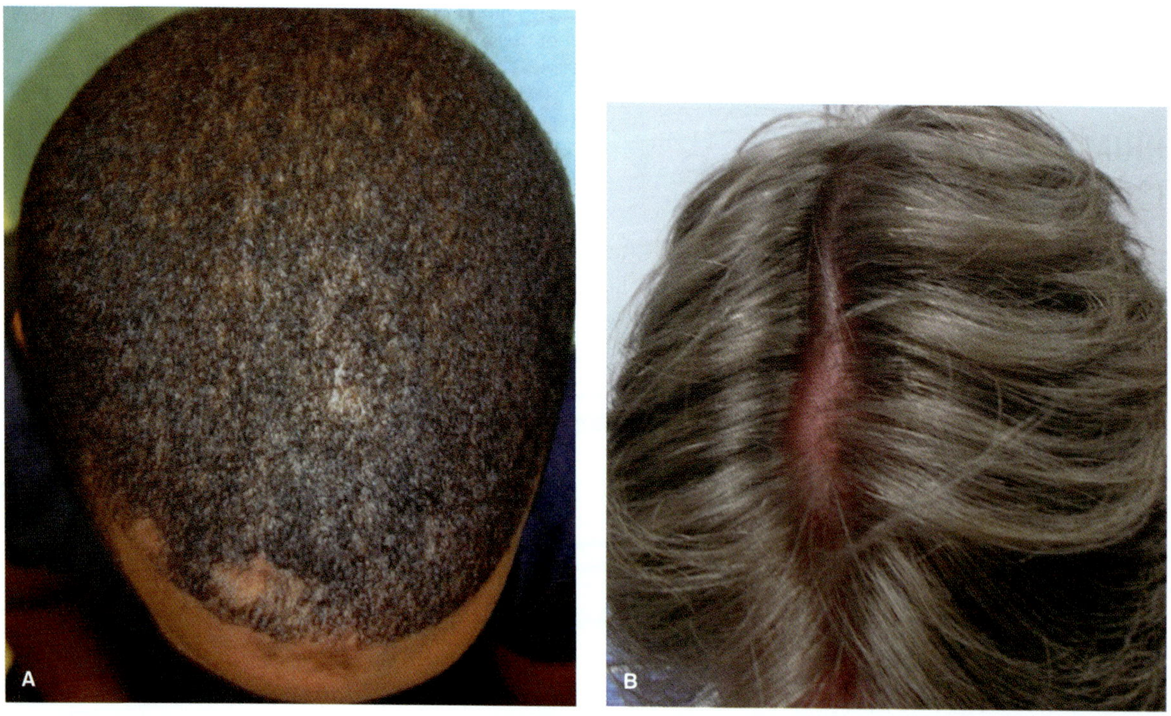

Figure 43-2 A. Discoid lupus erythematosus with typical hyper/hypopigmented plaques with scarring alopecia. **B.** Brightly erythematous plaques on scalp, previously mistaken for seborrheic dermatitis, which on close inspection demonstrated early scarring alopecia. Histopathology and direct immunofluorescence confirmed the diagnosis of cutaneous lupus erythematosus.

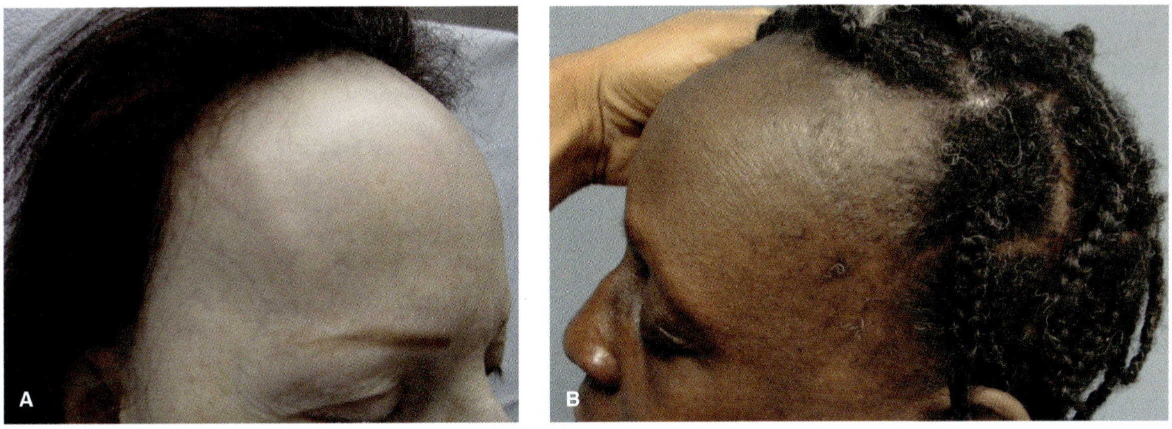

Figure 43-3 **A.** Classic presentation of frontal fibrosing alopecia with recession of the frontal hairline and eyebrow loss. **B.** African American woman originally diagnosed with traction alopecia. However, on closer inspection, she had symmetric frontal hairline recession with skin atrophy, perifollicular papules, and eyebrow loss. The diagnosis of frontal fibrosing alopecia was confirmed with biopsy.

late stages, perifollicular fibrosis, scar, and polytrichia may be present. DIF of LPP lesions shows grouped globular IgM immunofluorescence and shaggy fibrin deposition adjacent to the follicular epithelium.[11]

CENTRAL CENTRIFUGAL CICATRICIAL ALOPECIA

Central centrifugal cicatricial alopecia (CCCA) is a progressive, expanding, symmetric scarring hair loss on the crown of the scalp, most commonly seen in African American women (Fig. 43-4). Because of the symmetric, progressive nature of the hair loss, it can often be mistaken for androgenetic alopecia during a hair transplant consultation. On scalp examination, the involved area may appear shiny and atrophic, and tiny "doll hairs" may be present. CCCA has been variably associated with the use of chemical relaxers and traumatic hairstyling practices such as tight braids, weaves, and use of "hot combs." Histologic examination demonstrates lymphohistiocytic inflammation at the upper portions of the follicle with variable loss of the sebaceous glands, concentric lamellar fibroplasia and premature desquamation of the inner root sheath. In late stages, perifollicular fibrosis and polytrichia may be present.[12]

TRACTION ALOPECIA

Traction alopecia is a "biphasic alopecia" in that in its early stages this entity is considered nonscarring; however, with chronic involvement the hair loss can become permanent. Traction alopecia is caused by chronic pulling and tension on the hair because of prolonged tight hairstyling practices, such as tight braids, ponytails, weaves, extensions, curlers, or dreadlocks. It is most commonly seen in African

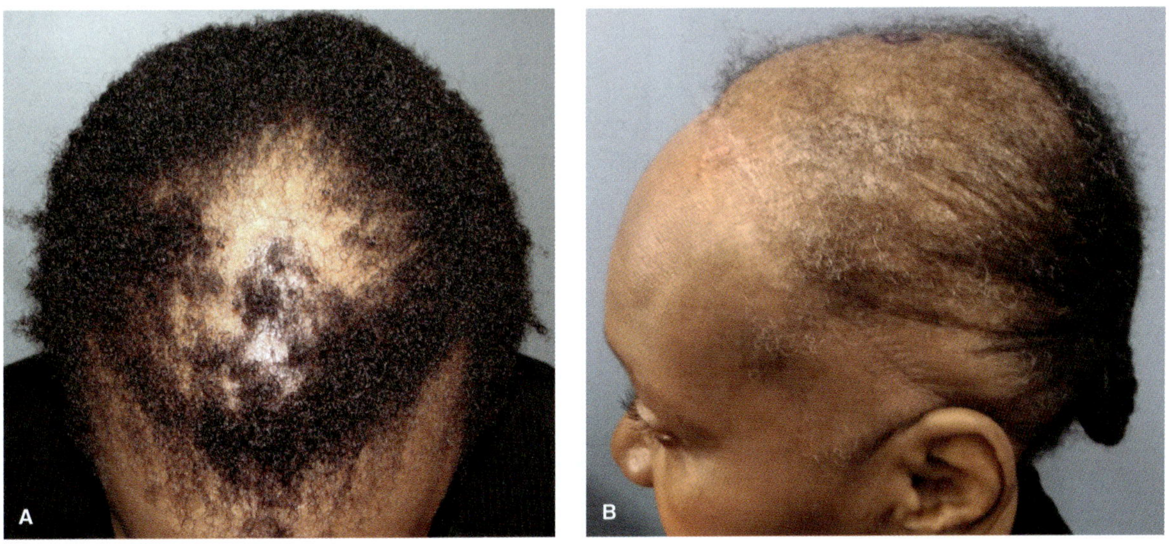

Figure 43-4 **A** and **B.** Two patients demonstrating traction alopecia of the frontotemporal hairline and CCCA, which can often coexist.

TABLE 43-4
Examples of Secondary Cicatricial Alopecias

Secondary Cicatricial Alopecias			
Trauma	Infection	Postinflammatory	Neoplastic
Pressure-induced	Tinea capitis	Sarcoid	Basal cell carcinoma
Postsurgical scars		Morphea	Squamous cell carcinoma
Burns		Graft-versus-host disease	Alopecia neoplastica
Radiation			

American women. If the hair styling practice is discontinued and treatment is sought early on, hair regrowth is possible. However, chronic traction on the hair will lead to permanent loss in that area. Clinically, patchy areas of nonscarring alopecia are seen most commonly around the hairline with no associated evidence of perifollicular papules or scale (Fig. 43-4).[13] Histopathologic findings can mimic trichotillomania in its early stages. End-stage traction alopecia shows a marked reduction in terminal hairs with columns of connective tissues replacing the follicular epithelium.[14]

SECONDARY CICATRICIAL ALOPECIAS

As stated earlier, with secondary cicatricial alopecias, the hair follicle is not the inflammatory target, but is simply in the same area as disease activity or trauma (Table 43-4).

POSTSURGICAL ALOPECIA

Cosmetic surgeries, such as a face or brow lift, or excision on the scalp can leave visible scars. In addition, hairlines may be altered and/or pulled posteriorly (Fig. 43-5). Hair transplantation can provide cosmetically pleasing correction of these postsurgical alopecias with restoration of hair in the temporal and preauricular regions and/or placing hair into the scar itself.[15]

PRESSURE-INDUCED (POSTOPERATIVE) ALOPECIA

Pressure-induced alopecia can occur in individuals after long periods of pressure on the scalp during general anesthesia or in chronically ill individuals with persistent pressure on one area of the scalp. It is thought to be due to pressure-induced ischemia.[16] Histology can show thrombosis and dermal and subcutaneous perivascular inflammation in the early stages and epidermal and perieccrine necrosis if severe, with an increased number of telogen hairs.

TINEA CAPITIS

Tinea capitis is a dermatophyte infection of the hair shaft. Common causes include *Trichophyton tonsurans* and *Microsporum canis*. It is more commonly seen in African American children or their caregivers. Examination reveals annular, scaly, crusted patches of alopecia with variable occipital lymphadenitis. If infection persists chronically, the affected individual may develop permanent hair loss in the area (Fig. 43-6). The diagnosis can be

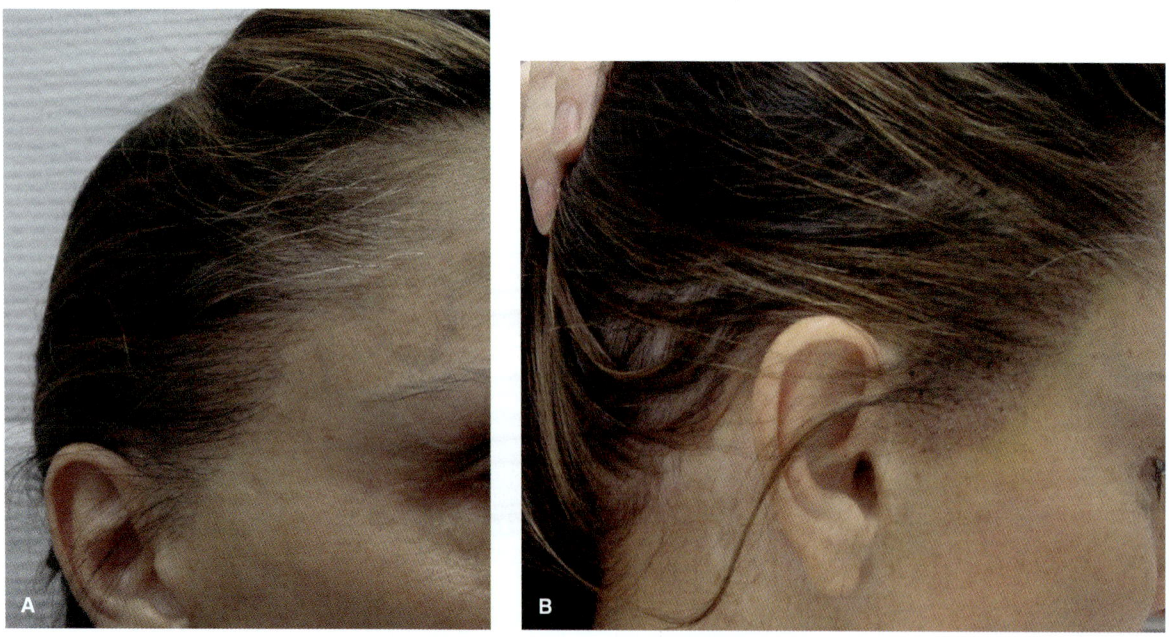

Figure 43-5 A. Immediate postoperative photograph of transplant into preauricular area after a facelift with the hairline pulled posteriorly. **B.** Restoration of the preauricular hairline and camouflaged scar.

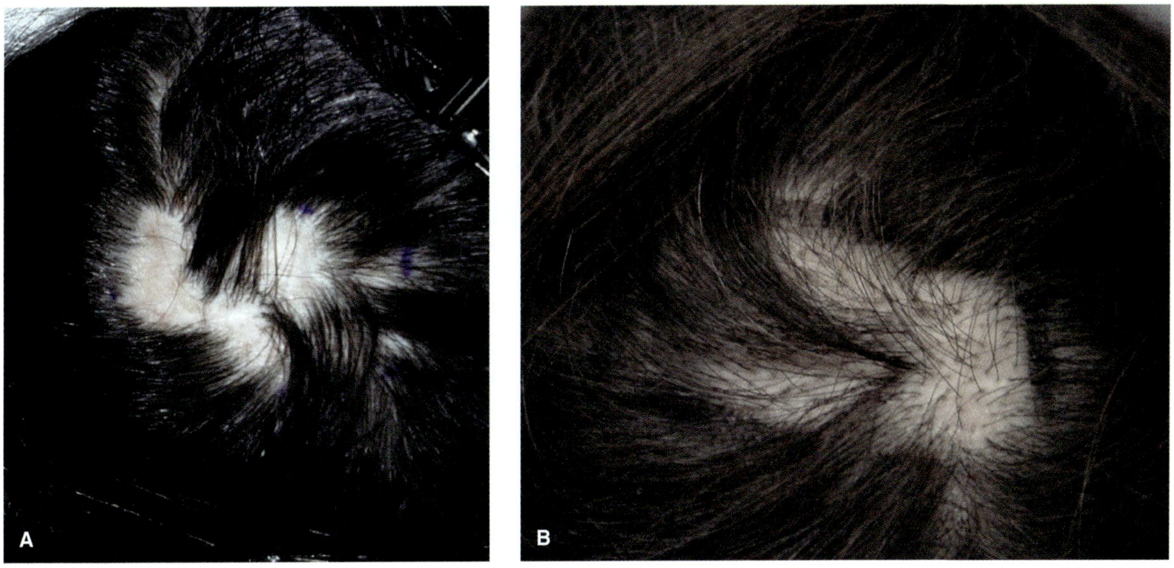

Figure 43-6 **A.** A 14 year-old girl with patchy scarring alopecia in the vertex scalp due to tinea capitis. **B.** Modest coverage after one session of 150 1 to 3 follicular unit grafts into the scarred areas.

confirmed with a fungal culture. KOH preparation of an involved hair follicle can reveal ectothrix (hyphal elements adjacent to the hair shaft) or endothrix (hyphal elements present within the hair shaft).[17]

TECHNICAL CONSIDERATIONS FOR HAIR TRANSPLANTATION IN CICATRICIAL ALOPECIA

The same general principles apply in scarring alopecias when performing hair transplantation as when tranplanting nonscarred scalp. This includes the instrumentation, anesthesia, graft creation, and postoperative care.[18] The major differences when transplanting into scarring alopecia lie in candidate selection, managing patient expectations, donor harvesting, recipient site creation, and the number of surgeries performed (Table 43-5).[15] Special consideration needs to be taken when determining whether the individual is a proper candidate, as candidate selection is one of the most important aspects of hair restoration surgery. When a patient seeks consultation for hair transplantation, it is important to perform a detailed history as well as a scalp examination. The history and scalp examination should be used to determine the type of alopecia the patient has, as well as details of the technical components of the surgery, such as donor supply and the caliber and density of hair. Transplants should only be performed into primary cicatricial alopecias if the involved areas have been inactive for 1 to 2 years; the disease should be quiescent, without anticipation of further disease progression.[19] This decreases the chance of the transplantation causing a disease flare and prevents the transplanted hairs from being targeted by the immune system. If the transplanted hairs do not grow as expected or have signs of inflammation, it is important to consider performing a biopsy postoperatively to evaluate for disease activity.

Areas of scarring alopecia often have decreased blood supply and thickened fibrotic tissue. For this reason, there is typically decreased graft survival. Therefore, scalp thickness and available blood supply should be determined preoperatively to the greatest degree possible.[9]

TABLE 43-5
Differences Between Performing Hair Transplantation in Patients With Scarring Alopecia Versus Nonscarring Alopecia.

	Scarring Alopecia	Nonscarring Alopecia
Number of Sessions	Consider test area, then two to four sessions	One to two sessions
Donor Area	More unpredictable	More predictable safe donor area
Recipient Area	Disease must be inactive for at least 1–2 years	May have ongoing disease activity
	Transplant with lower densities due to altered vascular supply and fibrotic tissue	Can transplant at higher densities
Outcomes	Decreased graft survival	Most grafts survive and grow
	Less coverage can be achieved with each surgery	More coverage can be achieved with greater cosmetic satisfaction

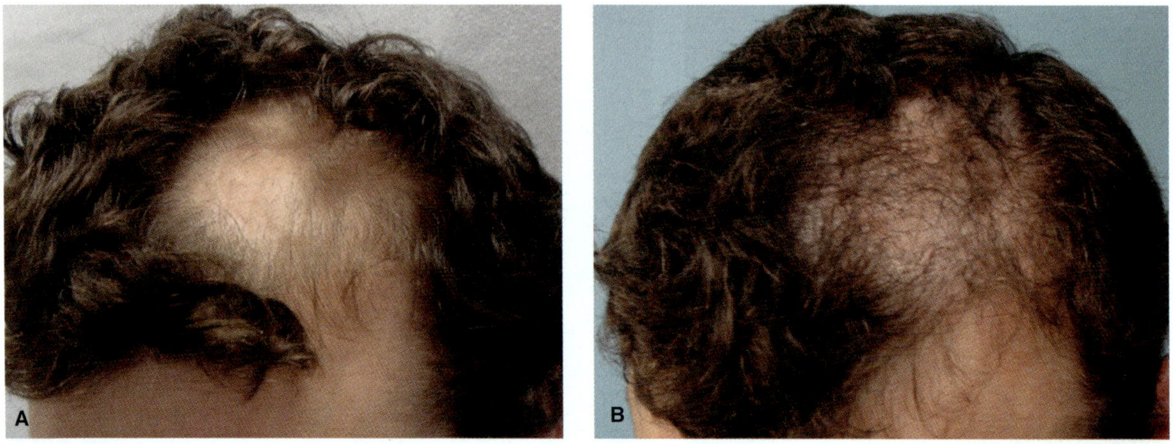

Figure 43-7 A. Large scarring defect on left frontal scalp secondary to craniotomy and radiation. B. With adequate cosmetic coverage after one session with 640 1 to 4 follicle unit grafts. Note the varied growth and graft survival within the scar tissue. The patient was unable to undergo a second session.

THE EFFECT OF VASCULAR SUPPLY ON HAIR TRANSPLANTATION

Vascular supply can be a major limitation of transplantation into scar tissue. Scar tissue tends to have a decreased blood supply compared to normal tissue. This difference can lead to poor graft survival (Fig. 43-7). Dense packing of transplanted hairs is not advisable in scar tissue because of poor blood supply. A test transplant to assess growth of transplanted hair in patients with a compromised vascular supply may be helpful (Fig. 43-8). Some recommend applying 2% to 5% minoxidil topically 1 week preoperatively or pentoxyphylline 400 mg 2 weeks preoperatively in order to increase blood supply to the area.[19]

SCALP THICKNESS AND FIBROSIS

Scars can be hypertrophic or atrophic; therefore, their thickness and texture can vary a great deal. Scar tissue can be tough and tacked down or inelastic and friable. Because hypertrophic scars tend to be thicker, the surgeon may want to consider making deeper incisions to reach the blood supply. Atrophic scars may have a poor blood supply and incisions may need to be performed more superficially in these areas, leading to poor graft survival. Incisions within atrophic scars should be made at a more acute angle to compensate for the lack of subcutaneous tissue to support the transplanted hair follicle.[15]

DONOR AREA

When surgically treating androgenetic alopecia, the optimal donor region is the midoccipital scalp.[18] This is considered the safe zone in anticipation that the hair will continue to thin to a greater degree over the rest of the scalp, as androgenetic alopecia is a progressive process. Placement of the donor site in the occipital region minimizes the risk of a visible donor scar in the future. With scarring alopecia, however, the horizontal zone in the occiput from which hair would typically be harvested may have been affected by disease activity. Therefore, it

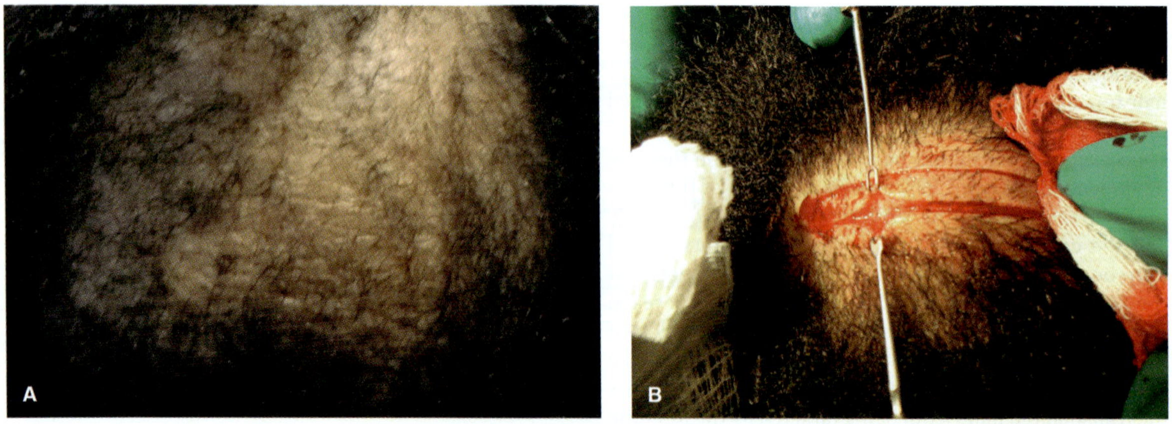

Figure 43-8 A. African American woman with diffuse scarring alopecia due to CCCA. Example of extension of scarring alopecia into occipital donor area. B. Diminished density in donor area due to involvement of scarring alopecia.

is important to individually assess each patient to determine where adequate follicular units may be available and whether the patient has adequate donor hair to produce a desirable cosmetic outcome.

As with hair transplantation for the treatment of androgenetic alopecia, evaluation of the caliber of hair as well as donor density should be performed. The caliber of the hair may become even more important when transplanting into scarring alopecia. Transplanting at higher densities into the scarred skin is inadvisable due to reduced blood supply[19]; therefore, with lower densities, larger-caliber hairs will achieve greater coverage than lower-caliber fine hairs.

Donor density is a major determinant of the success of transplantation into scarring alopecia, and may be even more limiting than in individuals affected by androgenetic alopecia alone. Certain scarring alopecias, such as CCCA, can lead to diffuse hair loss involving even the occiput, from which the grafts would normally be harvested (Fig. 43-8). Because of disease activity in the occipital region, donor hair density may be limited and surgery may not be possible. Density is determined by the number of follicular units per square centimeter as opposed to the number of hairs per square centimeter. Most surgeons generally aim to achieve at least 20 to 40 follicular units per square centimeter; however, with cicatricial alopecia, fewer units may be acceptable because the density of the transplanted hair is generally decreased.

DONOR HARVESTING

Similar to performing hair transplantation for androgenetic alopecia, there are two methods of donor harvesting: (1) strip excision and (2) follicular unit extraction (FUE).[18] When determining which method is preferred, a number of factors should be considered (Table 43-6). Patient preference can also dictate which method to choose.

The advantage of strip excision is that the surgeon can harvest more follicular units more quickly with lower transection rates. However, there is a visible scar present if a patient wears his/her hair short. Strip excision is, therefore, recommended for individuals who wear their hair longer in the back, those who require more follicular units to be harvested, and those who have contraindications to FUE or where FUE would be technically more difficult, such as in individuals with very curly hair.

FUE is recommended for patients with scarring alopecia in whom a linear scar in the occiput would be visible, who have a limited donor area or require a decreased number of follicular units, or those individuals who tend to heal with wider, thickened scars.

OTHER CONSIDERATIONS

A small test area can be performed in patients in whom growth of transplanted follicles is uncertain due to scarring (Fig. 43-9). A 1 to 2 square centimeter area can be transplanted initially. After 9 to 12 months, depending on the assessment of graft survival in the test area, a larger session can be performed.[19]

Due to reduced blood supply we suggest using fewer recipient sites per centimeter squared in patients with scarring alopecia (10–20 cm^2) versus male or female pattern hair loss (20–30 cm^2). The patient is counseled that two to four sessions may need to be performed every 9 to 12 months at a minimum, and that with each session higher densities can be achieved.

It is important to set expectations for hair transplantation patients with scarring alopecia. They must be aware that graft survival is decreased, that they may not achieve full coverage of the alopecic area, that the hairs may grow in kinky at first and then straighten with additional hair cycles, and that two to four surgical sessions may be necessary. Those who accept the limitations of the procedure are generally satisfied with any cosmetic improvement; therefore, all patients with end-stage cicatricial alopecia should be offered hair restoration surgery as an option for treatment of their cosmetically disfiguring condition (Figs. 43-10 and 43-11).

TABLE 43-6
Factors to Consider When Determining Donor Harvesting Method

	Strip	FUE
Duration of Surgery	Shorter time to harvest Longer time to trim grafts Same time for planting grafts	Longer harvesting time Less time to trim grafts Same time for planting grafts
Number of Grafts	Typically more grafts can be harvested in defined safe harvesting zone	Less grafts harvested, may need more than one session Robotic FUE may yield close to equal of an ellipse
Overall Cosmetic Outcome	Same	Same
Considerations for Scarring Alopecia	Because of unpredictable donor area, may have more variable density in linear area	Can choose areas of higher density and areas not involved with alopecia for harvesting
Scar	Visible linear scar	No visible linear scar, may see hypopigmented dots or risk moth-eaten look with over harvesting

SUMMARY CONSIDERATIONS FOR CICATRICIAL ALOPECIA

1. If caused by inflammatory alopecia, disease should be inactive without progression and inactive on biopsy for 1 to 2 years.
2. Consider starting with a test area with decreased density.

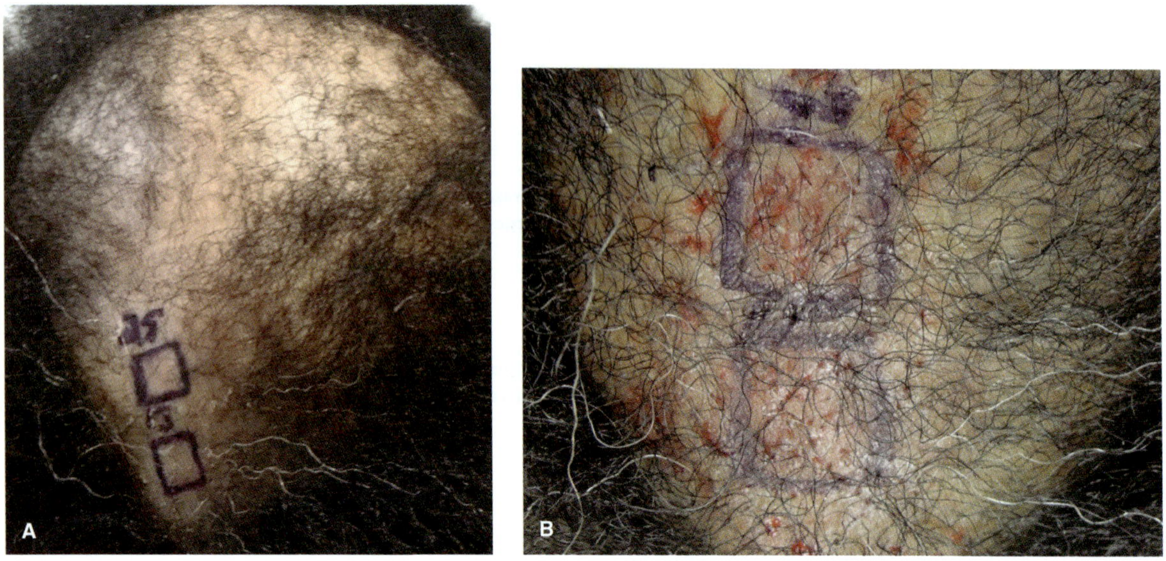

Figure 43-9 **A.** Diffuse scarring alopecia due to CCCA. Demonstrating two 1 cm^2 test areas with 15 grafts per square centimeter and 25 grafts per square centimeter. **B.** Immediately after transplantation into test areas.

3. Perform smaller, less dense sessions every 9 to 12 months.
4. Consider minoxidil to improve blood flow.
5. Consider making incisions at acute angle.

CORRECTIVE HAIR RESTORATION SURGERY

From the 1960s until the 1990s, hair transplantation was performed using 3 to 4 mm punch biopsies and later strip excisions to harvest hair from the donor areas. The donor grafts were dissected into large follicular groupings of 10 to 25 hairs per graft (Fig. 43-12). Incisions were then made into the alopecic areas with punch incisions and the large grafts were inserted into these areas. This led to very unnatural appearing, "pluggy" hair transplants that were not only unflattering cosmetically, but patients who received these procedures were also easily recognizable to the general public. In addition, natural appearing hairline design was less emphasized during this time period and led to very straight, unnatural appearing hairlines. Because of its unnatural, cosmetically unflattering results, hair restoration surgery as a whole endured a time period of negative public opinion.

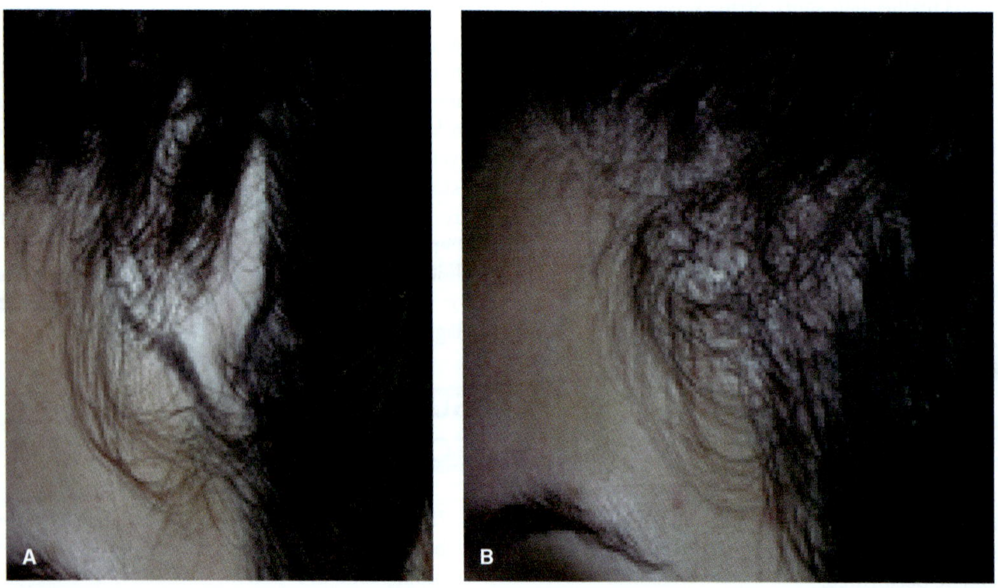

Figure 43-10 **A.** Scarring alopecia over left temporal scalp. **B.** Improved coverage after hair transplantation of 500 1 to 3 follicular unit grafts.

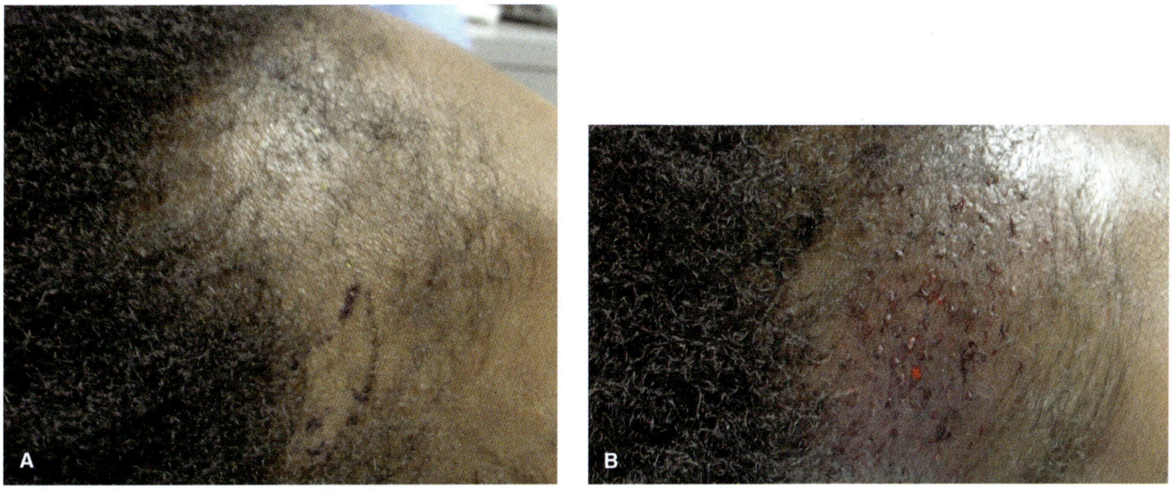

Figure 43-11 **A.** Traction alopecia. **B.** Immediate postoperative placement of grafts restoring the frontal hairline.

Some patients may be angry, depressed, or even devastated by the results of their previous surgery, so it is important to develop trust and aim to truly understand their concerns and goals with respect to corrective surgery. Their goal may be to simply achieve a "normal" appearance. That is a realistic goal. It may take multiple sessions to achieve the ultimate cosmetic outcome but improvement is possible.

Overall, corrective hair surgery should aim to conceal flaws from previous surgeries by adding hair strategically, to remove grafts that cannot be naturally concealed, and to further treat worsening areas of balding.[20–24]

Many hair transplant surgeons are now seeing patients from previous generations who are seeking out consultation for corrective surgery to create a more natural appearing, less recognizable hair transplant. Fortunately, there are now many options for correction of these patients' previous hair transplant surgeries. This can include a combination of softening the hairline and adding density to the affected areas, surgical removal of the larger, "pluggy" grafts, and/or partially thinning the larger grafts, using selective FUE or laser hair removal.[22]

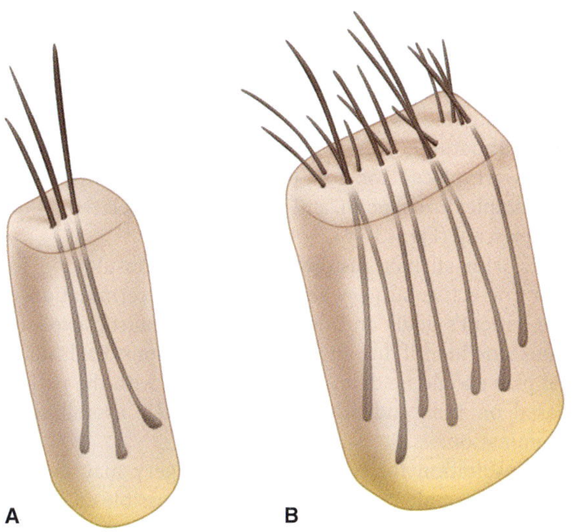

Figure 43-12 **A.** Follicular unit graft. **B.** 3 to 4 mm punch/plug with multiple follicular units.

CONSULTATION

REASONS FOR CONSULTATION

Previous methods of hair transplantation led to various complications, including unnatural hairline design, a "pluggy" appearance, scalp irregularities, or improper angling of transplanted hair (Figs. 43-13 and 43-14 and Table 43-7).[23]

UNNATURAL HAIRLINE DESIGN

A transplant may have been performed with a low or unnatural hairline design. These designs may have been too straight, and lack irregularity or single follicle grafts.

TABLE 43-7
Common Complications from Previous Hair Surgeries Leading to Consultation for Corrective Surgery

Common Reasons for Corrective Surgery
Unnatural hairline design
"Pluggy" appearance
Scalp irregularities
Improper angles
Poor anticipation for ongoing hair loss

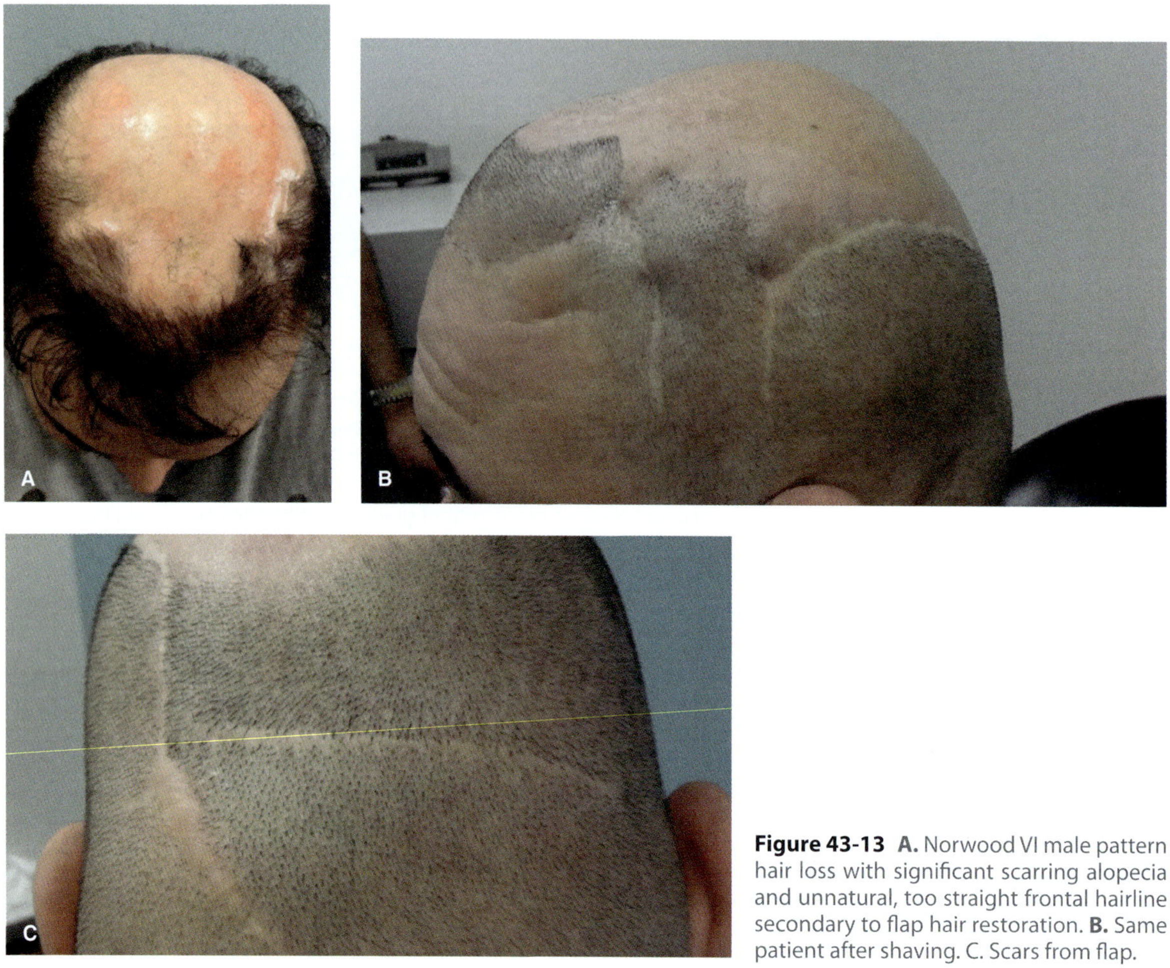

Figure 43-13 **A.** Norwood VI male pattern hair loss with significant scarring alopecia and unnatural, too straight frontal hairline secondary to flap hair restoration. **B.** Same patient after shaving. C. Scars from flap.

PLUGGY APPEARANCE

Larger, 10 to 25 follicular unit grafting produced a "corn row" or pluggy appearance along the grafted scalp. Large gaps between the grafts may also be present.

SCALP IRREGULARITIES

As previously mentioned, older techniques for site creation entailed multiple punch excisions. This often led to textural changes on the scalp including perifollicular scarring, cobblestoning, and hypo/hyperpigmentation (Fig. 43-15).

IMPROPER ANGLES

The previous transplant may have been performed with a natural appearing hairline design; however, the transplant may not appear natural due to improper angling of the hairs at the time of implantation.

INADEQUATE ANTICIPATION OF ONGOING HAIR LOSS

Even with use of smaller, 1 to 4 follicular unit grafts and natural hairline design, if the grafts were placed in areas without consideration of future, ongoing hair loss, the cosmetic outcome several years after the transplant can appear quite unnatural. This is most frequently seen when the grafts are placed too low on the frontal hairline, when the temples are filled in, and when grafts are placed on the vertex scalp (Fig. 43-16).

As with all hair restoration surgery, consultation for hair corrective surgery should include determination of the patient's goals and desires, setting realistic expectations, and identifying any possible limitations. Each surgical plan should be detailed and reviewed with the patient based on their individual goals and their overall scalp examination.

Consultation for hair corrective surgery may include correction or alteration of one or more possible complications. Therefore, a combination of approaches may need to be performed in order to provide the most natural appearing, cosmetically improved result. In addition, the

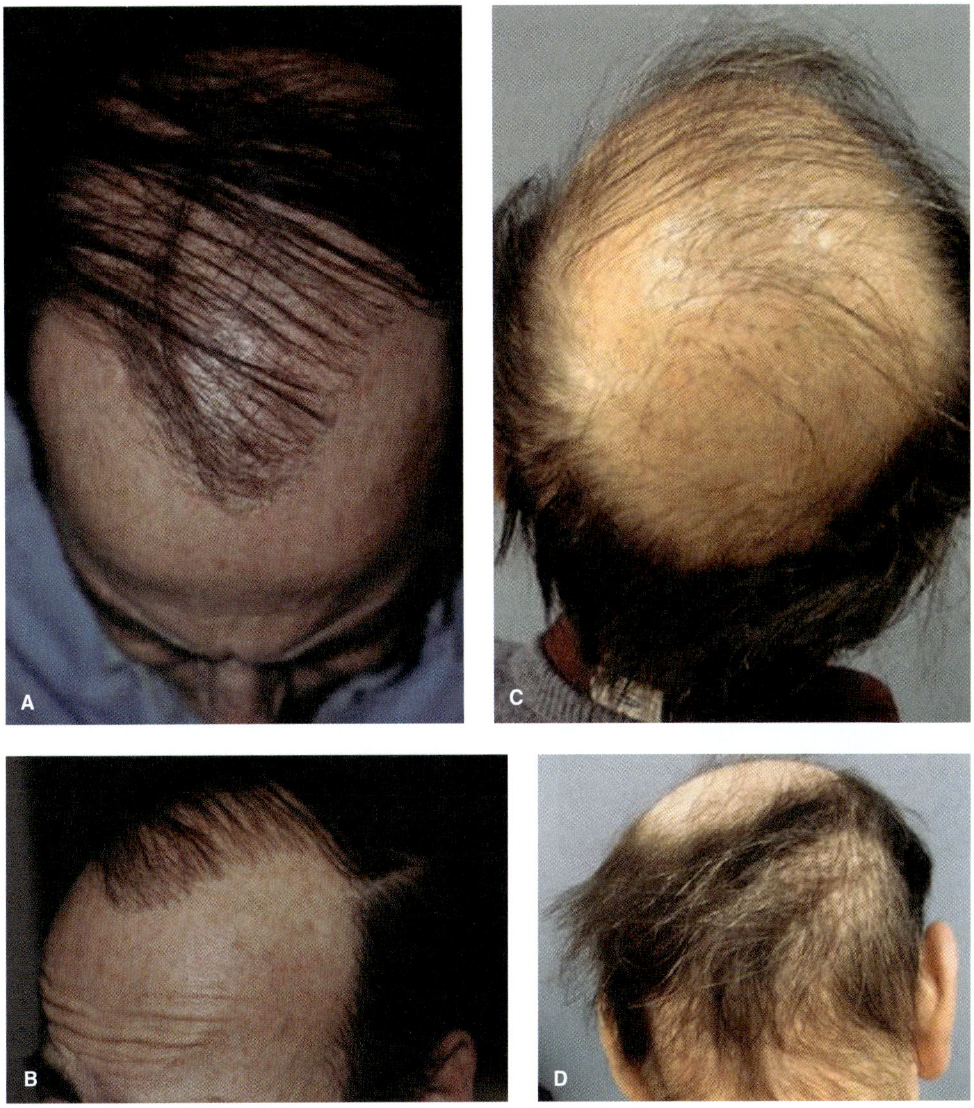

Figure 43-14 **A.** Demonstrating unnatural appearing, too straight, pluggy frontal hairline. **B.** Lateral view. **C.** Same patient 5 years later with ongoing hair loss demonstrating pluggy vertex scalp with ring of alopecia. **D.** Six years later with continued thin coverage in donor area, hypopigmented scars from excised plugs are now visible.

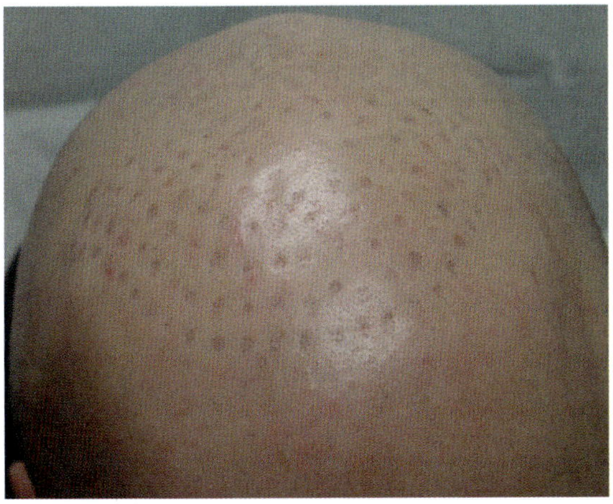

Figure 43-15 Demonstrating too regular, unnatural appearing, pluggy frontal hairline and scalp with atrophic, pitted scars.

transplant surgeon should assess donor availability from either newly harvested or already transplanted areas from which plugs will be removed. Ongoing hair loss or balding can also affect outcomes and selection of donor area, and must be taken into consideration.

PATIENT SELECTION

The most appropriate patient for hair corrective surgery is one with realistic expectations as to what can be achieved, with stable hair loss, who ideally is aged 40 years or older. Patients with unrealistic expectations or those with minimal donor hair availability should be excluded. If the patient is not a candidate for hair restoration, cosmetic camouflages, such as hairpieces or tattooing, may be discussed.

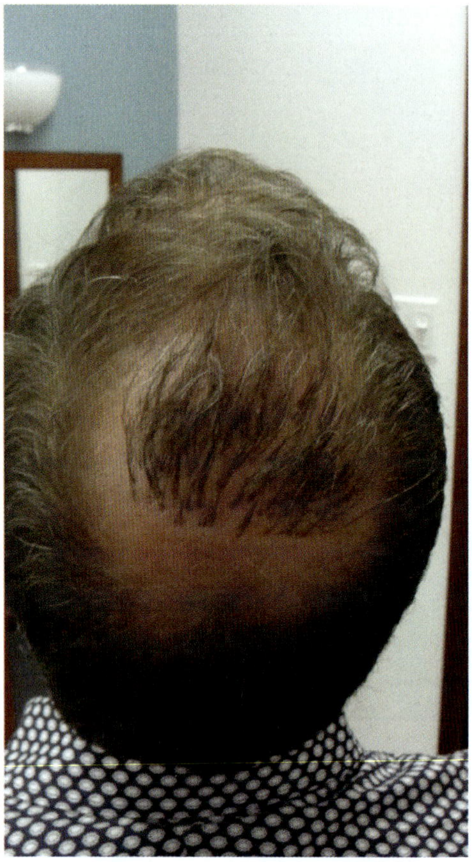

Figure 43-16 Demonstrating unnatural appearing, pluggy grafts in the vertex with ongoing hair loss leaving ring of alopecia surrounding grafts.

CONSULTATION ASSESSMENT

The caliber, density, wave pattern, and color of the donor hair are important to assess. In addition, assessing possible ongoing hair loss is pertinent as well. The patient can expect improved cosmetic outcomes based on increased density and coverage, as well as a more natural appearing hairline, covering the bald scalp.

GENERAL APPROACH TO CORRECTIVE HAIR SURGERY

In many instances, the hairline may have been created with a design that was too "regular," such as with straight lines, or it may have been placed too low (Table 43-8). To correct this problem, an elliptical excision may be performed to remove those grafts and relocate them on the scalp in a softer, more natural distribution, with 1 to 4 follicular units per graft.[24]

If the hairline is unnatural and designed with widely spaced, larger plugs, punch excision may be performed to relocate these grafts to other areas on the scalp, once again to create a more natural, denser appearing hairline.

To make large plugs less recognizable, a combination of methods may need to be pursued. The patient may simply want to get rid of the plugs, especially on the crown or vertex scalp. This can be achieved either with elliptical or punch excision or with laser hair removal. Otherwise, plugs may be selectively excised or debulked using FUE or punch excision and relocated with a combination of an FUT procedure to fill in the gaps, add density, and produce a more natural appearance. An additional FUT procedure would be again limited by donor supply and the potential for future ongoing hair loss.

TABLE 43-8
Strategies For Corrective Hair Restoration Surgery

FUT to soften, increase density, and create more natural appearing hair
Surgical removal with punch biopsy or elliptical excision of existing plugs +/– dissection into smaller follicular units and relocation
Laser hair removal of existing plugs
Strategic thinning or debulking of plugs
Combination of all of the above

Source: Reproduced with permission from Avram MR. Corrective hair transplantation. In: Avram MR, Rogers NE, eds. *Hair Transplantation.* New York, NY: Cambridge University Press, 2010. © Cambridge University Press 2010.

USING A COMBINATION OF FUT AND DISSECTION AND RELOCATION OF LARGER REMOVED PLUGS

Excised grafts can be dissected under magnification into smaller 1 to 4 follicular units per graft. Depending on donor supply in the occipital region, an additional FUT can be performed using strip excision or FUE depending on patient preference and the possibility of a visible scar. These additional grafts can be used to strategically fill in larger areas of balding scalp, as well as add density, soften, and recreate a more natural looking hairline (Fig. 43-17).

CORRECTIVE SURGERY OF THE VERTEX SCALP

If corrective surgery is needed to provide a more natural appearing vertex scalp, the frontal scalp is also likely to need revision. Therefore, because of limited donor availability, the vertex scalp may need special consideration. The exception occurs when the frontal scalp has been designed well, but ongoing hair loss was not anticipated on the vertex scalp, leading to a ring of alopecia surrounding the transplanted hair on the vertex.

The vertex scalp may be the area that is most amenable to complete removal of grafts with either laser hair removal or surgical removal to create a natural appearance (Fig. 43-18). Because there is a limited supply of donor hairs, the surgeon may be required to restore density to

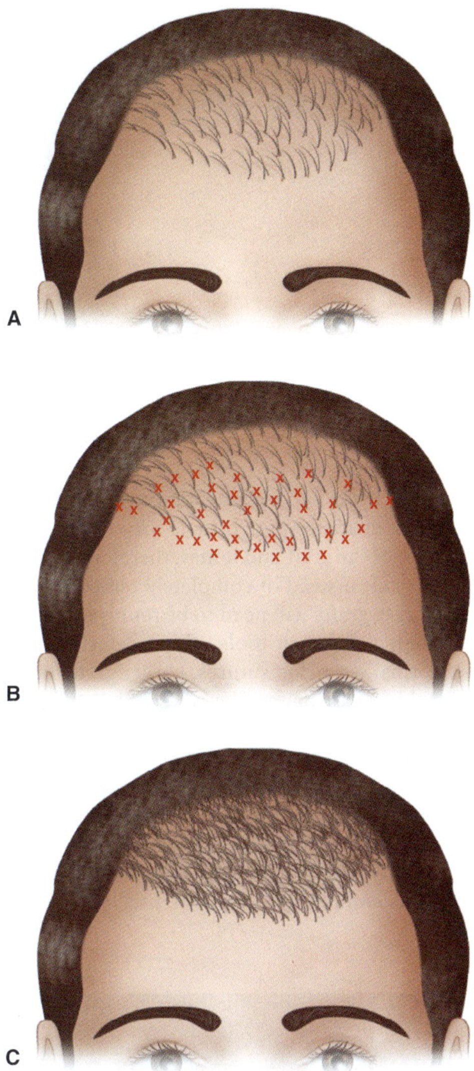

Figure 43-17 **A.** Large, pluggy, unnatural appearing grafts. **B** and **C.** Adding smaller follicular unit grafts to soften the cosmetic appearance.

the frontal scalp more than the vertex scalp to optimize the outcome of the corrective procedure.

TECHNICAL CONSIDERATIONS

FOLLICULAR UNIT TRANSPLANTATION

One treatment option for corrective hair restoration is to perform an additional hair transplant surgery using standard techniques and fill in the affected area with more natural appearing 1 to 4 hair follicular units. This approach can be used to soften and mask an unnatural appearing hairline, increase density overall and create a more natural look.

CAMOUFLAGING "PLUGS"

To correct poor hairline design, the surgeon can choose either to construct a more natural hair line anterior to the previous one, to fill in the gaps created by the plugs, or a combination of the two. The new hairline appears more natural with single hair follicular units and without lowering the hairline more than necessary. Adding smaller follicular unit grafts to the larger, pluggier grafts is advisable because of the appearance of increased density (Figs. 43-19 and 43-20). If the donor supply is insufficient to fill in spaces or gaps, strategically removing the larger plugs and simply relocating them along the hairline is advised.

REMOVAL OF TRANSPLANTED HAIR

This is typically the first step with any corrective hair surgery. However, there are many ways to go about removing the hair. First, it is important to discuss the choices with the patient as well as the goals he/she wishes to achieve with corrective surgery. The physician can decide with the patient which grafts to remove in order to achieve a more natural appearance. In general, it is best to remove the pluggier grafts at the hairline to soften its appearance and have it look more natural. It is important to be strategic about which grafts to remove; all grafts do not necessarily need to be removed to achieve a more natural appearing hairline.

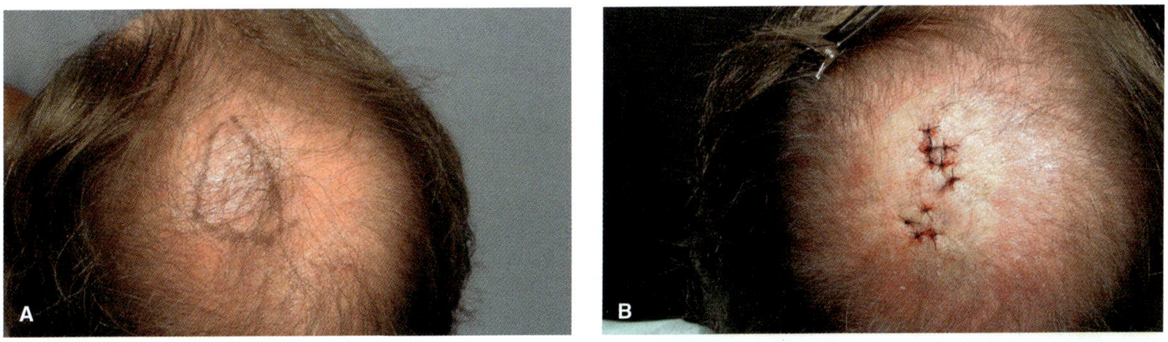

Figure 43-18 **A.** Demonstrating lack of anticipation of ongoing hair loss on vertex scalp with ring of alopecia surrounding grafts. **B.** Multiple 3 mm punch biopsies to excise previous grafts, leaving natural appearing balding vertex scalp.

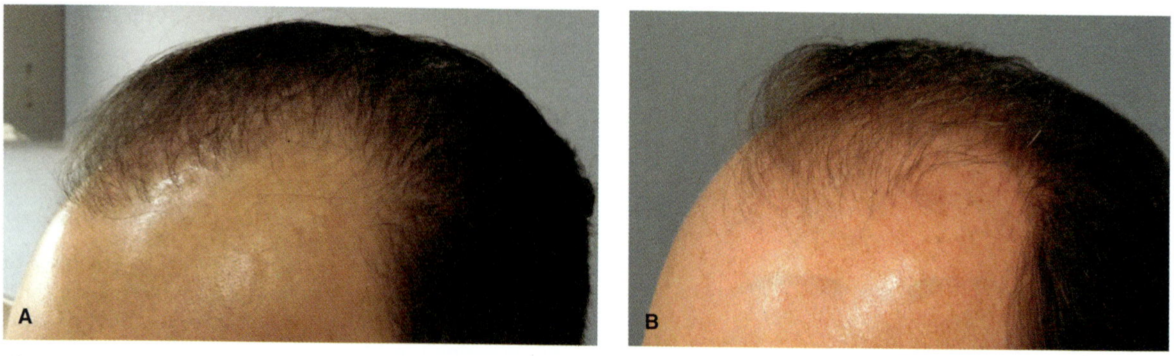

Figure 43-19 A. Demonstrating pluggy, unnatural appearing frontal hairline. B. Softening of frontal hairline after graft removal with punch excision and reimplantation of grafts after dissecting into smaller 1 to 4 follicular unit grafts.

Graft removal can be performed with a punch tool or with elliptical excision. If the goal is to completely remove the graft, the punch should be large enough to fit the entire graft. If the goal is to simply debulk the graft, a smaller punch diameter may be selected. With both techniques, care should be taken not to transect the follicles. The risk of this can be reduced by increasing punch diameter, angling in the direction of follicle growth, and using saline tumescence to increase tissue turgor. The holes that remain should be closed with 4-0 nylon suture.

If the patient chooses to use the excised hairs to retransplant in a more natural fashion, the larger grafts can be strategically excised. FUE with a 0.75 to 1 mm punch tool can be utilized as these smaller diameter punch tools are less likely to leave a visible scar and are less likely to leave perifollicular hypo/hyperpigmentation. However, often these smaller diameter punch tools may be smaller than the diameter of the graft and it may, therefore, make sense to thin the graft instead of completely removing it. Typically, the larger grafts will need to be removed with larger, >2 mm, diameter punch tools. These defects are closed with epidermal 4-0 nylon sutures. Larger grafts may leave unpredictable scarring and/or a cobblestoning effect. There is also a risk of postoperative erythema. In addition, there are visible sutures present in the postoperative period, which are removed in 5 to 7 days. If the diameter of the punch is less than 2 mm, these wounds may be left to heal by secondary intention. Excising multiple grafts in close proximity may reduce scalp laxity and make closure difficult. This complication can potentially be eliminated

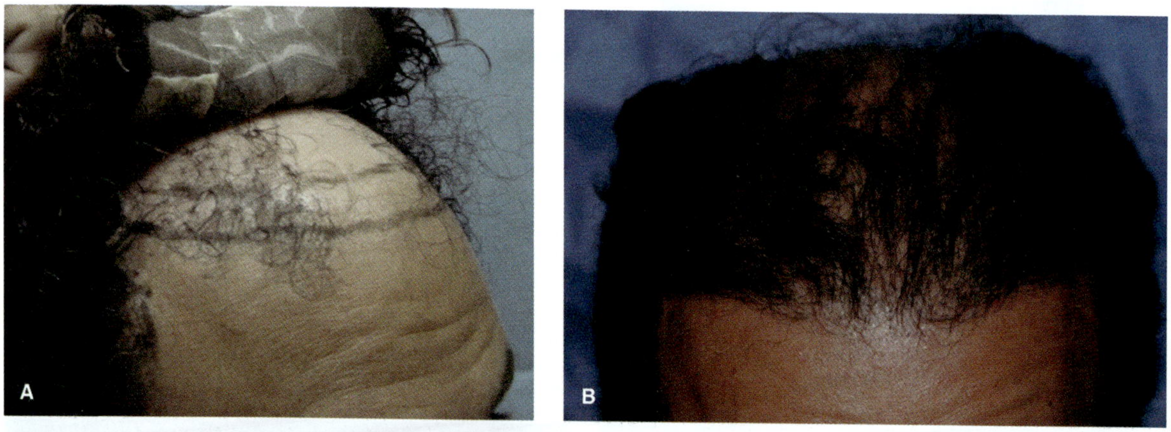

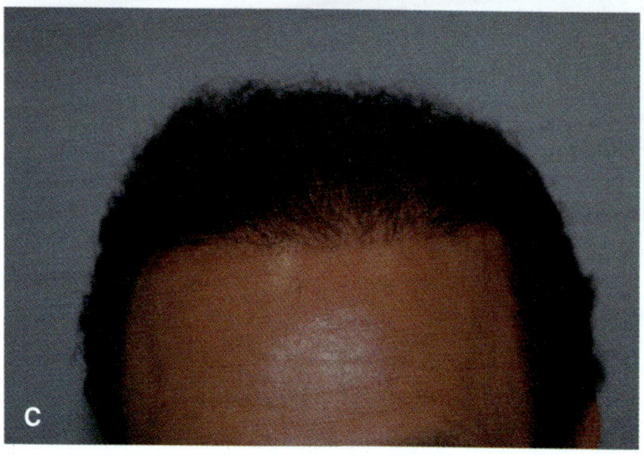

Figure 43-20 A. Demonstrating very unnatural appearing, too straight, pluggy frontal hairline and scalp with poor anticipation of ongoing hair loss and depleted donor supply. The patient masks the outcome of his previous transplant with a hair piece. **B.** Same patient after FUT, selective larger graft removal with punch excision and subsequent addition of 1000 1 to 4 follicle unit grafts to the frontal hairline and scalp in between the pluggy grafts. **C.** After second FUT, adding 350 additional 1 to 4 follicle unit grafts to frontal scalp and reinforcing the hairline. Patient was very satisfied and no longer needed his hair piece.

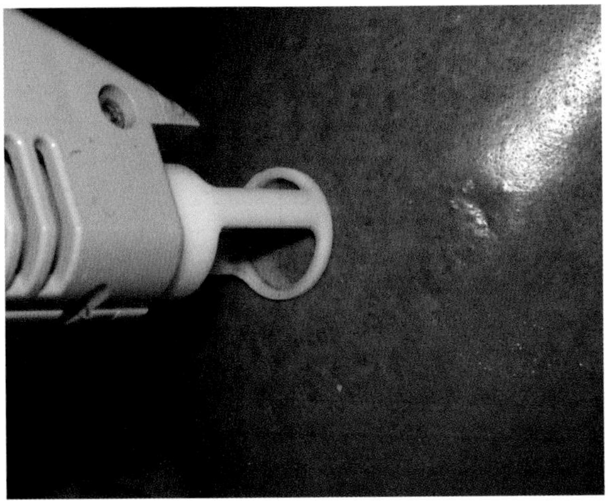

Figure 43-21 Demonstrating laser hair removal of plugs.

by performing an elliptical excision of more closely spaced grafts. Elliptical excision may be an important tool for cosmetically less important areas, and is less laborious than punching out individual grafts. Elliptical excisions may be closed in two layers with 4-0 vicryl interrupted vertical mattress sutures and then 4-0 nylon or 3-0 polypropylene interrupted superficial sutures.

After the grafts have been strategically excised, if the patient chooses, the hairs can be dissected into smaller one to four follicle groupings and retransplanted as mentioned previously to create a more natural look and add increased density. Otherwise, the patient's look will be restored to its pretransplantation appearance.

If the patient wants to permanently remove the hairs, one easy method without carrying the risk of additional scarring is to perform laser hair removal to the affected areas (Fig. 43-21). Permanent laser hair removal typically takes five to seven sessions and only works on pigmented hairs. The major disadvantage is that those hairs are permanently lost and cannot be retransplanted elsewhere on the scalp. However, laser hair removal is noninvasive and has a decreased risk of scar, cobblestoning, or pigmentary change. There is no recovery time and, in addition, because laser hair removal reduces the number of hair follicles by 50% to 80%, it can reduce larger grafts to smaller follicular units.

Depending on the patient's ultimate goals and donor and recipient site qualities, a combination of adding additional 1 to 4 follicular unit grafts, FUE of the pluggy grafts, and laser hair removal of the larger grafts may need to be performed in order to achieve the best, most natural appearing outcome.

CONCLUSION

Corrective hair restoration surgery is typically performed in individuals who have undergone outdated or poorly designed hair transplantations. During consultation, understanding the patient's goals, developing realistic expectations, and constructing a plan that all parties are comfortable with is essential. Depending on the patient's goals, a combination of strategic excision of grafts with relocation to the frontal scalp and additional FUT is likely to be required to achieve an optimal result.

REFERENCES

1. Somani N, Bergfeld WF. Cicatricial alopecia: classification and histopathology. *Dermatol Ther.* 2008;21:221–247.
2. Ross EK, Tan E, Shapiro J. Update on primary cicatricial alopecias. *J Am Acad Dermatol.* 2005;53:1–37.
3. Rongioletti F, Christana K. Cicatricial (scarring) alopecias: an overview of pathogenesis, classification, diagnosis, and trreatment. *Am J Clin Dermatol.* 2012;13(4);247–260.
4. Sperling LC, Cowper SE. The histopathology of primary cicatricial alopecia. *Semin Cutan Med Surg.* 2006;25:41–50.
5. McElwee KJ. Etiology of cicatriciai alopecias: a basic science point of view. *Dermatol Ther.* 2008;21:212–220.
6. Olson EA, Bergfeld WF, Costerelis G, et al. Summary of North American Hair Research Society (NAHRS)-sponsored Workshop on Cicatricial Alopecia, Duke University Medical Center. *J Am Acad Dermatol.* 2003;48:103–110.
7. Hordinsky M. Cicatricial Alopecia: discoid lupus erythematosus. *Dermatol Ther.* 2008;21:245–248.
8. Kang H, Alzolibani AA, Otberg N, Shapiro J. Lichen planopilaris. *Dermatol Ther.* 2008;21:249–256.
9. Tan KT, Messenger AG. Frontal fibrosing alopecia: clinical presentations and prognosis. *Br J Dermatol.* 2009;160:75–79.
10. Viglizzo G, Verrini AM, Rongioletti F. Familial Lassueur-Graham-Little-Piccardi syndrome. *Dermatology.* 2004;208:142–144.
11. Mehregan DA, Van Hale HM, Muller SA. Lichen planopilaris: clinical and pathologic study of forty-five patients. *J Am Acad Dermatol.* 1992;27:935–942.
12. Whiting DA, Olson EA. Central centrifugal cicatricial alopecia. *Dermatol Ther.* 2008;21:268–278.
13. Callender VD, McMichael AJ, Cohen GF. Medical and surgical therapies for alopecias in black women. *Dermatol Ther.* 2004;17(2):164–176.
14. Borovicka JH, Thomas L, Prince C, Mehregan DR. Scarring alopecia: clinical and pathologic study of 54 African-American women. *Int J Dermatol.* 2009;48(8):840–845.
15. Unger W, Unger R, Wesley C. The surgical treatment of cicatricial alopecia. *Dermtalogic Ther.* 2008;21(4):295–311.
16. Wiles JC, Hansen RC. Postoperative (pressure) alopecia. *J Am Acad Dermatol.* 1985;12:195–198.
17. Alvarez MS, Silverberg NB. Tinea Capitis. *Cutis.* 2006;78(3): 189–196.
18. Avram MR, Rogers NE. *Hair Transplantation.* New York, NY: Cambridge University Press; 2010.
19. Rose PT, Shapiro R. Transplanting into scar tissue and areas of cicatricial alopecia. In: Shapiro R, Unger W, eds. *Hair Transplantation.* New York, NY: Marcel Dekker; 2004:606–610.
20. Bernstein RM, Rassman WR, Rashid N, Shiell RC. The art of repair in surgical hair restoration–part II: the tactics of repair. *Dermatol Surg.* 2002;28(10):873–893.
21. Bernstein RM, Rassman WR, Rashid N, Shiell RC. The art of repair in surgical hair restoration part I: basic repair strategies. *Dermatol Surg.* 2002;28(9):783–794.
22. Avram MR. Corrective hair transplantation. In: Avram MR, Rogers NE, eds. *Hair Transplantation.* New York, NY: Cambridge University Press, 2010.
23. Unger WP. Recipient area hair direction and angle during transplanting. *Dermatol Surg.* 2004;30(6):829–836.
24. Knudsen RG. The donor area. *Facial Plast Surg Clin North Am.* 2004;12(2):233–240.

CHAPTER 44

Sclerotherapy

Karen L. Beasley & Robert A. Weiss

INTRODUCTION

Utilized in ancient Greece to alleviate painful leg varicosities, sclerotherapy, the therapeutic injection of sclerosant into veins, has been successfully practiced for thousands of years. Sclerotherapy is the treatment of choice for telangiectasias and reticular veins of the legs. The technique has undergone significant advancements in the development of foamed solutions to improve its efficacy and side-effect profile. It provides a rapid, effective, and safe treatment alternative that is particularly attractive for patients with extensive networks of small abnormal veins.

The appearance of telangiectatic vessels may be so disturbing to patients that they curtail their activities and modify their lifestyles to avoid situations in which their legs are visible. They may avoid the pool and the beach, as well as wearing shorts or skirts. Besides causing cosmetic embarrassment, spider veins can also produce symptoms of pain, burning, and fatigue. These symptoms may be worsened by prolonged standing or sitting and can be relieved by wearing support hose or by elevation of the legs.[1] Vein size alone does not predict the presence of symptoms. Vessels causing symptoms may be smaller than 1 mm in diameter.[2] Sclerotherapy not only offers remarkably good cosmetic results, but has also been reported to yield an 85% reduction in symptoms.[3] Many different techniques have been used in the treatment of small veins, but certain basic principles are universal and will be outlined later.[4–8]

CLASSIFICATION AND ANATOMY

To diagnose and treat telangiectasias in a logical way, a classification scheme is helpful (Table 44-1). A discussion of the classification of leg veins includes telangiectasias (tiny red vessels <1 mm), venulectasias (small dark red or purple veins 1–2 mm), and associated reticular veins (light blue vessels 2–4 mm). For the purposes of discussion of sclerotherapy of spider veins (types I–III), it will be assumed that the major primary varicose veins of types IV and V have already been eliminated or are absent.

TELANGIECTASIA FROM AXIAL REFLUX

Telangiectatic webs may be the result of axial reflux due to junctional or large perforator incompetence.[7] It is crucial to realize that axial reflux does not always result in large visible varicosities. A detailed history and physical examination are therefore essential to identify patients who require further noninvasive diagnostic evaluation prior to treatment. Common factors that would alert physicians to the possibility that further testing with ultrasound may be needed would include: leg pain and/or swelling; bulging veins, a prominent reticular vein network, history of varicose vein surgery, or a strong family history of varicose veins coupled with prominent telangiectasias in the areas supplied by the greater or small saphenous vein. All large sources of reflux must be detected and eliminated before any treatment of spider veins is undertaken. Failure to do so will cause a high rate of treatment failure and complications, including telangiectatic matting, hyperpigmentation, and early recurrence.[7]

TELANGIECTASIA FROM RETICULAR VEINS

Telangiectasia can develop due to reflux from reticular veins, thin-walled blue superficial venules that are part of an extensive network of subcuticular veins, otherwise referred to as the lateral subdermic venous system (LSVS). This lateral network typically does not have direct connections to the saphenous system. Although it is commonly being performed at vein treatment centers around the United States, endovenous saphenous vein ablation rarely has an effect on the appearance of telangiectasias associated with the LSVS. Small perforating veins may be present, particularly in the calf, which connect to the deep venous system. Reticular veins associated with telangiectasias are commonly called "feeder" veins and can be visually identified by the "arrowhead sign" (Fig. 44-1). With

TABLE 44-1
Classification of Veins[9]

Type I	Telangiectasia (spider veins)—0.1–1 mm diameter, usually red IA—telangiectatic matting (red network)
Type II	Venulectasia—1–2 mm diameter, violaceous IIA—venulectatic matting (violaceous network)
Type III	Reticular varicosities (feeder veins) 2–4 mm diameter, cyanotic blue to blue-green
Type IV	Varicosities (secondary saphenous branch or perforator related) 3–8 mm, blue to blue-green or colorless if deeper
Type V	Saphenous varicosities (truncal or axial varicosities including main saphenous trunks and first-generation branch varicosities) 5 mm or greater—blue to blue-green, colorless if deeper, may be palpable and not visible

Reproduced with permission from Weiss RA, Weiss MA. Sclerotherapy. In: Wheeland RG, ed. *Cutaneous Surgery*. Philadelphia: WB Saunders, 1994. Copyright Elsevier.

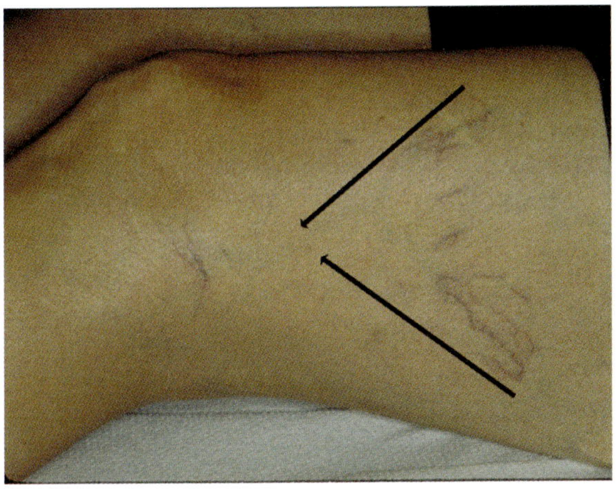

Figure 44-1 Arrowhead sign.

careful Doppler technique, free reflux with augmentation can be heard through these reticular veins, and ultrahigh-resolution duplex ultrasound may be used to map the path of transmission of venous hypertension from small reticular veins into telangiectasias.[10,11]

ISOLATED ARBORIZING WEBS

Reflux through failed valves is the source of nearly all telangiectatic webs associated with reticular veins. When diagnostic tests fail to identify a large vessel or a reticular network as a source of reflux, localized small-vein valve failure is usually the culprit. Flow within even the smallest of venules is normally regulated by valves[12] and localized valve failure can produce arborizing networks of dilated cutaneous venules that are direct tributaries of underlying larger veins.[13] Arborization occurs through a recruitment phenomenon in which high pressure causes dilatation of a venule, failure of its valves, and transmission of the high pressure across the failed valves into an adjacent vein. Angiogenesis may also play a role in formation of telangiectasias. Treatment of an arborizing system must be directed at the entire system, because if the point source of reflux is not ablated, the web will rapidly recur.

STEPS PRIOR TO TREATMENT

HISTORY AND PHYSICAL EXAMINATION

No matter how small and how localized the telangiectasias, every patient must initially be evaluated by a detailed history and physical examination, with noninvasive diagnostic vascular tests performed as needed. Even when the physical examination is normal, historical factors may suggest that further testing is necessary. Previous venous surgery is an indication for more extensive evaluation, as is a family history of large varicose veins, since such patients are likely to have early axial reflux even when presenting with telangiectasias alone.[14–16] The patient's leg veins should be evaluated with a 360 degree view while standing and supine to assess for bulging veins. Sclerotherapy patients should be in good health. Contraindications to sclerotherapy include pregnancy, inability to ambulate or comply with postsclerotherapy compression, clotting disorders, general poor health, or active immunodeficiency.

EDUCATION AND CONSENT

Once a diagnosis is made and the patient is judged to be a candidate for sclerotherapy, it is necessary to obtain informed consent. Possible complications such as hyperpigmentation, matting, and ulceration are discussed. The necessity for multiple treatment sessions is emphasized and the need for maintenance therapy is highlighted. If the treatment plan will include sclerosants that are used off-label or are not FDA approved, this fact must be clearly communicated. If the patient understands the plan, risks, benefits, and alternatives, the consent form is signed.

PHOTOGRAPHS

It is impossible to overemphasize the importance of photographs. As treatment progresses, patients invariably forget the original appearance of the treated areas. Pretreatment photographs are absolutely essential to help the physician evaluate treatment progress and to allow the patient to recognize improvement.

PRETREATMENT INSTRUCTIONS

Patients are told to wear shorts and not to use moisturizers or shave their legs on the day of treatment. Shaving the leg may cause erythematous streaks, making it difficult to visualize patterns of reticular and telangiectatic veins. Use of moisturizers causes poor adhesion of the tape used to secure compression following injections, but more importantly causes slower evaporation of the alcohol used to prep the leg. Patients are encouraged to eat at least a small meal beforehand to minimize vasovagal reactions.

TEST INJECTIONS

Test injections, which were standard practice with use of the sclerosant sodium tetradecyl sulfate (STS), are now optional if using the sclerosant polidocanol (POL). The package insert for STS (Sotradecol®) recommends a test site injection to assess for allergic reactions. The package insert for POL (Asclera®) does not require a test site injection. If utilizing STS as the sclerosant or if the patient is nervous, the first treatment session may be limited to a small number of sites to observe for any allergic reactions. It also serves to familiarize the patient with the treatment and treating physician, clinic surroundings, and the sensation of the fine needle. More extensive treatment can usually be undertaken on the second visit, as the patient is typically more relaxed. The effectiveness of the concentration and class of the sclerosing agent used during the test injections can also be evaluated at the following visit.

When the patient returns in 2 to 6 weeks, the test site or limited treatment area is compared with pretreatment photographs. Any side effects such as matting and pigmentation can be explained. Reasonable time intervals for clearance of treated vessels can be reinforced. At each session, all sites treated are noted in anatomic diagrams in the chart.

SCLEROSANT SELECTION

As sclerosing solution flows away from the point of injection, it is diluted by blood and becomes less potent. This problem has been alleviated with the advance of using foamed sclerosants. The foamed sclerosants displace the blood inside the vein, which maximizes contact with and subsequent damage to the endothelial surface. Foamed solutions are, therefore, stronger then liquid solutions, and a smaller sclerosant concentration is required for the same therapeutic effect. Decreased concentration logically leads to decreased potential side effects, such as inflammation, hyperpigmentation, necrosis, and systemic toxicity. Table 44-2 shows suggested volumes and concentrations of sclerosants for treating small reticular veins. Table 44-3 shows suggested volumes and concentrations of sclerosants for treating telangiectasias.

The volume injected should be only as much as is necessary to flush the visible segment of vein that is being treated to be clear of blood. Usually no more than 0.5 cc of sclerosing solution per injection site is necessary, although some larger or longer reticular veins may require up to 1 cc of solution. In many cases, spasm may be observed after injection of sclerosant. When this occurs, it is a desirable endpoint. The most commonly used sclerosing solutions include STS, POL, 72% glycerin compound, and hypertonic saline. In our practice, we have abandoned the use of hypertonic saline due to pain, the risk of necrosis and the inability to treat larger numbers of vessels in one session.

TABLE 44-2
Sclerosant Concentrations for Small Reticular Veins

Recommended Starting Concentration (%)	Maximum Recommended Concentration (%)	Sclerosant
0.2	0.5	Sodium tetradecyl sulfate (Sotradecol) liquid
0.5	1.0	Polidocanol (Asclera) liquid
0.1	0.2	Sodium tetradecyl sulfate (Sotradecol) foam
0.25	0.5	Polidocanol (Asclera) foam

TABLE 44-3
Sclerosant Concentrations for Telangiectasia

Minimum Effective Concentration	Maximum Recommended Concentration	Sclerosant
0.1%	0.2%	Sodium tetradecyl sulfate (Sotradecol) liquid
72%	Unchanged	Glycerin diluted with 1% lidocaine (1:100,000) in a 2:1 solution
0.25%	0.5%	Polidocanol (Asclera) liquid
11.7%	23.4%	Hypertonic saline
Not recommended	Not recommended	Any foamed solution

EQUIPMENT

- Cotton balls soaked with 70% isopropyl alcohol
- Protective gloves
- 3 cc disposable syringes
- 30 gauge ½ in disposable transparent hub needles
- Cotton balls or foam pads for compression
- Hypoallergenic tape (synthetic silk or paper)
- 2% nitroglycerin paste (for prolonged blanching or extravasation)
- Sclerosing solutions (sequestered from other injectables in the clinic and labeled)
- Magnifying loupes or lenses (2–5×)
- Sterile connector for foam production

The brand of syringe to be used for sclerotherapy is a personal choice. It is worth the effort to try a variety of syringes, as there is a marked difference in plunger friction between different kinds of syringes and between syringes from different manufacturers. When any detergent type of sclerosant is utilized, it is recommended to use latex-free syringes. In high enough concentrations (≥0.5%), STS or POL will dissolve the rubber from the plunger, thereby releasing rubber and rubber products into solution (data on file, Wyeth–Ayerst Laboratories). There is a relatively high and increasing incidence of latex allergy in the general population.[17] Theoretically, the risk of a severe allergic reaction may be increased with latex-containing syringes. We have not yet seen allergic reactions to STS in more than 400,000 injections we have performed since switching to latex-free syringes in 1994. Since POL was approved in the United States we have not encountered any allergic reactions with the use of latex-free syringes for POL injections. In a recent comparison study, no reaction to either POL or STS was observed.[18]

PATIENT PREPARATION

The patient is placed in a recumbent position that allows convenient access to the leg veins to be treated. If available, a motorized table with height adjustment will facilitate easy access to all regions of the leg. The areas to be treated may be cleansed with cotton balls saturated with 70% isopropyl alcohol, temporarily allowing better visualization of the vessels by increasing light transmission through reflective scale on the epidermal surface. Glycerin can also be used, which does not cause an evaporative cooling effect. When alcohol is used, it needs to evaporate completely or be wiped off to minimize pain of the needle pushing alcohol into the skin. Use of double-polarized lighting (Syris v600, Syris Scientific, Gray, ME) has also proven to be helpful. The neck and back position of the treating physician must be optimal to avoid injury to the physician over the long term. Indirect lighting is best, as harsh halogen surgical lights bleach out reticular veins and some telangiectasias.

TECHNIQUE

INJECTION OF RETICULAR VEINS

The same basic principle of treatment from the largest to the smallest varicosities holds true no matter the size of the vessels being treated. Sclerotherapy of small veins begins with injection of the feeding reticular veins, then venulectases, then telangiectatic webs or networks, and finally the smallest and most isolated telangiectasias.

HAND POSITION

The syringe is held in the dominant hand, which rests on the patient's leg, and the needle is advanced at a shallow angle through the skin and into the reticular vein. When the physician feels the typical "pop-through" sensation of piercing the vein, the plunger is gently pulled back until blood return is seen in the transparent plastic hub (Fig. 44-2). The pull back is important for solutions that could potentially cause skin necrosis. Typically one injects up to 0.5 cc of sclerosant and then massages the solution toward any associated telangiectasias. When injecting foam, enough foam is injected to visually fill the targeted reticular vein. Injection should be stopped immediately if any signs of leakage occur or if a bleb or bruising is noted.

CANNULATION OF THE VESSEL

A 3 cc syringe with a 30 gauge needle is used, which is bent to an angle of 10 to 30 degrees to facilitate cannulation (rather than transfixion) of the vein. A 1 cc syringe generates too much pressure and will most likely rupture the vein, so it should not be utilized. The cannulation of a reticular vein can be quite difficult at times because reticular veins can go into spasm, and may virtually disappear during an attempt at cannulation. Use of alcohol for cleansing may cause evaporative cooling, which may lead to reticular vein spasm. When this occurs, another injection site must be sought. During the injection of sclerosant, extravasation will result from the slightest movement of the injecting hand, and can also occur when the

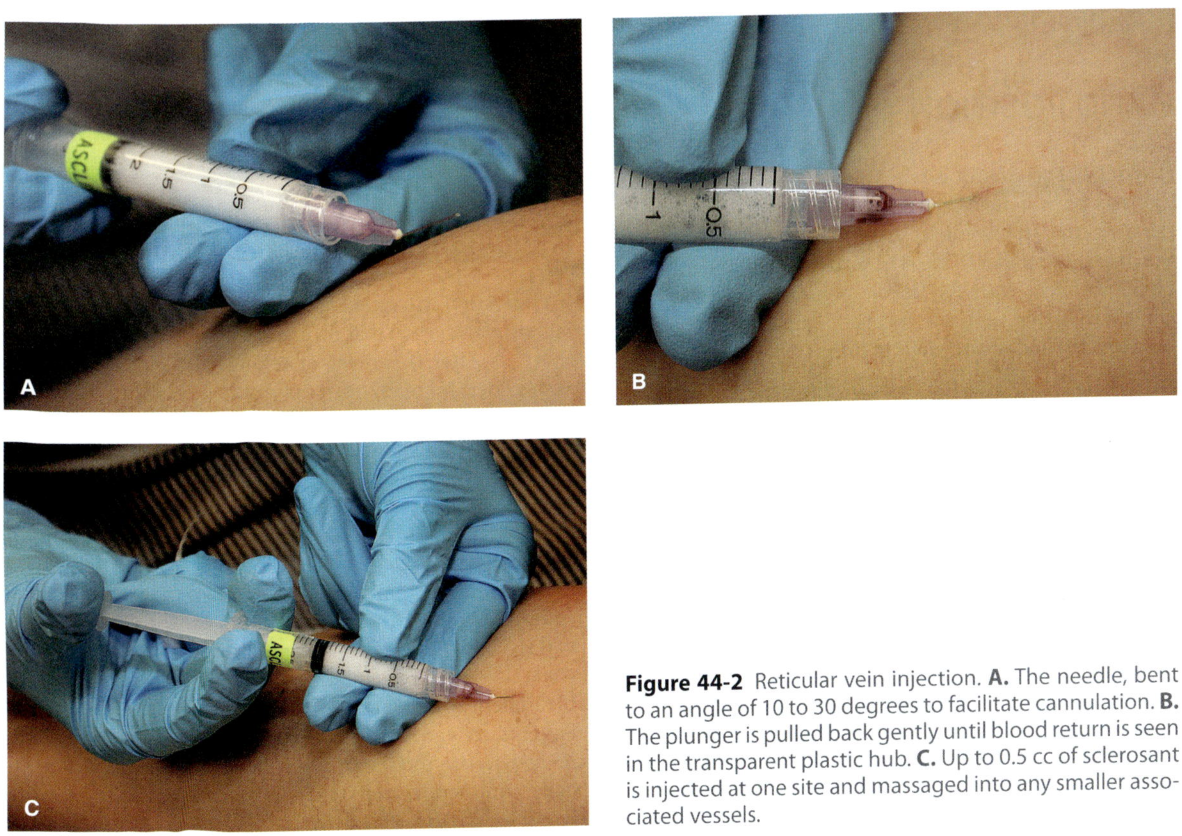

Figure 44-2 Reticular vein injection. **A.** The needle, bent to an angle of 10 to 30 degrees to facilitate cannulation. **B.** The plunger is pulled back gently until blood return is seen in the transparent plastic hub. **C.** Up to 0.5 cc of sclerosant is injected at one site and massaged into any smaller associated vessels.

vessel goes into spasm and pulls away from the cannulating needle. Until the physician gains experience with reticular veins, cautious injection with the gentlest sclerosants should be the rule, to avoid tissue necrosis and ulceration.

INJECTION OF SCLEROSANTS

When injecting a reticular vein, the sclerosing solution is sometimes seen flowing into the telangiectasias. When this happens, the telangiectasias often do not need to be injected directly. Similarly, sclerosing solution injected into a telangiectasia may be seen flowing into the feeder vein, but reticular veins usually still need to be injected directly, as it is difficult to deliver an effective volume and concentration of sclerosant to the reticular vein indirectly. Until the reticular vein has been adequately treated, telangiectasias will be resistant to treatment and will demonstrate early recurrence. For this reason, some prefer to treat reticular veins first, to wait and assess the results of treatment after a few weeks, and to treat remaining telangiectasias at a later time.[19–21] Others prefer to treat the entire refluxing system at one time, although treating reticular veins first theoretically minimizes pigmentation and matting in telangiectatic webs.[6,21]

INJECTION OF TELANGIECTASIAS

Injection of telangiectasias is performed after all sites of reflux, larger varicosities, and feeding vessels have been injected. The smaller the vein, the lower the initial volume and concentration of sclerosant needed for effective treatment. Foamed sclerosant is too strong to inject in most telangiectasias, especially those less than 1 mm in diameter, and may cause a higher incidence of matting and pigmentation.

HAND POSITION

A syringe of sclerosant is prepared with a 30 gauge needle that has been bent to an angle of 10 to 30 degrees with the bevel up. The needle is placed flat on the skin so that the needle is parallel to the skin surface. Most practitioners prefer to inject with the needle pointing away from the clinician. In this case, the syringe is held like a cigarette between the index and middle fingers, and the thumb is used to control the plunger.

CANNULATION OF THE VESSEL

The technique requires a gentle, precise touch, but with practice the beveled tip of the 30 gauge (0.3 mm diameter) needle may be used to cannulate vessels as small as 0.1 mm. The bevel of the needle usually can be seen within the lumen of the telangiectasias with use of 1.75× to 5× magnification. Needles smaller than 30 gauge or longer than ½ in are difficult to use because they tend to veer off course when advanced through the skin. Depending on the patient's skin type, needles can become dull rather quickly, and should be replaced whenever resistance to skin puncture is noted. This typically occurs within 3 to 10 punctures.

Once the needle tip is seen in the lumen of the vessel, a tiny bolus of air (<0.05 cc) may be injected to help demonstrate that the needle is within the vein. Some phlebologists recommend an "air block" technique in which a larger bolus of air is used to clear the arborizing vessels of blood before the sclerosing solution is infused.[22]

INJECTION OF SCLEROSANTS

Because solutions are not readily diluted in telangiectasias, the initial treatment of telangiectatic webs begins with the minimal effective concentration of sclerosant.[23] At the next visit, the same concentration is used if sclerosis was effective and a higher concentration is used if sclerosis was ineffective. The injection of telangiectasias is performed very slowly, with minimal pressure on the syringe (Fig. 44-3). A few drops of sclerosant are sufficient to fill the vein and maintain contact with the vessel wall for 10 to 15 seconds. The amount infused is approximately 0.1 to 0.2 cc per site, which is often sufficient to produce blanching in a radius of 2 cm from the site of injection. Rapid flushing of the vessels with larger volumes of sclerosant or with higher pressures leads to problems with extravasation, tissue necrosis, and ulceration, as well as an increased incidence of telangiectatic matting and hyperpigmentation.[24]

To minimize skin necrosis, especially with hypertonic saline, extravasation must be avoided. If there is resistance to the flow of sclerosant, or if a "bleb" begins to form at the injection site, the injection must be stopped immediately. Extravasation of low concentrations of POL does not cause tissue necrosis, but significant extravasation of higher concentration (>0.1%) STS or of hypertonic saline will cause necrosis and ulceration. A randomized study in animals found the incidence of ulceration to be greater when attempts were made to dilute the extravasated sclerosant by the injection of normal saline into the area.[25] Vigorous massage of any blebs is recommended to minimize the chance of necrosis.

COMPRESSION

Compression will speed vessel clearance and reduce staining from any vessel that protrudes above the surface of the skin.[26–28] After treatment of telangiectasias, compression is provided by ready-to-wear gradient compression hose (15–20 mm Hg) placed over cotton balls that are secured with tape at the sites of injection. If larger reticular veins (>3 mm) are treated at the same session, Class I 20 to 30 mm Hg compression is used (Table 44-4). Some authorities recommend that continuous compression be applied for as long as the patient will tolerate it (usually 1–7 days). However, in our practice, we ask the patient to wear the compression hose daily for 2 weeks, except when bathing and sleeping. There is ongoing debate about compression while sleeping. We believe that external compression while recumbent is not necessary as venous pressure is zero. Patients are encouraged to walk, and the only restrictions on activity are those that result in sustained forceful muscular contraction and venous pressure elevation, such as heavy weightlifting.

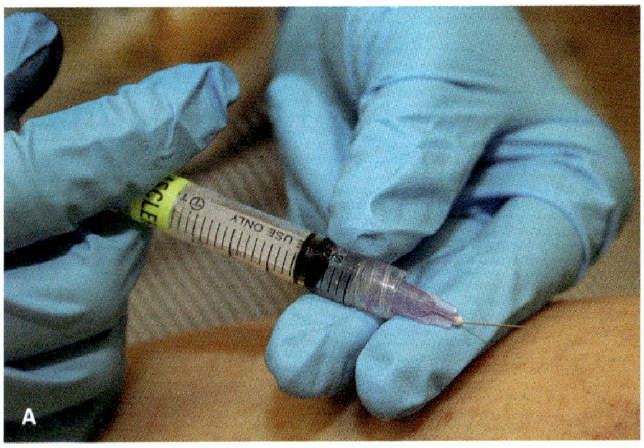
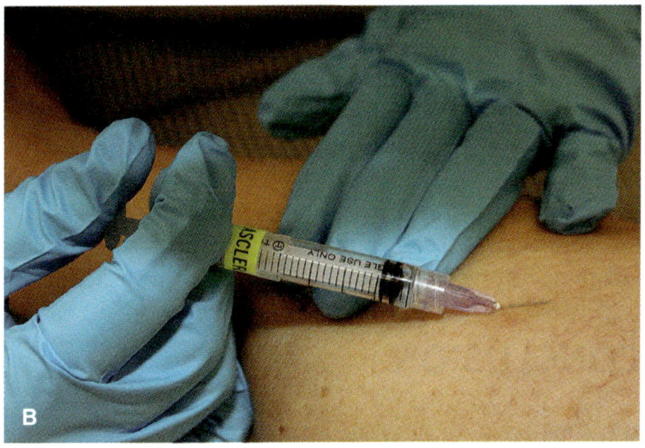
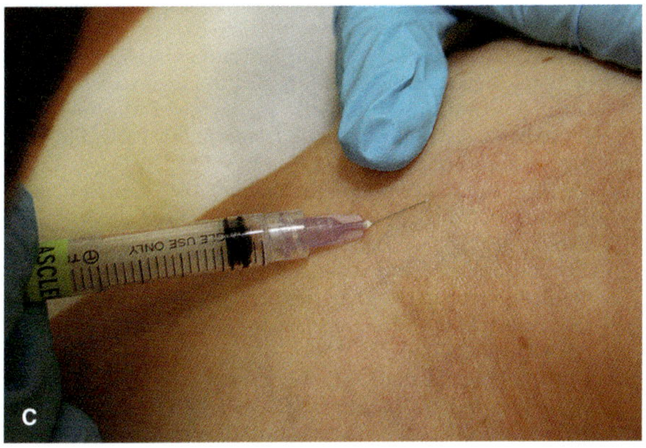

Figure 44-3 Telangiectatic web injection. **A.** A 30 gauge needle (bent to an angle of 10–30 degrees, bevel up) is placed flat on the skin so that the needle is parallel to the skin surface. **B.** The firmly supported needle pierces the top of the tiny vein sufficiently to allow infusion of solution with minimal pressure on the plunger. **C.** The amount slowly infused is approximately 0.1 cc to 0.2 cc per site, leading to visible blanching of the connected telangiectasias.

TREATMENT INTERVALS

Physician and patient preferences play a large role in determining treatment intervals. New areas may be treated at any time, but retreatment of the same areas should be deferred for several weeks because some telangiectasias will ultimately clear even after exhibiting no response within the first 2 weeks.[29] Patients often are anxious to speed their course of treatment, but allowing a longer time between treatment sessions may minimize the number of sessions needed. Some physicians recommend waiting as long as 4 to 8 weeks between treatments, while others may see their patients at weekly intervals. It is not uncommon for there to be small, firm areas of hyperpigmentation along the track of reticular veins and protuberant telangiectasias. On follow-up sessions, these areas are typically "nicked" with an 18 gauge needle to release the dark, liquid blood trapped in the developing fibrosis. This allows faster resolution of the pigmentation. The number of treatments needed depends on the extent of the problem and the extent of the areas treated at each session. Some patients are highly responsive to treatment, and can be treated with weak sclerosants in only a few sessions. Others are highly resistant, and may require more sessions and stronger sclerosants.

After the initial series of treatments, a "rest" period of 4 to 6 months will allow time for pigmentation and matting to clear, and for any remaining reticular veins to establish "new" routes of reflux or drainage. Approximately 80% of patients will clear to their satisfaction during the first course of treatment. Any remaining telangiectatic webs or new telangiectasias are then reassessed to determine the best approach for another round of treatment.

TABLE 44-4
Guidelines for Compression

Telangiectasias only—OTC 15–20 mm Hg
Telangiectasias and reticular veins—20–30 mm Hg
Reticular and small varicose veins—20–30 mm Hg
Truncal varicose veins—30–40 mm Hg
All compression for 2–3 wks, most critical in the first 3 days

POOR RESPONSE TO TREATMENT

When patients have had a poor response to the initial series of treatments, the original diagnosis must always be called into question. Failed treatment often means that a hidden source of reflux was overlooked. Evaluation with handheld Doppler or preferably color-flow duplex ultrasound is indicated to elucidate the patterns and sources of reflux that have led to a treatment failure. Unsuspected sources of reflux can include truncal varices, incompetent perforating veins, and unrecognized reticular vessels.

If no untreated source of reflux can be identified, the patient must be carefully questioned about proper compliance with compression. Many patients abandon compression immediately after sclerotherapy, and this can lead to treatment failures. The concentration and volume of sclerosant used should also be reexamined. It is not uncommon to find that the concentrations selected were ineffective for the size and type of vessel being treated. If no explanation for the treatment failure is found, the concentration of sclerosant may be increased or another class of sclerosants may be used.[30] Some women taking high doses of estrogen and progesterone may rarely improve the results of sclerotherapy by temporarily suspending hormonal supplementation.[31–33]

CONCLUSION

When based upon a correct diagnosis and an appropriate treatment plan, sclerotherapy is a highly effective method of treatment for telangiectasias. Formulating an effective treatment plan requires a detailed knowledge of venous anatomy, a thorough understanding of the principles and patterns of reflux, and an intimate familiarity with a range of volumes and concentrations of sclerosing solutions. The results obtained depend greatly on the experience of the clinician, but with care and attention to detail, clearing rates of 90% can be achieved in most patients.

Patient satisfaction is enhanced through education and informed consent, photographic documentation, and a measured approach to treatment. When the basic principles of diagnosis and treatment are followed meticulously, a successful outcome is highly likely. It is important to educate the patient that telangiectasias may be a lifelong problem. Development of new veins within a few months to years after successful treatment does not constitute treatment failure; rather, it demonstrates the chronicity of venous insufficiency. It also demonstrates an active wound healing response in which new capillaries and small vessels are generated in seemingly limitless capacity.

REFERENCES

1. Blättler W, Kreis N, Lun B, Winiger J, Amsler F. Leg symptoms of healthy people and their treatment with compression hosiery. *Phlebology.* 2008;23(5):214–221.
2. Weiss RA, Heagle CR, Raymond-Martimbeau P. The Bulletin of the North American Society of Phlebology. Insurance Advisory Committee Report. *J Dermatol Surg Oncol.* 1992; 18:609–616.
3. Weiss RA, Weiss MA. Resolution of pain associated with varicose and telangiectatic leg veins after compression sclerotherapy. *J Dermatol Surg Oncol.* 1990;16:333–336.
4. Beasley KL, Weiss RA. Leg Rejuvenation. In: Hirsh RJ, ed. *Aesthetic Rejuvenation A Regional Approach.* New York, NY: McGraw-Hill;2009:173–189.
5. Goldman MP, Bennett RG. Treatment of telangiectasia: a review. *J Am Acad Dermatol.* 1987;17:167–182.
6. Weiss RA, Weiss MA. Therapy of telangiectasia and varicose veins and their complications. In: Baran R, Maibach H, eds. *Textbook of Cosmetic Dermatology.* London: Martin Dunitz LTD; 2004:375–384.
7. Weiss RA, Weiss MA. Painful telangiectasias: diagnosis and treatment. In: Bergan JJ, Weiss RA, Goldman MP, eds. *Varicose Veins and Telangiectasias: Diagnosis and Treatment.* 2nd ed. St. Louis, MO: Quality Medical; 1999:389–406.
8. Goldman MP, Bergan JJ, Guex JJ. *Sclerotherapy, treatment of varicose and telangiectatic leg veins.* 4th ed. New York, NY: Elsevier Health Sciences; 2006.
9. Weiss RA, Weiss MA. Sclerotherapy. In: Wheeland RG, ed. *Cutaneous Surgery.* Philadelphia, PA: W.B. Saunders Co; 1994: 951–981.
10. Weiss RA, Weiss MA. Doppler ultrasound findings in reticular veins of the thigh subdermic lateral venous system and implications for sclerotherapy. *J Dermatol Surg Oncol.* 1993; 19(10):947–951.
11. Somjen GM, Ziegenbein R, Johnston AH, Royle JP. Anatomical examination of leg telangiectases with duplex scanning. *J Dermatol Surg Oncol.* 1993;19(10):940–945.
12. Braverman IM, Keh-Yen A. Ultrastructure of the human dermal microcirculation. IV. Valve-containing collecting veins at the dermal-subcutaneous junction. *J Invest Dermatol.* 1983; 81(5):438–442.
13. deFaria JL, Moraes IN. Histopathology of telangiectasias associated with varicose veins. *Dermatologica.* 1963;127:321–329.
14. Thibault P, Bray A, Wlodarczyk J, Lewis W. Cosmetic leg veins: evaluation using duplex venous imaging. *J Dermatol Surg Oncol.* 1990;16:612–618.
15. Komsuoglu B, Goldeli O, Kulan K, Cetinarslan B, Komsuoglu SS. Prevalence and risk factors of varicose veins in an elderly population. *Gerontology.*1994;40(1):25–31.
16. Schultz-Ehrenburg U, Weindorf N, Matthes U, Hirche H. New epidemiological findings with regard to initial stages of varicose veins (Bochum study I-III). In: Raymond-Martimbeau P, Prescott R, Zummo M, eds. *Phlebologie '92.* Paris, FR: John Libbey Eurotext; 1992:234–236.
17. Cheng L, Lee D. Review of latex allergy. *J Am Board Fam Pract.* 1999;12(4):285–292.
18. Rabe E, Schliephake D, Otto J, Breu FX, Pannier F. Sclerotherapy of telangiectases and reticular veins: a double-blind, randomized, comparative clinical trial of polidocanol, sodium tetradecyl sulphate and isotonic saline (EASI study). *Phlebology.* 2010;25(3):124–131.
19. Guex JJ. [The treatment of microvarices, varicosities and telangiectasis in 1992]. *Phlebologie.* 1992;45:401–404; discussion 405–407.
20. Guex JJ. Indications for the sclerosing agent polidocanol (aetoxisclerol dexo, aethoxisklerol kreussler). *J Dermatol Surg Oncol.* 1993;19:959–961.
21. Guex JJ. Microsclerotherapy. *Semin Dermatol.* 1993;12:129–134.
22. Bodian EL. Sclerotherapy: a personal appraisal. *J Dermatol Surg Oncol.* 1989;15:156–161.
23. Sadick NS. Sclerotherapy of varicose and telangiectatic leg veins. Minimal sclerosant concentration of hypertonic saline and its relationship to vessel diameter. *J Dermatol Surg Oncol.* 1991;17:65–70.
24. Ouvry PA, Davy A. The sclerotherapy of telangiectasia. *Phlebol.* 1982;35:349–359.
25. Zimmet SE. The prevention of cutaneous necrosis following extravasation of hypertonic saline and sodium tetradecyl sulfate. *J Dermatol Surg Oncol.* 1993;19:641–646.
26. Fegan WG. Continuing uninterrupted compression technique of injecting varicose veins. *Proc R Soc Med.* 1960;53:837–840.
27. Goldman MP, Beaudoing D, Marley W, Lopez L, Butie A. Compression in the treatment of leg telangiectasia: a preliminary report. *J Dermatol Surg Oncol.* 1990;16:322–325.
28. Weiss RA, Sadick NS, Goldman MP, Weiss MA. Post-sclerotherapy compression: controlled comparative study of duration of compression and its effects on clinical outcome. *Dermatol Surg.* 1999;25(2):105–108.
29. Goldman MP. My sclerotherapy technique for telangiectasia and reticular veins. *Dermatol Surg.* 2010;36(Suppl 2):1040–1045.
30. Sadick NS. Hyperosmolar versus detergent sclerosing agents in sclerotherapy.Effect on distal vessel obliteration. *J Dermatol Surg Oncol.* 1994;20(5):313–316.
31. Weiss RA, Weiss MA. Incidence of side effects in the treatment of telangiectasias by compression sclerotherapy: hypertonic saline vs. polidocanol. *J Dermatol Surg Oncol.* 1990;16: 800–804.
32. Sadick NS, Niedt GW. A study of estrogen and progesterone receptors in spider telangiectasias of the lower extremities. *J Dermatol Surg Oncol.* 1990;16:620–623.
33. Davis LT, Duffy DM. Determination of incidence and risk factors for postsclerotherapy telangiectatic matting of the lower extremity: a retrospective analysis. *J Dermatol Surg Oncol.* 1990; 16:327–330.

CHAPTER 45

Minimally Invasive Treatment of Varicose Veins

Karen L. Beasley & Robert A. Weiss

INTRODUCTION

The development of minimally invasive methods to heat, denature, and shrink varicose veins has been a major achievement in the field of phlebology and medicine. Minimally invasive endovenous occlusion techniques using radiofrequency (RF) or laser are now the standard of care in the United States. When saphenous venous system reflux is present, it must be addressed prior to the treatment of visible associated varicosities, reticular veins or telangiectasias. Without elimination of reflux, the patient will be doomed to recurrence of the varicosities and smaller vessels below the level of saphenous vein reflux. Previously, the only treatment option for these patients with varicose veins from saphenous insufficiency was surgical ligation and stripping of the vessels under general anesthesia. This procedure resulted in significant postoperative down time with surgical scars, swelling, bruising, and pain. The expense of a hospital stay and missed work, along with an unacceptable rate of recurrence, has greatly decreased the popularity of this procedure.

RF ablation started the minimally invasive varicose vein trend with its approval in March 1999 by the US FDA as the VNUS Closure™ procedure, now known as the Venefit™ procedure. Subsequently, endovenous ablation techniques utilizing lasers were filed as US FDA 510(k) applications as substantially equivalent procedures to RF ablation. The first laser FDA cleared by substantial equivalence to RF was the 810 nm diode laser, which was cleared for marketing in 2000.

The advances in endovenous ablation have revolutionized in-office varicose vein treatment for physicians and patients. RF energy, like a laser with a water absorption predominant wavelength, heats and contracts the collagen within the vein wall causing contraction of the varicose vein. Endovenous laser treatment of varicose veins can be divided into two categories: hemoglobin absorption predominant and water absorption predominant. The water absorption predominant wavelengths are primarily above 1100 nm, in which hemoglobin is no longer a chromophore (Fig. 45-1).

VENEFIT™ PROCEDURE (COVIDIEN, SAN JOSE, CA)

TARGETED ENDOVENOUS THERAPY

RF energy is delivered through a specially designed endovenous electrode to accomplish controlled resistive heating of the vessel wall. This causes vein shrinkage or occlusion by contraction of venous wall collagen to eliminate saphenous venous reflux. Although the concept of endovenous elimination of reflux is not new, previous

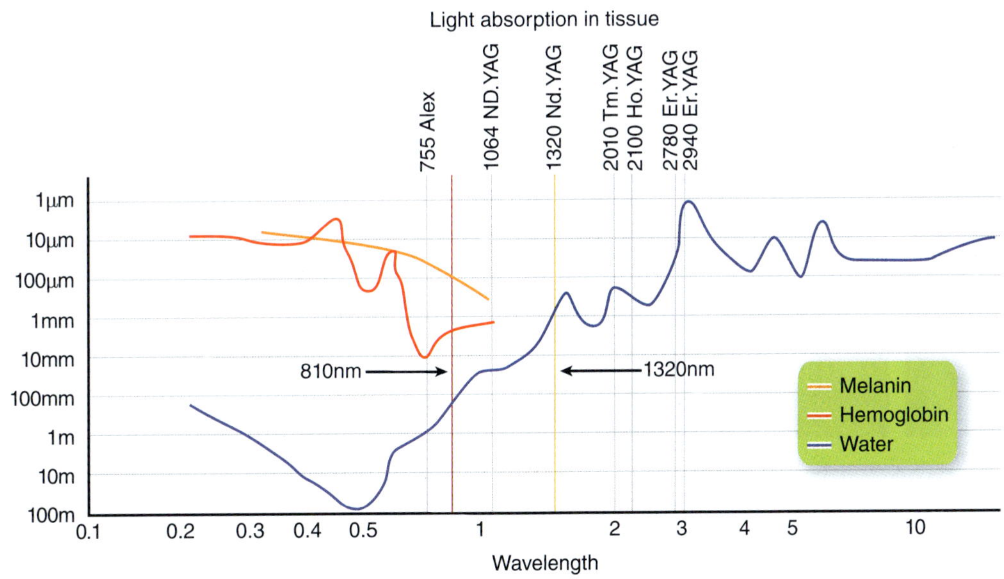

1320nm is absorbed uniformly in water, with little or no effect be melanin and hemoglobin

Figure 45-1 Absorption curves of light through infrared wavelengths. There is virtually no absorption by hemoglobin beyond 1100 nm. Water is the target of 1320 nm.

approaches have relied on electrocoagulation of blood. This resulted in thrombus occluding the venous structures, with the potential for recanalization of thrombus being very high. The concept of application of RF directly to tissue, rather than blood, has been effectively applied for ablation of abnormal conduction pathways for arrhythmias.[1] This concept was conceived and adapted for the treatment of varicose veins as well. The potential safety of this technique was supported by the fact that in animal studies there was no evidence of thrombus extension, while the zone of thermal damage had been limited to no more than 2 mm beyond the targeted vessel. A high acute success rate of 92% was followed by long-term vessel occlusion in the animal model.

ORIGINAL VNUS CLOSURE TECHNOLOGY™ VERSUS VENEFIT CLOSUREFAST™

Present ClosureFast™ technology utilizes a method for vein heating that evolved from the original version (Fig. 45-2). In the current model, RF energy is directed toward vein walls. The vein walls then shrink from the resultant denaturing of the vein wall protein. The previous mechanism by which RF current heated tissue was resistive (or ohmic) heating of a narrow rim (<1 mm) of tissue that was in direct contact with an electrode. This method was much more difficult to perform as electrodes were susceptible to coagulum, which would cut off the RF due to high resistance or impedance. The present system completely bypasses this problem. Temperature, not ohmic resistance, is the limiting factor for the feedback loop.

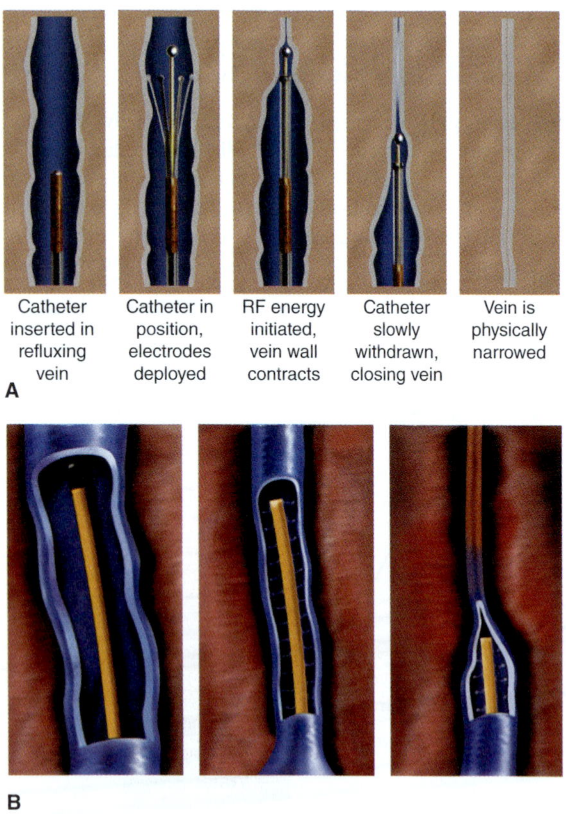

Figure 45-2 Comparison of original design of RF catheter versus the new ClosureFast™ design. **A.** Electrodes contact the vein wall. **B.** A wire coil heats up using RF energy, which then secondarily heats vein wall by direct contact as the catheter is pulled back. (Used with permission of Covidien, San Jose, CA. Venefit is a trademark of a Covidien company. © 2013 Covidien.)

It was thought that the optimal target temperature for vein closure was 70° to 90°C since tissue heated above 100°C begins to boil, but we now understand that this not the case.[2] All of the endovenous techniques heat the vessel at 120°C or beyond. A 7 cm long metal core at the tip of the catheter is heated to 120°F and allowed to transmit heat to the treated vessel for 20 seconds, which shrinks veins 7 cm at a time to allow for very fast ablation. The ClosureFast™ catheter and machine are shown in Figure 45-3. This catheter cannot treat segments shorter than 7 cm, with a rigid structure that also limits the treatment of more serpentine saphenous veins, but a new 3 cm metal core has been developed to treat shorter segments. The RF device requires close, stable contact between the active electrode and the vessel wall and requires tumescent anesthesia to allow contact of the vein wall with the metal coil. By controlling temperatures, boiling, vaporization, and carbonization of the tissues are avoided.[3] With the previous generation RF system, as shrinkage and compaction of tissue occurred, there was a decrease in impedance that decreased heat generation,[4] but this is no longer the case as only the temperature of the catheter's metal tip is monitored. Over 10 years of clinical experience suggest that the RF endovenous ablation procedures are highly effective at occluding saphenous veins and abolishing reflux. Studies of Closure Fast™, introduced in 2007, indicate that it is even more efficacious than the previous generation RF model.[5]

RESULTS OF RADIOFREQUENCY ENDOVENOUS ABLATION

For clinical symptoms, the RF endovenous occlusion procedure rapidly reduces patient pain, fatigue and aching correlating with a reduction in CEAP clinical class for symptoms and clinical severity of disease (Table 45-1). When patients have had surgical stripping on the opposite leg, the degree of pain, tenderness, and bruising have been far greater on the leg treated by stripping. Skin burns occurred prior to the tumescent anesthesia technique in 2.5%, but this has not been seen since 1998. Other side effects virtually eliminated by tumescent anesthesia included clinical phlebitis at 6 weeks in 5.7%, and temporary quarter-sized areas of paresthesia in 18%, with most of these occurring immediately above the knee and resolving within 6 months to a year. Endovenous RF occlusion has replaced traditional surgery, which consisted of ligation and stripping of similar size saphenous veins. Most importantly for patients, side effects of DVT and nerve injury are far lower with RF when used with tumescent anesthesia compared to traditional ligation and stripping. Endovenous ablation using the Closure-Fast™ catheter has been reported to maintain occlusion of 97.4% of treated vessels at 1 year[6] and 92% of treated

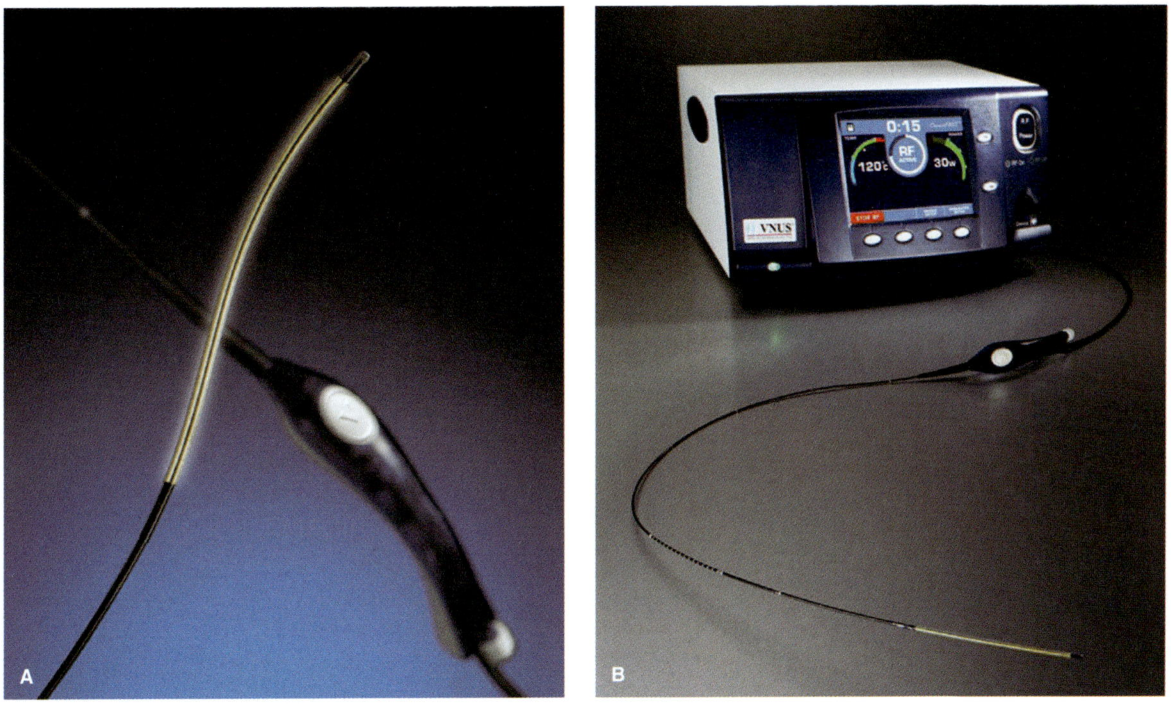

Figure 45-3 **A.** The ClosureFast™ catheter. **B.** The Venefit™ radiofrequency machine. (Used with permission of Covidien, San Jose, CA. Venefit is a trademark of a Covidien company. © 2013 Covidien.)

TABLE 45-1
CEAP Class Description with Findings after Endovenous RF Occlusion

CEAP Clinical Class	Description		
0	Asymptomatic		
1	Telangiectasia		
2	Varicose veins		
3	Edema		
4	Skin changes		
5	Healed venous ulcer		
6	Venous ulcer		
Mean CEAP Class			
Closure Study Population	**Pretreatment**	**6 Wk**	**6 Mo**
Pre-Tx CEAP class = 2	2.0	0.5	0.5
Pre-Tx CEAP class = 3	3.0	0.5	0.3
Pre-Tx CEAP class = 4	4.0	2.3	1.4
Total	2.4	0.8	0.6

vessels at 5 years.[7] A clinical example is shown in Figure 45-4. This is a more favorable outcome for varicose veins than traditional surgery, which has been reported to have long-term efficacy rates much lower than 90%.[8] Patients remain symptom free and patent GSVs are not visible under Duplex ultrasound. Clinical results observed at 6 months are indicative of the long-term results, so that if the GSV is ablated at 6 months, it is likely to remain ablated at 10 years.

The superior epigastric vein that continues to empty superiorly into the common femoral vein is a critical structure to preserve and endovenous techniques are now performed so as to preserve this vein. Energy is applied starting at 2 cm below the saphenofemoral junction below the superior epigastric tributary. We have always believed that a high margin of safety is maintained by maintaining flow through this tributary. Among the many reasons, the most important are that the high flow rate through the epigastric vein into the common femoral vein appears to diminish the possibility of extension of any thrombus (in the unlikely event that this would occur) from the GSV, as well as the fact that normal venous drainage from the lower abdomen is allowed to continue. In our experience, thrombus has never been observed in over 1000 cases of endovenous ablation, although it has been reported by others.[8,9]

LASERS WITH HEMOGLOBIN PREDOMINANT ABSORPTION

Endovenous laser treatment with these wavelengths is designed to produce endothelial and vein wall shrinkage

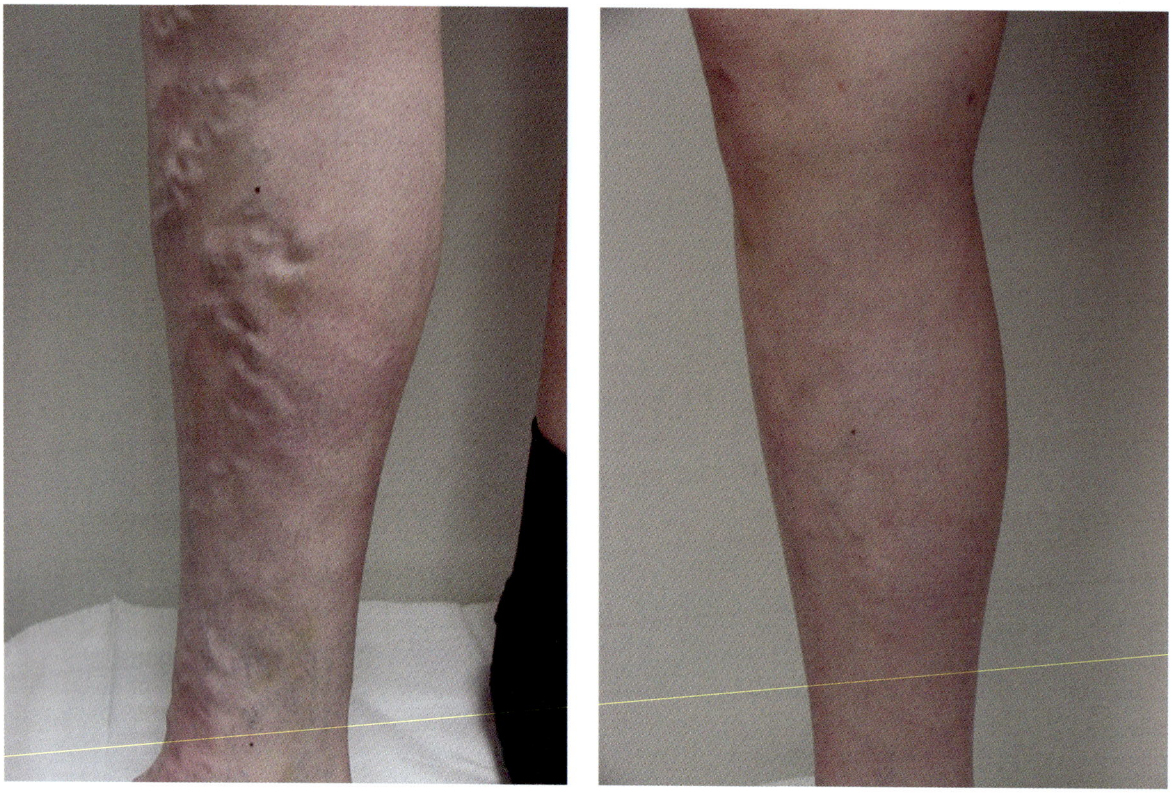

Figure 45-4 Clinical improvement after RF endovenous ablation. Pretreatment varicosities are prominent and 6 weeks postprocedure varicosities are undetectable.

by nonspecific heating of the vessel, often by a superheated coagulum at the fiber tip or by the heating of hemoglobin within red blood cells to create steam bubbles.[10] The target for lasers with 810, 940, 980, and 1064 nm wavelengths is the intravascular red blood cell. Without the presence of blood in the vein, such as in an experimental situation in which the vein is filled with saline, laser-induced vessel wall injury is confined to a small site of direct laser impact. By contrast, blood-filled veins exhibit thermal damage in more remote areas, including the vein wall opposite to the laser impact. Steam bubbles are generated in hemolytic blood by all four lasers, while no bubbles can be produced in normal saline or plasma.[10] Therefore the success of these lasers is highly dependent on correct placement of tumescent local anesthesia to have a thin layer of blood surrounding the laser fiber while having enough anesthesia present to protect the surrounding nerves and muscles from injury. This can be difficult to achieve and results in unpredictable pain and recurrence.

Direct thermal effects on the vein wall without the presence of blood may lead to small spots of wall injury with resulting pain and early recanalization of the treated vein.[11] Less consistent clinical results are seen than with RF ablation or with 1320 nm endovenous laser (see lasers with water predominant absorption). Considerable site variation in success rates and postoperative pain for these types of lasers has been reported.[12,13] This is understandable given that these lasers are dependent on so many different factors, including the amount of blood in the lumen, the rate of pullback, pulsed versus continuous laser output, and the amount of tumescent anesthesia placed around the vein. The overall long-term efficacy of hemoglobin-targeting lasers is less than that of water-absorbing lasers.

SUMMARY OF ENDOVENOUS LASERS WITH HEMOGLOBIN PREDOMINANT ABSORPTION

Wavelengths of 810, 940, and 980 nm endovenous lasers have short-term efficacy ranging from 90% occlusion during the first year of follow-up to 70% after 2 years.[13–17] Unfortunately, many patients experience significant degrees of postoperative ecchymosis and discomfort.[17–23] (Fig. 45-5) Saphenous nerve injury, skin burns, and deep venous thromboses have occurred due to the high temperatures of blood heating at these wavelengths (Fig. 45-6), although the overall safety and efficacy record is better with these laser endovenous ablations than with ligation and stripping.[22] Of all the wavelengths, 810 nm has the lowest long-term improvement at 70%.[23] Ideally, for a hemoglobin-absorbed wavelength to work most efficaciously, it is best to have a well-defined layer of hemoglobin between the fiber and the vein wall. Varicose veins are saccular, however, and irregular pockets of hemoglobin are frequently encountered, leading to sharp rises in temperature and vein perforations when using hemoglobin-absorbing wavelengths. When using tumescent anesthesia with a hemoglobin-targeting wavelength, it can be very difficult to gauge the correct amount of fluid to compress the vein since some hemoglobin is necessary for the mechanism of

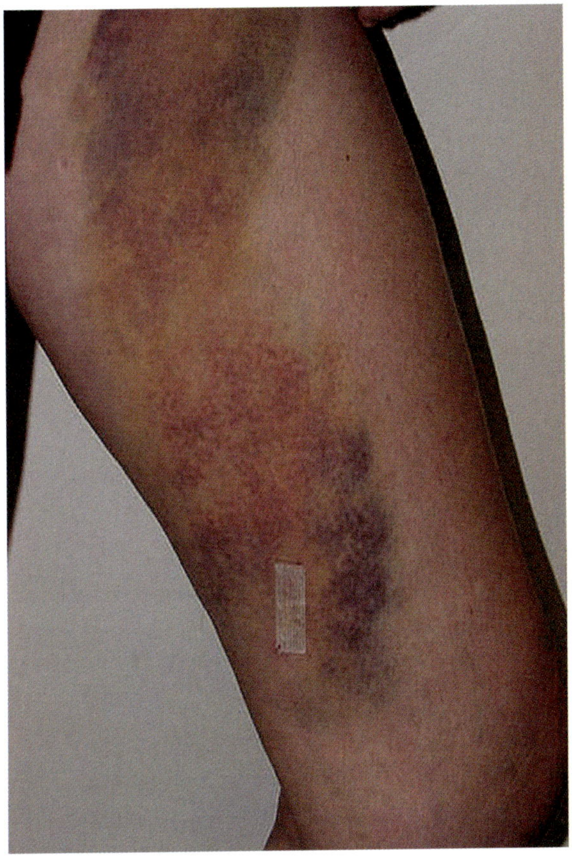

Figure 45-5 One day post endovenous 810 nm diode laser ablation demonstrates bruising.

action. If too much tumescence is used, there can be charring of the inner wall of the vein without heating of the outer vein wall, with resulting inter- and postoperative pain and failure to close the vein. With all of these potential obstacles to ideal treatment conditions for the hemoglobin-absorbing laser wavelengths, it makes far more sense to use a predominantly water-absorbing wavelength to treat incompetent varicose veins by endovenous laser. Tumescent anesthesia can then be employed using the preferred method of complete compression of the vein with exsanguination leading to uniform results and reduced side effects.

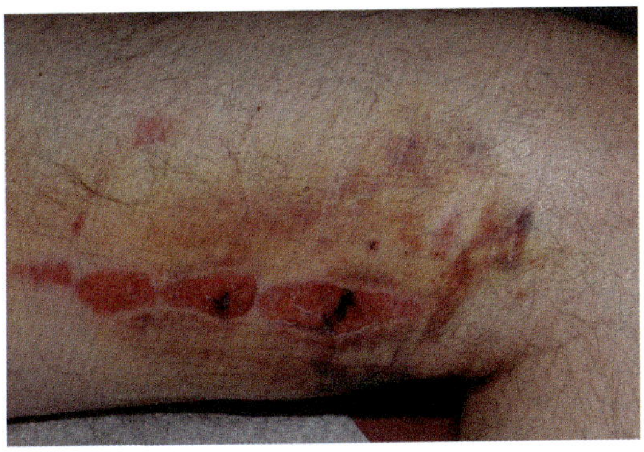

Figure 45-6 **A.** Skin burns caused by diffusion of heat from 810 nm diode endovenous laser seen at 4 days post-procedure.

LASERS WITH WATER PREDOMINANT ABSORPTION

COOLTOUCH ENDOVENOUS CTEV™ 1320 NM (COOLTOUCH, INC., ROSEVILLE, CA)

A variation of the endovenous laser with a wavelength of 1320 nm (CoolTouch CTEV™ Endovenous Treatment) was developed in 2003 by dermatologic surgeons, Robert A. Weiss and Mitchel P. Goldman, in an attempt to circumvent the problems associated with the wavelengths that absorb hemoglobin. Tissue water within the vein wall is the specific target of the 1320 nm laser, and the presence or absence of red blood cells within the vessels is, therefore, unimportant. For a more controlled release of laser energy, the laser is coupled with an automatic pullback device that can pull back the laser fiber at the rate of 0.5 or 1 mm/sec (Fig. 45-7). The penetration of the 1320 nm wavelength is unique in that it effectively heats and contracts the vein with far less heat generation and fewer risks than with the hemoglobin-absorbing wavelengths. The 1320 nm wavelength was explored for use in endovenous ablation and clinical trials performed resulting in FDA clearance in September 2004 for treatment of the greater saphenous vein. By August 2005, sufficient data had been accumulated that the FDA approved the 1320 nm device for obliteration of reflux in the small saphenous vein as well. Based on our experience, there is reduced pain reported with the 1320 nm versus the hemoglobin-absorbing wavelengths due to infrequent vein perforations and more uniform heating. This is likely due to the 1320 nm device targeting water in the vein wall combined with a defined pullback speed for uniform distribution of energy. Although patients may rarely experience mild pain after 1320 nm, this is related to heat dissipated into

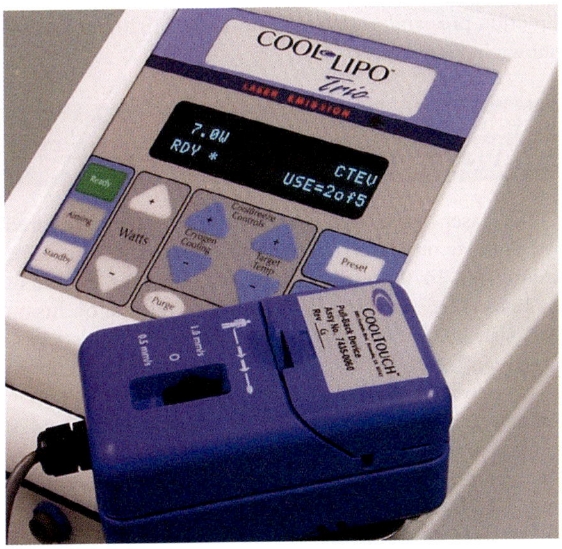

Figure 45-7 CTEV CoolTouch Trio laser with automatic pullback mechanism. (Used with permission of CoolTouch Inc., Roseville, CA.)

the surrounding tissue rather than vein perforations. This side effect can be virtually eliminated by the correct use of tumescent anesthesia. Our incidence of pain following 1320 nm is less than 1% and the vast majority of patients return to work within 24 hours of the procedure. Side effects are also kept to a minimum by using the minimal effective energy to shrink the vein. Energy treatment ranges from 5 to 8 W, with most veins requiring 7 to 8 W of energy. In our own unpublished observations, we have found that during emission of 5 W of 1320 nm energy through a 600 μ fiber moving at 1 mm/sec in a 2 mm thick vein wall, the highest temperature recorded on the exterior of the vein wall is 48°C. Typically, steam bubbles are observed on Duplex ultrasound during the procedure. In a saphenous vein, for effective sealing and shrinkage, higher energies must sometimes be utilized. Proebstle et al.[20] demonstrated a statistically reduced rate of postoperative pain accompanied by a higher initial success rate using 1320 nm versus 940 nm. With the 1320 nm group, treatment-related pain and the need for analgesics were significantly reduced ($p<0.005$) in comparison with treatment-related pain (81%) and the need for analgesics (67%) for the 940 nm laser group. Ecchymosis was also significantly reduced ($p<0.05$) using the 1320 nm wavelength. It has recently been shown that microsecond-pulsed wave lasers with high peak power densities may be the best choice to minimize soft thrombus formation during endovenous ablation treatments and reduce side effects and complications.[21]

The 1320 nm CTEV system is a microsecond-pulsed system. Our own experience has shown reduced side effects, with a reduction in pain and bruising of 80%, when switching from 810 nm endovenous to 1320 nm endovenous ablation. Having treated over 1000 greater saphenous veins with 1320 nm, with follow-up as long as 10 years, our incidence of mild pain lasting less than 24 hours is 5%. No significant pain interfering with walking has been observed with the 1320 nm laser although it has been observed in up to 50% of patients who underwent 810 nm laser treatment in our clinic. No deep venous thrombosis has been observed. A clinical example of varicose veins resulting from reflux at the saphenofemoral junction pre- and post-treatment with a 1320 nm laser is shown in Figure 45-8.

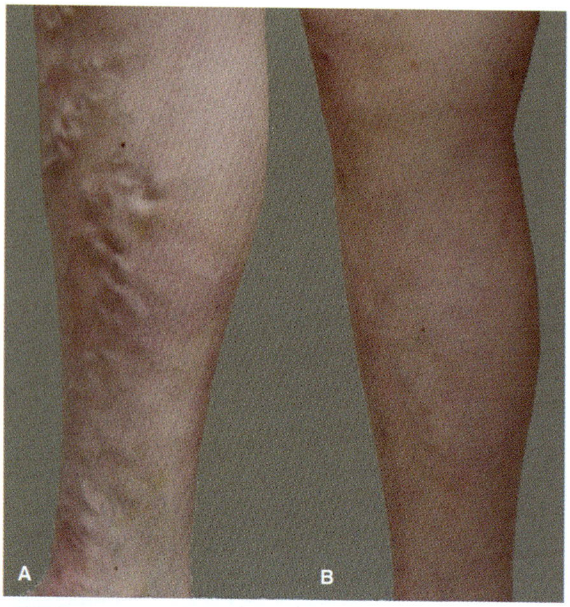

Figure 45-8 Clinical results with 1320 nm endovenous laser. **A.** Before treatment, varicosities are noted. **B.** 6 weeks post treatment demonstrates significant improvement in varicosities.

MISCELLANEOUS ENDOVENOUS WAVELENGTHS

Other laser wavelengths are currently being explored for endovenous laser obliteration of varicose veins. For example, a 1470 nm diode was studied in the treatment of 134 saphenous veins. It showed high rates of occlusion at 1 year but patients also had a 7.6% rate of paresthesias at 1 year.[24] An additional study concluded that closure of the varicose veins was possible with a marked reduction in energy, postoperative pain, and ecchymosis with the 1470 nm as compared to the 980 nm wavelength.[25] The 980 nm wavelength was also compared with another new laser with a 1500 nm wavelength in an animal model. This study found that use of the 1500 nm laser correlated with a more homogeneous vein wall destruction and less perivenous tissue destruction, which could possibly lead to less postoperative pain.[26] Further studies on a larger number of patients will determine the effectiveness of these newly reported wavelengths employed for endovenous ablation.

IMPORTANCE OF TUMESCENT ANESTHESIA FOR ENDOVENOUS TECHNIQUES

It is critical for all the endovenous techniques that tumescent local anesthesia be employed. General anesthesia should not be utilized for the endovenous ablation techniques as patient immobility after the procedure increases the risk of deep-vein thrombosis. Tumescent anesthesia is the technique for local anesthesia delivery that maximizes safety by using pharmacokinetic principles to achieve extensive regional anesthesia of skin and subcutaneous tissue. Initially described for liposuction, the subcutaneous infiltration of a large volume of very dilute lidocaine and epinephrine causes the fat tissue to become swollen and firm, or tumescent. The primary advantage of tumescent anesthesia is that it permits procedures to be performed on patients without subjecting them to the inherent risks of general anesthesia and blood loss.

When applied to endovenous techniques, the rationale for use of tumescent anesthesia is different from its rationale for use in liposuction. The fluid compresses the vein, allowing contact with the laser fiber or RF catheter. Furthermore it provides anesthesia and provides a heat sink for the rise in vein temperature to protect surrounding tissue. This application of tumescent anesthesia to endovenous ablation was considered unique enough to be issued the following patents: US 6258084 B1 Method for Applying Energy to Biological Tissue Including the Use of Tumescent Tissue Compression and US 6752803 B2 Method and Apparatus for Applying

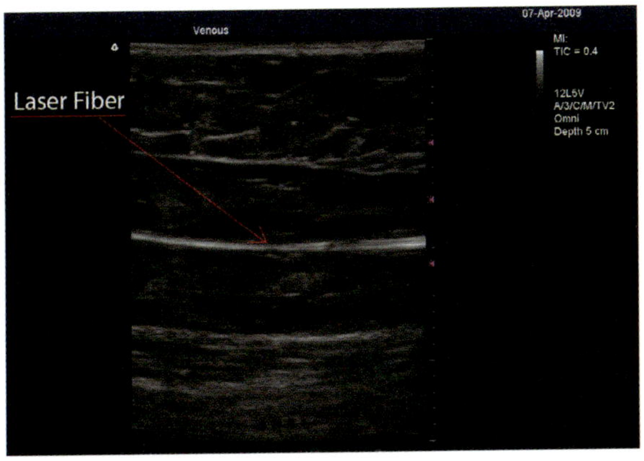

Figure 45-9 SUPT anesthesia seen in a longitudinal view. Dark, non-ultrasound reflective space is the tumescent fluid "space," which is created by instillation of 0.1% lidocaine. The fiber is in the center of the vein as indicated.

Energy to Biological Tissue Including the Use of Tumescent Tissue Compression.

A further refinement of tumescent anesthesia for endovenous techniques is its application under Duplex visualization. This allows the operator to instill the tumescent anesthesia fluid directly around the vein between the superficial and deep fascia, essentially isolating the vein from surrounding structures such as nerves and arteries. This has been named the SUPT technique, which stands for **S**ubfascial **U**ltrasound—Guided **P**erivenous **T**umescent anesthesia (Fig. 45-9). Since the application of this method in our practice, there have been virtually no incidences of paresthesias and the incidence of postoperative pain is virtually zero. This anesthesia is administered using the Klein tumescent pump and a tumescent mixture of 0.1% lidocaine with 1:1,000,000 epinephrine. The Klein pump makes the application of tumescent anesthesia far simpler than with the use of syringes. Since typical volumes range from 300 to 700 cc for the entire length of treated GSV, a pump is highly recommended. A recent report details the use of a syringe but we recommended against this as it slows down the procedure.[27] Tumescent anesthesia placement is even more critical to reduce side effects from small saphenous vein endovenous ablation. A safe total dose of lidocaine is achieved using the tumescent method.

CLINICAL TECHNIQUE

TARGETED ENDOVENOUS THERAPY VENEFIT™ PROCEDURE (RADIOFREQUENCY)

Patients with reflux in the great or small saphenous vein are candidates. We have treated veins as large as 2.5 cm when standing but which are compressed by tumescent anesthesia when the procedure is performed. Using Duplex ultrasound, the procedure begins with marking the vein to be treated on the skin. An appropriate entry point that is easily percutaneously cannulated is selected. This is usually just below where reflux is no longer seen in the GSV or SSV or where the vein becomes too small to cannulate with a standard introducer set. For the majority of patients in our series this is at a point just above or below the knee along the course of the GSV or just below the mid-calf with treatment of the SSV.

Before proceeding, the patient's feet are wrapped in thick socks to minimize vasoconstriction, a heating pad is placed under the thigh or around the foot and a small amount of 2% nitroglycerin paste may be rubbed onto the intended entry point to minimize vasoconstriction during the initial cannulation process. The patient is then prepped and draped, after which 0.2 cc of 1% lidocaine with or without epinephrine is injected at the ultrasound premarked site. It is important that the patient experience no pain during cannulation as the awareness or perception of pain will cause an immediate and rapid contraction of the saphenous vein. This makes cannulation almost impossible until the vein is no longer in spasm, which can take 30 minutes.

In order to place the sheath, a guidewire must be first inserted through the initial needle puncture. The guidewire is passed approximately 5 cm into the GSV. The sheath is then threaded along the guidewire, piercing the skin after a stab incision with a number 11 blade. Its progress is followed by Duplex ultrasound until it is seen firmly placed within the lumen of the GSV. After establishing the intraluminal placement of the sheath, the guidewire is carefully withdrawn. Once the sealed sheath is placed into the vein, the Closure™ catheter is then advanced. Others prefer initializing entry via a venous cutdown or pulling of the vein close to the surface with an ambulatory phlebectomy hook.

With the old design of the VNUS Closure™ catheter, diluted heparin solution or normal saline was required to slowly drip through a central lumen but the new ClosureFast™ design eliminates this concern. Passage of the RF catheter is monitored by duplex ultrasound. Once the RF catheter is in place, tumescent anesthesia is injected under ultrasound guidance primarily between the superficial fascia, the cannulated GSV and the deep fascia (so-called SUPT technique for **S**ubfascial **U**ltrasound—Guided **P**erivenous **T**umescent anesthesia). This is for the purpose of providing a heat sink, causing the vein to compress around the catheter and to provide a painless experience for the patient. Duplex monitoring of the anesthesia injection is not only recommended but is essential to insure that the tumescent fluid is injected into the perivenous space and that the fascial planes are pushed away from the vein.

The final check of the position of the catheter is made with Duplex ultrasound. The tip of the metal core of the 7 cm long energy delivery tip is carefully placed 2 cm below the base of the terminal valve cusps. The readout of temperature prior to initiation of heating to 120°C should be substantially lower than body temperature due to the subfascial tumescent anesthesia. If the temperature readout from the thermocouple is higher than 28°C, then insufficient tumescent fluid has been injected. We prefer to see a baseline temperature after tumescent infiltration of 25° to 26°C. If a body temperature of 37°C is measured at baseline, some aspect of setup is critically wrong and the procedure should not continue.

The RF is then applied; the physician monitors the temperature and impedance. Within 10 to 15 seconds the target temperature of 120°C should be reached. If this does not occur, the catheter has most likely been mistakenly advanced too far into the common femoral vein and the placement of the catheter needs to be carefully reassessed. After target temperature is achieved, the catheter is moved 7 cm down using the markings on the catheter as a guide and the second application of energy occurs. It is important to prevent application of energy to the skin by making sure that markings on the catheter for the final 7 cm of application are carefully observed. At the conclusion, duplex ultrasound of the SFJ should reveal no flow except within the superficial epigastric vein emptying into the common femoral vein. The GSV should be more echogenic with thicker appearing walls. Postoperative instructions are the same as those given after endovenous laser ablation and are discussed later.

ENDOVENOUS LASER ABLATION

As previously discussed in the RF ablation technique section, the leg to be treated should remain warm as veins tend to contract to conserve heat when skin temperature decreases. We often place a heating pad set on low around the foot and patients are encouraged to bring warm socks. If the vein remains too small to cannulate when the patient is supine, we apply gravitation pressure by tilting into reverse Trendelenburg position. A small amount of topical 2% nitrogen paste may be rubbed into the skin where percutaneous access will be initiated.

The patient's leg undergoes sterile preparation and a small catheter is threaded percutaneously into the incompetent vein. In the older technique, a sheath is placed along the entire length of the vein to be treated up to the saphenofemoral or saphenopopliteal junction. In the newer technique, this step is omitted by using specially developed blunt-tipped fibers that do not require a protective sheath. Tumescent anesthesia is then injected along the vein and injected subfascially to separate and dissect the targeted vein. Once tumescent anesthesia is achieved and totally surrounds the targeted vein, the CTEV™ 600 μm laser fiber is inserted. A helium neon aiming beam that is continuously illuminated when the laser is on ensures that the laser fiber is in the superficial venous system and can be used to monitor automatic pullback visually. The sheath acts to protect the vein from perforation during the insertion of a sharp-tipped optical fiber. However, the sheath must be completely removed from the vein prior to application of laser energy at 1320 nm. This is performed so that the automatic pullback device may retract the fiber unimpeded. Secondly, if the laser fiber retracts within the sheath, thermal destruction of the sheath occurs with no energy transmission to the vein wall. With the addition of a rounded or protected tip, such as the SaphFire™ tip, no sheath is required as there is minimal danger of puncturing the wall of a vein while advancing the fiberoptic (Fig. 45-10).

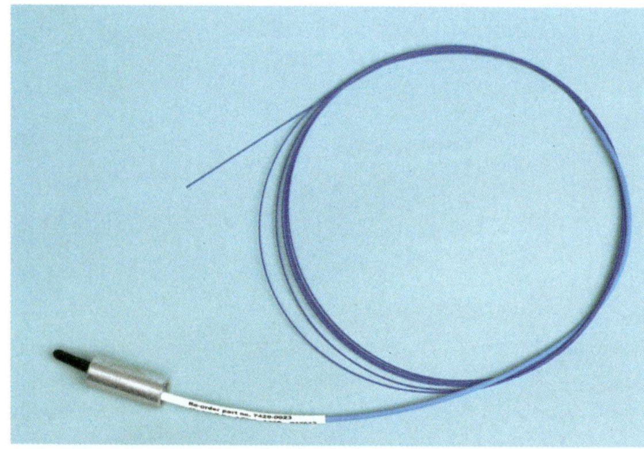

Figure 45-10 The SaphFire™ laser fiber has a rounded tip that requires no sheath during CTEV treatment since there is minimal danger of puncturing the wall of a vein while advancing the fiberoptic. (Used with permission of CoolTouch Inc., Roseville, CA.)

Correct placement of the laser fiber at least 2 cm distal to the saphenofemoral junction or 3 cm distal to the saphenopopliteal junction is confirmed with ultrasound. Tumescent anesthesia is critical to compress the vein. Under ultrasound guidance and with an automatic pullback system, the laser seals the varicose vein from the inside out. Pullback is set for 0.5 mm/sec for the first 2 to 3 cm of the GSV and then 1 mm/sec for the remainder of the treatment. The laser is set for 7 to 8 W at 50 Hz. Once tumescent anesthesia is complete and the tip of the fiber confirmed at 2 cm below the SFJ, the laser is fired for 2 to 3 seconds to visualize sealing of the targeted vein on Duplex. The laser is then stopped for a moment while the pullback device is turned on. Once the laser fiber starts to pull back, the laser is immediately switched on. The progress can be monitored by Duplex or visually by the aiming beam reaching the skin surface from within the vein. As the fiber approaches the entry site, the laser is stopped. Patients can return to work the next day, discomfort is minimal and the rate of successful long-term vein closure is 99% at 8 years. Side effects such as deep-vein thrombus and nerve damage are extremely rare. We have never seen deep-vein thrombosis in our clinic, although it has been reported elsewhere.[28] Please refer to postoperative instructions in Figure 45-11.

Venous Procedure Postoperative Instructions

1. Keep compression hose on until bedtime. Leave compression bandage on until the morning. If toes turn blue or feel numb, loosen the bandage. If symptoms persist, call the doctor immediately.
2. You can resume normal activities today (walking is encouraged).
3. You can resume exercising in 3 days (no weights with the legs for 1 week).
4. You can shower tomorrow but no hot baths for 1 week.
5. Wear your compression hose for the next 3 days, from first thing in the morning until last thing at night.
6. Schedule your next follow-up in 6 weeks.
7. Bruising, numbness, local swelling, and tenderness are normal after surgery, but please fell free to call the office if you have any questions. To help relieve symptoms, 400-mg ibuprofen may be taken in the morning and evening with food for 1–2 weeks.
8. Doctor's emergency phone number is _______________.

Figure 45-11 Venous procedure postoperative instructions.

COMPARISON OF RF TO ENDOVENOUS LASER ABLATION

Our experience is that postoperative pain is greatly reduced with the ClosureFast™ system compared with most laser systems that utilize wavelengths targeting hemoglobin. These include wavelengths of 810, 940, 980, and 1064 nm, but not 1320 and 1470 nm, which target water. Several recent reports of patient experiences kept via a diary indicate less postoperative discomfort with the ClosureFast™ system compared with the 980 nm wavelength.[29,30] In this report, 81 patients returned a home diary (RF ablation = 45, 980 nm laser = 36). Patients receiving RF reported less postoperative pain than those receiving 980 nm at 3 and 10 days. Most significantly those receiving RF via ClosureFast™ returned to work earlier than those receiving 980 nm endovenous ablation (median 5 vs. 9 days).[29] Clinical outcomes were similar at 6 weeks.[30]

When RF is compared to water targeting 1320 nm (CTEV) endovenous laser, postoperative pain is virtually nonexistent and most patients return back to work by the next day. Although these data are not yet published, this is our clinical experience, which we have utilized for hundreds of patients since 2004. Clinical outcomes are excellent with both RF and 1320 nm with successful saphenous occlusion in 90% of original RF, 97.4% ClosureFast™, and 99% of 1320 nm treated GSVs.

CONCLUSION

Endovenous ablation techniques have become the gold standard for the treatment of saphenous reflux. These methods are well proven to offer a less invasive alternative to ligation and stripping. Endoluminal targeting of water rather than hemoglobin is recommended for decreasing patient discomfort as well as obtaining the best possible long-term outcomes. Our clinical experience with endovenous techniques in thousands of patients shows a high degree of success with minimal side effects using RF and 1320 nm laser. Most patients return to work the next day. Tumescent anesthesia is critical to the safety and efficacy of endovenous techniques. Endovenous RF and laser ablation side effects and downtime are reduced with proper wavelength selection for targeting water. Excellent long-term results are achieved with success rate of nonsurgical elimination of saphenous veins in over 98% of patients when proper technique and wavelengths are utilized.

REFERENCE

1. Olgin JE, Kalman JM, Chin M, et al. Electrophysiological effects of long, linear atrial lesions placed under intracardiac ultrasound guidance. *Circulation.* 1997;96(8):2715–2721.
2. Haines DE. The biophysics of radiofrequency catheter ablation in the heart: the importance of temperature monitoring. *Pacing Clin Electrophysiol.* 1993;16(3 Pt 2):586–591.
3. Haines DE, Verow AF. Observations on electrode-tissue interface temperature and effect on electrical impedance during radiofrequency ablation of ventricular myocardium. *Circulation.* 1990;82(3):1034–1038.
4. Lavergne T, Sebag C, Ollitrault J, et al. [Radiofrequency ablation: physical bases and principles]. *Arch Mal Coeur Vaiss.* 1996;89 Spec No 1:57–63.
5. Proebstle TM, Alm J, Gockeritz O, et al; European Closure Fast Clinical Study Group. Three-year European follow-up of endovenous radiofrequency-powered segmental thermal ablation of the great saphenous vein with or without treatment of calf varicosities. *J Vasc Surg.* 2011;54(1): 146–152.
6. Dietzek A, Two-Year Follow-Up Data From A Prospective, Multicenter Study Of The Efficacy Of The ClosureFAST Catheter, 35th Annual Vein Symposium. November 19, 2008. New York.
7. Proebstle T. ClosureFast Long-Term European Multi-Center Study in patients with Chronic Venous Insufficiency (CVI). American College of Phlebology 26th Annual Congress. November 15, 2012 Heidelberg, Germany.
8. Hach-Wunderle V, Hach W. Invasive therapeutic options in truncal varicosity of the great saphenous vein. *Vasa.* 2006;35(3):157–166.
9. Komenaka IK, Nguyen ET. Is there an increased risk for DVT with the VNUS closure procedure? *J Vasc Surg.* 2002; 36(6):1311.
10. Proebstle TM, Sandhofer M, Kargl A, et al. Thermal damage of the inner vein wall during endovenous laser treatment: key role of energy absorption by intravascular blood. *Dermatol Surg.* 2002;28(7):596–600.
11. Weiss RA. Comparison of endovenous radiofrequency versus 810 nm diode laser occlusion of large veins in an animal model. *Dermatol Surg.* 2002;28(1):56–61.
12. de Medeiros CA, Luccas GC. Comparison of endovenous treatment with an 810 nm laser versus conventional stripping of the great saphenous vein in patients with primary varicose veins. *Dermatol Surg.* 2005;31(12):1685–1694.
13. Navarro L, Min RJ, Bone C. Endovenous laser: a new minimally invasive method of treatment for varicose veins–preliminary observations using an 810 nm diode laser. *Dermatol Surg.* 2001;27(2):117–122.
14. Min RJ, Zimmet SE, Isaacs MN, Forrestal MD. Endovenous laser treatment of the incompetent greater saphenous vein. *J Vasc Interv Radiol.* 2001;12(10):1167–1171.
15. Min RJ, Khilnani N, Zimmet SE. Endovenous laser treatment of saphenous vein reflux: long-term results. *J Vasc Interv Radiol.* 2003;14(8):991–996.
16. Bush RG. Regarding "Endovenous treatment of the greater saphenous vein with a 940-nm diode laser: thrombolytic occlusion after endoluminal thermal damage by laser-generated steam bubbles". *J Vasc Surg.* 2003;37(1):242.
17. Desmyttere J, Grard C, Wassmer B, Mordon S. Endovenous 980-nm laser treatment of saphenous veins in a series of 500 patients. *J Vasc Surg.* 2007;46(6):1242–1247.
18. Proebstle TM, Lehr HA, Kargl A, et al. Endovenous treatment of the greater saphenous vein with a 940-nm diode laser: thrombotic occlusion after endoluminal thermal damage by laser-generated steam bubbles. *J Vasc Surg.* 2002;35(4): 729–736.
19. Sharif MA, Soong CV, Lau LL, Corvan R, Lee B, Hannon RJ. Endovenous laser treatment for long saphenous vein incompetence. *Br J Surg.* 2006;93(7):831–835.
20. Proebstle TM, Moehler T, Gül D, Herdemann S. Endovenous treatment of the great saphenous vein using a 1320 nm Nd:YAG laser causes fewer side effects than using a 940 nm diode laser. *Dermatol Surg.* 2005;31(12):1678–1683.
21. Hennings T, Hennings D, Lindsay C. Thrombus formation using endovenous lasers: an in vitro experiment. *Phlebology.* 2013;29(3):1–8.
22. Chang CJ, Chua JJ. Endovenous laser photocoagulation (EVLP) for varicose veins. *Lasers Surg Med.* 2002;31(4): 257–262.
23. Weiss R, Weiss M, Beasley K. *Sclerotharapy and Vein Treatment.* 2nd ed. New York, NY: McGraw Hill; 2011. Chapter 21;p.165.
24. Pannier F, Rabe E, Maurins U. First results with a new 1470-nm diode laser for endovenous ablation of incompetent saphenous veins. *Phlebology.* 2009;24(1):26–30.
25. Almeida J, Mackay E, Javier J, Mauriello J, Raines J. Saphenous laser ablation at 1470 nm targets the vein wall, not blood. *Vasc Endovascular Surg.* 2009;43(5):467–472.

26. Vuylsteke M, Van DJ, Roelens J, De BT, Mordon S. Endovenous laser treatment: a morphological study in an animal model. *Phlebology*. 2009;24(4):166–175.
27. Lapid O. Syringe-Delivered tumescent anesthesia made easier. *Aesthetic Plast Surg*. 2011;35(4):601–602.
28. Knipp BS, Blackburn SA, Bloom JR, et al.; Michigan Venous Study Group. Endovenous laser ablation: venous outcomes and thrombotic complications are independent of the presence of deep venous insufficiency. *J Vasc Surg*. 2008;48(6):1538–1545.
29. Shepherd AC, Gohel MS, Lim CS, Hamish M, Davies AH. Pain following 980-nm endovenous laser ablation and segmental radiofrequency ablation for varicose veins: a prospective observational study. *Vasc Endovascular Surg*. 2010;44(3):212–216.
30. Shepherd AC, Gohel MS, Brown LC, Metcalfe MJ, Hamish M, Davies AH. Randomized clinical trial of VNUS ClosureFAST radiofrequency ablation versus laser for varicose veins. *Br J Surg*. 2010;97(6):810–818.

CHAPTER 46

Phototherapy and Photodynamic Therapy for the Treatment of Acne Vulgaris

Michael H. Gold

INTRODUCTION

Acne vulgaris, by all accounts, is the most common skin concern seen regularly by dermatologists in their clinical practices. By some estimates, patient visits for treating acne vulgaris and dealing with its associated sequelae make up roughly one-third of all visits to dermatology offices in the United States.[1] This is a very high percentage, and for this reason alone, we, as dermatologists, need to stay at the forefront of new therapeutic options and ideas, to foster new medical approaches for our patients when appropriate, and to offer alternative forms of therapy to best manage those suffering from acne vulgaris. These "other" forms of therapy may involve non-medical therapy for our patients, including the use of lasers and light sources, and may at times involve use of photosensitizers that sensitize the pilosebaceous glands to an appropriate laser or light source.

Why care about treating acne vulgaris, especially in a procedural manner, when there are many other procedures that make patients look and feel younger and more beautiful? Why care about a skin condition that occurs predominantly in children and in young adults? And why care about a skin disease that, more and more, is being cared for by our primary care colleagues so we can concentrate on the more glamorous cosmetic concerns?

Acne vulgaris affects almost all individuals at some point in their lifetime, with reports noting that as many as 94% of all females in the United States will suffer from acne vulgaris.[2] The percentage in men is slightly lower than that in women but is still significant. It is important for dermatologists to be at the forefront of new therapies and modalities to enhance those therapeutic options. As a point of reference, it can be noted that 20 years ago, the dermatologist was the usual first point of contact care for those suffering with acne vulgaris. Over the past 20 years, many acne patients have first been treated by non-dermatologists, whether the pediatrician or family physician for the younger group of patients, or by a host of other physicians in the older patient population, including the family physician, the internist, and the gynecologist, among others. More recently, a variety of over-the-counter skin care and acne products have emerged as "wonder" products, which have become first-line therapy for patients who attempt to avoid a medical visit to their dermatologist.

Dermatologists need to embrace the care of those suffering from and with acne vulgaris. We need to be at the forefront of treating and counseling those with this skin concern and realize that the number of patients who will be helped by our skills is remarkable. With many of the newer therapeutic modalities now available, including the use of photosensitizers with lasers and light sources, we have incredible "tools" at our disposal to help almost every patient who suffers from acne vulgaris.

ETIOLOGY AND PATHOGENESIS OF ACNE VULGARIS

Acne vulgaris is considered a multifactorial skin condition with both genetic and hormonal influences playing a role in the origin of this disease and its progression over time.

Most patients with acne have a strong family history of acne vulgaris in their parents or close relatives. Hormonal influences are also strongly involved in the pathogenesis of acne. The formation of sebum in the pilosebaceous glands begins at or shortly before puberty, which leads to overproduction of sebum in the follicular unit. This overproduction leads to the formation of what is typically called the follicular "plug," one of the earliest events in the formation of the acne vulgaris skin lesion.

In addition to genetics and hormonal influences, environmental concerns, on occasion, also play a role in the development of acne vulgaris.[3] We all have had patients who note that stress is causing their breakouts or that eating this food or drinking that soft drink causes their acne to flare. Although there is much more study to be done, most dermatologists believe that the environment can influence the course of acne, but it is not a direct reason for our patients to develop it, especially without the other factors already in place. Readers are encouraged to seek out other references to learn more about how hormones and environmental factors can influence the course of acne vulgaris, which will not be covered further in this chapter.

Acne vulgaris is a disorder of the pilosebaceous unit. Detailed descriptions are available elsewhere on the current understanding of this process. When the production of sebum increases, this causes the follicular unit to become dilated, which is then followed by obstruction of the sebaceous glands, resulting in the first phase of the acne lesion, known as the comedone. This non-inflammatory acne lesion takes the form of the open comedone, or whitehead, or the closed comedone, the blackhead. With obstruction of the sebaceous gland, there is proliferation and production of bacterial species within the gland itself. The most common bacterium in the sebaceous gland associated with acne vulgaris is known as *Propionobacterium acnes*. With the proliferation of *P. acnes* comes an associated inflammatory response within the gland, resulting in acne lesions, commonly known as papules, pustules, and cysts. It is during this crucial phase that many cytokines and inflammatory mediators, which are the means by which some of our new therapeutic modalities benefit our patients, come into play.[4]

MEDICAL THERAPY FOR ACNE VULGARIS

Despite the hype for lasers and light sources in dermatology, the gold standard for the treatment of acne vulgaris remains medical therapy. There are a variety of medical therapies that have proven worthwhile in the treatment of acne. Guidelines of care regarding how these medicines should be used assure the most appropriate outcomes for our patients suffering from non-inflammatory acne vulgaris and inflammatory acne vulgaris.[5,6] The aim of this section is to give an overview of the most common therapeutic modalities. Lasers and light therapies and photodynamic therapy (PDT) also have their places and their roles in the treatment armamentarium and will be explained shortly.

Topical therapy has been a mainstay for the treatment of acne vulgaris for many years and numerous therapies exist, which, when used appropriately, can truly be of benefit to our patients. Most of the current guidelines for the treatment of acne recommend that all patients utilize a topical retinoid in their regimens. Topical retinoids are known to reverse follicular keratinization and improve comedones. They come as stand-alone products or as combination products, either with the addition of benzoyl peroxide or a topical antibiotic. All of these newer combination products have shown superiority compared to a topical retinoid alone in clinical trials, supporting their increased use in dermatology. Topical antibiotics and benzoyl peroxides still have their place in the treatment of acne vulgaris as well, although benzoyl peroxides have recently gone over the counter and are not being promoted as they once were. A topical dapsone has also been recently introduced. Dapsone is known as an oral anti-inflammatory agent but this has been shown to be the case topically as well. Clinical trials with topical dapsone have shown that female acne vulgaris patients actually respond better than their male counterparts, so this therapy has gained widespread use among dermatologists for treating female acne vulgaris sufferers.[3]

One of the more interesting facets of topical therapy recently has been the vehicle in which newer medicines and combination medicines are being placed. We are finding that the vehicles elicit their own effects in many instances; these enhanced vehicles may themselves play a future role in topical therapy. Several new research initiatives are looking at some of these more unique vehicles to understand their future potential in dermatology.

Systemic therapy also is commonly used, especially when we have patients presenting with inflammatory acne or mixed non-inflammatory and inflammatory acne lesions. Once again, guidelines of care exist, which the reader is encouraged to read to further enhance their understanding of the rationale for proper use of these therapies.[5,6] Systemic agents utilized early on to treat acne vulgaris were oral erythromycin and tetracycline. These medicines are rarely used today and have been replaced by oral minocycline and doxycycline, the most commonly prescribed systemic agents used for acne vulgaris. In order to differentiate themselves from one another and from generic equivalents, many dose forms and extended release formulations have become available. As dermatologists, we must know the differences between the various brand and generic equivalents and determine whether the generic formulations are appropriate or whether should we utilize brand name pharmaceuticals. Dermatologists also sometimes use systemic sulfonamides, which are useful in cases when other systemic agents are not effective. Oral contraceptives and antiandrogenic medications are also used by many in treating what is sometimes described as hormonal acne in the young adult female patient. Again, the reader is encouraged to learn more about these medicines, their clinical indications, and their supporting evidence, outside of this chapter.[5,6]

The treatment of severe inflammatory acne vulgaris changed dramatically with the discovery and availability of oral isotretinoin. Isotretinoin is indicated for the treatment of recalcitrant cystic acne vulgaris. Many patients and for that matter, many dermatologists, have found this drug to be a wonder drug in the treatment of acne vulgaris and again, dermatologists are fortunate to have this drug at the ready when needed. One must remember that isotretinoin use is currently under the auspices of the iPledge program and that all patients and physicians prescribing isotretinoin utilize this program to assure that patients are being properly monitored throughout their course of treatment. Most patients require isotretinoin in doses of 1 mg/kg/day and continue therapy for 20 weeks, with monitoring done every 4 weeks. Isotretinoin may be teratogenic in women who become pregnant while on the drug and has an associated potential for psychiatric effects in a small percentage of patients, necessitating the need for strict and accurate monitoring.[3]

The use of systemic medicines for those suffering from inflammatory acne is crucial when needed. Unfortunately, several recent developments and reports have made the use of these medications to be considered somewhat suspect. This includes reports of systemic antibiotic resistance to the *P. acnes* lesions, with some noting antibiotic resistance as high as 60% to current medical regimens.[7,8] Other interesting reports that are important to mention include one linking an increase in breast cancer to long-term antibiotic use[9] and another linking long-term antibiotic use to an increased risk of pulmonary infections in some individuals.[10] The restrictions and mandates of the iPledge system, designed to reduce the risks from the use of isotretinoin, are also associated with more paperwork than some offices are willing to accept.

Once again, medical therapy remains the gold standard for the treatment of both non-inflammatory and inflammatory acne vulgaris. Dermatologists are fortunate to have medicines that are tried and true for their patients, as well as newer combination compounds that have synergistic effects to combat acne vulgaris. Pharmaceutical companies are also working diligently on new formulations and compounds that will aid our patients even more in the future.

However, not every patient responds to the therapies just described. Some are interested in other therapeutic modalities. Others may not want to endure the mandatory waiting period that can exist for the iPledge program—especially those who are not on a contraceptive medicine. One of the options that has become more and more popular in the past several years is the use of lasers and light sources in the treatment of acne. The remainder of this chapter will deal with the use of lasers, light therapy, and PDT in the treatment of acne vulgaris.

LASERS AND LIGHT SOURCES FOR THE TREATMENT OF INFLAMMATORY ACNE VULGARIS

When using lasers and light therapy for the treatment of inflammatory acne, we need to consider the varied mechanisms of action used by these medical devices to make lesions improve. One mechanism of action is by selective destruction of the *P. acnes* bacterium itself. This process occurs from light that penetrates into the sebaceous gland and causes selective destruction of bacteria and their associated gland. The second mechanism that has been commonly used in the past is destruction of the sebaceous gland through a thermal reaction using light or laser energy that targets water as a chromophore. A third mechanism of action is partial destruction of the sebaceous gland, which is the mechanism most commonly described with PDT, as will be discussed later.[4]

LASERS AND LIGHT SOURCES THAT DESTROY *PROPIONOBACTERIUM ACNES*

Several light sources and lasers may be used for the selective destruction of *P. acnes*. These include both the blue and red light sources, green light lasers, yellow light lasers, and the intense pulsed light source, commonly known as the IPL. These lasers and light sources work through what is known as an endogenous PDT response.

Propionobacterium acnes demonstrates a PDT response that naturally occurs in the skin. During its growth cycle, *P. acnes* produces porphyrins, predominantly protoporphyrin IX (PpIX) and coproporphyrin III. These porphyrins have an absorption spectrum of light that is demonstrated in Figure 46-1 for PpIX. Coproporphyrin III has a similar absorption spectrum. From the graph, we can see that the major peak for PpIX is in the blue range of light at 415 nm, and this peak is commonly referred to as the Soret band of absorption. A second major absorption peak is also seen at about 630 nm, corresponding to red light. Both blue and red light sources have been used routinely over the past 10 years to treat inflammatory acne vulgaris and will be reviewed later. One should appreciate, however, from the absorption spectrum, that other, smaller peaks also exist, explaining why other lasers and light sources can be useful for the treatment of acne vulgaris. These include, as noted earlier, the green light lasers at 532 nm, the yellow light lasers at 585 to 595 nm, and the IPL, which emits energies via flashlamps and a series of "cut-off" filters in the range typically between 400 to 1200 nm. Based on the filters being used, light below the "cut-off" filter will be blocked.[3]

Blue light therapy for the treatment of inflammatory acne vulgaris has been reviewed extensively in the medical literature.[11–17] There have been three major blue light

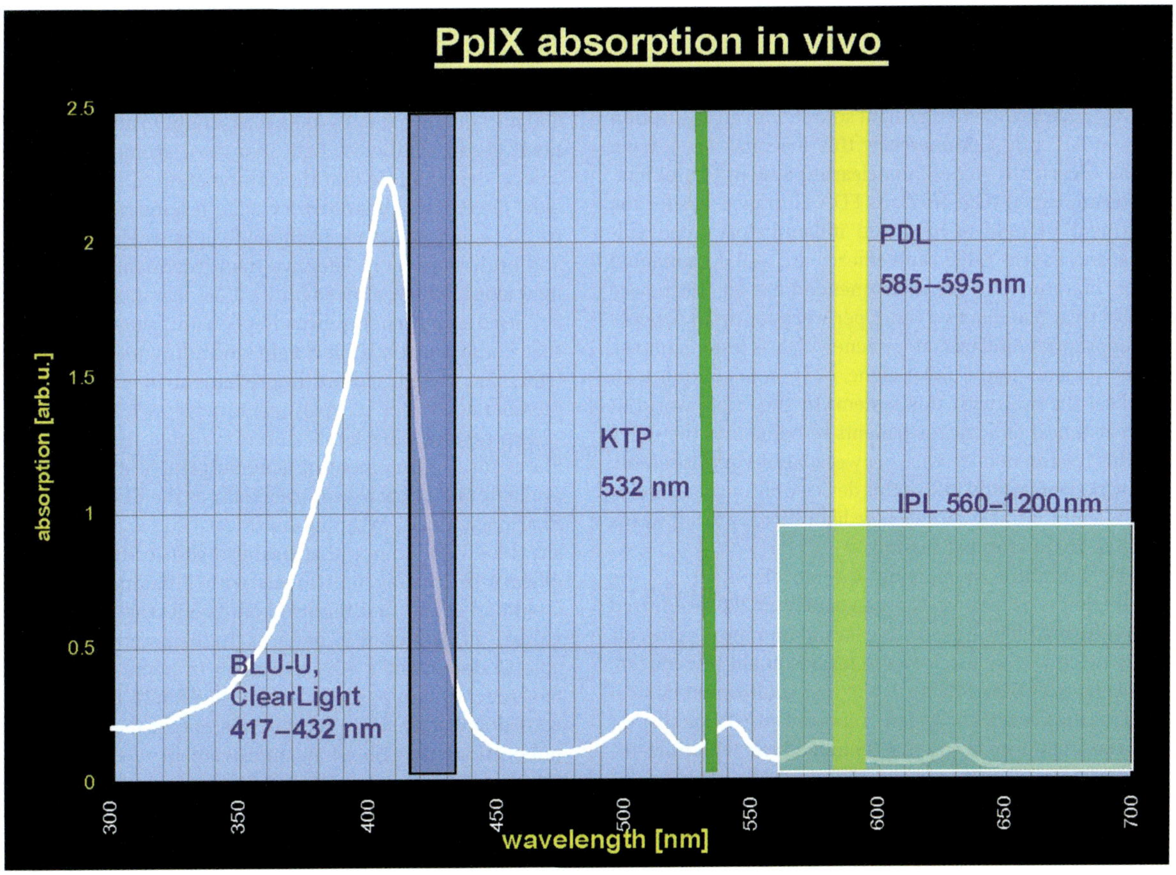

Figure 46-1 Absorption spectrum of PpIX. (Used with permission from Michael H. Gold, M.D.)

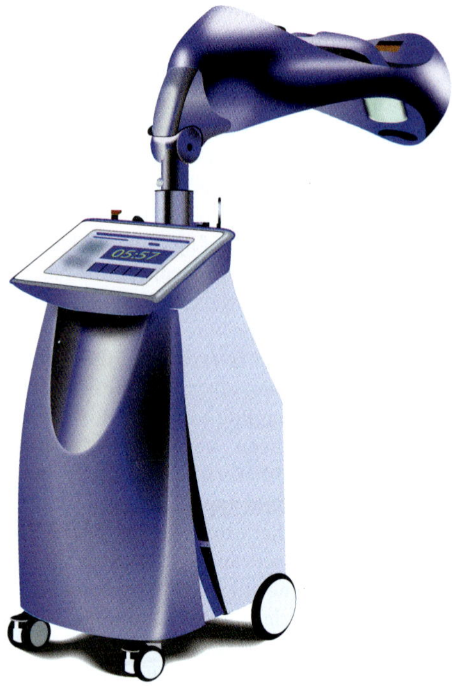

Figure 46-2 ClearLight acne clearing device. (Used with permission from Michael H. Gold, M.D.)

systems available for the treatment of inflammatory acne in the United States. The reader should be aware that other blue light systems have since come and gone throughout the years and although they may be comparable to what is described later, each system is unique and should be studied on its own.

The first FDA-approved, blue light source was a high-intensity, narrow-band blue light source with an absorption peak at 417 nm. Commercially this machine was known as the ClearLight Acne Photoclearing System (CureLight, Yokneam, Israel) (Fig. 46-2). Its FDA clearance was for the treatment of mild-to-moderate inflammatory acne vulgaris, and its use, safety, and efficacy are well documented in the literature.[12,13] The recommended use for this device was to treat patients two times per week for up to 4 weeks for appropriate inflammatory acne vulgaris lesion control. Many patients found relief alone, or in combination with medical therapy, with this system. In the "real" world, it was, at times, difficult for patients to come into the office for this treatment on a twice per week basis. For this reason, many patients would utilize this device only once per week, and would routinely receive blue light therapy for upwards of 15 to 20 minutes per session.

The literature supporting the development of the ClearLight is as follows. Kawada et al.,[11] in 2002, reported that by using a blue light source for inflammatory acne vulgaris twice weekly for 5 weeks, lesions could be reduced, on average, by 64%. Shalita et al.,[12] in a multicenter clinical trial for the ClearLight system, reported an 80% significant improvement rate in treating 35 individuals with mild-to-moderate inflammatory acne twice weekly for 4 weeks. Of note was that following therapy, further acne improvement was noted in many of the patients who entered into this study. Adverse events were not seen and all skin types were successfully treated.

Gold reported on 40 individuals treated with the ClearLight system for mild-to-moderate inflammatory acne vulgaris.[13] The patients in this clinical trial also received blue light therapy twice weekly for 4 weeks and were followed-up 1 and 3 months after their final treatment. A 43% reduction in acne lesions was noted in this trial. Adverse events, similar to the previous work, were not seen and lesions continued to improve in many patients during the follow-up period. When comparing the clinical trials of both Gold and Shalita, Gold's data included both "responders" and "nonresponders," something that was not done in Shalita's clinical trial. It has been noted that upwards of 20% of individuals treated with the blue light system are nonresponders. Adding them into the total percentage of clearance would certainly have brought the two clinical trials closer together in terms of the percentage clearance. From these clinical trials, the safety and efficacy of this blue light system was confirmed and it became one of the most popular light-based acne treatment systems in the United States in the 2000s.

For a variety of reasons, the ClearLight, high-intensity, blue light system is currently not available commercially, and its replacement device, known commercially as the IClear, is also no longer available. Many still utilize these light sources in their clinical practices, and they have made a major difference for many patients suffering from inflammatory acne who either had not been adequately controlled with medical therapy or who were looking for a faster path to lesion clearance. Clinical examples of the use of the ClearLight system are shown in Figures 46-3 and 46-4.

Several other clinical trials regarding blue light are worth reviewing for the sake of completeness, and several other blue light sources are also worthy of mention for the treatment of inflammatory acne vulgaris. Papageorgiou et al.[14] used a mixed blue and red light system (415 nm and 660 nm) in one patient group, a blue light in another treatment group, and white light in a third group. They were able to demonstrate that the combination of blue and red light decreased inflammatory acne lesions by 76% compared to 58% clearance in the blue light treatment group, and both were more effective than treatment with white light alone, which showed only a 25% clearance. Meffert et al.[15] used a high-energy, broad-spectrum, blue light source that combined both blue light and ultraviolet A (UVA) light, and noted marked improvement in patients with pustular acne after 10 treatments.

The second blue light source available in the United States for the treatment of acne vulgaris is still currently available and is known commercially as the BLU-U (DUSA Pharmaceuticals, Wilmington, MA). This is a low-intensity, blue light source that has also shown its safety and efficacy in treating individuals with inflammatory acne. Goldman et al.[16] first reported on its effectiveness in acne vulgaris in a series of 12 patients. In their study, they were able to document a 40% reduction in papular lesions, a 65% reduction in pustular lesions, and a 62% reduction in comedonal acne. Of note, this was one of the first major publications that noted an improvement not only in the inflammatory component of acne vulgaris with blue light but also in the non-inflammatory lesions. The improvements described were seen as early as 2 weeks of therapy, similar to what had been reported with the high-intensity blue light systems. Gold et al.[17] followed up on the previous

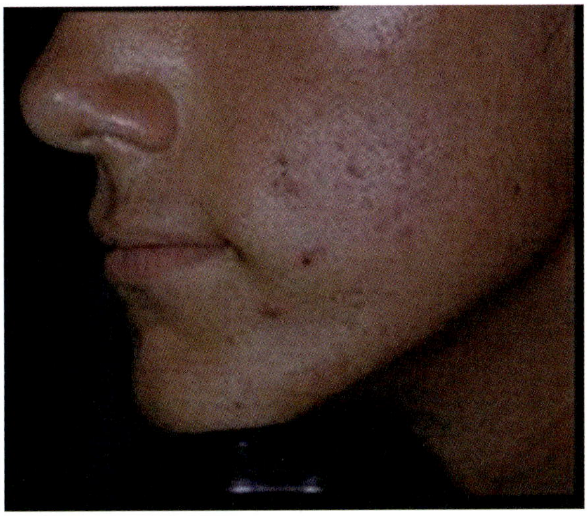

Figure 46-3 Patient before treatment with the ClearLight. (Used with permission from Michael H. Gold, M.D.)

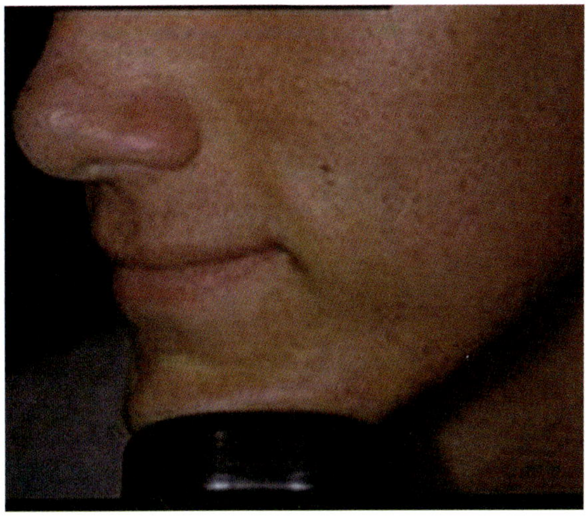

Figure 46-4 Patient after treatment with the ClearLight. (Used with permission from Michael H. Gold, M.D.)

report and did a comparison clinical trial of topical 1% clindamycin solution versus blue light therapy in patients with mild to moderate inflammatory acne vulgaris. They demonstrated that blue light therapy was more effective than topical clindamycin in reducing inflammatory acne vulgaris lesions. The BLU-U device available commercially is shown in Figure 46-5. A recent clinical evaluation looking at blue light therapy with the BLU-U and its effect on acne vulgaris with or without a topical photosensitizer demonstrated that blue light alone was statistically significant in improving severe inflammatory acne vulgaris, leading to a supplemental FDA filing, which was granted

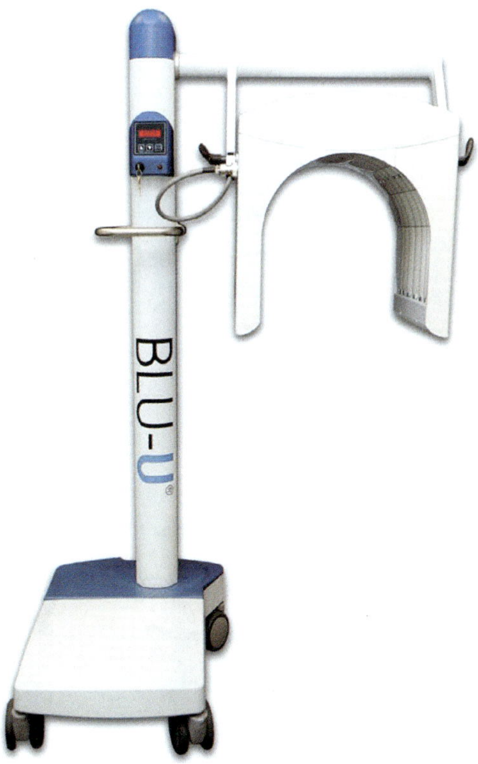

Figure 46-5 BLU-U device. (Used with permission from DUSA Pharmaceuticals, Inc.)

for this claim.[18] Clinical examples utilizing the BLU-U for inflammatory acne vulgaris are shown in Figures 46-6 and 46-7. Patients utilize this system in a fashion similar to that of the high-intensity, blue light system—once or two times per week for 4 to 6 weeks is the norm, with patients receiving 15 to 20 minutes of blue light therapy per treatment.

A third blue light source developed for the treatment on inflammatory acne vulgaris is called the OmniLux Blue Phototherapeutics System (OmniLux, Manchester, UK). Clinical studies have also shown its effectiveness in treating inflammatory acne vulgaris. It used LED blue light arrays with a peak irradiance of 410 to 420 nm and has shown lesion reductions of up to 74% in clinical trials.[19]

It should be noted that there are a variety of home-use blue light sources available for patients. The home-use blue light devices will not be discussed here; there are other reviews that are readily available. Many patients find these devices useful and are using them on a regular basis.[20]

Clinical studies with red light alone are not widely available in the medical literature,[21,22] but a variety of red light sources are also available commercially, which can be utilized for the treatment of inflammatory acne vulgaris. The use of red light devices, however, is quite widespread, especially in association with the methyl form of aminolevulinic acid (ALA), which will be discussed later in this chapter. Zane et al.[21] performed a split-face randomized red light trial in 28 patients on a home-use red light source device. Statistical improvement was noted with acne vulgaris lesions improving more on the treated side versus the non-treated side. Red light, because of its longer wavelength as compared to blue light, penetrates more deeply than blue light, including within the follicular unit, and thus may have benefits beyond those of blue light alone. Blue light has been shown, through clinical studies, to be virtually painless for patients receiving treatment; red light, however, can be painful, which may limit its overall use for patients with acne vulgaris. Greater study of this phenomenon needs to be performed.[23]

Green and yellow light lasers also have been reported to improve inflammatory acne vulgaris.[24–26] Bowes et al.[24] treated 11 patients with mild-to-moderate inflammatory acne in a split-face, prospective, randomized clinical trial

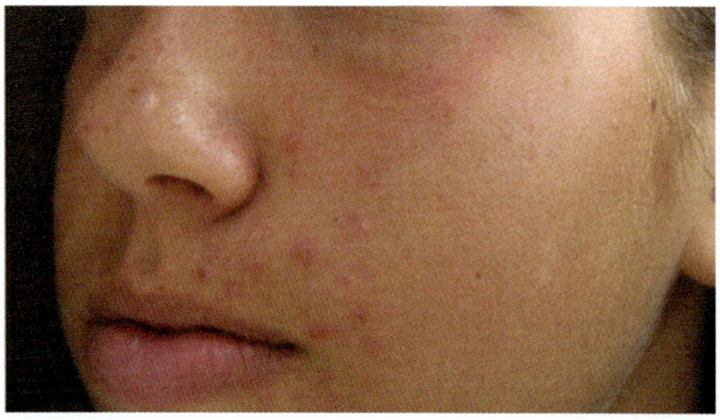

Figure 46-6 Patient before treatment with the BLU-U for acne. (Used with permission from Michael H. Gold, M.D.)

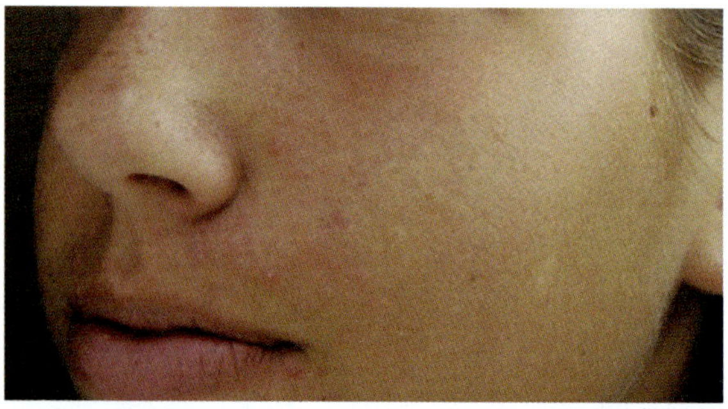

Figure 46-7 Patient after treatment with the BLU-U for acne. (Used with permission from Michael H. Gold, M.D.)

with a 532 nm laser system. Four treatments were given, at monthly intervals, and there was a 1 month follow-up visit. Lesion counts decreased by 35.9% on the treated side versus 11.8% on the controlled, non-treated side. Sebum measurements were also made and were shown to have decreased by 28.1% on the treated side versus 6.4% on the control side. KTP laser systems are used regularly in many clinics for the treatment of telangiectasias, but can also be used for the treatment of inflammatory acne vulgaris.

Yellow light pulsed dye lasers (PDLs) can also effectively treat inflammatory acne vulgaris. PDLs were developed to treat vascular lesions, predominantly port-wine stains and hemangiomas. Since their introduction into the market, a variety of cutaneous disorders have been shown to be treatable with PDLs, including hypertrophic scars, keloids, and recalcitrant verrucous lesions. Several PDLs are currently available on the US market and the reader can find out more about them in other sections of this textbook. Seaton et al.[25] evaluated 41 individuals with inflammatory acne treated with a low-fluence PDL. In this double-blind, randomized clinical trial 31 patients received PDL treatments and 10 patients received sham treatments. One treatment was given to all patients. Acne severity decreased from 3.8 to 1.9 in the PDL group versus 3.6 to 3.5 in the sham treatment group (using a modified Leeds grading system). The second clinical trial, by Orringer et al.,[26] did not confirm these results and, in fact, found no improvement with this particular low-fluence device. As noted, there are several PDLs available. When utilized with appropriate settings, these devices can be used to treat inflammatory acne. More research, however, is required before definitive answers can be given with respect to the effectiveness of these devices in treating inflammatory acne vulgaris.

IPLs also have been studied for the treatment of acne.[27,28] There are a myriad of systems available and the reader must decide which system works best for them and whether to use these devices for the treatment of inflammatory acne. These devices were first developed for the treatment of leg veins, then hair removal, and then pigment. In 2000, IPL became known as the therapy of choice for photorejuvenation.[29] In photorejuvenation, IPLs can effectively treat the vascular components and pigment associated with aging and have an effect on the collagen and elastic tissues that improves the texture and tone of the skin. The first clinical use of IPL in the treatment of inflammatory acne vulgaris used a low-powered device known as the ClearTouch (Radiancy Inc., Orangeburg, NY) or the SkinStation. This IPL device used light and heat energy, known as "LHE technology," to trigger destruction of the *P. acnes* bacteria. Elman et al.[27] treated 19 patients with twice weekly therapy for 4 weeks and demonstrated that 85% of the individuals had a greater than 50% improvement in their inflammatory acne. In another study, Dierickx et al. reported on the use of the LuxV handpiece (Palomar Medical Technologies, Burlington, MA) IPL system known at the time as the EsteLux. Newer models have included the MediLux and the StarLux systems. Fourteen patients with mild-to-moderate inflammatory acne vulgaris each received five treatments, given every 2 to 4 weeks. Two to three passes were performed in each treatment with an average fluence of 10 J/cm^2. Six months after the last treatment, 73% improvement was noted in the inflammatory acne lesions and 72% in the non-inflammatory lesions.

Of note is the recent development of IPL systems with an associated vacuum apparatus that are now popular in

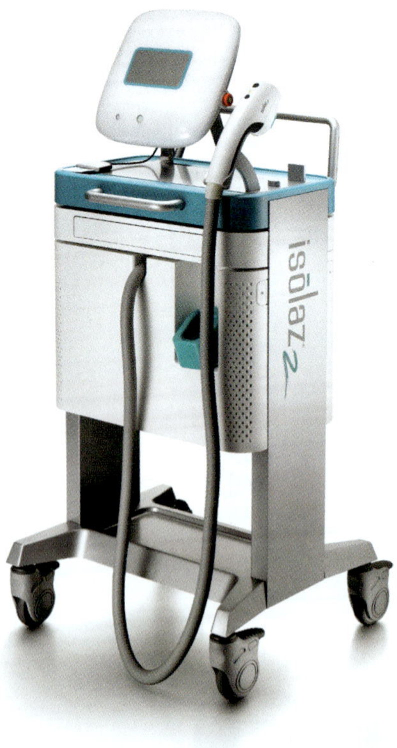

Figure 46-8 Isolaz®. (Reproduced with permission of Solta Medical, Inc.; courtesy of Solta Medical Aesthetic Center.)

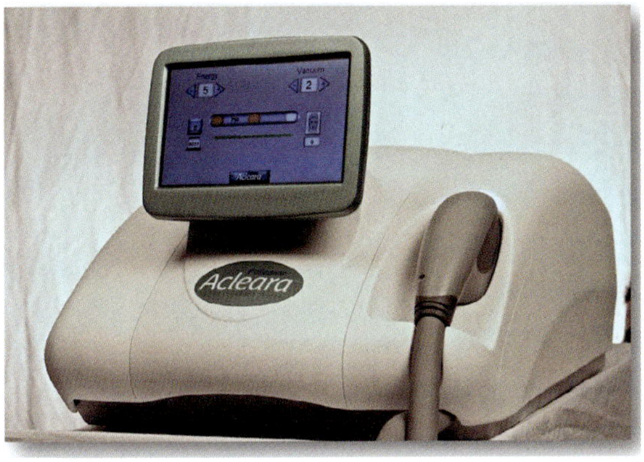

Figure 46-9 Acleara. (Used with permission of Cynosure, Inc.)

treating both inflammatory and non-inflammatory acne lesions, for which they now have FDA clearance. Two such devices are currently on the market. The first device, shown in Figure 46-8, is known as the Isolaz (Solta Medical, Hayward, CA) and the second device is called the Acleara (Palomar Medical, Boston, MA), shown in Figure 46-9. Several clinical trials have shown their effectiveness in the treatment of acne.[30–32] Their mechanism is quite interesting—by using the vacuum, one can essentially clean out the acne pore and its accompanying sebum. The light then selectively destroys the *P. acnes* in the sebaceous gland, thus generating both inflammatory and non-inflammatory acne improvement. This mechanism of action is shown schematically in Figure 46-10.

In the first report on the use of this device, Munavalli and Weiss reported their experience in 10 patients treated with the Isolaz. Patients received four treatments at one-week intervals and were given two to four passes with the device per session. Treatment sessions lasted no more than 15 minutes and no topical anesthesia was given. The patients were followed for 1 month after their last treatment. The median time for improvement was 5 days, with some patients noting improvement in as little as 2 days. Lesion counts for papules decreased 50% to 60%, for pustules 70% to 80%, and for comedones 40% to 50%. There were no adverse events noted. Shamban et al.[31] carried out a retrospective evaluation of 56 individuals and showed a 50% reduction after the first treatment, which increased to 90% after four treatments. In a study published in 2008,[32] Gold et al. treated 11 individuals with the Isolaz at 3 week intervals for four treatments. The patients were followed for 3 months after their last treatment. The study found that a 78% reduction (p = 0.0137) was achieved in inflammatory acne lesions and a 57.8% reduction (p = 0.0383) in non-inflammatory acne lesions. Pain was minimal and was most likely associated with the vacuum itself. Side effects were not seen. Patients treated with the Isolaz are shown in Figures 46-11 and 46-12. A second-generation device, known as the Acleara, is also now available (Palomar Medical); this device has a cooling system built for added safety.

LASERS THAT DESTROY SEBACEOUS GLANDS

The second group of lasers that has been used in treating acne vulgaris consists of lasers that destroy the sebaceous glands themselves. These include the near-infrared lasers and possibly the radiofrequency (RF) devices. Although all seem to have been effective in the treatment of acne vulgaris, it is not clear how many of these devices are still in use for the treatment of acne. Pain with treatment was significant and for that reason alone, many clinicians stopped using these therapies. However, the literature does support their effectiveness.[33–39]

The near-infrared lasers used to treat acne vulgaris include the 1064 nm lasers, the 1319 nm Sciton Profile (Sciton, Palo Alto, CA), the 1320 nm CoolTouch CT3 (CoolTouch Inc., Roseville, CA), the 1450 nm SmoothBeam (Candela,

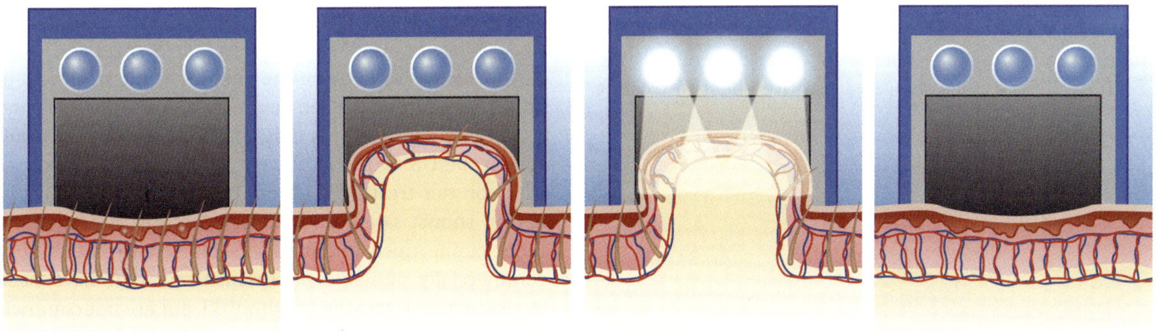

Figure 46-10 Mechanism of action of PPX. (Used with permission from Michael H. Gold, M.D.)

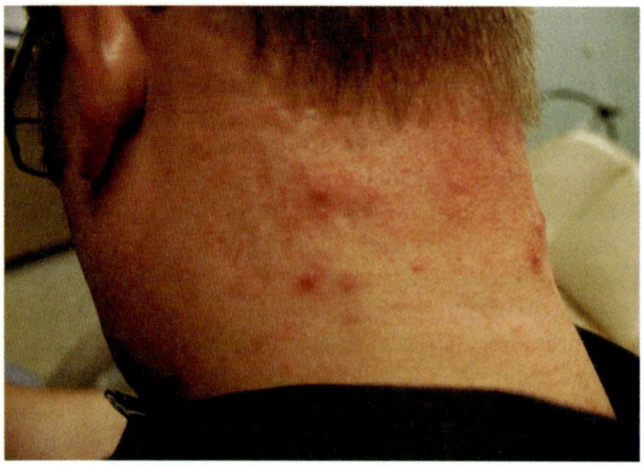

Figure 46-11 Patient before treatment with the Isolaz. (Used with permission from Michael H. Gold, M.D.)

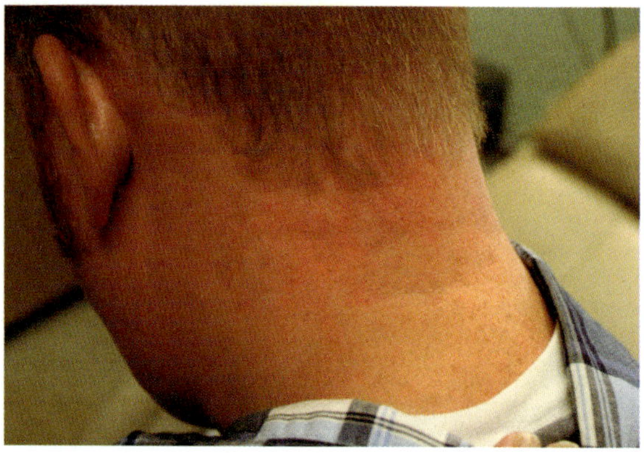

Figure 46-12 Patient after treatment with the Isolaz. (Used with permission from Michael H. Gold, M.D.)

Wayland, MA), and the 1540 nm erbium glass Aramis (WaveLight-Quantel, Clermont-Ferrant, France).

Of all the laser systems noted earlier, the Smooth-Beam has the most literature supporting its effectiveness in destroying sebaceous glands and for the treatment of inflammatory acne. Paithankar et al.[33] reported their experience with this device and its associated patented dynamic cooling device (Fig. 46-13) in treating 27 individuals with inflammatory acne vulgaris on the back. Four treatments were given at 3 week intervals and the patients were followed for 6 months after their last treatment. A 98% reduction in inflammatory acne lesions was demonstrated after the four treatment sessions and at 6 months, all but one of the patients demonstrated 100% lesion clearance. Friedman et al.[34] evaluated 19 patients with facial acne vulgaris and noted a 37% reduction in acne lesions after one treatment, a 58% reduction after two treatments, and an 83% reduction after three treatments. Transient erythema and edema were seen; topical anesthesia was needed to reduce discomfort from the therapy. Newer protocols and a new handpiece were introduced to reduce the pain component,[35] but most clinics have stopped treating patients with this device at the time of this writing.

Other clinical studies have evaluated the use of photosensitizers and laser systems in treating inflammatory acne vulgaris. Tuchin et al.[36] and Lloyd et al.[37] used indocyanine green and a diode laser to destroy sebaceous glands. Both of these studies showed a positive effect in treating inflammatory acne. Indocyanine green is not readily available so this photosensitizer is not commonly used in clinical practice. The 1540 nm laser has been used by Kassir et al.[38] in treating patients with inflammatory acne vulgaris. They evaluated 20 patients, treating with this device every 2 weeks for four sessions, and noted a 70% improvement over 3 months. No adverse effects were reported. Ruiz-Esparza et al.[39] reported an observation using a monopolar RF device in the treatment of inflammatory acne vulgaris. In 22 patients, excellent responses were noted in 82%, moderate responses in 9%, and no response in 9%. Further work is needed to see what further potential RF devices may have for the treatment of inflammatory acne.

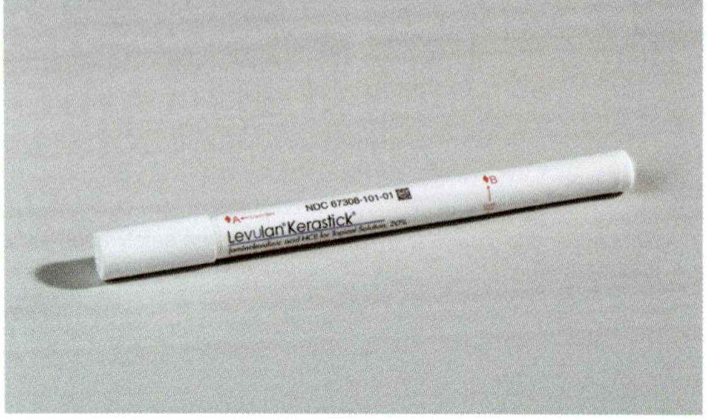

Figure 46-13 Levulan Kerastick. (Used with permission from DUSA Pharmaceuticals, Inc.)

PHOTODYNAMIC THERAPY IN THE TREATMENT OF ACNE VULGARIS

PDT with either 5-aminolevulinic acid (ALA) or methyl aminolevulinate (MAL) applied topically has shown efficacy in the treatment of acne vulgaris in small, investigator-initiated clinical trials. Although neither photosensitizing agent is FDA-cleared for the treatment of acne by PDT, both—ALA as Levulan® Kerastick® (DUSA Pharmaceuticals, Wilmington, MA) and MAL cream as Metvix™ (PhotoCure ASA, Norway, Galderma, Lausanne, Switzerland)—are cleared by the US FDA for the photodynamic treatment of nonhyperkeratotic actinic keratoses (AK) of the face and scalp. At the time of this writing, MAL is no longer available in the US market, although it is used in many countries for the treatment of non-melanoma skin cancers, having shown safety and efficacy for this indication.[40,41] Indocyanine green and methylene blue are two other non-commercially available photosensitizers that have been studied for acne treatment with PDT but are not commercially available at this time. This section will focus on ALA and MAL for the treatment of acne vulgaris.

ALA is FDA-approved for the treatment of nonhyperkeratotic AKs of the face and scalp utilizing a blue light source for 16 minutes and 40 seconds. ALA, once in the skin, acts as a prodrug, is converted to its active metabolite, PpIX, and accumulates in specific cells within the skin, mainly actinically damaged cells, nonmelanoma skin cancer cells, and the pilosebaceous unit itself. The only

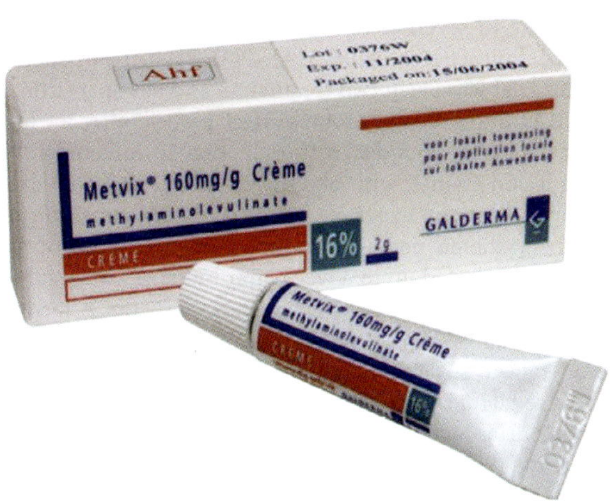

Figure 46-14 Galderma—Metvix Package (Used with permission from Galderma.)

product available in the United States is known as the Levulan Kerastick (DUSA Pharmaceuticals, Wilmington, MA), shown in Figure 46-13. MAL, available in Europe (Galderma), is shown in Figure 46-14.

Hongcharu et al.[42] reported the first clinical trial utilizing ALA-PDT in the treatment of inflammatory acne vulgaris. Their group evaluated 22 patients with inflammatory acne treated with ALA and a 550 to 570 nm broadband light source. The ALA used in this clinical trial was incubated on the skin for 3 hours prior to light exposure. Significant clearance of the acne lesions was evident after four weekly treatments. The patients experienced downtime prior to healing, known commonly today as the "PDT effect," as has been previously described by this author. The PDT effect in this trial consisted of an acneiform folliculitis, post-inflammatory hyperpigmentation, superficial peeling, and crusting, which lasted upwards of a week post-therapy. The mechanism of action for the improvement seen was documented through skin biopsies and immunofluorescence staining to be via destruction of the *P. acnes* bacteria as well as partial destruction of the sebaceous glands.

Many others have reported their clinical experiences with ALA-PDT. Itoh et al.[43] first utilized a 635 nm pulsed excimer dye laser as well as a 4 hour ALA drug incubation in a single patient with intractable acne vulgaris on the face. Following the therapy, the treated area remained disease free for 8 months. The authors did report a PDT effect, manifested by erythema, edema, and crusting immediately after the therapy. In a subsequent study, Itoh et al.[44] reported experiences with 13 patients utilizing ALA-PDT and a 600 to 700 nm halogen light source. All of the patients in this trial showed improvement in their acne and they were able to demonstrate that the formation of new lesions was reduced at 1, 3, and 7 months following therapy. A PDT effect was seen and some recurrence was noted during the following 6 months.

Further investigations utilizing ALA for the treatment of inflammatory acne vulgaris soon appeared in the medical literature. As was the case with AKs and ALA-PDT, these investigators utilized a short-contact, full-face therapeutic approach in their clinical trials, an off-label use of the approved FDA indications. Goldman[16] was the first of these investigators to look at short-contact, full-face ALA-PDT therapy for acne vulgaris when he reported his experience treating inflammatory acne vulgaris and sebaceous gland hyperplasia. He utilized a 1 hour ALA incubation with either an IPL source or blue light for drug activation. The report noted "relative" clearing of the acne vulgaris lesions after two to four once weekly ALA-PDT treatments. Patients noted the therapy to be pain free and no PDT effects were seen.

Gold[13] then reported his experience using a 30 to 60 minute ALA drug incubation and a high-intensity blue light source to evaluate moderate to severe inflammatory acne vulgaris lesions in 10 individuals. The study used once-weekly ALA-blue light treatments and patients were evaluated at 1 and 3 months following their final therapies. Response rates of 60% were found. The treatments were well tolerated and no adverse events were observed in any of the treated patients.

Goldman et al.[45] then treated 22 patients with moderate-to-severe inflammatory acne vulgaris using a blue light with and without ALA. They found a greater response rate in those treated with ALA-PDT and blue light in comparison to those treated with blue light alone. No adverse events were seen in this patient population. Taub[46] reported her experience with short-contact, full-face therapy utilizing blue light sources (ClearLight or BLU-U) or IPL with RF (Aurora®, Syneron, Yokneam, Israel) in 18 individuals. The patients received two to four treatments over a 4 to 8 week time period. Improvement was noted 4 months following the last treatment; this included 11 of 18 patients showing 50% improvement and five patients showing greater than 75% improvement in their lesions.

Gold et al.[47] reported their experience with short-contact, full-face therapy utilizing ALA and an IPL device (Harmony, Alma Lasers, Buffalo Grove, IL). Patients received once weekly ALA-IPL treatments for up to four treatments and were followed for up to 3 months after their final treatment. A 72% reduction in acne lesions was seen. No PDT effects were observed.

There have been at least two split-face IPL treatments with ALA-PDT reported in the literature for the treatment of inflammatory acne vulgaris. Santos et al.[48] reported their experience with ALA-PDT in moderate-to-severe inflammatory acne utilizing ALA-PDT and the Quantum IPL device (Lumenis, Santa Clara, CA). Thirteen patients were treated with short-contact, full-face therapy. In this split-face analysis, 10 of 13 patients showed a marked response on the ALA-IPL treated side versus the IPL side alone after a single treatment. A second split-face clinical trial, performed by Rojanamatin et al.[49] confirmed the results previously described. Their group evaluated 14 patients in a split-face fashion with the same kind of IPL described by Santos et al.[48] They found that ALA-IPL treatment was superior to treatment with the IPL alone.

Lasers have also been reported to be effective in treating inflammatory acne vulgaris with ALA-PDT. Alexiades-Armenakas[50] reported her experience with the long pulsed dye (PDL) laser utilizing ALA in patients with inflammatory acne. She utilized a drug incubation time period that averaged 45 minutes and reported that with an average of three PDL sessions, she cleared all of the 14 patients treated. Miller and Van Camp[51] reported on the successful use of ALA and the KTP laser in patients with inflammatory acne vulgaris. Examples of patients treated with ALA-PDT are shown in Figures 46-15 and 46-16.

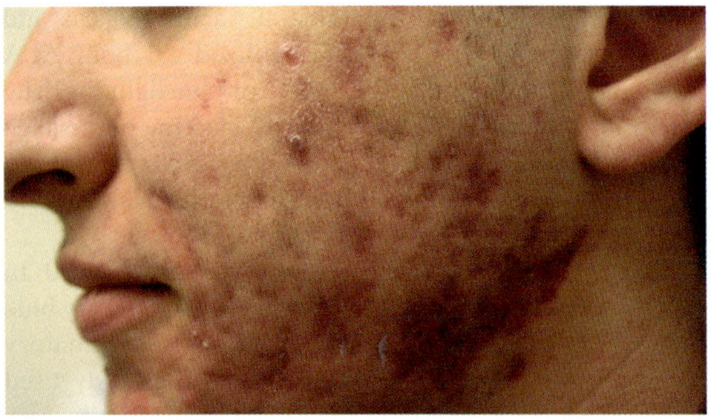

Figure 46-15 Patient before treatment with ALA-PDT. (Used with permission from Michael H. Gold, M.D.)

A large multicenter controlled FDA clinical trial in the United States evaluated the use of ALA in the treatment of moderate-to-severe inflammatory acne. The trial studied the effectiveness of blue light versus blue light plus ALA to determine the effect of adding ALA to the already FDA-approved blue light source. Unfortunately, the study did not show clinical significance[18] and thus the US acne vulgaris program for ALA-PDT was halted.

Many in the United States still feel that the use of ALA-PDT is warranted for moderate-to-severe acne vulgaris, despite the failings of the FDA clinical trial. Many clinicians are utilizing ALA in their acne vulgaris treatment armamentarium. There is no set "algorithm" that exists, so clinicians will need to determine how best to use ALA-PDT in their practices. In our clinical practice, which tries to keep patient comfort at the forefront and downtime to a minimum, we normally incubate the ALA for 15 to 30 minutes at the first visit and give blue light for 10 minutes. We treat our patients every 2 weeks and increase the drug incubation by 15 minutes at each subsequent visit as well as increasing the light treatment by 2 to 3 minutes per session, as tolerated. We have found that treatments are well tolerated and our patients do not have any significant downtime, which is important for students and younger patients who have to go to school or to work and cannot afford the downtime that occurs with longer drug incubations and longer light periods.

In Europe, MAL-PDT has been studied in several clinical trials for the treatment of inflammatory acne. Wiegell and Wulf[52] were the first to evaluate 21 patients with moderate-to-severe acne vulgaris in a randomized, controlled clinical trial utilizing MAL-PDT. Each of the patients in this trial was given two treatments 2 weeks apart utilizing MAL and a red light source. Twelve weeks after the last treatment they found a 68% reduction in inflammatory acne lesion counts, with no changes noted in the control group. All patients experienced a "PDT effect" consisting of severe erythema, pustular eruptions, and exfoliation of the skin, which lasted up to a week after therapy. Moderate to severe pain was also noted during the treatments. A second clinical trial by Horfelt et al.[53] evaluated 30 patients with moderate-to-severe inflammatory acne lesions using MAL and a red light source. This was a split-face analysis, with a 3 hour drug incubation under occlusion, exposure to red light, and two treatments given at 2 week intervals. Twelve weeks after the last treatment, there was a statistical reduction in acne lesions of 54% versus 20% in the control group. Pain and a "PDT effect" were once again seen. Further clinical trials are underway in Europe to further evaluate the role of the methyl ester of ALA in the treatment of moderate-to-severe inflammatory acne vulgaris and whether varying protocols (such as drug incubation times) can lead to more acceptable results, especially in relation to PDT effects. It seems that with shorter contact, non-occlusion MAL to acne vulgaris lesions and shorter light doses with the red light source, a more tolerable approach for patients will be achieved. It should be noted that others are evaluating longer drug incubations and longer light times to "blast" the acne vulgaris lesions—this approach may have efficacy, but we still need to be aware of the potential morbidity associated with this approach.

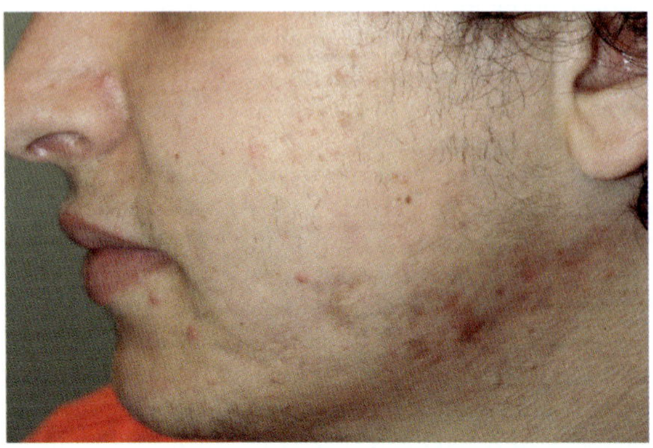

Figure 46-16 Patient after treatment with ALA-PDT. (Used with permission from Michael H. Gold, M.D.)

COMPARISON OF ALA-PDT AND MAL-PDT

Several reports have appeared in the medical literature trying to determine whether ALA-PDT is more effective than MAL-PDT and vice-versa, as well as looking at pain associated with each of the therapies.[54,55] In these evaluations, MAL was studied utilizing the recommended lesion preparations and drug incubation under occlusion. ALA used in these evaluations used the recommended FDA protocols but with compounded ALA, rather than the standard FDA-approved product, and was not used in the manner currently considered to be the "standard of care," which is short contact, full-face therapy. Pain was associated with the treatments performed in this manner. An editorial by this author[23] pointed out that there has not been a comparison of the standard US and European methods for PDT and that, for the most part, ALA-PDT in this country has been performed with minimal downtime and usually with no PDT effects.

CONCLUSION

Lasers and light sources as well as ALA-PDT can be effective therapies for inflammatory acne vulgaris. Dermatologists are at the forefront of the treatment of this disease and must remain the leaders in this field. We are also the leaders in the use of lasers and light sources in skin disease. Topical and systemic medications remain the first line of treatment for our acne patients, but many lasers and light sources, as well as ALA-PDT, have also been shown to be safe and effective for the treatment of acne vulgaris. When appropriate, these devices should be utilized for our patients with inflammatory acne after treatment with topical and systemic medications, both to help minimize the extent of their lesions as well as the sequelae of their disease.

REFERENCES

1. Leyden JJ. Therapy for acne vulgaris. *N Engl J Med.* 1997; 336:1156–1162.
2. Leyden JJ. Oral isotretinoin. How can we treat difficult acne patients? *Dermatology.* 1997;195(S1):29–33.
3. Gold MH. Acne and PDT: New techniques with lasers and light sources. *Lasers Med Sci.* 2007;22:67–72.
4. Gold MH. Phototherapy for acne: What is the best approach? *Expert Rev Dermatol.* 2010;5(2):159–172.
5. Strauss JS, Krowchuk DP, Leyden JJ et al. Guidelines of care for acne vulgaris management. *J Am Acad Dermatol.* 2007;56:651–663.
6. http://emedicine.medscape.com/article/1069804-treatment
7. Gollnick H, Cunliffe W, Berson D et al. Management of acne: A report from a global alliance to improve outcomes in acne. *J Am Acad Dermatol.* 2003;49(S1):S1–S37.
8. Coates P, Vyakrnam S, Eady EA et al. Prevelance of antibiotic-resistance propionibacteria on the skin of acne patients: 10-year surveillance data and snapshot distribution study. *Br J Dermatol.* 2002;146:840–848.
9. Velicer CM, Heckbert SR, Lampe JW et al. Antibiotic use in relation to the risk of breast cancer. *JAMA.* 2004;291:827–835.
10. Ellis CN, Krach KJ. Uses and complications of isotretinoin therapy. *J Am Acad Dermatol.* 2001;45:S150–S157.
11. Kawada A, Aragane Y, Kameyama H, Sangen Y, Tezuka T. Acne phototherapy with a high-intensity, enhanced narrow-band, blue light source: An open study and in vitro investigation. *J Dermatolog Sci.* 2002;30:129–135.
12. Shalita AR, Harth Y, Elman M. Acne photoclearing using a novel, high-intensity, enhanced, narrow-band blue light source. *Clin Application Notes.* 2003;9:1
13. Gold MH. The utilization of ALA-PDT and a new photoclearing device for the treatment of severe inflammatory acne vulgaris—Results of an initial clinical trial. *J Lasers Surg Med.* 2003; 15(Suppl):46.
14. Papageorgiou P, Katsambas A, Chu A. Phototherapy with boule (415 nm) and red (660 nm) light in the treatment of acne. *Br J Dermatol.* 2000;142:973–978.
15. Meffert H, Gaunitz K, Gutewort T, Amlong UJ. [Therapy of acne with visible light; decreased irradiation time by using a blue-light high energy lamp]. *Dermatol Monatssehr.* 1990;176:597–560.
16. Goldman MP, Atkin D, Kincad S. PDT/ALA in the treatment of actinic damage; real world experience. *J Lasers Surg Med.* 2002;14(Suppl):24.
17. Gold MH, Goldman MP. A multi-center investigatory study of the treatment of mild to moderate inflammatory acne vulgaris with visible blue light in comparison to topical 1% clindamycin antibiotic solution. *J Am Acad Dermatol.* 2004;50 (Suppl):56.
18. http://www.clinicaltrials.gov/ct2/show/results/NCT00706433?term=DUSA+Pharmaceuticals&rank=1
19. Dierickx CC, Capezzera R, Pedretti A, et al. Lasers, light, and radiofrequency for treatment of acne. *Med Laser Appl.* 2004; 19:196–204.
20. Gold MH. Blue light for the treatment of acne vulgaris. *Prime.* 2013;1(3):19–25.
21. Zane C, Capezzera R, Pedretti A, Facchinetti E, Calzavara-Pinton P. Non-invasive diagnostic evaluation of phototherapeutic effects of red light phototherapy of acne vulgaris. *Photodermatol Photoimmunol Photomed.* 2008;24(5):244–248.
22. Na JI, Suh DH. Red light phototherapy alone is effective for acne vulgaris: randomized, single-blinded clinical trial. *Dermatol Surg.* 2007;33(10):1228–1233.
23. Gold MH. 5-Aminolevulinic acid photodynamic therapy versus methyl aminolevulinate photodynamic therapy for inflammatory acne vulgaris. *J Am Acad Dermatol.* 2008;58(2):S60–S62.
24. Bowes LE, Manstein D, Anderson RR. Effect of 532 nm KTP laser on exposure on acne and sebaceous glands. *Lasers Med Sci.* 2003;18:S6–S7.
25. Seaton ED, Charakida A, Mouser PE, Grace I, Clement RM, Chu AC. Pulsed dye laser treatment for inflammatory acne vulgaris: a randomized controlled trial. *Lancet.* 2003;362:1347–1352.
26. Orringer JS, Kang S, Hamilton T, et al. Treatment of acne vulgaris with a pulsed dye laser: a randomized controlled trial. *JAMA.* 2004;291:2834–2839.
27. Elman M, Lask G. The role of pulsed light and heat energy (LHE) in acne clearance. *J Cosmet Laser Ther.* 2004;6:91–95.
28. Dierickx CC. Treatment of acne vulgaris with a variable-filtration IPL system. *Lasers Surg Med.* 2004;34(S16):66.
29. Bitter PH. Noninvasive rejuvenation of photodamaged skin using serial, full-face intense pulsed light treatments. *Dermatol Surg.* 2000;26:835–843.
30. Munavalli GS, Weiss RA. Rapid acne regression using photopneumatic (ppx) therapy. *Lasers Surg Med.* 2007;39(S19):22.
31. Shamban AT, Enokibori M, Narurkar V, Wilson D. Photoneumatic technology for the treatment of acne vulgaris. *J Drugs Dermatol.* 2008;7(2):139–145.
32. Gold MH, Biron J. Efficacy of a novel combination of pneumatic energy and broadband light for the treatment of acne. *J Drugs Dermatol.* 2008;7(2):639–645.
33. Paithankar DY, Ross EV, Saleh BA, Blair MA, Graham BS. Acne treatment with a 1,450 nm wavelength laser and cryogen skin cooling. *Lasers Surg Med.* 2002;31:106–114.
34. Friedman PM, Jih MH, Kimyai-Asadi A, Goldberg LH. Treatment of inflammatory acne vulgaris with a 1450 nm diode laser: A pilot study. *Dermatol Surg.* 2004;30:147–151.
35. Friedman PM, Marquez D, Kunishige J. Evaluation of large spot 1450 nm diode laser for the treatment of facial acne vulgaris. *Lasers Surg Med.* 2008;40(S20):32.
36. Tuchin VV, Genina EA, Bashkatov AN, et al. A pilot study of ICG laser therapy of acne vulgaris: photodynamic and photothermolysis treatment. *Lasers Surg Med.* 2003;33:296–310.
37. Lloyd JR, Mirkov M. Selective photothermolysis of the sebaceous glands for acne treatment. *Lasers Surg Med.* 2002;31: 115–120.
38. Kassir M, Newton D, Maris M, Euwer R, Servell P. Er: glass (1.54 nm) laser for the treatment of facial acne vulgaris. *Lasers Surg Med.* 2004;34(S16):S65.
39. Ruiz-Esparza J, Gomez JB. Nonablative radiofrequency for active acne vulgaris: the use of deep dermal heat in the treatment of moderate to severe active acne vulgaris (thermotherapy): A report of 22 cases. *Dermatol Surg.* 2003;29:333–339.
40. Gold MH. Aminolevulinic acid photodynamic therapy: Medical evidence for its expanded use. *Expert Rev Med Devices.* 2006;3(3):357–371.
41. Gold MH. Novel treatment options for severe inflammatory acne vulgaris. *Expert Rev Dermatol.* 2006;1(1):13–23.
42. Hongcharu W, Taylor CR, Chang Y, Aghassi D, Suthamjariya K, Anderson RR. Topical ALA-photodynamic therapy for the treatment of acne vulgaris. *J Invest Dermatol.* 2000;115(2):183–192.
43. Itoh Y, Ninomiya Y, Tajima S, Ishibashi A. Photodynamic therapy for acne vulgaris with topical 5-aminolevulinic acid. *Arch Dermatol.* 2000;136(9):1093–1095.
44. Itoh Y, Ninomiya Y, Tajima S, Ishibashi A. Photodynamic therapy of acne vulgaris with topical delta aminolevulinic acid and incoherent light in Japanese patients. *Br J Dermatol.* 2001;144:575–579.
45. Goldman MP, Boyce SM. A single-center study of aminolevulinic acid and 417 NM photodynamic therapy in the treatment of moderate to severe acne vulgaris. *J Drugs Dermatol.* 2003;2(4);393–396.
46. Taub AF. Photodynamic therapy for the treatment of acne: a pilot study. *J Drugs Dermatol.* 2004;3: S10–S14.
47. Gold MH. The use of a novel intense pulsed light and heat source and ALA-PDT in the treatment of moderate to severe inflammatory acne vulgaris. *J Drugs Dermatol.* 2004;3(6): S14–S18.

48. Santos AV, Belo VG, Santos G. Effectiveness of photodynamic therapy with topical 5-Aminolevulinic acid and intense pulsed light versus intense pulsed light along in the treatment of acne vulgaris: comparative study. *Dermatol Surg.* 2005;31(8 Pt 1):910–915.
49. Rojanamatin J, Choawawanich P. Treatment of inflammatory facial acne vulgaris with intense pulsed light (IPL) and short contact of topical 5-aminolevulinc acid (ALA): a pilot study. *Dermatol Surg.* 2006;32:991–997.
50. Alexiades-Armenakas MR. Long pulsed dye laser-mediated photodynamic therapy combined with topical therapy for mild-to-severe comedonal, inflammatory and cystic acne. *J Drugs Dermatol.* 2006;5:45–55.
51. Miller A, Van Camp A. "Treatment of cane vulgaris with photodynamic therapy: the use of aminolevulinic acid and green light". *Cosm Derm.* 2006;19(10): 624–627.
52. Wiegell SR, Wulf HC. Photodynamic therapy of acne vulgaris using methyl aminolaevulinate: a blinded, randomized controlled trial. *Br J Dermatol.* 2006;154:969–976.
53. Horfelt C, Funk J, Frohm-Nilsson M, Wiegleb Edstrom D, Wennberg AM. Topical methyl aminolaevuninate photodynamic therapy for treatment of facial acne vulgaris: results of a randomized controlled study. *Br J Dermatol.* 2006;155:608–613.
54. Wiegell SR, Wulf HC. Photodynamic therapy of acne vulgaris using 5-aminolevulinic acid versus methyl aminolevulinate. *J Am Acad Dermatol.* 2006;54(4):647–651.
55. Kasche A, Luderschmidt S, Ring J, Hein R. Photodynamic therapy induces less pain in patients treated with methyl aminolevulinate compared to aminolevulinic acid. *J Drugs Dermatol.* 2006;5(4):353–356.

CHAPTER 47

Acne Scarring

Snehal Amin

CLINICAL OVERVIEW

Acne vulgaris affects almost 80% of the population at some point in life and leads to scarring in up to 95% of patients with acne.[1,2] Many patients suffer long-term psychological and social effects from the complications of acne.[3] The prevalence of acne scarring in the general population has been estimated to be 1% but is much higher in the dermatology clinic population.[4] Even though the treatment of acne scarring has greatly improved in the last decade with respect to safety and efficacy, many patients are unaware of their options regarding potential therapies. The proliferation of devices and techniques for improving acne scarring present a challenge for the clinician who must often apply several treatments for an individual patient with multiple types of acne scars.

Most patients with acne report that prevention of acne scarring is one of the main reasons for seeking professional dermatologic care, especially in severe cases. However, many patients specifically seek out the dermatologist or dermatologic surgeon to address acne scarring long after the active lesions have subsided. Only in the last few decades has improvement of acne scarring become a significant practice area for dermatologists with the development of new modalities such as lasers, surgical devices, chemical peels, and fillers.

Most patients with acne scarring have limited areas of involvement on the temples or cheeks. Some have more widespread involvement on the face, chest, and back. There is no correlation between the Fitzpatrick skin type and gender with acne scar severity.[5] Although most acne scarring is atrophic, there are several subtypes and clinical variations. In addition, while the underlying pathophysiology of various types of acne scars may be similar, the treatment options vary for each type, so it is worth classifying acne scarring from a clinical perspective.

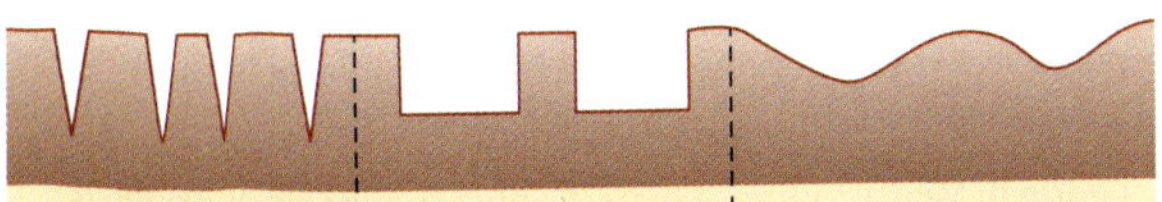

Icepick	Boxcar	Rolling
Punch excision	Punch elevation	Fillers
--	Laser resurfacing	Laser resurfacing
Dermabrasion	Dermabrasion	--
--	--	Subcision
Pinpoint TCA	Chemical peels	--

Figure 47-1 Three types of atrophic acne scars. Appropriate therapy selection depends on the type of scars present.

CLASSIFICATION: TYPE AND SEVERITY

Acne scars are either depressed (atrophic) or elevated (hypertrophic). There are three clinical subtypes of *atrophic* acne scars: icepick, boxcar, and rolling (Fig. 47-1). The *elevated* type acne scars can be hypertrophic or keloidal. Macular acne scars may also have associated vascular and pigment changes even if the skin texture is unchanged. Finally, it is important to note severity and distribution in selecting the appropriate treatment modality (Table 47-1).

In the dermatology clinic, the most common form of acne scarring is the atrophic type, with most patients exhibiting features of two or more subtypes. The most common subtype of atrophic acne scar is the crateriform or boxcar type (Fig. 47-2). This lesion often presents as a cluster of scars on the temples or cheeks. Individual lesions are 3 to 4 mm in diameter and about 0.5 mm deep. Eventually

TABLE 47-1
Clinical Classification of Acne Scarring and Associated Skin Changes

- Major types of acne scarring
  - Atrophic or depressed scars
    - Icepick scars
    - Boxcar scars
    - Rolling scars
  - Elevated or protruding scars
    - Hypertrophic scars
    - Keloidal scars
- Macular changes +/− scarring
  - Vascularity and erythema
  - Postinflammatory pigment changes
- Severity
  - Depth
    - Superficial (epidermal)
    - Moderate (papillary dermis)
    - Deep (deep dermis)
- Distribution
  - Localized
  - Generalized

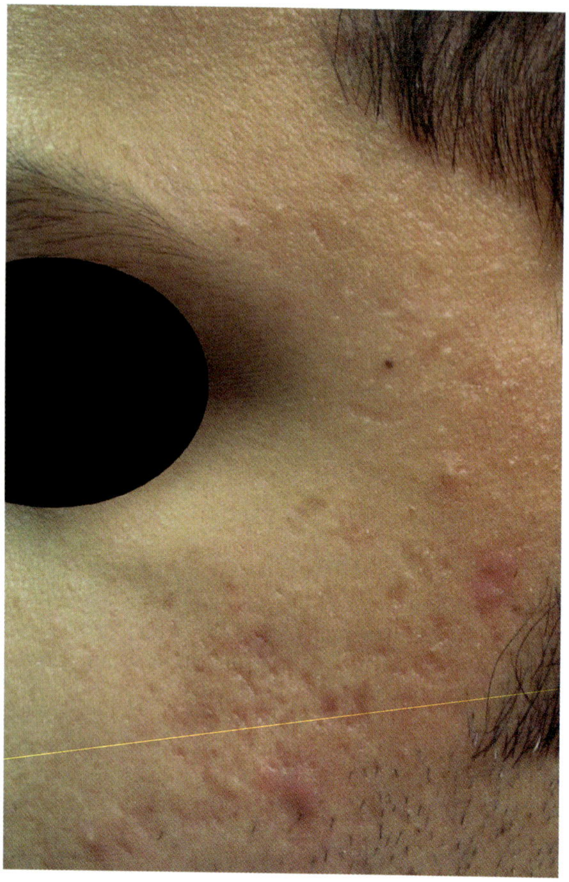

Figure 47-2 Active inflammatory acne with icepick- and boxcar-type scars in a patient with Fitzpatrick type 4 skin.

after 3 to 12 months, acne scars assume a slightly hypopigmented or more often a normal skin tone. Most patients exhibit multiple subtypes of acne scar (Fig. 47-3).

The cosmetic impact of an acne scar is dependent on the depth of the scar as well as the angle of the border or wall at the edge of the scar (Fig. 47-4). A vertical wall with a deeper base will create a more pronounced shadow and, therefore, have a greater cosmetic impact. Rolling scars are less problematic cosmetically because of edges that minimize shadow formation. The angle of incident light will also have a significant impact on the appearance of the scar in photographs; overhead spot-lighting tends to exacerbate the appearance of acne scars, whereas ambient natural light tends to minimize scar severity. The angle and quality of lighting is especially important to note when photographing acne scars for clinical or research purposes. A useful clinical grading system is described in Table 47-2.[4,6]

DIFFERENTIAL DIAGNOSIS

Although the clinical diagnosis of acne scars is usually obvious, several skin conditions produce scarring that can mimic localized or even generalized acne scarring. Varicella scars in solitary and generalized forms can mimic acne scarring. A solitary varicella scar is often better defined at the edges with nearly vertical walls (Fig. 47-3). Discoid lupus scars tend to coalesce with central areas of violaceous pigment and are usually much larger. Smallpox scars tend to be deeper, more evenly distributed on the face and are often the rolling type of scars (Fig. 47-4). Scarring from self-traumatization tends to have irregular patterns of distribution as well as very well-defined borders (Fig. 47-5). Scarring induced by herpes simplex and varicella viruses often appear in clusters and arrays and has a punched-out border. Solitary keloidal or hypertrophic acne scars on the torso in the appropriate clinical context may be differentiated from dermatofibrosarcoma protuberans with a punch biopsy.

PATHOPHYSIOLOGY

The pathogenesis of the initial inflammatory acne lesion has been studied in detail.[5,7] However, the pathogenesis of acne scarring is less well understood.[4] The initial follicular inflammatory process around a comedone leads to follicular rupture, perifollicular abscess formation, and eventually wound healing. The cascade of events involved in wound healing that lead to acne scarring are complex and involve inflammation, granulation tissue formation, and matrix remodeling. Matrix remodeling during the final stages of wound healing may involve fibrosis, atrophy, pigment, and vascular changes.[8] Atrophic or hypertrophic fibrosis may be temporary or permanent. Occasionally, acne scars are elevated or thickened, especially on the chest, shoulders, and back. Although not confirmed in controlled studies, traumatization, superinfection by staphylococcus or proprionibacterium, long-standing duration, or large size of acne cysts can predispose patients to severe acne scarring. The type of initial lesion does not seem to determine the clinical type or level of acne scarring.[2] Cell-mediated immunity, which is genetically influenced, may determine the severity level of acne scarring.[9]

The role of oral medications in preventing or possibly exacerbating acne scarring has been debated. Given the

TABLE 47-2
Clinical Severity Grading System

Grade I: Macular changes only with erythema, hyperpigmentation, or hypopigmentation. Patients may perceive this to be severe despite having minimal texture changes in the skin.
Grade II: Mild atrophic or hypertrophic changes not obvious at conversational distance. Slight textural changes with associated collagen disorganization. Patients note lack of *"glowing skin."* Easily covered with makeup or cosmetic products.
Grade III: Moderate atrophic or hypertrophic changes easily visible at conversational distance. Not easily covered up with makeup. Distensible or flattened with manual traction.
Grade IV: Severe atrophic or hypertrophic changes that are non-distensible or do not improve by stretching the skin. Deep icepick- or boxcar-type scars obvious in any lighting.

Source: Data from Goodman[28] and Fabbrocini[4]

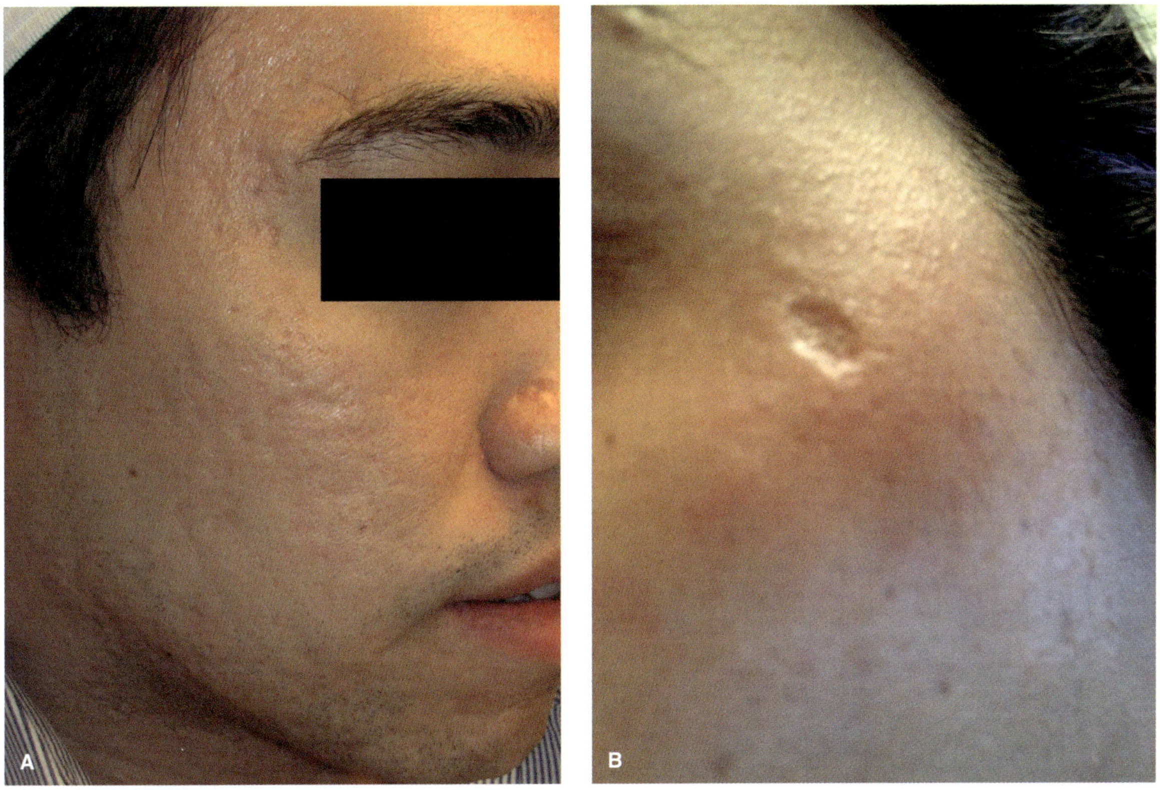

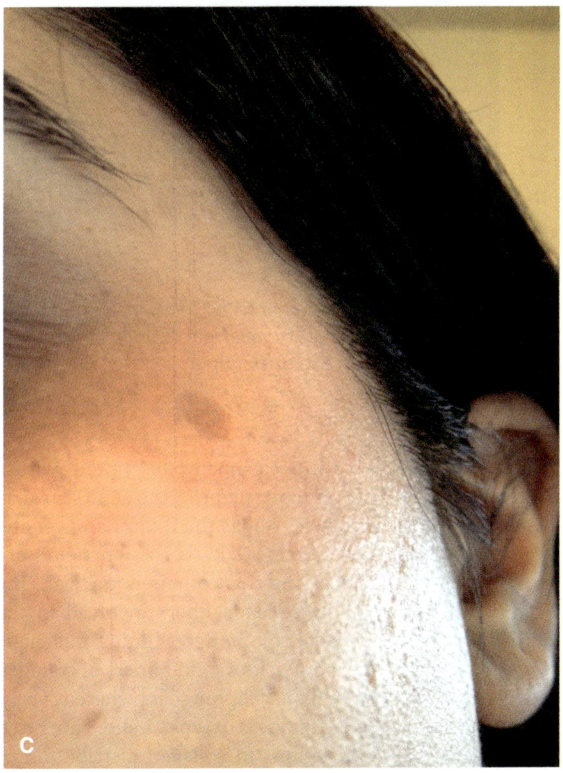

Figure 47-3 **A.** East-Asian patients with Fitzpatrick type 3 skin exhibiting boxcar and rolling scars on the temples, cheeks, and neck. **B.** Solitary varicella scar with side-lighting on the left. C. Ambient light on the right.

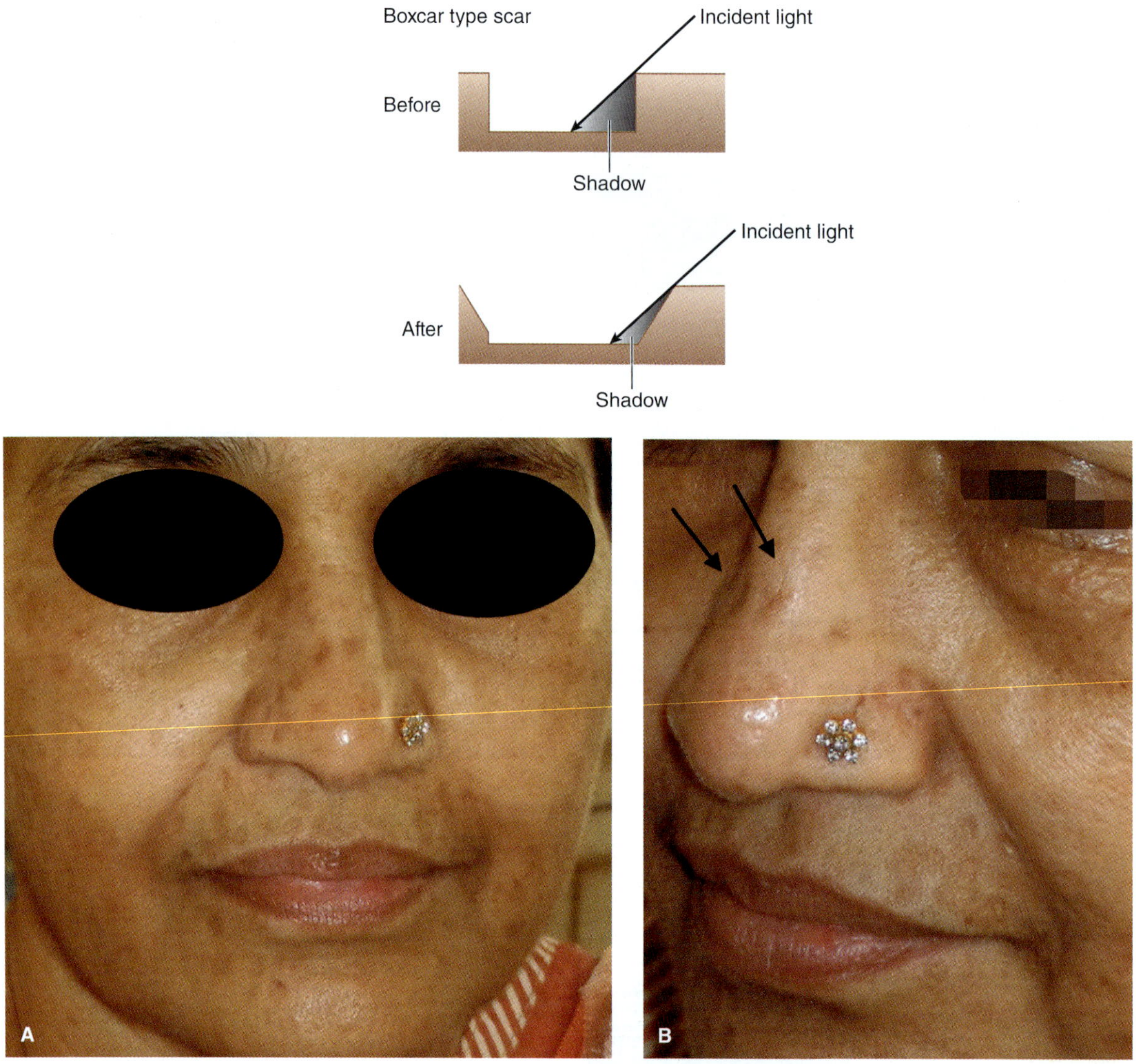

Figure 47-4 Boxcar-type scar. Boxcar-type acne scars appear dark because of shadows created by incident light. Dermabrasion or any other epidermal resurfacing softens the sharp edges of epidermal scars. After dermabrasion, the shadow length decreases even if the depth of the scar remains the same. **A.** Smallpox scars on the upper lip and nose with hyperpigmentation and atrophy. **B.** Note the severe atrophy within individual lesions.

long history of oral antibiotics in treating active acne vulgaris, it is unlikely that these medications exacerbate acne scarring. Several studies have analyzed acne scarring as a clinical endpoint; they support the use of oral antibiotics to prevent the occurrence of acne scarring and do not show any increased scarring.[10] The role of oral retinoids is less certain in exacerbation of acne scarring; therefore, concomitant use of oral steroids is often recommended to decrease the inflammation that is often seen during initiation of oral retinoid therapy.[5] Whether either of these medications ultimately reduces the level of acne scarring often depends on early initiation of therapy. Delayed initiation of treatment was strongly correlated with increased severity of scarring.[10,11]

The pathophysiology of acne scarring has also been studied on a histologic level and is characterized by fibrosis in the dermis.[11] This dermal neo-collagenesis results in a depression in the overlying epidermis, which is more often atrophic and rarely sclerotic. A parchment paper–like change can occasionally be noted within larger acne scars. The ultimate shape of the acne scar may depend on other factors as well as the underlying genetic predisposition of the patient. Why certain patients are more prone to acne scarring than others is unclear. The orientation and types of collagen fibers involved in the fibrosis may play a central role in determining the shape of the acne scar. For example, horizontal fibers of collagen type 4 are often seen in hypertrophic scars whereas vertical and horizontal collagen fibers of types 1 and 3 are often seen in keloids.[12,13] Variations in collagen distribution as well as matrix enzymes and healing responses, which are likely to be genetically determined, may predispose acne patients to scarring.

Acne vulgaris may also lead to changes in epidermal and dermal pigmentation without palpable skin surface changes. This color change may or may not be associated with scarring or fibrosis. Because patients often associate color change with scarring, the management

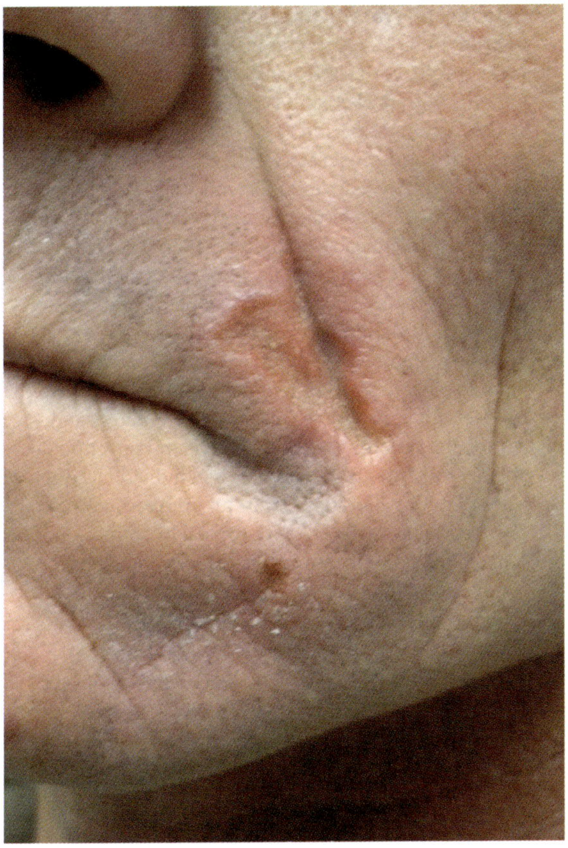

Figure 47-5 Coalescing boxcar-type scars on the left angle of the mouth in a patient with HSV exacerbated by excoriations.

of postinflammatory pigment changes after resolution of acne vulgaris is an important aspect of treating acne scarring. Postinflammatory hyperpigmentation consisting of red-brown to violaceous macules is often noted, especially in darker skinned patients, and can persist for 12 months.[14] Isolated erythema usually resolves sooner unless hypervascularity within acne scars is present.

TREATMENT PLANNING

Given the proliferation of treatment modalities for acne scarring in the past few decades, an increasing number of patients are visiting their dermatologist for cosmetic improvement of these skin changes. Treatment selection should take into consideration important factors listed in Table 47-3. A brief discussion of each factor follows.

TABLE 47-3
Factors in Therapy Selection

1. Current acne involvement and likelihood of future flares
2. Distribution, location, severity of acne scarring
3. Type of acne scarring, i.e., dermal vs. epidermal, icepick vs. boxcar
4. Differentiating scar from pigment and vascular changes
5. Medication history, especially oral and topical retinoids
6. Psychological and social history, i.e., compliance, picking
7. Gender, i.e., presence of beard hair, use of makeup, etc.
8. Recent surgical, laser, or ultraviolet light exposure
9. Fitzpatrick skin type, i.e., postprocedure pigment changes
10. Keloid and surgical scar history
11. Patient expectations, i.e., results, pain, healing period

1. Current acne involvement and likelihood of future flares will determine the timing and selection of acne scar therapy. During active acne flares, medical therapies including oral and topical retinoids as well as strategies to decrease the severity of acne should be employed. Patients should be advised to avoid excoriating their lesions and maintain an aggressive medical regimen to decrease acne scarring. Treatment modalities such as non-ablative lasers and chemical peels may be initiated to treat active inflammatory or comedonal acne as well as acne scarring.
2. The distribution, location, and severity of acne scarring will strongly influence therapeutic selection. Surgical treatments that are safe on facial skin are often contraindicated on the chest or shoulders due to risk of keloid formation. The advent of fractional laser treatments has allowed for safer resurfacing on non-facial locations of acne scars. Solitary lesions often respond well to scalpel-based treatments, whereas widely distributed lesions will respond well to laser-based treatments.
3. Perhaps the most important factor in treatment selection is the type of acne scar present. Figure 47-1 describes the three main types of acne scars and also lists the typical treatments for each type of acne scar. Icepick scars respond well to focal surgical treatments. Since most icepick scars involve deep fibrosis, 2 mm punch excision is an ideal treatment, especially when followed with a series of non-ablative fractional resurfacing treatments; pinpoint trichloracetic acid (TCA) is also very effective for these lesions. Deep icepick scars do not respond to dermabrasion or non-ablative laser resurfacing. Ablative laser resurfacing, if done at the appropriate settings, can result in partial improvement. Because of their epidermal involvement, boxcar scars respond to multiple modalities. Superficial boxcar scars respond to mechanical and laser resurfacing. Multiple chemical peels and dermabrasion can also correct these mostly epidermal defects. Deeper boxcar scars respond very well to punch excision for narrow scars and punch elevation for wider scars. The ideal approach for boxcar scars may involve initial surgery for focal lesions followed by multiple fractional resurfacing sessions for generalized pigment and textural improvements. Subcision is the ideal treatment for rolling scars because of the associated dermal fibrosis. Subcision followed by filler therapy has become a standard approach for deep rolling scars. Surgical approaches that involve cutting into the epidermis are not indicated for rolling scars since the skin surface appears normal in this subtype of acne scars. Non-ablative laser and light treatments such as the 1064 nm Nd:YAG laser are often

prescribed for rolling scars; however, the cosmetic improvement is usually very subtle.

4. Differentiating permanent scarring involving fibrosis (either atrophic or hypertrophic) from other long-lasting complications of acne such as hyperpigmentation is important in treatment selection. Many patients use the term "acne scars" to describe the presence of postinflammatory hyperpigmentation and/or erythema even if there is no fibrosis. Treatment of postinflammatory pigmentation differs from treatment of true acne scars. Many patients have both, so a detailed discussion about risks and expectations is very important as well as an explanation of fibrotic versus pigmentary changes. Any treatment for patients with type 4 skin or higher should not be initiated without an experienced dermatologist present. Many patients have multiple types of acne scars in various anatomic locations and therefore require multiple modalities to achieve an optimal cosmetic outcome.
5. Most dermatologists recommend abstaining from any laser or surgical treatments for a period of 6 to 12 after oral isotretinoin therapy to avoid excessive or abnormal scarring. Concurrent oral isotretinoin is strongly associated with delayed wound healing and hypertrophic scarring.[15] Anecdotal evidence suggests that such a long waiting period may be unnecessary.[16] Patients should be advised to avoid application of any topical retinoid products or similarly irritating agents such as glycolic acids for at least 2 weeks prior to and following any skin procedure.
6. The patient's psychosocial assessment will strongly impact therapy selection. Compliance level including tendency toward picking should be thoroughly evaluated in the acne scar patient. Elements of body dysmorphic syndromes and obsessive-compulsive disorders are often noted in acne scar patients who have anxiety, habitual picking, or an exaggerated sense of their scar severity. Because acne scar improvement often involves long-term therapies, a high-quality doctor–patient communication strategy will facilitate clinical outcomes. Asking about upcoming social events will facilitate therapeutic planning. Compliance with physician directives is essential for more invasive therapies. Avoidance of over-the-counter anticoagulants and retinoids should be strongly advised. Preoperative treatment with antiviral and antibiotic therapy may be necessary when using ablative modalities such as laser resurfacing or deep chemical peels. Postoperative care instructions, which may include pressure dressings, antibiotics, and occlusive ointments, should be reviewed with the patient and caregivers. The operating physician should assess the likelihood of compliance with sun avoidance and sunblock application.
7. Patient gender will impact the specific therapies chosen. Some women may not mind using cover-up for persistent erythema after resurfacing treatments. Hair styling may be used to cover sutures or dressing material.
8. Patients should be given at least a month to heal from previous laser or surgical therapies before initiating new treatments. Patients should be instructed not to tan for at least 1 month prior to most surgical or laser treatments—longer for those patients with darker skin types who retain their tans for a longer period of time. Postoperative sun avoidance and sunscreen application should be included in any instruction sheet.
9. As with any other dermatologic treatment, acne scar patients with Fitzpatrick skin types 3 or greater should be treated only by experienced operators. Subcision or filler therapies carry little risk of pigmentation changes and should be strongly favored in dark-skinned patients. The potential for postoperative pigment changes with fractional laser treatments can be low with appropriate treatment parameters and compliant patients, whereas surgical or conventional ablative treatments in dark-skinned individuals often leave pigment alterations. Careful pretreatment and posttreatment regimens with topical hydroquinone, oral or topical steroids, and possibly retinoids have been suggested for these patients with dark skin undergoing cosmetic procedures.[17]
10. All patients should be informed of the risk for keloids with surgical therapy. It is unclear whether acne scar patients are actually at higher risk for keloid development.[18]
11. As with any cosmetic treatment, the patient's expectations about the level of improvement, the duration of healing periods, and risk of complications should be discussed. The operating physician must elicit specific understanding of these issues with the acne scar patient before selecting any therapies.

Preoperative and postoperative planning are essential to the success of any cosmetic treatment. Every cosmetic patient should complete a detailed and specific procedure consent form highlighting the individual procedure as well as the specific risks associated with the procedure. Preoperative and postoperative operative photography are crucial in treating the cosmetic patient. Because acne scar severity can vary with the angle of incident light, standardized and professional photography by the dermatologist is strongly suggested. Use of a camera flash, position of the patient relative to the camera, camera exposure settings, ambient colors, room lighting, and location in the examination room can all affect the appearance of acne scars on digital photography.

TREATMENTS

On the basis of the clinical classification of acne scarring, there are several approaches to the cosmetic improvement of acne scars. Specifically, these lesions can be treated by the following approaches, which are explained in more detail in the next section:

- Surgically excising or recountouring the lesions (punch excision, subcision)
- Resurfacing the epidermis (lasers and dermabrasion)
- Changing the lesion color (vascular lasers and medical therapy)
- Increasing the lesion volume (fillers and fat)
- Decreasing the lesion volume (steroid injections)
- Relaxing the surrounding skin (botulinum toxins)

SURGICAL TREATMENTS

Given that some physicians think that predisposition to acne scarring can be seen more often in patients who suffer hypertrophic scarring after scalpel surgery, any surgical approach must evaluated carefully for the acne scar patient. However, a retrospective study showed no correlation between a previous history of non-acne scarring and subsequent development of acne scarring.[2] Over the last decade, fractional laser resurfacing has overtaken scalpel-based approaches to treating acne scarring. However, surgical treatments such as subcision and punch excision remain simple and effective treatments for certain types of scarring. Moreover, these therapies can be combined in a sequential manner with laser therapy. Once the therapy has been selected, application of appropriate anesthetic techniques is essential for patient comfort. Most of the surgical modalities can be performed with injectable anesthetic, whereas the laser treatments can be performed with topical anesthetics.[19,20] Extensive subcision or conventional resurfacing or dermabrasion may require tumescent or regional anesthesia and, in some cases, general anesthesia.[21]

Subcision is indicated for depressed or atrophic-type acne scars that have a rolling surface. Icepick- and boxcar-type acne scars, which have a well-demarcated or vertical wall at the edges, should not be treated with subcision. A simple test of the potential utility of subcision involves stretching the skin with the thumb and index finger around the scars. If the scars improve, then subcision may be helpful. If the scar persists during the maneuver, then the epidermal change in the scar negates the utility of subcutaneous subcision. The term itself is derived by shortening the phrase *subcutaneous incisionless* surgery.[22]

Various instruments including 20 gauge needles, Nokor needles, mini-Beaver blades, and iris needles have been used to cut the vertical fibers that tether the epidermis to the deep dermis and subcutaneous tissue. After local or even tumescent anesthesia, the needle is inserted into the skin a few millimeters adjacent to the scar perpendicular to the skin surface. The needle is then angled nearly parallel to the skin and inserted further and swept back and forth to cut the subcutaneous tissue under the scars. The subcision needle can also be introduced under the skin after an initial puncture with an 18 gauge needle. Once the subcision device is in place, fanning and stabbing techniques are applied to release the dermis from the subcutaneous tethers and occasionally the deep dermis (Fig. 47-6). The area being treated should be firmly stretched by the non-dominant hand of the operator, and tenting the skin away from the patient with the tip of the needle may facilitate the severing of subcutaneous bands. Bruising may occur despite firm pressure for at least 10 minutes. No after care is necessary. Injection of fibrin foam or volumizing fillers can be performed after the subcision taking care not to over-correct the defect.[23] Steroid injections are occasionally necessary for hypertrophic scarring after subcision. Following subcision, vertically oriented fibrotic bands are released and clot formation and fibrosis lead to recontouring of the scarred skin. Formation of additional scar tissue in the dermis and subcutis may also elevate the scar.[24]

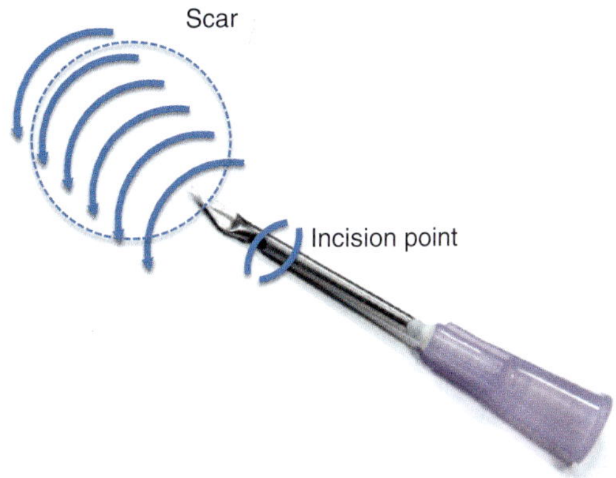

Figure 47-6 Subcision technique with Nokor needle.

Scalpel excision includes conventional elliptical excision as well as punch biopsy–type excision. Deep linear scars or round scars that have coalesced are good candidates for conventional excision. Meticulous suturing technique combined with postsurgical laser treatments with fractional resurfacing or pulsed dye lasers can achieve significant cosmetic improvement (Fig. 47-7).

Small icepick scars that are less than 1 mm in diameter may be excised with a 2 mm punch biopsy tool, which creates a very small surgical defect and a nearly scar-less outcome. This simple yet effective technique can be performed on multiple lesions during a single visit (Fig. 47-8). Increased efficacy is seen when punch excisions are followed shortly thereafter by a series of non-ablative fractional resurfacing treatments.

Boxcar-type acne scars that are approximately 3 mm in diameter can be excised using a 3 to 4 mm punch tool. Orienting the final defect along the skin folds is very important for larger scars. These larger scars can also be treated with punch elevation and punch grafting. In either case, meticulous suturing with 6-0 nylon is suggested. Dermal suturing with 5-0 vicryl may be necessary if the surgical defect is greater than 2.5 mm. It is important to orient the punch excision along the relaxed skin tension lines. Specifically, the skin is stretched perpendicular to the relaxed skin tension lines with the thumb and index finger in order to achieve an elliptical surgical defect with a round punch tool (Fig. 47-9).

A related technique, punch elevation, is used for circular boxcar type or crateriform acne scars greater than 4 mm in diameter (Fig. 47-10). In this technique, a punch tool exactly the same diameter as the base of the crater is inserted into the skin to the subcutis. The partially attached plug of tissue is elevated slightly above the level of the surrounding skin. This plug of skin is fixed into place with Steri-Strips, cyanoacrylate adhesive, or suturing with 6.0 nylon. Superficial skin resurfacing is usually required for residual epidermal scarring. Punch grafting is a similar technique with the exception that donor skin for the central plug is acquired from a distance site rather than the base of the scar. Skin color, thickness, and texture matching are difficult with punch grafting and also require postsurgical resurfacing for optimal cosmetic appearance.

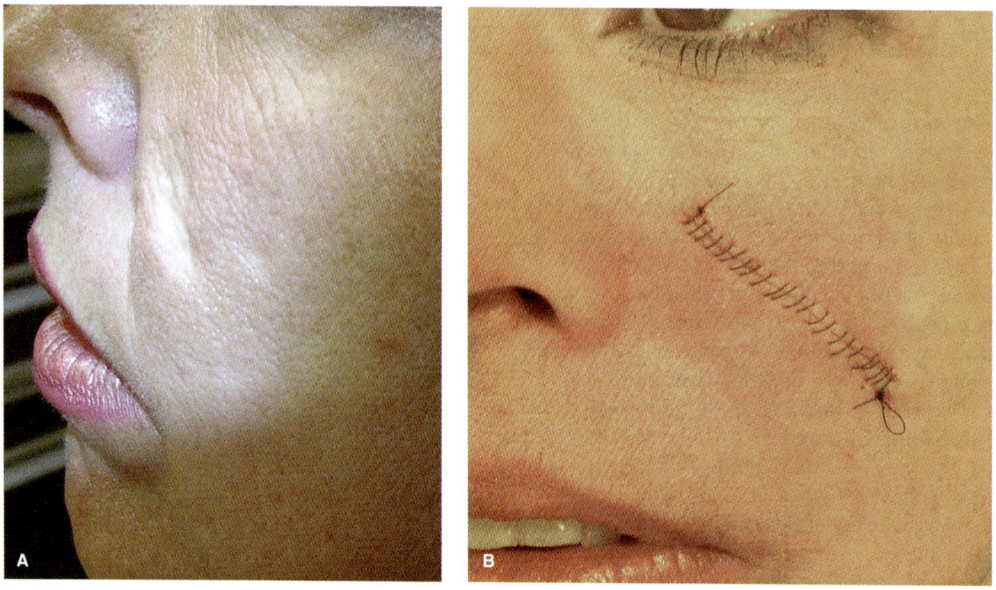

Figure 47-7 Deep atrophic acne scar treated with surgical excision. **A.** Presurgical photograph shows depth of scar with side-lighting. **B.** Following conventional excision, surgical scars can be treated with pulse dye laser or fractional resurfacing for further cosmetic improvement.

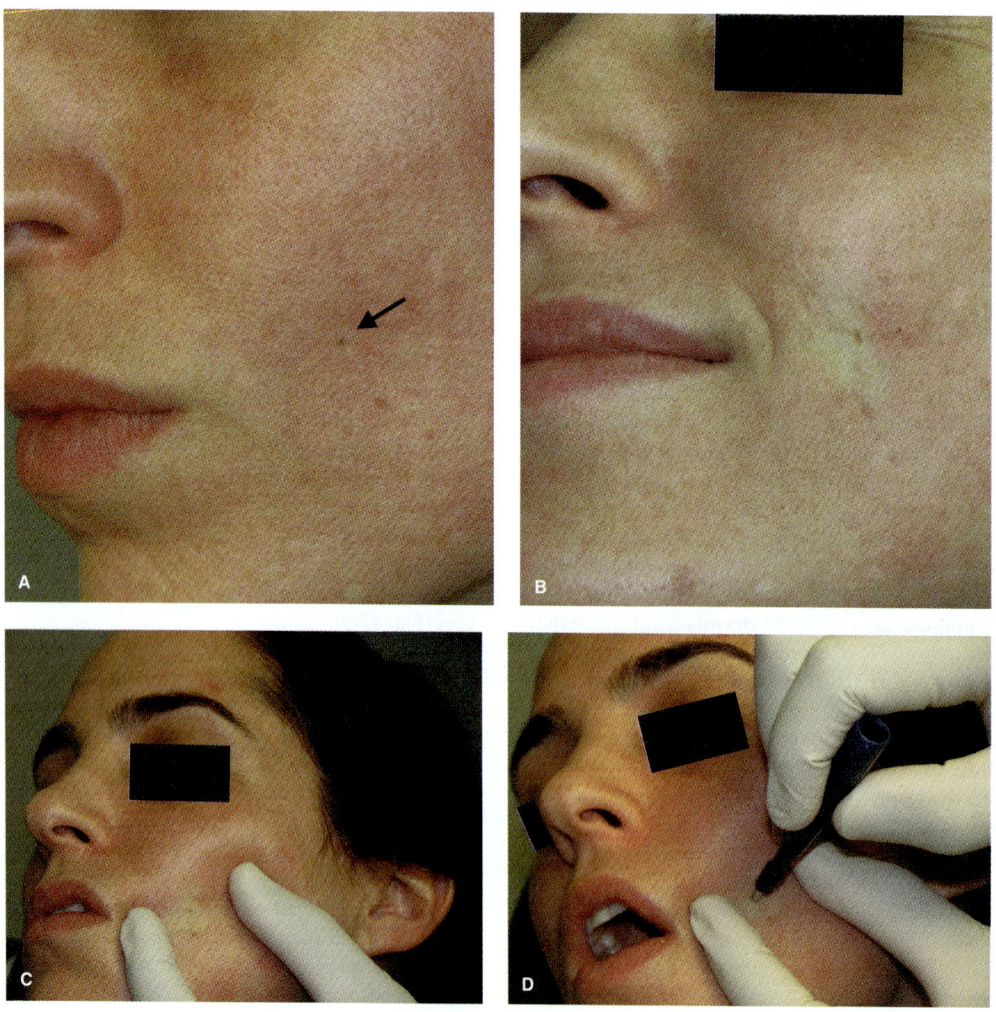

Figure 47-8 **A.** Punch excision of a small dilated pore or icepick scar. **B.** Mobilizing the skin will help define the relaxed skin tension lines (RSTL). **C.** and **D.** Stretching the skin perpendicularly to the RSTL will create an oval surgical incision with a round punch device.

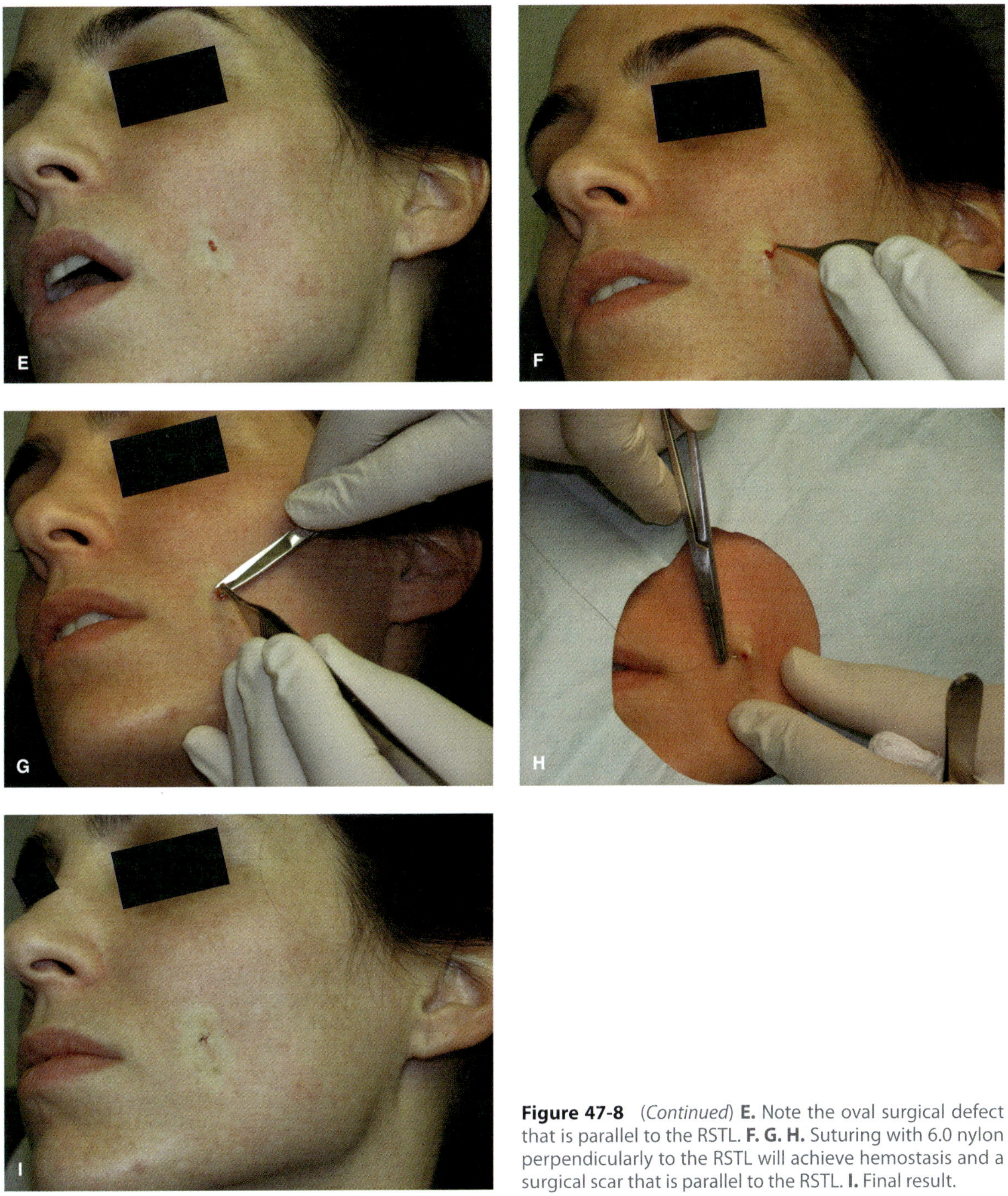

Figure 47-8 (*Continued*) **E.** Note the oval surgical defect that is parallel to the RSTL. **F. G. H.** Suturing with 6.0 nylon perpendicularly to the RSTL will achieve hemostasis and a surgical scar that is parallel to the RSTL. **I.** Final result.

Dermabrasion with various instruments including sterile sandpaper, circular knives, rasps, wire brushes, and circular sanding drills have been described over the last 100 years. One of the earliest insights into this cosmetic technique involved the precise regulation of the depth of injury by the operating surgeon.[25] If the reticular dermis was not injured during the mechanical abrasion of the epidermis, there was limited or no scarring after re-epithelialization. The correct clinical endpoint can be achieved by looking for pinpoint bleeding, which implies that the papillary dermis has been abraded. Acne scars that have sharp epidermal borders respond well to dermabrasion. The shadow created by a boxcar-type scars will be greatly reduced if the border of the scar is rounded or softened (Fig. 47-4). Rolling scars may improve slightly with dermabrasion techniques but deep icepick scars should not be treated aggressively with this technique. As with any surgical or laser procedure, patient selection should take into account pigmentation, potential for further scarring, and other factors listed in Table 47-3. Hypopigmentation is a major complication with dermabrasion and may be worsened with cryoanesthesia used prior to dermabrading the skin.[26] Tumescent anesthesia may decrease the risk of hypopigmentation.[27]

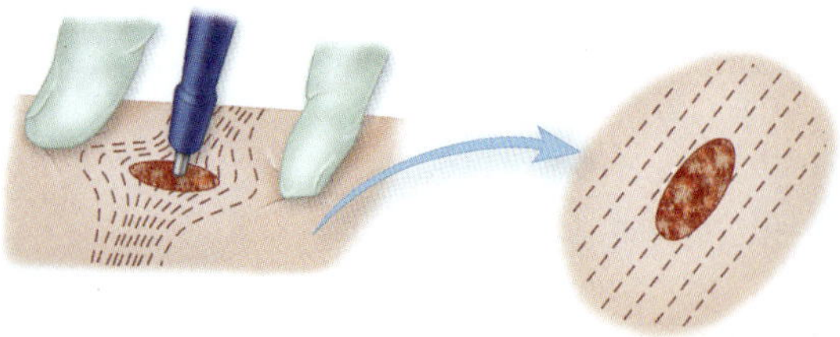

Figure 47-9 Prior to the insertion of a punch into the skin, stretching the skin perpendicular to the relaxed skin tension lines will create a surgical defect that is elliptical. The avoidance of standing cones and orientation parallel to skin tension lines will result in a more cosmetically acceptable scar.

Microdermabrasion should be differentiated from conventional dermabrasion. Microdermabrasion involves the application of a vacuum tip with high-pressure aluminum oxide or silica crystals to the skin. Only the epidermis is abraded with this technique resulting in temporary erythema of the skin. The depth of abrasion is dependent on the vacuum pressure as well as the concentration and type of crystals applied. With multiple sessions of microdermabrasion, histologic studies have revealed slight fibrosis in the upper dermis as well as a significantly smoother epidermis.[28] All skin types can undergo this procedure without significant or permanent postinflammatory pigment changes.

Microneedling is a simple and possibly effective treatment for many types of acne scarring. A small observational study showed significant improvement without resultant hyperpigmentation in 32 patients with rolling acne scars treated with two sessions of microneedling.[29] A sample device is shown in Figure 47-11. In a related technique, small areas of scarring can be treated with a 30 gauge needle that is repeatedly stabbed to a depth of 2 to 3 mm. In either technique, dermal punctures trigger collagen formation, edema, fibrosis, bleeding, and ultimately collagen remodeling. Microneedling, unlike fractional or conventional laser resurfacing, does not create any thermal injury and therefore may have less efficacy but also fewer side effects. The risk for injury to the operator with some of the more aggressive devices may be high; reusing the rollers is not advised.

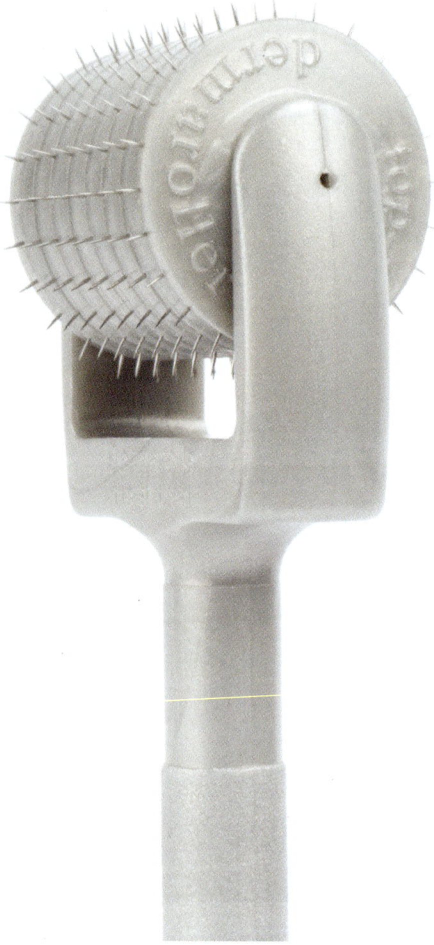

Figure 47-11 Microneedling device. (Dermaroller, LLC, Thousand Oaks, CA.)

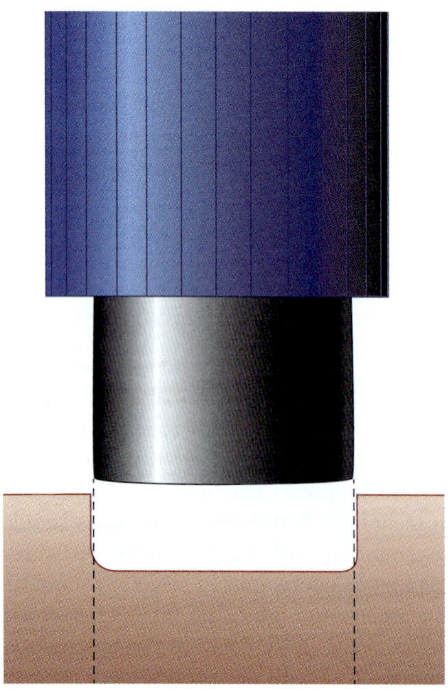

Figure 47-10 Punch elevation. Punch tool must be the same diameter as the inner crater of a boxcar-type scar when performing punch elevation.

FILLER TREATMENTS

Filler therapy for acne scarring is appropriate for rolling or depressed scars but not icepick or boxcar-type scars. Various materials have been employed for improving depressed scars including autologous fat, collagen, hyaluronic acid, calcium hydroxyapatite gel, silicone, and poly-L-lactic acid.[12] Combining subcision techniques with filler therapy results in an optimal clinical appearance. Selection of the right filler for an individual patient involves evaluation of the acne scars as well the patient's risk tolerance. Patients who are new to the dermatologist should not receive permanent fillers without extensive operator experience. Superficial or thin lesions should be treated with hyaluronic gel products, whereas deeper lesions that require a thicker or more viscous product can be treated with calcium hydroxylapatite gels.[30] Poly-L-lactic acid gel is indicated for rolling acne scars after subcision and not recommended for superficial scars. Injection into the papillary dermis may create visible persistent papules in a few months after injection of poly-L-lactic acid, which can be treated with simple excision.[31]

A simple maneuver to assess the appropriateness of filler therapy for acne scars involves stretching the scarred skin with the thumb and forefinger. If the scar improves, then the area is an appropriate site for filler therapy. The same maneuver can be used to assess for appropriateness of subcision. Combining subcision and filler therapy can be more effective than the use of either alone.[32] The mechanism of cosmetic improvement depends on the specific filler utilized. For example, autologous fat transfer involves not only volume replacement with mature adipocytes but also subsequent fibrosis associated with dead adipocytes and possibly stem cell transfer and stimulation.[33] Taking care not to inject into facial vessels is crucial. Vascular occlusion can lead to ulceration and scar. Additional details regarding fillers and injection techniques are described elsewhere in this textbook.

CHEMICAL PEEL TREATMENTS

Chemical peeling involves the application of a caustic substance to the skin, which destroys the epidermis and part of the dermis in order to stimulate epidermal and dermal regeneration. Chemical peels have been utilized for a variety of acne scars in all Fitzpatrick skin types. The most common agents used include phenolic, trichloroacetic, salicylic, and glycolic acids. The particular agent utilized as well as its concentration determines the effective depth of treatment. Deeper peels such as phenolic acids when used in darker skin types often result in medium- to long-term hyperpigmentation.[34] The same approaches used to minimize postinflammatory hyperpigmentation with laser treatments can be applied to chemical peels such as pretreatment hydroquinone and posttreatment sun avoidance. Repeat sessions on a monthly basis with mild-to-moderate depth chemical peels can also avoid pigmentary alteration while achieving significant improvement.

Glycolic acid treatments are probably the most commonly used and best-tolerated alpha-hydroxy acid peels. The duration of application and the concentration of glycolic acid peel determine the depth of epidermal damage. A typical treatment course involves monthly sessions of 50% to 70% glycolic acid. In addition to causing epidermolysis in the stratum corneum and dispersing basal layer melanin, glycolic acids have also been shown to increase hyaluronic acid and collagen production in the dermis.[35] This treatment is contraindicated in patients with an active skin dermatitis, hypersensitivity, or pregnancy.

Several other compounds are also used for chemical peels in patients with active acne vulgaris as well as acne scarring. Jessner's solution is composed of salicylic acid, lactic acid, and resorcinol. The components of this peel act synergistically to disrupt the stratum corneum and enhance absorption into the epidermis. Tolerability is similar to other superficial alpha hydroxyl peels. Thirty percent salicylic acid is a beta hydroxy acid peel that has been used effectively in darker skin types without complications.[36] Salicylism, characterized by tinnitus, abdominal pain, and dizziness, can be avoided by use of this agent on a limited skin surface area. TCA causes immediate epidermal protein denaturation, which is manifested as frosting of the skin. A superficial dermal peel can be performed with 10% TCA; concentrations higher than 35% can cause dermal injury and therefore possible scarring. The use of TCA for acne scar treatment should be avoided in patients with Fitzpatrick skin type 4 and higher due to the risk of hyperpigmentation and hypopigmentation.[37]

A variant of TCA chemical peeling was specifically developed to address icepick-type acne scars. Pinpoint application of 50% to 100% trichloroacetic acid with a sharp tool such as the broken end of a cotton-tipped applicator directly into the center of the icepick scar can essentially close the epidermal defect.[38] Carving the wooden end of the applicator stick with a surgical blade to approximate the shape of the icepick scar has been suggested to improve clinical results. Care should be taken to avoid application to the surrounding normal skin by preapplication of petrolatum. Due to the risk of hyperpigmentation and depigmentation, TCA treatments should be avoided in patients with dark skin. No anesthesia is required for focal and limited treatment. This procedure can be repeated monthly to achieve optimal results.

LASER TREATMENTS

Over the last few decades, many types of lasers and energy devices have been introduced to treat acne scarring (Table 47-4). Initially, conventional ablative lasers such as carbon dioxide and erbium:YAG lasers were used for general

TABLE 47-4
Lasers and Devices for Acne Scarring

	Device	Indication	Fractionated
Ablative lasers	Carbon dioxide Er:YAG	Resurfacing Resurfacing	Available Available
Non-ablative	Pulsed dye laser LED Infrared lasers (i.e., 1320 nm) Er:YAG (i.e., 1550/1927 nm)	Erythema reduction Photomodulation Thermal effects Non-ablative resurfacing	N/A N/A N/A Available
Mixed	Radiofrequency	Resurfacing, collagen remodeling	Available

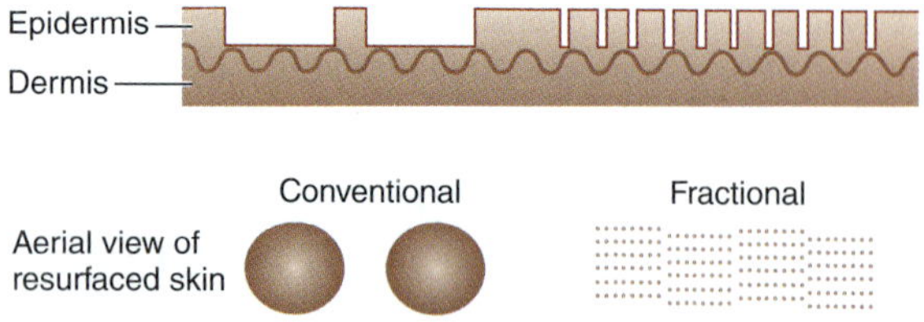

Figure 47-12 Conventional and fractional ablation of the skin.

resurfacing of the skin.[39] Non-ablative lasers such as the 1320 nm infrared lasers were later introduced to improve skin texture without actually disrupting the epidermis.[40] The overall clinical effect of non-ablative lasers in long-term studies was subtle as best.[23] In the last decade, a new class of lasers described as pixelated, scanning, or fractional has been developed (Fig. 47-12). Essentially, a wider laser beam is split or fractionated into many smaller beams; the resultant spot size for the fractionated beam is small enough that scarless healing occurs while achieving significant depth of penetration into the dermis. Alternatively, a laser with a very narrow spot size can be scanned across the skin in a controlled manner to achieve the same result. In between the pulses is normal undamaged skin, which promotes quick re-epitheilization. The immediate clinical result of fractionated ablative resurfacing with a scanning carbon dioxide laser is shown in Figure 47-13. More recently, radiofrequency devices have utilized the principles of fractional resurfacing to achieve remodeling with minimal tissue damage. More detailed descriptions of these modalities are found elsewhere in this text.

Conventional ablative treatments include carbon dioxide (10,600 nm) and Er:YAG (2940 nm) lasers. These lasers have been proven to be effective in treating all types of moderate-to-severe acne scarring. The infrared laser energy is absorbed by water and vaporizes tissue to a precise depth dependent on the fluence, dwell time, and the number of passes. The superficial epidermis and dermis are vaporized while skin appendages are left intact. The regenerated epidermis is smoother and more evenly pigmented after the skin heals. Thermal effects in the dermis

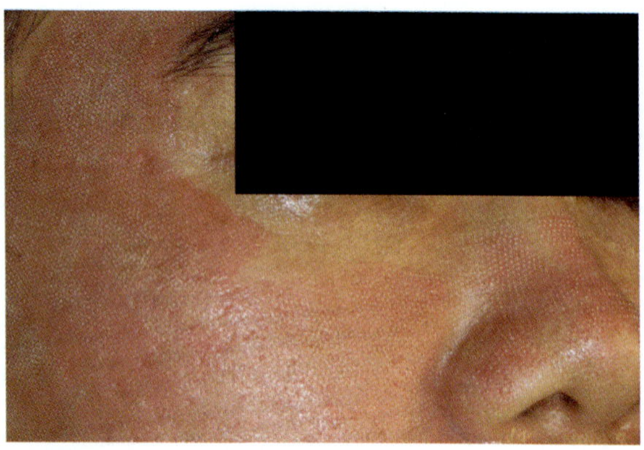

Figure 47-13 A patient with icepick scars immediately after fractional carbon dioxide ablative laser treatment. Note the individual areas of ablation with white frosting are approximately 350 μm in diameter with normal skin in between.

stimulate collagen and myofibroblast remodeling. In general, icepick and deep acne scars have demonstrated poor responses to conventional laser resurfacing. In order to ensure an optimal cosmetic outcome, the whole face should be treated when using conventional laser resurfacing for acne scarring.

Er:YAG lasers can be used alone or in combination with carbon dioxide lasers to treated depressed scars. Er:YAG lasers produce less thermal injury to surrounding tissue than carbon dioxide lasers despite more avid absorption by water in the vaporized tissue. Multiple passes are performed until pinpoint bleeding is noted.[41] As is the case with all conventional laser resurfacing treatments, there is a significant risk of edema, pruritus, transient and persistent erythema, hypopigmentation, hypertrophic scarring, and superinfection with bacteria and herpes virus. Careful patient selection is required to avoid these complications. Most patients with Fitzpatrick skin types 4 or greater should not be treated with conventional resurfacing without extensive operator experience. Detailed instruction on ablative laser resurfacing is discussed elsewhere in this text.

Fractionated or pixelated lasers are available in ablative, non-ablative, and radiofrequency modalities for acne scarring. The advantages of these lasers stem from the spot size of the individual laser beam. The area of thermal damage and/or ablation in both ablative and non-ablative fractional devices is approximately 100 to 350 μm. Between these individual areas of thermal damage is normal skin. Both the regeneration of adjacent epidermis and dermis as well as the trans-epidermal extrusion of necrotic dermis promote fast healing, which is essentially free of noticeable scar even though the depth of penetration of the necrosis is up to 1500 μm.[42] The fractionated devices leave most of the skin intact; the small areas of thermal damage slough off as flaky skin for a few days after the treatment. With fractional resurfacing, there are usually fewer areas of pinpoint bleeding than are usually seen with conventional resurfacing. Therefore, the healing time is significantly accelerated to just 5 to 7 days. Improvement was noted in 90% of patients without subsequent dyspigmentation or scarring in a large prospective study of atrophic acne scar patients treated with a fractional laser.[43] However, ablative fractional devices have been reported to produce hypertrophic scarring—particularly at higher fluences and when treating off the face.

Conventional resurfacing lasers should generally not be used on non-facial acne scars. The use of conventional carbon dioxide and erbium lasers can result in depigmentation and hypertrophic scarring on the neck and chest. Even on the face, the incidence of a porcelain-like appearance after carbon dioxide resurfacing is so high that many dermatologists limit the use of conventional carbon dioxide lasers to patients with Fitzpatrick skin types 1 and 2. However, the fractionated class of resurfacing lasers has allowed dermatologists to treat non-facial lesions safely and effectively.[44] Deeper resurfacing involving high fluences, high laser dwell times, and high density of individual ablation zones (pitch or coverage) must still be avoided on non-facial sites. Additionally, it is possible that fractionated lasers, including the thulium laser (1927 nm, designed more for the treatment of pigmentation than acne scars) will largely replace conventional carbon dioxide resurfacing.

Non-ablative tissue remodeling may also be undertaken without epidermal disruption with lasers that target water as a chromophore.[45] Mid-infrared lasers such as the 1320 nm Nd:YAG and the 1415 nm diode laser target dermal water to create thermal injury and stimulate collagen remodeling. Repeated treatments are required and clinical efficacy is highly variable.[46] Since these lasers are not pigment-specific, they are safe for use in all skin types and especially useful for rolling scars. With appropriate caution, pigment-specific lasers such as the 595 nm pulsed dye laser, the 1064 nm Nd:YAG laser, and the 755 nm alexandrite laser have also been used for non-ablative dermal remodeling with variable and mostly short-term results.

A significant component of acne scarring involves erythema and hypertrophic scars. KTP and pulsed dye lasers are commonly used to reduce both of these problems without epidermal disruption. Most commonly used is the 595 nm pulsed dye laser that targets hemoglobin as a chromophore. Macular erythema and telangiectasias are easily treated with this modality. Keloidal or hypertrophic acne scars also respond but require many treatment sessions. Purpura is a common short-term side effect; blistering and depigmentation can occur, especially in highly pigmented patients.

Because the pigment deposition in acne scarring is dermal as well as epidermal, ultra-short-pulsed lasers used for solar lentigines or tattoos should generally not be used on acne scars. Medical treatments are more likely to benefit patients with hyperpigmentation associated with acne scars.

An alternative to carbon dioxide or erbium laser resurfacing is plasma skin resurfacing.[43] High-energy ionized nitrogen is used to heat and vaporize the epidermis and superficial dermis. Because nitrogen is an inert gas, very little oxidation occurs, resulting in less carbonization or charring. Since there is no open wound formation, there is a quicker healing and less risk for infection and scarring. There is very little published research regarding this modality; however, plasma skin resurfacing may be equivalent to non-ablative laser surfacing.[47]

MEDICAL TREATMENTS

For grade 1 acne scarring, which includes macular and mild contour changes, medical treatments are often adequate therapies. Patients with severe scarring should be advised of the potential benefit from simple and effective medical treatments. Multiple topical medications can improve epidermal and dermal hyperpigmentation. These include retinoids, dapsone, hydroquinone, azelaic acid, adapalene, and hydroxy acids. Sunscreen should be recommended for patients who develop hyperpigmentation along with acne scarring. Hypertrophic acne scars can be easily treated with intralesional steroid injections. Deep scars that fall into areas of dynamic rhytides such as the perioral and periorbital areas often appear accentuated with muscle activity. Botulinum toxin injections can temporarily improve the cosmetic appearance of these areas by relaxing the surrounding skin.

CONCLUSION

The proliferation of treatments for acne scarring has given patients options for what was once a permanent cosmetic problem. The dermatologist now has numerous therapeutic options to draw from; however, a thorough understanding of the pathophysiology and classification of acne scarring is required in order to properly match patients with appropriate therapy. Aggressive management to prevent acne scarring should always be combined with regimens to treat acne scarring to optimize effectiveness and cosmesis.

REFERENCES

1. Ghodsi SZ, Orawa H, Zouboulis CC. Prevalence, severity, and severity risk factors of acne in high school pupils: A community-based study. *J Invest Dermatol.* 2009;129(9):2136–2141.
2. Layton AM, Henderson CA, Cunliffe WJ. A clinical evaluation of acne scarring and its incidence. *Clin Exp Dermatol.* 1994;19:303–308.
3. Capitanio B, Sinagra JL, Bordignon V, Cordiali Fei P, Picardo M, Zouboulis CC. Underestimated clinical features of post-adolescent acne. *J Am Acad Dermatol.* 2010;63(5):782–788.
4. Fabbrocini G, Annunziata MC, D'Arco V, et al. Acne scars: Pathogenesis, classification and treatment. *Dermatol Res Pract.* 2010;2010:893080. doi: 10.1155/2010/893080.
5. Rivera AE. Acne scarring: A review and current treatment modalities. *J Am Acad Dermatol.* 2008;59(4):659–676.
6. Goodman GJ, Baron JA. Post acne scarring: A qualitative global scarring grading system. *Dermatol Surg.* 2006;32:1458–1466.
7. Goodman GJ. Post-acne scarring: A short review of its pathophysiology. *Australas J Dermatol.* 2001;42(2):84–90.
8. Sato T, Kurihara H, Akimoto N, Noguchi N, Sasatsu M, Ito A. Augmentation of gene expression and production of promatrix metalloproteinase 2 by Propionibacterium acnes-derived factors in hamster sebocytes and dermal fibroblasts: a possible mechanism for acne scarring. *Biol Pharm Bull.* 2011;34(2):295–299.
9. Holland DB, Jeremy AH, Roberts SG, Seukeran DC, Layton AM, Cunliffe WJ. Inflammation in acne scarring: A comparison of the responses in lesions from patients prone and not prone to scar. *Br J Dermatol.* 2004;150(1):72–81.
10. Layton AM. Optimal management of acne to prevent scarring and psychological sequelae. *Am J Clin Dermatol.* 2001; 2(3):135–141.
11. Shalita A. The integral role of topical and oral retinoids in the early treatment of acne. *J Eur Acad Dermatol Venereol.* 2001;15:43–49. doi: 10.1046/j.0926-9959.2001.00012.x
12. Alam M, Hsu TS, Dover JS, Wrone DA, Arndt KA. Nonablative laser and light treatments: Histology and tissue effects—A review. *Lasers Surg Med.* 2003;33:30–39.
13. Tsao SS, Dover JS, Arndt KA, et al. Scar management. In: Kaminer MS, Dover JS, Arndt KA, et al., eds. *Atlas of Cosmetic Surgery*. Philadelphia, PA: W.B. Saunders Company; 2002.
14. Shah S, Alster TS. Laser treatment of dark skin: An update. *Am J Clin Dermatol.* 2010;11(6):389–397.
15. Mandy SH. Tretinoin in the preoperative and postoperative management of dermabrasion. *J Am Acad Dermatol.* 1986;15 (4):888–889.
16. Kingsley M, Graber E, Soo Y, Bae-Harboe C. Treatment of acne scarring with ablative fractionated laser resurfacing following isotretinoin therapy. *J Am Acad Dermatol.* 2012; 66(4):AB216.
17. West TB, Alster TS. Effect of pretreatment on the incidence of hyperpigmentation following cutaneous CO2 laser resurfacing. *Dermatol Surg.* 1999;25(1):15–17.
18. Fife D. Practical evaluation and management of atrophic acne scars. Tips for the general dermatologist. *J Clin Aesthet Dermatol.* 2011;4(8):50–57.

19. Amin SP, Goldberg DJ. Topical anesthetics for cosmetic and laser dermatology. *J Drugs Dermatol.* 2005;4(4):455–461.
20. Sobanko JF, Miller CJ, Alster TS. Topical anesthetics for dermatologic procedures: A Review. *Dermatol Surg.* 2012;38: 709–721.
21. Harahap M, Abadir A, eds. *Anesthesia and Analgesia in Dermatologic Surgery.* New York: Informa Health Care; 2008.
22. Orentreich DS, Orentreich N. Subcutaneous incisionless (subcision) surgery for the correction of depressed scars and wrinkles. *Dermatol Surg.* 1995;21(6):543–549.
23. Gottlieb SK. Soft tissue augmentation. The search for implantation materials and techniques. *Clin Dermatol.* 1987; 5(4):128–134.
24. Koranda FC. Treatment and modalities in facial acne scars. In: Holt T, Jr., (ed.) *Facial scars.* Saint Louis: Mosby; 1989:278–289.
25. Kromayer E. *Cosmetic Treatment of Skin Complaints.* London: Oxford University Press; 1930.
26. Harmon CB, Mandy SH. Dermabrasion. In: Nouri K, Leal-Khouri S, eds. *Techniques in Dermatologic Surgery.* New York: Mosby; 2003:163–169.
27. Goodman GJ. Dermabrasion using tumescent anaesthesia. *J Dermatol Surg Oncol.* 1994;20:802–807.
28. Freedman BM, Rueda-Pedraza E, Earley RV. Clinical and histologic changes determine optimal treatment regimens for microdermabrasion. *J Dermatolog Treat.* 2002;13(4):193–200.
29. Fabbrocini G, Fardella N, Monfrecola A, Proietti I, Innocenzi D. Acne scarring treatment using skin needling. *Clin Exp Dermatol.* 2009;34(8):874–879.
30. Goldberg DJ, Amin S, Hussain M. Acne scar correction using calcium hydroxylapatite in a carrier-based gel. *J Cosmet Laser Ther.* 2006;8(3):134–136.
31. Burgess CM, Quiroga RM. Assessment of the safety and efficacy of poly-L-lactic acid for the treatment of HIV-associated facial lipoatrophy. *J Am Acad Dermatol.* 2005;52(2):233–239.
32. Goodman GJ. Treatment of acne scarring. *Int J Dermatol.* 2011;50(10):1179–1194.
33. Shiffman MA, ed. *Autologous Fat Transfer: Art, Science, and Clinical Practice.* Berlin; Heidelberg: © Springer-Verlag; 2010.
34. Park JH, Choi YD, Kim SW, Kim YC, Park SW. Effectiveness of modified phenol peel (Exoderm) on facial wrinkles, acne scars and other skin problems of Asian patients. *J Dermatol.* 2007;34:17–24.
35. Bernstein EF, Lee J, Brown DB, Yu R, Van Scott E. Glycolic acid treatment increases type I collagen mRNA and hyaluronic acid content of human skin. *Dermatol Surg.* 2001;27(5):429–433.
36. Grimes PE. The safety and efficacy of salicylic acid chemical peels in darker racial-ethnic groups. *Dermatol Surg.* 1999;25(1): 18–22.
37. Al-Waiz MM, Al-Sharqi AI.Medium-depth chemical peels in the treatment of acne scars in dark-skinned individ- uals. *Dermatol Surg.* 2002;28(5):383–387.
38. Lee JB, Chung WG, Kwahck H, Lee KH. Focal treatment of acne scars with trichloroacetic acid: Chemical reconstruction of skin scars method. *Dermatol Surg.* 2002;28:1017–1021.
39. Alster TS, West TB. Resurfacing of atrophic facial acne scars with a high-energy, pulsed carbon dioxide laser. *Dermatol Surg.* 1996;22(2):151–154; discussion 154–155.
40. Rogachefsky AS, Hussain M, Goldberg DJ. Atrophic and a mixed pattern of acne scars improved with a 1320-nm Nd:YAG laser. *Dermatol Surg.* 2003;29(9):904–908.
41. Kye YC. Resurfacing of pitted facial scars with a pulsed Er:YAG laser. *Dermatol Surg.* 1997;23(10):880–883.
42. Hantash BM, Bedi VP, Sudireddy V, Struck SK, Herron G, Chan K. Laser-induced transepidermal elimination of dermal content by fractional photothermolysis. *J Biomed Opt.* 2006;11(4):041115.
43. Alster TS, Konda S. Plasma skin resurfacing for regeneration of neck, chest, and hands: Investigation of a novel device. *Dermatol Surg.* 2007;33(11):1315–1321.
44. Tierney EP, Hanke CW. Ablative fractionated CO2, laser resurfacing for the neck: Prospective study and review of the literature. *J Drugs Dermatol.* 2009;8:723–731.
45. Tanzi EL, Alster TS. Comparison of a 1450-nm diode laser and a 1320-nm Nd:YAG laser in the treatment of atrophic facial scars: A prospective clinical and histologic study. *Dermatol Surg.* 2004;30:152–157.
46. Bhatia AC, Dover JS, Arndt KA, Stewart B, Alam M. Patient satisfaction and reported long-term therapeutic efficacy associated with 1,320 nm Nd:YAG laser treatment of acne scarring and photoaging. *Dermatol Surg.* 2006;32:346–352.
47. Kono T, Groff WF, Sakurai H, Yamaki T, Soejima K, Nozaki M. Treatment of traumatic scars using plasma skin regeneration (PSR) system. *Lasers Surg Med.* 2009;41:128–130.

CHAPTER 48

Management of Dyschromias

Claire Marie Reyes-Habito & Molly Wanner

Dyschromia is a broad term used for disorders of pigmentation. Three common pigmentary issues are melasma, postinflammatory hyperpigmentation (PIH), and dermatoheliosis. All are characterized by increased melanin deposition in the skin, although the pathogenesis of each increase is distinct.

The treatment of dyschromia is accomplished with topical therapies, chemical peels, and lasers. Dermatoheliosis is the most easily treatable of the forms of dyschromia. Melasma and PIH are far more challenging. This chapter will review the treatment options for each of these disorders.

MELASMA

Melasma is hyperpigmentation of the face, usually seen in women with Fitzpatrick skin types III to IV and typically distributed on the central face, malar, or mandibular areas. This chronic disorder occurs in 50% of pregnant women and 10% of men.[1] The prevalence has been reported to be 40% in Southeast Asia and to range from as low as 8% to as high as 80% among Latina females.[2,3]

Melasma is caused by increased melanin pigment deposition in the skin triggered by ultraviolet light, visible light, and hormones such as in pregnancy, oral contraception, and hormone replacement therapy.[1,4] Thyroid disorders, genetic predisposition, and antiseizure and phototoxic medications are other risk factors that may affect melasma.[1] Epidermal barrier dysfunction may also play a role.[5]

The pigmentation in melasma is due to enlarged melanocytes, increased melanosomes, increased melanin content in keratinocytes, and melanin deposition in melanophages.[5,6] Traditionally, melasma has been classified as epidermal, dermal, or mixed type[2,7]; however, confocal microscopy has demonstrated that most melasma is mixed, with epidermal hyperpigmentation playing the primary role.[5,8] Dermal pigmentation contributes less to the clinical manifestations; however the dermal fibroblasts may be involved in signaling pathways that lead to melasma.[5] Wood's light examination, historically used to distinguish epidermal and dermal melasma, has not been found to be clinically accurate.[6,9,10]

Therapies for melasma include topical lightening creams, chemical peels, and lasers. Even oral treatments have been tried, although the utility of this approach needs to be further elucidated.[11] Treatment can be challenging and is often characterized by recurrence. Long-term remission can be difficult to achieve.

TOPICAL TREATMENTS

Lightening agents. Hydroquinone (1,4 dihydroxybenzene) is the most commonly used lightening agent for melasma. It inhibits the enzyme tyrosinase and prevents the conversion of L-3,4 dihydroxyphenylalanine to melanin, leading to altered melanosome production and increased melanosome destruction.[1,12] In combination with sun protection, this medication can improve the epidermal component of melasma. Hydroquinone 4% may be used twice a day on a regular basis for short periods of time. The recommended treatment time varies and ranges from 8 weeks to 6 months, depending on the hydroquinone formulation.[13]

Although generally well tolerated, hydroquinone can be associated with adverse effects. It can cause redness and irritation, and as a result, once daily use is often recommended initially. The medication has been reported to cause eye damage and should be used cautiously near the eye.[14] Contact dermatitis has also been reported.[15] There is a risk of exogenous ochronosis or blue-black skin macules caused by local inhibition of homogentisic acid oxidase by hydroquinone. Exogenous ochronosis is commonly seen with prolonged use, usually within 6 to 60 months in concentrations as low as 1% to 2%.[16] This side effect is reported to be common in South Africa, where high concentrations of hydroquinone were available and used for long-term periods.[16] Occupational vitiligo in photographic developers handling hydroquinone has been reported.[17,18]

In 2006, the FDA raised questions about the safety of hydroquinone[19] due to concerns about side effects and potential carcinogenicity.[20] In laboratory rodent studies, hydroquinone given systemically caused bone marrow toxicity and benign renal adenomas. At this time, there is inadequate evidence to support carcinogenicity in humans.[12] In Europe, hydroquinone has been banned from all cosmetic products and is only available by prescription. The US FDA is considering a similar approach.[12]

Hydroquinone is prescribed both alone and in combination with other medications. One of the first combination creams was the Kligman–Willis formula, which contains hydroquinone 5%, tretinoin 0.1%, and dexamethasone 0.1%.[12] The addition of tretinoin enhances hydroquinone's lightening effect by preventing its oxidation and improving its epidermal penetration. Corticosteroids, on the other hand, reduce irritation from the two ingredients and decrease cellular metabolism, which inhibits melanin synthesis.[12] An FDA-approved triple combination cream for melasma is composed of hydroquinone 4%, tretinoin 0.05%, and fluocinolone acetonide 0.01%. This combination cream yielded clearance of melasma in 35% of patients compared to 5% of patients who used hydroquinone 4% alone.[21]

Triple combination cream is indicated for the short term treatment of melasma, and should be used for no more than 8 weeks due to the risk of exogenous ochronosis and steroid-induced skin atrophy.[22] However, a review of intermittent or continuous use of triple combination therapy for longer durations of up to a year demonstrated a relatively safe profile with only two cases of mild atrophy.[23] In another study, no statistically significant histopathologic signs of epidermal or dermal atrophy were seen after 6 months of use of triple combination creams.[24]

Other lightening agents include topical retinoids, azelaic acid, kojic acid, glycolic acid (GA), ascorbic acid, ellagic acid, arbutin, rucinol, oligopeptides, licorice extract, mequinol, and soy.[1,12,25] Mequinol and soy, however, have been mainly studied for pigmentation in lentigines. Mequinol has been used effectively for melasma in a case series of five patients[26] and no trials in melasma have been done using soy.

Retinoids, particularly tretinoin 0.05% and adapalene 0.1%, have produced a decrease in the Melasma Area and Severity Index (MASI) score by 37% and 41%, respectively after 14 weeks of use.[27] Azelaic acid 20% has also shown to be as effective as hydroquinone 4% in a 24 week double-blind trial for melasma.[28] Similarly, a study comparing kojic acid + GA preparation with hydroquinone + GA found improvement of melasma in both preparations with no statistical difference between the two.[29] In a split-face randomized study comparing ascorbic acid 5% cream and hydroquinone 4% cream, subjective improvement was found to be 62% and 93%, respectively.[30]

Ellagic acid 1%, arbutin 1%, and the plant extract ellagic acid were compared in a randomized, prospective, open label study. All three showed a significant decrease in mexameter pigment density of melasma with no significant difference among the groups.[31] Rucinol 0.3% has also shown significant improvement of melasma in a randomized, double-blind placebo controlled study.[32] Oligopeptides and topical liquiritin (licorice) have also shown clinical improvement of melasma compared to vehicle cream in split-face studies.[33,34]

Maintenance therapy is often needed as the risk of recurrence is high, particularly in sunny climates. Lightening agents can be used once or twice a week and increased to daily when necessary.[7,35] Alternatively, daily use of a nonhydroquinone topical such as tretinoin, azelaic acid, kojic acid, or GA may be also used for a maintenance regimen.

Photoprotection. Melasma is stimulated by ultraviolet and visible light and as such, sun protection is important. The use of hats, protective clothing, and sunscreen with a high UVA and UVB sun protection factor is a critical part of treatment. Without sun protection, most therapies will be marginally effective.

Titanium dioxide and zinc oxide are often recommended in the treatment of melasma[36] because they can protect against visible light. However, these sunscreens appear white on the skin and micronized versions do not offer the same protection.[37,38] Many sunscreen formulations have the disadvantage of offering low UVA1 protection and visible light protection[38,39] making the use of a hat all the more important. Iron oxide, as an alternative, is shown to decrease visible light penetration.[38] Some formulations combine hydroquinone with a sunscreen. A double-blind study showed that hydroquinone 4% combined with broad-spectrum sunscreen cleared melasma in 96% of patients compared to hydroquinone alone.[40]

CHEMICAL PEELS

While topical products alone can be effective, improvement of melasma may be enhanced with superficial or medium depth chemical peels. Chemical peels remove melanin and can increase penetration of lightening agents. The depth of peel and concentration of peeling agents are individualized according to the patient's history and skin type. Patient considerations are listed in Table 48-1. Skin phototype will impact peel choice. In lighter skin types, more aggressive peels can be used. In darker skin types, it is recommended to start cautiously with superficial peels.

Generally, peels are contraindicated for patients who are pregnant or nursing, who have taken isotretinoin within 6 months or have active herpes simplex infection. For those who had herpes simplex in the past, prophylactic antivirals are given. Other factors to consider include connective tissue disorders or the presence of a systemic disease that impacts healing.[41] Smoking will impact healing after peels as well.

Concurrent treatments will alter peel results. Sun avoidance and use of a sunscreen for the month prior to a peel is a key part of the treatment. Tretinoin helps enhance penetration and peel intensity, and pretreatment 2 to 4 weeks prior to a peel may be helpful. Discontinuation of tretinoin 1 week prior will lessen the intensity of the subsequent peel and increase the safety margin, and is recommended with medium depth peels. Hydroquinone decreases PIH and is a useful adjunct in darker phototypes at higher risk for hyperpigmentation. Starting hydroquinone 1 to 4 weeks prior to peeling and continuing postpeel will be helpful in most patients with melasma, but particularly those with darker skin.

After peels, strict sun protection is required for at least 1 month. Patients should be advised to use gentle cleansers and skin care products and to avoid electrolysis and waxing for the week following the peel.[42] Hydroquinone may be restarted as soon as several days after the peel, depending on peel intensity. Patients should not attempt

TABLE 48-1
Patient Considerations Prior to Cosmetic Procedures

Skin phototype
Pregnancy
Nursing
Isotretinoin use
HSV history
Current topical treatments
Recent laser or surgery
Hypertrophic scar history
Connective tissue disorder
Systemic disease
Smoking
Sun exposure/tan
History of Vitiligo

to peel their skin after the procedure and should be instructed to expect that a maintenance peel protocol may be necessary.[43] Postpeel patients can expect slight dryness with very superficial peels, or redness, scaling and even crusting lasting 1 to 2 weeks with deeper peels.

Superficial peels. The most commonly used peels are superficial. Superficial peels affect part or all of the epidermis and accelerate epidermal turnover.[44] Peels facilitate a more uniform epidermal structure and more evenly distributed melanin. Superficial peels include alpha and beta hydroxy acids, amino fruit peels, Jessner's peel, and low concentrations of trichloroacetic acid (TCA) (10%–30%).

GA is the most studied chemical peel used for melasma. GA peels accelerate the turnover of the epidermis by decreasing the adhesion of corneocytes at the lower levels of the stratum corneum.[45] GA also reduces melanin formation in melanocytes through inhibition of tyrosinase.[46] Serial GA peels are performed every 4 to 6 weeks with increasing concentrations as tolerated by the patient. The typical starting point ranges from 20% to 35% with a 2 to 3 minute application. The depth of the peel depends on the concentration and length of time it is left on the skin before it is neutralized with bicarbonate. One study found clinical improvement of melasma with GA 52.3% applied for 3 minutes, but not at lower concentrations.[43]

GA peels may enhance the penetration of depigmenting agents for melasma. Serial GA peels combined with modified Kligman's cream (hydroquinone 4% + tretinoin 0.05% + hydrocortisone 1%) were compared to GA peels alone, and showed decreases in MASI score of 79.9% and 63.1%, respectively, after 21 weeks.[47]

There are many other superficial chemical peels that can be used for melasma that may have similar effects to GA peels according to some studies. Tretinoin 1% peeling has been shown to be comparable to GA 70% peeling in a randomized, double-blind clinical trial involving 63 patients with bilateral melasma treated with four sessions done biweekly.[48]

Amino fruit acids (AFAs) are carboxylated amino acids. A study that compared serial GA peels (20%–70%) with AFA peels (20%–60%) done every 2 weeks for 6 months in a split-face trial showed no significant difference between the two in treating melasma. In this study, AFA peels were less irritating and better tolerated.[49]

TCA, another commonly used peel for melasma, is a derivative of acetic acid. TCA causes epidermal protein denaturation and necrosis causing subsequent reepithelialization from epidermal appendages. Histologic findings after a series of TCA peels showed an acanthotic epidermis with a marked decrease in the amount of melanin within the epidermal cells, as well as an increase in the amount of collagen.[50]

Protein denaturation is responsible for the skin frosting observed after one to two coats of TCA. The intensity of the peel is related to concentration. Low TCA concentrations (10%–30%) produce a superficial peel.[51] In a study comparing serial chemical peels of GA (20%–35%) and TCA (10%–20%) applied every 2 weeks for 12 weeks, the reductions to MASI scores were 79% and 73%, respectively, with no significant difference between the two.[52]

Jessner's peel, a combination of lactic acid 14%, salicylic acid (SA) 14%, and resorcinol 14% in an alcohol base, has also been found to improve melasma. Like TCA, it results in frosting of the skin. In a study comparing Jessner's solution to GA peel in a split-face treatment of melasma, colorimeter analysis showed an average lightening of 2.93 and 3.14 light reflectance (L value), respectively, with no significant difference between the two.[53]

Less frequently used for melasma is SA, a keratolytic beta-hydroxy acid. Compared with GA, SA is lipophilic and removes the intercellular lipids. This results in flattening of residual epidermal cells and facilitates regeneration of the epidermis and the papillary dermis.[54] In a study comparing SA 30% with Jessner's solution, both solutions produced a significant reduction in melasma and MASI scores ($p < 0.0001$) with no significant difference between the two.[55] However, in a split-face study using four serial peels of SA 20% to 30% + hydroquinone 4% twice a day on one side of the face and hydroquinone 4% alone on the other half of the face twice a day, reduction in pigmentation using narrowband reflectance spectrophotometry showed no significant difference.[56] Hence, SA peels seemed to offer minimal advantage compared with topical treatment alone.

Medium depth peels. Medium depth peels treat the epidermis and part of the papillary dermis, and may be useful to improve dermal melasma. Solutions used to achieve a medium depth peel are TCA 35% to 50%, Jessner's solution + TCA 35%, GA 70% + TCA 35%, and GA 70%.[51] Skin desquamation and reepithelialization may take up to 7 to 10 days. Patients should be advised that they will have at least a week of downtime. Gentle skin care with avoidance of sun and make-up is required. These peels are more uncomfortable than superficial ones, and premedication is used for some patients.[41]

For darker-skinned individuals with Fitzpatrick phototypes IV-VI, medium depth full face peels are not advised due to the risk of PIH. However, medium depth focal peels of TCA 30% to 50% for light to dark brown melasma and focal peels of TCA 10% to 20% for periocular melasma have been evaluated in 20 dark-skinned patients.[57] After a mean of 3.2 peel sessions done 1 to 2 months apart, 55% of patients had a good clinical response, with no significant complications. Since frequent superficial peels may induce hyperpigmentation in some dark-skinned patients,[58] focal medium depth TCA peels may be another option for these patients with a reduced number of cautiously used as peel sessions.

LASERS

Lasers are not considered to be a first-line treatment for melasma, since there is a large degree of variability in response. All patients should be counseled about the high risk of recurrence and partial response. There are multiple lasers and light treatments that have been tried for melasma including the Q-switched ruby, alexandrite and Nd:YAG lasers, intense pulsed light (IPL), fractional laser, pulsed dye laser, Er:YAG, and carbon dioxide laser, with varying levels of success.[12,59] There is minimal evidence that ablative resurfacing lasers should be used for melasma.[12,60–62]

In planning for a laser procedure, a thorough history of medical conditions and medications should be documented. Lasers are contraindicated for patients who have used isotretinoin in the previous 6 months, have active herpes simplex infection or have vitiligo.[63] Antiviral prophylaxis can be considered depending on the type of laser to be used, and fractional laser is such an indication. Other patient considerations are laser dependent. Q-switched lasers are contraindicated in patients with a history of gold injections, for example. Strict sun avoidance and use of broad-spectrum sunscreens is important for every patient with every laser. The use of lightening agents before and after a procedure should be discussed with the patient, especially if they are prone to PIH.

Fractional resurfacing. Fractional lasers create islands of damage surrounded by normal skin.[64] Wavelengths of fractional lasers include 1540 nm, 1550 nm, 1927 nm, 2790 nm, 2940 nm, or 10,600 nm. Fractional lasers have been shown to improve melasma,[65–67] but recurrence has been reported with long-term follow-up.[68]

The 1550 nm fractional laser is FDA cleared for treatment of melasma and has been reported to improve this condition.[65,66] A consensus paper described melasma as the most difficult to treat of the FDA-cleared indications.[63] Histologic and ultrastructural analysis of melasma before and after four treatments with the 1550 nm fractional laser confirmed a decrease in the number of epidermal melanocytes and fewer enlarged melanocytes on electron microscopy.[67] However, a randomized study comparing the 1550 nm fractional laser to a triple combination hydroquinone cream found both modalities to be effective with no significant difference between the two. Six months posttreatment, recurrence of melasma occurred in half of the subjects in both groups.[69] Similarly, fractional photothermolysis and TCA 15% peels have been shown to have comparable rates of improvement and recurrence.[70] A study of fractional laser in Asian skin reported diminishing efficacy over time as well as PIH in some subjects.[71] Paradoxical worsening of melasma with diffuse hyperpigmentation over the entire face has been reported after fractional laser treatment.[69]

The 1927 nm and 10,600 nm wavelengths have been evaluated for melasma. These wavelengths have a higher absorption coefficient for water, conferring greater ability to target pigment in the epidermis. Significant improvement in MASI has been shown after 1 month posttreatment using the 1927 nm laser in several studies.[72–74] In one study, the 1927 nm laser elicited a 51% reduction in MASI that decreased to a 34% reduction 6 months after three to four treatments.[74] Fractional ablative laser at 10,600 nm has also been shown to improve melasma with a lower recurrence rate if used in combination with Kligman's cream.[75] Fractional ablative laser has been anecdotally reported to have a higher incidence of recurrence and PIH than nonablative fractional lasers.[76]

Q-switched lasers. The 1064, 755, and 694 nm Q-switched lasers have been studied for melasma. These lasers treat pigmentary conditions by targeting melanosomes. The Q-switched Nd:YAG laser in particular can target melanosomes well into the dermis. Electron microscopy has revealed a decrease in melanocyte volume, fewer dendritic melanocytes, and a decrease in stage IV melanosomes after Q-switched Nd:YAG laser.[77]

There is little evidence for treating melasma with the Q-switched 694 and 755 nm lasers, and these lasers have resulted in worsening of the condition.[60,78,79] The Q-switched Nd:YAG laser has been reported to improve melasma, but has resulted in both hyperpigmentation and punctate hypopigmentation in multiple studies, even at low fluences and especially after multiple treatments.[80–83]

Low fluence Q-switched Nd:YAG laser in combination with microdermabrasion, hydroquinone, tretinoin, and L-ascorbic acid yielded improvement in melasma in 27 subjects in an observational study.[75] The lack of PIH or hypopigmentation in this study was attributed to the use of very low fluences, the treatment interval, and a limited number of treatments. Although this study evaluated subjects with refractory melasma who failed topical treatments, it is unclear how much of the improvement can be attributed to the laser or microdermabrasion plus a topical regimen. More data is needed to fully elucidate the additive value of the Q-switched Nd:YAG.

Intense pulsed light (IPL). IPL is a nonlaser light source that emits wavelengths between 515 nm and 1200 nm. As with laser treatments, IPL can improve melasma, but carries a risk of PIH and recurrence. In a study of 89 patients with recalcitrant melasma who underwent four treatments of IPL, the mean MASI decreased from 15.2 to 5.2 and after 3 months to 4.5.[84] Side effects included edema, erythema, microcrusting, and PIH in three patients. A study of hydroquinone and sunscreen with and without IPL found more improvement in the IPL arm with a decrease in melanin index of 39.8% versus 11.6% after 16 weeks.[85] At 6 months posttreatment, the IPL treated side showed some recurrence with a decreased melanin index of 24.5%.

Vascular lasers. The rationale for the use of vascular lasers for pigmentary conditions is twofold. First, pulsed dye lasers can target melanin if used in conjunction with compression. Compression removes the more highly absorbed target (hemoglobin) and allows pigmentation to be treated. Second, there may be a connection between altered vasculature and melasma.[86,87] In a small, randomized controlled study, the pulsed dye laser with compression was used in combination with Tri-Luma® cream versus Tri-Luma® alone.[59] There was a statistically significant reduction in the MASI score with the combination treatment; however, PIH was noted in some subjects. In another small study of 578 and 511 nm lasers, a statistically significant reduction in MASI was seen.[72]

SUMMARY

Melasma is a challenging condition to treat, and every patient should be counseled to expect recurrence. First line should be the use of topical therapies and sun avoidance. In treatment resistant patients, chemical peels and lasers can be considered. Multiple studies support the use of glycolic peels, although other peel formulations have shown efficacy as well. While low fluence Q-switched Nd:YAG in combination with microdermabrasion and hydroquinone has shown recent promise, caution should be exercised with the use of any laser, since all of them carry risk with this difficult to treat condition.

POSTINFLAMMATORY HYPERPIGMENTATION

PIH is another skin disorder common among Fitzpatrick skin types III to VI, and appears as brown macules or patches in areas of previous skin irritation. PIH is caused by inflammatory mediators that stimulate melanocyte synthesis and transfer of pigment to surrounding keratinocytes. In addition, inflammation can lead to breakdown of the basal layer of the epidermis, releasing melanin into the dermis. This melanin is engulfed by dermal melanophages and leads to further discoloration and PIH at the site of injury.[88]

Inflammatory processes that may induce PIH include infection, inflammatory skin conditions or in some cases, treatment of skin disorders. Cutaneous injuries, papulosquamous disorders, allergic reactions, and acne are common causes of PIH. One study estimated that 65.3% of African Americans, 52.7% of Hispanics, and 47.4% of Asians have acne-induced PIH.[89] The occurrence of PIH after cosmetic and laser procedures is not uncommon, with an incidence varying from 3.8% to 92% depending on the type of treatment.[90]

The management of PIH generally involves early and effective treatment of the underlying skin condition to reduce further inflammation. Application of topical lightening agents may be used to decrease melanin and achieve uniform skin color. Resurfacing procedures such as chemical peels or lasers may be added to hasten skin normalization.

PREVENTION OF PIH

PIH can be prevented by early treatment of the inflammatory skin condition and reducing the risk of irritation from topical medications and procedures. Irritation from acne medications and subsequent acne-induced PIH may be minimized by using topical treatments with the lowest effective concentration, drug combinations with moisturizing vehicles and use of moisturizers concurrently with medications.[91] Avoidance of mechanical irritation, including scratching, rubbing, or picking, should also be emphasized to prevent hyperpigmentation.[92]

Laser procedures and chemical peels can lead to PIH, as well as sun exposure after treatment.[93] The risk of PIH can be reduced by avoiding these procedures in patients who have a tan, and advising strict sun protection with the use of sunscreen and hats for one month prior to and after the treatment.[94] Matching procedure to skin phototype is also critical. For example, the risk of PIH after fractional ablative laser has been reported to be 92% in patients with skin type IV compared with 23% in patients with skin types I to III.[95,96]

The use of hydroquinone prior to laser treatment has been advocated as a means to decrease PIH risk; however, hydroquinone can cause irritation and may contribute to PIH in some cases.[97] Topical steroids may also decrease the risk of PIH if used after laser treatments, but should be used sparingly to avoid steroid-induced side effects.[98] In addition, PIH is reduced by exercising caution when selecting treatment parameters in dark-skinned individuals. Aggressive chemical peels or lasers that are highly selective for epidermal melanin are riskier.

Lasers can cause PIH. Those that heat the epidermis less intensely and allow time for epidermal cooling are preferred to minimize that risk. Long-pulsed lasers have a lower risk of PIH compared with Q-switched lasers.[99,100] The choice of laser endpoint may influence the risk as well. The endpoint of Q-switched lasers is whitening of the skin in the area of treatment and corresponds to the gas bubbles produced by cavitation and rupture of melanosomes.[101–103] A randomized study of Q-switched laser (ruby laser and frequency doubled ND:YAG laser) treatments for lentigines found that slight whitening produced less PIH compared with complete whitening in Asian patients.[104] The use of high-density fractional laser treatments has a higher risk of PIH compared with low-density treatments.[94] Cooling of the skin, especially in small anatomical areas, is important as well to help decrease bulk tissue heating and prevent PIH.

TOPICAL TREATMENTS

Lightening agents. Topical hydroquinone 2% to 4% is commonly used to treat PIH and can be combined with tretinoin or α-hydroxy acids to increase penetration and efficacy. Care should be applied when spreading lightening agents over areas with pigmentation because normal skin can be "bleached," causing a side effect called "hydroquinone halo."[105] However, for patients with many PIH macules in whom spot treatment is not feasible, hydroquinone may be applied over the entire affected area.[106]

In some patients with irritant or allergic dermatitis to hydroquinone, further inflammation and PIH may occur. Testing a small area such as on the upper inner arm for several days is advisable. Alternative lightening agents such as mequinol, azelaic acid, kojic acid, arbutin, soy, and niacinamide can be applied.

Retinoids have also demonstrated lightening of PIH by increasing epidermal turnover.[107] In a randomized placebo controlled trial, tretinoin 0.1% used for 40 weeks showed lightening of PIH lesions by 40% compared to 18% in the placebo group. Epidermal melanin content also decreased by 23% in the tretinoin group compared to 3% in the placebo group.[108] Likewise, tazarotene 0.1% cream and adapalene 0.1% gel have shown significant improvement of acne-induced PIH in patients with dark skin after 12 to 18 weeks of once daily application.[109,110]

Photoprotection. Sun exposure can exacerbate or cause PIH after cosmetic treatments. Use of broad-spectrum sunscreen is important to prevent the worsening of PIH through UV-induced melanogenesis. Photoprotection before and after dermatologic procedures such as laser is critical to reduce the risk of pigmentation.

CHEMICAL PEELS

Adjunctive chemical peels can be done for PIH lesions not responding to topical creams. Peels can be applied to a localized pigmented patch or over a generalized area with scattered pigmented macules. However, care should be taken in selecting the appropriate chemical peel to avoid irritation, which can worsen PIH. Prepeel and postpeel instructions include strict daily use of broad-spectrum sunscreens and avoidance of sun exposure to prevent additional postinflammatory lesions.

Superficial peels. Superficial peels are generally well tolerated by all skin types. A series of peels may be beneficial for those patients, including dark-skinned patients, who have postinflammatory pigmentary changes. However, chemical peels should be used cautiously so as not

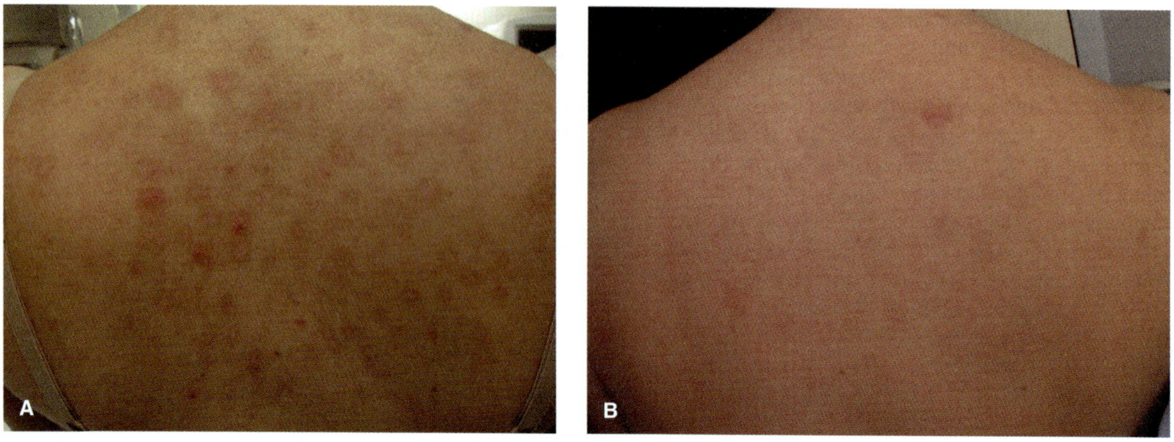

Figure 48-1 Before (**A**) and after (**B**) seven treatments of fractional photothermolysis (1550 nm) for acne scarring and postinflammatory hyperpigmentation.

to worsen PIH, especially in dark-skinned patients. For patients with acne-induced PIH, chemical peels can act both as comedolytic and lightening agents.

Beta hydroxy acid peels, such as SA 20% to 30% and its derivative lipohydroxy acid (LHA) 5% to 10%, induce keratolysis by disrupting intercellular linkages between epidermal cells.[42] Beta hydroxyl peels are lipophilic and, therefore, are particularly useful in treating acne-induced PIH. In a study of 24 Asian subjects with acne-induced PIH, SA peels done biweekly for 3 months showed an increase in lightening of lesions, although it was not statistically significant.[111] In another study, SA 20% combined with a mandelic acid 10% peel showed statistically significant improvement in PIH compared with GA 35% peels done biweekly for 6 months (59.8% and 46.3%, respectively).[112]

GA peels may also be used as adjuncts in treating PIH. Given that chemical peels can also induce PIH, it is advisable to start treatment with a low GA concentration, particularly in skin of color patients. In a study of 16 African American subjects with facial PIH, GA peels (50%–68%) with a topical regimen of 2% hydroquinone + 10% GA and 0.05% tretinoin were compared to topical regimen use alone. The peel group showed that the addition of six GA peels done every 3 weeks reduced hyperpigmentation more rapidly than topicals alone, although there was no statistically significant difference between the two groups.[113]

TCA 10% to 30% and Jessner's peel may also be effectively used as light surface peels but lack studies supporting treatment for PIH.

Medium depth peel. Medium depth peels may cause further PIH, especially in patients with dark skin. Medium peels are usually done as a single treatment, causing redness for several days and significant desquamation. Medium depth peels may be useful for acne-induced PIH with associated dermal pigmentation or depressed scars. However, because of the risk of hyperpigmentation, strict sun avoidance, daily sunscreen, and potentially hydroquinone are advised.

LASERS

Studies and case reports have shown variable success in using different lasers for PIH. In a retrospective analysis of the treatment of acne-induced PIH, the use of topical treatments (triple combination cream, azelaic acid with steroid and hydroquinone 4%–6%), lasers (595 nm long-pulsed dye laser and/or 1064 nm QS ND:YAG) or a combination of all three showed significant global improvement in PIH (50%, 55.6%, and 70.6%, respectively) with no significant difference between the groups.[114]

A small case series reported improvement in PIH with the 1064 nm Q-switched Nd:YAG at low fluence.[115] The Q-switched Nd:YAG was also shown to be effective in the treatment of acne-induced PIH in Asian patients in one prospective study. Subjects given five weekly 1064 nm QS ND:YAG laser treatments with concomitant benzoyl peroxide twice daily were compared to subjects treated with weekly comedone extraction and intralesional injection procedures in addition to benzoyl peroxide twice daily. After 1 and 3 months, blinded evaluator assessments showed improvement in PIH in the laser group and little to no improvement in PIH in the nonlaser group.[116]

Fractional resurfacing has also been reported to improve PIH (see Fig. 48-1). In one case report, PIH was reduced by 50% to 75% after five sessions of fractional 1550 nm erbium-doped laser over a 2 month period.[117] In another report using the same device, PIH improved by 95% after three sessions.[118]

SUMMARY

Prevention of PIH by choosing the treatment that best matches skin phototype is important. The choice of treatment should not exacerbate inflammation or pigmentation. Topical treatment can improve PIH, and in nonresponders, peels and lasers can be considered.

DERMATOHELIOSIS

Dermatoheliosis is a term used to describe ultraviolet light-induced changes or "photoaging." It is induced by chronic ultraviolet light exposure, as opposed to intrinsic aging, which is due to genetic factors.[119] Characteristics can include uneven pigmentation, elastosis, wrinkles, erythema, telangiectasia, actinic keratosis, and textural changes.

The dyschromia of dermatoheliosis in part is caused by solar lentigines. Solar lentigines, or liver spots, are well-demarcated macules in sun-exposed areas that vary in size from a few millimeters to more than a centimeter, and vary in color from yellow and light brown to dark brown.[120] They have been shown to be strongly associated with age and cumulative and intermittent sun exposure. In a study of risk factors in Caucasian women, solar lentigines were associated with darker skin color, tanning capacity, a history of freckles, sun exposure behavior, and current intake of oral contraceptive or progesterone treatments.[121]

Histologically, solar lentigines have an increased number of melanocytes with two epidermal patterns: (1) a flattened epidermis with basal melanosis and (2) epidermal hyperplasia with budding rete ridges composed of deeply pigmented basaloid cells.[122] Reflectance confocal microscopy studies of solar lentigines show that their edges present with more active melanocytes, which produce more melanin and have horizontally spreading dendrites. This finding may explain the central lightening observed when using bleaching agents and the occurrence of PIH at the edges of solar lentigines after laser therapy.[123]

In addition to solar lentigines, the presence of seborrheic keratoses adds to the uneven pigmentation in photoaged skin. Seborrheic keratoses are benign yellow- or brown-raised papules that appear "stuck on." Ultraviolet light contributes to the growth of these keratoses. In a split-face study of 148 truck drivers, solar lentigines, seborrheic keratoses, and actinic keratoses were found to be increased on the more sun-exposed "driver's side" of the face.[124]

The treatment of dyschromia is central to the treatment of dermatoheliosis. However, the treatment may also improve telangiectasias, wrinkles, and texture. Topical therapy, chemical peeling, and laser may be done to improve all of the features of dermatoheliosis and are particularly helpful for the dyschromic component.

TOPICAL TREATMENTS

Photoprotection. As with the management of other dyschromias, photoprotection is a critical part of the treatment program for dermatoheliosis. Ultraviolet light induces skin pigmentation by directly and indirectly influencing melanocytes and keratinocytes. Chronic ultraviolet light has been associated with solar lentigines, pigmented actinic keratoses, and hypopigmented spots.[125] In skin-grafted mouse models, ultraviolet B has also been shown to stimulate keratinocyte production of interleukin-1 alpha, which leads to increased pigment production and solar lentigo formation.[126]

Sun protection through the use of broad-spectrum sunscreens of at least SPF 30, sun avoidance between 10 AM and 2 PM and use of protective wear such as long-sleeved shirts and wide-brimmed hats are important to prevent photodamage and maintain treatment results.

Retinoids. Retinoids have been proven histologically and clinically to improve aging skin. Topical retinoids include retinol, retinaldehyde, tretinoin, isotretinoin, tazarotene, and adapalene. Among these, tretinoin is the most studied, and the histologic changes associated with it are epidermal hyperplasia, compaction of the stratum corneum, thickening of the granular layer, reduced melanocytic hypertrophy, increased collagen formation, and normalization of the appearance of elastic tissue.[127] Long-term use of tretinoin may reduce epidermal and melanocyte atypia, decrease perivascular inflammation, and increase epidermal mucin.[128,129]

Tretinoin-induced epidermal desquamation and tyrosinase inhibition improve dyschromia.[130,131] Improvement of photodamaged skin and lightening of solar lentigines have been reported with the use of tretinoin in multiple studies (see Fig. 48-2).[130–138] In a 24 month randomized placebo controlled trial, significant improvement in rhytides and lentigines in the tretinoin 0.05% group was seen by the fourth month and sustained throughout the 24 month study.[139] Local irritation, scaling, and erythema can limit the use of topical tretinoin, and as a result, specialized emollient formulations have been developed.

Other retinoids studied for the treatment of solar lentigines are adapalene and tazarotene. In a study on the treatment of actinic keratosis and solar lentigines using adapalene, patients (75% of whom had solar lentigines) were randomized to receive adapalene 0.1% or 0.3% or vehicle gel once daily for a month then twice daily for up to 9 months. After 9 months, adapalene 0.1% and 0.3% showed significant lightening of lesions in 57% and 59%

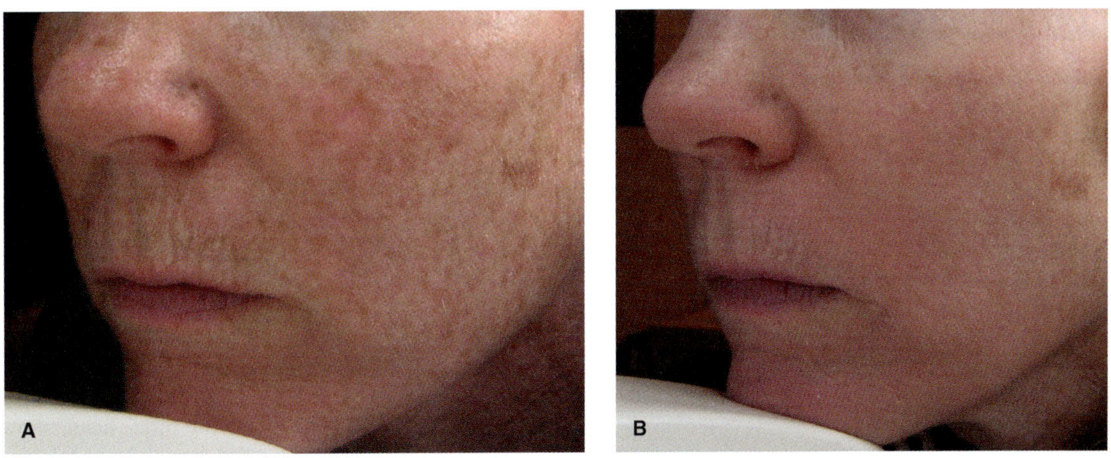

Figure 48-2 Before (**A**) and after (**B**) 16 weeks of tretinoin cream 0.05% at night.

of patients, respectively and an improvement in wrinkles based on photograph evaluations.[140] Tazarotene 0.1% gel has also been shown to yield some improvement in fine wrinkling, mottled pigmentation, lentigines, and other signs of photodamage after 24 weeks in two large multicenter trials.[141,142]

Lightening agents. Hydroquinone has been widely used for the treatment of sun-induced hyperpigmentation. In a treatment study of forearm solar lentigines, hydroquinone 2% with cyclodextrin, an absorption enhancer applied twice daily for 2 months, reduced melanin, thereby decreasing the size of the lentigines.[143] In another study, hydroquinone 5% combined with varying concentrations of tretinoin (0.1% on the face, 0.2% on the trunk, and 0.4% on the extremities) was used in Asian patients with hyperpigmentation disorders, including 90 with solar lentigines. After 2 months of twice daily application, lightening of lesions was observed in 82.2% of patients based on narrowband reflectance spectrophotometry.[144]

Another well-studied lightening agent for solar lentigines is mequinol or 4-hydroxyanisole combined with tretinoin. Mequinol is a phenolic agent that is believed to act as a competitive inhibitor of tyrosinase.[12] In two randomized, controlled, double-blind multicenter clinical studies involving 1175 subjects, mequinol 2%/tretinoin 0.01% was compared with its active components and vehicle for the treatment of solar lentigines. After 24 weeks of twice daily application, a higher proportion of subjects in the mequinol 2%/tretinoin 0.01% group had at least moderate improvement on both the forearm and face (52.6% and 56.3%) compared to mequinol 2% alone (24% and 33%), tretinoin 0.01% alone (35% and 43%), and vehicle (17% and 19%). Benefit was maintained posttreatment in both trials after 4 and 24 months. As with hydroquinone and tretinoin, mequinol can result in local irritation.[145]

Mequinol 2%/tretinoin 0.01% has been compared with hydroquinone 3% in a randomized, double-blind study.[146] A greater proportion of patients in the mequinol 2%/tretinoin 0.01% group showed significant improvement in forearm lentigines compared to the hydroquinone 3% group based on the physician's global assessment (60% vs. 38%). More patients in the mequinol 2%/tretinoin 0.01% group also had improvement in facial lentigines, but this finding was not statistically significant.

CRYOTHERAPY

Liquid nitrogen can be used to treat lentigines and seborrheic keratoses. Melanocytes and keratinocytes are susceptible to cold injury at –4° to –7°C and –20° to –30°C, respectively.[147] Side effects include redness, swelling, crusting, edema, bulla formation, hyperpigmentation, and hypopigmentation, which can be permanent.[130]

Cryotherapy has been compared to chemical peeling. In lightening solar lentigines, several studies have shown cryotherapy to be superior to TCA 30% to 35%,[148,149] but not to medium depth peel with TCA 35% + GA 70%.[150] Cryotherapy was found to be superior to early generation lasers,[151] but inferior to newer technologies such as Q-switched lasers.[152]

Similar to lentigines, seborrheic keratosis lesions generally respond to cryotherapy. Longer freeze times may be required for raised growths.[153] For large raised lesions curettage may be helpful, or these lesions may require several sessions of cryotherapy.

CHEMICAL PEELS

Chemical peels improve dermatoheliosis by both decreasing wrinkles and lightening pigmentation. Characteristic histologic and ultrastructural features of the skin after peeling include decreased epidermal intracytoplasmic vacuoles, decreased solar elastosis, increased activated fibroblasts, and organized parallel arrays of collagen.[154,155]

The type and depth of peel depends on the histologic depth of the clinical changes of dermatoheliosis treated. Epidermal pigmentation, fine wrinkling, and rough texture can be managed by superficial peels. Solar lentigines, characterized by pigmented basal cells, will be treated more effectively when using medium depth peels reaching the papillary dermis, while deep wrinkles can be treated with deeper peels reaching the reticular dermis.[51]

Superficial peels. GA 50% peels, done weekly for 4 weeks, have been shown to improve texture, decrease fine wrinkles and actinic keratoses and slightly lighten solar lentigines in a randomized double-blind controlled trial.[156] Single or multiple monthly SA 30% peels have also been reported to fade pigmented spots, decrease surface roughness and reduce fine lines.[157] SA derivative LHA 5% to 10% and GA 20% to 50% peels were compared in a randomized, single-blinded, split-face study. After 12 weeks of biweekly peel sessions, both LHA and GA peels demonstrated significant reduction of fine lines (41% and 30% of subjects, respectively) and hyperpigmentation (46% and 34% of subjects, respectively) with no significant difference between the two.[158]

Medium depth peels. Medium depth peels reaching the papillary dermis treat dyschromia in dermatoheliosis effectively, especially in patients with light skin. TCA peels 35% to 50% can be used alone and TCA 35% can be used in combination with Jessner's solution or GA 70%.

TCA peels may be used as a full face peel or focally as a localized spot peel for target areas. TCA 40% has been shown to moderately improve solar lentigines and skin texture, but not wrinkles in one study on photoaged skin.[159] Focal use of TCA 50% to 65% has also been studied for the treatment of solar lentigines and has shown to be effective in 42 of 49 patients with dark skin.[57]

Combination peels may allow deeper penetration of TCA 35% without producing severe complications. Jessner's solution or GA 70% peeling is done first followed by application of TCA 35%.

Several studies have shown that a combination of GA 70% + TCA 35% to 40% successfully lighten irregular pigmentation and solar lentigines in nonfacial photoaged skin.[150,160] In a split-face study, GA 70% + TCA 35% and Jessner's + TCA 35% were compared in photoaged skin. Both peels equally lightened lentigines. However more organized elastic fibers and wider papillary dermis were observed using GA + TCA suggesting deeper penetration. Jessner's + TCA peel, on the other hand, showed prolonged erythema in some patients, and a histologically greater inflammatory response.[161]

LASERS

Lasers and light sources effectively treat dermatoheliosis, and a variety of treatment options exist. Some lasers can target a specific component of dermatoheliosis such as lentigines, while others may improve more than one component.[162] Q-switched ruby, alexandrite, and Nd:YAG as well as long-pulsed dye lasers and alexandrite lasers all can treat lentigines via targeting of the chromophore melanin. IPL, fractional photothermolysis, and ablative lasers such as CO_2 erbium lasers will treat dyschromia in a more nonspecific manner.

Q-switched lasers. Q-switched ruby laser, Q-switched Nd:YAG laser, and Q-switched alexandrite lasers are melanin-specific lasers and have been shown to improve lentigines.[101,163–165] QS ruby laser has been shown to improve solar lentigines in 91 patients after one to two sessions by at least 75%.[163] A retrospective study of the QS alexandrite laser found that at least 50% of lentigines cleared in half of the subjects after at least three treatments.[164] QS Nd:YAG (532 nm) has also been shown to effectively clear 60% of solar lentigines treated by at least 75% in a study involving 37 patients after a single treatment.[165]

Immediately after laser exposure, whitening of epidermal pigmented lesions is seen.[166] This whitening resolves several minutes after exposure. Redness and swelling are expected, and over the course of the next several days, darkening of the area will occur. After 1 to 2 weeks, there is desquamation of the crusted area, and in some cases mild redness remains, which dissipates over time. Patients should be warned about the risks of hyperpigmentation and hypopigmentation, and advised to avoid sun exposure to minimize these risks. Scarring and blisters are rare side effects.

Long-pulsed lasers. The long-pulsed dye laser and alexandrite 755 nm laser can be used to treat pigmented lesions. Long-pulsed lasers typically require more treatments to clear lentigines compared with Q-switched lasers, but are associated with a lower risk of PIH in studies of Asian skin.[97,99] Several minutes after laser exposure, there will be darkening of the lentigo. As with the Q-switched lasers, redness, swelling, hyperpigmentation, hypopigmentation, scarring, and blisters are all potential side effects.

A study of long-pulsed alexandrite laser improved solar lentigines after one treatment in 16 patients by at least 50%.[167] A split-face study comparing Q-switched and long-pulsed alexandrite lasers for the treatment of freckles and solar lentigines showed no statistically significant difference between the two in improving pigmentation. PIH, however, occurred more frequently in the Q-switched treatment (22%) than in the long-pulsed treatment (6%). Patients also reported more severe pain, erythema, and edema during the Q-switched alexandrite treatment.[168]

Long-pulsed dye laser with compression has also been compared with Q-switched ruby laser in a study of 18 Japanese patients with solar lentigines. The addition of glass compression eliminates hemoglobin absorption, thus allowing the treatment of pigmentation. The degree of clearance was 83.3% for long-pulsed dye laser and 70.3% for Q-switched ruby laser. Complications were substantially decreased for the long-pulsed dye laser. Only four patients developed erythema and none developed hyperpigmentation after long-pulsed dye treatment, while all patients developed erythema and four patients developed hyperpigmentation after Q-switched ruby laser.[97]

Intense pulsed light (IPL). IPL sources are nonspecific and can target the dyschromic component of dermatoheliosis as well as the telangiectasias. Cutoff filters are provided with some IPL devices to allow slightly more specific targeting of lentigines. Similar to long-pulsed lasers, treatment of lentigines results in lesion darkening after several minutes as well as erythema and swelling in the treatment.[169] During the week after treatment, and as epidermal turnover occurs, patients should expect the lentigines to slowly resolve. Typically, several treatments are needed.

An open study performed on patients with facial lentigines treated with IPL three to five times showed that 40% of patients had more than 50% clearance and 16% of patients had more than 75% clearance of lesions.[170] Patients with small solar lentigines responded well to IPL, but patients with large or a combination of small and large lesions showed a poor response. Solar lentigines of the hands have also been shown to improve with IPL after five treatments in an open study. Among the 31 patients, 62% had more than 50% improvement and 23% had more than 75% improvement.[171]

Fractional resurfacing. Fractional photothermolysis treats dermatoheliosis and dyschromia via nonspecific microscopic columns of injury in the epidermis and dermis. These zones of damage contain melanin and degenerated dermal material, and are extruded through the epidermis. Epidermal and dermal repair occurs in the areas of damage.[172] The benefit of fractional photothermolysis is that several components of dermatoheliosis can be improved, including lentigines, texture, rhytides, and telangiectasia. Multiple different wavelengths are used in fractional devices, which can result either in thermal damage or ablation in the zones of injury.

Fractional resurfacing using the 1550 nm erbium-doped fiber laser has been studied in 50 patients with moderate photodamage, rhytides, and dyspigmentation. Three monthly laser treatments were done on facial and nonfacial skin and clinical improvement based on photographs was graded by two blinded assessors using quartile scoring scales. Clinical improvement by at least 51% to 75% was seen in 73% and 55% of patients with facial and nonfacial treated skin, respectively after 9 months.[173] Nonablative fractional 1540 nm laser has also been studied for treatment of photodamaged skin and actinic keratoses in 17 patients. Three months posttreatment there was 51% to 75% clinical improvement in 12 patients and >75% improvement in three patients after two to three treatments.[174]

In general, multiple treatments are needed to improve dermatoheliosis. Patients should expect redness and swelling after treatment for several days and may notice small dark dots in the area of treatment. Patients may experience a tan-like appearance that resolves over 1 to 2 weeks following treatment.

The 1927 nm fractional thulium fiber laser has also been evaluated for the treatment of nonfacial photodamage. Twelve treatment areas in nine patients who underwent three monthly laser procedures were evaluated. Clinical improvement was graded by a blinded assessor on a scale of 0 to 4 one month from the last treatment. Mean improvement in photodamage was 3.25 and mean improvement in lentigines was 3.3 representing a 51% to 75% improvement (see Fig. 48-3).[175]

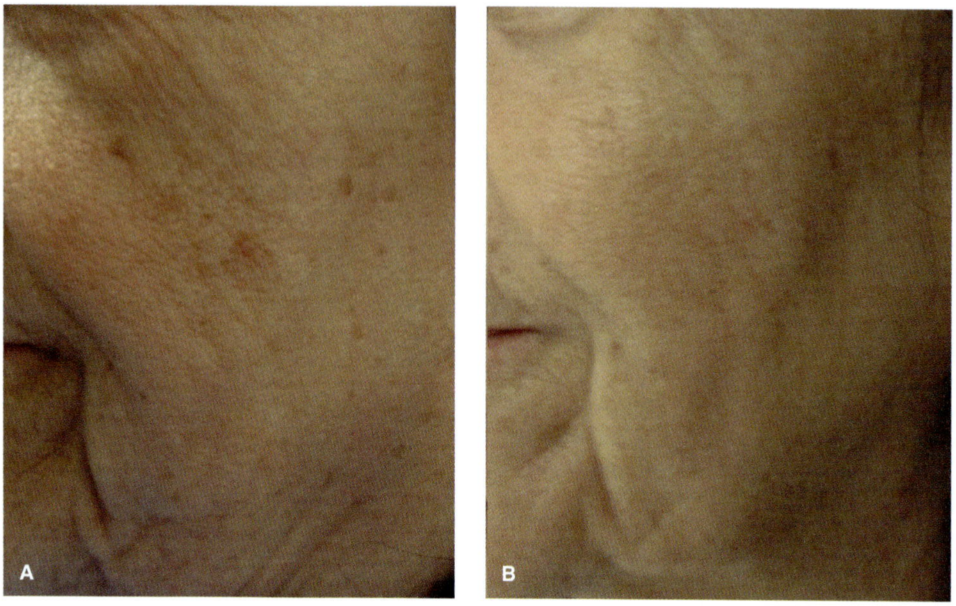

Figure 48-3 Before (**A**) and after (**B**) one treatment fractional photothermolysis 1927 nm and one treatment Q-switched ruby laser.

The 1927 nm laser may be able to target dyschromia with fewer treatments, but has more downtime compared to nonablative modalities. It can also be used to treat actinic keratoses and macular seborrheic keratoses.[176,177] Patients should expect redness, swelling, and darkening of lentigines followed by epidermal peeling that lasts approximately 1 week and redness that can last approximately 1 month. During healing, patients are advised to apply plain petrolatum or another bland moisturizer two to three times per day.

Fractional ablative lasers such as the CO_2, erbium, and YSGG lasers have shown efficacy in treating photodamaged skin. The ablative fractional lasers are particularly suited for treatment of rhytides, but can treat all aspects of dermatoheliosis including dyschromia. The 2790 nm Er:YSGG laser has been evaluated for treatment of photodamage and wrinkles in 11 subjects.[178] Most subjects showed improvement in tone/texture (93%), dyschromia (82%), and wrinkles (54%) after two facial treatments. Ablative Er:YAG laser (2940 nm) has also been studied in 28 patients with mild to moderate actinic damage. Two months after the last treatment, all subjects had improvement.[179] In a prospective single-blinded study of the fractional ablative CO_2 laser, 45 patients received two to three laser treatments. Mean improvement was 48.5% for skin texture, 50.3% for skin laxity, 53.9% for dyschromia, and 52.4% for overall cosmetic outcome.[180]

Fractional ablative lasers have the most downtime of the fractional devices. In general, patients should anticipate 1 to 2 treatments, and should expect redness, swelling, and oozing after treatment. Healing can be augmented through the use of cool soaks. Every 3 to 4 hours, patients are advised to apply water-soaked gauze to the face followed by application of petrolatum. The majority of the healing process is accomplished in a week, but redness and in some cases swelling can last a month.

Ablative lasers. CO_2 lasers followed by erbium lasers were some of the first devices used for the treatment of dyschromia.[151,181–184] Ablative lasers can lead to substantial improvement in rhytides as well as dermatoheliosis. Resurfacing the skin with CO_2 laser obliterates the epidermis and partially ablates the upper papillary dermis. Ablative resurfacing promotes epidermal and dermal remodeling with formation of collagen and elastin.[181] Although excellent cosmetic outcomes can be achieved with the ablative lasers, these devices are operator and technique dependent with greater risks and downtime for the patient. The risks for postprocedure complications such as erythema, infection, PIH, hypopigmentation, and scarring are higher with the CO_2 laser compared with the fractional devices.[175]

SUMMARY

Dermatoheliosis is responsive to most treatment modalities. Although topical medications can work, laser treatments and peels provide more substantial results. The choice of tool depends on the patient and his or her preferred balance between ease of recovery and speed of improvement.

CONCLUSION

Disorders of dyschromia are common. Chemical peels, lasers, and topical treatments are all effective for dychromia. However, each subtype is treated somewhat differently, and prognosis is etiology dependent. Topical treatments can be used for melasma, PIH, and dermatoheliosis, and are often first line in these disorders, particularly for melasma and PIH. Chemical peels are helpful in dyschromia, with glycolic peels better studied for melasma and SA peels for acne-induced PIH. Dermatoheliosis is highly responsive to laser treatment, but may not be as effective in PIH and melasma. In addition to the etiology of the dyschromia, choice of treatment will be influenced by the patient's skin type, with more aggressive treatments used more cautiously in darker skin types. Regardless of the treatment, skin type, or subtype of dyschromia, sun protection is recommended for all forms of dyschromia and should be a part of every treatment recommendation.

REFERENCES

1. Ball Arefiev KL, Hantash BM. Advances in the treatment of melasma: a review of the recent literature. *Dermatol Surg.* 2012;38:971–984.
2. Sheth VM, Pandya AG. Melasma: a comprehensive update: part I. *J Am Acad Dermatol.* 2011;65(4):689–697.
3. Pawaskar MD, Parikh P, Markowski T, et al. Melasma and its impact on health-related quality of life in Hispanic women. *J Dermatol Treat.* 2007;18:5–9.
4. Passeron T: Melasma pathogenesis and influencing factors-an overview of the latest research. *J Eur Acad Dermatol Venereol.* 2013;27(Suppl 1):5–6.
5. Kang HY, Suzuki I, Lee DJ, et al. Transcriptional profiling shows altered expression of wnt pathway- and lipid metabolism-related genes as well as melanogenesis-related genes in melasma. *J Invest Dermatol.* 2011;131(8):1692–1700.
6. Kang HY, Bahadoran P, Suzuki I, et al. In vivo reflectance confocal microscopy detects pigmentary changes in melasma at a cellular level resolution. *Exp Dermatol.* 2010;19:e228–e233.
7. Sanchez NP, Pathak MA, Sato S, et al. Melasma: a clinical, light microscopic, ultrastructural, and immunofluorescence study. *J Am Acad Dermatol.* 1981;4(6):698–710.
8. Ardigo M, Cameli N, Berardesca E, Gonzalez S. Characterization and evaluation of pigment distribution and response to therapy in melasma using in vivo reflectance confocal microscopy: a preliminary study. *J Eur Acad Dermatol Venereol.* 2010;24(11):1296–1303.
9. Grimes PE, Yamada N, Bhawan J. Light microscopic, immunohistochemical, and ultrastructural alterations in patients with melasma. *Am J Dermatopathol.* 2005;27:96–101.
10. Sarvjot V, Sharma S, Mishra S, Singh A. Melasma: a clinicopathological study of 43 cases. *Indian J Pathol Microbiol.* 2009;52:357–359.
11. Wu S, Shi H, Wu H, et al. Treatment of melasma with oral administration of tranexamic acid. *Aesth Plast Surg.* 2012;36:964–970.
12. Sheth VM, Pandya AG. Melasma: a comprehensive update: part II. *J Am Acad Dermatol.* 2011;65(4):699–714.
13. Grimes PE, Bhawan J, Guevara IL, et al. Continuous therapy followed by a maintenance therapy regimen with a triple combination cream for melasma. *J Am Acad Dermatol.* 2010; 62(6):962–967.
14. DeCaprio AP. The toxicology of hydroquinone–relevance to occupational and environmental exposure. *Crit Rev Toxicol.* 1999;29(3):283–330.
15. Lyon CC, Beck MH. Contact hypersensitivity to monobenzyl ether of hydroquinone used to treat vitiligo. *Contact Dermatitis.* 1998;39(3):132–133.
16. Tse TW. Hydroquinone for skin lightening: safety profile, duration of use and when should we stop? *J Dermatolog Treat.* 2010;21(5):272–275.
17. Frenk E, Loi-Zedda P. Occupational depigmentation due to a hydroquinone-containing photographic developer. *Contact Dermatitis.* 1980;6(3): 238–239.
18. Kersey P, Stevenson CJ. Vitiligo and occupational exposure to hydroquinone from servicing self-photographing machines. *Contact Dermatitis.* 1981;7(5):285–287.
19. Levitt J. The safety of hydroquinone: a dermatologist's response to the 2006 Federal Register. *J Am Acad Dermatol.* 2007;57(5):854–872.
20. Food and Drug Administration: Hydroquinone Studies Under The National Toxicology Program. http://www.fda.gov/AboutFDA/CentersOffices/ OfficeofMedicalProductsandTobacco/ CDER/ ucm203112.htm. Silver Spring, MD 2010. Accessed September 1, 2012.
21. Cestari T, Adjadj L, Hux M, Shimizu MR, Rives VP. Cost-effectiveness of a fixed combination of hydroquinone/tretinoin/fluocinolone cream compared with hydroquinone alone in the treatment of melasma. *J Drugs Dermatol.* 2007;6(2):153–160.
22. Food and Drug Administration: Triluma FDA final printed labeling. http://www.accessdata.fda.gov/drugsatfda_docs/label/2002/21112lbl.pdf. Silver Spring, MD 2002. Accessed September 1, 2012.
23. Torok HM. A comprehensive review of the long-term and short-term treatment of melasma with a triple combination cream. *Am J Clin Dermatol.* 2006;7(4):223–230.
24. Bhawan J, Grimes P, Pandya AG, et al. A histological examination for skin atrophy after 6 months of treatment with fluocinolone acetonide 0.01%, hydroquinone 4%, and tretinoin 0.05% cream. *Am J Dermatopathol.* 2009;31(8):794–798.
25. Draelos ZD. Skin lightening preparations and the hydroquinone controversy. *Dermatol Ther.* 2007;20(5):308–313.
26. Keeling J, Cardona L, Benitez A, Epstein R, Rendon M. Mequinol 2%/tretinoin 0.01% topical solution for the treatment of melasma in men: a case series and review of the literature. *Cutis.* 2008;81(2):179–183.
27. Dogra S, Kanwar AJ, Parsad D. Adapalene in the treatment of melasma: a preliminary report. *J Dermatol.* 2002; 29(8):539–540.
28. Baliña LM, Graupe K. The treatment of melasma. 20% azelaic acid versus 4% hydroquinone cream. *Int J Dermatol.* 1991;30(12):893–895.
29. Garcia A, Fulton JE Jr. The combination of glycolic acid and hydroquinone or kojic acid for the treatment of melasma and related conditions. *Dermatol Surg.* 1996;22(5):443–447.
30. Espinal-Perez LE, Moncada B, Castanedo-Cazares JP. A double-blind randomized trial of 5% ascorbic acid vs. 4% hydroquinone in melasma. *Int J Dermatol.* 2004;43(8):604–607.
31. Ertam I, Mutlu B, Unal I, Alper S, Kivçak B, Ozer O. Efficiency of ellagic acid and arbutin in melasma: a randomized, prospective, open-label study. *J Dermatol.* 2008;35(9):570–574.
32. Khemis A, Kaiafa A, Queille-Roussel C, Duteil L, Ortonne JP. Evaluation of efficacy and safety of rucinol serum in patients with melasma: a randomized controlled trial. *Br J Dermatol.* 2007;156(5):997–1004.
33. Hantash BM, Jimenez F. A split-face, double-blind, randomized and placebo-controlled pilot evaluation of a novel oligopeptide for the treatment of recalcitrant melasma. *J Drugs Dermatol.* 2009;8(8):732–735.
34. Amer M, Metwalli M. Topical liquiritin improves melasma. *Int J Dermatol.* 2000;39(4):299–301.
35. Arellano I, Cestari T, Ocampo-Candiani J, et al. Preventing melasma recurrence: prescribing a maintenance regimen with an effective triple combination cream based on long-standing clinical severity. *J Eur Acad Dermatol Venereol.* 2012;26(5):611–618.
36. Wolf R, Matz H, Orion E, Lipozencić J. Sunscreens–the ultimate cosmetic. *Acta Dermatovenerol Croat.* 2003;11(3): 158–162.
37. Moseley H, Cameron H, MacLeod T, Clark C, Dawe R, Ferguson J. New sunscreens confer improved protection for photosensitive patients in the blue light region. *Br J Dermatol.* 2001;145(5):789–794.
38. Bissonnette R, Nigen S, Bolduc C, Méry S, Nocera T. Protection afforded by sunscreens containing inorganic sunscreening agents against blue light sensitivity induced by aminolevulinic acid. *Dermatol Surg.* 2008;34(11):1469–1476.
39. Wang SQ, Stanfield JW, Osterwalder U. In vitro assessments of UVA protection by popular sunscreens available in the United States. *J Am Acad Dermatol.* 2008;59:934–942.
40. Vázquez M, Sánchez JL. The efficacy of a broad-spectrum sunscreen in the treatment of melasma. *Cutis.* 1983;32(1):92, 95–96.
41. Fischer TC, Perosino E, Poli F, Viera MS, Dreno B; Cosmetic Dermatology European Expert Group. Chemical peels in aesthetic dermatology: an update 2009. *J Eur Acad Dermatol Venereol.* 2010;24(3):281–292.
42. Rendon MI, Berson DS, Cohen JL, Roberts WE, Starker I, Wang B. Evidence and considerations in the application of

chemical peels in skin disorders and aesthetic resurfacing. *J Clin Aesthet Dermatol.* 2010;3(7):32–43.
43. Gupta RR, Mahajan BB, Garg G. Chemical peeling–evaluation of glycolic acid in varying concentrations and time intervals. *Indian J Dermatol Venereol Leprol.* 2001;67(1):28–29.
44. Zakopoulou N, Kontochristopoulos G. Superficial chemical peels. *J Cosmet Dermatol.* 2006;5(3):246–253.
45. Van Scott EJ, Yu RJ. Hyperkeratinization, corneocyte cohesion, and alpha hydroxy acids. *J Am Acad Dermatol.* 1984; 11(5 Pt 1):867–879.
46. Usuki A, Ohashi A, Sato H, Ochiai Y, Ichihashi M, Funasaka Y. The inhibitory effect of glycolic acid and lactic acid on melanin synthesis in melanoma cells. *Exp Dermatol.* 2003;12(Suppl 2):43–50.
47. Sarkar R, Kaur C, Bhalla M, Kanwar AJ. The combination of glycolic acid peels with a topical regimen in the treatment of melasma in dark-skinned patients: a comparative study. *Dermatol Surg.* 2002;28(9):828–832.
48. Faghihi G, Shahingohar A, Siadat AH. Comparison between 1% tretinoin peeling versus 70% glycolic acid peeling in the treatment of female patients with melasma. *J Drugs Dermatol.* 2011;10(12):1439–1442.
49. Ilknur T, Biçak MU, Demirtaşoğlu M, Ozkan S. Glycolic acid peels versus amino fruit acid peels in the treatment of melasma. *Dermatol Surg.* 2010;36(4):490–495.
50. El-Domyati MB, Attia SK, Saleh FY, Ahmad HM, Uitto JJ. Trichloroacetic acid peeling versus dermabrasion: a histometric, immunohistochemical, and ultrastructural comparison. *Dermatol Surg.* 2004;30(2 Pt1):179–188.
51. Clark E, Scerri L. Superficial and medium-depth chemical peels. *Clin Dermatol.* 2008;26(2):209–218.
52. Kumari R, Thappa DM. Comparative study of trichloroacetic acid versus glycolic acid chemical peels in the treatment of melasma. *Indian J Dermatol Venereol Leprol.* 2010;76(4): 447.
53. Lawrence N, Cox SE, Brody HJ. Treatment of melasma with Jessner's solution versus glycolic acid: a comparison of clinical efficacy and evaluation of the predictive ability of Wood's light examination. *J Am Acad Dermatol.* 1997;36(4):589–593.
54. Isoda M, Ueda S, Imayama S, Tsukahara K. New formulation of chemical peeling agent: histological evaluation in sun-damaged skin model in hairless mice. *J Dermatol Sci.* 27(Suppl 1):S60–S67.
55. Ejaz A, Raza N, Iftikhar N, Muzzafar F. Comparison of 30% salicylic acid with Jessner's solution for superficial chemical peeling in epidermal melasma. *J Coll Physicians Surg Pak.* 2008;18(4):205–208.
56. Kodali S, Guevara IL, Carrigan CR, et al. A prospective, randomized, split-face, controlled trial of salicylic acid peels in the treatment of melasma in Latin American women. *J Am Acad Dermatol.* 2010;63(6):1030–1035.
57. Chun EY, Lee JB, Lee KH. Focal trichloroacetic acid peel method for benign pigmented lesions in dark-skinned patients. *Dermatol Surg.* 2004;30(4 Pt1):512–516.
58. Grimes PE. Melasma. Etiologic and therapeutic considerations. *Arch Dermatol.* 1995;131(12):1453–1457.
59. Passeron T, Fontas E, Kang HY, Bahadoran P, Lacour JP, Ortonne JP. Melasma treatment with pulsed-dye laser and triple combination cream: a prospective, randomized, single-blind, split-face study. *Arch Dermatol.* 2011;147(9): 1106–1108.
60. Angsuwarangsee SA, Polnikorn N. Combined ultrapulse CO_2 laser and Q-switched alexandrite laser compared with Q-switched alexandrite laser alone for refractory melasma: split-face design. *Dermatol Surg.* 2003;29:59–64.
61. Nouri K, Bowes L, Chartier T, Romagosa R, Spencer J. Combination treatment of melasma with pulsed CO_2 laser followed by Q-switched Alexandrite laser: a pilot study. *Dermatol Surg.* 1999;25:494–497.
62. Manaloto RM, Alster T. Erbium:YAG laser resurfacing for refractory melasma. *Dermatol Surg.* 1999;25:121–123.
63. Sherling M, Friedman PM, Adrian R, et al. Consensus recommendations on the use of an erbium-doped 1550-nm fractionated laser and its applications in dermatologic laser surgery. *Dermatol Surg.* 2010;36(4):461–469.
64. Manstein D, Herron GS, Sink RK, Tanner H, Anderson RR. Fractional photothermolysis: a new concept for cutaneous remodeling using microscopic patterns of thermal injury. *Lasers Surg Med.* 2004;34:426–438.
65. Rokhsar CK, Fitzpatrick RE. The treatment of melasma with fractional photothermolysis: a pilot study. *Dermatol Surg.* 2005;31(12):1645–1650.
66. Tannous ZS, Astner S. Utilizing fractional resurfacing in the treatment of therapy-resistant melasma. *J Cosmet Laser Ther.* 2005;7:39–43.
67. Goldberg DJ, Berlin AL, Phelps R. Histologic and ultrastructural analysis of melasma after fractional resurfacing. *Lasers Surg Med.* 2008;40(2):134–138.
68. Katz TM, Glaich AS, Goldberg LH, Firoz BF, Dai T, Friedman PM. Treatment of melasma using fractional photothermolysis: a report of eight cases with long-term follow-up. *Dermatol Surg.* 2010;36(8):1273–1280.
69. Kroon MW, Wind BS, Beek JF, et al. Nonablative 1550-nm fractional laser therapy versus triple topical therapy for the treatment of melasma: a randomized controlled pilot study. *J Am Acad Dermatol.* 2011;64(3):516–523.
70. Hong SP, Han SS, Choi SJ, et al. Split-face comparative study of 1550 nm fractional photothermolysis and trichloroacetic acid 15% chemical peeling for facial melasma in Asian skin. *J Cosmet Laser Ther.* 2012;14(2):81–86.
71. Lee HS, Won CH, Lee DH, et al. Treatment of melasma in Asian skin using a fractional 1550-nm laser: an open clinical study. *Dermatol Surg.* 2009;35:1499–1504.
72. Ho SG, Yeung CK, Chan NP, Shek SY, Chan HH. A retrospective study of the management of Chinese melasma patients using a 1927 nm fractional thulium fiber laser. *J Cosmet Laser Ther.* 2013:15(4):200–206.
73. Niwa Massaki AB, Eimpunth S, Fabi SG, Guiha I, Groff W, Fitzpatrick R. Treatment of melasma with the 1927-nm fractional thulium fiber laser: A retrospective analysis of 20 cases with long-term follow-up. *Lasers Surg Med.* 2013;45(2):95–101.
74. Polder KD, Bruce S. Treatment of melasma using a novel 1927-nm fractional thulium fiber laser: a pilot study. *Dermatol Surg.* 2012;38(2):199–206.
75. Trelles MA, Velez M, Gold MH. The treatment of melasma with topical creams alone, CO2 fractional ablative resurfacing alone, or a combination of the two: a comparative study. *J Drugs Dermatol.* 2010;9(4):315–322.
76. Kauvar AN. The evolution of melasma therapy: targeting melanosomes using low-fluence Q-switched neodymium-doped yttrium aluminium garnet lasers. *Semin Cutan Med Surg.* 2012;31(2):126–132.
77. Mun JY, Jeong SY, Kim JH, Han SS, Kim IH. A low fluence Q-switched Nd:YAG laser modifies the 3D structure of melanocyte and ultrastructure of melanosome by subcellular-selective photothermolysis. *J Electron Microsc (Tokyo).* 2011;60:11–18.
78. Taylor CR, Anderson RR. Ineffective treatment of refractory melasma and postinflammatory hyperpigmentation by Q-switched ruby laser. *J Dermatol Surg Oncol.* 1994;20:592–597.
79. Tse Y, Levine VJ, McClain SA, Ashinoff R. The removal of cutaneous pigmented lesions with the Q-switched ruby laser and the Q-switched neodymium: yttrium-aluminum-garnet laser: A comparative study. *J Dermatol Surg Oncol.* 1994;20:795–800.
80. Suh KS, Sung JY, Roh HJ, Jeon YS, Kim YC, Kim ST. Efficacy of the 1064-nm Q-switched Nd: YAG laser in melasma. *J Dermatolog Treat.* 2011;22:233–238.
81. Chan NP, Ho SG, Shek SY, Yeung CK, Chan HH. A case series of facial depigmentation associated with low fluence Q-switched 1064 nm Nd: YAG laser for skin rejuvenation and melasma. *Lasers Surg Med.* 2010;42:712–719.
82. Kim MJ, Kim JS, Cho SB. Punctate leucoderma after melasma treatment using 1064-nm Q-switched Nd: YAG laser with low pulse energy. *J Eur Acad Dermatol Venereol.* 2009;23:960–962.
83. Wattanakrai P, Mornchan R, Eimpunth S. Low-fluence Q-switched neodymium-doped yttrium aluminum garnet (1064 nm) laser for the treatment of facial melasma in Asians. *Dermatol Surg.* 2010;36(1):76–87.

84. Li YH, Chen JZ, Wei HC, et al. Efficacy and safety of intense pulsed light in treatment of melasma in Chinese patients. *Dermatol Surg.* 2008;34(5):693–700.
85. Wang CC, Hui CY, Sue YM, Wong WR, Hong HS. Intense pulsed light for the treatment of refractory melasma in Asian persons. *Dermatol Surg.* 2004;30(9):1196–200.
86. Kim EH, Kim YC, Lee ES, Kang HY. The vascular characteristics of melasma. *J Dermatol Sci.* 2007;46(2):111–116.
87. Lee HI, Lim YY, Kim BJ, et al. Clinicopathologic efficacy of copper bromide plus/yellow laser (578 nm with 511 nm) for treatment of melasma in Asian patients. *Dermatol Surg.* 2010;36(6):885–893.
88. Callender VD, St Surin-Lord S, Davis EC, Maclin M. Postinflammatory hyperpigmentation: etiologic and therapeutic considerations. *Am J Clin Dermatol.* 2011;12(2):87–99.
89. Davis EC, Callender VD. Postinflammatory hyperpigmentation: a review of the epidemiology, clinical features, and treatment options in skin of color. *J Clin Aesthet Dermatol.* 2010;3(7):20–31.
90. Eimpunth S, Wanitphadeedecha R, Manuskiatti W. A focused review on acne-induced and aesthetic procedure-related postinflammatory hyperpigmentation in Asians. *J Eur Acad Dermatol Venereol.* 2013;27(Suppl 1):7–18.
91. Zeichner J. Strategies to minimize irritation and potential iatrogenic post-inflammatory pigmentation when treating acne patients with skin of color. *J Drugs Dermatol.* 2011;10(Suppl 12):s25–s26.
92. Lacz NL, Vafaie J, Kihiczak NI, Schwartz RA. Postinflammatory hyperpigmentation: a common but troubling condition. *Int J Dermatol.* 2004;43(5):362–365.
93. Hasan AT, Eaglstein W, Pardo RJ. Solar-induced postinflammatory hyperpigmentation after laser hair removal. *Dermatol Surg.* 1999;25(2):113–115.
94. Chan HH, Manstein D, Yu CS, Shek S, Kono T, Wei WI. The prevalence and risk factors of post-inflammatory hyperpigmentation after fractional resurfacing in Asians. *Lasers Surg Med.* 2007;39(5):381–385.
95. Manuskiatti W, Triwongwaranat D, Varothai S, Eimpunth S, Wanitphakdeedecha R. Efficacy and safety of a carbon-dioxide ablative fractional resurfacing device for treatment of atrophic acne scars in Asians. *J Am Acad Dermatol.* 2010; 63:274–283.
96. Chapas AM, Brightman L, Sukal S, et al. Successful treatment of acneiform scarring with CO_2 ablative fractional resurfacing. *Lasers Surg Med.* 2008;40:381–386.
97. Momosawa A, Yoshimura K, Uchida G, et al. Combined therapy using Q-switched ruby laser and bleaching treatment with tretinoin and hydroquinone for acquired dermal melanocytosis. *Dermatol Surg.* 2003;29(10):1001–1007.
98. Uaboonkul T, Nakakes A, Ayuthaya PK. A randomized control study of the prevention of hyperpigmentation post Q-switched Nd:YAG laser treatment of Hori nevus using topical fucidic acid plus betamethasone valerate cream versus fucidic acid cream. *J Cosmet Laser Ther.* 2012;14(3):145–149.
99. Ho SG, Chan NP, Yeung CK, Shek SY, Kono T, Chan HH. A retrospective analysis of the management of freckles and lentigines using four different pigment lasers on Asian skin. *J Cosmet Laser Ther.* 2012;14(2):74–80.
100. Kono T, Manstein D, Chan HH, Nozaki M, Anderson RR. Q-switched ruby versus long-pulsed dye laser delivered with compression for treatment of facial lentigines in Asians. *Lasers Surg Med.* 2006;38(2):94–97.
101. Anderson RR, Margolis RJ, Watenabe S, Flotte T, Hruza GJ, Dover JS. Selective photothermolysis of cutaneous pigmentation by Q-switched Nd:YAG laser pulses at 1064, 532, and 355 nm. *J Invest Dermatol.* 1989;93:28–32.
102. Taylor CR, Anderson RR. Treatment of benign pigmented epidermal lesions by Q-switched ruby laser. *Int J Dermatol.* 1993;32:908–912.
103. Polla LL, Margolis RJ, Dover JS, et al. Melanosomes are primary target of Q-switched ruby laser irradiation in guinea pig skin. *J Invest Dermatol.* 1987;89:281–286.
104. Negishi K, Akita H, Tanaka S, Yokoyama Y, Wakamatsu S, Matsunaga K. Comparative study of treatment efficacy and the incidence of post-inflammatory hyperpigmentation with different degrees of irradiation using two differentquality-switched lasers for removing solar lentigines on Asian skin. *J Eur Acad Dermatol Venereol.* 2013;27(3):307–312.
105. Woolery-Lloyd H, Kammer JN. Treatment of hyperpigmentation. *Semin Cutan Med Surg.* 2011;30(3):171–175.
106. Chandra M, Levitt J, Pensabene CA. Hydroquinone therapy for post-inflammatory hyperpigmentation secondary to acne: not just prescribable by dermatologists. *Acta Derm Venereol.* 2012;92(3):232–235.
107. Rossi AB, Leyden JJ, Pappert AS, et al. A pilot methodology study for the photographic assessment of post-inflammatory hyperpigmentation in patients treated with tretinoin. *J Eur Acad Dermatol Venereol.* 2011;25(4):398–402.
108. Bulengo-Ransby SM, Griffiths CE, Kimbrough-Green CK, et al. Topical tretinoin (retinoic acid) therapy for hyperpigmented lesions caused by inflammation of the skin in black patients. *N Engl J Med.* 1993;328(20):1438–1443.
109. Grimes P, Callender V. Tazarotene cream for postinflammatory hyperpigmentationand acne vulgaris in darker skin: a double-blind, randomized, vehicle-controlled study. *Cutis.* 2006;77(1):45–50.
110. Jacyk WK, Mpofu P. Adapalene gel 0.1% for topical treatment of acne vulgaris in African patients. *Cutis.* 2001;68(Suppl 4):48–54.
111. Ahn HH, Kim IH. Whitening effect of salicylic acid peels in Asian patients. *Dermatol Surg.* 2006;32(3):372–375.
112. Garg VK, Sinha S, Sarkar R. Glycolic acid peels versus salicylic-mandelic acid peels in active acne vulgaris and post-acne scarring and hyperpigmentation: a comparative study. *Dermatol Surg.* 2009;35(1):59–65.
113. Burns RL, Prevost-Blank PL, Lawry MA, Lawry TB, Faria DT, Fivenson DP. Glycolic acid peels for postinflammatory hyperpigmentation in black patients. A comparative study. *Dermatol Surg.* 1997;23(3):171–174.
114. Ho SG, Yeung CK, Chan NP, Shek SY, Kono T, Chan HH. A retrospective analysis of the management of acne post-inflammatory hyperpigmentation using topical treatment, laser treatment, or combination topical and laser treatments in oriental patients. *Lasers Surg Med.* 2011;43(1):1–7.
115. Kim S, Cho KH. Treatment of procedure-related postinflammatory hyperpigmentation using 1064-nm Q-switched Nd:YAG laser with low fluence in Asian patients: report of five cases. *J Cosmet Dermatol.* 2010;9(4):302–306.
116. Kim S, Cho KH. Treatment of facial postinflammatory hyperpigmentation with facial acne in Asian patients using a Q-switched neodymium-doped yttrium aluminum garnet laser. *Dermatol Surg.* 2010;36(9):1374–1380.
117. Rokhsar CK, Ciocon DH. Fractional photothermolysis for the treatment of postinflammatory hyperpigmentation after carbon dioxide laser resurfacing. *Dermatol Surg.* 2009;35(3):535–537.
118. Katz TM, Goldberg LH, Firoz BF, Friedman PM. Fractional photothermolysis for the treatment of postinflammatory hyperpigmentation. *Dermatol Surg.* 2009;35(11):1844–1848.
119. Tierney EP, Hanke CW. Recent advances in combination treatments for photoaging: review of the literature. *Dermatol Surg.* 2010;36(6):829–840.
120. Castanet J, Ortonne JP. Pigmentary changes in aged and photoaged skin. *Arch Dermatol.* 1997;133(10):1296–1299.
121. Ezzedine K, Mauger E, Latreille J, et al. Freckles and solar lentigines have different risk factors in Caucasian women. *J Eur Acad Dermatol Venereol.* 2013;27(3):345–356.
122. Yonei N, Kaminaka C, Kimura A, Furukawa F, Yamamoto Y. Two patterns of solalentigines: A histopathological analysis of 40 Japanese women. *J Dermatol.* 2012;39(10):829–832.
123. Nakajima A, Funasaka Y, Kawana S. Investigation by in vivo reflectanceconfocal microscopy: melanocytes at the edges of solar lentigines. *Exp Dermatol.* 2012;21(Suppl 1):18–21.
124. Kavak A, Parlak AH, Yesildal N, Aydogan I, Anul H. Preliminary study among truck drivers in Turkey: effects of ultraviolet light on some skin entities. *J Dermatol.* 2008; 35(3):146–150.
125. Ortonne JP, Schwarz T [Clinical aspects and pathogenesis of UV-induced pigmentary disorders]. *J Dtsch Dermatol Ges.* 2003;1(4):274–284.

126. Chen N, Hu Y, Li WH, Eisinger M, Seiberg M, Lin CB. The role of keratinocyte growth factor in melanogenesis: a possible mechanism for the initiation of solar lentigines. *Exp Dermatol.* 2010;19(10):865–872.
127. Bhawan J. Short- and long-term histologic effects of topical tretinoin onphotodamaged skin. *Int J Dermatol.* 1998;37(4):286–292.
128. Cho S, Lowe L, Hamilton TA, Fisher GJ, Voorhees JJ, Kang S. Long-term treatment of photoaged human skin with topical retinoic acid improves epidermal cell atypia and thickens the collagen band in papillary dermis. *J Am Acad Dermatol.* 2005;53(5):769–774.
129. Bhawan J, Olsen E, Lufrano L, Thorne EG, Schwab B, Gilchrest BA. Histologic evaluation of the long term effects of tretinoin on photodamaged skin. *J Dermatol Sci.* 1996; 11(3):177–182.
130. Ortonne JP, Pandya AG, Lui H, Hexsel D. Treatment of solar lentigines. *J Am Acad Dermatol.* 2006;54:S262–S271.
131. Romero C, Aberdam E, Larnier C, Ortonne JP. Retinoic acid as modulator of UVB-induced melanocyte differentiation. Involvement of the melanogenic enzymes expression. *J Cell Sci.* 1994;107(Pt 4):1095–1103.
132. Rafal ES, Griffiths CE, Ditre CM, et al. Topical tretinoin (retinoic acid) treatment for liver spots associated with photodamage. *N Engl J Med.* 1992;326:368–374.
133. Weinstein GD, Nigra TP, Pochi PE, et al. Topical tretinoin for treatment of photodamaged skin. *Arch Dermatol.* 1991;127:659–665.
134. Olsen EA, Katz I, Levine N, et al. Tretinoin emollient cream: a new therapy for photodamaged skin. *J Am Acad Dermatol.* 1992;26:215–224.
135. Lever L, Kumar P, Marks R. Topical retinoic acid for the treatment of solar damage. *Br J Dermatol.* 1990;122:91–98.
136. Leyden JJ, Grove MJ, Thorne EG, Lufrano L. Treatment of photodamaged skin with topical tretinoin. *J Am Acad Dermatol.* 21:638–644, 1989
137. Gilchrest BA, Fitzpatrick TB, Anderson RR, Parrish JA. Localization of melanin pigmentation in the skin with Wood's lamp. *Br J of Dermatol.* 1977;96:245–248.
138. Gilchrest B. Treatment of photodamage with topical tretinoin: an overview. *J Am Acad Dermatol.* 1997;36:S27–S36.
139. Kang S, Bergfeld W, Gottlieb AB, et al. Long-term efficacy and safety of tretinoin emollient cream 0.05% in the treatment of photodamaged facial skin: a two-year,randomized, placebo-controlled trial. *Am J Clin Dermatol.* 2005;6(4):245–253.
140. Kang S, Goldfarb MT, Weiss JS, et al. Assessment of adapalene gel for the treatment of actinic keratoses and lentigines: a randomized trial. *J Am Acad Dermatol.* 2003; 49(1):83–90.
141. Kang S, Krueger GG, Tanghetti EA, et al. Tazarotene Cream in Photodamage Study Group. A multicenter, randomized,double-blind trial of tazarotene 0.1% cream in the treatment of photodamage. *J Am Acad Dermatol.* 2005;52(2):268–274.
142. Phillips TJ, Gottlieb AB, Leyden JJ, et al; Tazarotene Cream Photodamage Clinical Study Group. Efficacy of 0.1% tazarotene cream for the treatment of photodamage: a 12-month multicenter, randomized trial. *Arch Dermatol.* 2002;138(11):1486–1493.
143. Petit L, Piérard GE. Analytic quantification of solar lentigines lightening by a 2% hydroquinone-cyclodextrin formulation. *J Eur Acad Dermatol Venereol.* 2003;17(5):546–549.
144. Yoshimura K, Harii K, Aoyama T, Iga T. Experience with a strong bleaching treatment for skin hyperpigmentation in Orientals. *Plast Reconstr Surg.* 2000;105(3):1097–1108.
145. Fleischer AB Jr, Schwartzel EH, Colby SI, Altman DJ. The combination of 2% 4-hydroxyanisole (Mequinol) and 0.01% tretinoin is effective in improving the appearance of solar lentigines and related hyperpigmented lesions in two double-blind multicenter clinical studies. *J Am Acad Dermatol.*42(3):459–467.
146. Jarratt M. Mequinol 2%/tretinoin 0.01% solution: an effective and safe alternative to hydroquinone 3% in the treatment of solar lentigines. *Cutis.* 2004;74(5):319–322.
147. Vujevich JJ, Goldberg LH. Cryosurgery and electrosurgery. In: Wolff K, Goldsmith LA, Katz SI, Gilchrest BA, Paller AS, Laffell DJ, eds. *Fitzpatrick's Dermatology in General Medicine.* 7th ed. USA: McGraw Hill Companies; 2008: 2330.
148. Lugo-Janer A, Lugo-Somolinos A, Sanchez JL. Comparison of trichloroacetic acid solution and cryosurgery in the treatment of solar lentigines. *Int J Dermatol.* 2003;42(10): 829–831.
149. Raziee M, Balighi K, Shabanzadeh-Dehkordi H, Robati RM. Efficacy and safety of cryotherapy vs. trichloroacetic acid in the treatment of solar lentigo. *J Eur Acad Dermatol Venereol.* 2008;22(3):316–319.
150. Sezer E, Erbil H, Kurumlu Z, Taştan HB, Etikan I. A comparative study of focal medium-depth chemical peel versus cryosurgery for the treatment of solar lentigo. *Eur J Dermatol.* 2007;17(1):26–29.
151. Stern RS, Dover JS, Levin JA, Arndt KA. Laser therapy versus cryotherapy of lentigines: a comparative trial. *J Am Acad Dermatol.* 1994;30(6):985–987.
152. Todd MM, Rallis TM, Gerwels JW, Hata TR. A comparison of 3 lasers and liquid nitrogen in the treatment of solar lentigines: a randomized, controlled, comparative trial. *Arch Dermatol.* 2000;136(7):841–846.
153. Thai KE, Sinclair RD. Cryosurgery of benign skin lesions. *Australas J Dermatol.* 1999;40(4):175–184.
154. Nelson BR, Fader DJ, Gillard M, Majmudar G, Johnson TM. Pilot histologic and ultrastructural study of the effects of medium-depth chemical facial peels on dermal collagen in patients with actinically damaged skin. *J Am Acad Dermatol.* 1995;32(3):472–478.
155. El Samahy MH, Ghoz MM, Ramzy N. Morphological investigation of chemical peel on photodamaged facial skin. *Int J Cosmet Sci.* 1998;20(5):269–282.
156. Newman N, Newman A, Moy LS, Babapour R, Harris AG, Moy RL. Clinical improvement of photoaged skin with 50% glycolic acid. A double-blind vehicle-controlled study. *Dermatol Surg.* 1996;22(5):455–460.
157. Kligman D, Kligman AM. Salicylic acid peels for the treatment of photoaging. *Dermatol Surg.* 1998;24(3):325–328.
158. Oresajo C, Yatskayer M, Hansenne I. Clinical tolerance and efficacy of capryloyl salicylic acid peel compared to a glycolic acid peel in subjects with fine lines/wrinkles and hyperpigmented skin. *J Cosmet Dermatol.* 2008;7(4):259–262.
159. Humphreys TR, Werth V, Dzubow L, Kligman A. Treatment of photodamaged skin with trichloroacetic acid and topical tretinoin. *J Am Acad Dermatol.* 1996;34(4):638–644.
160. Cook KK, Cook WR Jr. Chemical peel of nonfacial skin using glycolic acid gel augmented with TCA and neutralized based on visual staging. *Dermatol Surg.* 2000;26(11):994–999.
161. Tse Y, Ostad A, Lee HS, et al. A clinical and histologic evaluation of two medium-depth peels. Glycolic acid versus Jessner's trichloroacetic acid. *Dermatol Surg.* 1996; 22(9):781–786.
162. Polder KD, Landau JM, Vergilis-Kalner IJ, Goldberg LH, Friedman PM, Bruce S. Laser eradication of pigmented lesions: a review. *Dermatol Surg.* 2011;37(5):572–595.
163. Sadighha A, Saatee S, Muhaghegh-Zahed G. Efficacy and adverse effects of Q-switched ruby laser on solar lentigines: a prospective study of 91 patients with Fitzpatrick skin type II, III, and IV. *Dermatol Surg.* 2008;34(11):1465–1468.
164. Kagami S, Asahina A, Watanabe R, et al. Treatment of 153 Japanese patients with Q-switched alexandrite laser. *Lasers Med Sci.* 2007;22(3):159–163.
165. Kilmer SL, Wheeland RG, Goldberg DJ, Anderson RR. Treatment of epidermal pigmented lesions with the frequency-doubled Q-switched Nd:YAG laser. A controlled, single-impact, dose-response, multicenter trial. *Arch Dermatol.* 1994;130(12):1515–1519.
166. Watanabe S. Basics of laser application to dermatology. *Arch Dermatol Res.* 2008;300(1):S21–S30.
167. Trafeli JP, Kwan JM, Meehan KJ, et al. Use of a long-pulse alexandrite laser in the treatment of superficial pigmented lesions. *Dermatol Surg.* 33(12):1477–1482.
168. Ho SG, Yeung CK, Chan NP, Shek SY, Chan HH. A comparison of Q-switched and long-pulsed alexandrite laser for

the treatment of freckles and lentigines in oriental patients. *Lasers Surg Med.* 2011;43(2):108–113.

169. Goldberg DJ. Current trends in intense pulsed light. *J Clin Aesthet Dermatol.* 2012;5(6):45–53.
170. Kawada A, Shiraishi H, Asai M, et al. Clinical improvement of solar lentigines and ephelides with an intense pulsed light source. *Dermatol Surg.* 2002;28(6):504–508.
171. Sasaya H, Kawada A, Wada T, Hirao A, Oiso N. Clinical effectiveness of intense pulsed light therapy for solar lentigines of the hands. *Dermatol Ther.* 2011;24(6):584–586.
172. Tierney EP, Kouba DJ, Hanke CW. Review of fractional photothermolysis: treatment indications and efficacy. *Dermatol Surg.* 2009;35(10):1445–1461.
173. Wanner M, Tanzi EL, Alster TS. Fractional photothermolysis: treatment of facial and nonfacial cutaneous photodamage with a 1550-nm erbium-doped fiber laser. *Dermatol Surg.* 2007;33(1):23–28.
174. Lapidoth M, Adatto M, Halachmi S. Treatment of actinic keratoses and photodamage with non-contact fractional 1540-nm laser quasi-ablation: an ex vivo and clinical evaluation. *Lasers Med Sci.* 2012;28(2):537–542.
175. Polder KD, Harrison A, Eubanks LE, Bruce S. 1927-nm fractional thulium fiber laser for the treatment of nonfacial photodamage: a pilot study. *Dermatol Surg.* 2011;37(3):342–348.
176. Weiss ET, Brauer JA, Anolik R, et al. 1927-nm fractional resurfacing of facial actinic keratoses: a promising new therapeutic option. *J Am Acad Dermatol.*68(1):98–102.
177. Polder KD, Mithani A, Harrison A, Bruce S. Treatment of macular seborrheic keratoses using a novel 1927-nm fractional thulium fiber laser. *Dermatol Surg.* 2012;38(7 Pt 1):1025–1031.
178. Walgrave SE, Kist DA, Noyaner-Turley A, Zelickson BD. Minimally ablative resurfacing with the confluent 2790 nm erbium:YSGG laser: a pilot study on safety and efficacy. *Lasers Surg Med.* 44(2):103–111.
179. Lapidoth M, Yagima Odo ME, Odo LM. Novel use of erbium:YAG (2940-nm) laser for fractional ablative photothermolysis in the treatment of photodamaged facial skin: a pilot study. *Dermatol Surg.* 2008;34(8):1048–1053.
180. Tierney EP, Hanke CW. Fractionated carbon dioxide laser treatment of photoaging: prospective study in 45 patients and review of the literature. *Dermatol Surg.* 2011;37(9):1279–1290.
181. Alster TS. Cutaneous resurfacing with CO2 and erbium: YAG lasers: preoperative, intraoperative, and postoperative considerations. *Plast Reconstr Surg.* 1999;103(2):619–632.
182. Alster TS. Clinical and histologic evaluation of six erbium:YAG lasers for cutaneous resurfacing. *Lasers Surg Med.* 24:87–92.
183. Alster TS, Lupton JR. Erbium:YAG cutaneous laser resurfacing. *Dermatol Clin.* 2001;19(3):453–466.
184. Somoano B, Hantash MB, Fincher EF, Wu P, Gladstone HB. The erbium micropeel: a prospective, randomized trial of the effects of two fluence settings on facial photoaging. *J Drugs Dermatol.* 10(2):179–185.

CHAPTER 49

Laser and Light Treatment of Pigmented Lesions

Mussarrat Hussain, Suzanne L. Kilmer, & Omar A. Ibrahimi

INTRODUCTION

One of the earliest applications of lasers in medicine was Leon Goldman's use of the ruby laser to treat pigmented lesions in 1963. At that time, the ability of a normal-mode ruby laser with a 0.5 ms pulse duration was noted to selectively destroy pigmented structures in the skin.[1] Although seemingly ironic in hindsight, the field of laser dermatology then shifted to the use of continuous wave modalities such as the carbon dioxide laser (10,600 nm) and the argon laser (418 nm), which were used in a non-selective fashion to treat pigmented lesions. Needless to say, the results were often unpredictable, with complications such as scarring and dyspigmentation.

A new era in the laser treatment of pigmented lesions arrived when R. Rox Anderson and John Parrish of Massachusetts General Hospital described the theory of selective photothermolysis,[2] which provided laser surgeons with a platform on which to perform the selective treatment of pigmented lesions. More recently, fractional photothermolysis has been introduced to non-selectively improve the appearance of certain types of undesirable pigment,[3–7] but this time without the risks and downsides of the continuous wave lasers.

LASERS AND IPL SOURCES USED TO TREAT BENIGN PIGMENTED LESIONS

Q-SWITCHED LASERS

Melanosomes have a size range of roughly 0.5 to 1.0 μm, which translates into a thermal relaxation time in the nanosecond to microsecond range. Clinically these structures can be targeted through the use of Q-switched lasers (QSLs). QSLs store large amounts of energy in the optical cavity through the use of an optical shutter. When the laser is fired, it releases high-powered pulses of extremely short duration, in the nanosecond range,[8] resulting in a photomechanical tissue reaction. QSLs are the current modality of choice in the treatment of pigmented lesions. While most lesions can be significantly improved, complete clearance may be difficult to achieve and there is no guarantee that the skin will appear normal after treatment. In addition, the operator's ability, clinical knowledge, and training in the laser device are major factors affecting the outcome of treatment.

Currently, six wavelengths of QSL are available, which include the Q-switched ruby laser (694 nm), the Q-switched alexandrite laser (755 nm), the Q-switched Nd:YAG laser (1064 nm), the Q-switched frequency-doubled (FD) Nd:YAG laser (532 nm), and the Q-switched Nd:YAG laser with dye handpieces (585 and 650 nm). Many QSLs are also capable of operating in a microsecond mode, which can be used to target melanosomes.

LONG-PULSED LASERS

Although long-pulsed (LP) lasers (pulsed dye laser [PDL] at 585–595 nm, LP ruby at 694 nm, LP alexandrite at 755 nm, LP Nd:YAG at 1064 nm, and LP diode at 800 nm) have pulse durations that are in the millisecond domain, they are capable of targeting melanosomes in clinical practice because melanosomes have a tendency to cluster together, particularly in Caucasians and Asians. Thus, the overall size of the clustered melanosomes may enable confined spatial damage with a millisecond laser pulse. Treatment with LP lasers may be done in combination with diascopy to remove competing chromophores such as hemoglobin.

INTENSE PULSED LIGHT SYSTEMS

Intense pulsed light (IPL) systems are high-intensity pulsed sources that emit polychromatic light in a broad wavelength spectrum of 515 to 1200 nm. The wavelength determines not only the absorption behavior but also the penetration depth of the light. With the aid of different cut-off filters (515–755 nm), the wavelength spectrum can be optimized to filter out light that does not correspond to the type and depth of the target structures.[9,10] Similarly, the wavelength spectrum can be adapted to suit the patient's skin type, thereby minimizing adverse effects in those with darker skin types.[9] The pulse duration of IPL systems is in the millisecond domain.

FRACTIONAL PHOTOTHERMOLYSIS

Fractional photothermolysis is the treatment of the skin with an array of laser beams that create vertical columns of thermal damage or tissue ablation[3] (see Chapters 35 and 36). It has been observed that melanin may also be eliminated in the microscopic epidermal necrotic debris that is formed with fractional photothermolysis.[4]

TYPES OF PIGMENTED LESIONS

PROPER LESION CLASSIFICATION

Prior to any laser treatment, proper evaluation of the pigmented lesion must be performed. It is the opinion of the authors that every lesion, but especially one that is new or changing, should be evaluated by a dermatologist prior to treatment. Because of the increasing prevalence of melanoma, there are numerous ethical and medicolegal implications that must be considered when performing laser treatment on pigmented lesions.[11] Lesion classification will assist the laser surgeon in determining a treatment approach to each individual pigmented lesion. In particular, understanding the depth of the target pigment distribution, epidermal, dermal, or a combination of both, is essential to selecting a treatment regimen.

LASER TREATMENT OF EPIDERMAL PIGMENTED LESIONS. Epidermal pigmented lesions can be approached with multiple laser modalities due to their superficial location. The 532 nm (FD Nd:YAG) and 694 nm (ruby) wavelengths are the preferred wavelengths for epidermal lesions, followed by the 755 nm (alexandrite) and, the least effective, the 1064 nm wavelength (Nd:YAG). The shorter wavelengths are particularly attractive because they have relatively greater melanin absorption and, given the superficial location of epidermal pigmented lesions, depth of penetration is not a significant issue. These lesions are amenable to treatment with pulse durations ranging from nanoseconds to milliseconds. Ablative and non-ablative fractional photothermolysis lasers are also capable of treating epidermal pigmented lesions, although use of this technology would be more appropriate in the context of a diffuse epidermal pigmentary aberration.

Lentigines. Lentigines are small, sharply demarcated, round- to oval-shaped, light- to dark-brown macules. They can be from a few millimeters to a few centimeters in diameter and found on any area of the body including mucous membranes. Senile lentigines are acquired lesions resulting from sun exposure. They are found on sun-exposed areas, such as the back of the hands, face, and neck. The number of lesions increases with age. Histologically, the basal cell layer often shows an increase in the number of melanocytes in the epidermis with increased levels of melanin.[12] Lentigo simplex can often be found on younger patients without a predilection for sun exposure and is histologically similar to a senile lentigo. Lentigines can also be a component of various cutaneous syndromes, such as lentiginosis profusa, Peutz–Jeghers syndrome, Moynahan syndrome, and Leopard syndrome.

Nanosecond QSLs (Fig. 49-1), LP lasers, and IPL devices have demonstrated efficacy in the clearance of lentigines.[13–21] The desired treatment endpoint with QSLs

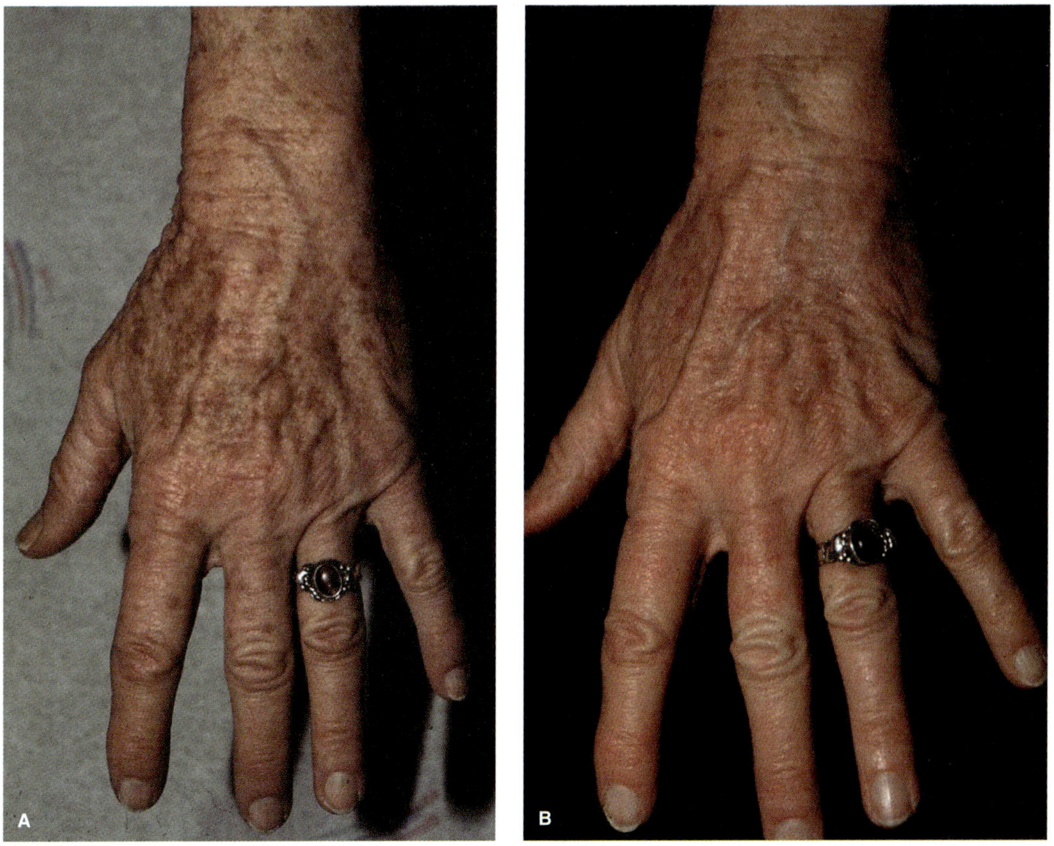

Figure 49-1 **A.** Lentigines on the dorsum of the hand. **B.** Appearance following two treatments with a QS alexandrite laser.

would be to use a fluence that produces brisk whitening without epidermolysis. LP lasers and IPL devices have a much more subtle clinical endpoint that includes lesion graying or darkening.

Ephelides or Freckles. Ephelides or freckles are 1 to 3 mm tan-brown macules, which are present in sun-exposed areas and not on mucous membranes. They not only darken but almost always recur on exposure to ultraviolet (UV) rays. Histologically, the number of melanocytes is unchanged from that of neighboring skin, although the melanosomes are typically larger.[22] Axillary freckling, the only type of ephelide that appears on non–sun-exposed skin, is seen in von Recklinghausen's disease (neurofibromatosis).

The treatment algorithm and desired endpoints for treatment of ephelides are analogous to those for lentigines.[17,18] Recurrence is high without strict UV protection following treatment. Postlaser treatment, sun exposure and tanning booths should be avoided for at least 6 weeks and sunblocks should be used extensively.

Café-au-Lait Macules. Café-au-lait macules (CALMs) are well-circumscribed, light- to dark-brown, hypermelanotic flat lesions which may be 1 to 20 cm in diameter. CALMs may be found in the normal population as an isolated finding or may be part of various syndromes, especially when multiple, such as von Recklinghausen's disease, or neurofibromatosis, Marfan syndrome, and McCune–Albright syndrome.[11] There are no malignant tendencies in CALM.[12,23] Histologically, hypermelanosis is present within the epidermis. Giant melanosomes are present only in patients with neurofibromatosis, in both basal melanocytes and keratinocytes.

Although CALMs are thin epidermal lesions that are in theory amenable to treatment with pigment-specific lasers, in clinical practice they are notoriously difficult to treat. Multiple treatments over a period of months or even years may be required. Lesions may remain clear for up to a year with spontaneous or UV-induced recurrences in more than 50% of cases. QSLs have been reported to have some success at improving CALMs.[24,25] The authors have also used the LP alexandrite laser with good success with the hypothesis that the longer pulse width allows for collateral thermal damage to non–pigment-containing melanocytes.

Nevus Spilus. Nevus spilus is a lesion characterized by darkly pigmented macules or papules within a field that corresponds clinically to a CALM. These lesions are mostly present on the trunk or lower extremities.[26] There are reports of melanoma arising within the nevi of the nevus spilus, but in general, it is not considered to be a precursor of malignant melanoma.[27–29] When treating these lesions, careful clinical assessment is important and any suspicious changes should be evaluated by biopsy.[29]

Pigment-specific QSLs have been successfully used to treat the nevus spilus.[30,31] Many studies have reported good responses to IPL treatments as well.[32] We have also found LP lasers to be beneficial in improving the appearance of these lesions, particularly the more darkly pigmented speckled areas.

Seborrheic Keratoses. Seborrheic keratosis (SK) is a benign epidermal proliferation of keratinocytes with a normal or slightly increased number of melanocytes, increased melanization of keratinocytes, and a thickened hyperkeratotic epidermis. These lesions range from tan to black in color. There are several histopathologic variants but the acanthotic type is the most common one. Dermatosis papulosa nigra is an entity that is clinically and histologically similar to SK and occurs on the face in patients with darker skin types.

Lasers reported to treat SKs successfully include QSLs (Fig. 49-2), LP lasers and UltraPulse CO_2 laser, fractional erbium-doped fiber laser, fractional CO_2 laser, and the 1927 nm thulium fiber laser.[33–38] Multiple treatment sessions may be needed for thicker lesions. It is important to note laser therapy has not been shown to be any more effective than treatment with non-laser destructive methods (cryotherapy and electrodesiccation).[20,21] for these lesions

LASER TREATMENT OF EPIDERMAL/DERMAL PIGMENTED LESIONS

Becker's Nevus. Becker's nevus is an organoid hamartoma, i.e., a developmental anomaly consisting of abnormalities in pigmentation, hair follicles, and smooth muscle. The lesion is predominantly flat but can have a papular verrucous surface. Becker's nevus usually arises in males around the age of 15 years. It is usually a light to medium brown patch that may be 2 to 30 cm in diameter. Increased hair growth follows the onset of pigmentation and is localized to the area of the patch. Histologically, there is hyperpigmentation in the basal layer with variable acanthosis and hyperkeratosis. Although there is an increased number of melanocytes, no nevus cells are found.[39,40]

When treating a Becker's nevus, one should consider both of its components, i.e., the hair and the pigmented patch. Test spots are recommended before treatment is commenced. For hair removal, longer-pulsed lasers should be considered.[41] Treatment with Q-switched or millisecond lasers or IPLs have variable success, whether used alone or in combination. High recurrence rates and hyperpigmentation have been reported, probably due to the pathophysiology of this entity.[42,43] We have found in our experience that the LP alexandrite lasers can be used for the simultaneous treatment of both the hair and pigment components (Fig. 49-3). Fractional photothermolysis has been reported to non-selectively improve the undesirable pigment component, but long-term study data from a larger number of patients are needed.[5]

Melasma. Melasma is an acquired disorder of hyperpigmentation, usually symmetric, that occurs most often on the face. Melasma has a genetic predisposition, with over 50% having a family history,[44–48] and can be exacerbated by sun exposure, hormonal fluctuations, and other less defined factors. Melasma appears to be more common in females, people with constitutive brown skin color, and those who have greater sun exposure. Additionally, patients with endocrine disorders or cancers, nutritional disorders, and hepatic diseases may also present with melasma.

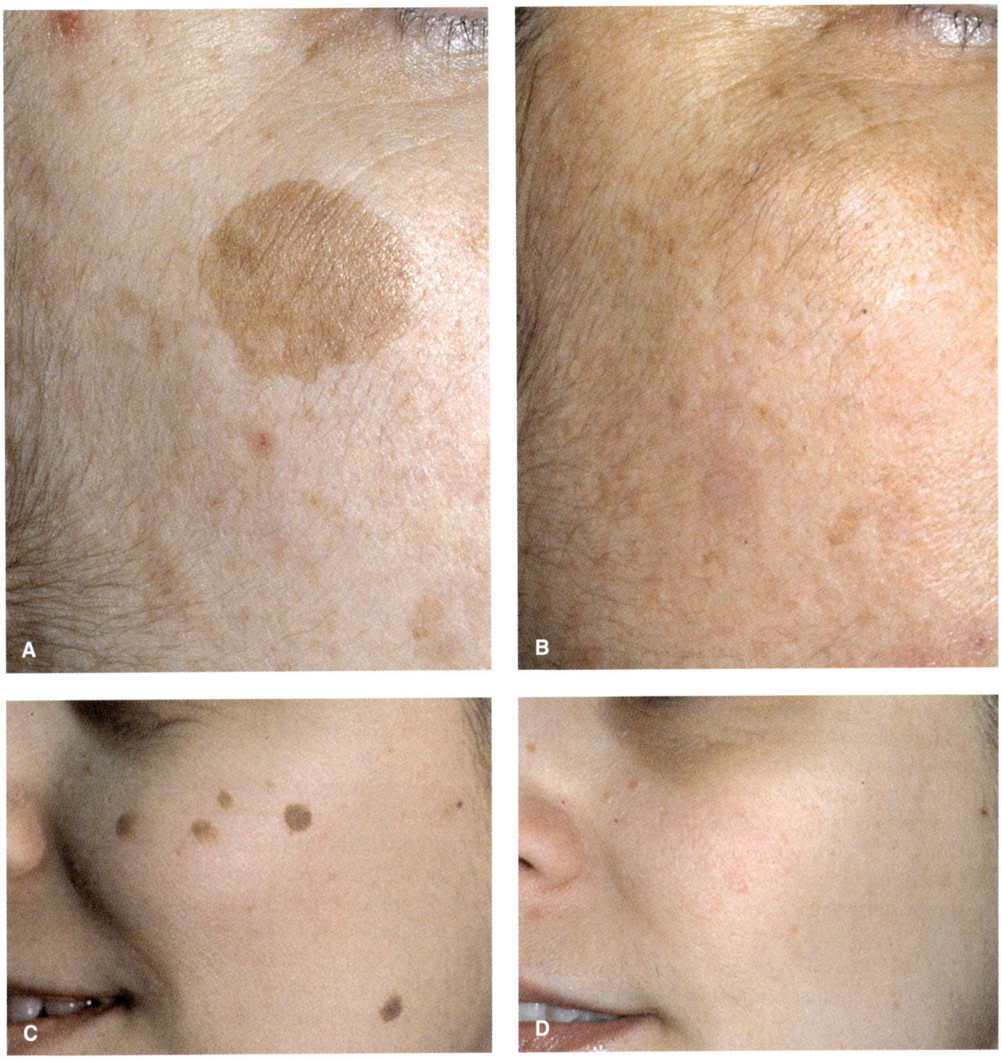

Figure 49-2 **A.** Seborrheic keratosis prior to treatment. **B.** Following one treatment with a QS alexandrite laser. **C.** A cluster of seborrheic keratoses. **D.** Following three treatments with a 532 nm KTP laser.

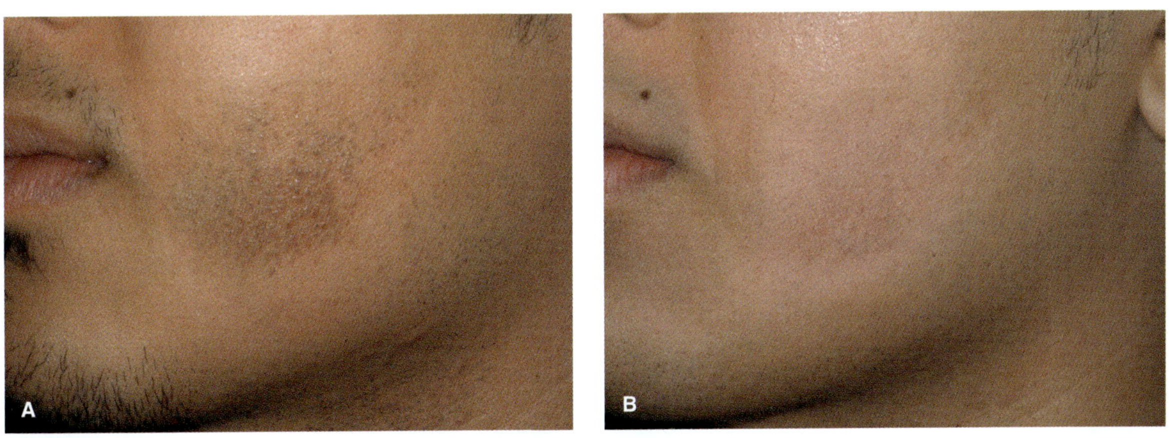

Figure 49-3 **A.** Becker's nevus **B.** Following three treatments with an LP alexandrite laser, improvement in both the hypertrichosis and the pigmented portion is noted.

Clinically three patterns are recognized on the basis of their distribution:

i. A centrofacial pattern
ii. A mandibular pattern
iii. A malar pattern

There are three histologic types that are recognized:

i. Epidermal (70%)
ii. Dermal (10%–15%)
iii. Mixed—occurring in both epidermis and dermis (20%)

Histologically, in the epidermal type, melanin deposition occurs in all layers of the epidermis. In the dermal type, melanin-laden macrophages are present in a perivascular distribution in both superficial and deep dermis. Subtypes of melasma are best identified by examination under a Wood's lamp. Epidermal melasma exhibits enhancement of color contrast when examined with a Wood's lamp, while no enhancement of color contrast is observed in patients with dermal melasma.[49]

QSLs, LP lasers, and IPL sources have been evaluated in the treatment of melasma.[50–58] In our experience, melasma is a challenging condition to treat with lasers. Strict sun precaution and inhibitors of pigmentation (such as hydroquinone) must be part of any treatment regimen. In addition, we find the recurrence rate and appearance of postinflammatory hyperpigmentation (PIH) to be high with laser therapy.[43,59–63] A recent study using a low-fluence QS Nd:YAG laser in combination with microdermabrasion has been reported to result in >75% improvement in 22 of 27 patients.[64]

Fractional lasers (Fig. 49-4) have also been approved by the Food and Drug Administration (FDA) for the treatment of melasma, and successful treatment has been reported.[6] However, despite low treatment parameters and well-spaced treatment intervals, PIH occurs in 50% of treated patients.

Postinflammatory Hyperpigmentation. Any cutaneous condition associated with inflammation or injury to the skin may result in PIH, characterized by the deposition of either melanin or hemosiderin or both. Histologically, PIH can have both epidermal and dermal components.

Treatment of PIH with QSLs and IPL devices is mostly unsatisfactory with little improvement, or even the possibility of exacerbation of the PIH. Strict sun avoidance and topical bleaching creams should considered first-line therapies. Epidermal PIH has been reported to respond better than dermal PIH.[59] Before commencing laser treatment, test spots are recommended.

Nevomelanocytic Nevi

Acquired Nevomelanocytic Nevi. Acquired nevomelanocytic nevi begin to appear in early childhood and can manifest throughout life.[65] They are mostly asymptomatic, acquired pigmented lesions, usually <1 cm in size, and can present as macules, papules, or nodules.

They are subdivided into junctional, compound, and intradermal nevi based on the location of melanocytic nevus cells. Nevi often have a natural course of evolution starting as junctional nevi, and maturing to compound nevi and ultimately intradermal nevi. The exact factors influencing the natural history of acquired nevomelanocytic nevi are not fully known, although sun exposure is likely a factor in the induction of nevi in exposed areas.[66–69]

Laser treatment of nevi should be undertaken with caution. All nevi should be evaluated by a dermatologist prior to treatment to ensure that there is a low level of suspicion for atypia or malignancy. Nevi can be treated with both QSL and LP laser that are melanin-specific. In our experience, smaller and thinner nevi respond better to QSLs. All three QSL systems (QS ruby, alexandrite, and Nd:YAG lasers) are effective with minimal side effects, although recurrence rates are high. LP lasers have been shown to more efficiently eradicate these nevi, but hypertrophic scarring can occur.[70] Skin cooling may be turned off to increase efficacy but carries the risk of excessive thermal damage to the epidermis. Ablative resurfacing with an Er:YAG laser has been reported in a small cohort to result in cosmetically satisfactory results.[71]

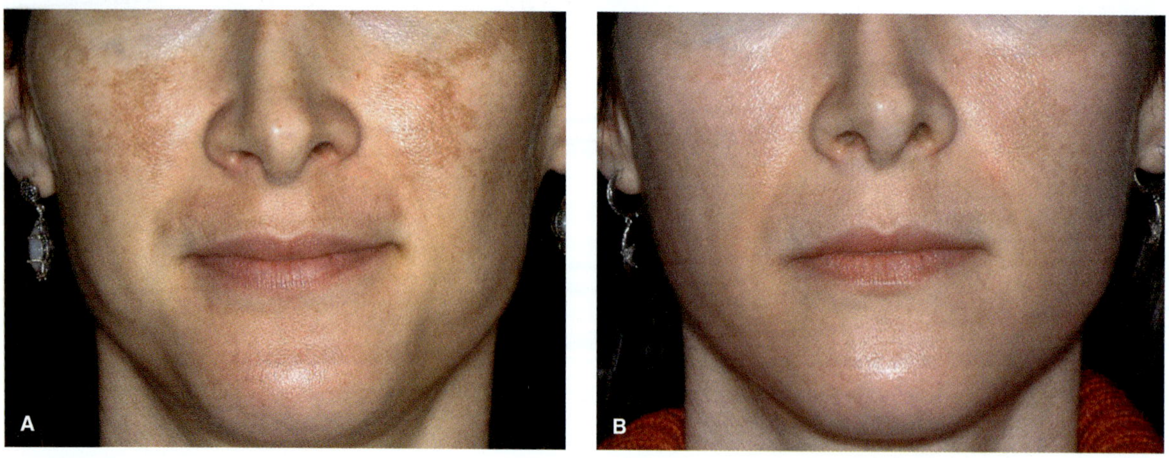

Figure 49-4 **A.** Melasma. Test spots with QSL and LP laser did not yield improvement, while non-ablative fractional resurfacing test spots were found to be helpful. **B.** Appearance following three non-ablative fractional resurfacing treatments with low densities.

Congenital Nevomelanocytic Nevi (CMN). By definition, CMN appear at birth, but they may arise during infancy. They are mostly light or dark brown in color and are classified by size. Small CMN are <1.5 cm, medium CMN are between 1.5 to 20 cm, and large/giant CMN are >20 cm in size.[72,73] It has been reported that congenital melanocytic nevi, in particular large/giant CMN, demonstrate an increased potential for the development of melanoma,[74–77] but pooled data suggest that the risk for malignant transformation is significantly lower at ~2.5% for large/garment-sized congenital nevi.[78] Interestingly, nearly half of patients with a large/garment-sized CMN have psychological or social difficulties.[79] Arguments have been made both for and against treatment of CMN. Laser irradiation of CMN continues to be controversial, as opponents of laser treatment argue that it can theoretically induce a neoplastic change in the cellular behavior of the lesion. However, no direct correlation has been made linking laser treatment and malignant transformation of CMN. Proponents of laser treatment of CMN argue that laser treatment can reduce the burden of nevomelanocytes, thereby reducing the risk of melanoma transformation, while also improving the appearance of these lesions and lessening their psychosocial burden.

A variety of lasers have been used to treat CMN. QSLs have been popular for treatment because their nanosecond pulse durations closely match the thermal relaxation time of melanosomes. Responses range from poor to excellent. Multiple treatments are needed, and it has been noted in one study[80] that after a single initial laser treatment of CMN, repopulation of the initially depleted layers usually occurs within 3 to 6 months. While QSL treatments may improve the cosmetic appearance, they are unlikely to remove all the nevus cell nests, in particular the non-pigmented nests in the deeper dermis. LP lasers have also been used to treat CMN due to their potential to better target nests of melanocytes. Like QSLs, results have been too variable to draw definitive conclusions. Combination treatment (Fig. 49-5) with both QSLs and LP lasers has also been reported with promising results.[81] Ablative lasers such as the CO_2 and Er:YAG lasers have been used alone or in combination with QSLs. Arguing against any role for lasers in promoting malignant degeneration, a long-term histologic study of patients with congenital nevi treated with normal mode ruby laser failed to show any malignant changes after 8 years.[82]

LASER TREATMENT OF DERMAL PIGMENTED LESIONS

Nevus of Ota and Nevus of Ito. Nevus of Ota is a congenital dermal pigmented lesion. Although most commonly unilateral, a rare bilateral variant form known as Hori's nevus can also occur.[83] It is a confluent mixture of blue and brown hyperpigmented patches on the skin and mucous membranes and is innervated by the ophthalmic or maxillary divisions of the trigeminal nerve. The conjunctiva, sclera, external auditory canal, tympanic membrane, oral and nasal mucosa, and hard palate may also be involved. Occasionally, there are papular, or even nodular portions in the pigmented patch.[83] The blue hue of the lesion results from the presence of ectopic melanocytes in the deep dermis, which produce a Tyndall effect. Histologically, dermal melanocytes are scattered in the upper and deep reticular dermis.[84,85] Rare cases of melanoma arising in the nevus of Ota have been reported,[86] but these lesions are generally considered benign.

Clinically and histologically, the nevus of Ito is quite similar to the nevus of Ota, except that it occurs in the areas innervated by the supraclavicular and cutaneous brachii lateralis nerves, i.e., the scapular, supraclavicular, or deltoid areas.

Pigment-specific QSLs have excellent clearance rates in the treatment of these lesions. Q-switched ruby, Q-switched alexandrite (Fig. 49-6), and Q-switched Nd:YAG lasers have been used and tend to be the best able to treat these conditions.[87–89] Laser treatments in patients with the nevus of Ota or Ito can be safely initiated at any age, but children usually respond better and

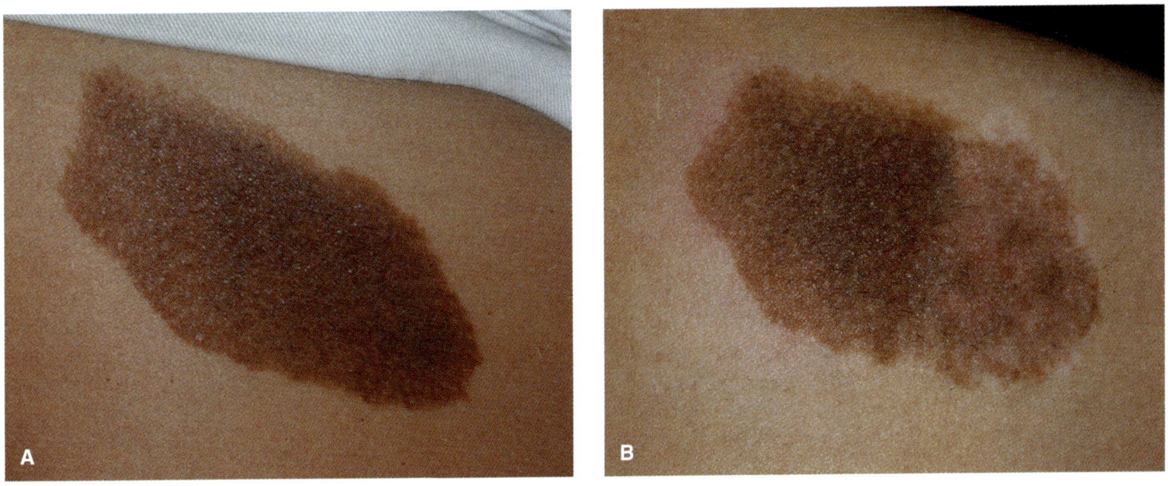

Figure 49-5 **A.** Congenital nevus on the right thigh of a young woman. **B.** Appearance of lesion following one treatment of combination LP and QS alexandrite lasers to right half of lesion.

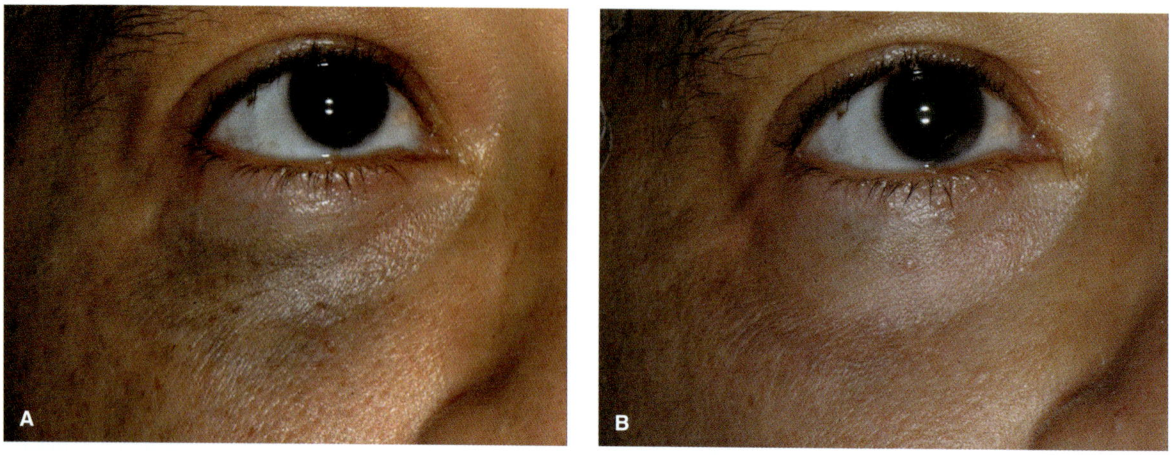

Figure 49-6 **A.** Nevus of Ota. **B.** Appearance following six treatments with a QS alexandrite laser.

need fewer treatment sessions.[90] Response is usually gradual and patients may require four to six treatment sessions. Periorbital lesions may require more treatments,[91] and ocular shields must be used to minimize the risk of damage to retinal melanin. Treatment with non-ablative fractional photothermolysis has also been reported to successfully clear these lesions.[7] However, larger studies are needed to establish these results. Post-treatment, strict sun protection, and the use of bleaching agents can help minimize the risk of pigmentary complications.

Nevus of Hori. Nevus of Hori is also termed acquired bilateral nevus of Ota-like macules. Clinically, it is characterized by speckled or confluent blue-brown or slate gray macules in the malar, temple, or forehead regions. Unlike the nevus of Ota, these lesions are acquired, bilateral, and without scleral or mucosal involvement. Histologically, melanocytes are largely present in the upper dermis.[92] Although promising results in the treatment of Hori's nevus with pigment-specific QSLs (Q-switched ruby, Q-switched alexandrite, and Q-switched Nd:YAG) have been reported, complete clearance rates are slightly lower than those for the nevus of Ota, and lesions may require more treatment sessions.[93] A higher rate of PIH is also observed following laser treatments compared to the nevus of Ota.[94]

Blue Nevus. Blue nevi are acquired, solitary, well-circumscribed papules or nodules. They are mostly asymptomatic and benign and arise spontaneously, usually in children and young adults. These nevi result from ectopic proliferation of melanin-producing melanocytes within the dermis, and their dark color results from the Tyndall light scattering effect of the overlying tissues.

The deep dermal melanocytes of blue nevi respond well to the pigment-specific QSL (Q-switched ruby, Q-switched alexandrite, and Q-switched Nd:YAG) treatments, as long as the lesion does not extend into deep subcutaneous tissue.

PATIENT SELECTION AND TREATMENT APPROACH

INITIAL PATIENT CONSULTATION

The initial patient consultation/evaluation is important, both for patients, who must leave with realistic expectations of treatment efficacy and downtime, and also for physicians, to identify those patients at risk of complications. Written informed consent, including a discussion of possible risks and adverse events, should be obtained prior to any treatment. Patients should understand that multiple treatments may be required, depending on the type of lesion being treated, and that complete clearance cannot be guaranteed. Usually, there is a 4 to 6 week interval between treatments.

A focused medical history including recent sun exposure, pregnancy, breast-feeding, intake of photosensitizing medications, photosensitive diseases, and genetic conditions,[9] information regarding wound healing and scarring tendencies and history of infectious diseases is important. Patients with a history of herpes simplex virus require antiviral prophylaxis[10] if laser treatment is occurring in the vicinity of the mouth. Patients who have received gold salts for diseases such as rheumatoid arthritis should be approached with caution, as laser-induced chrysiasis after treatment with QSL has been reported in individuals with a history of gold salt use.[95,96]

Laser treatment in individuals who have taken isotretinoin therapy in the previous 6 months is controversial because there have been reports of keloid formation in these individuals after laser treatment,[97] although there is increasing evidence that these individuals may not have a higher incidence of scarring.[98] The importance of avoiding tanning prior to any laser treatments should be emphasized, as it elevates the risk for temporary and permanent dyspigmentation.

Expected sequelae of therapy, such as blistering, purpura, or crusting, as well as potential side effects, such as infection, prolonged erythema, hypopigmentation, hyperpigmentation, atrophy, scarring, hypertrophic scarring, or keloid formation, should be discussed prior to treatment.

Photographic documentation should also be obtained prior to treatment. Additionally, inspection and documentation of pre-existing pigment disturbances, textural changes, or scarring may be beneficial when evaluating patients for treatment.

PROCEDURE

Prior to treatment, basic laser safety measures should be observed in the procedure room. Every person in the room should wear protective eyeglasses with the proper optical density, including the patient. The treatment site should be free of any make-up, lotions, or creams. Topical or intralesional anesthesia may be necessary to thwart procedural pain. Topical anesthetic creams are often applied under occlusion for 30 to 60 minutes before laser irradiation.

It is always advisable to perform a test spot. An immediate ash-white color[99] is the desired treatment endpoint with a QSL for most pigmented lesions. Some pinpoint bleeding may also be observed, which is acceptable. Subtle darkening of the lesion is the desired endpoint with a LP or IPL device.

Skin tissues and blood can splatter and be aerosolized during treatment, particularly with QSL. This is likely because of the photomechanical effect of QSLs resulting in rapid heating of the chromophore and generation of shock waves. The use of protective shields for mucosal surfaces is recommended, particularly in situations where patients have hepatitis or HIV. A smoke evacuator can help minimize the amount of laser-induced plume that is inhaled.

POSTTREATMENT

Appropriate posttreatment wound care is critical to optimize good cosmetic results and minimize the risk for complications. After completion of laser treatment, a clean dressing with an occlusive ointment such as petrolatum is recommended. Occasionally, large blisters can occur. Patients should avoid lancing the blisters. If they are uncomfortable enough, they can be lanced by the treating physician in the office. The patient should expect the area to develop crusting and scabbing that will last for 3 to 10 days after treatment.

Patient should avoid sun exposure during the treatment period and for at least a month after the final treatment to minimize PIH.

FUTURE DIRECTIONS

A greater understanding of the underlying biology of pigmented lesions will undoubtedly help clinicians to treat them more effectively. The use of fractional photothermolysis, either in combination or in isolation, for pigmented lesions will be forthcoming. Importantly, newer laser technology, such as picosecond pulsed lasers, will likely improve our ability to treat pigmented lesions as well.

REFERENCES

1. Goldman L, Igelman JM, Richfield DF. Impact of the laser on nevi and melanomas. *Arch Dermatol.* 1964;90:71–75.
2. Anderson RR, Parrish JA. Selective photothermolysis: precise microsurgery by selective absorption of pulsed irradiation. *Science.* 1983;220:524–527.
3. Lauback HJ, Tannous Z, Anderson RR, Monstein D. Skin responses to fractional photothermolysis. *Laser Surg.* 2006; 36:142–149.
4. Hantash BM, Bedi VP, Sudireddy V, Struck SK, Herron GS, Chan KF. Laser-induced transepidermal elimination of dermal contents by fractional photothermolysis. *J Biomed Opt.* 2006;27:1104–1115.
5. Glaich AS, Goldberg LH, Dai T, Kunishige JH, Friedman PM. Fractionated resurfacing: a new therapeutic modality for Becker's nevus. *Arch Dermatol.* 2007;143:1488–1490.
6. Kroon MW, Wind BS, Beck JF, et al. Non-ablative 1550-nm fractional laser therapy versus triple topical therapy for the treatment of melasma: a randomized, controlled pilot study. *J Am Acad Dermatol.* 2011;64:516–523.
7. Kouba DJ, Fincher EF, Moy RL. Nevus of Ota successfully treated by fractional photothermolysis using a fractionated 1440 nm Nd:YAG laser. *Arch Dermatol.* 2008;144: 156–158.
8. Duke D, Byers R, Sober AJ, Anderson RR, Greevelink JM. Treatment of benign and atypical nevi with the normal-mode ruby laser and the Q-switched ruby laser. *Arch Dermatol.* 1999;135:290–296.
9. Raulin C, Greeve B, ed. *Lasers and IPL-technologie in der Dermatologie und Asthetschen Medizin.* 1st ed. New York, NY: Schattaur Stuttgart; 2001.
10. Goldman MP. Treatment of benign vascular lesions with the PhotoDerm VL, high intensity pulsed light source. *Adv Dermatol.* 1998;13:503–521.
11. Stankiewicz K, Chuang G, Avram M. Lentigines, laser, and melanoma: a case series and discussion. *Lasers Surg Med.* 2012;44(2):112–116.
12. Braun-Falco O, Schoefinias HH. Lentigosenilis. *Hautarzt.* 1971;22:277–283.
13. Kilmer SL, Garden JM. Laser treatment of pigmented lesions and tattoos. *Semin Cutan Med Surg.* 2000;19(4):232–244.
14. Watanabe S, Anderson RR, Brorson S, Dalickas G, Fujimoto JG, Flotte TJ. Comparative studies of femtosecond to microsecond laser pulses on selective pigmented cell injury in skin. *Photochem Photobiol.* 1991;53:757–762.
15. Goldberg DJ. Laser treatment of pigmented lesions. *Dermatol Clin.* 1997;15:397–407.
16. Kilmer SL, Wheeland RG, Goldberg DJ, Anderson RR. Treatment of epidermal pigmented lesions with the frequency-doubled Q switched Nd:YAG laser: a controlled, single-impact, dose-response, multicenter trial. *Arch Dermatol.* 1994;130:1515–1519.
17. Taylor CR, Anderson RR. Treatment of benign pigmented epidermal lesions by QS ruby laser. *Int J Dermatol.* 1993;32:908–912.
18. Kawada A, Shiraishi H, Asai M, et al. Clinical improvement of solar lentigines and ephelides with an intense pulsed light source. *Dermatol Surg.* 2002;28:504–508.
19. Ho SG, Yeung CK, Chan NP, Shek SY, Chan HH. A comparison of Q-switched and long-pulsed alexandrite laser for the treatment of freckles and lentigines in oriental patients. *Lasers Surg Med.* 2011;43:108–113.
20. Kundu RV, Joshi SS, Suh KY, et al. Comparison of electrodesiccation and potassium-titanyl-phosphate laser for treatment of dermatosis papulosa nigra. *Dermatol Surg.* 2009;35:1079–1083.
21. Garcia MS, Azari R, Eisen DB. Treatment of dermatosis papulosa nigra in 10 patients: a comparison trial of electrodesiccation, pulsed dye laser, and curettage. *Dermatol Surg.* 2010;36:1968–1972.
22. Breathnach AS. Melanocyte distribution in forearm epidermis of freckled human subjects. *J Invest Dermatol.* 1957; 29:253–261.

23. Duray TH. Café-au-Lait spots. In: Demis DJ, ed. *Clinical Dermatology*. 19th ed. Philadelphia, PA: JB Lippincott; 1992.
24. Carpo GB, Grevelink JM, Grevelink SV. Laser treatment of pigmented lesions in children. *Semin Cutan Med Surg.* 1999;18:233–243.
25. Shimbashi T, Kamide R, Hashimoto T. Long-term follow-up in treatment of solar lentigo and café-au-lait macules with Q-switched ruby laser. *Aesthetic Plast Surg.* 1997;21:445–448.
26. Kopf AW, Levine IJ, Rigel DS, Friedman RJ, Levenstein M. Congenital nevus-like nevi, nevi spili, and Café-au-Lait spots in patients with malignant melanoma. *J Dermatol Surg Oncol.* 1985;11:275–280.
27. Stern JB, Haupt HM, Aaronson CM. Malignant melanonma in a speckled zosteriform lentiginous nevus. *Int J Dermatol.* 1990;29:583–584.
28. Rutten A, Goos M. Nevus spilus with malignant melanoma in a patient with neurofibromatosis. *Arch Dermatol.* 1990;126:539–540.
29. Abecassis S, Spatz A, Cazeneuve C, et al. Melanoma within nevus spilus: 5 cases. *Ann Dermatol Venereol.* 2006;133: 323–328.
30. Moreno-Arias GA, Bull F, Vilata-Corell JJ, Camps-Fresneda A. Treatment of wide-spread segmental nevus spilus by Q-switched alexandrite laser (755-nm, 100 nsec). *Dermatol Surg.* 2001;27:841–843.
31. Grevelink JM, Gonzalez S, Bonoan R, Vibhagool C, Gonzalez E. Treatment of nevus Spilus with the Q-switched ruby laser. *Dermatol Surg.* 1997;23:365–369.
32. Gold MH, Foster TD, Bell MW. Nevus spilus successfully treated with an intense pulsed light source. *Dermatol Surg.* 1999;25:254–255.
33. Fitzpatrick RE, Goldman MP, Ruiz-Esparza J. Clinical advantage of the CO_2 laser superficial mode. Treatment of verruca vulgaris, seborrheic keratoses and actinic cheilitis. *J DermatolSurg Oncol.* 1994;20:449–456.
34. Khatri KA. Ablation of cutaneous lesions using an erbium: YAG laser. *J Cosmet Laser Ther.* 2003;5:150–153.
35. Mehrabi D, Brodell RT. Use of alexandrite laser for treatment of seborrheic keratoses. *Dermatol Surg.* 2002;28:437–439.
36. Winstanley D, Blalock T, Houghton N, Ross EV. Treatment of benign pigmented lesions using a long-pulse alexandrite laser. *J Drugs Dermatol.* 2012;11(11):1327–1330.
37. Raulin C, Schonermark MP, Breve B Werner S. Q-switched ruby laser treatment of tattoos and benign pigmented skin lesions: a critical review. *Ann Plast Surg.* 1998;41(5): 555–565.
38. Polder KD, Mithani A, Harrison A, Bruce S. Treatment of macular seborrheic keratoses using a novel 1927 nm fractional thalium fiber laser. *Dermatol Surg.* 2012;38(7 Pt 1): 1025–1031.
39. Chapel TA, Tavafoghi V, Mehregan AH. Becker's melanosis: an organoid hamartoma. *Cutis.* 1981;27:405–406.
40. Heneke E. The dermal component in melanosis naeviformis Becker. *J Cutan Pathol.* 1979;6:53–58.
41. Nanni CA, Alster TS. Treatment of a Becker's nevus using a 694 nm log-pulsed ruby laser. *Dermatol Surg.* 1998;24:1032–1034.
42. Kopera D, Hohenleutner U, Landthaler M. Quality-switched ruby laser treatment of solar lentigens and Becker's nevus: a histological and immunohistochemical study. *Dermatology.* 1997;194:338–343.
43. Tse Y, Levine VJ, McClain SA, Ashinoff R. The removal of cutaneous pigmented lesions with Q-switched ruby laser and the Q-switched Nd:YAG laser: a comparative study. *J Dermatol Surg Oncol.* 1994;20:795–800.
44. Kimbrough-Green CK, Griffiths CE, Finkel IJ, et al. Topical retinoic acid (tretinoin) for melasma in black patients: A vehicle-controlled clinical trial. *Arch Dermatol.* 1994;130: 727–731.
45. Hassan I, Kaur I, Sialy R, Dash RJ. Hormonal milieu in maintenance of melasma in fertile women. *J Dermatol.* 1998;25(8):510–512.
46. Lawrence N, Cox SE, Brody HJ. Treatment of melasma with Jessner's solution versus glycolic acid: a comparison of clinical efficacy and evaluation of the predictive ability of Wood's light examination. *J Am Acad Dermatol.* 1997;36(4): 589–593.
47. Kodali S, Guevara IL, Carrigan CR, et al. A prospective, randomized, split-face, controlled trial of salicylic acid peels in the treatment of melasma in Latin American women. *J Am Acad Dermatol.* 2010;63(6):1030–1035.
48. Balina LM, Graup K. The treatment of melasma: 20% azelaic acid versus 4% hydroquinone cream. *Int J Dermatol.* 1991;30(12):893–895.
49. Sanchez NP, Pathak MA, Sato S, Fitzpatrick TB, Sanchez JL, Mihm MC Jr. Melasma: A clinical, light microscopic, ultrasructural, and immunofluorescenece study. *J Am Acad Dermatol.* 1981;4:698–710.
50. Yoshimura K, Sato K, Aiba-Kojima E, et al. Repeated treatment protocols for melasma and acquired dermal melanocytosis. *Dermatol Surg.* 2006;32:365–371.
51. Suh KS, Sung JY, Roh HJ, Jeon YS, Kim YC, Kim ST. Efficacy of the 1064-nm Q-switched Nd:YAG laser in melasma. *J Dermatolog Treat.* 2011;22:233–238.
52. Cho SB, Kim JS, Kim MJ. Melasma treatment in Korean women using a 1064-nm Q-switched Nd:YAG laser with low pulse energy. *Clin Exp Dermatol.* 2009;34:e847–e850.
53. Jeong SY, Shin JB, Yeo UC, Kim WS, Kim IH. Low-fluence Q-switched neodymium-doped yttrium aluminum garnet laser for melasma with pre- or post-treatment triple combination cream. *Dermatol Surg.* 2010;36:909–918.
54. Angsuwarangsee S, Polnikorn N. Combined ultrapulse CO_2 laser and Q-switched alexandrite laser compared with Q-switched alexandrite laser alone for refractory melasma: split-face design. *Dermatol Surg.* 2003;29:59–64.
55. Nouri K, Bowes L, Chartier T, Romagosa R, Spencer J. Combination treatment of melasma with pulsed CO_2 laser followed by Q-switched alexandrite laser: a pilot study. *Dermatol Surg.* 1999;25:494–497.
56. Trelles MA, Velez M, Gold MH. The treatment of melasma with topical creams alone, CO_2 fractional ablative resurfacing alone, or a combination of the two: a comparative study. *J Drugs Dermatol.* 2010;9:315–322.
57. Manaloto RM, Alster T. Erbium:YAG laser resurfacing for refractory melasma. *Dermatol Surg.* 1999;25:121–123.
58. Wanitphakdeedecha R, Manuskiatti W, Siriphukpong S, Chen TM. Treatment of melasma using variable square pulse Er:YAG laser resurfacing. *Dermatol Surg.* 2009;35: 475–481.
59. Taylor CR, Anderson RR. Ineffective treatment of refractory melasma and post-inflammatory hyperpigmentation by Q-switched laser. *J Dermatol Surg Oncol.* 1994;20:592–597.
60. Goldberg GJ. Benign pigmented lesions of the skin. Treatment with Q-switched ruby laser. *J Dermatol Surg Oncol.* 1993;19:376–379.
61. Grekin RC, Shelton RM, Geisse JK, Frieden I. 510-nm pigmented lesion dye laser, its characteristics and clinical uses. *J Dermatol Surg oncol.* 1993;19:380–387.
62. Moreno-Arias GA, Ferrando J. Intense pulsed light for melanocytic lesions. *Dermatol Surg.* 2001;27:397–400.
63. Wang CC, Hui CY, Sue YM, Wong WR, Hang HS. Intense pulsed light for the treatment of referactory melasma in Asian persons. *Dermatol Surg.* 2004;30:1196–1200.
64. Kauvar AN. Successful treatment of melasma using a combination of microdermabrasion and Q-switched Nd:YAG lasers. *Lasers Surg Med.* 2012;44(2):117–124.
65. Rhodes AR. Neoplasm: benign neoplasma, hyperplasias, and dysplasias of melanocytes. In: Fitzpatrick TB, Eisen AZ, Wolff E, et al., eds. *Dermatology in general medicine.* 3rd ed. New York, NY: McGraw Hill; 1987.
66. Beral V, Evans S, Shaw H, Milton G. Cutaneous factors related to the risk of malignant melanoma. *Br J Dermatol.* 1983;109:165–172.
67. Osterlind A, Tucker MA, Hou-Jensen K, Stone BJ, Engholm G, Jensen OM. A Danish case-control study of cutaneous malignant melanoma.1 Importance of host factors. *Int J Cancer* 1988;42:200–206.
68. Mackie RM, Watt D, Doherty V, Aitchison T. Malignant melanonma occurring in those aged under 30 in the west of Scotland, 1979–1986: a study of incidence, clinical features, and survival. *Br J Dermatol.* 1991;124:560–564.

69. Trozak DJ, Rowland WD, Hu F. Metastatic melanoma in prepubertal children. *Pediatrics.* 1975;55:191–204.
70. Reda AM, Taha IR, Riad HA. Clinical and histological effect of a single treatment of normal mode alexandrite (755 nm) laser on small melanocytic nevi. *J Cutan Laser Ther.* 1999;1:209–215.
71. Baba M, Bal N. Efficacy and safety of the short-pulse erbium:YAG laser in the treatment of acquired melanocytic nevi. *Dermatol Surg.* 2006;32:256–260.
72. Alikhan A, Ibrahimi OA, Eisen DB. Congenital melanocytic nevi: where are we now? Part I. Clinical presentation, epidemiology, pathogenesis, histology, malignant transformation, and neurocutaneous melanosis. *J Am AcadDermatol.* 2012;67(4):495. e1–e17.
73. Ibrahimi OA, Alikhan A, Eisen DB. Congenital melanocytic nevi: where are we now? Part II. Treatment options and approach to treatment. *J Am Acad Dermatol.* 2012;67(4):515. e1–e13.
74. Rhodes AR, Weinstock MA, Fitzpatrick TB, Mihm MC Jr, Sober AJ. Risk factors for cutaneous melanoma: a practical method of recognizing predisposed individuals. *JAMA.* 1987;258:3146–3154.
75. Illig L, Weidner F, Hundeiker M, et al. Congenital nevi <10 cm as precursor to melanoma: 52 cases, a review, and a new conception. *Arch Dermatol.* 1985;121:1274–1281.
76. Rhodes AR, Sober AJ, Day CL, et al. The malignant potential of small congenital nevocellular nevi: an estimate of association based on a histologic study of 234 primary cutaneous melanomas. *J Am Acad Dermatol.* 1982;6: 230–241.
77. Rhodes AR, Melski JW. Small congenital nevocellular nevi and the risk of cutaneous melanoma. *J Pediatr.* 1982;100: 219–224.
78. Krengel S, Hauschild A, Schafer T. Melanoma risk in congenital melanocytic naevi: a systematic review. *Br J Dermatol.* 2006;155:1–8.
79. Pers M. Naevuspigmentosusgiganticus: indikationer for operative behandling. *Ungeskrift Laeger.* 1963;125:63.
80. Greevelink JM, van Leeuwen RL, Anderson RR, Byers HR. Clinical and histological responses of congenital melanocytic nevi after single treatment with QSL. *Arch Dermatol.* 1997;133:349–352.
81. Kono T, Erçöçen AR, Nozaki M. Treatment of congenital melanocytic nevi using the combined (normal-mode plus Q-switched) ruby laser in Asians: clinical response in relation to histological type. *Ann Plast Surg.* 2005;54: 494–501.
82. Imayama S, Ueda S. Long and short-term histological observations of congenital nevi, treated with the normal-mode ruby laser. *Arch Dermatol.* 1999;135:1211–1218.
83. Turnbull JR, Assaf Ch, Zouboulis C, Tebbe B. Bilateral nevus of Ota: a rare manifestation in a Caucasian. *J Eur Acad Dermatol Venereol.* 2004;18:353–355.
84. Hori Y, Kawashima M, Oohara K, Kukita A. Acquired bilateral nevus of Ota-like macules. *J Am Acad Dermatol.* 1984;10:961–964.
85. Mizoguchi M, Murakami F, Ito M, et al. Clinical, pathological and etiologic aspects of acquired dermal melanocytosis. *Pigment Cell Res.* 1997;10:176–183.
86. Dorsey CS, Mongomery H. Blue nevus and its distinction from Mongolian spot in the nevus of Ota. *J Invest Dermatol.* 1954;22:225–236.
87. Lowe NJ, Winder JM, Sawcer D, Burrows P, Chalet M. Nevus of Ota: treatment with high energy fluencies of the Q-switched ruby laser. *J Am Acad Dermatol.* 1993;29:997–1001.
88. Chan HH, Leung RS, Ying SY, et al. A retrospective analysis of complications in the treatment of nevus of Ota with the Q-switched alexandrite and Q-switched Nd: YAG lasers. *Dermatol Surg.* 2000;26:1000–1006.
89. Moreno-Arias GA, Camps-Fresneda A. Treatment of nevus of Ota with the Q-switched alexandrite laser. *Laser Surg med.* 2001;28:451–455.
90. Kono T, Chan HH, Ercocen AR, et al. Use of Q-switched ruby laser in the treatment of nevus of Ota in different age groups. *Laser Surg Med.* 2003;32:391–395.
91. Chan HH, Lam LK, Wong DS, et al. Nevus of Ota: a new classification based on the response to laser treatment. *Laser Surg Med.* 2001;28:267–272.
92. Lam AY, Wong DS, Lam LK, Ho WS, Chan HH. A retrospective study on the efficacy and complications of Q-switched alexandrite laser in the treatment of acquired bilateral nevus of Ota-like macules. *Dermatol Surg.* 2001;27:937–942.
93. Polnikorn N, Tanrattanakorn S, Goldberg DJ. Treatment of Hori's nevus with the Q-switched Nd: YAG laser. *Dermatol Surg.* 2000;26:477–480.
94. Lee B, Kim YC, Kang WH, Lee ES. Comparison of characteristics of acquired bilateral nevus of Ota-like macules and nevus of Ota, according to therapeutic outcome. *J Korean Med Sci.* 2004;19:554–559.
95. Vergas G, Chan K, Thomsen S, Welch A. Use of osmotically active agents to alter optical properties of tissues: effects on the detected fluorescence signal measured through skin. *Lasers Surg Med.* 2001;29(3):213–220.
96. McNicholas R, Fox M, Gowda A, Fox MA, Tuya S, Bell B, Motamedi M. Temporary dermal scatter reduction quantitative assessment and implications for improved laser tattoo removal. *Lasers Surg Med.* 2005;36(4):289–296.
97. Kobayashi H, Togashi K. CT of tattoos removed with laser therapy. *Am J Roentgenol.* 2000;174:1468–1469.
98. Baumler W, Eibler ET, Hohenleuter U, Sens B, Sauer J, Landthaler M. Q-switced laser and tattoo pigments: first results of the chemical and photophysical analysis of 41 compounds. *Lasers Surg Med.* 2000;26:13–21.
99. Taylor CR, Gange RW, Dover JS, et al. Treatment of tattoos by Q-switched ruby laser. A dose response study. *Arch Dermatol.* 1990;126:893–899.

SECTION 5

Aesthetic Problems

CHAPTER 50

Tattoos

Mussarrat Hussain, Suzanne L. Kilmer, & Omar A. Ibrahimi

HISTORY

Humans have marked their bodies with tattoos for millennia. These designs have always been personal and functioned as amulets, status symbols, declarations of love, signs of religious beliefs, and adornment. Often their uses extended beyond the decorative and were utilized as a form of therapy or even punishment.[1]

"Otzi the Iceman," discovered on the Italian-Austrian border in 1991, became the earliest known example in terms of tattoos on the actual body; he was carbon-dated at around 5,200 years old. His body was found to harbor 57 tattooed dots and small crosses on his lower spine, right knee, and ankle joints, likely suggestive of his tattoos holding therapeutic significance.[2] Ancient Egyptian women had tattoos on their bodies and limbs and were present on several female mummies dating back to c2000 BC. Numerous figurines depicting tattooing on their bodies have also been discovered from up to c4000 to 3500 BC, many with tattoos on their thighs.[3] Crude needles and pigmented bowls used in early tattooing have also been found in Egypt, France, Spain, and Portugal.[3,4]

In the late 1800, the invention of the electric tattooing machine revolutionized the art of tattooing.[1] This advance brought tattooing into the mainstream culture in many countries. In the United States, it is estimated that up to one-quarter of young to middle-aged adults have at least one tattoo.[5,6] However, despite the popularity of tattooing in the United States, it is still poorly regulated.

TYPES OF TATTOOS

Tattoos result from the exogenous deposition of micron-sized ink or other pigment-containing particles into the dermis, deliberately or as result of trauma. Instruction on how to administer a tattoo were published as early as 6th century, in a book entitled "Medicae Artis Principes," written by the Greek Physician Aetius.[7] Tattoos can be classified as decorative, cosmetic, medical, traumatic, and iatrogenic.

a. **DECORATIVE TATTOOS:** Decorative tattoos are most common and are further subdivided into professional and amateur. Professional tattoos are typically placed more deeply in the dermis by the vibrating needle of a tattoo machine, along with a greater density of pigment. Professional tattoo pigments are mostly dyes used in chemical industry, which incorporate different kinds of organic and inorganic pigments. Inorganic pigments may be composed of cadmium, chromium, mercury, iron, titanium, aluminum, silica, copper, bromine, sulfur, carbon, and magnesium.[8] The number of organic materials used is even more impressive, with most classified as either azo or non-azo, or polycyclic compounds.[9] One study[10] has shown photodecomposition of two widely used azo-containing tattoo pigments into known carcinogenic and cytotoxic products.

   Amateur tattoos are often homemade carbon-rich mixtures that are often mixed with chipped automobile paints or other industrial sources to boost the color. Both professional and amateur tattoo pigments are composed of non-homogeneous granules size as well of unknown purity and composition.

b. **COSMETIC TATTOOS:** Cosmetic tattoos have become increasingly popular in recent years. They are applied for a variety of reasons, including to improve or create the appearance of normal anatomical structures or to disguise scars. Some cosmetic tattoos are related to medical conditions, such as tattoos that mimic an areola in breast reconstruction following mastectomy, whereas others are used to thicken the appearance of thinning eyebrows, eyelashes, or the lip vermilion. The colors that are used most frequently are brown, pink, red, and dull orange.[11]

c. **TRAUMATIC TATTOOS:** Traumatic tattoos can occur following different types of injury that breach the epidermal barrier of the skin, such as abrasions, avulsions, and lacerations. These pigments become trapped in the dermis after re-epithelialization of the wound and result in tattoos.

   Traumatic tattoo particles vary in size from very fine microscopic particles to large masses of gravel, carbon, road tar, asphalt, and dirt from motor vehicle accidents, graphite from pencils, surgical pens, or glass. Amalgam tattoos are traumatic in origin and typically follow implantation of metal particles into the oral mucosa during dental procedures. On occasion, explosion of particulate matter such as gun powder, fireworks, or petroleum products can drive foreign bodies into the skin and result in traumatic tattoos.

d. **MEDICAL TATTOOS:** Tattoos may also be created for medical purposes. In radiation therapy, tattoos are often placed to designate a radiation port. India ink is commonly used in most cases.

e. **IATROGENIC TATTOOS:** Iatrogenic tattoos may result from implantation of pigmented particles into a wound during surgery or another medical procedure, such as with the use of Monsel's solution.[12]

TATTOO BIOLOGY

Tattoo particles reside at various depths in the skin, ranging from 1.1 to 2.9 mm in depth, from the granular layer of the epidermis to the reticular dermis. Professional tattoos tend to reside more deeply in the dermis, whereas amateur tattoos are more superficial. In older tattoos, all pigment granules are intracellular and are found within lysosomes of mononuclear cells, such as fibroblasts and macrophages. The distribution of such cells is typically perivascular or periadnexal.[13]

The size of pigment granules can vary from 10 to 100 μm[14] and is critical to the tattoo's appearance, and also correlates with the ease of subsequent removal. Larger granules provide more visible color and greater longevity, whereas smaller granules provide greater homogeneity in the tattoo's appearance, but are more prone to migration.[15]

HISTORY OF TATTOO REMOVAL

Regardless of the initial motivation for acquiring tattoos, the desire to remove them is probably as old as their existence. Although reasons for tattoo acquisition vary between populations, the motivation for tattoo removal appears quite similar.[16,17] Patient surveys have shown that these decorative tattoos are sometimes obtained impulsively.[3] The reasons stated for tattoo removal in one study[18] included: enhancement of self-esteem (70%), social reasons (35%), family pressure (19%), improving employment prospects (18%), and change of partner (6%).

The earliest documentation of tattoo removal was by the Greek physician Aetius in 543 AD.[19]

Historically, all methods used in tattoo removal involved some element of destruction (traumatizing) of the superficial dermis. The best results were obtained in patients with prolonged/delayed wound healing and an increased inflammatory response, which elicits an exudative phase, and promotes an accumulation of macrophages in the injured area with their increased phagocytic activity. These responses promote the loss of additional pigment in post-operative phase of healing.[20,21]

Many techniques have been tried to achieve the goal of successful tattoo removal, including chemical, mechanical and thermal treatment, infrared coagulation, surgical excision, and laser treatment. Even today, with the development of nanosecond and picosecond pulsed lasers, the quest for complete tattoo removal remains unfulfilled.

CHEMICAL TREATMENT OF TATTOOS

a. **SALABRASION:** Salabrasion is the process of abrading the skin followed by the application of salts and was first described by the Greek physician Aetius in 543 A.D.[19] Salabrasion has been recently studied by a number of research groups.[19,22–24] After adequate local anesthesia, a rotary motor with a felt wheel is lightly applied to remove the superficial layer of the skin. Moist sponges dipped in normal table salt are then rubbed lightly with even pressure over the treatment area for a total of 10 to 11 minutes for the first treatment. The absence of the superficial skin layer allows the salt to penetrate into the dermis. The skin appears a bright red color after 5 to 6 minutes. After the procedure, a dressing may be applied that also contains salts, which stimulates additional cell injury that can result in even more tattoo pigment being removed, or the wound is covered with a dry, sterile dressing and the patient is placed on antibiotics until the wound is healed. The dressing is changed daily and wound healing usually occurs on 21st day. Repeat treatments can be performed 2 to 3 months later. Disadvantages of salabrasion include the significant risk of hypertrophic scarring or keloid formation, and overtreatment may result in loss of pigment and full-thickness skin loss.[25]

b. **CAUSTIC CHEMICALS:** Caustic chemicals have been used for tattoo removal for centuries.[26] A standard deep chemical peel solution, such as phenol, used to be painted on the tattoo with Q-tips. For tattoos on the extremities, a gentler peel solution would be used. Following 24 to 48 hours, a 2% aqueous gentian violet solution would be painted on the wound and then covered with gauze. The dressings were changed daily until epithelialization occurred. This method was beneficial for very superficial tattoos, but was a difficult procedure to tolerate. Professional tattoos did not respond well and hyper- and hypopigmentation occurred frequently.[25]

c. **TANNIC ACID:** The use of tannic acid introduced into the skin with reciprocating needles was published by Scutt.[27] After tannic acid application, a dry, sterile dressing is applied. An eschar forms in a few days and sloughs off in about 7 to 10 days. Following this, the wound is allowed to epithelialize. Good results have been reported with a low incidence of scarring but hyperpigmentation has been observed.

MECHANICAL TREATMENTS

Mechanical irritation as a treatment for tattoo removal has also been an old remedy, and can be performed either by over-tattooing or with dermabrasion. A number of studies suggest that the key to mechanical treatment is prolonged healing and increasing the inflammatory response.[25,28]

a. **DERMABRASION**: Dermabrasion uses a wire brush or diamond fraise to abrade the skin and the tattoo pigments within it. Dermabrasion can also be done in combination with cryotherapy to create a rigid skin surface to abrade. Following dermabrasion, the wound can be coated with 2% aqueous gentian violet and covered with a layer of Adaptic gauze followed by a compression dressing of sterile pads and gauze wrap. The dressings are changed daily and repainted with gentian violet.

   Dermabrasion for the removal of tattoos is usually administered in a single treatment or sometimes in a series of treatments in an attempt to decrease the scarring that may occur from a single more aggressive treatment. Even with multiple, less aggressive sessions of dermabrasion, there is virtually always some scarring, loss of normal skin pigment, and residual tattoo. When used on non-facial skin, the risk of scarring from dermabrasion is significant. Additionally, this procedure aerosolizes blood and tissue particles, which can be a hazard to the treating physician and other staff in the treatment room.[21,23,24,29,30]

THERMAL TREATMENTS FOR TATTOO REMOVAL

Virtually any source of heat has been used at one point or another to remove tattoos. Patients have used fire, hot coals, heated metal objects, cigarettes and cigars, and other sources of heat to remove tattoos by destroying the superficial layer of the skin with resulting inflammation and resultant tattoo removal. These thermal methods of tattoo removal inevitably almost always leave a scar.[28]

a. **Electrodesiccation and electrocautery** with low wattage settings used to remove tattoos by damaging the superficial skin have resulted in unpredictable benefits and scarring in a good number of patients.
b. **Infrared coagulation** was developed to remove a variety of skin lesions by thermally coagulating the skin. It has also been used for tattoo removal.[31–34]
c. **Liquid nitrogen:** On the opposite end of the thermal spectrum, liquid nitrogen (–196°C), has been used to destroy a number of superficial skin lesions including tattoos, in a non-specific manner, with a lower risk of scarring.[35,36] Cryotherapy, however, can cause atrophy and hypopigmentation.[25]

SURGICAL EXCISION

Surgical excision has also been used to remove tattoos. Prior to the development of pulsed lasers (see below), excision was the treatment of choice for small, surgically amenable tattoos. This treatment has the advantage of immediate removal without the need for multiple patient visits, typically at a far lower cost than laser tattoo removal. Larger tattoos require more complex or multiple staged surgeries that held the potential to be disfiguring. Surgical removal of tattoos can be done either by full thickness excision or split-thickness excision with over-grafting or split-thickness tangential excision techniques.[25]

Although surgical excision can remove a tattoo in a single treatment with the possibility of leaving a linear scar, scarring can be quite significant or tattoo removal incomplete. Tattoos requiring multiple procedures take place over many months in a staged removal process.[37–39]

Excision and grafting often give poor cosmetic results because the patient receives two blemished areas. The grafted area wrinkles and contracts, whereas its border usually forms a hypertrophic scar, and the donor site may be visible as well. Furthermore, the skin graft frequently does not cover all of the deep pigment.

LASER TREATMENT FOR TATTOO REMOVAL

On the basis of Einstein's quantum theory of light, Maiman[40] developed the first operating laser in 1960. Exploration of possible medical applications of this device immediately followed, and in 1963, Leon Goldman and his colleagues[41] reported the ability of laser light to selectively destroy targets in the skin. They noted highly selective injury of pigmented structures shortly thereafter. Goldman also reported the use of a normal-mode ruby laser with 0.5 ms pulse duration and 5 J energy as the first laser to treat tattoos.[42]

Later in the 1960s and 1970s, a number of continuous-wave lasers such as the carbon dioxide laser (10,600 nm wavelength), the argon-ion (Ar-ion) laser (488 and 514 nm wavelengths), and the Nd:YAG laser (1064 nm wavelength) were developed. These lasers could vaporize and coagulate tissue with greater precision than electrosurgical tools and were incorporated into surgical and dermatologic practices as vaporization and coagulation devices.

The use of these continuous-wave lasers during the 1970s and early 1980s resulted in clinically significant new dermatologic laser treatment techniques, including their non-selective use for tattoo removal. In hindsight, it is not surprising that these devices usually left a scar, but the scars they left were preferable in many cases to the scars left by excisional surgery or dermabrasion.

a. **CARBON DIOXIDE LASER:** Carbon dioxide (CO_2) lasers emit energy at 10,600 nm in the infrared region. The primary chromophore for CO_2 laser is water, which undergoes instantaneous vaporization on exposure to laser energy. In 1978, the first reports regarding the successful removal of tattoos using continuous-wave CO_2 laser were published.[43,44]

It appears that the CO_2 laser removes tattoo pigments by means of thermal tissue coagulative effects, with the laser surgeon relying on visual feedback to confine the depth of tissue necrosis to the precise level of tattoo pigments. Variation of the pigment depth in different tattoos corresponds to thermal wounds of varying depths, the deepest of which can often cause significant inflammation, prolonged healing, and the development of hypertrophic scars.[45] No specific effects on tattoo ink particles were seen.[46]

Although tattoo removal by CO_2 laser was skillfully developed over the years and later combined with topical gentian violet and topical 50% urea paste dressings, with improved results[47], residual tattoo pigment and a significant incidence of atrophic and hypertrophic scarring were still seen.

b. **ARGON LASER:** The argon laser emits a blue or green continuous laser beam at 488 and 514 nm wavelengths and vaporizes tissue by non-selective heating. Although black tattoos selectively absorb green light, the continuous-wave delivery of the beam results in bulk heating to the surrounding skin and results in scarring.[45,48]

THEORY OF SELECTIVE PHOTOTHERMOLYSIS

Although excitement was initially generated by the early use of continuous-wave lasers for tattoo removal, ultimately these lasers proved to be too destructive with a high incidence of scarring.

In 1983, Anderson and Parrish of Harvard Medical School's Department of Dermatology published their landmark article describing the principle of selective photothermolysis,[49] which revolutionized cutaneous laser surgery. The theory elegantly explained that targets in the skin such as hemoglobin, melanin, and water were chromophores that had a defined light absorption spectrum. Selective damage of a target could be achieved by choosing a laser wavelength that was maximally absorbed by the chromophore of which the target consisted. The damage could be confined to that target by limiting the pulse duration to less than the thermal relaxation time of the cutaneous chromophore. The thermal relaxation time is the time that it takes for the target tissue to lose 50% of its incident heat without conducting heat to the surrounding tissue. In this way, selective non-scarring surgery could be performed on targeted tissue without damage to surrounding structures.

PHOTOREACTIONS INVOLVED IN LASER TATTOO TREATMENT

The mechanism of laser tattoo removal has been analyzed and studied extensively.

Clinically this is accomplished through the use of Q-switched lasers. Q-switched lasers store large amounts of energy in their optical cavity through the use of an optical shutter. When the laser is fired, it releases high-powered pulses of extremely short duration, in the nanosecond range,[50] resulting in a photomechanical tissue reaction.

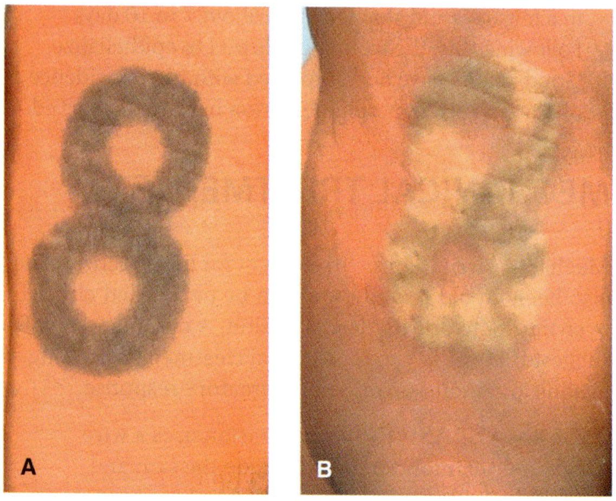

Figure 50-1 A. Tattoo pre-laser treatment. **B.** The appropriate clinical endpoint of whitening for laser tattoo removal is seen.

Photomechanical effects rely on the generation of plasma, a process called optical breakdown, followed by shock wave generation, cavitation, and if the reaction occurs near a solid boundary, jet formation.[51] The end result is the desired clinical end point of tissue whitening over the tattoo (Fig. 50-1).

MECHANISM OF TATTOO LIGHTENING/TATTOO ELIMINATION

The process of tattoo lightening or in some cases tattoo clearance after treatment with Q-switched lasers is not yet fully understood. In a sense, laser tattoo removal is actually a misnomer as it appears that the tattoo ink is not completely removed from the body.[52] Furthermore, complete clinical clearance cannot always be achieved.

Possible mechanisms for tattoo lightening may include:

a. Redistribution of ink particles to the lymphatic system.
b. External transdermal elimination.
c. Alteration of the optical properties of the tattoo to make it less visibly apparent.

Clinically and histologically, the first of these appears to be the dominant mechanism.

TYPES OF LASERS CURRENTLY USED FOR TATTOO REMOVAL

Tattoo pigment particles vary from less than 10 to 100 nm in diameter.[14] These very small structures (particles) require very rapid heating, and the laser pulse duration must be shorter (nanosecond or picosecond range) than the thermal relaxation time of the target pigment particles to selectively destroy them. Clinically, this is accomplished through the use of Q-switched lasers. Tattoo removal by Q-switched lasers is the current gold standard for unwanted tattoos.[53,54] However, complete clearance is not always possible and there is no guarantee that the skin will appear normal after treatment. Clinical efficacy depends on the type of tattoo, the depth and density of the

TABLE 50-1
Possible Adverse Events

Adverse Event	Possible Reason/Reasons
Darkening	Pure chemical transformation or laser-induced reduction of metallic compounds such as ferric oxide and titanium oxide
Allergy	Mercuric sulfide is considered to be the most common cause, which may trigger an immediate or delayed, localized or systemic allergic reaction
Chrysiasis	Q-switched laser can induce structural alteration of the gold deposits, leading to blue-gray discoloration within the treated area
Hypopigmentation	Partially a wavelength-dependent phenomenon. Increased melanin absorption with shorter wavelength
Hyperpigmentation	Mostly related to patients' skin type. Darker skin types are more prone, no matter which wavelength is used
Scarring	Retattooing, high density of pigment, strong absorption of energy. Higher fluences produce intense heat, causing damage to the surrounding dermis
Textural changes	Mostly transient. These changes have been noted with excessive fluences, re-tattooing, or multiple treatments
Pin-point bleeding	Higher fluences
Blistering	Higher fluences, darker skin types
Infection	Inadequate post-treatment care
Itching	Early sign of allergy or can be part of healing process

pigments injected in the dermis, and the chemical nature of the pigments used.[53,55,56] In addition, the operator's ability, clinical knowledge, and adequate training in laser device are factors that contribute to the outcome.[57]

Laser tattoo removal currently requires several sessions, usually at 4 to 6 week intervals. Because many tattoos are multicolored, they often necessitate treatment with multiple laser devices or a device that has multiple wavelength output (Table 50-1).

Currently, six wavelengths of Q-switched lasers for tattoo removal are available: the Q-switched ruby laser at 694 nm wavelength, the Q-switched alexandrite laser at 755 nm wavelength, the Q-switched Nd:YAG laser at 1064 nm wavelength, the Q-switched frequency-doubled Nd:YAG laser at 532 nm wavelength, the Q-switched dye laser at 585 nm wavelength, and the Q-switched Nd:YAG laser at 650 nm wavelength. These lasers are made by a variety of commercial entities.

a. **Q-SWITCHED RUBY 694 nm LASER:** Presently, the Q-switched ruby laser remains one of the most useful lasers in the treatment of amateur, professional, traumatic, and medical tattoos.

   A study by Taylor et al.[58] reported removal of amateur and professional tattoos using the Q-switched ruby laser, demonstrating substantial lightening or complete removal in 78% of amateur tattoos but only 23% of professional tattoos.

   Of 57 tattoos treated in this study, only one developed scarring.

   Scheibner et al.[59] published a study in which a Q-switched ruby laser was used to treat 163 tattoos, including 101 amateur and 62 professional tattoos. On average, three treatments were administered to each tattoo. In this study too, amateur tattoos responded well with complete removal in 4 cases, and almost complete removal in 84, with significant pigment removal in 11, and minimal removal in 2. Of the professional tattoos that were treated, 2 achieved complete removal, nearly complete removal was achieved in 5, 18 had significant removal, minimal removal was seen in 25, and little removal in 12. Professional tattoos that had yellow, red, or green pigments faded less than the black tattoos. No scarring was reported in any of the treated patients.

   Additional clinical studies[60] confirmed these pioneering clinical studies, showing substantial lightening and clearing of the amateur and improvement in the professional tattoos treated with Q-switched ruby lasers.

   Q-switched ruby lasers are quite effective at removing black and dark-blue tattoo pigments. However, Anderson et al. have shown that these lasers also effectively remove not only black pigment but also blue and green pigments.[61]

b. **Q-SWITCHED Nd:YAG 1064 nm LASER:** The Q-switched Nd:YAG laser was developed in 1989, and is a solid-state, high-fluence laser containing a crystal rod of yttrium-aluminum-garnet doped with 1% to 3% neodymium ions. The 1064 nm wavelength of light is invisible to the human eye. The laser emission can be doubled in frequency by placing a potassium-titanyl-phosphate (KTP) crystal inside the laser cavity and focusing the beam through the crystal, producing a green light at 532 nm.

   In addition, many Q-switched Nd:YAG lasers offer handpieces that contain a dye-impregnated polymer that converts 532 nm wavelength light to 585 nm or 650 nm light, thus enabling the variety of tattoo colors that we often see in today's multicolored tattoos to be targeted (Table 50-2).[62]

   Kilmer et al.[63] published their findings after treating 39 tattoos using the Q-switched Nd:YAG laser with

TABLE 50-2
Optimal Absorption Based on Pigment Color[62]

Dark Brown	Laser
Black/Dark blue	QS ruby (694 nm), QS alexandrite (755 nm), QS Nd:YAG (1064 nm)
Green	QS ruby (694 nm), QS alexandrite (755 nm)
Purple/Orange/Red/Yellow/Light brown/Tan	Frequency-doubled QS Nd:YAG (532 nm)

fluences ranging from 6 to 12 J/cm^2. In their study, greater than 75% removal of black pigment was accomplished in 77% of patients, and 90% clearance was noted in 28% of patients after four treatments. Colors other than black were removed less effectively in the study.

Greevelink and Anderson[64] showed that the Q-switched Nd:YAG laser with fluences of 6 J/cm^2 was as effective as the Q-switched ruby laser in removing black tattoo ink. It was associated with less blistering and pain, fewer textural changes, and no hypopigmentation. Although blue-black pigment responded well, green and red pigmentation did not show significant response to the Q-switched ND:YAG.

Jones et al.[65] reported on the treatment of 15 tattoos with the Q-switched Nd:YAG laser in patients with Fitzpatrick skin type VI. More than half the tattoos treated in this study were rated as being 75% to 95% improved after 3 to 4 treatments. Slight skin lightening was noted in only two patients in this study, and no scarring or textural changes were reported.

c. **Q-SWITCHED ALEXANDRITE 755 nm LASER:** In 1993, the Q-switched alexandrite laser was introduced for the treatment of tattoos. The alexandrite crystal emits energy at a wavelength of 755 nm, which is in the visible to near-infrared spectrum. This wavelength is longer than that of the Q-switched ruby laser and significantly shorter than that of the Nd:YAG laser at 1064 nm.

In a study published by Fitzpatrick et al.,[66] 25 patients with both amateur and professional tattoos were treated with a Q-switched alexandrite laser and reported 95% removal of tattoo pigment in an average of 8.9 treatment sessions. Temporary hypopigmentation was noted in 50% of patients, and 12% noted transient textural changes. The Q-switched alexandrite laser has been shown to be better than the Q-switched ruby and Q-switched Nd:YAG lasers in the removal of green tattoos.[67] Unfortunately, like the 694 nm wavelength of Q-switched ruby laser, the Q-switched Alexandrite laser's 755 nm wavelength is well absorbed by melanin, which results in hypopigmentation following treatment.[68]

COMPARISON BETWEEN THE THREE Q-SWITCHED LASERS

Comparative studies[67,68] for the effectiveness of these lasers have been published. However, because many companies make laser devices with identical wavelengths that may differ in spot size, pulse duration, and fluence ranges, comparative studies are difficult to perform and interpret.

Zelickson et al.,[67] using an animal model, studied the clinical, histopathologic, and ultrastructural effects of the three types of Q-switched lasers (Q-switched ruby, Q-switched alexandrite, and Q-switched Nd:YAG). According to the study, red-brown, dark-brown, and orange pigments responded best to the Nd:YAG laser, whereas the Q-switched alexandrite laser was most effective for removing blue and green pigments, and the Q-switched ruby laser was more effective for removing purple and violet pigments. The 532 nm wavelength of the frequency-doubled, Q-switched Nd:YAG laser was considered best for removing red pigment. All of these lasers were found to be relatively equivalent for removing black tattoo pigment.

LASER TATTOO TREATMENT

a. **INITIAL PATIENT CONSULTATION**: The initial patient consultation/evaluation is important for both the physician and patient. The patient should leave the consultation with realistic expectations, mindful of possible adverse outcomes (Table 50-2), a realistic expectation of the range in number of treatments required, an awareness of the limitations of treatment, as well as the treatment cost. The consultation allows the physician to identify those patients who have unrealistic expectations, who will be non-compliant or who may be at a risk for an adverse event.

Unfortunately, while tattoos are far more difficult to remove than they are to acquire, there is a common misconception that lasers can easily remove tattoos, which is driven in part by the media, advertisements, wishful thinking and the proliferation of medical spas and laser tattoo removal shops with untrained and uninformed practitioners.

Following the consultation, the patient should understand that multiple treatments will be required and that complete clearance cannot be guaranteed. Often it takes 6 to 15 treatments or even more to remove the tattoo depending on the tattoo color(s), age, location, patient's skin type, and mechanism of placement (Fig. 50-2). Treatments are usually performed at 4 to 6 week intervals, so patients are looking at a commitment of 6 months to 1 to 2 years or more to complete treatment. Patients should also be

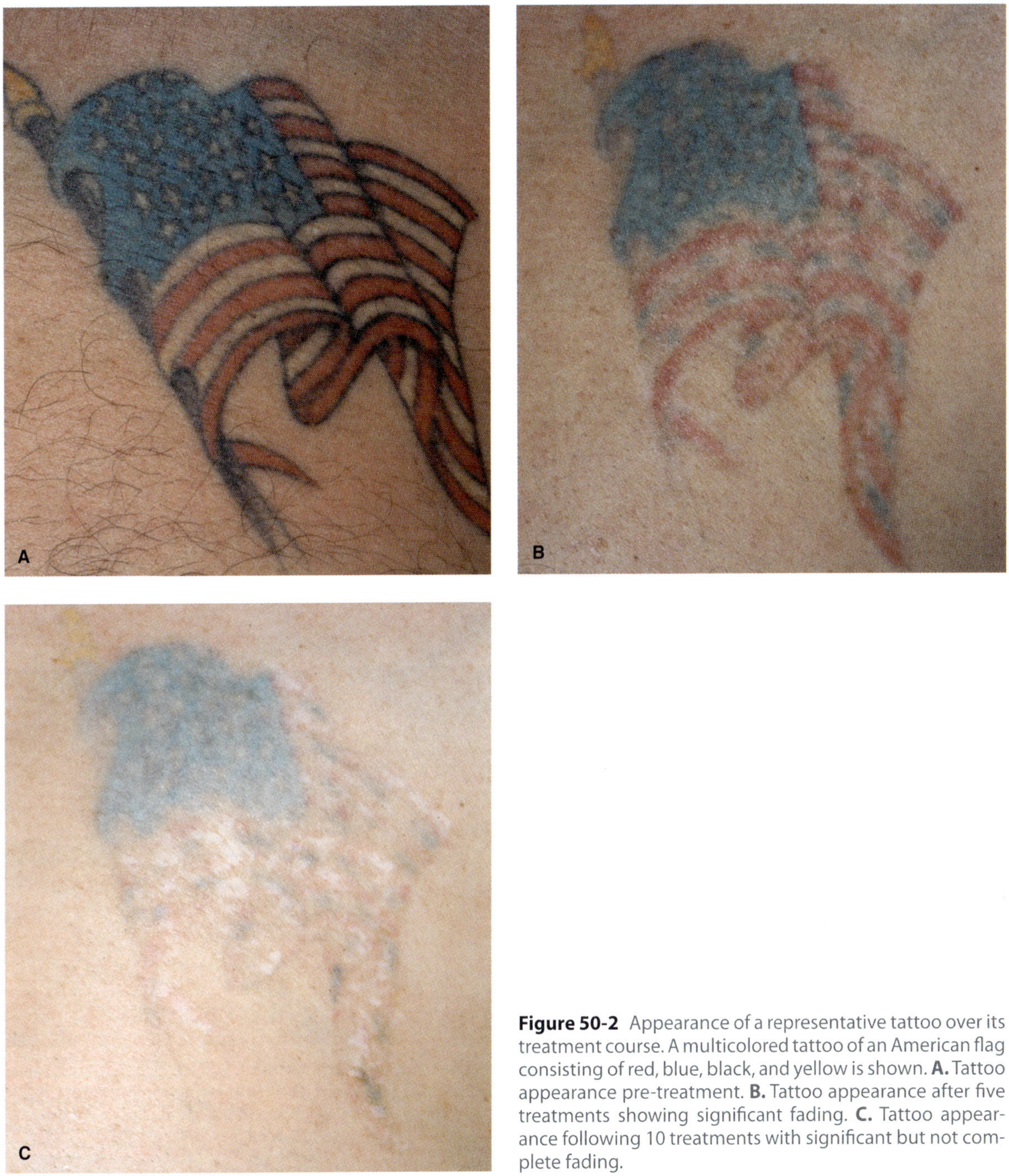

Figure 50-2 Appearance of a representative tattoo over its treatment course. A multicolored tattoo of an American flag consisting of red, blue, black, and yellow is shown. **A.** Tattoo appearance pre-treatment. **B.** Tattoo appearance after five treatments showing significant fading. **C.** Tattoo appearance following 10 treatments with significant but not complete fading.

advised that if they think they will be unsatisfied with only partial removal of their tattoo, they should not pursue treatment.

A focused medical history including medication history, information regarding wound healing and scarring tendencies and history of infectious diseases is important. Importantly, patients who have received gold salts for diseases such as rheumatoid arthritis, should be approached with caution, as laser-induced chrysiasis has been reported in individuals with a history of gold salt use after treatment with Q-switched lasers.[69,70] Chrysiasis is a characteristic blue-black discoloration of the skin that is very difficult to treat. Laser treatment in individuals who have taken isotretinoin therapy in the previous 6 months is controversial because there have been reports of keloid formation in these patients after laser treatment,[71] although there is increasing evidence that these individuals may not have a higher incidence of scarring.[72] In addition, the importance of avoiding excessive sun exposure both before and after treatment should be emphasized, as this raises the likelihood of dyspigmentation, which has the potential to be permanent (Fig. 50-3).

Written information regarding the procedure is useful and should be given to the patient pre-operatively. Photographic documentation and

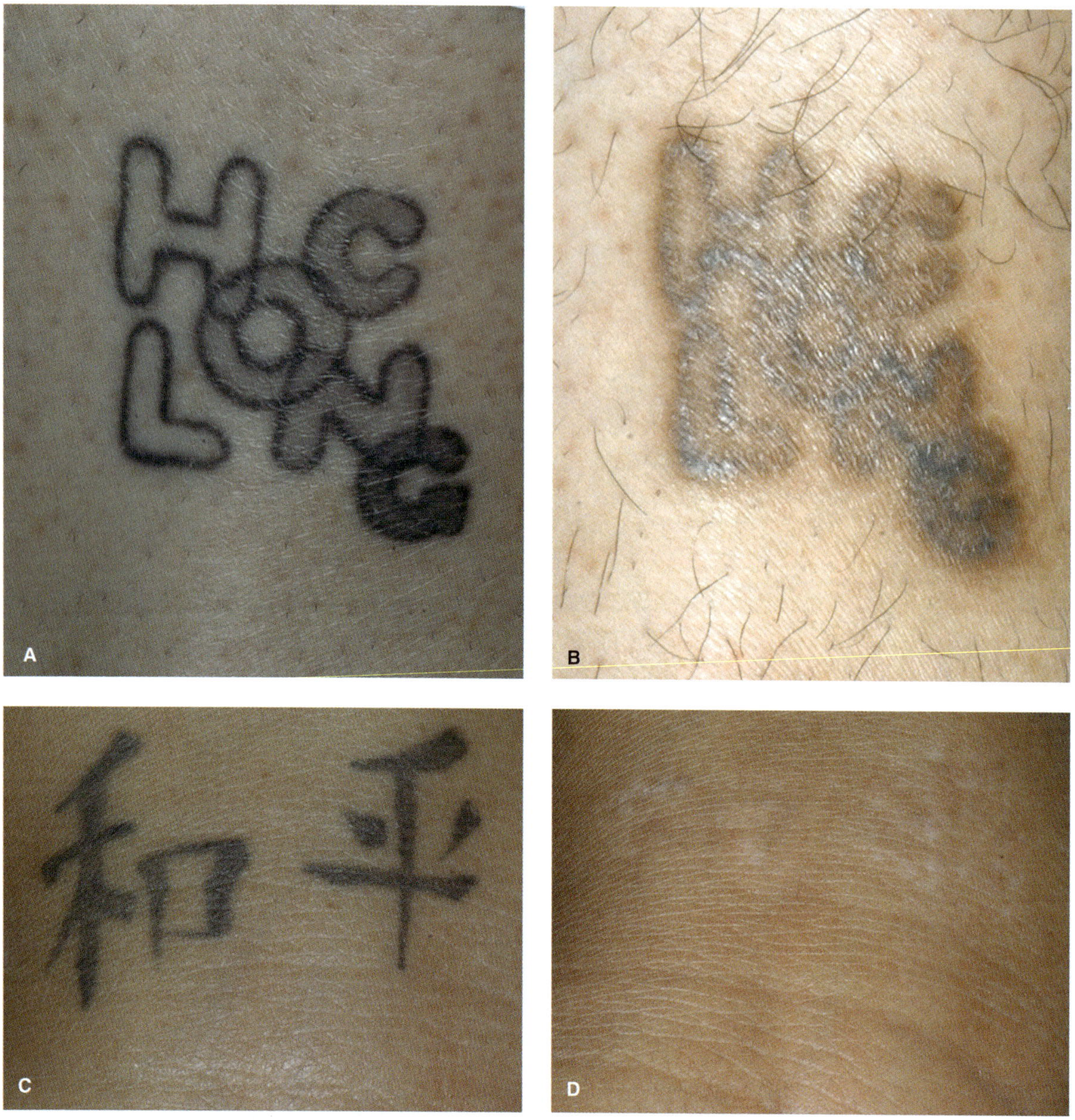

Figure 50-3 Examples of dyspigmentation with laser tattoo removal. **A.** Pre-laser treatment. **B.** Post-laser hyperpigmentation following treatment with a QS Nd:YAG 1064 nm laser. **C.** Pre-laser treatment. **D.** Post-laser hypopigmentation following treatment with a QS Nd:YAG 1064 nm laser.

written informed consent should be obtained prior to the treatment. Inspection and documentation of pre-existing pigment disturbances, prior tattoos, textural changes, or scarring is important.

Observation of various colors in the tattoo/tattoos is important not only to plan treatment but also to anticipate the possibility of ink darkening on exposure to Q-switched laser irradiation for tattoos containing iron or titanium dioxide particles (Fig. 50-4). Furthermore, tattoos placed over prior existing tattoos should be treated at lower fluences in order to avoid a higher potential for scar due to the abundance of tattoo ink particles.

b. **TREATMENT PEARLS:** Before commencing treatment, safety protocols should be cross-checked in the procedure room. Every person in the procedure room should wear protective eye-glasses that are specific for the laser wavelength being used. The patient should be provided with protective eyewear or intraocular shields, if needed.

The treatment site should be kept dry after proper cleansing to remove any make-up, lotions, or creams. Topical or intralesional anesthesia may be necessary to minimize the sharp needle-like pricking sensation felt with Q-switched lasers. The most commonly used topical anesthetic compounds are EMLA cream (Astra Pharmaceuticals, Westborough, MA), a eutectic mixture of lidocaine 2.5% and prilocaine 2.5%, within an oil-in-water emulsion, Ela-Max (Ferndale Laboratories, Ferndale, MI), a lidocaine-containing liposomal cream, and LMX-5 (Ferndale Laboratories, Ferndale, MI) a 5% lidocaine cream.[73,74]

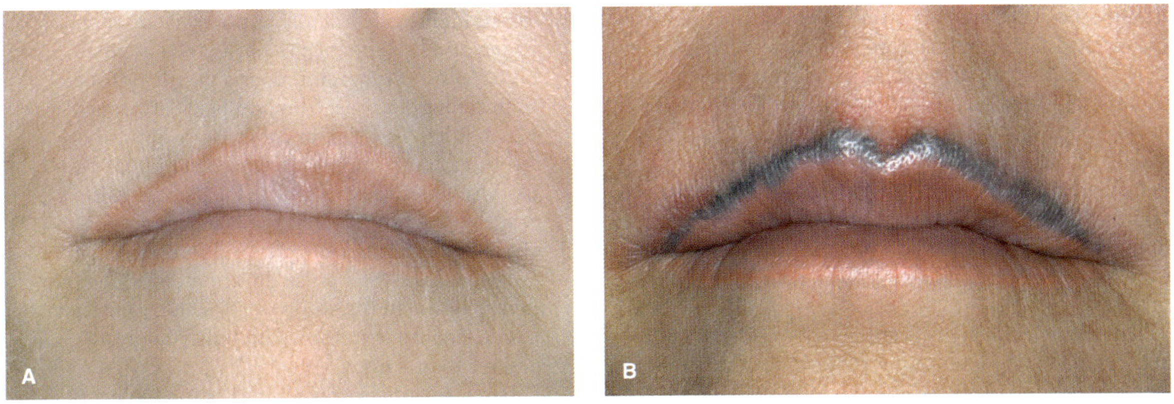

Figure 50-4 **A.** Red lip liner tattoo pre-laser treatment. **B.** Ink darkening of the upper vermilion border post-laser treatment

The topical anesthetic creams are often applied under occlusion for 30 to 60 minutes before laser irradiation. For intralesional anesthesia, local infiltration of 1% to 2% lidocaine with or without epinephrine is generally used.

Removal of different colors within tattoos can theoretically be accomplished when lasers are used in accordance with the absorption spectra of their pigments. This, however, is complicated in clinical practice.

Each of the available Q-switched lasers has its benefits and determining the appropriate laser for a given patient depends upon the type and color of tattoo (Table 50-1) and the patient's Fitzpatrick skin type. The longer wavelength of Q-switched Nd:YAG laser (1064 nm) interacts less with epidermal melanin and is preferable for use in darker skin–type individuals. It is always prudent to perform a test spot, particularly if the tattoo to be removed is on the face or another cosmetically sensitive area or when a tattoo pigment is suspected of containing ferric oxide or titanium dioxide. An immediate ash-white color at the site of impact will resolve in 20 minutes.[58] This should be considered a treatment endpoint known as "tissue whitening" (Fig. 50-1). If it is not observed, it is likely that the laser exposure fluence is not sufficient or that an ineffective wavelength was used. Some pinpoint bleeding may also be observed, which is acceptable. Before completing the treatment, the test spot should be carefully observed for an immediate paradoxical darkening reaction.

Tissue and blood can splatter and be aerosolized during tattoo removal, and thus protective garb covering the eyes and mucosal surfaces of the laser surgeon and staff is recommended.[61] Tissue splatter occurs because of rapid heating of the skin surface and generation of shock waves due to very short pulses and high peak powers delivered by Q-switched lasers.

The fluences chosen depend on the laser used and are also based on the physician operator's clinical observation during the initial laser pulses or the test spot. Tissue observation during Q-switched laser impact shows immediate whitening of the tissue, with at most pinpoint bleeding. Whitening of the tissue is due to the formation of gas as water is vaporized by heating. Tissue loss or excessive bleeding is not required to obtain a satisfactory response. If they occur, pigmentation disturbances or textural changes may result.

The greater the amount of tattoo ink present, the more impressive the clinical response and the less energy required to achieve a proper tissue response during therapy.

c. **POST-TREATMENT**: Appropriate post-treatment wound care is critical to optimize good cosmetic results. After completion of laser treatment, a non-stick dressing (Telfa, Kendall Medical Device Co., Mansfield, MA) with an occlusive ointment that does not contain antibiotics, such as Aquaphor ointment (Beiersdorf Inc., Wilton, CT), is recommended. In the absence of Aquaphor ointment, simple hydrated petrolatum can be used.

Often large blisters can occur, especially when the tattoo is treated with the relatively short wavelength ruby laser or higher fluences. Patients should avoid breaking the blisters, if possible. If they are uncomfortable, they should be lanced in the office with sterile or clean technique. The patient should expect the area to develop crusting and scabbing that will last for 7 to 10 days after treatment.

Free pigments will be intracellular again at approximately 4 weeks after treatment, so subsequent treatments should be scheduled at 4 to 6 week intervals[56] to maximize the removal of tattoo ink particles by macrophages.[75] Patients should avoid sun exposure during the treatment period and for at least a month before and after treatment (longer for higher Fitzpatrick skin types), to minimize post-inflammatory hyperpigmentation.

LASER TREATMENT OF TRAUMATIC TATTOOS

Treatment of traumatic tattoos is essentially similar to that of amateur and professional tattoos. Most often, tattoos containing carbon and graphite have been shown to respond well to treatment with Q-switched lasers.[76–78]

If tattoo particles are very large, the ultrashort pulses of Q-switched lasers may not be able to treat them effectively. In this situation, an ablative laser may be an option to remove large embedded particles.[79,80] Additionally, if the origin of the traumatic tattoo is unclear, a biopsy should be considered.

If traumatic tattoos are the result of explosive accidents, treatments should be approached with caution, because fragments of gunpowder or firework may ignite upon exposure to nanosecond laser pulses, potentially resulting in explosions.[81,82]

Traumatic tattoos typically respond more quickly and completely to laser tattoo removal than professional tattoos.

TREATMENT OF MEDICAL TATTOOS

Medical tattooing is commonly used by radiation oncologists to localize areas of treatment. India ink is commonly used in most instances, which can be successfully treated by any of the available Q-switched lasers.[60] They respond quickly and completely to laser tattoo removal. Prior to removal, communication with the patient's radiation oncologist is recommended.

TREATMENT OF TATTOO ALLERGIES

Treatment of allergic tattoo reactions is challenging. Simple surgical excision can be the treatment of choice for small allergic reactions. One study[83] found that frequency-doubled, Q-switched Nd:YAG laser (532 nm) is effective in patients with allergic reactions, particularly to the red pigment. Importantly, allergic precautions should be implemented prior to any Q-switched laser treatment in order to avoid a systemic allergic reaction.

The authors have recently described the treatment of tattoo allergy successfully treated with ablative fractional resurfacing.[84]

COMPLICATIONS ASSOCIATED WITH LASER TATTOO TREATMENTS

a. **PIGMENT DARKENING:** Following treatment with Q-switched lasers, pigment darkening can occur in certain tattoos, primarily cosmetic tattoos. (Fig. 50-4). The mechanism is not completely understood, but laser-induced reduction of metallic compounds used in carbon dyes may result in immediate or progressive darkening. Tattoos containing ferric oxide, a brown-red ingredient widely used in red, pink, and flesh-colored tattoos, have been reputed to result in a black discoloration upon treatment with Q-switched lasers. The mechanism is thought to involve the reduction of ferric oxide to ferrous oxide, which is jet black in color.[85]

   Titanium dioxide is another potential offender, widely used to enhance the brilliance of green, blue, yellow, flesh-colored, and purple tattoos.[86,87] In untreated tattoos, titanium is in TiO_2 form, which is bright white in color. High-intensity laser irradiation results in the reduction of Ti_4+ to Ti_3+, which is responsible for its blue color.[88,89] A study[90] has shown that the laser-induced changes in titanium dioxide and ferrous oxide are wavelength and pulse duration dependent. Investigators of the study were unable to induce ink darkening in tattoos with pulse durations greater than 1 ms.

   Laser-treatment of darkened tattoo pigment must be approached with extreme caution. This generally but not always can be removed with successive treatments.[67]

   It is, therefore, highly advisable to perform a test spot when dye within a tattoo is suspected of containing ferric oxide or titanium dioxide, especially when treating permanent make-up.

b. **POST-LASER TREATMENT ALLERGIC REACTIONS TO TATTOO PIGMENT AND TRANSIENT IMMUNOREACTIVITY:** Metal salts used in tattoo pigments can cause allergic, granulomatous, lichenoid, photoallergic, and pruritic reactions. Red ink containing mercuric sulfide (cinnabar) is the most common cause of allergic reactions. However, these reactions are also well-documented to cadmium sulfide, chromium sulfate, and cobalt manganese present in different tattoos.[91]

   It may be because of the antigenic properties of red and yellow tattoo pigments that they are noticed more by the immune system and often fade more quickly than other tattoo pigments in patients who do not experience an allergic reaction.[28]

   Additionally, some patients may experience transient immunoreactivity following laser tattoo removal treatment.[92] Symptoms may include lymphadenopathy, which may be mistaken for cellulitis by those unaware of this phenomenon.[93–98]

c. **PIGMENTARY CHANGES:** Despite Q-switched lasers' ability to target tattoo ink precisely, epidermal melanin pigment is often a competing chromophore during laser treatment. As a result, some transient or permanent pigmentary changes, either hypopigmentation or hyperpopigmentation, are not uncommon (Fig. 50-3). These changes are partially a wavelength-dependent phenomenon. Q-switched ruby laser at 694 nm wavelength; frequency-doubled, Q-switched Nd:YAG laser at 532 nm wavelength; and Q-switched alexandrite laser at 755 nm wavelength are strongly absorbed by melanin and, therefore, cause injury to pigmented cells including melanocytes. Permanent hypopigmentation can be seen with repetitive treatment sessions, particularly at higher fluences. Often, much of the hypopigmentation improves over a period of 1 to 2 years.

   Q-switched laser-induced transient hyperpigmentation has been reported in up to 15% of cases, and is more common in darker-skinned or suntanned individuals.

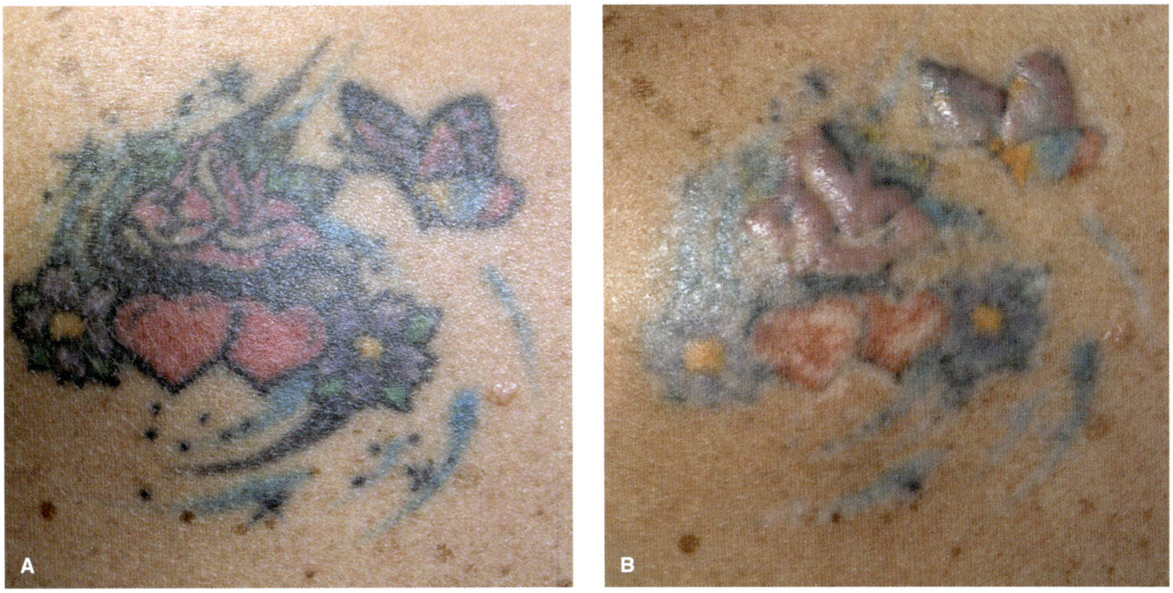

Figure 50-5 **A.** Tattoo prior to laser treatment. **B.** Patchy hypertrophic scar formation post-laser treatment

Hyperpigmentation can be caused by deposition of either melanin or hemosiderin.

Animal studies[99,100] in Q-switched laser–induced epidermal hyperpigmentation have suggested that melanocyte stimulation leading to transiently increased melanin formation occurs.

d. **TEXTURAL CHANGES:** Textural changes or scarring are not common after treatment with Q-switched lasers (Fig. 50-5). The incidence of scarring is less than 0.5% .[101] Microscopically, the absence of disruption or necrosis of collagen suggests that vacuolation causes reversible collagen deformation without significantly altering its dermal architecture.

However, transient textural changes such as fine cigarette paper-like wrinkling, mild erythema or a waxy, shiny surface, as well as hypertrophic and atrophic scarring have been noted, when excessive fluences are used. The use of excessive fluences cause the epidermis to absorb a greater amount of energy, which may result in blistering, skin sloughing, and a higher likelihood of scarring.

Scarring or textural changes may also be associated with the original placement of tattoos, very strong absorption of laser energy by high-density pigments in "double tattoos," or with the healing response seen after multiple treatments.[75,102]

To reduce the risk of textural changes or scarring, areas that are known to be prone to hypertrophic scars, such as the chest, neck, upper back, arms, and ankles, should be treated with lower fluences.

Larger laser handpiece spot sizes tend to minimize epidermal damage, penetrate more deeply into the dermis, and are associated with fewer textural changes.[103]

e. **PRURITUS:** Twenty-five percent of Q-switched laser treated patients complain of pruritus. It is significant during the healing phase and usually resolves within 2 to 3 days of its onset. Topical corticosteroids may be helpful to avoid excessive scratching and subsequently minimize local trauma.[67,104]

PEARLS

a. Patients undergoing laser therapy for tattoo removal should not have a tan at the time of treatment. If any significant tan is present, treatment should be postponed, since these patients will have a much higher risk of post-operative hyperpigmentation because of stimulation of their melanocytes. A bleaching cream may be prescribed to hasten the resolution of the suntan.
b. Q-switched lasers are the current treatment of choice for all types of tattoos. The use of continuous or long-pulsed lasers or intense pulsed light (IPL) systems is contraindicated as a pulse duration in milliseconds or longer is associated with a high risk of scarring.[105]
c. The lowest fluences required to invoke the tissue whitening response should be used. Although higher fluences may clear tattoos more effectively,[62] they may also be associated with a higher incidence of adverse events.
d. Patients with darker skin types have a higher risk of pigmentary alteration and possible scarring. For these patients, longer wavelength lasers, such as the Q-switched Nd:YAG laser (1064 nm), may be more appropriate because of their decreased interference with melanin.[106]
e. Selection of proper spot size or beam diameter is important. It is better to use the largest spot size that elicits a clinically relevant tissue whitening response. Larger spot size results in decreased peripheral scatter; subsequently a higher percentage of energy is delivered to the target.
f. Increasing the laser fluence by reducing the spot size is a mistake and should be avoided, as it results in the deposition of maximum total beam energy in the

upper layer of the skin, resulting in potential scarring.

g. When treating a tattoo with colors that may darken, a single laser pulse test spot should be placed to asses for immediate darkening. The test area is best visualized after the initial whitening clears. If darkening is not observed, the treatment may be continued. If darkening is observed, the same test area should be retreated, to reobserve it after a few weeks for its lightening, before completing the treatment.

FUTURE DIRECTIONS

Despite the tremendous advances which Q-switched lasers provide in the treatment of unwanted tattoos, there is still considerable room for improvement in terms of enhancing the efficacy of laser tattoo removal. Recent advances in the treatment of unwanted tattoos include a study by Kossida et al.,[107] in which the authors found that repeated treatments at 20 minute intervals for a total of four treatments in the same day led to enhanced clearance of tattoos. Additionally, Ibrahimi et al.[84] found that the use of ablative fractional resurfacing resulted in the ability to remove ink particles faster and even provided the ability to treat colors that are resistant to commercially available Q-switched laser wavelengths. Finally, the most promising advance in the treatment of tattoos is the development of picosecond laser technology. Picosecond lasers have a pulse duration that is shorter than that of the current nanosecond lasers and thereby have the potential to more accurately target the smaller tattoo ink particles than nanosecond lasers. The Wellman Center for Photomedicine at Massachusetts General Hospital pioneered the use of picosecond lasers for tattoo treatment over 14 years ago. Ross et al.[14] reported the first data on a picosecond laser for tattoo removal in 1988 and demonstrated the superiority of picosecond laser pulses over nanosecond laser pulses. Unfortunately, the availability of these devices was hampered by an inability to produce a commercially viable and stable version of a picosecond laser. Recently, Izikson et al.[108] demonstrated the safety and effectiveness of an initial commercial model of a picosecond laser that has been followed with small pilot trials showing enhanced clearance of tattoo ink particles. Further study will elucidate the promising potential of this technology.

REFERENCES

1. Gilbert S. *Tattoos History: A source Book.* New York, NY: Juno Books; 2000.
2. Lineberry C. *Tattoos, Smithsonian.* 2007. http://www.smithsonianmag.com/history-archeology/tattoo.html. Accessed April 27, 2012.
3. Scutt RWB, Gotch C. *Art, Sex and Symbol.* London: Cornwall Books; 1985.
4. Goldstein N, Sewall M. III. Tattoos in different cultures. *J Dermatol Surg Oncol.* 1979;5(11):857–864.
5. Laumann A, Derick A. Tattoo and body piercing in the United States: A national data set. *J Am Acad Dermatol.* 2006;55(3):413–421.
6. Armstrong M, Roberets A, Owen D. Contemporary college students and body piercing. *J Adolesc Health.* 2004;35(1):58–61.
7. Berchon E. *Histoire Medicale Du Tatuage.* Paris: Baillière; 1869:454–455.
8. Timko AL, Miller CH, Ross EV. In vitro quantitative chemical analysis of tattoo pigments. *Arch Dermatol.* 2001;137:143–147.
9. Baumler W, Eibler ET, Hohenleutner U. Q-switched laser and tattoo pigments: First results of the chemical and photophysical analysis of 41 compounds. *Laser Surg Med.* 2000;26:13–21.
10. Vasold R, Naarmann N, Ultrich H, et al. Tattoo pigments are cleaved by laser light—the chemical analysis in vitro provides evidence for hazardous compounds. *Photochem Photobiol.* 2004;80(2):185–190.
11. Suchin KR, Greenbaum SS. Successful treatment of a cosmetic tattoo using a combination of lasers. *Dermatol Surg.* 2004;30:105–107.
12. Amazon K, Robinson MJ, Rywlin AM. Ferrugination caused by Monsel's solution. Clinical observations and experimentations. *Am J Dermatopathol.* 1980;2:197–205.
13. Ferguson JE, Andrew SM, Jones CJ. The Q-switched neodymium: YAG laser and tattoos: A microscopic analysis of laser-tattoo interactions. *Br J Dermatol.* 1997;137:405–410.
14. Ross EV, Naseef G, Lin G, et al. Comparison of responses of tattoos to picoseconds and nanosecond Q-switched neodymium: YAG lasers. *Arch Dermatol.* 1998;134:167–171.
15. Tierney EP, Golgberg DJ. Laser hair removal pearls. *J Cosmet Laser Ther.* 2008;10:17–23.
16. Wohlrab S, Stahl J, Kappeler PM. Modifying the body: Motivation for getting tattooed and pierced. *Body Image.* 2007;4:87–95.
17. Harris Interactive Inc. Three in ten Americans with a tattoo say having one makes them feel sexier. 2009. http://www.harrisinteractive.com/harris_poll/index.asp?PID=868. Accessed May 24, 2010.
18. Verma S, Lanigan SW. Reasons for requesting laser removal of unwanted tattoos. *Br J Dermatol.* 1999;140:483–485.
19. Manchester G. Tattoo removal. A new simple technique. *Calif Med.* 1973;118(3):10–12.
20. Boo-Chai K. The decorative tattoo—its removal by dermabrasion. *Plast Reconstr Surg.* 1963;32:559–563.
21. Clabauch W. Removal of tattoos by superficial dermabrasion. *Arch Dermatol.* 1968;98:515–521.
22. Crittenden FM. Salabrasion—removal of tattoos by superficial abrasion with table salt. *Cutis.* 1971;7:295–300.
23. Manchester GH. The removal of commercial tattoos by abrasion with table salts. *Plast reconstr.* 1974;53:517–521.
24. Strong AM, Jackson JT. The removal of amateur tattoos by salabrasion. *Br J Dermatol.* 1979;101:693–696.
25. Apfelberg DB, Manchester GH. Decorative and traumatic tattoo biophysics and removal. *Clin Plast Surg.* 1987;14(2):243–251.
26. Roenig HH Jr. Tattooing—history, techniques, complications, removal. *Clev Clin Q.* 1971;38:179–186.
27. Scutt RWB. The chemical removal of tattoos. *Br J Plast Surg.* 1972;25:189–194.
28. Bernstein EF. Laser tattoo removal. *Semin Plast Surg.* 2007;21:175–192.
29. Alster T, Apfelberg D. *Cosmetic Laser Surgery.* New York, NY: Wiley-Liss; 1996.
30. Johannesson A. A simplified method of focal salabrasion for removal of linear tattoos. *J Dermatol Surg Oncol.* 1985;11:1004–1005.
31. Goldmn MP, Fitzpatrick RE. *Cutaneous Laser Therapy: The Aret and Science of Selective Photothermolysis.* St. Louis, MO: Mosby-Year Book; 1994.
32. Groot DW, Arlette JP, Johnston PA. Comparison of the infrared and the carbon dioxide laser in the removal of decorative tattoos. *J Am Acad Dermatol.* 1986;15:518–522.
33. Colver GB, Cherry GW, Dawber RP, Ryan TJ. Tattoo removal using infrared coagulation. *Br J Dermatol.* 1985;112:481–485.
34. Venning VA, Clover GB, Millard PR, Ryan TJ. Tattoo removal using infrared coagulation: A dose comparison. *Br J Dermatol.* 1987;117:99–105.
35. Leopold PJ. Cryosurgery for facial skin lesions. *Proc R SOC Med.* 1975;68:606–608.

36. Zacarian SA. Cryosurgery for cutaneous carcinoma. *Dermatol Dig.* 1970;9:49–56.
37. Goldstein N, Penoff J, Price N, et al. Techniques of removal of tattoos. *J Dermatol Surg Oncol.* 1979;5:901–910.
38. Morgan BD. Tattoos. *BMJ.* 1974;3:34–36.
39. Gupta SC. An investigation into a method for the removal of dermal tattoos: Aa report on animals and clinical studies. *Plast Reconstr Surg.* 1965;36:354–361.
40. Maimann TH. Stimulated optical stimulation in ruby. *Nature.* 1960;187:493–494.
41. Goldman L, Blaney DJ, Kindel DJ Jr, Franke EK. Effect of the laser beam on the skin. *J Invest Dermatol.* 1963;40:121–123.
42. Goldman L, Rockwell RJ, Meyer R, Otten R, Wilson RG, Kitzmiller KW. Laser treatment of tattoos: A preliminary survey of three years clinical experience. *JAMA.* 1967;201: 841–844.
43. Brady SC, Blockmanis A, Jewett L. Tattoo removal with the carbon dioxide laser. *Ann Plast Surg.* 1978;2:482–490.
44. McBurney EI. Carbon dioxide laser treatment of dermatologic lesions. *South Med J.* 1978;71:795–797.
45. Reid R, Muller S. Tattoo removal by CO_2 laser dermabrasion. *Plast Recosntr Surg.* 1980;65:717–728.
46. Kent KM, Graber EM. Laser tattoo removal: A review. *Dermatol Surg.* 2012;38:1–13.
47. Dvir E, Hirshowitz B. Tattoo removal by cryosurgery. *Plast Reconstr Surg.* 1980;66:373–379.
48. Apfelberg D, Maser M, Lash H. Argon laser treatment of decorative tattoos. *Br J Plast Surg.* 1979;32(2):141–144.
49. Anderson RR, Parrish JA. Selective photothermolysis: precise microsurgery by selective absorption of pulsed radiation. *Science.* 1983;220(4596):524–527.
50. Graber E, Iyengar V, Rohrer T, Arndt K. Laser treatment of tattoos and pigmented lesions. In: Robinson JK, Hanke CW, Siegel DM, Fratila A, eds. *Surgery of the Skin: Procedural Dermatology.* 2nd ed. China: Mosby; 2010:537–548.
51. Neimz M. *Laser-Tissue Interactions: Fundamentals and Applications.* 3rd ed. Berlin: Springer; 2007.
52. Anderson RR. Tattoos. In: Arndt KA, Dover JS, eds. *Controversies & Conversations in Cutaneous Laser Surgery.* Chicago, IL: AMA Press; 2002:317–318.
53. Adatto MA. Laser tattoo removal: Benefits and caveats. *Med Laser Appl.* 2004;19:175–185.
54. Bernstein FF. Laser treatment of tattoos. *Clin Dermatol.* 2006;24:43–55.
55. Vasold R, Engel E, Konig B, Landthaler M, Bäumler W. Health risks of tattoo colors. *Anal Bioanal Chem.* 2008;391:9–13.
56. Pfirmann G, Karsai S, Roos S, Hammes S, Raulin C. Tattoo removal—state of the art. *J Dtsch Dermatol Ges.* 2007;5: 889–897.
57. Karsai S, Krieger G, Raulin C. Tattoo removal by non-professionals—medical and forensic considerations. *J Eur Acad Dermatol Venereol.* 2010;24:756–762.
58. Taylor CR, Gange RW, Dover JS, et al. Treatment of tattoos by Q-switched ruby laser. A dose response study. *Arch Dermatol.* 1990;126:893–899.
59. Sheibner A, Kenny G, White W, et al. A superior method of tattoos removal using the Q-switched ruby laser. *J Dermatol Surg Oncol.* 1990;16:1091–1098.
60. Ashinoff R, Geronemus RG. Rapid response of traumatic and medical tattoos to treatment with the Q-switched ruby laser. *Plast Reconstr Surg.* 1993;91:841–845.
61. Kilmer SL, Anderson RR. Clinical use of the Q-switched Nd:YAG (1064 nm and 532 nm) lasers for treatment of tattoos. *J Dermatol Surg Oncol.* 1993;19:330–338.
62. Hodersdal M, Bech-Thomsen N, Wulf HC. Skin reflectance-guided laser selections for treatment of decorative tattoos. *Arch Dermatol.* 1996;132:403–407.
63. Kilmer SL, Lee MS, Grevelink JM, Flotte TJ, Anderson RR. The Q-switched Nd:YAG laser effectively treats tattoos. A controlled, dose response study. *Arch Dermatol.* 1993;129: 971–978.
64. Grevelink JM, Duke D, van Leeuwen RL, Gonzalez E, DeCoste S, Anderson RR. Laser treatment of tattoos in darkly pigmented patients: Efficacy and side effects. *J Am Acad Dermatol.* 1996;34(4):653–656.
65. Jones A, Roddey P, Orengo I, Rosen T. The Q-switched Nd:YAG laser effectively treats tattoos in darkly pigmented skin. *Dermatol Surg.* 1996;22:999–1001.
66. Fitzpatrick RE, Goldman MP. Tattoo removal using the Alexandrite laser. *Arch Dermatol.* 1994;130:1508–1514.
67. Zelickson B, Mehregan D, Zarrin A, et al. Clinical, histological, and ultrastructural evaluation of tattoos treated with three laser systems. *Lasers Surg Med.* 1994;15(4);364–372.
68. Leunberger M, Mulas M, Hata T, Goldman MP, Fitzpatrick RE, Grevelink JM. Comparison of the Q-switched alexandrite, Nd:YAG, and ruby lasers in treating blue-black tattoos. *Dermatol Surg.* 1999;25(1):10–14.
69. Yun P, Arndt KA, Anderson RR. Q-switched laser-induced chrysiasis treated with long-pulsed laser. *Arch Dermatol.* 2002;138(8):1012–1014.
70. Almoallium H, Klinkhoff A, Arthur A, Rivers JK, Chalmers A. Laser-induced chrysiasis: Disfiguring hyperpigmentation following Q-switched laser therapy in a woman previously treated with gold. *J Rheumatol.* 2006;33(3):620–621.
71. Bernstein L, Geronemus R. Keloid formation with the 585 nm pulsed dye laser during isotretinoin treatment. *Arch Dermatol.* 1997;133(1):111–112.
72. Alissa A. *Concomitant Use of Laser and Isotretinoin, How Safe.* Grapevine, TX: American Society for Laser Medicine and Surgery; 2011.
73. Friedman PM, Mafong EA, Friedman ES, Geronemus RG. Topical anesthetics update: EMLA and beyond. *Dermatol Surg.* 2001;27:1010–1018.
74. Ashinoff R, Geronemus RG. Effect of the topical anesthetic EMLA on the efficacy of the pulsed dye laser treatment of portwine stains. *J Dermatol Surg Oncol.* 1990;16:1008–1011.
75. Adatto MA. *Living Skin—Decorative Tattooing and Dermatology.* Basel: Editions Roche; 1993:84–86.
76. Moreno-Arias G, Casals-Andreu M, Camps-Fresneda A. Use of Q-switched alexandrite laser (755 nm, 100 nsec) for removal of traumatic tattoos of different origin. *Laser Surg Med.* 1999;25(5):445–450.
77. Bernstein L, Palaia DA, Bank D, Geronemus RG. Tattoo formation from absorbable synthetic suture and successful removal with Q-switched ruby laser. *Dermatol Surg.* 1996;22(12):1040–1042.
78. Miles B, Ellis E 3rd. The neodymium:YAG laser in the treatment of traumatic tattoo: A case report. *J Oral Maxillofac Surg.* 2006;64(5):850–855.
79. Kunzi-Rapp K, Krahn G, Wortmann S, Peter R. Early treatment of traumatic tattoo by erbium:YAG laser. *Br J Dermatol.* 2001;144(1):219–221.
80. Cambier B, Rogge F. Traumatic tattoos: Use of the variable pulsed erbium:YAG laser. *Photomed Laser Surg.*2006; 24(5):605–609.
81. Fusade T, Toubel G, Grognard C, Mazer JM. Treatment of gun-powder traumatic tattoo by Q-switched Nd:YAG laser: An unusual adverse effect. *Dermatol Surg.* 2000;26:1057–1059.
82. Taylor CR. Laser ignition of traumatically embedded firework debris. *Laser Surg Med.* 1998;22:157–158.
83. Antony FC, Harland CC. Red ink tattoo reactions: Successful treatment with the Q-switched 532 nm Nd:YAG laser. *Br J Dermatol.* 2003;149(1):94–98.
84. Ibrahimi OA, Syed Z, Sakamoto FH, Averam MM, Anderson RR. Treatment of tattoo allergy with ablative fractional resurfacing: A novel paradigm for tattoo removal. *J Am Acad Dermatol.* 2011;64:1111–1114.
85. Anderson RR, Geronemus RG, Kilmer SL, Ferinelli W, Fitzpatrick RE. Cosmetic tattoo ink darkening: A complication of Q-switched and pulsed laser treatment. *Arch Dermatol.* 1993;129:1010–1014.
86. Lehmann G, Pierchalla P. Tattooing dyes. [in German]. *Dermatosen Beruf Umwelt.* 1988;36:152–156.
87. Verma S, Swanson NA, Lee KK. Tattoo ink darkening of a yellow tattoo after Q-switched laser treatment. *Clin Exp Dermatol.* 2002;27:461–463.
88. Torimoto T, Fox R III, Fox M. Photoelectric electrochemical doping of TiO_2 particles and the effects of charged carrier density on the photocatalytic activity of microporous semiconductor electrode film. *J Electrochem Soc.* 1996;143:3712–3717.

89. Ross EV, Yashar S, Michaud N, et al. Tattoo darkening and non-response after laser treatment: A possible role for titanium dioxide. *Arch Dermatol.* 2001;137:33–37.
90. Tope W, Tsoukas M, Farinelli W, Anderson RR. Tattoo ink darkening: The effect of wavelength, fluence and pulse duration. *Lasers Surg Med.* 1994;15:364(abstract).
91. Jacob CI. Tattoo-associated dermatoses: A case report and review of the literature. *Dermatol Surg.* 2002;28: 962–965.
92. Ashinoff R, Levine VJ, Soter NA. Allergic reactions to tattoo pigment after laser treatment. *Dermatol Surg.* 1995;21: 291–294.
93. Izkison L, Avram M, Anderson RR. Transient immunoreactivity after laser tattoo removal: Report of two cases. *Lasers Surg Med.* 2008;40(4):231–232.
94. England RW, Vogal P, Hagan L. Immediate cutaneous hypersensitivity after treatment of tattoo with Nd:YAG laser: A case report and review of the literature. *Ann Allergy Asthma Immunol.* 2002;89:215–217.
95. Dave R, Mahaffey PJ. Successful treatment of an allergic reaction in a red tattoo with the Nd:YAG laser. *Br J Plast Surg.* 2002;55:456.
96. Kuperman-Beade M, Levine VJ, Ashinoff R. Laser removal of tattoos. *Am J Clin Dermatol.* 2001;2(1):21–25.
97. Jimenez G, Weiss E, Spencer JM. Multiple color changes following laser therapy of cosmetic tattoos. *Dermatol Surg.* 2002;28:177–179.
98. Nelson JS, Applebaum J. Treatment of superficial cutaneous lesions by melanin-specfic selective photothermolysis using the Q-switched ruby laser. *Ann Plast Surg.* 1992;29:231–237.
99. Dover JS, Margolis RJ, Polla LL, et al. Pigmented guinea pig skin irradiated with Q-switched ruby laser pulses. Morphologic and histologic findings. *Arch Dermatol.* 1989; 125:43–49.
100. Polla LL, Margolis RJ, Dover JS, et al. Melanosomes are a primary target of Q-switched ruby laser irradiations in guinea pig skin. *J Invest Dermatol.* 1987;89:281–286.
101. Levine PC, Anderson RR. Q-switched ruby laser treatment of pigmented lesions and tattoos. *Clin Dermatol.* 1995;13(1):75–79.
102. Alora MB, Arndt KA, Taylor CR. Scarring following Q-switched laser treatment of 'double tattoos'. *Arch Dermatol.* 2000;136:269–270.
103. Kilmer SL, Farinelli W, Tearney G, et al. Use of a large spot size for the treatment of tattoos enhances clinical efficacy and decreases potential side effects. *Laser Surg Med Suppl.* 1994;6:5.
104. Ferguson J, August P. Evaluation of the Nd:YAG laser for treatment of amateur and professional tattoos. *Br J Dermatol.* 1996;135(4):586–591.
105. Anderson RR. Dermatologic history of the ruby laser: The long story of the short pulse. *Arch Dermatol.* 2003;139: 70–74.
106. Kilmer SL. Laser treatment of tattoos. *Dermatol Clin.* 1997; 15(3):409–417.
107. Kossida T, Riqopoulos D, Katsambas A, Anderson RR. Optimal tattoo removal in a single laser session based on the method of repeated exposures. *J Am Acad Dermatol.* 2012;66(2):271–277.
108. Izikson L, Farinelli W, Sakamoto F, Tannous Z, Anderson RR. Safety and effectiveness of black tattoo clearance in a pig model after a single treatment with a novel 758 nm 500 picosecond laser: A pilot study. *Laser Surg Med.* 2010;42(7): 640–646.

CHAPTER 51

Noninvasive Scar Treatment

Anna Chacon, Katlein Franca, Jennifer Ledon, Jessica Savas, & Keyvan Nouri

INTRODUCTION

Scars are the result of connective tissue that has replaced lost substance in the dermis or deeper tissue due to injury or disease as part of a normative process. Scar characteristics, such as shape and size, are determined by previous damage. Scars can be thin or atrophic, boxcar, or may develop into a hypertrophic scar or keloid.

TOPICAL TREATMENT OF SCARS

Topical therapies for scars have gained popularity among both physicians and patients for their ease of use, widespread availability, and relatively low cost. This section will review pressure therapy, silicone sheeting, onion-extract gels, topical vitamin preparations, imiquimod cream, and topical corticosteroids for the treatment of scars.

PRESSURE THERAPY

Despite a paucity of controlled studies supporting its efficacy, pressure dressings have long been a mainstay in the prevention and minimization of hypertrophic scars and keloids.[1] The proposed mechanism of action of pressure dressings centers upon the acceleration of wound maturation through several pressure-related effects, including thinning of the dermis, decreased edema, and reduction of blood flow and oxygen through the compression of small vessels.[2] The hypoxic environment created by continuous pressure is thought to decrease collagen formation and increase collagen lysis through the induction of enzymes and cytokines that promote extracellular matrix remodeling.[3]

Pressure dressings provide the most clinical benefit in the early, active stages of scarring, becoming less efficacious after 6 months.[2] These custom-made elastic garments are worn for approximately 1 year, with replacement dressings applied every 6 to 8 weeks. While inexpensive, the disadvantages of this form of therapy are primarily related to patient compliance due to discomfort and inconvenience. The dressings must be worn at all times and are cumbersome in areas of anatomic depression or associated with frequent motion, such as flexural areas. In addition, they carry the potential for skin breakdown and ulceration if the pressure is too great or unevenly distributed. Furthermore, there is no consensus on the optimal pressure to achieve maximal efficacy while maintaining minimal adverse effects. Current thought asserts that a pressure of 25 mm Hg is sufficient; however, recent evidence has shown that pressures much lower than this have been associated with improved clinical outcomes.[4]

SILICONE ELASTOMER SHEETING

Silicone elastomer sheeting has been used in scar management since the early 1980s.[5] The exact mechanism by which silicone sheeting improves hypertrophic scars and keloids has not yet been completely elucidated. It is hypothesized that its beneficial effects occur primarily through occlusion and hydration. Resultant decreases in capillary activity, hyperemia, and fibroblast-induced collagen deposition aid in extracellular matrix remodeling and improvement in the clinical appearance of scars.[6]

Silicone gel sheeting should be worn for 12 to 24 hours a day for at least 2 to 3 months to be effective. Daily cleaning may be required to prevent irritation, rash, skin maceration, and pruritus.[7]

Although large, controlled, clinical trials supporting the efficacy of silicone sheeting are lacking, several smaller studies have documented its scar-reducing benefits. Investigation into its utility for scar prophylaxis is also currently ongoing. Clinically, silicone sheeting appears to be an effective means of treating and possibly preventing mature scars while posing minimal risk to the patient. Silicone gel sheeting is, therefore, almost always a part of the therapeutic regimen for hypertrophic scars and keloids.

ONION EXTRACT

Onion-extract–based gel (Mederma, Merz Pharmaceuticals, Greensboro, NC) is an over-the-counter, inexpensive, easy to use, natural option for wound management. *Allium cepa*, the active ingredient derived from quercetin, possesses inherent anti-inflammatory, bacteriostatic, and collagen down regulatory properties that aid in scar remodeling.[8]While previous studies have been unable to find significant clinical benefit from onion extract–based products, a recent randomized, double-blinded study showed a statistically significant difference in mean improvement of lesion induration, pigmentation, tenderness, and overall cosmetic appearance when compared to placebo.[9] Because of its potential efficacy, low cost, ease of use, and low risk for adverse effects, onion-extract–based gels can be considered for the topical treatment of scars.

CONTRACTUBEX®

When onion extract is combined with heparin and allantoin, the product is called Contractubex®. Contractubex® is a commercial preparation that has been clinically and experimentally proven to improve scars through the inhibition of fibroblast proliferation and downregulation of glycosaminoglycan synthesis.[10] A 2006 study showed that Contractubex® was significantly more effective than topical corticosteroids with respect to normalization of scar erythema, pruritus, and consistency. Moreover, a more favorable side effect profile and decrease in the amount of time to normalization of these parameters was found with Contractubex® when compared to the corticosteroid-treated group.[11]

VITAMINS

VITAMIN A

Vitamin A functions to maintain the integrity of mucosal and epithelial surfaces and, therefore, may be of some benefit in the prevention and/or management of scars. Studies conducted to investigate this theoretical benefit used vitamin A in the form of 0.5% retinoic acid applied daily. This topical therapy reduced scar size and associated pruritus and resulted in skin softening, flattening, and improved color.[12] The disadvantages of topical vitamin A therapy include the risks of teratogenicity and hypervitaminosis, which limit its utility in the treatment of scars.

VITAMIN E

Vitamin E is a lipid-soluble antioxidant that exerts its effects primarily within the reticular dermis by preventing reactive oxygen species-mediated damage to DNA, cell membranes, and lipids. It also functions to stabilize membranes through alteration of collagen and glycosaminoglycan production as well as inhibition of cellular membrane lipid peroxidation.[12] Baumann et al. looked at the improvement in the appearance of scars with topical vitamin E versus a standard emollient. New surgical scars after Mohs surgery were found not to differ significantly in cosmetic outcome between the topical vitamin E and placebo groups. Furthermore, a significant amount of patients in the group treated with vitamin E developed contact dermatitis.[13] Because of its lack of proven efficacy and potential for irritation and scar worsening, topical vitamin E is not recommended for the treatment of scars.

VITAMIN D

Vitamin D has also been investigated for use in hypertrophic scar treatment and prevention. Its anti-inflammatory properties and modulation of keratinocytes and Langerhans cells may offer a benefit in wound maturation. However, a recent randomized controlled trial found no difference in scar thickness or prevalence of hypertrophic scars after treatment with topical calcipotriol when compared to placebo.[14]

IMIQUIMOD 5%

Imiquimod is a topical immunomodulatory agent that stimulates pro-inflammatory cytokines, namely interferon-α. Interferon-α promotes collagen breakdown and alters the expression of genes involved in apoptosis, which is helpful in preventing keloid recurrence after excision. Preliminary studies investigating the efficacy of topical imiquimod for hypertrophic scars and keloids have shown promising results.[15] Side effects are consistent with a local inflammatory response and are characterized by erythema, pain, and pinpoint bleeding.[15]

CORTICOSTEROIDS

Intralesional corticosteroid delivery is widely used in the treatment of mature scars; however, corticosteroids are occasionally applied topically, either with or without occlusion. While associated with fewer adverse effects when compared to intralesional or systemic therapy, cutaneous use in isolation has not been shown to be effective.[16] A recent study found that a popular over-the-counter 0.5% hydrocortisone, silicone, and vitamin E preparation yielded the highest mean percent improvement in almost all scar parameters when compared to an onion-extract–based product and placebo.[9] Topical corticosteroid combination preparations, therefore, may play a role in the treatment of hypertrophic scars and keloids; however their use is not recommended as monotherapy.

INTRALESIONAL TREATMENT OF SCARS

The majority of intralesional scar therapies are designed for the reduction of hypertrophic and keloidal scars, with varying success. Many forms of intralesional therapy are currently available, including, but not limited to steroids, cryotherapy, chemotherapeutic agents, and fillers. Intralesional therapy for hypertrophic and keloid scars is aimed at altering this abnormal cell signaling and proliferation.

CORTICOSTEROIDS

Considered the gold standard for intralesional treatment of hypertrophic and keloidal scars, corticosteroids are thought to improve the appearance of these lesions by inhibiting fibroblast growth and promoting collagen degradation.[17] Triamcinolone, the most frequently used corticosteroid for this technique, is typically injected into the mid-dermis to avoid scar atrophy. Unfortunately, effective treatment is not guaranteed, typically requiring many sessions, and it is not unusual for patients to prematurely stop treatment secondary to pain.[18]

Of the possible side effects secondary to intralesional triamcinolone therapy, pain, atrophy, and changes in pigmentation are most common. Although rare, systemic effects such as iatrogenic Cushing's syndrome are also possible.[19] To minimize pain associated steroid administration, a 1:1 mixture of 2% lidocaine and 0.5% bupivacaine can be injected subcutaneously beneath and around the keloid edge 3 minutes prior to treatment, with special care to avoid piercing normal skin, thus inducing new lesions.[20] Topical lidocaine application may be of benefit as well.[21]

Given the requirement for many sessions, the large size of many lesions, and the tendency for these lesions to recur, intralesional steroid therapy may become costly. When evaluating the cost-effectiveness of this procedure, one study showed that by initially starting treatment with low-dose steroids and then advancing to high-dose steroids in later sessions, treatment is most cost effective with the lowest risk of recurrence.[22]

CRYOTHERAPY

Because of clinical improvement seen in some scars following topical cryotherapy, it has been suggested that intralesional cryotherapy may be more efficacious in larger, bulkier scars. Weshahy first attempted intralesional application of cryosurgery in 1993 with the use of cryosurgery needles.[23] By directly targeting the deeper layers of keloids and hypertrophic scars with extreme cold, intralesional cryotherapy can reduce the number of fibroblasts and mast cells and thus revert scars' collagen structure to a more normal organization.[24]

The clinical efficacy of intralesional cryotherapy has ranged from 20% to greater than 75% scar volume reduction.[25–28] Reported side effects include pain, edema, mild epidermolysis, and temporary hypopigmentation, but pain may be less than that of contact cryotherapy.[26,29] Decreased skin surface temperature during intralesional cryotherapy, as opposed to contact, may also spare melanocyte destruction thus explaining the reduced incidence of hypopigmentation.[30]

5-FLUOROURACIL

Shown to inhibit fibroblast proliferation in rabbit cell culture, 5-fluorouracil (5-FU) has been more recently demonstrated to induce fibroblast apoptosis without necrosis, an important factor in scar prevention, via G2/M cell cycle arrest.[31,32] Furthermore, 5-FU is known to inhibit transforming growth factor-beta (TGF-β) signaling in collagen I production, a pathway that is considered to be awry in keloid genesis.[33]

Although 5-FU is typically used for triamcinolone refractory scars, there is a paucity of studies directly comparing the two modalities. Success rates with 5-FU are variable, with greater improvement in younger scars.[34] Pain and hyperpigmentation are common side effects.[32,34,35]

BLEOMYCIN

Bodokh and Brun[36] first studied the effects of intralesional bleomycin on keloids or hypertrophic scars in 1996. 36 scars were treated with three to five sessions of intralesional bleomycin within a 1 month period with total regression seen in 80% of lesions. These promising results subsequently led to several studies evaluating bleomycin for this purpose. Complete or significant scar flattening has been reported in 66% to 100% of lesions.[37–39] Furthermore, bleomycin was found to be better than contact cryotherapy plus intralesional triamcinolone for lesions greater than 100 mm^2.[2,38–40]

Although resulting in DNA damage similar to that following X-irradiation, local administration of low-dose bleomycin is not associated with systemic effects and is considered safe in human skin.[41,42] At the cellular level, intralesional bleomycin was found to result in necrosis and dyskeratosis of keratinocytes as well as reduced collagen synthesis by fibroblasts.[42,43] This dose-dependent inflammatory response resolves after several days with residual post-inflammatory hyperpigmentation.[42]

OTHER CHEMOTHERAPEUTICS

Intralesional interferon-α 2b, mitomycin C, and tumor necrosis factor-alpha (TNF-α) have also been studied to determine their role in the improvement of keloidal or hypertrophic scars. Interferons are thought to improve hypertrophic or keloidal scars by inhibition of collagen synthesis by fibroblasts, specifically collagens I and III.[44,45] Interferon-alpha 2 is also known to increase collagenase production.[46] Success with this modality varies, however, and side effects may be systemic, including flu-like symptoms.[47,48]

Although topical mitomycin C after scar excision was found to improve the appearance of hypertrophic or keloidal scars, intralesional mitomycin C may not be as promising, as it was found to worsen lesions and cause ulcerations.[49] In addition, while TNF-α was effective in reducing pruritus associated with scars, intralesional triamcinolone was more efficacious in scar improvement overall.[50]

VERAPAMIL

Several mechanisms have been implicated for verapamil's role in the improvement of keloid or hypertrophic scars. Calcium antagonists have been shown to reduce extracellular matrix production, induce fibroblast procollagenase synthesis, and inhibit interleukin-6, vascular endothelial growth factor and cellular proliferation of fibroblasts.[51–53] In addition, as mentioned previously, quantities of decorin may be decreased in hypertrophic and keloid scars. As such, the calcium channel blocker verapamil has been shown to augment decorin expression in animal models.[54] Finally, verapamil was shown to inhibit proliferation and TGF-β1 expression in fibroblasts and induce apoptosis.[55] Clinically, verapamil has shown to be of benefit following surgical excision of hypertrophic and keloidal scars.[56–58] In a head-to-head analysis with triamcinolone, although both improved the appearance of proliferative scars, verapamil had a reduced incidence of adverse effects.[59]

FILLERS

Although most of the intralesional therapies for scars are aimed at hypertrophic or proliferative scars, fillers may replace lost volume in large atrophic areas or depressed scars. Used for mild, moderate, and severe acne scarring, dermal fillers can be comprised of bovine or human collagen, hyaluronic acid, silicones, or numerous polyacrylamides.[60]

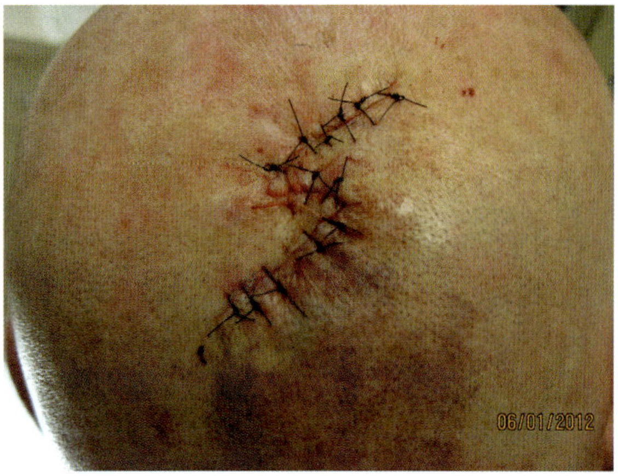

Figure 51-1 A patient's scalp status posttransposition flap with a Z-plasty after Mohs micrographic surgery.

In mild scarring, human collagen or hyaluronic acid is preferred over more permanent options. With severe and diffuse atrophic scarring, fat replacement may be the best option.[61] Fillers such as hyaluronic acid or calcium hydroxyapatite may also be used for atrophic scars that result from indicated surgical procedures, such as Mohs micrographic surgery (Figs. 51-1 and 51-2).[62] Taking care to avoid injection into vessels is essential to avoid vascular occlusion and ulceration.

COMBINATION THERAPY

Several combinations of intralesional therapies for the treatment of scars have been studied. Contact cryotherapy, 5-FU, interferon-alpha 2b, and topical steroids have all been considered as adjuvant therapies to intralesional triamcinolone, with varying success. As mechanisms of action differ for each of these modalities, it may be that targeting different aberrant pathways can lead to greater clinical efficacy.

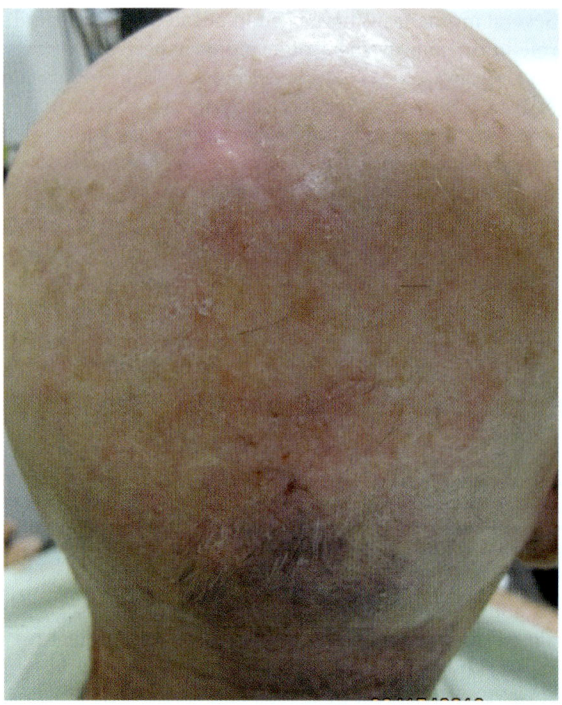

Figure 51-2 The patient has developed a pink, raised scar 6 weeks after suture removal.

FUTURE DIRECTIONS

It is important to note that these are only some of the more common intralesional therapies for hypertrophic scars. Botulinum toxin A has been shown to minimize scar tension and improve erythema, pruritus, and pliability.[63,64] Pentoxifylline, a methylxanthine derivative, has also been shown to improve the elasticity of hypertrophic scars.[65] In animal models, minocycline reduced hypertrophy by 85% and collagen-glycosaminoglycan copolymers have been used as adjuvant therapy in human chest keloids with success.[47,66,67] Finally, due to its success in treating cutaneous hemangiomas, intralesional propranolol is being considered as well.[68]

DERMABRASION

Dermabrasion is a facial resurfacing technique that mechanically ablates aged or damaged skin to promote re-epithelialization.[69] It allows the epidermis to regenerate as a smooth surface after the defective dermis and epidermis have been removed. The procedure involves the use of a device that scrapes off the scarred outer layers of skin so that new skin growth is encouraged. The epidermis will regenerate from the epidermal appendages located in the remaining dermis. This process may improve the skin surface and appearance of scars. The re-epithelialization process is usually complete in 5 to 7 days and residual erythema is common for up to 4 weeks.[70] Several methods and instruments are currently being employed for dermabrasion, which are detailed below.[71]

Small, portable hand-held dermabraders are the most popular units available and are able to generate rotation speeds of 18,000 to 35,000 revolutions per minute. End pieces, including wire brushes, diamond fraises, and serrated wheels, are attached to the end of the dermabrader to allow precise resurfacing and treatment. The surgeon can usually control speed with a foot pedal.[70]

Dermabrasion should be performed by a trained and skilled surgeon and can be associated with other dermatologic procedures including chemical exfoliation, soft tissue augmentation and laser procedures.[70]

INDICATIONS

Dermabrasion was initially developed to treat acne scars and traumatic facial scars. Other indications are partial-thickness Mohs surgical defects and rhinophyma, improvement of actinic keratoses, seborrheic keratoses, angiofibromas, syringomas, solar elastosis, epidermal nevi, and tattoo removal.[70,72] Nowadays it is primarily used for cosmetic facial resurfacing.[73]

Dermabrasion remains an important tool when used in combination for treating acne scarring, especially cystic acne.[74] Cai et al. performed a study in 2005 to investigate the application of dermabrasion in the treatment of acne scars. A total of 110 patients were treated with dermabrasion and postoperatively, curative results were achieved in 45 cases; good results in 40 cases, and effective results in 25 cases.[75]

For surgical and traumatic scars, the contour, thickness, and overall appearance are routinely improved with postoperative dermabrasion. The procedure is best performed 6 to 8 weeks after the initial surgery or wounding event.[74] In 2003, Poulos et al.[76] suggest an improvement of surgical scars of the face in 80% of patients after 6 months of treatment.

CONTRAINDICATIONS

Dermabrasion is contraindicated for patients who have had recent facial surgery, those using isotretinoin within the last 6 to 12 months, and with those active herpes or other skin infections. Anti-viral prophylaxis may be appropriate. The presence of active inflammatory skin disease, or immune disorders that could affect the healing process, as well as active acne, are also contraindications for this procedure.[74]

CONCLUSION

Dermabrasion is one of many techniques that can be used to treat scars. It is indicated for surgical or traumatic scarring, acne scars, chickenpox scars, rhinophyma, premalignant actinic damage, and perioral rhytides. When performed correctly, the procedure has minimal complications. Dermabrasion does not require expensive equipment and should be performed by a trained and skilled surgeon.[70] It is an inexpensive technique that can be combined with other treatments, such as lasers and chemical peels for optimization of results.

CHEMICAL PEELS

A chemical peel is a technique in which a chemical solution is applied to the skin. It represents accelerated exfoliation by caustic agents that cause controlled damage, followed by the release of inflammatory mediators and cytokines. The result is thickening of the epidermis, deposition of collagen, reorganization of structural elements, and increases in dermal volume.[77] The strength of the peel performed is dependent on skin condition and desired results. For patients who cannot afford the costly alternatives for deep scars, repeated peeling will help reduce the visibility and depth of the scars.

Chemical peels are classified by their depth of action into superficial, medium, and deep peels. Specific peeling agents should be selected based on the disorder to be treated and used with an appropriate peel depth, determined by the severity of skin pathology, histological level, or to maximize success.[78,79] Deeper peels target deeper pathologic processes whereas more superficial peels address more superficial pathology, such as pigment.

INDICATIONS

Chemical peels are used to improve the appearance of fine lines and wrinkles, sun damage, skin discoloration, and mild acne scars. Chemical peels with both α- and β-hydroxy acids have been used to improve acne scarring with pigmentation.[80]

TYPES

The most common chemical peels used to treat scars include glycolic acid, lactic acid, salicylic acid, and trichloroacetic acid (TCA).

GLYCOLIC ACID

Glycolic acid (20%–70%) is commonly used in the treatment of active acne vulgaris and postacne scarring and hyperpigmentation.[81] The mechanism of action of α-hydroxy acid is a chemical reaction with the upper layer of the epidermis, thereby weakening the cohesion of the intercellular material of the stratum corneum (SC). The result is a uniform exfoliation of its outermost layers (the stratum disjunctum).[82] This agent can help enhance delivery of topical medications more deeply into the skin.

LACTIC ACID

Lactic acid percentages range from 10% to 70%. This agent tends to be less irritating than glycolic acid. It is a molecule that penetrates the skin slowly, reducing treatment-induced inflammation. Its mechanism of action is to dissolve the intercellular desmosomes to promote exfoliation. It is, therefore, useful to treat superficial scars.[80]

TRICHLOROACETIC ACID

TCA is a synthetically derived peeling agent made of acetic acid and chlorine. Percentages range from 5% to 100%. The mechanism of action of TCA is coagulation of proteins and necrosis of cells. In higher concentrations (50%–100%), it is considered a good method of chemical improvement for skin scars. The use of the cross technique has been reported as an effective method for treating acne scars. This method consists of focal application of TCA using a sharpened wooden applicator. It is pressed down firmly over the entire depressed area of the scar, producing multiple, frosted white spots on each scar. The recovery period and healing process are faster when this technique is used.[83,84]

SALICYLIC ACID

Salicylic acid is a β-hydroxy acid. Although available in higher percentages, salicylic acid is typically applied in 20% to 30% formulations.[80] It is a hydroxyl derivative of benzoic acid and is a carboxylic acid attached to an aromatic alcohol, phenol.[80,85] Salicylic acid is a lipophilic keratolytic agent and is useful for the treatment of superficial scars.[80,85] Some formulations produce a characteristic whitening indicating that the peel has self-neutralized.

COMPLICATIONS

Complications such as hyper- or hypopigmentation, erythema, hypertrophic and keloid scars, infections, and milia may occur.[78]

CONCLUSION

Chemical peels are widely used in dermatological practice. Several sessions are usually needed to improve the appearance and depth of scars. More superficial scars have a better response to this treatment.

MICRONEEDLING

Medical microneedling or collagen induction therapy is a procedure in which microneedles, arranged on a drum-shaped instrument, are passed (rolled) along the skin. They produce channels in the dermis, stimulating neocollagenesis. A minimum of 6 weeks is recommended between treatments as it takes that long for new collagen to form.[86] The most common device used by dermatologists is the dermaroller. The microneedles are available in a variety of shapes and sizes.

INDICATIONS

Microneedling is used for the treatment of scars especially acne scars, burn scars, surgical scars, and for rejuvenation.

RISKS AND SIDE EFFECTS

Side effects are minimal and include stinging, itching, redness, and slight peeling, which usually subside within 24 hours.[87,88] Infection is also a risk associated with microneedling.

CONCLUSION

Microneedling is a simple and inexpensive office procedure, and is safe in all skin types.[87] This procedure can be used in association with other treatments like chemical peels, microdermabrasion and subcision-a surgical technique that aims to sever fibrous attachments beneath a depressed scar in order to lift up the scar and induce formation of connective tissue through normal wound healing. The ability to use microneedling with other treatments allows the procedure to be individualized to maximize benefits to patietns.[86,89]

LASERS FOR SCARS

BACKGROUND

The management of keloids and hypertrophic scars is challenging because of the well-known high rates of recurrence ranging from 45% to 100% and often encountered side effects.[90,91] The ablative Er:YAG (Erbium:YAG) and CO_2 lasers were initially used for hypertrophic scars and subsequently discontinued due to the advent of new and improved laser techniques. The pulsed dye laser (PDL) is currently the gold standard for hypertrophic scars, with less effective outcomes noted in keloids.[92] PDLs deliver results through selective photothermolysis of blood vessels. Blood vessels contain a large amount of oxyhemoglobin, which has peak chromophore absorption peaks at 418, 542, and 577 nm. Although the exact mechanism of how the PDL causes improvement in scars is not well characterized, recent work by Yang et al.[93] has suggested that PDL treatment of keloids significantly downregulates connective tissue growth factor (CTGF) expression in most cases. PDL is thought to cause microvascular damage to the blood supply resulting in ischemia and subsequent decrease in scarring.[94]

INDICATIONS AND CONTRAINDICATIONS FOR LASER SCAR TREATMENT

Common indications for laser treatment of cutaneous scars include functional impairment, adverse effects, aesthetic desirability, and symptomatic discomfort. Therefore, indications for laser treatment of hypertrophic scars usually include pruritus, dysesthesias, functional impairment, and issues regarding appearance. The expected outcome of laser treatment is a reduction in redness and height of the scar, greater pliability, and symptomatic relief of associated symptoms, such as pruritus. As mentioned previously, other items to strongly consider include scar type and skin type. This is important because patients with fairer skin types (Fitzpatrick skin types I–III) tend to fare better with more positive outcomes and fewer side effects from laser therapy. On the other hand, patients with Fitzpatrick skin types IV to VI have an increased risk of laser light absorption by melanin in the epidermis, resulting in less effective targeting of the skin and greater risk of postoperative hyper- or hypopigmentation. The type of scar also plays an important role in successful management. For example, newer lesions (i.e., <1 year old) and scars that are red and elevated are better suited for laser treatment.[94] Lasers may also be useful as a preventive measure against scars in some cases. For example, the 585/595 nm PDL laser may prevent development of hypertrophic scars in wounds due to burns. Furthermore, treatment of surgical scars on day 0, the day of suture removal, has proven beneficial.[95]

PRE- AND POSTOPERATIVE TECHNIQUES

PREOPERATIVE MANAGEMENT

When considering laser treatment of hypertrophic scars or keloids, it is important to inquire about scar age, changes, and previous therapy to determine prognosis. When assessing the scar, one should take note of size, color, height, pliability, and associated symptoms. Treatment within the first few months after onset is ideal because of the numerous blood vessels that are present during this time. Previous treatments (i.e., cryotherapy) may induce fibrosis; thus adjustments of laser parameters and settings may be required, such as the use of higher fluences and/or a greater number of treatment sessions.[96] The location of the scar is also important. According to Dierickx et al.[97] facial scars respond better to laser therapy. Nouri et al.[95] also found that facial, shoulder, and arm scars responded better to treatment than those on the anterior chest wall, while other investigators have found no relationship between the location of a scar and its response to therapy.[92]

PROCEDURE

Everyone present during the procedure must wear protective eyewear at all times corresponding to the specific wavelength of laser used. PDL for keloids and hypertrophic scars is typically carried out as an outpatient procedure and usually does not require anesthesia unless specifically requested. If necessary, a topical anesthetic cream may be placed upon the affected area 30 to 60 minutes before laser therapy.

OPERATIVE TECHNIQUE

As with all lasers, the device should be appropriately calibrated and parameters selected before commencing therapy. For the PDL, the ideal setting is 585 nm at 450 μs pulse duration, using a spot size of 7 to 10 mm, with a fluence range of 3.5 to7.5 J/cm^2. Initial therapy should begin with a lower fluence, but when using a smaller spot size, the fluence should be increased. Lower fluences (3–3.5 J/cm^2 with a 10 mm spot size) are preferable for darker skin types to reduce complications. A 10% overlap is acceptable.

Lasers may be used alone or in conjunction with medical therapy, such as intralesional steroids or 5-FU. When comparing PDL alone to laser therapy combined with intralesional corticosteroids, Alster found no significant difference and similar efficacy rates.[98] However, it is important to keep in mind that if intralesional steroids are going to be used, they should be injected immediately following laser therapy at a dose of 10 to 40 mg/mL. If injected before therapy, blanching of the scar may occur and there is considerable risk of losing the laser target. Finally, multiple treatments may be needed for optimal results. Subsequent laser therapy sessions may be carried out within 4 to 6 weeks.

ADVERSE EFFECTS OF LASER SCAR TREATMENT

A commonly reported complaint from the patient during treatment with the PDL is pain akin to being hit by a snapped rubber band. Other associated symptoms include burning sensations or pruritus in the affected area, but these typically subside within a few days. The most commonly expected side effect is purpura, which appears immediately after the procedure and lasts 7 to 10 days. The development of purpura is dependent on both the fluence and the pulse duration that are selected for treatment. Lower fluences and longer pulse durations both decrease the chance of purpura. Changes in pigmentation may also

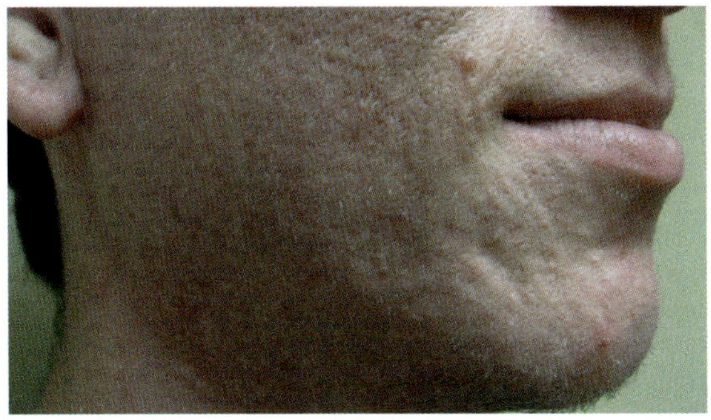

Figure 51-3 Photograph of a 16 year-old patient with multiple facial acne scars before laser therapy.

occur. If hyperpigmentation results, a bleaching cream, such as topical hydroquinone cream or gel may be prescribed. Strict sun avoidance is also recommended. Furthermore, subsequent sessions may be delayed in order to ensure effective targeting of the lesion. Uncommon complications include crusting, oozing, and development of vesicles.

An atrophic scar is a depression in the skin due to destruction of the architecture of dermis and subcutaneous tissue by inflammatory, infectious, or traumatic precursors.[99] These scars result from acne, varicella infection, trauma, or striae; nevertheless, they may be treated with laser therapy once the underlying etiology has resolved. Laser resurfacing for acne scars may be classified as follows: ablative, nonablative, and/or fractional.

Ablative lasers are effective, but side effects including excess scarring, infection, changes in pigmentation, lines of demarcation, prolonged redness, and dryness limit its use. The most common types of ablative lasers are CO_2 and Er:YAG lasers. Fractional ablative lasers are now considered the treatment of choice for acne scars and offer promising results (Figs. 51-3 and 51-4). Still, these methods have several disadvantages.

- The need for antibiotic prophylaxis to prevent superimposed bacterial, viral, or fungal infections.
- The need for appropriate anesthesia and sedation; some are administered systemically and combined with locally injected anesthesia.
- Necessary postoperative care including analgesia, dressings, and antibiotic coverage.
- Increased risk of postoperative bleeding with Er:YAG lasers due to high water absorption; in comparison to CO_2 lasers, this prevents deep penetration, which prevents the production of sufficient heat for blood vessel coagulation.

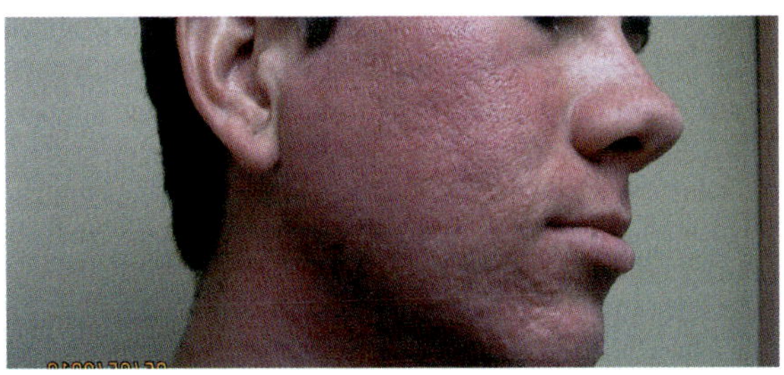

Figure 51-4 Acne scars after immediately after treatment with a fractional nonablative laser.

- There is a considerable tendency for postoperative erythema and changes in pigmentation, which may prolong down time. This is especially relevant to patients with darker skin types who may experience permanent hypo- or hyperpigmentation.

To minimize the disadvantages, some methods that have been employed are preoperative bleaching agents, topical anesthesia combined with a regional nerve block, oral analgesia, and sedation for pain management. In addition, several modalities have been introduced to reduce complications.

- The high-energy short-pulsed CO_2 laser offers less tissue damage compared to the conventional continuous-mode CO_2 laser.
- The variable-pulsed or dual-modality Er:YAG laser has a long pulse duration, which allows deeper penetration than short-pulse alone; this results in an optimal reaction to stimulate regeneration of the skin and sealing of vessels, which reduces bleeding.[100,101] For dual advantage, the combined-mode Er:YAG and CO_2 laser system offers ablation from Er:YAG laser as well as coagulation from the CO_2 laser.[102]

Although it is a safe alternative, nonablative laser resurfacing may not be as effective as ablative resurfacing. Nonablative resurfacing became popular due to low complication rates and low downtime compared to other treatment modalities such as ablative resurfacing, chemical peels, or dermabrasion.

Several laser options that have shown significant improvement of acne scars include the following: 1064 nm Q-switched Nd:YAG laser,[103] 1064 nm long-pulsed Nd:YAG laser,[104,105] 1320 nm Nd:YAG laser,[106,107] 1450 nm diode laser,[108] and 1540 nm erbium-doped phosphate glass laser.[109] The 585 nm flash lamp-pumped PDL and intense pulse light systems have proven to be beneficial for post-acne erythema.[110,111] These options are helpful for patients who desire less aggressive forms of treatment.

FRACTIONAL RESURFACING

Nonablative fractional resurfacing is nearly as effective as fully ablative lasers and as safe as nonablative lasers. After enduring the high complications of ablative laser options and the limited benefits of nonablative techniques, fractional resurfacing was introduced as a technique that offered the best of both worlds. Fractional resurfacing delivers promising results for facial rejuvenation, melasma, and acne scarring. Its mechanism of action utilizes the concept of fractional photothermolysis through the creation of microscopic zones of thermal injury of controlled width, depth, and density surrounded by normal skin that serves as a reservoir for rapid healing of tissue.[112]

Other benefits include less downtime and fewer complications than conventional ablative lasers as well as greater efficacy for tissue regeneration than nonablative lasers. Many fractional resurfacing devices have been launched, both nonablative and ablative. The most popular options include erbium-doped, Er:YAG, CO_2, and Xenon lights.

Several sources have described how efficacious the 1550 laser system can be for acne scars. In a study on 53 patients with Fitzpatrick types I to IV, Alster et al. used the 1550 nm erbium-doped fiber at fluences of 8 to 16 J/cm^2 and densities of 125 to 250 MTZ/in 8 to 10 passes in atrophic acne scars. Although multiple treatments were needed, almost 90% of patients achieved clinical improvement, with an average improvement of 50% to 75%.[113] In a similar study by Lee et al., 27 patients of Asian extraction with Fitzpatrick skin types IV to V were treated for moderate to severe acne scars. Patients received three to five laser sessions every 3 to 4 weeks. Patients demonstrated significant improvement 3 months after the final treatment session. According to patient ratings regarding improvement, 30% were excellent; 59% were significant; and 11% were moderate.[114] In a separate investigation by Emmy et al., 961 patients treated with the 1550 nm erbium-doped laser were reviewed. Complications included temporary erythema, pain, and swelling. Only 7.6% of patients developed complications, most frequently acneiform eruptions in 1.87% and episodes of herpes simplex virus in 1.77%. Rare complications included prolonged erythema, swelling, dermatitis, purpura, and postoperative infections such as impetigo.[115] Other fractional resurfacing options include fractional CO_2 and fractional Er:YAG lasers.

Investigations have shown improvement of scars with fractional resurfacing; however, a small subset of patients have experienced adverse effects.[116] Still, optimal laser parameters to achieve improvement of acne scars with minimal side effects need to be investigated further. Fractional photothermolysis technology induces microthermal zones of injury, which stimulate rapid wound healing, resulting in improvement of various skin conditions including aesthetic, inflammatory, and pre-neoplastic disorders.[117] Further investigation regarding the proper spacing of microthermal zones within the context of scar management is also warranted.

CONCLUSIONS AND FUTURE DIRECTIONS

As mentioned earlier, using PDL or intralesional steroid therapy may prevent formation of hypertrophic scars. Evidence-based medicine suggests that laser therapy, particularly PDL, is most effective for hypertrophic scars and keloids if used early and in conjunction with other techniques.[118]

However, these methods have their own disadvantages. Both 5-FU and intralesional steroids may cause pain, pruritus, and purpura at the site of injection, although studies that combine these modalities with PDL have shown promising results thus far. The 585/595 nm PDL may be used for improving surgical scars on the day of suture removal, and in some instances, hypertrophic and keloid scars as well. The fractional ablative and nonablative lasers have emerged as the standard of care for treating acne and surgical scars. Novel research is demonstrating that the fractional CO_2 laser is effective for treating burn scars, especially contractures.[119]

Many patients with scars suffer physical and emotional challenges that may be compounded by ineffective treatment results and unrealistic expectations. How to address these factors while minimizing adverse effects for all patients is one of the primary goals of scar management. Still, combining therapy may be the optimal choice for future treatment of scars. In addition, further studies that evaluate combination therapy with short- and long-pulsed lasers may show interesting findings and may lead to new directions in scar treatment.

REFERENCES

1. Tolhurst DE. Hypertrophic scarring prevented by pressure: a case report. *Br J Plast Surg*. 1977;30(3):218–219.
2. Staley MJ, Richard RL. Use of pressure to treat hypertrophic burn scars. *Adv Wound Care*. 1997;10(3):44–46.
3. Kischer CW, Shetlar MR, Shetlar CL. Alteration of hypertrophic scars induced by mechanical pressure. *Arch Dermatol*. 1975;111(1):60–64.
4. Ward RS. Pressure therapy for the control of hypertrophic scar formation after burn injury. A history and review. *J Burn Care Rehabil*. 1991;12(3):257–262.
5. Perkins K, Davey RB, Wallis KA. Silicone gel: a new treatment for burn scars and contractures. *Burns Incl Therm Inj*. 1983;9(3):201–204.
6. Quinn KJ, Evans JH, Courtney JM, Gaylor JD, Reid WH. Non-pressure treatment of hypertrophic scars. *Burns Incl Therm Inj*. 1985;12(2):102–108.
7. Fette A. Influence of silicone on abnormal scarring. *Plast Surg Nurs*. 2006;26(2):87–92.
8. Augusti KT. Therapeutic values of onion (Allium cepa L.) and garlic (Allium sativum L.). *Indian J Exp Biol*. 1996; 34(7):634–640.
9. Perez OA, Viera MH, Patel JK, et al. A comparative study evaluating the tolerability and efficacy of two topical therapies for the treatment of keloids and hypertrophic scars. *J Drugs Dermatol*. 2010;9(5):514–518.
10. Willital GH, Heine H. Efficacy of Contractubex gel in the treatment of fresh scars after thoracic surgery in children and adolescents. *Int J Clin Pharmacol Res*. 1994;14(5–6):193–202.
11. Beuth J, Hunzelmann N, Van Leendert R, Basten R, Noehle M, Schneider B. Safety and efficacy of local administration of contractubex to hypertrophic scars in comparison to corticosteroid treatment. Results of a multicenter, comparative epidemiological cohort study in Germany. *In Vivo*. 2006;20(2):277–283.
12. Zurada JM, Kriegel D, Davis IC. Topical treatments for hypertrophic scars. *J Am Acad Dermatol*. 2006;55(6):1024–1031.
13. Baumann LS, Spencer J. The effects of topical vitamin E on the cosmetic appearance of scars. *Dermatol Surg*. 1999; 25(4):311–315.
14. van der Veer WM, Jacobs XE, Waardenburg IE, Ulrich MM, Niessen FB. Topical calcipotriol for preventive treatment of hypertrophic scars: a randomized, double-blind, placebo-controlled trial. *Arch Dermatol*. 2009;145(11):1269–1275.
15. Prado A, Andrades P, Benitez S, Umaña M. Scar management after breast surgery: preliminary results of a prospective, randomized, and double-blind clinical study with aldara cream 5% (imiquimod). *Plast Reconstr Surg*. 2005;115 (3):966–972.
16. Jenkins M, Alexander JW, MacMillan BG, Waymack JP, Kopcha R. Failure of topical steroids and vitamin E to reduce postoperative scar formation following reconstructive surgery. *J Burn Care Rehabil*. 1986;7(4):309–312.
17. McCoy BJ, Diegelmann RF, Cohen IK. In vitro inhibition of cell growth, collagen synthesis, and prolyl hydroxylase activity by triamcinolone acetonide. *Proc Soc Exp Biol Med*. 1980;163(2):216–222.
18. Muneuchi G, Suzuki S, Onodera M, Ito O, Hata Y, Igawa HH. Long-term outcome of intralesional injection of triamcinolone acetonide for the treatment of keloid scars in Asian patients. *Scand J Plast Reconstr Surg Hand Surg*. 2006;40(2):111–116.
19. Liu MF, Yencha M. Cushing's syndrome secondary to intralesional steroid injections of multiple keloid scars. *Otolaryngol Head Neck Surg*. 2006;135(6):960–961.
20. Mishra S. Safe and less painful injection of triamcenolone acetonide into a keloid–a technique. *J Plast Reconstr Aesthet Surg*. 2010;63(2):e205.
21. Tosa M, Murakami M, Hyakusoku H. Effect of lidocaine tape on pain during intralesional injection of triamcinolone acetonide for the treatment of keloid. *J Nihon Med Sch*. 2009;76(1):9–12.
22. Anthony ET, Lemonas P, Navsaria HA, Moir GC. The cost effectiveness of intralesional steroid therapy for keloids. *Dermatol Surg*. 2010;36(10):1624–1626.
23. Weshahy AH. Intralesional cryosurgery. A new technique using cryoneedles. *J Dermatol Surg Oncol*. 1993;19(2):123–126.
24. Har-Shai Y, Brown W, Labbé D, et al. Intralesional cryosurgery for the treatment of hypertrophic scars and keloids following aesthetic surgery: the results of a prospective observational study. *Int J Low Extrem Wounds*. 2008;7 (3):169–175.
25. Zouboulis CC, Rosenberger AD, Forster T, Beller G, Kratzsch M, Felsenberg D. Modification of a device and its application for intralesional cryosurgery of old recalcitrant keloids. *Arch Dermatol*. 2004;140(10):1293–1294.
26. Har-Shai Y, Amar M, Sabo E. Intralesional cryotherapy for enhancing the involution of hypertrophic scars and keloids. *Plast Reconstr Surg*. 2003;111(6):1841–1852.
27. Har-Shai Y, Sabo E, Rohde E, Hyams M, Assaf C, Zouboulis CC. Intralesional cryosurgery enhances the involution of recalcitrant auricular keloids: a new clinical approach supported by experimental studies. *Wound Repair Regen*. 2006;14(1):18–27.
28. Gupta S, Kumar B. Intralesional cryosurgery using lumbar puncture and/or hypodermic needles for large, bulky, recalcitrant keloids. *Int J Dermatol*. 2001;40(5):349–353.
29. Mirmovich O, Gil T, Goldin I, Lavi I, Mettanes I, Har-Shai Y. Pain evaluation and control during and following the treatment of hypertrophic scars and keloids by contact and intralesional cryosurgery–a preliminary study. *J Eur Acad Dermatol Venereol*. 2012;26(4):440–447.
30. Har-Shai Y, Dujovny E, Rohde E, Zouboulis CC. Effect of skin surface temperature on skin pigmentation during contact and intralesional cryosurgery of keloids. *J Eur Acad Dermatol Venereol*. 2007;21(2):191–198.
31. Blumenkranz MS, Claflin A, Hajek AS. Selection of therapeutic agents for intraocular proliferative disease. Cell culture evaluation. *Arch Ophthalmol*. 1984;102(4):598–604.
32. Huang L, Wong YP, Cai YJ, Lung I, Leung CS, Burd A. Low-dose 5-fluorouracil induces cell cycle G2 arrest and apoptosis in keloid fibroblasts. *Br J Dermatol*. 2010;163(6): 1181–1185.
33. Wendling J, Marchand A, Mauviel A, Verrecchia F. 5-fluorouracil blocks transforming growth factor-beta-induced alpha 2 type I collagen gene (COL1A2) expression in human fibroblasts via c-Jun NH2-terminal kinase/activator protein-1 activation. *Mol Pharmacol*. 2003; 64(3):707–713.
34. Gupta S, Kalra A. Efficacy and safety of intralesional 5-fluorouracil in the treatment of keloids. *Dermatology*. 2002;204(2): 130–132.
35. Kontochristopoulos G, Stefanaki C, Panagiotopoulos A, et al. Intralesional 5-fluorouracil in the treatment of keloids: an open clinical and histopathologic study. *J Am Acad Dermatol*. 2005;52(3 Pt 1):474–479.
36. Bodokh I, Brun P. [Treatment of keloid with intralesional bleomycin]. *Ann Dermatol Venereol*. 1996;123(12):791–794.
37. Aggarwal H, Saxena A, Lubana PS, Mathur RK, Jain DK. Treatment of keloids and hypertrophic scars using bleom. *J Cosmet Dermatol*. 2008;7(1):43–49.
38. Saray Y, Gulec AT. Treatment of keloids and hypertrophic scars with dermojet injections of bleomycin: a preliminary study. *Int J Dermatol*. 2005.44(9):777–784.
39. Espana A, Solano T, Quintanilla E. Bleomycin in the treatment of keloids and hypertrophic scars by multiple needle punctures. *Dermatol Surg*. 2001;27(1):23–27.

40. Naeini FF, Najafian J, Ahmadpour K. Bleomycin tattooing as a promising therapeutic modality in large keloids and hypertrophic scars. *Dermatol Surg.* 2006;32(8):1023–1029; discussion 1029–1030.
41. Kuo MT, Haidle CW. Characterization of chain breakage in DNA induced by bleomycin. *Biochimica et Biophysica Acta (BBA) - Nucleic Acids and Protein Synthesis.* 1974;335(2):109–114.
42. Templeton SF, Solomon AR, Swerlick RA. Intradermal bleomycin injections into normal human skin. A histopathologic and immunopathologic study. *Arch Dermatol,* 1994; 130(5):577–583.
43. Hendricks T, Martens MF, Huyben CM, Wobbes T. Inhibition of basal and TGF beta-induced fibroblast collagen synthesis by antineoplastic agents. Implications for wound healing. *Br J Cancer.* 1993;67(3):545–550.
44. Jimenez SA, Freundlich B, Rosenbloom J. Selective inhibition of human diploid fibroblast collagen synthesis by interferons. *J Clin Invest.* 1984;74(3):1112–1116.
45. Granstein RD, Flotte TJ, Amento EP. Interferons and collagen production. *J Invest Dermatol.* 1990;95(Suppl 6):75S–80S.
46. Duncan MR, Berman B. Differential regulation of glycosaminoglycan, fibronectin, and collagenase production in cultured human dermal fibroblasts by interferon-alpha, -beta, and -gamma. *Arch Dermatol Res.* 1989;281(1):11–18.
47. Davison SP, Mess S, Kauffman LC, Al-Attar A. Ineffective treatment of keloids with interferon alpha-2b. *Plast Reconstr Surg.* 2006;117(1):247–252.
48. Lee JH, Kim SE, Lee AY. Effects of interferon-alpha2b on keloid treatment with triamcinolone acetonide intralesional injection. *Int J Dermatol.* 2008;47(2):183–186.
49. Seo SH, Sung HW. Treatment of keloids and hypertrophic scars using topical and intralesional mitomycin C. *J Eur Acad Dermatol Venereol.* 2012;26(5):634–638.
50. Berman B, Patel JK, Perez OA, et al. Evaluating the tolerability and efficacy of etanercept compared to triamcinolone acetonide for the intralesional treatment of keloids. *J Drugs Dermatol.* 2008;7(8):757–761.
51. Lee RC, Ping JA. Calcium antagonists retard extracellular matrix production in connective tissue equivalent. *J Surg Res.* 1990;49(5):463–466.
52. Doong H, Dissanayake S, Gowrishankar TR, LaBarbera MC, Lee RC. The 1996 Lindberg Award. Calcium antagonists alter cell shape and induce procollagenase synthesis in keloid and normal human dermal fibroblasts. *J Burn Care Rehabil.* 1996;17(6 Pt 1):497–514.
53. Giugliano G, Pasquali D, Notaro A, et al. Verapamil inhibits interleukin-6 and vascular endothelial growth factor production in primary cultures of keloid fibroblasts. *Br J Plast Surg.* 2003;56(8):804–809.
54. Yang JY, Huang CY. The effect of combined steroid and calcium channel blocker injection on human hypertrophic scars in animal model: a new strategy for the treatment of hypertrophic scars. *Dermatol Surg.* 2010;36(12):1942–1949.
55. Xu SJ, Teng JY, Xie J, Shen MQ, Chen DM. [Comparison of the mechanisms of intralesional steroid, interferon or verapamil injection in the treatment of proliferative scars]. *Zhonghua Zheng Xing Wai Ke Za Zhi.* 2009;25(1):37–40.
56. D'Andrea F, Brongo S, Ferraro G, Baroni A. Prevention and treatment of keloids with intralesional verapamil. *Dermatology.* 2002;204(1):60–62.
57. Skaria AM. Prevention and treatment of keloids with intralesional verapamil. *Dermatology.* 2004;209(1):71.
58. Lawrence WT. Treatment of earlobe keloids with surgery plus adjuvant intralesional verapamil and pressure earrings. *Ann Plast Surg.* 1996;37(2):167–169.
59. Margaret Shanthi FX, Ernest K, Dhanraj P. Comparison of intralesional verapamil with intralesional triamcinolone in the treatment of hypertrophic scars and keloids. *Indian J Dermatol Venereol Leprol.* 2008;74(4):343–348.
60. Goodman GJ, Baron JA. The management of postacne scarring. *Dermatol Surg.* 2007;33(10):1175–1188.
61. Coleman SR. Structural fat grafting: more than a permanent filler. *Plast Reconstr Surg.* 2006;118(Suppl 3):108S–120S.
62. Kasper DA, Cohen JL, Saxena A, Morganroth GS. Fillers for postsurgical depressed scars after skin cancer reconstruction. *J Drugs Dermatol.* 2008.7(5):486–487.
63. Liu RK, Li CH, Zou SJ. Reducing scar formation after lip repair by injecting botulinum toxin. *Plast Reconstr Surg.* 2010;125(5):1573–1574; author reply 1575.
64. Xiao Z, Zhang F, Cui Z. Treatment of hypertrophic scars with intralesional botulinum toxin type A injections: a preliminary report. *Aesthetic Plast Surg.* 2009;33(3):409–412.
65. Isaac C, Carvalho VF, Paggiaro AO, de Maio M, Ferreira MC. Intralesional pentoxifylline as an adjuvant treatment for perioral post-burn hypertrophic scars. *Burns.* 2010;36 (6):831–835.
66. Henry SL, Concannon MJ, Kaplan PA, Diaz-Arias AA. The inhibitory effect of minocycline on hypertrophic scarring. *Plast Reconstr Surg.* 2007;120(1):80–88; discussion 89–90.
67. Davison SP, Sobanko JF, Clemens MW. Use of a collagen-glycosaminoglycan copolymer (Integra) in combination with adjuvant treatments for reconstruction of severe chest keloids. *J Drugs Dermatol.* 2010;9(5):542–548.
68. de Mesquita CJ, About strawberry, crab claws, and the Sir James Black's invention. Hypothesis: can we battle keloids with propranolol? *Med Hypotheses.* 2010;74(2):353–359.
69. Alkhawam L, Alam M. Dermabrasion and microdermabrasion. *Facial Plast Surg.* 2009;25(5):301–310.
70. Gold MH. Dermabrasion in dermatology. *Am J Clin Dermatol.* 2003;4(7):467–471.
71. Emsen IM. An update on sandpaper in dermabrasion with a different and extended patient series. *Aesthetic Plast Surg.* 2008. [Epub ahead of print].
72. Coleman WP 3rd, Yarborough JM, Mandy SH. Dermabrasion for prophylaxis and treatment of actinic keratoses. *Dermatol Surg.* 1996;22(1):17–21.
73. Kirkland EB, Gladstone HB, Hantash BM. What's new in skin resurfacing and rejuvenation? *G Ital Dermatol Venereol.* 2010;145(5):583–596.
74. Harmon C, PC Dermabrasion procedures. 2011.
75. Cai GB, Li HD, Zhang Y, et al. [Full face dermabrasion for acne scars]. *Zhonghua Zheng Xing Wai Ke Za Zhi.* 2005; 21(3):192–193.
76. Poulos E, Taylor C, Solish N. Effectiveness of dermasanding (manual dermabrasion) on the appearance of surgical scars: a prospective, randomized, blinded study. *J Am Acad Dermatol.* 2003;48(6):897–900.
77. Fabbrocini G. Chemical peels. *Medscape.* 2012.
78. Camacho FM. Medium-depth and deep chemical peels. *J Cosmet Dermatol.* 2005;4(2):117–128.
79. Rendon MI, Berson DS, Cohen JL, Roberts WE, Starker I, Wang B. Evidence and considerations in the application of chemical peels in skin disorders and aesthetic resurfacing. *J Clin Aesthet Dermatol.* 2010;3(7):32–43.
80. Sachdeva S. Lactic acid peeling in superficial acne scarring in Indian skin. *J Cosmet Dermatol.* 2010;9(3):246–248.
81. Garg VK, Sinha S, Sarkar R. Glycolic acid peels versus salicylic-mandelic acid peels in active acne vulgaris and post-acne scarring and hyperpigmentation: a comparative study. *Dermatol Surg.* 2009;35(1):59–65.
82. Fartasch M, Teal J, Menon GK. Mode of action of glycolic acid on human stratum corneum: ultrastructural and functional evaluation of the epidermal barrier. *Arch Dermatol Res.* 1997;289(7):404–409.
83. Fabbrocini G, Cacciapuoti S, Fardella N, Pastore F, Monfrecola G. CROSS technique: chemical reconstruction of skin scars method. *Dermatol Ther.* 2008;21(Suppl 3):S29–S32.
84. Bhardwaj D, Khunger N. An assessment of the efficacy and safety of CROSS technique with 100% TCA in the management of ice pick acne scars. *J Cutan Aesthet Surg.* 2010;3(2):93–96.
85. Fung W, Orak D, Re TA, Haughey DB. Relative bioavailability of salicylic acid following dermal application of a 30% salicylic acid skin peel preparation. *J Pharm Sci.* 2008;97(3):1325–1328.
86. Doddaballapur S. Microneedling with dermaroller. *J Cutan Aesthet Surg.* 2009;2(2):110–111.

87. Sharad J. Combination of microneedling and glycolic acid peels for the treatment of acne scars in dark skin. *J Cosmet Dermatol.* 2011;10(4):317–323.
88. Majid I. Microneedling therapy in atrophic facial scars: an objective assessment. *J Cutan Aesthet Surg.* 2009;2(1):26–30.
89. Badran MM, Kuntsche J, Fahr A. Skin penetration enhancement by a microneedle device (Dermaroller) in vitro: dependency on needle size and applied formulation. *Eur J Pharm Sci.* 2009;36(4–5):511–523.
90. Berman B, Bieley HC. Keloids. *J Am Acad Dermatol.* 1995;33(1):117–123.
91. Rockwell WB, Cohen IK, Ehrlich HP. Keloids and hypertrophic scars: a comprehensive review. *Plast Reconstr Surg.* 1989;84(5):827–837.
92. Alster TS, Nanni CA. Pulsed dye laser treatment of hypertrophic burn scars. *Plast Reconstr Surg.* 1998;102(6): 2190–2195.
93. Yang Q, Ma Y, Zhu R, Huang G, Guan M, Avram M, Lu Z. The effect of flashlamp pulsed dye laser on the expression of connective tissue growth factor in keloids. *Lasers Surg Med.* 2012;44(5):377–383.
94. Vejjabhinanta V, Patel S, Elsaie M, Nouri K. Laser for scars. In: Nouri K, ed. *Lasers in Dermatology and Medicine.* London:Springer-Verlag; 2011;45–51.
95. Nouri K, Jimenez GP, Harrison-Balestra C, et al. 585-nm pulsed dye laser in the treatment of surgical scars starting on the suture removal day. *Dermatol Surg.* 2003;29(1):65–73; discussion 73.
96. Alster T. Laser revision of scars and striae. In: Alster T, ed. *Manual of Cutaneous Laser Techniques.* Philadelphia, PA: Lippincott; 2000:89–107.
97. Dierickx C, Goldman MP, Fitzpatrick RE. Laser treatment of erythematous/hypertrophic and pigmented scars in 26 patients. *Plast Reconstr Surg.* 1995;95(1):84–90; discussion 91–92.
98. Alster T. Laser scar revision: comparison study of 585-nm pulsed dye laser with and without intralesional corticosteroids. *Dermatol Surg.* 2003;29(1):25–29.
99. Bayat A, McGrouther DA, Ferguson MW. Skin scarring. *BMJ.* 2003;326(7380):88–92.
100. Pozner JM, Goldberg DJ. Histologic effect of a variable pulsed Er:YAG laser. *Dermatol Surg.* 2000;26(8):733–736.
101. Tanzi EL, Alster TS. Treatment of atrophic facial acne scars with a dual-mode Er:YAG laser. *Dermatol Surg.* 2002;28 (7):551–555.
102. Goldman MP, Marchell N, Fitzpatrick RE. Laser skin resurfacing of the face with a combined CO2/Er:YAG laser. *Dermatol Surg.* 2000;26(2):102–104.
103. Friedman PM, Jih MH, Skover GR, Payonk GS, Kimyai-Asadi A, Geronemus RG. Treatment of atrophic facial acne scars with the 1064-nm Q-switched Nd:YAG laser: six-month follow-up study. *Arch Dermatol.* 2004;140(11):1337–1341.
104. Keller R, Belda Júnior W, Valente NY, Rodrigues CJ. Nonablative 1064-nm Nd:YAG laser for treating atrophic facial acne scars: histologic and clinical analysis. *Dermatol Surg.* 2007;33(12):1470–1476.
105. Yaghmai D, Garden JM, Bakus AD, Massa MC. Comparison of a 1064 nm laser and a 1320 nm laser for the nonablative treatment of acne scars. *Dermatol Surg.* 2005;31(8 Pt 1):903–909.
106. Rogachefsky AS, Hussain M, Goldberg DJ. Atrophic and a mixed pattern of acne scars improved with a 1320-nm Nd:YAG laser. *Dermatol Surg.* 2003;29(9):904–908.
107. Sadick NS, Schecter AK. A preliminary study of utilization of the 1320-nm Nd:YAG laser for the treatment of acne scarring. *Dermatol Surg.* 2004;30(7):995–1000.
108. Chua SH, Ang P, Khoo LS, Goh CL. Nonablative 1450-nm diode laser in the treatment of facial atrophic acne scars in type IV to V Asian skin: a prospective clinical study. *Dermatol Surg.* 2004;30(10):1287–1291.
109. Lupton JR, Williams CM, Alster TS. Nonablative laser skin resurfacing using a 1540 nm erbium glass laser: a clinical and histologic analysis. *Dermatol Surg.* 2002;28(9):833–835.
110. Alster TS, McMeekin TO. Improvement of facial acne scars by the 585 nm flashlamp-pumped pulsed dye laser. *J Am Acad Dermatol.* 1996;35(1):79–81.
111. Cartier H. Use of intense pulsed light in the treatment of scars. *J Cosmet Dermatol.* 2005;4(1):34–40.
112. Jih MH, Kimyai-Asadi A. Fractional photothermolysis: a review and update. *Semin Cutan Med Surg.* 2008;27(1): 63–71.
113. Alster TS, Tanzi EL, Lazarus M. The use of fractional laser photothermolysis for the treatment of atrophic scars. *Dermatol Surg.* 2007;33(3):295–299.
114. Lee HS, Lee JH, Ahn GY, et al. Fractional photothermolysis for the treatment of acne scars: a report of 27 Korean patients. *J Dermatolog Treat.* 2008;19(1):45–49.
115. Graber EM, Tanzi EL, Alster TS. Side effects and complications of fractional laser photothermolysis: experience with 961 treatments. *Dermatol Surg.* 2008;34(3):301–305; discussion 305–307.
116. Avram MM, Tope WD, Yu T, Szachowicz E, nelson JS. Hypertrophic scarring of the neck following ablative fractional carbon dioxide laser resurfacing. *Lasers Surg Med.* 2009;41(3):185–188.
117. Tierney EP, Kouba DJ, Hanke CW. Review of fractional photothermolysis: treatment indications and efficacy. *Dermatol Surg.* 2009;35(10):1445–1461.
118. Alster TS. Improvement of erythematous and hypertrophic scars by the 585-nm flashlamp-pumped pulsed dye laser. *Ann Plast Surg.* 1994;32(2):186–190.
119. Cho SB, Lee SJ, Chung WS, Kang JM, Kim YK. Treatment of burn scar using a carbon dioxide fractional laser. *J Drugs Dermatol.* 2010;9(2):173–175.

CHAPTER 52

Laser and Light-Based Treatment of Vascular Lesions

Kathryn Serowka & Kristen M. Kelly

INTRODUCTION

Vascular lesions are a commonly encountered problem in procedural dermatology, and patients frequently desire their removal. Light-based devices such as lasers and intense pulsed light (IPL) are among the most utilized technologies for removal of these lesions. This chapter will discuss the evolution of light-based therapies, the treatment of vascular lesions using the principles of photothermolysis, and will review diagnostic criteria and suggested treatments for many vascular lesions including port wine stain (PWS) birthmarks, infantile hemangiomas (IHs), venous malformations (VMs), telangiectasias and rosacea, cherry and spider angiomas, poikiloderma of Civatte, and angiokeratomas.

LIGHT DEVICES USED TO TREAT VASCULAR LESIONS

One of the first indications for the use of lasers in dermatologic surgery was for the treatment of vascular lesions. In 1968, the argon laser was one of the first lasers used to treat PWS and IH.[1] The argon laser is a continuous wave laser that produces blue-green light from 488 to 514 nm. The blue-green light is preferentially absorbed by its complementary color, red. It is thus absorbed by hemoglobin in the superficial vessels of vascular lesions.[2] It is this heating of the blood vessels that leads to thermal damage and thrombosis, which can be demonstrated on histology.[3] Although the argon laser, and other continuous and quasi-continuous wave lasers such as the copper vapor, krypton-ion, argon-pumped dye, and carbon dioxide lasers, improved the color of the vascular lesions, they also caused a large amount of nonselective heating due to long pulse durations and unwanted absorption by epidermal melanin. Scarring and dyspigmentation were common. These lasers are no longer used for treatment of vascular lesions, as the theory of selective photothermolysis revolutionized the use of lasers for treatment of skin lesions.

The theory of selective photothermolysis, defined in 1983 by Anderson and Parrish, comprises three governing principles.[4] The first principle is to select a wavelength that has a greater optical absorption by the target chromophore than by the surrounding tissue. Secondly, the pulse duration should be matched to the thermal relaxation time of the target chromophore. The thermal relaxation time is defined as the time required for the heat, which is generated within the chromophore by the absorbed light, to cool to one-half of the original temperature. The thermal relaxation time is directly proportional to the square of the diameter of the target and inversely proportional to the thermal diffusivity of the tissue. Larger target chromophores should be targeted with longer pulse durations, whereas smaller chromophores necessitate shorter pulse durations. Pulse durations that are longer than the thermal relaxation time of the target chromophore tend to create more heat than can be absorbed by the target chromophore. This extra heat diffuses away from the target chromophore and creates generalized nonselective heating of the surrounding tissue. The final principle is the need for a fluence that will treat the target chromophore, but will minimize nonspecific thermal related injury.[4] The chromophore classically targeted in selective photothermolysis of vascular lesions is oxyhemoglobin. Oxyhemoglobin has its peak absorptions at 418, 542, and 577 nm (Fig. 52-1). By targeting oxyhemoglobin, it is possible to transfer heat to the vessel walls, causing subsequent coagulation and destruction of the vessels.

The flashlamp-pumped pulsed-dye laser (PDL) was the first laser developed to treat vascular lesions on the basis of selective photothermolysis.[5] The first generations of PDLs had wavelengths of 577 or 585 nm and pulse durations of 0.3 to 0.5 ms.[6] The wavelength of 577 nm was originally chosen to correspond with the last peak in the absorption spectrum of the target chromophore, oxyhemoglobin (418, 542, and 577 nm).[4,7] This wavelength was found preferable to both lower absorption peaks, 418 and 542 nm, because it imparted a better penetration depth and less competi-

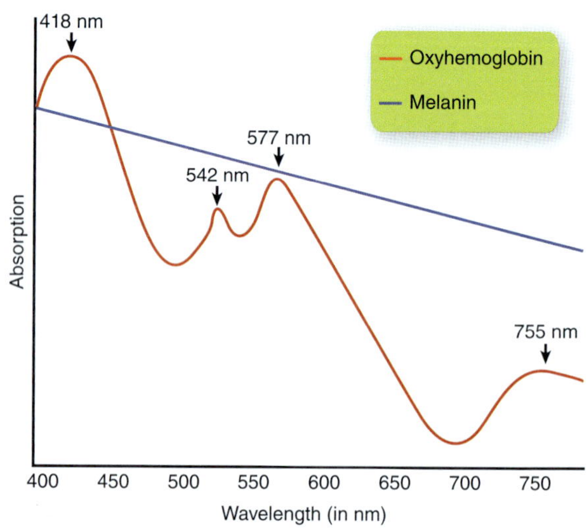

Figure 52-1 Schematic drawing of the absorption curve for oxyhemoglobin and melanin.

tive absorption with melanin. Melanin, the major competing chromophore, has its peak absorption in the UV range with decreasing absorption as the wavelength of light increases through the visible spectrum (Fig. 52-1).[8] Using shorter wavelengths that fall in the melanin absorption spectrum not only increases the risk of adverse events such as dyspigmentation secondary to melanin absorption, but also decreases efficacy by decreasing the amount of light that reaches the vessels in the dermis (longer wavelengths penetrate more deeply).[4]

Modification of the original PDL design gave rise to a number of later generation models that incorporated more flexible settings and included larger spot sizes, epidermal cooling, higher fluences, varying pulse durations, and longer wavelengths.[9] Spot size refers to the diameter of the emitted beam of light that hits the surface of the skin. Increasing spot size decreases the amount of scattering, allowing more light energy to penetrate to the target chromophore. Larger spot sizes also allow for faster treatment of large lesions.[10]

The addition of epidermal cooling to current generation PDLs allows for the use of higher fluences. Epidermal cooling decreases the temperature of the skin surface allowing light energy to pass through the epidermis without causing injury. Ideally the blood vessels in the dermis are not cooled and this allows light absorption with subsequent damage of the targeted vessels. Initially ice bags were applied to the skin in an attempt to impart epidermal cooling.[11] These attempts were messy and not very successful because the skin quickly reached a steady-state temperature, at which any decrease in the epidermal temperature was offset by a similar decrease in the temperature of the dermal blood vessels, preventing the desired injury to the target. In 1994, Nelson et al.[12] first introduced the concept of cryogen spray cooling. By applying a cryogen spray to the epidermis for a millisecond period of time, it is possible to cool the epidermis without affecting the temperature of the deeper vessels. Epidermal cooling allows for use of increased fluences without injury and thus, increased efficacy of laser treatment of vascular lesions. In addition, epidermal cooling improves patient comfort. Types of cooling devices now available include cryogen sprays,[12] contact cooling, and chilled air cooling.[13]

Current PDLs can have pulse durations which vary between 0.45 and 40 ms. Having the option to use longer pulse durations offers the advantage of being able to treat without purpura. Short pulse durations lead to rapid heating and can result in vessel rupture with associated bruising. The use of longer pulse durations, but not so long as to allow heating of tissue surrounding blood vessels, prolongs the delivery of energy over an extended period of time, allowing for more gentle heating of target vessels without sudden vessel rupture.[14] It was discovered that for selective photothermolysis to occur, wavelength does not have to correspond exactly with the absorption peak of the target chromophore, as long as preferential absorption is still present. Longer wavelengths such as 585 nm and subsequently 595 nm became preferable as these wavelengths penetrate more deeply and are more effective.[8]

One important limitation to the treatment of vascular lesions with PDL is that, even with longer wavelengths, yellow light cannot reach deep dermal vessels, as its maximum penetration ranges from 1 to 2 mm.[8] To treat these deeper vessels, near-infrared lasers, such as the alexandrite, diode and the neodymium:yttrium–aluminum–garnet (Nd:YAG) lasers, can be utilized. Each of these near-infrared lasers penetrates 50% to 75% more deeply in the skin than the PDL.[15] The 755 nm alexandrite laser has selective absorption peaks that correspond more closely with deoxyhemoglobin than with oxyhemoglobin, allowing the selective targeting of veins rather than arteries.[15] The 1064 nm Nd:YAG laser targets oxyhemoglobin in a manner similar to that of the PDL.[16] For these more deeply penetrating lasers, very high energies have to be used as they target a lower peak on the hemoglobin absorption curve (from 700 to 1200 nm). The energies required to obtain adequate oxyhemoglobin absorption at these wavelengths and the depth of penetration of these devices increase the risk for scarring, especially with the 1064 nm Nd:YAG laser.

An additional laser which may be used for the treatment of vascular lesions is the frequency doubled Nd:YAG laser, also known as the potassium titanyl phosphate (KTP) laser. To create the KTP laser, the light from the Nd:YAG laser is passed through a KTP crystal. Its wavelength of 532 nm can be used to target oxyhemoglobin at its 542 nm absorption peak (Fig. 52-1); however, its short wavelength limits its depth of penetration to less than that of the PDL. 532 nm also has higher melanin absorption, increasing the risk of dyspigmentation, especially in patients with darker skin types.

IPL is a noncoherent flashlamp device that produces light with wavelengths from 515 to 1200 nm with varying pulse durations. By using a selective light filter, it is possible to screen out shorter wavelengths of light and these devices may also be used to treat vascular lesions.

In the next section, we will review diagnostic criteria and suggested treatments for some specific vascular lesions.

CATEGORIZATION OF INFANT AND CHILDHOOD VASCULAR ANOMALIES

Mulliken and Glowacki[17] first categorized the differences between vascular anomalies of childhood and infancy in 1982 on the basis of differences in cell turnover, natural history, and histology. Using these criteria they were able to define two unique categories: vascular malformations and vascular tumors. In 1996, the International Society for the Study of Vascular Anomalies (ISSVA) updated this classification system (Table 52-1).[18]

Vascular malformations are vascular lesions comprised of dysplastic vessels which never involute or regress and have endothelium which shows normal mitotic activity.[19] They are categorized by a predominant vessel type, which can be any of the following: capillaries, veins, arteries, or lymphatics. However, many lesions have more than one type of vessel. Examples of capillary malformations include PWS are capillary malformations. These lesions may thicken over time. Progression is often gradual but may be accelerated by certain conditions such as pregnancy or trauma.

TABLE 52-1
Comparison of Vascular Tumors and Vascular Malformations

Vascular Tumors	Vascular Malformations
Infantile hemangioma Kaposiform Hemangioendothelioma	Port wine stains Venous malformation Lymphatic malformation Arterial malformation Arteriovenous malformation
Increased mitotic activity in endothelial cells	Normal endothelial cell mitotic activity
May be present at birth or arise shortly after	Present at birth
Rapid growth followed by rapid involution phase	Growth proportional with growth of child

Lesions that fall under the classification of "vascular tumors" are characterized by a growth phase of proliferating endothelial cells that can be seen as increased mitotic figures on pathology.[19] The prototypical vascular tumor is the IH. In IH, but not in all vascular tumors, this growth phase is subsequently followed by an involutional phase. This involution is due in part to a rapid decrease in the density of the endothelial cells. Once the tumor has completed its involution, only a few capillaries with thickened basement membranes remain. Other examples of vascular tumors include Kaposiform hemangioendothelioma and tufted angioma.

PORT WINE STAINS

PWSs are vascular malformations comprised of ectatic capillaries and postcapillary venules of the superficial capillary plexus. The greatest density of dilated vessels is in the upper 0.46 mm of the dermis.[20] The vessels range in size from 10 to 300 μm, and tend to increase in size as the patient ages.[20,21] These vessels are characterized by decreased vascular tone, and decreased density of autonomic nerves.[22]

PWSs occur in 0.3% of live births and are equally distributed among both sexes and all racial groups.[23] They usually arise sporadically, but familial cases and rare acquired cases have been described.[24] There are approximately 900,000 people in the United States and 20 million people worldwide with PWS.[23] While PWSs may be found anywhere on the body or in a segmental distribution, they are most commonly found on the head and neck. Their association with many congenital syndromes pinpoints their development to within the first 5 to 8 weeks of gestation.[25] Some of the syndromes that are associated with PWS, which are important to identify, include Sturge–Weber syndrome (SWS) (encephalotrigeminal angiomatosis) and Klippel–Trenaunay syndrome.

SWS is defined as a facial PWS, usually in the V1 distribution, in association with ipsilateral leptomeningeal vascular anomalies and ipsilateral choroidal vascular lesions with resultant glaucoma. The pathogenesis is incompletely understood at this time. Neurological presenting symptoms include seizures, which may be resistant to anticonvulsant therapy, hemiparesis, and hemiplegia.[26] Infants with a V1 distributed PWS should be evaluated by a neurologist familiar with this syndrome if SWS is suspected. Early testing may include ultrasound or electroencephalogram (EEG) and eventually magnetic resonance imaging (MRI) with and without contrast. If MRI is performed early, it should be repeated after 1 year of age to provide definitive information. Ocular involvement can present as glaucoma at birth, but pressures may also increase over time, so it is important to continue ophthalmologic examinations and monitor eye pressures, even if an initial examination is negative. Patients with bilateral PWS have a higher risk of SWS and a worse prognosis.[27]

Klippel–Trenaunay syndrome is a congenital syndrome characterized by the triad of an extremity PWS, lymphatic/venous malformation, and hypertrophy of soft tissues and/or bone.[28] Klippel–Trenaunay syndrome is considerably more common on the lower extremities as compared to the upper extremities, occurring there 85% of the time and only 15% of the time on the upper extremity. Eighty-five percent of cases are unilateral. As many as 10% of patients may have involvement of both the upper and lower extremities.[29] Evaluation may be done with ultrasonography, Doppler ultrasonography, MRI, and sometimes lymphoscintigraphy.

PWSs begin as well-demarcated, flat, light pink to red patches that tend to progressively darken to purple as the individual ages. By adulthood, they will often become raised and take on a more cobblestoned appearance due to the formation of vascular papules and nodules. These changes in color and texture may be attributed to the progressive ectasia of the dysplastic vascular plexus. One large study demonstrated that two-thirds of patients will have hypertrophy and nodularity by age 46 years.[30] The exact mechanisms for the progressive ectasia of PWS remain unclear. The most likely hypothesis suggests that it may result from an abnormality in neuronal control of the vasculature, which can be demonstrated by a decrease in neuronal mass found within these lesions. As a result of decreased neuronal control, the dysplastic vessels are unable to contract appropriately and therefore dilate over time. There are several medical complications that accompany the progressively dilating vessels of an aging PWS. These can include spontaneous bleeding and/or bleeding with minimal trauma, development of glaucoma, and hypertrophy of the underlying soft tissues.

In addition to medical complications, PWS can be associated with long-lasting detrimental effects on a child's psychological, social, interpersonal, and cognitive development.[31–33] Personality development can be adversely affected in children with PWS, secondary to the negative reaction of others.[34] For the above reasons, treatment should be initiated early and continued until acceptable cosmesis is achieved.

Many modalities for the treatment of PWS have been tried in the past, but most have met with only limited success. With advances in selective photothermolysis, laser therapy has become the gold standard for the treatment of PWS and is essentially the only acceptable treatment option for the vast majority of cases.

The PDL is the most commonly used laser to treat PWS. The goals of treatment are to decrease the red/violaceous color of the lesion, to prevent spontaneous bleeding, to prevent and reverse bleb formation, and to improve psychological discomfort. PDL is considered safe and effective with 80% of lesions showing improvement with treatment, although only 20% completely clear. Multiple treatments are needed.[35–37] One characteristic that makes a PWS less likely to respond to therapy is older patient age.[35,38,39] In a retrospective study of 133 patients, Fitzpatrick et al.[40] found 89.4% and 90% of patients with PWS aged 0 to 5 years and 6 to 10 years, respectively, had good or excellent responses as compared with 66.7% of those older than 50 years. We start treatments as soon as possible, ideally within a few weeks of age. The optical advantages to treating earlier in life include the presence of less melanin to compete for laser light absorption; less dermal collagen to cause backscattering of light out of the skin, and a thinner dermis which allows more light to reach the PWS vessels. Other predictors of poorer response include location on the trunk, distal extremity, or central face (medial cheek, upper lip, nose); violaceous color; and nodular surface.

To treat a PWS with PDL, the laser handpiece is guided across the affected area in a systematic fashion delivering pulses evenly across the surface using spot size of 7 to 12 mm. A variety of factors go into selection of treatment parameters, including lesion location, patient skin type, and the number and effect of previous treatments. As noted above, the larger the spot size the deeper the laser light will penetrate.[10] Therefore, using the largest spot size that allows sufficient fluence to achieve the desired endpoint is recommended. The thermal relaxation time for PWS blood vessels, which have a diameter of 50 to 300 μm, is calculated to be approximately 1 to 10 ms.[41,42] We generally use 0.45 or 1.5 ms. It is most important to watch tissue response and adjust settings based on observations. The outcome desired is immediate purpura (Fig. 52-2). A confluent gray color is a warning sign that the fluence is too high and epidermal injury may be occurring. Using a standard formula to determine settings is not recommended and can lead to complications.

PWSs are characterized by a large amount of vessel heterogeneity.[20] Using a variety of pulse durations, spot sizes and increasing radiant exposures with time (as long as epidermal injury is not occurring) will help to improve treatment response. When initiating therapy in a child, pulse durations and wavelengths should be shorter to target the small (30–50 μm) diameter vessels seen in pediatric PWS. Settings to consider include a 7 to 10 mm spot size, a pulse duration of 0.45 to 6 ms, and a fluence of 5.5 to 9.5 J/cm^2 with appropriate epidermal cooling. Lower energies are used with larger spot sizes. Longer pulse durations can improve safety in darker skin types, but may also limit lesion response. Parameters vary by device.

Short-term side effects that are expected after treatment include postoperative edema, erythema, and purpura. While edema and erythema generally resolve within 48 hours after treatment, the "bruising effect" may take up to 2 weeks to resolve completely. The decrease in the blood volume in the dermis that is achieved when treating PWS is seen clinically as lesional blanching. Unwanted side effects, such as dyspigmentation, may occur. Hyperpigmentation usually resolves in weeks or months. Hypopigmentation may indicate more serious damage to melanocytes, and while it may resolve, it can be permanent and should be avoided. Using longer pulse durations and appropriate epidermal cooling can help minimize pigmentary changes. Treatment intervals may need to be increased in patients with darker skin, to allow for resolution of pigmentary changes prior to additional procedures. Hair loss can occur and while it often resolves, it can be permanent, especially in pediatric patients with dark hair. Surgilube can be placed over eyebrows and eyelashes to prevent removal with the laser.

Almost all PWSs will lighten to some extent, but few will achieve complete clearance with PDL (Fig. 52-3). One study noted a 79% improvement with an average of 9 treatments.[43] Sessions are spaced 4 to 8 weeks apart.[44] It is common to require many (15 or more) sessions before reaching a plateau in fading or achieving the desired response. Even lesions that initially respond well to PDL may reach a plateau at which they become unresponsive to

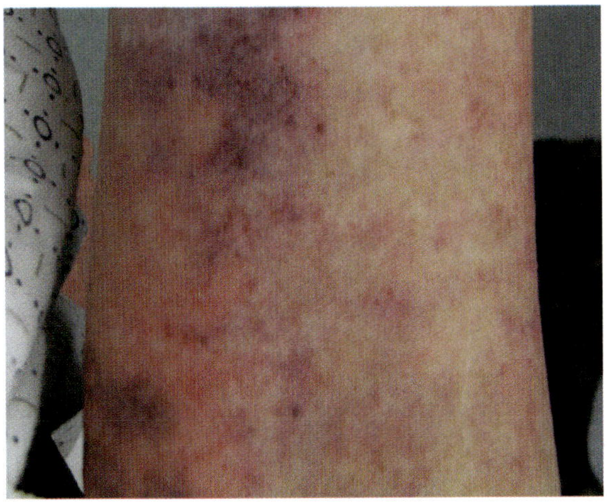

Figure 52-2 Appropriate immediate purpura with PDL.

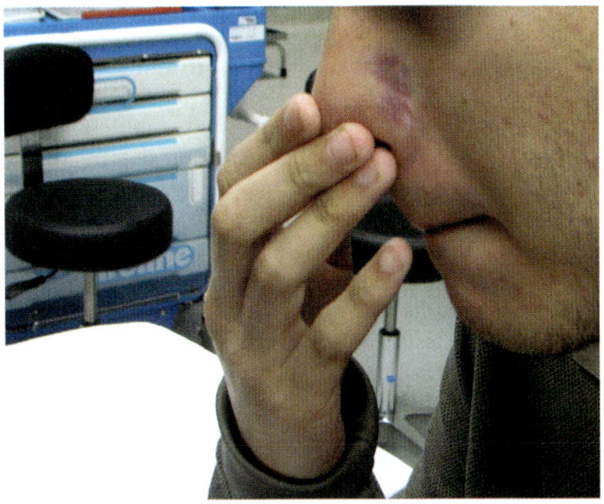

Figure 52-3 PWS resistant to PDL, some improvement with alexandrite laser, treatment ongoing.

further treatments, a phenomenon known as "treatment resistance."[16] Treatment resistance can be partially attributed to optical absorption and scattering which limits the penetration depth of the PDL to 1 to 2 mm, whereas many PWS can extend as deep as 3 to 5 mm.[8] In addition, hypertrophic and thickened PWS in adults may be less responsive to PDL.

Hypertrophic and thickened PWS may respond better to a long-pulsed 755 nm alexandrite laser. The 755 nm wavelength is preferentially absorbed by deoxyhemoglobin over oxyhemoglobin, allowing targeting of veins over arteries.[45] The desired end point is a subtle blue-gray discoloration that is followed after several minutes by a deeper purpura. A sustained gray color indicates that the fluence is too high with an associated risk of scarring. Side effects of the alexandrite laser are similar to those of the PDL with increased risk for permanent hair reduction and scarring due to deeper penetration. Clinicians using this laser to treat vascular lesions must be aware of the desired tissue response and must watch the treated areas closely to avoid complications.

The long-pulsed Nd:YAG laser (i.e., 1064 nm), another near-infrared laser, has a higher absorption coefficient for blood compared to the surrounding dermis. This property allows for laser penetration to blood vessels deeper in the dermis (>2 mm), making it another treatment option for hypertrophic PWS. However, unlike the 755 nm wavelength, the 1064 nm wavelength preferentially targets arteries over veins and has a narrow therapeutic window. Fluences of only 1.2 times that of the minimal purpuric dose can produce extensive deep dermal damage and result in scarring.[16] This narrow therapeutic window may be explained by the partial conversion of oxyhemoglobin to methemoglobin by the 1064 nm wavelength. Methemoglobin has a high absorption for light at 1064 nm and leads to a steep fluence–response curve. These devices should be used with caution for PWS.

Long-pulsed frequency doubled Nd:YAG lasers (i.e., 532 nm), also known as KTP lasers, have been shown to be effective for PDL-resistant PWS.[46] Dual wavelength systems combining 532 and 1064 nm lasers have also been proposed as treatment options. By using both wavelengths at fluences lower than their therapeutic thresholds, there is a lower-risk profile. Thus far, equivalent efficacy to KTP has been demonstrated with these lasers, with 30% less irradiant exposure at 532 nm.[47]

IPL has also been studied for the treatment of PDL-resistant PWS. In theory, IPL could achieve good results because longer pulse durations and multiple pulse sequences can be applied, allowing for the treatment of larger blood vessels which may be resistant to other devices. Furthermore, the range of IPL wavelengths should allow for the targeting of all the absorption peaks of oxyhemoglobin and the simultaneous treatment of both superficial and deep vessels.[48] Despite these theoretical considerations, a side-to-side study concluded that a single treatment of PDL remains superior to a single treatment of IPL for inducing lesion clearance.[49] However, one study did show that in treatment-resistant PWS not in the V2 distribution, approximately 50% of patients had greater than 50% reduction in their lesions with IPL.[50]

There are several other modalities being evaluated for treatment of PWS. Photodynamic therapy (PDT) has been utilized, especially in China. A vascular specific photosensitizer is administered intravenously to the patient and after a preselected time interval, during which the photosensitizer reaches the target tissue, light is applied that allows for specific absorption by the photosensitizer. A photochemical reaction occurs that results in generation of free radical species, causing irreversible damage to the target tissue. An advantage of PDT is the ability to treat all skin types. One disadvantage is that administration of the photosensitizer leads to skin photosensitization for 3 to 30 or more days, depending on the photosensitizer used. Combining photodynamic and photothermal injury has also been explored experimentally and may offer an improved treatment approach.[51]

Most recently, the combination of PDL therapy with posttreatment administration of agents that modify the wound healing response has been investigated. Imiquimod 5% cream applied 3 times per week for 8 weeks immediately after PDL therapy was shown to enhance treatment response. Therapy was well tolerated with only minor irritation reported.[52] Rapamycin (RPM) is a specific inhibitor of mammalian mTOR, which has antiangiogenic properties via the downregulation of hypoxia-inducible factor (HIF-1α). Phase I trials with oral RPM plus PDL showed promising results,[53] leading to the development of topical formulations to reduce risks associated with systemic drug exposure. Topical formulations used in combination with PDL on normal skin also demonstrated inhibition of regrowth and neo-angiogenesis of blood vessels.[54]

INFANTILE HEMANGIOMAS

IH is the most common benign vascular tumor of children. These lesions arise in 1% to 3% of neonates,[23] and can affect up to 10% of infants within the first year of life.[55,56] While some IH may be present at birth, most arise within the first 2 to 3 weeks of life and then rapidly enlarge (Fig. 52-4). This is in contrast to vascular malformations, which are present at birth and expand only in concordance with the child's growth. They may be either superficial (capillary), deep (cavernous), or a mixture of the two. Superficial lesions, which involve the papillary dermis, appear as bright

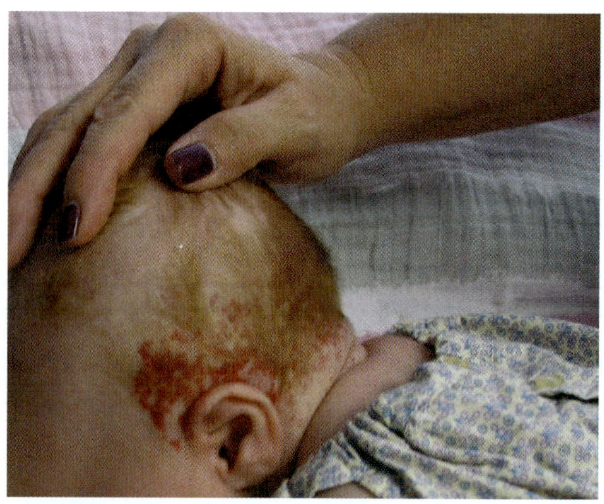

Figure 52-4 Infantile hemangioma in a 1 month-old infant.

red papules, plaques, or nodules. Deeper lesions, occurring in the reticular dermis or subcutaneous fat, with little to no involvement of the overlying papillary dermis, appear as flesh colored or bluish subcutaneous nodules. The incidence of IHs is inversely proportional to gestational age at birth, with higher incidences occurring in premature infants.[57,58] They are also much more commonly found in females with almost a 3:1 ratio over males. They may occur anywhere on the skin but the head and neck are the most common locations. IHs can be differentiated from other vascular tumors and vascular malformations by their GLUT-1 expression. GLUT-1 is a fetal-type endothelial glucose transporter.[59] Two rare types of GLUT-1 negative hemangiomas, which may also be present at or soon after birth are noninvoluting hemangiomas (NICHs) and rapidly involuting hemangiomas (RICHs).

The natural history of IH is to progress through three stages: a growth stage which generally occurs over the first 5 to 6 months of life, a stable phase, and a slower regression phase. As a general rule of thumb, IHs regress at a rate of approximately 10% per year. For example, 30% will have regressed by age 3, 50% by age 5, and 90% by age 9.[60] Speed of regression has not been found to correlate with lesion size, number of lesions, site, or age at first appearance.[60] The earliest sign of regression is white streaks of fibrosis appearing on the surface of the lesion. After regression, many IHs will leave behind fibro-fatty tissue, atrophy, and telangiectasia.[19]

Most patients have only a single lesion, but up to 15% to 20% of patients will have multiple lesions. The presence of three or more IHs has been associated with visceral involvement, and has been referred to as diffuse neonatal hemangiomatosis.[61] Ultrasound and MRI imaging may be useful for detecting visceral lesions in a patient with multiple cutaneous lesions. It may also be useful to check a fecal occult blood, which can detect GI tract involvement. The organs most commonly affected are the gastrointestinal tract, brain, liver, and lung. Complications include high-output cardiac failure, gastrointestinal bleeding, hydrocephalus, and consumption coagulopathy. The mortality rate remains very high for these patients and usually results from high-output cardiac failure. Some infants may have multiple cutaneous IHs, but no evidence of visceral involvement, in which case benign neonatal hemangiomatosis can be diagnosed.[62] These infants tend to follow a benign course.

In patients with large facial hemangiomas, PHACE syndrome must be considered. PHACE is an acronym for a neurocutaneous syndrome consisting of posterior fossa malformations of the brain, large facial hemangiomas, arterial anomalies, cardiac anomalies, aortic coarctation, and eye abnormalities. If the child also has ventral midline defects, such as sternal clefting and/or a supraumbilical raphe, then PHACE syndrome becomes PHACES syndrome.[63] PHACE syndrome has a striking female predominance. Approximately 70% of the infants with PHACE syndrome have no more than one extracutaneous malformation.[64,65] Children with large facial hemangiomas should have, at minimum, appropriate CNS imaging studies and a cardiac evaluation.

Many questions have been raised about the need to treat IHs due to their natural tendency to involute.[66] Historically, most lesions have been treated conservatively with watchful waiting, reserving aggressive treatments for lesions that develop complications, such as infection, ulceration, or bleeding, and for those that impair vital functions (blocking vision, obstructing the airway, obstructing the auditory canal), and for those at sites that may develop significant deformity following involution. More recently, however, it has been shown that early treatment may prevent scarring as well as the psychological consequences that may arise if the lesions are allowed to run their natural course. Lesions in cosmetically sensitive areas should be strongly considered for early treatment and include lesions on the nose, glabella, lips, and especially in females, the chest. Treatment should be tailored to each patient by taking into consideration the depth and size of the lesion, as well as any functional impairment that it may cause. Treatment options include topical treatments, intralesional corticosteroids, β-blocker systemic therapy, laser, and surgical excision. Some combination of the above may provide the best overall response.

Topical treatments for IHs include high-potency topical steroids, topical timolol, and possibly topical imiquimod. Superpotent topical steroids have shown some efficacy for the treatment of small, superficial IH and have mostly been studied in the periocular region. Disadvantages include possible systemic absorption, cutaneous atrophy, and limited penetration limiting effectiveness (especially if the lesion has a deep component).[67] Topical timolol gel, twice a day for 16 weeks, has recently been reported to be effective in the treatment of superficial IHs of the head and neck.[68,69] Rare reports of systemic adverse events, including wheezing, respiratory distress, and bradycardia, have been noted. These events are more likely to occur when using topical timolol over an extended time period or over a widespread area.[70] In addition, the ophthalmic solution has significantly higher systemic bioavailability when compared to gel formulation.[71] Imiquimod has shown some efficacy for the treatment of superficial uncomplicated hemangiomas, but its use is controversial. Efficacy has not been studied in mixed or complicated hemangiomas.[72]

Ulceration is the most common complication in IHs and occurs in 5% to 15% of lesions, generally during the proliferative phase.[73,74] Ulcerated hemangiomas may be treated with topical wound care, topical barrier creams, topical antibiotics, topical becaplermin gel (a recombinant human platelet–derived growth factor),[75] and occlusive dressings. Lasers may also be very useful for treatment of ulcerated hemangiomas (see next page).

Systemic treatments are indicated when functions are threatened (for example vision, breathing), when lesion progression will be disfiguring, when there is significant ulceration or there is associated morbidities such as congestive heart failure. Historically, oral steroids were the treatment of choice for these IHs; however, they are associated with many side effects including adrenal suppression, growth suppression, cataract development, osteoporosis, and increased infection risk.[76] Propranolol was first reported as efficacious for the treatment of IHs by Léauté-Labrèze et al.[77] in 2008; since this time it has become a first-line option for the treatment of IH. However, close monitoring for bradycardia, hypotension, bronchospasm, and hypoglycemia is required.In addition, β-blockers may blunt the signs of high-output cardiac failure that can be associated with large or miliary hemangiomas.[78] The level of monitoring required when starting propranolol is controversial, and hospitalization for the first 48 to 72 hours of therapy is standard at some centers.[79] Contraindications for use include history of bronchospasm or asthma, cardiac disease, and CNS vascular anomalies (such as those associated with PHACE syndrome). Propranolol can be used but should be approached with caution in patients with diabetes mellitus and chronic renal insufficiency.[80,81]

The role of lasers for the treatment of IHs is controversial and accurate efficacy rates are difficult to determine. Superficial lesions respond better to laser treatment than mixed and deeper lesions. PDL is the most commonly used device for treatment of IHs. The long-pulsed PDL at 595 nm showed, in several uncontrolled studies, quicker resolution and improved clinical clearance with significantly lower rates of adverse events when compared to the 585 nm.[82,83] A randomized trial compared a group treated with a 585 nm PDL without epidermal cooling to a group treated with a 595 nm PDL with cryogen spray cooling. In this trial, while almost the same number of children had complete to almost complete clearing at 1 year (~60%), children in the group treated with the 595 nm PDL with dynamic cooling were found to have significantly shorter times of maximum proliferation (106 vs. 177 days) and lower risk for laser-induced adverse events such as hyperpigmentation, hypopigmentation, and atrophy.[84] More recently, a retrospective study noted that combination propranolol and PDL demonstrated greater improvement over propranolol alone. Patients who were treated with combination therapy demonstrated greater overall fading and obtained clearance over a shorter period of time (150 vs. 228 days) than those treated with propranolol alone. In addition, propranolol alone tended to leave residual superficial hemangioma that responded well to PDL therapy, either concurrently or subsequently to propranolol treatment.[85]

Settings for the treatment of IHs with the 595 nm PDL should be selected based on multiple patient factors. First, the stage of the lesion, proliferating versus involuting, will affect the settings selected. PDL treatment for proliferating IHs should be approached cautiously, with lower fluences, as this will minimize risk for ulceration that can result in scarring. Lower fluences and longer pulse durations should be used in darker skinned patients. Epidermal cooling should always be used. Parameters vary by device. Multiple treatments are usually required. For proliferating and ulcerated lesions, treatments can be spaced approximately 2 to 4 weeks apart. For stable and involuting lesions, treatments can be every 4 to 6 weeks.

The most common side effect of treatment is bruising and/or temporary local swelling. Other risks of treatment include ulceration, scarring, and hypopigmentation. Using appropriate epidermal cooling and avoiding excessively high fluences minimize the risk of ulceration and bleeding.[86] In addition, patients with diffuse segmental hemangiomas should be approached with extra caution as they may be at increased risk for adverse effects.[67,86]

The use of PDL for the treatment of ulceration has been supported by several uncontrolled trials and is generally regarded as effective. Goals of treatment for ulcerated IHs include decreasing pain, decreasing bleeding, and decreasing risk of infection by inducing re-epithelialization of the skin. PDL has even been shown to induce healing as early as after one treatment session.[87,88] Pain levels were shown to dramatically improve in these studies; for example all nine patients treated by Morelli et al.[87] showed improvement in their pain levels. David et al.[89] showed 91% improvement with a mean of 2 treatments in 78 patients with ulcerated hemangiomas.

Laser treatment is also used to improve the appearance of involuted hemangiomas with residual lesion. PDL may help to improve the redness and telangiectasia that remains after involution.[90] Fractionated ablative and nonablative lasers can be added to improve the appearance of remaining fibro-fatty residua and epidermal atrophy, and to reduce redundant skin.[91,92]

Other light-based devices which have been used to treat IHs include the frequency doubled Nd:YAG (KTP) and IPL. The KTP laser was compared to the PDL in 50 infants with superficial IHs and was found to have fewer side effects and to cause less pain, but also demonstrated lower efficacy than the PDL.[93] IPL has demonstrated efficacy for the treatment of both centrofacial hemangiomas and ulcerated hemangiomas.[94] One case report noted re-epithelialization and pain control in an ulcerated hemangioma after one IPL treatment.[95]

VENOUS MALFORMATIONS

Venous malformations clinically present as soft, compressible, nonpulsatile blue-violaceous papules and nodules. They are slow-flow malformations that are present at birth (although not always clinically apparent at birth) and slowly enlarge throughout life. Venous malformations are nonproliferating, vascular birthmarks caused by localized errors in the embryologic formation of the venous system. Histologically, there are collections of abnormal venous channels with vessel walls that are commonly calcified. Most are solitary, but 1% of patients will have multiple lesions, especially if they are associated with familial venous malformation syndromes, including familial cutaneous and mucosal venous malformation syndrome and blue rubber bleb nevus syndrome, which are caused by a mutation in VMCM1 on chromosome 9p21, resulting in a gain of function in the tyrosine kinase receptor, TIE2.[96] Symptoms are related to the size and the location of the lesion and can include pain, functional impairment, and bleeding. MRI can be utilized to determine the extent of the lesion.[97]

Treatment options include surgical resection, sclerotherapy, and percutaneous or intralesional laser therapy. Recurrence rates with sclerotherapy and laser therapy alone are high; thus, if feasible, these treatments should be followed by surgical excision of all or large parts of the remaining lesion.[98] Due to the deep nature of these lesions, lasers in the infrared spectrum which have deeper penetration, such as diode or Nd:YAG lasers, are utilized when laser therapy is pursued. Benefits of the Nd:YAG laser include increased fibrosis in the upper dermis, tissue shrinkage, and improved color, all of which may increase the effectiveness of subsequent sclerotherapy and/or surgical excision, while decreasing side effects, include tissue swelling, blistering, scarring, and discoloration.[99] Treatment of these lesions should be approached by an experienced multidisciplinary team.

Fitzpatrick skin type	
I	Always burns, never tans
II	Usually burns, minimally tans
III	Sometimes burns, moderately tans
IV	Seldom burns, tans easily
V	Rarely burns, tans profusely
VI	Never burns, deeply pigmented

For darker skin types consider: hydroquinone 4% QHS prior to procedure (hold for irritation)

Step 1: Initial consultation - At the initial consultation make diaganosis, discuss treatment options, and determine skin type. Before treatment appointment, patient should use good sun protection. If patient has a tan, treament should be delayed as this increases risk for hyperpigmentation, blistering and scarring.

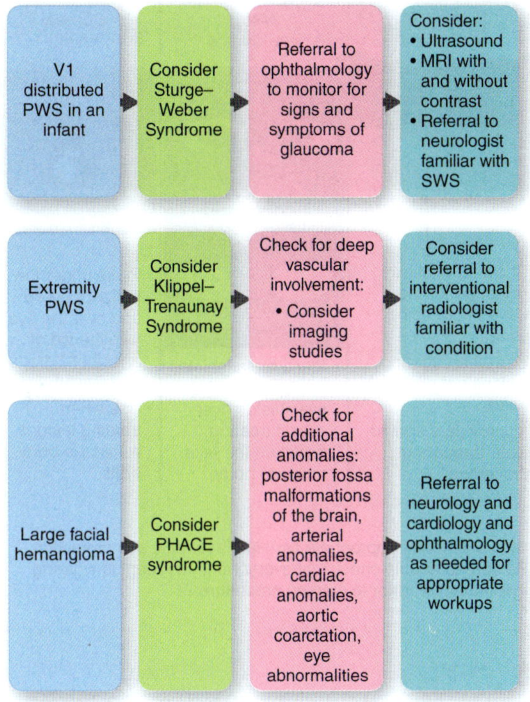

Step 2: If at the initial workup there is concern for a syndrome or additional abnormalities, initiate additional workup.

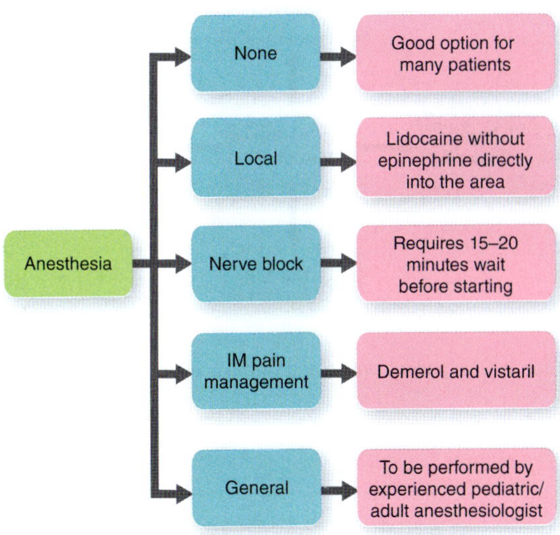

Step 3: Discuss and personalize anethesia for patient

Expected tissue response
Sunburn type pain
Bruising
Swelling

Unexpected tissue response
Infection
Blistering
Hypopigmentation
Scarring

Step 4: Consent for treatment

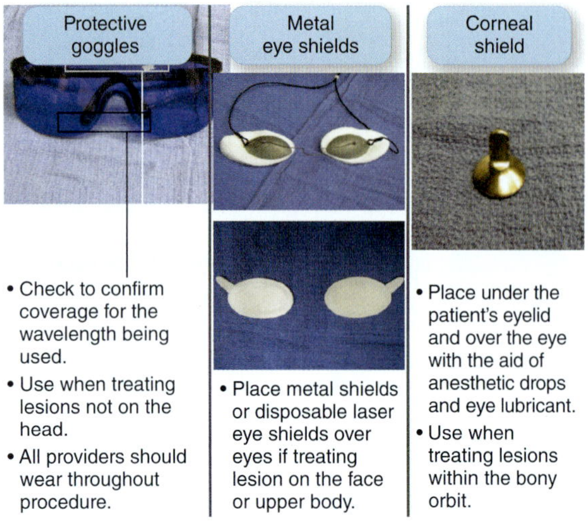

Step 5: Choose appropriate certified laser safe eye protection. Be sure to double check that everyone in the room is wearing eye protection prior to starting procedure.

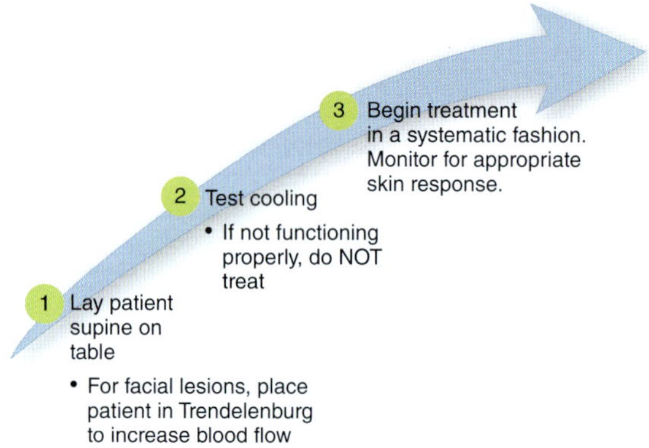

Step 6: Starting treatment

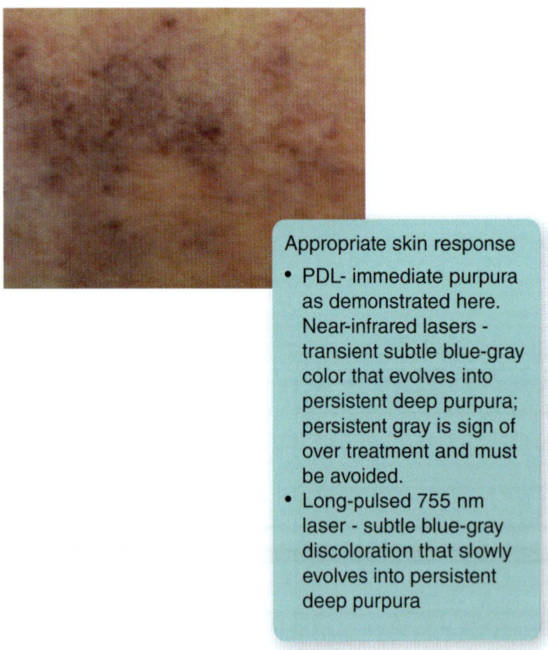

Step 7: Guide handpiece over lesion in a systematic fashion, being sure to treat the lesion evenly. Monitor for appropriate skin response.

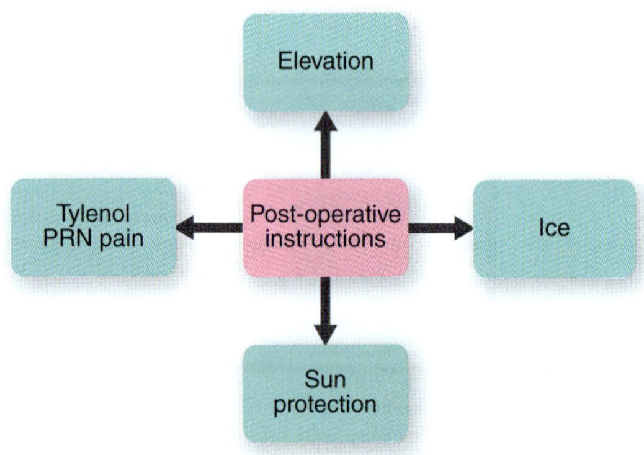

Step 8: Give patient written and verbal post-operative instructions

TELANGIECTASIAS AND ROSACEA

Telangiectasias are small 0.1 to 1 mm superficial dilated vessels visible on the skin. They can appear spontaneously, but they most often arise secondary to other conditions. Causes of telangiectasias include chronic photodamage, rosacea, connective tissue disease, liver disease, radiation, genodermatoses (i.e., hereditary hemorrhagic telangiectasia syndrome, ataxia–telangiectasia) and chronic topical steroid use. Patients with large numbers of telangiectasias and patients with rosacea will often present with complaints of diffuse facial redness.

Treatment is not required for telangiectasias unless they are cosmetically distressing for the patient. Removal is most effectively accomplished with electrocautery, IPL, and lasers. Commonly used lasers include PDL and KTP. Spot sizes and shapes (round vs. elliptical) can be adjusted and treatment should be tailored to each patient taking into consideration the vessel caliber, patient's skin type, and the patient's tolerance of purpura. In the cosmetic patient, purpura may be unacceptable. However, subpurpuric fluences are less effective than purpuric fluences for the treatment of facial telangiectasias[100,101] and more treatments are generally required. Multiple passes and carefully used pulse stacking can improve the efficacy of treatment with subpurpuric fluences.[102,103] By delivering additional pulses before the target has time to cool to its original temperature, target temperature is slowly increased without causing vessel rupture. Pulse stacking can be used with some settings but clinician should watch skin carefully for evidence of epidermal injury. PDL settings to consider include a 7 to 10 mm spot size, 6 ms pulse duration, and fluence of 6 to 9 J/cm^2 with epidermal cooling. Lower energies are used with larger spot sizes. Lower fluences should be used in patients with intense facial erythema and in patients with darker skin types. Longer pulse durations should also be selected in patients with darker skin types. Parameters vary by device. End points to look for on the skin when treating telangiectasias include vessel clearance, bluish coagulum, transient purpura, or purpura. Expected side effects include erythema and facial swelling. A cold pack can be applied post treatment to minimize swelling, and the patient can be instructed to sleep with their head elevated to minimize swelling.

KTP and IPL lasers have also demonstrated efficacy for the treatment of facial telangiectasias. Multiple studies have supported the efficacy of KTP for the treatment of these lesions, which also causes less swelling, pain, bruising, and redness than PDL.[104,105] KTP can be used to trace individual vessels. Because of the greater competition with melanin at 532 nm, caution must be taken in patients with darker skin types. Nd:YAG may also be used to treat larger vessels, reticular facial veins, and refractory telangiectasias, but the therapeutic window is narrow and there is a greater risk of scarring.

The background erythema associated with rosacea may be treated before or after the telangiectasias. Laser treatment of rosacea may relieve symptoms of burning and stinging[106] and may also decrease the papular and pustular components of rosacea.[107] In some patients, antibiotic doses may be decreased after 1 to 3 PDL sessions.[108] Intermittent maintenance treatments are necessary to maintain improvement, as light therapy tends to be effective, but is not a cure.

CHERRY ANGIOMAS

Cherry angiomas are the most common vascular lesions of the skin. They are benign lesions that are highly responsive to laser therapy, although they may also be treated with electrodesiccation or shave excision. They are most commonly treated with PDL; however, IPL and KTP may also be used. Only one treatment is usually required to achieve complete clearance (purpura is the end point) but large or resistant lesions may require multiple treatments. To improve efficacy for larger lesions, the first pulse can be delivered while performing diascopy (compressing the lesion with a glass slide). This will allow for treatment of the deeper component of the lesion. If purpura does not develop after the first pulse, a second pulse may then be delivered without diascopy to treat the more superficial vasculature. Spider angiomas may also be treated in this manner. Settings to consider for the PDL include a 5 to 7 mm spot size, 1.5 ms pulse duration, and fluences from 7 to 10 J/cm^2 with appropriate epidermal cooling. Settings vary by device used, and should be adjusted for patients with darker skin types.

POIKILODERMA OF CIVATTE

Poikiloderma of Civatte is a variant of telangiectasia presenting in sun-exposed skin that is associated with symmetrical atrophy and pigmentary irregularities, usually affecting the upper chest, lateral neck, and occasionally the lateral cheeks. Characteristically, it spares the area shaded by the chin. When treating poikiloderma of Civatte, it is important to treat the pigmentary and textural changes in addition to the telangiectasias. PDL has shown acceptable results,[109] but the neck is a sensitive area and needs to be approached with caution and experience, as there is the risk of mottling of the skin due to uneven overlap of the circular spots, and rarely, scarring. Multiple treatment sessions are almost always needed.[110,111] IPL may be a more appropriate choice in patients with significant hyperpigmentation and erythema, since it can simultaneously target both the vascular and pigmentary components.

ANGIOKERATOMAS

Angiokeratomas are superficial ectatic vessels with overlying hyperkeratosis. They commonly appear as asymptomatic 2 to 5 mm blue to red papules. They can be categorized into localized and systemic forms. Localized forms include: (1) solitary lesions usually found on the lower extremities, (2) the Fordyce type localized to the genitals, (3) angioma circumscriptum, and (4) the Mibelli type inherited in an autosomal dominant manner and occurring primarily on the dorsal hands and feet. The generalized systemic type, known as angiokeratoma corporis diffusum, is usually associated with metabolic disorders, most commonly Fabry disease, an X-linked recessive syndrome secondary to a deficiency of α-galactosidase

A, and fucosidosis. These lesions generally do not require treatment; however, patients may request removal secondary to bleeding, discomfort, or for cosmesis. PDL, IPL, and Nd:YAG have all been found to be effective for angiokeratomas, although it is important to note that scarring may occur and several sessions may be required to penetrate the hyperkeratotic epidermis overlying these lesions.[112,113] To overcome this hyperkeratosis, ablative lasers such as the CO_2 or the erbium laser may be utilized but will result in scarring. Ablative lasers followed by PDL can also be utilized.[114]

CONCLUSIONS

There are many different types of vascular lesions, and knowledge of diagnostic criteria and of the characteristics of the vessels composing these lesions is imperative to determine the best treatment options and ensure good outcomes. Many advances have been made in the removal of vascular lesions, and light-based therapy is a good option in many cases. Clinicians using lasers to treat vascular lesions must be aware of laser–tissue interactions, appropriate settings for the device they are utilizing, and desired tissue endpoints. Larger prospective, comparative, and controlled clinical studies are still needed to lead to better solutions for recalcitrant vascular lesions.

ACKNOWLEDGMENT

Dr. Kelly has received research equipment from Light Sciences Oncology, CoolTouch and Asclepion and has served as a consultant for Pierre Fabre.

REFERENCES

1. Arndt KA. Treatment techniques in argon laser therapy. *J Am Acad Dermatol.* 1984;11(1):90–97.
2. Cosman B. Experience in the argon laser therapy of port wine stains. *Plast Reconstr Surg.* 1980;65(2):119–129.
3. Apfelberg DB, Kosek J, Maser MR, Lash H. Histology of port wine stains following argon laser treatment. *Br J Plast Surg.* 1979;32(3):232–237.
4. Anderson RR, Parrish JA. Selective photothermolysis: precise microsurgery by selective absorption of pulsed radiation. *Science.* 1983;220(4596):524–527.
5. Garden JM, Polla LL, Tan OT. The treatment of port-wine stains by the pulsed dye laser. Analysis of pulse duration and long-term therapy. *Arch Dermatol.* 1988;124(6):889–896.
6. Levine VJ, Geronemus RG. Adverse effects associated with the 577- and 585-nanometer pulsed dye laser in the treatment of cutaneous vascular lesions: a study of 500 patients. *J Am Acad Dermatol.* 1995;32(4):613–617.
7. Anderson RR, Parrish JA. The optics of human skin. *J Invest Dermatol.* 1981;77(1):13–19.
8. Tan OT, Murray S, Kurban AK. Action spectrum of vascular specific injury using pulsed irradiation. *J Invest Dermatol.* 1989;92(6):868–871.
9. Lanigan SW, Taibjee SM. Recent advances in laser treatment of port-wine stains. *Br J Dermatol.* 2004;151(3):527–533.
10. Keijzer M, Pickering JW, van Gemert MJ. Laser beam diameter for port wine stain treatment. *Lasers Surg Med.* 1991;11(6):601–605.
11. Gilchrest BA, Rosen S, Noe JM. Chilling port wine stains improves the response of argon laser thearpy. *Plast Reconstr Surg.* 1982;69:278–283.
12. Nelson JS, Milner TE, Anvari B, et al. Dynamic epidermal cooling during pulsed laser treatment of port-wine stain. A new methodology with preliminary clinical evaluation. *Arch Dermatol.* 1995;131(6):695–700.
13. Raulin C, Greve B, Hammes S. Cold air in laser therapy: first experiences with a new cooling system. *Lasers Surg Med.* 2000;27(5):404–410.
14. Garden JM, Tan OT, Kerschmann R, et al. Effect of dye laser pulse duration on selective cutaneous vascular injury. *J Invest Dermatol.* 1986;87(5):653–657.
15. Izikson L, Nelson JS, Anderson RR. Treatment of hypertrophic and resistant port wine stains with a 755 nm laser: a case series of 20 patients. *Lasers Surg Med.* 2009;41(6):427–432.
16. Yang MU, Yaroslavsky AN, Farinelli WA, et al. Long-pulsed neodymium: yttrium-aluminum-garnet laser treatment for port-wine stains. *J Am Acad Dermatol.* 2005;52(3 Pt 1):480–490.
17. Mulliken JB, Glowacki J. Hemangiomas and vascular malformations in infants and children: a classification based on endothelial characteristics. *Plast Reconstr Surg.* 1982;69 (3):412–422.
18. Enjolras O, Mulliken JB. Vascular tumors and vascular malformations (new issues). *Adv Dermatol.* 1997;13:375–423.
19. Enjolras O. Vascular tumors and vascular malformations: are we at the dawn of a better knowledge? *Pediatr Dermatol.* 1999;16(3):238–241.
20. Barsky SH, Rosen S, Geer DE, Noe JM. The nature and evolution of port wine stains: a computer-assisted study. *J Invest Dermatol.* 1980;74(3):154–157.
21. Lever WF, Elder DE. *Lever's Histopathology of the Skin.* 10th ed. Philadelphia, PA: Lippincott Williams & Wilkins; 2009.
22. Smoller BR, Rosen S. Port-wine stains. A disease of altered neural modulation of blood vessels? *Arch Dermatol.* 1986; 122(2):177–179.
23. Jacobs AH Walton RG. The incidence of birthmarks in the neonate. *Pediatrics.* 1976.58(2):218–222.
24. Adams BB, Lucky AW. Acquired port-wine stains and antecedent trauma: case report and review of the literature. *Arch Dermatol.* 2000;136(7):897–899.
25. Thomas-Sohl KA, Vaslow DF, Maria BL. Sturge-Weber syndrome: a review. *Pediatr Neurol.* 2004;30(5):303–310.
26. Mazereeuw-Hautier J, Syed S, Harper JI. Bilateral facial capillary malformation associated with eye and brain abnormalities. *Arch Dermatol.* 2006;142(8):994–998.
27. Enjolras O, Riche MC, Merland JJ. Facial port-wine stains and Sturge-Weber syndrome. *Pediatrics.* 1985;76(1):48–51.
28. Redondo P, Aguado L, Martinez-Cuesta A. Diagnosis and management of extensive vascular malformations of the lower limb: part I. Clinical diagnosis. *J Am Acad Dermatol.* 2011; 65(5):893–906; quiz 907–908.
29. Gloviczki P, Hollier LH, Telander RL, Kaufman B, Bianco AJ, Stickler GB. Surgical implications of Klippel-Trenaunay syndrome. *Ann Surg.* 1983;197(3):353–362.
30. Geronemus RG, Ashinoff R. The medical necessity of evaluation and treatment of port-wine stains. *J Dermatol Surg Oncol.* 1991;17(1):76–79.
31. Wagner KD, Wagner RF Jr. The necessity for treatment of childhood port-wine stains. *Cutis.* 1990;45(5):317–318.
32. Malm M, Carlberg M. Port-wine stain–a surgical and psychological problem. *Ann Plast Surg.* 1988;20(6):512–516.
33. Lanigan SW, Cotterill JA. Psychological disabilities amongst patients with port wine stains. *Br J Dermatol.* 1989;121(2): 209–215.
34. Heller A, Rafman S, Zvagulis I, Pless IB. Birth defects and psychosocial adjustment. *Am J Dis Child.* 1985;139(3):257–263.
35. Reyes BA, Geronemus R. Treatment of port-wine stains during childhood with the flashlamp-pumped pulsed dye laser. *J Am Acad Dermatol.* 1990;23(6 Pt 1):1142–1148.
36. Orten SS, Waner M, Flock S, Roberson PK, Kincannon J. Port-wine stains. An assessment of 5 years of treatment. *Arch Otolaryngol Head Neck Surg.* 1996;122(11):1174–1179.
37. Fiskerstrand EJ, Svaasand LO, Kopstad G, Dalaker M, Norvang LT, Volden G. Laser treatment of port wine stains: therapeutic outcome in relation to morphological parameters. *Br J Dermatol.* 1996;134(6):1039–1043.
38. Tan OT, Sherwood K, Gilchrest BA, Treatment of children with port-wine stains using the flashlamp-pulsed tunable dye-laser. *N Engl J Med.* 1989;320(7):416–421.

39. Morelli JG, Weston WL, Huff JC, Yohn JJ. Initial lesion size as a predictive factor in determining the response of port-wine stains in children treated with the pulsed dye-laser. *Arch Pediatr Adolesc Med*. 1995;149(10):1142–1144.
40. Fitzpatrick RE, Lowe NJ, Goldman MP, Borden H, Behr KL, Ruiz-Esparza J. Flashlamp-pumped pulsed dye laser treatment of port-wine stains. *J Dermatol Surg Oncol*. 1994;20(11):743–748.
41. Van Gemert MJ, Welch AJ, Amin AP. Is there an optimal laser treatment for port wine stains? *Lasers Surg Med*. 1986;6(1):76–83.
42. Van Gemert MJ, Welch AJ. Treatment of port-wine stains - analysis. *Med Instrum*. 1987;21(4):213–217.
43. Alster TS, Wilson F. Treatment of port-wine stains with the flashlamp-pumped pulsed dye laser: extended clinical experience in children and adults. *Ann Plast Surg*. 1994;32(5):478–484.
44. Katugampola GA, Lanigan SW. Five years' experience of treating port wine stains with the flashlamp-pumped pulsed dye laser. *Br J Dermatol*. 1997;137(5):750–754.
45. Li L, Kono T, Groff WF, Chan HH, Kitazawa Y, Nozaki M. Comparison study of a long-pulse pulsed dye laser and a long-pulse pulsed alexandrite laser in the treatment of port wine stains. *J Cosmet Laser Ther*. 2008;10(1):12–15.
46. Chowdhury MM, Harris S, Lanigan SW. Potassium titanyl phosphate laser treatment of resistant port-wine stains. *Br J Dermatol*. 2001;144(4):814–817.
47. Ahcan U, Zorman P, Recek D, Ralca S, Majaron B. Port wine stain treatment with a dual-wavelength Nd:Yag laser and cryogen spray cooling: a pilot study. *Lasers Surg Med*. 2004;34(2):164–167.
48. Raulin C, Schroeter CA, Weiss RA, Keiner M, Werner S. Treatment of port-wine stains with a noncoherent pulsed light source: a retrospective study. *Arch Dermatol*. 1999;135(6):679–683.
49. Faurschou A, Togsverd-Bo K, Zachariae C, Haedersdal M. Pulsed dye laser vs. intense pulsed light for port-wine stains: a randomized side-by-side trial with blinded response evaluation. *Br J Dermatol*. 2009;160(2):359–364.
50. Bjerring P, Christiansen K, Troilius A. Intense pulsed light source for the treatment of dye laser resistant port-wine stains. *J Cosmet Laser Ther*. 2003;5(1):7–13.
51. Tournas JA, Lai J, Truitt A, et al. Combined benzoporphyrin derivative monoacid ring photodynamic therapy and pulsed dye laser for port wine stain birthmarks. *Photodiagnosis Photodyn Ther*. 2009;6(3–4):195–199.
52. Tremaine AM, Armstrong J, Huang YC, et al. Enhanced port-wine stain lightening achieved with combined treatment of selective photothermolysis and imiquimod. *J Am Acad Dermatol*. 2012;66(4):634–641.
53. Nelson JS, Jia W, Phung TL, Mihm MC Jr. Observations on enhanced port wine stain blanching induced by combined pulsed dye laser and rapamycin administration. *Lasers Surg Med*. 2011;43(10):939–942.
54. Loewe R, Oble DA, Valero T, Zukerberg L, Mihm MC Jr, Nelson JS. Stem cell marker upregulation in normal cutaneous vessels following pulsed-dye laser exposure and its abrogation by concurrent rapamycin administration: implications for treatment of port-wine stain birthmarks. *J Cutan Pathol*. 2010;37(Suppl 1):76–82.
55. Holmdahl K. Cutaneous hemangiomas in premature and mature infants. *Acta Paediatr*. 1955;44(4):370–379.
56. Jacobs AH. Strawberry hemangiomas; the natural history of the untreated lesion. *Calif Med*. 1957;86(1):8–10.
57. Amir J, Metzker A, Krikler R, Reisner SH. Strawberry hemangioma in preterm infants. *Pediatr Dermatol*. 1986;3(4):331–332.
58. Powell TG, West CR, Pharoah PO, Cooke RW. Epidemiology of strawberry hemangioma in low birthweight infants. *Br J Dermatol*. 1987;116(5):635–641.
59. North PE, Waner M, Mizeracki A, Mihm MC Jr. GLUT1: a newly discovered immunohistochemical marker for juvenile hemangiomas. *Hum Pathol*. 2000;31(1):11–22.
60. Bowers RE, Graham EA, Tomlinson KM. The natural history of the strawberry nevus. *Arch Dermatol*. 1960;82(5):667–680.
61. Golitz LE, Rudikoff J, O'Meara OP. Diffuse neonatal hemangiomatosis. *Pediatr Dermatol*. 1986;3(2):145–152.
62. Stern JK, Wolf JE Jr, Jarratt M. Benign neonatal hemangiomatosis. *J Am Acad Dermatol*. 1981;4(4):442–445.
63. Metry DW, Dowd CF, Barkovich AJ, Frieden IJ. The many faces of PHACE syndrome. *J Pediatr*. 2001;139(1):117–123.
64. Frieden IJ, Reese V, Cohen D. PHACE syndrome. The association of posterior fossa brain malformations, hemangiomas, arterial anomalies, coarctation of the aorta and cardiac defects, and eye abnormalities. *Arch Dermatol*. 1996;132(3):307–311.
65. Wong CH, Wright JG, Silove ED, Willetts R, Brawn WJ. A new syndrome of multiple hemangiomas, right dominant double aortic arch, and coarctation. *J Thorac Cardiovasc Surg*. 2001;121(6):1207–1209.
66. Smolinski KN, Yan AC. Hemangiomas of infancy: clinical and biological characteristics. *Clin Pediatr (Phila)*. 2005;44(9):747–766.
67. Maguiness SM, Frieden IJ. Current management of infantile hemangiomas. *Semin Cutan Med Surg*. 2010;29(2):106–114.
68. Pope E, Chakkittakandiyil A. Topical timolol gel for infantile hemangiomas: a pilot study. *Arch Dermatol*. 2010;146(5):564–565.
69. Guo S, Ni N. Topical treatment for capillary hemangioma of the eyelid using beta-blocker solution. *Arch Ophthalmol*. 2010;128(2):255–256.
70. Chakkittakandiyil A, Phillips R, Frieden IJ, et al. Timolol maleate 0.5% or 0.1% gel-forming solution for infantile hemangiomas: a retrospective, multicenter, cohort study. *Pediatr Dermatol*. 2012;29(1):28–31.
71. Shedden AH, Laurence J, Barrish A, Olah TV. Plasma timolol concentrations of timolol maleate: timolol gel-forming solution (TIMOPTIC-XE) once daily versus timolol maleate ophthalmic solution twice daily. *Doc Ophthalmol*. 2001;103(1):73–79.
72. Mao XH, Wang JY, Yan JL. Topical imiquimod treatment of cutaneous vascular disorders in pediatric patients: clinical evaluation on the efficacy and safety. *J Zhejiang Univ Sci B*. 2012;13(9):745–750.
73. Bruckner AL, Frieden IJ. Hemangiomas of infancy. *J Am Acad Dermatol*. 2003;48(4):477–493; quiz 494–496.
74. Achauer BM, Chang CJ, Vander Kam VM. Management of hemangioma of infancy: review of 245 patients. *Plast Reconstr Surg*. 1997;99(5):1301–1308.
75. Metz BJ, Rubenstein MC, Levy ML, Metry DW. Response of ulcerated perineal hemangiomas of infancy to becaplermin gel, a recombinant human platelet-derived growth factor. *Arch Dermatol*. 2004;140(7):867–870.
76. Frieden IJ, Haggstrom AN, Drolet BA, et al. Infantile hemangiomas: current knowledge, future directions. Proceedings of a research workshop on infantile hemangiomas, April 7–9, 2005, Bethesda, Maryland, USA. *Pediatr Dermatol*. 2005;22(5):383–406.
77. Leaute-Labreze C, Dumas de la Roque E, Hubiche T, Boralevi F, Thambo JB, Taïeb A. Propranolol for severe hemangiomas of infancy. *N Engl J Med*. 2008;358(24):2649–2651.
78. Siegfried EC, Keenan WJ, Al-Jureidini S. More on propranolol for hemangiomas of infancy. *N Engl J Med*. 2008;359(26):2846; author reply 2846–2847.
79. Enjolras O, Brevière GM, Roger G, et al. [Vincristine treatment for function- and life-threatening infantile hemangioma]. *Arch Pediatr*. 2004;11(2):99–107.
80. Maturo S, Hartnick C. Initial experience using propranolol as the sole treatment for infantile airway hemangiomas. *Int J Pediatr Otorhinolaryngol*. 2010;74(3):323–325.
81. Manunza F, Syed S, Laguda B, et al. Propranolol for complicated infantile haemangiomas: a case series of 30 infants. *Br J Dermatol*. 2010;162(2):466–468.
82. Rizzo C, Brightman L, Chapas AM, et al. Outcomes of childhood hemangiomas treated with the pulsed-dye laser with dynamic cooling: a retrospective chart analysis. *Dermatol Surg*. 2009;35(12):1947–1954.
83. Hunzeker CM, Geronemus RG. Treatment of superficial infantile hemangiomas of the eyelid using the 595-nm pulsed dye laser. *Dermatol Surg*. 2010;36(5):590–597.

84. Kono T, Sakurai H, Groff WF, et al. Comparison study of a traditional pulsed dye laser versus a long-pulsed dye laser in the treatment of early childhood hemangiomas. *Lasers Surg Med.* 2006;38(2):112–115.
85. Abstracts of the American Society for Laser Medicine and Surgery. April 18–22, 2012. Kissimmee, Florida, USA. *Lasers Surg Med.* 2012;44(Suppl 24):1–94.
86. Witman PM, Wagner AM, Scherer K, Waner M, Frieden IJ. Complications following pulsed dye laser treatment of superficial hemangiomas. *Lasers Surg Med.* 2006;38(2):116–123.
87. Morelli JG, Tan OT, Weston WL. Treatment of ulcerated hemangiomas with the pulsed tunable dye-laser. *Am J Dis Child.* 1991;145(9):1062–1064.
88. Wananukul S, Chatproedprai S. Ulcerated hemangiomas: clinical features and management. *J Med Assoc Thai.* 2002;85(11):1220–1225.
89. David LR, Malek MM, Argenta LC. Efficacy of pulse dye laser therapy for the treatment of ulcerated hemangiomas: a review of 78 patients. *Br J Plast Surg.* 2003;56(4):317–327.
90. Poetke M, Philipp C, Berlien HP. Flashlamp-pumped pulsed dye laser for hemangiomas in infancy: treatment of superficial vs mixed hemangiomas. *Arch Dermatol.* 2000;136(5):628–632.
91. Blankenship CM, Alster TS. Fractional photothermolysis of residual hemangioma. *Dermatol Surg.* 2008;34(8):1112–1114.
92. Brightman LA, Brauer JA, Terushkin V, et al. Ablative fractional resurfacing for involuted hemangioma residuum. *Arch Dermatol.* 2012;148(11):1–5.
93. Raulin C, Greve B. Retrospective clinical comparison of hemangioma treatment by flashlamp-pumped (585 nm) and frequency-doubled Nd:YAG (532 nm) lasers. *Lasers Surg Med.* 2001;28(1):40–43.
94. Angermeier MC. Treatment of facial vascular lesions with intense pulsed light. *J Cutan Laser Ther.* 1999;1(2):95–100.
95. Jorge BF, Del Pozo J, Castiñeiras I, Mazaira M, Fernández-Torres R, Fonseca E. Treatment of ulcerated haemangiomas with a non-coherent pulsed light source: brief initial clinical report. *J Cosmet Laser Ther.* 2008;10(1):48–51.
96. Vikkula M, Boon LM, Carraway KL 3rd, et al. Vascular dysmorphogenesis caused by an activating mutation in the receptor tyrosine kinase TIE2. *Cell.* 1996;87(7):1181–1190.
97. Dubois J, Garel L. Imaging and therapeutic approach of hemangiomas and vascular malformations in the pediatric age group. *Pediatr Radiol.* 1999;29(12):879–893.
98. Garzon MC, Huang JT, Enjolras O, Frieden IJ. Vascular malformations - Part I. *J Am Acad Dermatol.* 2007;56(3):353–370.
99. Scherer K, Waner M. Nd : YAG lasers (1064 nm) in the treatment of venous malformations of the face and neck: challenges and benefits. *Lasers Med Sci.* 2007;22(2):119–126.
100. Alam M, Dover JS, Arndt KA. Treatment of facial telangiectasia with variable-pulse high-fluence pulsed-dye laser: comparison of efficacy with fluences immediately above and below the purpura threshold. *Dermatol Surg.* 2003;29(7):681–685.
101. Tanghetti EA. More effects of double-pass intervals on purpuric threshold and depth of tissue injury in extended pulse dye laser (PhotoGenica V-Star). *Lasers Surg Med*; 2003;32:27.
102. Tanghetti E, Sherr EA, Sierra R, Mirkov M. The effects of pulse dye laser double-pass treatment intervals on depth of vessel coagulation. *Lasers Surg Med.* 2006;38(1):16–21.
103. Rohrer TE, Chatrath V, Iyengar V. Does pulse stacking improve the results of treatment with variable-pulse pulsed-dye lasers? *Dermatol Surg.* 2004;30(2):163–167.
104. Goldberg DJ, Marcus J. The use of the frequency-doubled Q-switched Nd:YAG laser in the treatment of small cutaneous vascular lesions. *Dermatol Surg.* 1996;22(10):841–844.
105. Clementoni MT, Gilardino P, Muti GF, et al. Facial teleangectasias: our experience in treatment with IPL. *Lasers Surg Med.* 2005;37(1):9–13.
106. Tan SR, Tope WD. Pulsed dye laser treatment of rosacea improves erythema, symptomatology, and quality of life. *J Am Acad Dermatol.* 2004;51(4):592–599.
107. Clark SM, Lanigan SW, Marks R. Laser treatment of erythema and telangiectasia associated with rosacea. *Lasers Med Sci.* 2002;17(1):26–33.
108. Lowe NJ, Behr KL, Fitzpatrick R, Goldman M, Ruiz-Esparza J. Flash lamp pumped dye laser for rosacea-associated telangiectasia and erythema. *J Dermatol Surg Oncol.* 1991;17(6):522–525.
109. Ross BS, Levine VJ, Ashinoff R. Laser treatment of acquired vascular lesions. *Dermatol Clin.* 1997;15(3):385–396.
110. Wheeland RG, Applebaum J. Flashlamp-pumped pulsed dye laser therapy for poikiloderma of civatte. *J Dermatol Surg Oncol.* 1990;16(1):12–16.
111. Sommer S, Sheehan-Dare RA. Atrophie blanche-like scarring after pulsed dye laser treatment. *J Am Acad Dermatol.* 1999;41(1):100–102.
112. Varshney S. Angiokeratoma circumscriptum of the tongue. *Int J Dermatol.* 2005;44(10):886–888.
113. Ergun S, Mete O, Yeşil S, Tanyeri H. Solitary angiokeratoma of the tongue treated with diode laser. *Lasers Med Sci.* 2009;24(1):123–125.
114. Kar HK, Gupta L. A case of angiokeratoma circumscriptum of the tongue: response with carbon dioxide and pulsed dye laser. *J Cutan Aesthet Surg.* 2011;4(3):205–207.

CHAPTER 53

Laser Hair Removal

Omar A. Ibrahimi & Suzanne L. Kilmer

INTRODUCTION

The ability of lasers to nonspecifically damage hair follicles was noted nearly 50 years ago in the first reports on the use of lasers on human skin.[1,2] It was not until the theory of selective photothermolysis was proposed by Rox Anderson and John Parrish at the Wellman Center for Photomedicine at Harvard Medical School, however, that the concept of selectively targeting a particular chromophore based on its absorption spectrum and size was realized.[3] Several years later, this group also reported one of the first successful uses of a normal-mode ruby laser for long-term and permanent hair removal.[4,5]

Today, removing unwanted body hair is a worldwide trend, and photoepilation by laser or other light-based technology is one of the most highly requested procedures in cosmetic dermatology.[6] Alternative methods for removing unwanted hair include bleaching, plucking, shaving, waxing, and chemical depilatories. Threading is a common practice in some cultures. Unfortunately, these methods do not provide a permanent solution to unwanted hair, and can be inconvenient and tedious.[7,8] Electrolysis is a method for hair removal in which a fine needle is inserted deep into the hair follicle and uses electrical current, thereby destroying the hair follicle and allowing for permanent hair removal of all types of hair.[9,10] However, this technique is extremely operator dependent and efficacy in achieving permanent hair removal is variable among patients.[9,10] It is also impractical in terms of treating large areas. Eflornithine is a topical inhibitor of ornithine decarboxylase that slows the rate of hair growth, which can be effective for decreasing unwanted facial hair,[8] and is currently indicated for the removal of unwanted facial hair in women. Eflornithine can be combined with lasers and intense pulsed light (IPL) for hair removal.[11,12] In this chapter, we provide a detailed overview of laser hair removal (LHR) including a discussion of hair follicle biology, the science behind LHR, key factors in optimizing treatment, and future directions.

THE HAIR FOLLICLE

The hair follicle is a complex, hormonally active structure with a programmed growth pattern (Fig. 53-1). It is anatomically divided into the infundibulum (hair follicle orifice to insertion of the sebaceous gland), isthmus (insertion of the sebaceous gland to the insertion of the arrector pili muscle), and inferior (insertion of the arrector pili to the base of the hair follicle) segments. The dermal papilla, a neurovascular structure that supplies the cells of the proliferating matrix at the base of the follicle, helps form the hair shaft.

Each hair follicle consists of a permanent (upper) and nonpermanent (lower) part, with the follicular bulge forming the lowermost aspect of the permanent part. In periods of active growth (anagen) the rapidly developing bulbar matrix cells differentiate into the hair shaft and the hair lengthens. A transition period follows in which

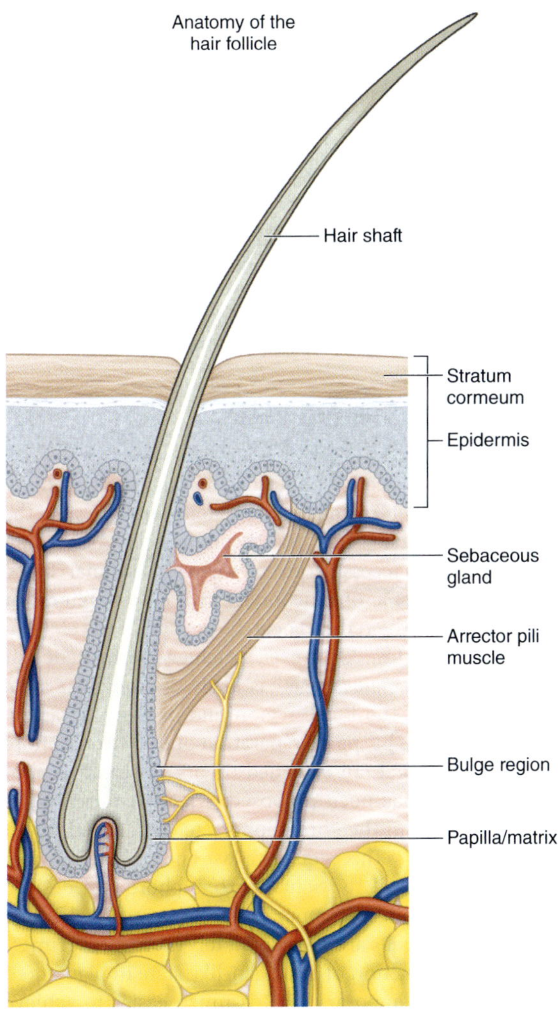

Figure 53-1 Hair follicle anatomy. (Reproduced with permission from Tsao SS, Hruza GJ. Laser hair removal. In: Robinson JK, Hanke CW, Sengelmann RD, Siegel DM, eds. *Surgery of the Skin*. Philadelphia, PA: Elsevier Mosby; 2005: 575–588. Copyright Elsevier.)

the bulbar part of the hair follicle undergoes degradation through apoptosis (catagen). A resting period (telogen) phase ensues, and regrowth is started once again in early anagen. Stem cells within the hair follicle regenerate the follicle within or near the hair bulb matrix. Slow-cycling stem cells have also been found in the follicular bulge arising from the outer root sheath at the site of arrector pili muscle attachment. The duration of each growth phase is body site dependent.

There are three main types of hair: lanugo, vellus, and terminal hairs. Lanugo hairs are fine hairs that cover a fetus and are shed in the neonatal period. Vellus hairs are usually nonpigmented, and have a diameter of roughly 30 to 50 μm. Terminal hair shafts range from 150 to 300 μm in cross-sectional diameter. The type of hair produced by an individual follicle is capable of change (e.g., vellus to terminal hair at puberty or terminal to vellus hair in androgenic alopecia). Only terminal hair follicles are responsive to LHR.

Hair color is determined by the amount of pigment in the hair shaft. Melanocytes produce two types of melanin—eumelanin, a brown-black pigment; and pheomelanin, a red pigment. Melanocytes are located in the upper portion of the hair bulb and outer root sheath of the infundibulum.

Excessive and unwanted body hair ranges in severity, depending on cultural mores, and can usually be classified as either hypertrichosis or hirsutism.[13] Hirsutism is defined as the abnormal growth of terminal hair in women in male-pattern (androgen-dependent) sites, such as the face and chest. Hypertrichosis refers to excess hair growth at any body site that is not androgen dependent.[13] In addition, the use of grafts and flaps in dermatologic and reconstructive surgery can often introduce hair to an area that causes a displeasing appearance or functional impairment.

MECHANISM OF LHR

The theory of selective photothermolysis enables one to selectively target pigmented hair follicles by using the melanin of the hair shaft as a chromophore.[3] As a result, LHR is only successful on pigmented terminal hairs. Melanin is capable of functioning as a chromophore for wavelengths in the red and near-IR portion of the electromagnetic spectrum.[14] However, to achieve permanent hair removal the biologic "target" is likely the follicular stem cells located in the bulge region and/or dermal papilla. Based on the slight spatial separation of the chromophore and desired target, an extended theory of selective photothermolysis has been proposed, which requires diffusion of heat from the chromophore to the desired target for destruction.[15] This requires a laser pulse that is longer in duration than if the actual chromophore and desired target were identical. Temporary LHR can result when the follicular stem cells are not completely destroyed, primarily through induction of a catagen-like state in pigmented hair follicles. Temporary LHR is much easier to achieve than permanent removal, using lower fluences. Long-term hair removal depends on hair color, skin color, and tolerated fluence. Roughly 15% to 30% long-term hair loss may be observed with each treatment when optimal treatment parameters are used.[16] Remaining hairs are also thinner and lighter in color. A list of laser and light devices that are commercially available at the time of this publication for hair removal are summarized in Table 53-1.

KEY FACTORS IN OPTIMIZING TREATMENT

The ability to selectively target hair follicles with lasers and light sources has revolutionized the ability to eliminate unwanted hair both temporarily and permanently in many individuals. As laser technology advances, the ability to treat individuals of all skin types and all hair colors broadens. Proper patient selection, preoperative preparation, informed consent, understanding of the principles of laser safety, and laser and light source selection are key to the success of laser treatment. An understanding of hair anatomy, growth and physiology, together with a thorough understanding of laser–tissue interaction, in particular within the context of choosing optimal laser parameters for effective LHR, should be acquired before using lasers for hair removal.

PATIENT SELECTION

Despite the seemingly cosmetic nature of LHR, a complete medical history, physical examination and informed consent, including setting realistic patient expectations and discussing potential risks, should be performed prior to any laser treatment (Table 53-2). Any patient with evidence of endocrine or menstrual dysfunction should be appropriately worked up by an endocrinologist or gynecologist. Similarly, patients with an explosive onset of hypertrichosis should be evaluated for paraneoplastic etiologies. Treatment of a pregnant woman for nonurgent conditions is discouraged, although there is no evidence suggesting a potential risk to pregnant women undergoing LHR. The past medical history should be reviewed to identify patients with photosensitive conditions, such as the autoimmune connective tissue disorders, or disorders prone to the Koebner phenomenon. A history of recurrent cutaneous infections such as HSV at or in the vicinity of the treatment area might warrant the use of prophylactic medications. Previous methods of hair removal, including any past laser treatments, should be reviewed. Any methods of epilation, such as waxing or tweezing, that entirely remove the target chromophore, render LHR less effective for at least 2 weeks. Although there is little evidence to confirm the time frame a patient must wait after complete epilation of the hair shaft and laser treatment, we recommend a minimum of 6 weeks. Shaving and depilatory creams can be used up to the day of laser treatment as they do not remove the entire hair shaft.

A thorough medication history should be obtained. Any history of gold intake is a contraindication for laser therapy. The use of any photosensitizing medications or over-the-counter supplements should also delay treatment until these medications can be safely discontinued. There is controversy as to whether patients on isotretinoin should be treated with lasers, although most practitioners recommend a 6 month to 1 year washout period prior to ablative resurfacing.[17–19] Whether this recommendation

TABLE 53-1

Commercially Available Lasers and Light Sources for Hair Removal[a]

Laser/ Light Source	Wavelength (nm)	System Name	Pulse Duration (ms)	Fluence (J/cm^2)	Spot Size (mm)	Other Features
Long-pulsed ruby	694	RubyStar and Ruby Star+	4	Up to 24	8, 10, 12, 18	Contact cooling
Long-pulsed alexandrite	755	Apogee (Cynosure)	0.5–300	25–50	5–15	Cold air or integrated cooling, can add 1064 nm Nd:YAG module to form Apogee Elite
		Arion (Quantel Derma)	5–140	Up to 40	6–16	Cold air unit
		ClearScan YAG (Sciton)	Up to 200	Up to 140	3, 6, and 30 × 30	Contact cooling
		Coolglide (Cutera)	0.1–300	5–300	10	Contact cooling
		Elite (Cynosure)	0.5–300	25–50	5–15	Cold air cooling, available with 1064 nm Nd:YAG, EliteMPX model can simultaneously treat with 755 nm Alexandrite and 1064 nm Nd:YAG
		EpiCare LP/LPX (Light Age)	3–300	22–40	7–16	
		GentleLASE, (Candela)	3	Up to 100	6–18	Dynamic cooling
		GentleMax (Candela)	0.25–300	Up to 600	1.5–18	Dynamic cooling, comes with 1064 nm Nd:YAG
		Ultrawave 755/II/III (AMC Aesthetics and Advanced Aesthetic Concepts)	Up to 100	up to 125	Up to 16	Available with 532, 1064, and 1320 nm Nd:YAG
Diode	805	Advantage (Lutronic, Freemont, California, USA)	5–400	Up to 100	10 × 10, 10 × 30	Contact cooling
	800–810	F1 Diode (Opusmed)	15–40	Up to 40	5, 7	Chiller tip
	808, 980	Leda (Quantel Derma)	6–60	Up to 60	50 × 12, 10 × 12	Contact cooling
	810, 940	MeDioStar XT (Aesclepion)	5–500	Up to 90	6, 12	Integrated scanner with cold air cooling device
	800	LightSheer Duet (Lumenis)	5–400	10–100, 4.5–12	9 × 9, 22 × 35	Chill tip for smaller handpiece, vacuum skin flattening for larger handpiece
	810	Soprano XL (Alma Lasers)	10–1350	Up to 120	12 × 10	Contact cooling
Long-pulsed Nd:YAG	1064	Acclaim (Cynosure)	0.4–300	35–600	1.5–15	Cold air or integrated cooling, can add 755 nm Alexandrite module to form Apogee Elite (Cynosure)
		ClearScan YAG (Sciton)	0.3–200	Up to 400	3, 6, and 30 × 30	Contact cooling
		CoolGlide CV/XEO/ Excel/Vantage (Cutera)	0.1–300	Up to 300	3–10	Contact cooling
		Cynergy (Cynosure)	0.3–300	Up to 600	1.5–15	Cold air
		Dualis XP, XP Plus, and XS Max (Fotona)	5–200	Up to 600	2–10	n/a
		GentleYAG (Candela, Wayland, MA)	0.25–300	Up to 600	1.5–18	Dynamic cooling
		Gemini (Iridex)	1–100	Up to 990	2, 10	Available with 532 nm KTP
		LightPod Neo (Aerolase)	0.65–1.5	Up to 312	2	Built-in cooling system
		Lyra (Iridex)	20–100	5–900	1–5, 10	Contact cooling

(Continued)

TABLE 53-1 (*Continued*)

Commercially Available Lasers and Light Sources for Hair Removal[a]

Laser/ Light Source	Wavelength (nm)	System Name	Pulse Duration (ms)	Fluence (J/cm²)	Spot Size (mm)	Other Features
		MultiFlex (Ellipse, Atlanta, GA)	n/a	Up to 600	1.5–5	Equipped with IPL device
		Mydon (Quantel)	0.5–90	10–450	1.5–10	Integrated air cooling
		NaturaLase 1064/LP (Focus Medical)	0.5–100	Up to 400	3–15	Integrated air cooling
		Profile (Sciton)	0.1–10,000	Up to 75	n/a	Contact cooling, 2940 nm Er:YAG and 410–1400 nm flashlamp in same device
		SmartEpil (Deka)	Up to 20	11	2.5, 4, 5, 6	
		SP Plus (Fotona)	Up to 300	Up to 600	1–42	
		Synchro_FT (Deka)	2–30	Up to 50	2.5–13	Available with IPL handpiece
		Ultrawave II/III (AMC Aesthetics, and Advance Aesthetic Concepts)	Up to 300	5–500	Up to 12	Pulsed cryogen cooling
		Varia (CoolTouch)	0.6	Up to 500	2–10	Dynamic cryogen cooling
Intense pulsed light sources	520–1200	Axiom (Viora)	25–75 and 2.2–12.5	Up to 39	50 × 25, 35 × 15, 20 × 10	Built-in cooling system
	420–1400	BBL (Sciton)	Up to 200	Up to 30	15 × 45	Built-in cooling system
	560–590	Cynergy (Cynosure)	0.3–300	Up to 600	n/a	Built-in cooling system
	400–1200	Duet/SkinStation/ SpaTouch II (Radiancy)	3–10	35	22 × 55	
	600–950	Ellipse I2 PL/ MultiFlex (Ellipse)	2.5–88.5	4–26	10 × 48	MultiFlex model with long-pulsed Nd:YAG
	400–1400	EsteLux (Palomar Medical Technologies)	10–100	up to 28	n/a	
	650–950	Harmony XL (Alma Lasers)	30–50	up to 40	30 × 30	Available with 755 nm alexandrite and 1064 and 1320 nm Nd:YAG
	530–1200	iPulse (Dermavista)	5–120	Up to 20	89 sq	Air cooling
	390–1200	Med Flash II (General Project)	Up to 100	Up to 45	n/a	
	525–1200	MediLux/StarLux Y, Ys, R, Rs (Palomar)	5–500	Up to 70	28 × 12, 46 × 16	1064 nm Nd:YAG handpiece for StarLux 500
	500–1200	MiniSilk_FT (Deka)	3–8	Up to 160	48 × 13, 23 × 13	Contact cooling
	400–1200	Mistral (Radiancy)	Up to 80	4–15	25 × 50, 13 × 50, 13 × 35, 12 × 12	
	640–1400	NannoLight MP50 (Sybaritic)	1–30	2.8–50	40 × 8	Nd:YAG handpiece, optional cooling
	640–1200	NaturaLight (Solamed)	Up to 500	Up to 50	10 × 40	
	750–1100	Solera Opus (Cutera)	Auto	3–24	10 × 30	
	550–950	PhotoSilk/ PhotoLight/MiniSilk (Cyanosure)	Up to 30	10–340	21 × 10, 46 × 10, 46 × 18	Nd:YAG handpiece
	770–1100	ProWave (Cutera)	Auto	5–35	10 × 30	
	500–1200	Quadra Q4 (DermaMed)	48	10–20	33 × 15	Built-in cooling system
	695–1200	Quantum HR (Lumenis)	15–100	25–45	34 × 8	
	560–950	SmoothCool (Eclipse)	1–60	10–45	8 × 34	Automatic temperature control system
	530–1200	Trios (Viora)	25	up to 22	15 × 50	

TABLE 53-1 (*Continued*)

Commercially Available Lasers and Light Sources for Hair Removal[a]

Laser/ Light Source	Wavelength (nm)	System Name	Pulse Duration (ms)	Fluence (J/cm²)	Spot Size (mm)	Other Features
Fluorescent pulsed light	615–920	OmniLight/ NovaLight (Medical Bio Care)	2–500	Up to 90	7 × 15, 10 × 20, 30 × 30	Sapphire tip cooling
Optical energy combined with RF electrical energy	580–980	eMax/eLight (Syneron)	Up to 100	Up to 50 optical; up to 50 J/cm³ RF	12 × 15	Contact cooling
Diode combined with RF electrical energy	800	eLaser (Syneron)	Up to 100	Up to 50 optical; up to 50 J/cm³ RF	12 × 15	Contact cooling
	810	MeDioStar Effect (Aesclepion, Jena, Germany)	UP to 500	Up to 90	10, 12, 14	Acoustic wave technology, integrated scanner with cold air cooling device, 940 nm simultaneously

[a]This table is intended only as a reference aid. The authors have made every attempt to provide an exhaustive list of available devices for laser hair removal but do not guarantee comprehensiveness.

TABLE 53-2

Pertinent History for Laser/Light Device Hair Removal

Presence of conditions that may cause hypertrichosis Hormonal Familial Drug (i.e., corticosteroids, hormones, immunosuppressives, self or spousal use of minoxidil) Tumor
History of local or recurrent skin infection
History of herpes simplex, especially perioral
History of herpes genitalis, important when treating the pubic or bikini area
History of keloids/hypertrophic scarring
History of koebnerizing skin disorders such as vitiligo and psoriasis
Previous treatment modalities—method, frequency, and date of last treatment, as well as response
Recent suntan or exposure to tanning or light cabinet
Onset of hair regrowth (recent)
Tattoos or nevi present
Patient's expectations
Patient's hobbies or habits that might interfere with treatment
Present medications Photosensitizing medications Isotretinoin intake within the past year Gold therapy

is appropriate for other laser procedures is speculative at best. Topical retinoids used in the treatment area should be discontinued 1 to 2 days prior to treatment to minimize postlaser erythema.

The physical examination should evaluate the patient's Fitzpatrick skin phototype. This will help determine which lasers and light sources are safe to use for that patient (Table 53-1), because epidermal melanin in darkly pigmented patients can compete with the melanin within hair follicles as the target chromophore. Importantly, every patient should always be evaluated for the presence of a tan, and if present, laser treatment should be delayed or the treatment parameters appropriately adjusted until the tan has faded. If a patient with a tan is treated, the risk of side effects is increased. Finally, the patient's hair color should be noted, as the chromophore for LHR is melanin. Terminal black and brown hairs usually contain sufficient amounts of melanin to serve as a chromophore for LHR. In contrast, the lack of melanin, paucity of melanin or presence of eumelanin in the hair follicle, which clinically correlates to white, gray, or red/blonde hair is predictive of, at best, a poor response to LHR and the procedure should not be performed. For patients with little to no melanin in their hair follicles, attempts have been made to use an exogenous chromophore that can be topically delivered to the hair follicles, thereby making the removal of white, gray, red, and blonde hair hypothetically possible. This concept was first demonstrated with a topical carbon solution dissolved in mineral oil.[20] However, we have noticed very little efficacy of topical chromophores in our experience.

INFORMED CONSENT

An explanation of the potential risks of LHR should be reviewed as part of the informed consent process. The risks include but are not limited to temporary and permanent hypo/hyperpigmentation, blister formation, scar formation, ulceration, hive-like response, bruising, infection, acne flare, and folliculitis. For those patients with Fitzpatrick skin type IV or greater or of Mediterranean, Middle Eastern, Asian, or South Asian descent, the low risk of paradoxical hypertrichosis (conversion of vellus hairs to terminal hairs), especially when treating the lateral face and jaw, should be reviewed.[21–24] Patients should be counseled that permanent and complete hair removal is not likely but that with multiple treatments, significant long-term reduction can be achieved. Hirsute women with hormonal abnormalities may require continued maintenance therapy and should be advised of this possibility. Procedural pain is expected with LHR but can be minimized with topical anesthetics and the use of cold air cooling. It is vital that a minimal amount of local anesthesia be applied to avoid risk of lidocaine toxicity. Erythema and edema are also expected with treatment and may rarely last up to 1 week. Patients should be made aware of the need for strict sun avoidance for a minimum of 6 weeks before and after each treatment.

PREOPERATIVE PREPARATION AND LASER SAFETY. The need for topical anesthesia is variable among patients and anatomic sites. Various topical anesthetics including lidocaine, lidocaine/prilocaine, and other amide/ester anesthetic combinations can be used to diminish the procedural discomfort, and should be applied 30 minutes to 1 hour before treatment under occlusion. Care should be taken when using lidocaine or prilocaine to apply these medications to a limited area to diminish the risk of lidocaine toxicity or methemoglobulinemia, respectively. Use of topical anesthesia over large body surface areas can be fatal.

Patients should be placed in a room with a treatment chair that makes the desired treatment area easily accessible. The room should be adequately cooled to keep the laser device from overheating and be free of any hanging mirrors or uncovered windows. A fire extinguisher should be readily available, especially if oxygen is being used. Having a vacuum device on hand during treatment can minimize the plume and unpleasant odor created by each laser pulse. Because the retina contains melanin, which can be damaged by all LHR devices, proper eye protection is absolutely critical for both the patient and laser surgeon. Each device requires the use of protective goggles that are unique to the device's particular wavelengths. Goggles cannot be interchangeably used with laser or IPL devices of other wavelengths. Furthermore, because of the risk of retinal damage, it is the authors' strong opinion that one should never treat a patient for LHR within the bony orbit.

DEVICE VARIABLES

WAVELENGTH. The chromophore for LHR is melanin. Within the hair follicle, melanin is principally located within the hair shaft, although the outer root sheath and matrix area also contain melanin. Melanin is capable of functioning as a chromophore for wavelengths in the red and near-IR portion of the electromagnetic spectrum,[14] and can be targeted by ruby, alexandrite, diode, and Nd:YAG lasers, as well as IPL devices.

The long-pulsed ruby laser (694 nm) was the first device used to selectively target hair follicles,[5] and to produce long-term (follow-up at 2 years) hair loss (6 mm spot size, 270 ms pulse duration, and fluences 30–60 J/cm^2).[4] The long-pulsed ruby laser can be safely used in Fitzpatrick skin phototypes I to III. A large multicenter trial of nearly 200 patients showed that the majority of patients had >75% hair loss at 6 months follow-up after an average of four treatments.[25] Table 53-1 lists the long-pulsed ruby lasers that are commercially available.

The long-pulsed alexandrite (755 nm) laser has been shown to be effective for hair removal in multiple studies.[26] The long-pulsed alexandrite laser can be safely used in Fitzpatrick skin phototypes I to IV, although some experts limit its use to Fitzpatrick skin phototypes I to III. A few studies have demonstrated the safety of the long-pulsed alexandrite laser in a large cohort of patients with Fitzpatrick skin phototypes IV to VI.[27,28] A randomized, investigator-blinded clinical trial[29] of subjects with skin phototypes III to IV treated with a long-pulsed alexandrite laser (12 and 18 mm spot size, 1.5 ms pulse duration, and fluences of 20 or 40 J/cm^2) for four sessions at 8 week intervals showed 76% to 84% hair reduction 18 months after the last treatment and provides the best evidence for long-term hair removal efficacy with the alexandrite laser. A randomized controlled trial of 144 Asian subjects with Fitzpatrick skin types III to V with a long-pulsed alexandrite laser (12.5 mm spot size, pulse duration of 40 ms, fluences of 16–24 J/cm^2) found that subjects undergoing three treatments had a 55% hair reduction compared to subjects treated two times, with a 44% hair reduction, and subjects treated one time, with a 32% hair reduction at 9 months follow-up.[30] Combination treatment with alexandrite and Nd:YAG lasers provides no added benefit over the alexandrite laser alone.[31] The commercially available long-pulsed alexandrite devices are summarized in Table 53-1.

The long-pulsed diode (800–810 nm) laser has also been extensively used for LHR.[26,32] The diode laser can be safely used in patients with Fitzpatrick skin phototypes I to V. Two long-term nonrandomized controlled studies showing roughly 40% hair reduction at a mean follow-up of 20 months after one or two treatments (9 mm spot size, pulse duration of 5–30 ms, fluences of 15–40 J/cm^2),[33] and 84% hair reduction at 1 year follow-up after four treatments (9 mm spot size, pulse duration of 5–30 ms, fluences of 12–40 J/cm^2)[34] demonstrate the efficacy of the diode laser for long-term hair removal.

The long-pulsed Nd:YAG laser has been thought to offer the best combination of safety and efficacy for Fitzpatrick skin phototype VI patients. We have found the Nd:YAG to offer good efficacy but with higher relative fluences relative to the above wavelengths. A nonrandomized trial reported a 70% to 90% reduction of facial, axillary, and leg hair growth 1 year after three monthly treatments with an Nd:YAG laser (5 mm spot size, pulse duration of 50 ms, fluences of 40–50 J/cm^2).[35] A small study of axillary LHR comparing long-pulsed alexandrite, diode, and Nd:YAG lasers showed that both the alexandrite and diode lasers were significantly more efficacious than the Nd:YAG laser for LHR.[36]

IPL is composed of polychromatic, noncoherent light ranging from 400 to 1200 nm. Various filters can be used to target particular chromophores, including melanin, using IPL. However, long-term (>1 year) hair removal has not been convincingly demonstrated to date. Various reports have demonstrated some short-term efficacy.[37,38] One study of patients treated with a single IPL session reported 75% hair removal 1 year after treatment.[39] Studies providing a head-to-head comparison of IPL versus either the long-pulsed alexandrite laser,[40] Nd:YAG laser,[41] or diode laser[66] all found the IPL to be inferior to laser devices for hair removal. In contrast, a study of hirsute women, some with a diagnosis of polycystic ovarian syndrome, who underwent a split face treatment with six IPL or long pulsed diode laser (LPDL), showed statistically equivalent reductions in hair counts at 1 (77% vs. 68%, respectively), 3 (53% vs. 60%, respectively), and 6 months (40% vs. 34%, respectively) after the final treatment.[42]

FLUENCE. Fluence is defined as the amount of energy delivered per unit area and is expressed as J/cm^2. Higher fluences have been correlated with greater permanent hair removal,[5,44] but are also more likely to cause untoward side effects. Recommended treatment fluences are often provided with each individual laser device for inexperienced operators. However, a more appropriate method of determining the optimal treatment fluence for a given patient is to evaluate for the desired clinical end point of perifollicular erythema and edema (Fig. 53-2). The highest possible tolerated fluence, which yields this end point without any adverse effects, is often the best fluence for treatment.

PULSE DURATION. Pulse duration is defined as the duration in seconds of laser exposure. The theory of selective photothermolysis[3] enables the laser surgeon to select an optimal pulse duration based on the thermal relaxation time (TRT). Higher TRTs require longer pulse durations for optimal efficacy. Terminal hairs are roughly 300 µm in diameter, and thus the calculated TRT of a terminal hair follicle is roughly 100 ms. However, unlike many other laser applications, the hair follicle is distinct in that there is a spatial separation of the chromophore (melanin) within the hair shaft and the biologic "target" stem cells in the bulge and bulb areas of the follicle. The expanded theory of selective photothermolysis[15] takes this spatial separation into account and proposes a thermal damage time (TDT), which is thought to be longer than the TRT. Shorter pulse widths are also capable of removing hair, and it is unclear which is more effective in producing permanent hair removal. Longer pulse widths are likely more selective for melanin within the hair follicle and can minimize epidermal damage as the pulse widths are greater than the TRT of the melanosomes and melanocytes within the epidermis.

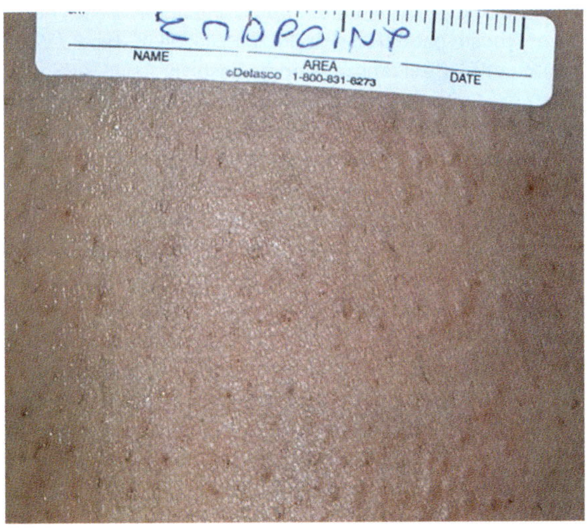

Figure 53-2 Appropriate clinical end point of perifollicular erythema and edema.

SPOT SIZE. The spot size is the diameter in millimeters of the laser beam. As photons within a laser beam penetrate the dermis, they are scattered by collagen fibers, and those that are scattered outside the area of the laser beam are essentially wasted. Photons are more likely to be scattered outside of the beam area for smaller spot sizes, whereas in a larger spot size, the photons are likely to remain within the beam area following scatter. A double-blind, randomized control trial of a long-pulsed alexandrite device for LHR of the axillary region comparing 18 and a 12 mm spot sizes at otherwise identical treatment parameters showed a 10% greater reduction in hair counts with the larger spot size.[44] Recently, a prospective study[45] using a LDPL with a large 22 × 35 mm handpiece at low fluences and no skin cooling was shown to have similar long-term hair removal efficacy to published studies of LPDLs using a smaller spot size, higher fluences, and skin cooling. Thus, larger spot sizes are preferable to smaller spot sizes.

SKIN COOLING. The presence of epidermal melanin, particularly in darker skin types, presents a competing chromophore to hair follicle melanin, which can be damaged during LHR. Cooling of the skin surface can be used to minimize epidermal damage, while permitting treatment with higher fluences.[46,47] All skin cooling methods function by acting as a heat sink and removing heat from the skin surface. The least effective type of cooling is the use of an aqueous cold gel, which passively extracts heat from the skin and is not capable of further skin cooling. Alternatively, cooling with forced chilled air can provide cooling to the skin before, during, and after a laser pulse. Today, most of the commercially LHR devices have a built-in skin cooling system, which either consists of contact cooling or dynamic cooling with a cryogen spray. Contact cooling, usually with a sapphire tip, provides skin cooling just before and during a laser pulse. It is most useful for treatments with longer pulse durations (>10 ms).[48] During the course of a treatment, it is advised that the operator touch the contact cooling tip to ensure it is cooled appropriately. Dynamic cooling with cryogen liquid spray[47] precools the skin with a millisecond spray of cryogen just before the laser pulse. A second spray can be delivered just after the laser pulse for postcooling, but parallel cooling during the laser pulse is not possible as the cryogen spray interferes with the laser beam. Dynamic cooling is best suited for use with pulse durations shorter than 5 ms.

POSTPROCEDURE CARE

It is expected for the patient to have perifollicular erythema and edema in the treatment area following LHR (Figure 53-2). This generally persists for 2 days but rarely can last for up to 1 week. Ice and application of a topical corticosteroid can be used to shorten the duration of these desired clinical findings. Patients will often find that a single treatment of LHR with shorter pulse durations results in nearly total epilation of the hair follicles in the treatment area. It is important to counsel the patient that a majority of these hairs will likely regrow, and that this is not considered a treatment failure. Generally, only about 15% of hairs are permanently removed with each laser treatment. On the other hand, LHR treatments with longer pulse durations may leave behind many hairs, which appear to "grow" following treatment. It is important to reassure the patient that these "growing" hairs are dislodged from the hair follicle and require 1 to 2 weeks to be completely shed. Nearly any method of epilation can be used to hasten their removal.

The importance of strict sun precautions following LHR treatments cannot be overemphasized. This can be achieved by the use of topical sunscreens, hats, ultraviolet light impermeable garments, and strict sun avoidance.

LONG-TERM EFFICACY

Dierickx et al.,[5] followed up 7 of 13 subjects from the seminal study demonstrating the first example of LHR, 2 years after a single treatment with the normal mode ruby laser. Of the seven subjects, four had evidence of persistent permanent hair reduction at 2 year follow-up, whereas three subjects experienced complete regrowth. Lou et al.[33] reported that 18 out of 50 original study subjects showed roughly a 25% to 33% and 36% to 46% hair reduction at a mean follow-up of 20 months after one or two treatments (9 mm spot size, pulse duration of 5–20 ms, fluences of 15–40 J/cm^2, single or triple pulsed), respectively, with a LPDL device. Eremia et al.,[34] in a head-to-head trial comparing a LPDL to a long-pulsed alexandrite laser, found a 49% to 94% hair reduction at 1 year follow-up after four treatments (9 mm spot size, pulse duration of 20 ms, fluences of 12–40 J/cm^2) with the LPDL in 15 subjects. Similar results were achieved with the alexandrite laser used in this study. Fifteen of 20 subjects with Fitzpatrick skin phototypes III to IV treated with a long-pulsed alexandrite laser (12 and 18 mm spot size, 3 ms pulse duration, and fluences of 20 or 40 J/cm^2) or a long-pulsed Nd:YAG laser (12 mm spot size, 3 ms pulse duration, and fluence of 40 J/cm^2) for four sessions at 8 week intervals showed 76% to 84% and 74% hair reduction, respectively, 18 months after the last treatment.[29] Braun[49] reported a head-to-head trial of a high-fluence LPDL (9 mm spot size, pulse duration of 30 ms, fluences of 20–50 J/cm^2) versus a low-fluence LPDL (12 × 10 mm spot size, pulse duration of 20 ms, fluences of 5–10 J/cm^2) in 22 subjects and showed similar, 94% and 90% hair reduction respectively, at 18 months' follow-up following five treatments spaced 6 to 8 weeks apart. Finally, we recently reported statistically significant hair clearance, 54% and 42%, at 6 and 15 month follow-up visits following three monthly treatments using a LPDL using a large handpiece in the largest prospective trial to date.[45] Remaining hairs were also found to be less thick and lighter when they grew back.

SIDE EFFECTS AND MANAGEMENT OF COMPLICATIONS. LHR was FDA cleared in 1996 and has an excellent safety and efficacy profile when performed by highly trained individuals. Complications are rare if treatments are done carefully and with the patient's skin type in mind. However, a recent analysis of publically available legal documents from the past 27 years relating to cutaneous laser surgery found that LHR was the most common litigated procedure, with a majority of cases involving nonphysician operators.[67]

LHR is not a painless procedure. Most patients experience some discomfort during and immediately after treatment. A topical or local anesthetic can be used before treatment as well as cold air cooling before, after, and during treatment to reduce this effect. Perifollicular erythema and edema are expected in many patients treated with significant laser fluences. The intensity and duration depend on hair color and hair density. This usually lasts a few hours (Fig. 53-2).

Epidermal damage occurs if excessive fluences are used, so appropriate epidermal cooling techniques (i.e., firm and full contact with the contact cooling device) are imperative. Epidermal damage is also more common in patients with a tan. Herpes simplex outbreaks are uncommon but may occur. There is a higher risk among patients with a previous history of herpes simplex and when the perioral, pubic, or bikini areas are treated. The risk of bacterial infection is extremely low. Folliculitis may also occur in areas treated after excessive sweating or vigorous exercise. An additional risk is posed by swimming or using a hot-tub around the time of treatment sessions. The most common side effects are transient pigmentary changes such as hyperpigmentation (Fig. 53-3), which can be prevented if the appropriate treatment fluences are chosen for each skin type. Pigmentary abnormalities are mostly seen in patients with darker skin types or in patients with a recent tan.[43,50–52] Permanent pigmentary changes are unlikely except in dark-skinned individuals (Fig. 53-4).[53]

For those patients with Fitzpatrick skin type IV or greater, of Mediterranean, Middle Eastern, Asian, or South Asian descent, or hirsutism in the "beard" and lateral face distribution, treatment with laser may result in paradoxical hypertrichosis[21–24] (conversion of vellus hairs to terminal hairs). The incidence of paradoxical hypertrichosis is not clear, although the aforementioned factors are thought to place the patient at risk for this rare and poorly understood phenomenon. Nonetheless, this phenomenon has also been observed on the back of Caucasian males when treated with hair removal lasers. One mechanistic explanation for paradoxical hypertrichosis is that the scattering of photons that occurs at the periphery of a laser beam lowers the effective fluence at the edges and that this low level of energy at the beam periphery may actually be stimulatory to hair growth rather than resulting in thermal destruction of the hair follicle stem cells.

Scarring is unlikely except in cases of overaggressive treatment, treatment of a tanned patient, failure to protect

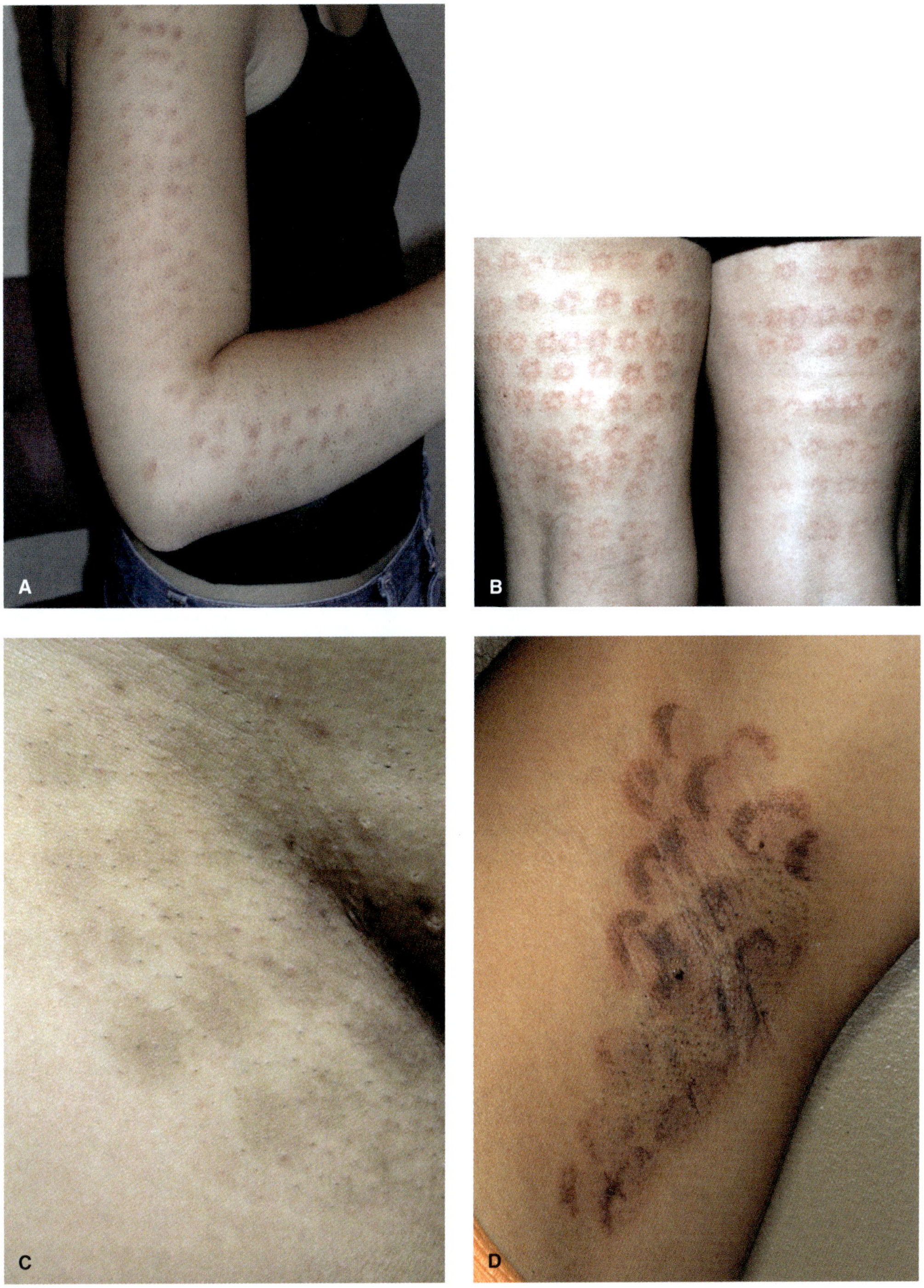

Figure 53-3 Examples of LHR-induced hyperpigmentation.

the epidermis, or postoperative infection. Loss of freckles or lightening of tattoos or pigmented lesions is not uncommon. Patients should be aware of this possibility. Poor operator technique with insufficient amounts of overlap between laser pulses can create zones of untreated skin that may leave a displeasing appearance (Fig. 53-5).

Temporary or permanent leukotrichia has been said to develop following laser or IPL hair removal.[54] This finding may be explained by the difference in the TRTs of melanocytes and germinative cells. The light absorbed and the heat produced by melanin may be sufficient to destroy or impair the function of melanocytes but insufficient to damage the hair follicle cells.

A case of lichen planus triggered by long-pulsed ruby-laser treatment for hair removal has been reported.[55] Logic would suggest that all patients with a history of skin diseases known to show a Koebner phenomenon, such as psoriasis vulgaris, vitiligo, lichen planus, and Darier's disease, should be informed about this possible adverse effect of treatment; clinically this is rarely seen.

Livedo reticularis,[56] intense pruritus, and urticaria[57] have been reported, including a case of intense swelling

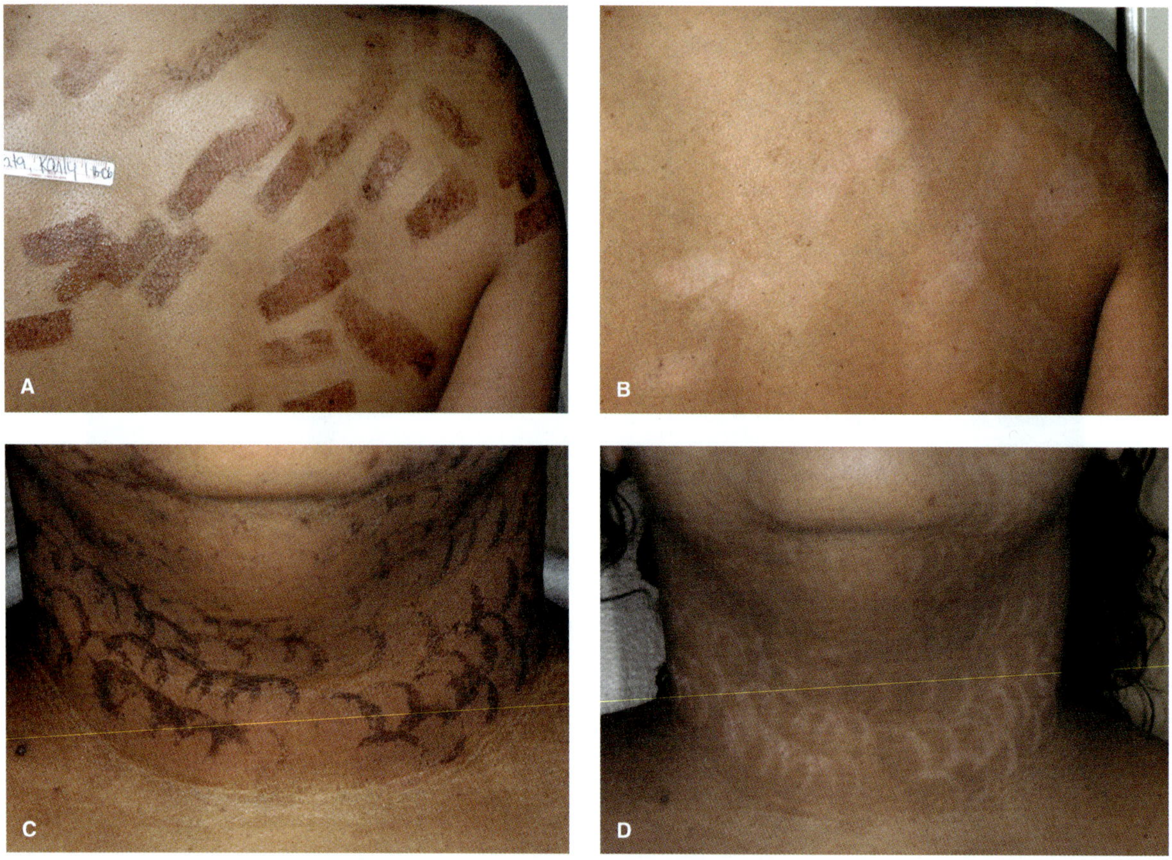

Figure 53-4 Permanent pigmentation changes resulting from LHR. **A.** Temporary hyperpigmentation in a Fitzpatrick skin phototype IV treated with an IPL device for hair removal. **B.** One month later, the hyperpigmented patches were replaced with persistent hypopigmented patches. **C.** Temporary hyperpigmentation in a Fitzpatrick skin phototype VI patient treated with an Nd:Yag device. **D.** Two weeks later, the annular hyperpigmented patches were replaced with persistent hypopigmented patches.

and erythema. The pathophysiology of these phenomena is not known. Management included topical corticosteroids, antihistamines, and discontinuing treatment. Several cases of induction of hair growth following LHR in young female patients with darker skin types have been reported.[21–24] Two different phenomena have been observed: conversion of fine vellus hair to dark, coarse terminal hair at the site of treatment or induction of growth of long fine hairs in the immediate vicinity of the treatment area. Repetitive, low-fluence treatments with hair removal devices have also been reported to induce hair growth. Further study is ongoing to assess the mechanisms for this response. Treatment of this side effect has included continued treatment in some cases.

Light-based hair removal devices are designed for strong absorption by melanin and deep tissue penetration. These systems are, therefore, capable of causing retinal injury and proper eye protection must be worn by the patient and operating personnel. Treatment near or on the surface of an eye is not recommended. All other body sites can be treated safely.

The "plume" generated by the vaporized hair shafts has a typical sulfuric smell and in large quantities, can be irritating to the respiratory tract. A smoke evacuator is recommended.

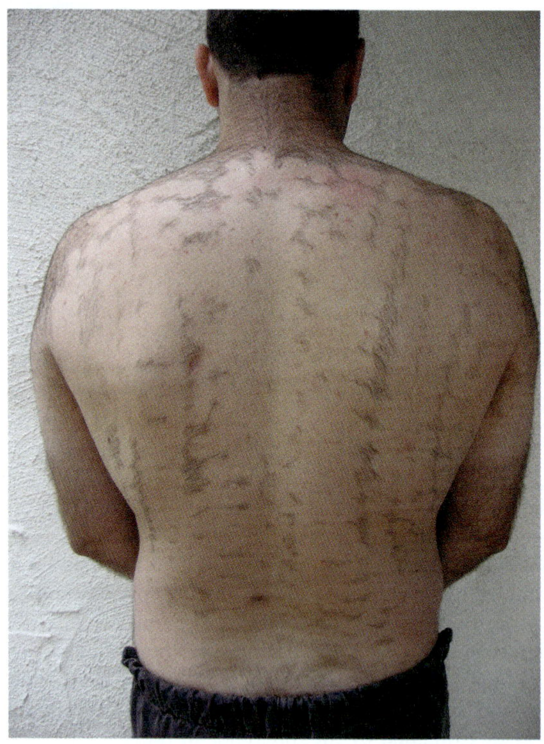

Figure 53-5 Zones of untreated skin resulting from poor operator technique.

CONCLUSION

FUTURE DIRECTIONS

ADVANCES IN PAIN CONTROL.

A novel technique to reduce LHR-associated pain is pneumatic skin flattening (PSF).[58] PSF works by coupling a vacuum chamber to generate negative pressure and flatten the skin against the handpiece treatment window. Based on the gate theory of pain transmission, this technique stimulates pressure receptors in the skin immediately prior to firing of the laser pulse, thereby blocking activation of pain fibers. PSF is just beginning to be incorporated into commercially available lasers (Table 53-1). A recent study of LHR using a LPDL with a large spot size and vacuum-assisted suction showed that the majority of subjects reported feeling no pain at all or up to moderate pain without the use of skin cooling or topical anesthetics.[45] Notably, none of the subjects in the study reported experiencing severe or intolerable pain.

HOME USE LASER AND LIGHT SOURCE DEVICES FOR HAIR REMOVAL.

In recent years, a number of devices have been developed that seek to provide patients with the ability to achieve hair removal at home. These devices are based on IPL, laser, and thermal technologies that target the hair follicle for destruction. These devices include Spa Touch (Radiancy), Tria (SpectraGenics), and no!no! (Radiancy).

The evidence behind such devices is scant and limited to small noncontrolled studies.[59–61] One recent small trial of 13 subjects showed 44% to 65% hair reduction at 12 months after eight monthly treatments, thereby suggesting that there is potential for long-term hair removal, albeit with much lower efficacy than traditional laser devices.[68] In addition, the risk for devastating eye injuries with improper use of laser- and IPL-based devices and lack of medical training raises a dilemma of how much autonomy a patient should have when using potentially harmful devices. Nonetheless, the appeal of having a personal device to remove unwanted hair in the privacy of one's home without the expense and inconvenience of multiple dermatologist or spa visits will likely drive the development of additional home use devices.

ALTERNATIVE TECHNOLOGIES FOR HAIR REMOVAL.

Photodynamic therapy (PDT) with aminolevulinic acid (ALA) has been shown in a small pilot study to result in up to 40% hair loss with a single treatment, although wax epilation was performed prior to treatment in this study.[62]

Electro-Optical Synergy (ELOS) technology combines electrical (conducted radiofrequency [RF]) and optical (laser/light) energies.[63] A handful of devices based on this technology have been produced (Table 53-1). The theory behind ELOS is based on the optical component (laser or IPL) heating the hair shaft, which then is thought to concentrate the bipolar RF energy to the surrounding hair follicle. Based on this combination, lower fluences are needed for the optical component, thereby suggesting that it might be well tolerated in all Fitzpatrick skin phototypes, and potentially effective in the removal of white and poorly pigmented hair. A study of 40 patients (Fitzpatrick skin phenotypes II to V) with varied facial and nonfacial hair colors were treated with combined IPL/RF ELOS technology. An average clearance of 75% was observed at 18 months following four treatments. No significant adverse sequelae were noted and there were no treatment differences between patients of varying skin types or hair color.[64] Pretreatment with ALA prior to use of a combined IPL and RF device has been shown to further augment the removal of terminal white hairs.[65]

In conclusion, hair removal has made a dramatic shift from an art to a science based on the theory of selective photothermolysis. Since the first reports of selective hair removal in 1996 by Anderson et al,[5] there has been a tremendous explosion in the number of devices used for LHR, making it the most commonly requested cosmetic procedure in the world. This review provides the reader with the fundamentals of hair follicle anatomy and physiology, pearls for patient selection and preoperative preparation, principles of laser safety, an introduction to the various laser/light devices and a discussion of laser–tissue interactions that are vital to optimizing treatment efficacy while minimizing complications and side effects.

REFERENCES

1. Goldman L, Blaney DJ, Kindel DJ Jr, Franke EK. Effect of the laser beam on the skin. Preliminary report. *J Invest Dermatol.* 1963;40:121–122.
2. Goldman L, Blaney DJ, Kindel DJ Jr, Richfield D, Franke EK. Pathology of the effect of the laser beam on the skin. *Nature.* 1963;197:912–914.
3. Anderson RR, Parrish JA. Selective photothermolysis: precise microsurgery by selective absorption of pulsed radiation. *Science.* 1983;220(4596):524–527.
4. Dierickx CC, Grossman MC, Farinelli WA, Anderson RR. Permanent hair removal by normal-mode ruby laser. *Arch Dermatol.* 1998;134(7):837–842.
5. Grossman MC, Dierickx C, Farinelli W, Flotte T, Anderson RR. Damage to hair follicles by normal-mode ruby laser pulses. *J Am Acad Dermatol.* 1996;35(6):889–894.
6. Ibrahimi OA, Avram MM, Hanke CW, Kilmer SL, Anderson RR. Laser hair removal. *Dermatol Ther.* 2011;24(1):94–107.
7. Lanigan SW. Management of unwanted hair in females. *Clin Exp Dermatol.* 2001;26(8):644–647.
8. Shapiro J, Lui H. Treatments for unwanted facial hair. *Skin Therapy Lett.* 2005–2006;10(10):1–4.
9. Richards RN, McKenzie MA, Meharg GE. Electroepilation (electrolysis) in hirsutism. 35,000 hours' experience on the face and neck. *J Am Acad Dermatol.* 1986;15(4 Pt 1):693–697.
10. Richards RN, Meharg GE. Electrolysis: observations from 13 years and 140,000 hours of experience. *J Am Acad Dermatol.* 1995;33(4):662–666.
11. Hamzavi I, Tan E, Shapiro J, Lui H. A randomized bilateral vehicle-controlled study of eflornithine cream combined with laser treatment versus laser treatment alone for facial hirsutism in women. *J Am Acad Dermatol.* 2007;57(1):54–59.
12. Smith SR, Piacquadio DJ, Beger B, Littler C. Eflornithine cream combined with laser therapy in the management of unwanted facial hair growth in women: A randomized trial. *Dermatol Surg.* 2006;32(10):1237–1243.
13. Rosenfield RL. Clinical practice. Hirsutism. *N Engl J Med.* 2005;353(24):2578–2588.
14. Anderson RR, Parrish JA. The optics of human skin. *J Invest Dermatol.* 1981;77(1):13–19.
15. Altshuler GB, Anderson RR, Manstein D, Zenzie HH, Smirnov MZ. Extended theory of selective photothermolysis. *Lasers Surg Med.* 2001;29(5):416–432.

16. Grossman MC. Long term comparison of different lasers and light sources for hair removal. *Lasers Surg Med.* 2000;12(suppl):89.
17. Cassano N, Arpaia N, Vena GA. Diode laser hair removal and isotretinoin therapy. *Dermatol Surg.* 2005;31(3):380–381.
18. Khatri KA. Diode laser hair removal in patients undergoing isotretinoin therapy. *Dermatol Surg.* 2004;30(9):1205–1207; discussion 1207.
19. Khatri KA, Garcia V. Light-assisted hair removal in patients undergoing isotretinoin therapy. *Dermatol Surg.* 2006;32(6): 875–877.
20. Goldberg DJ, Littler CM, Wheeland RG. Topical suspension-assisted Q-switched Nd:YAG laser hair removal. *Dermatol Surg.* 1997;23(9):741–745.
21. Bernstein EF. Hair growth induced by diode laser treatment. *Dermatol Surg.* 2005;31(5):584–586.
22. Desai S, Mahmoud BH, Bhatia AC, Hamzavi IH. Paradoxical hypertrichosis after laser therapy: A review. *Dermatol Surg.* 2010; 36(3):291–298.
23. Moreno-Arias G, Castelo-Branco C, Ferrando J. Paradoxical effect after IPL photoepilation. *Dermatol Surg.* 2002;28 (11):1013–1016; discussion 1016.
24. Willey A, Torrontegui J, Azpiazu J, Landa N. Hair stimulation following laser and intense pulsed light photoepilation: Review of 543 cases and ways to manage it. *Lasers Surg Med.* 2007; 39(4):297–301.
25. Anderson RR, Burns AJ, Garden J, et al. Multicenter study of long-pulse ruby laser hair removal. *Lasers Surg Med.* 1999;11 (suppl):14.
26. Wanner M. Laser hair removal. *Dermatol Ther.* 2005;18(3): 209–216.
27. Garcia C, Alamoudi H, Nakib M, Zimmo S. Alexandrite laser hair removal is safe for Fitzpatrick skin types IV-VI. *Dermatol Surg.* 2000;26(2):130–134.
28. Galadari I. Comparative evaluation of different hair removal lasers in skin types IV, V, and VI. *Int J Dermatol.* 2003;42(1):68–70.
29. Davoudi SM, Behnia F, Gorouhi F, et al. Comparison of long-pulsed alexandrite and Nd:YAG lasers, individually and in combination, for leg hair reduction: An assessor-blinded, randomized trial with 18 months of follow-up. *Arch Dermatol.* 2008;144(10):1323–1327.
30. Hussain M, Polnikorn N, Goldberg DJ. Laser-assisted hair removal in Asian skin: Efficacy, complications, and the effect of single versus multiple treatments. *Dermatol Surg.* 2003; 29(3):249–254.
31. Khoury JG, Saluja R, Goldman MP. Comparative evaluation of long-pulse alexandrite and long-pulse Nd:YAG laser systems used individually and in combination for axillary hair removal. *Dermatol Surg.* 2008;34(5):665–670; discussion 670–671.
32. Campos VB, Dierickx CC, Farinelli WA, Lin TY, Manuskiatti W, Anderson RR. Hair removal with an 800-nm pulsed diode laser. *J Am Acad Dermatol.* 2000;43(3):442–447.
33. Lou WW, Quintana AT, Geronemus RG, Grossman MC. Prospective study of hair reduction by diode laser (800 nm) with long-term follow-up. *Dermatol Surg.* 2000;26(5):428–432.
34. Eremia S, Li C, Newman N. Laser hair removal with alexandrite versus diode laser using four treatment sessions: 1-year results. *Dermatol Surg.* 2001;27(11):925–929; discussion 929–930.
35. Alster TS, Bryan H, Williams CM. Long-pulsed Nd:YAG laser-assisted hair removal in pigmented skin: A clinical and histological evaluation. *Arch Dermatol.* 2001;137(7):885–889.
36. Rao J, Goldman MP. Prospective, comparative evaluation of three laser systems used individually and in combination for axillary hair removal. *Dermatol Surg.* 2005;31(12):1671–1676; discussion 1677.
37. Weiss RA, Weiss MA, Marwaha S, Harrington AC. Hair removal with a non-coherent filtered flashlamp intense pulsed light source. *Lasers Surg Med.* 1999;24(2):128–132.
38. Sadick NS, Shea CR, Burchette JL Jr, Prieto VG. High-intensity flashlamp photoepilation: A clinical, histological, and mechanistic study in human skin. *Arch Dermatol.* 1999;135(6):668–676.
39. Gold MH, Bell MW, Foster TD, Street S. One-year follow-up using an intense pulsed light source for long-term hair removal. *J Cutan Laser Ther.* 1999;1(3):167–171.
40. McGill DJ, Hutchison C, McKenzie E, McSherry E, Mackay IR. A randomised, split-face comparison of facial hair removal with the alexandrite laser and intense pulsed light system. *Lasers Surg Med.* 2007;39(10):767–772.
41. Goh CL. Comparative study on a single treatment response to long pulse Nd:YAG lasers and intense pulse light therapy for hair removal on skin type IV to VI–is longer wavelengths lasers preferred over shorter wavelengths lights for assisted hair removal. *J Dermatolog Treat.* 2003;14(4):243–247.
42. Haak CS, Nymann P, Pedersen AT, et al. Hair removal in hirsute women with normal testosterone levels: A randomized controlled trial of long-pulsed diode laser vs. intense pulsed light. *Br J Dermatol.* 2010;163(5):1007–1013.
43. Campos VB, Dierickx CC, Farinelli WA, Lin TY, Manuskiatti W, Anderson RR. Ruby laser hair removal: Evaluation of long-term efficacy and side effects. *Lasers Surg Med.* 2000;26(2):177–185.
44. Nouri K, Chen H, Saghari S, Ricotti CA Jr. Comparing 18- versus 12-mm spot size in hair removal using a gentlease 755-nm alexandrite laser. *Dermatol Surg.* 2004;30(4 Pt 1):494–497.
45. Ibrahimi OA, Kilmer SL. Long-term clinical evaluation of a 800 nm long-pulsed diode laser with a large spot size and vacuum-assisted suction for hair removal. *Dermatol Surg.* 2012;38(6):912–917.
46. Zenzie HH, Altshuler GB, Smirnov MZ, Anderson RR. Evaluation of cooling methods for laser dermatology. *Lasers Surg Med.* 2000;26(2):130–144.
47. Nelson JS, Milner TE, Anvari B, et al. Dynamic epidermal cooling during pulsed laser treatment of port-wine stain. A new methodology with preliminary clinical evaluation. *Arch Dermatol.* 1995;131(6):695–700.
48. Battle EF Jr, Suthamjariya KK, Alora MB, Palli K, Anderson RR. Very long-pulsed (20–200 ms) diode laser for hair removal on all skin types. *Lasers Surg Med.* 2000;12(suppl):85.
49. Braun M. Comparison of high-fluence, single-pass diode laser to low-fluence, multiple-pass diode laser for laser hair reduction with 18 months of follow up. *J Drugs Dermatol.* 2011;10 (1):62–65.
50. Nanni CA, Alster TS. Laser assisted hair removal: Side effects of Q-switched Nd:YAG, long-pulsed ruby and alexandrite lasers. *J Am Acad Dermatol.* 1999;141:165–171.
51. Haedersdal M, Egekvist H, Efsen J, Bjerring P. Skin pigmentation and texture changes after hair removal with the normal-mode ruby laser. *Acta Derm Venereol.* 1999;79(6):465–468.
52. Hasan AT, Eaglstein W, Pardo RJ. Solar-induced postinflammatory hyperpigmentation after laser hair removal. *Dermatol Surg.* 1999;25(2):113–115.
53. Moreno-Arias GA, Tiffon T, Marti T, Camps-Fresneda A. Long-term hypopigmentation induced by diode laser photo-epilation. *J Cutan Laser Ther.* 2001;3(1):9–10.
54. Radmanesh M, Mostaghimi M, Yousefi I, et al. Leukotrichia developed following application of intense pulsed light for hair removal. *Dermatol Surg.* 2002;28(7):572–574.
55. Wimmershoff MB, Hohenleutner U, Landthaler M. Isomorphic phenomenon: Adverse effect after epilation with the long-pulsed ruby laser. *Arch Dermatol.* 2000;36(12):1570–1571.
56. Lapidoth M, Shafirstein G, Ben Amitai D, Hodak E, Waner M, David M. Reticulate erythema following diode laser-assisted hair removal: A new side effect of a common procedure. *J Am Acad Dermatol.* 2004;51(5):774–777.
57. Moreno-Arias GA, Tiffon T, Marti T, Camps-Fresneda A. Urticaria vasculitis induced by diode laser photo-epilation. *Dermatol Surg.* 2000;26(11):1082–1083.
58. Lask G, Friedman D, Elman M, Fournier N, Shavit R, Slatkine M. Pneumatic skin flattening (PSF): a novel technology for marked pain reduction in hair removal with high energy density lasers and IPLs. *J Cosmet Laser Ther.* 2006;8(2):76–81.
59. Rohrer TE, Chatrath V, Yamauchi P, Lask G. Can patients treat themselves with a small novel light based hair removal system? *Lasers Surg Med.* 2003;33(1):25–29.
60. Spencer JM. Clinical evaluation of a handheld self-treatment device for hair removal. *J Drugs Dermatol.* 2007;6(8):788–792.
61. Wheeland RG. Simulated consumer use of a battery-powered, hand-held, portable diode laser (810 nm) for hair removal: A

safety, efficacy and ease-of-use study. *Lasers Surg Med.* 2007; 39(6):476–493.
62. Grossman M, Dwyer P, Wimberley J, Flotte TJ. PDT for hirsutism. *Lasers Surg Med.* 1995;7(suppl):44.
63. Waldman A, Kreindle M. New technology in aesthetic medicine: ELOS electro optical synergy. *J Cosmet Laser Ther.* 2003;5 (3–4):204–206.
64. Sadick NS, Shaoul J. Hair removal using a combination of conducted radiofrequency and optical energies—an 18-month follow-up. *J Cosmet Laser Ther.* 2004;6(1):21–26.
65. Goldberg DJ, Marmur ES, Hussain M. Treatment of terminal and vellus non-pigmented hairs with an optical/bipolar radiofrequency energy source-with and without pretreatment using topical aminolevulinic acid. *J Cosmet Laser Ther.* 2005; 7(1):25–28.
66. Klein A, Steinert S, Baeumler W, Landthaler M, Babilas P. Photoepilation with a diode laser vs. intense pulsed light (IPL): A randomized, intrapatient left-to-right trial. *Br J Dermatol.* 2013;168(6):1287–1293. doi:10.1111/bjd.12182.
67. Jalian HR, Jalian CA, Avram MM. Common causes of injury and legal action in laser surgery. *JAMA Dermatol.* 2013; 149(2):188–193.
68. Wheeland RG. Permanent hair reduction with a home-use diode laser: Safety and effectiveness 1 year after eight treatments. *Lasers Surg Med.* 2012;44(7):550–557.

This chapter is modified and updated from Ibrahimi OA, Avram MM, Hanke CW, Kilmer SL, Anderson RR. Laser hair removal. *Dermatol Ther.* 2011;24(1):94–107.

CHAPTER 54

Eyelid Rejuvenation

Robyn Sackeyfio, Robert Silich, & Henry M. Spinelli

ANATOMY

The eyelid is composed of three distinct anatomic layers, similar to those found in the nose: the external skin, a middle supportive layer, and an internal lining (Fig. 54-1). One should view the eyelids as trilamellar structures, which are supported in space across the orbital rim by medial and lateral anchors, namely, the medial and lateral canthal tendons. The three lamellae include an outside layer of skin that is especially thin over the tarsus and preseptal areas with minimal to no subcutaneous fat. The middle, or supportive, layer includes the orbicularis muscles with the pretarsal portion lying in front of the tarsal plate and the preorbital portion lying anterior to the orbital septum. The tarsal plate is a rigid cartilaginous-like structure that measures 4 to 6 mm on the lower eyelid and 8 to 10 mm on the upper eyelid. This structural layer is pierced by glands that drain posterior to the eyelashes, or ciliary line, and number approximately 10 on the lower lid and 20 on the upper lid. These Meibomian glands and ducts are responsible for oil secretion, and when they become inspissated they may be responsible for hordeola or styes (acute inflammation), chalazia (chronic noncaseating granulomas), and other inflammatory processes. These are also the sites for inflammation in the postcosmetic blepharoplasty, including meibomianitis and blepharitis. The tarsal plate is particularly important for vertical support of the eyelid, which is fundamental to maintaining the lower eyelid position 1 to 2 mm above the corneoscleral junction or limbus. The internal lining of the eyelid is mucosa, which reflects off the globe and onto the posterior surface of the eyelids, including the posterior surfaces of the medial and lateral canthal tendons. The conjunctival surface, rich in secretory glands, is a virtually frictionless surface for the lids and globe to move against one another.

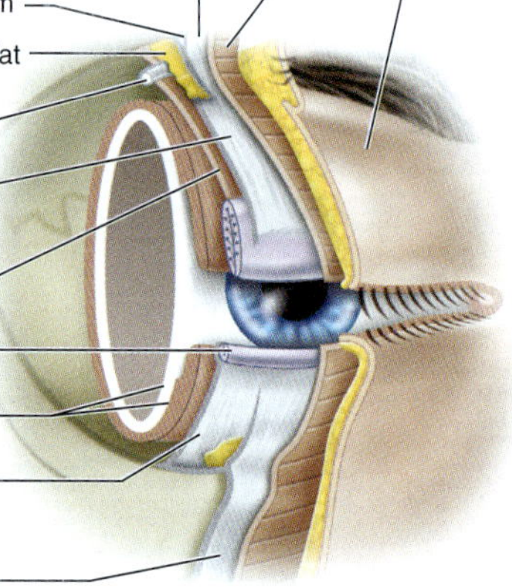

Figure 54-1 Oblique cross-section of the right orbit and adnexa beginning anteriorly with the skin and ending posteriorly with the conjuctiva covering the anterior sclera. The orbicularis muscle is contiguous with the frontalis, occipitalis, and superficial musculoaponeurotic (SMAS) layer. The orbital septum is confluent with the periosteum of the skull and orbit, as well as the periorbita. The orbital septum is also fused to the levator palpebrae and therefore serves as a complete boundary between the anterior and deep orbit. One cannot access the preaponeurotic fat without violating the superior septum. Analogously, the inferior orbital septum is intimately linked to the periosteum and the capsulopalpebral fascial system. The main retractors of the upper and lower lids are the levator and capsulopalpebral fascia, respectively. The levator is suspended from the superior orbit by Whitnall's ligament. This structure allows the muscle to change vector forces from anterior to posterior and superior to inferior, thus serving as a pulley. The preaponeurotic and precapsulopalpebral fat is loosely but definitely linked to the respective retractors; hence, dehiscence of the levator fascia from the tarsal plate will lead to a superior sulcus deformity. The tarsal plates are the end point for retractor insertion and provide lid stability and orientation.

The medial canthal tendon envelops the lacrimal sac and is tripartite, with anterior, posterior, and superior limbs. Like the lateral canthal tendon, its limbs are continuous with the tarsal plate. The components of this tendon, along with its lateral counterpart, are enveloped by the deep and superficial aspects of the orbicularis muscle, which is important in maintaining a functional, active lacrimal drainage system. The upper, lower, and common canaliculi closely approximate this tendinous system, and care should be taken to preserve their integrity when altering any aspect of the medial canthal tendon. Generally, the medial canthal apparatus is not directly addressed in cosmetic approaches to the eyelids; however, it may require an elective tightening procedure, especially in cases in which a lateral canthal procedure alone would produce punctual and lacrimal dystopia. The lateral canthal tendon is more commonly addressed surgically than the medial canthal apparatus. Topographically, it should be inclined 10 to 15 degrees superiorly with respect to the medial canthal tendon, which is the most anatomic and aesthetically pleasing position. It splits into an anterior and posterior leaflet, the anterior being continuous with the orbital rim periosteum and the posterior element inserting on Whitnall's tubercle. The lateral horn of the levator aponeurosis also inserts on Whitnall's tubercle, resulting in a coalescence of support and suspensory structures serving as anchor points for the eyelids. It also contains a coalescence of the inferior suspensory ligament of Lockwood. Thus, simply dividing the lateral canthal tendon will not sufficiently mobilize the complex in a repositioning and/or tightening procedure.

As demonstrated in Figure 54-2, the lower and upper eyelids and periocular structures are quite similar. Both the upper and lower eyelids are composed of the three aforementioned structural layers with the tarsal plate of the upper lid being a little wider. Both lids have a cul-de-sac that forms the junction between the parietal and visceral conjunctiva and are surrounded by orbicularis muscle that is continuous with the superficial musculo-aponeurotic system (SMAS), platysma, and frontalis muscles. The orbicularis functions as a sphincter or protractor and is divided into the pretarsal, preseptal, and preorbital areas. It is innervated by the seventh cranial nerve, and hence, with facial nerve paralysis, the cornea and globe can be exposed secondary to an atonic eyelid with unopposed retractor action. The eyelid retractors are made up of the levator palpebrae superioris muscle and a secondary sympathomimetically innervated Müller's muscle. Müller's muscle is responsible for approximately 2 mm of lid elevation during sympathetic stimulation, the so-called fight or flight responses. The levator palpebrae superioris is responsible for the remainder of voluntary lid elevation and measures approximately 37 mm in length and 4 mm in width at the apex of the orbit. It gradually widens anteriorly until it fans out into an approximately 20 mm long aponeurosis that expands from 6 mm at the distal end of the levator to a width of 30 mm where it inserts onto the tarsal plate. The levator muscle will send some fibers to the dermal surface of the upper lid creating the lid fold. Surgical manipulation can be a powerful tool for manipulating upper lid height, which can be achieved through plication, advancement, or recession. A normal upper eyelid lies midway between the upper aspect of the pupillary aperture and the upper corneal scleral junction/limbus, with the apex of its arch lying just medial to the pupil, and is an important landmark in any ptosis correction.

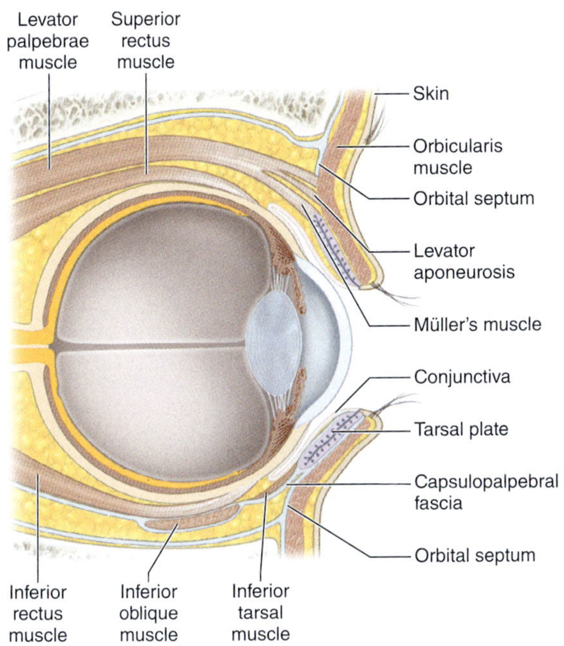

Figure 54-2 On the lateral view, the analogy between upper and lower eyelids is clear. The upper and lower septa merge with the periosteum externally and the periorbita internally. The levator aponeurosis merges with the septum, and the preaponeurotic fat is linked to the levator and only accessible by violating the septum. Müller's muscle is sympathomimetically innervated and is the flight/fright elevator of the upper lid, responsible for 1 to 2 mm of excursion. The capsulopalpebral fascia of the lower eyelid retractor system arises off the inferior oblique and rectus muscles. Therefore, the lower eyelid "gets out of the way" when the globe is depressed, as when reading the newspaper. The conjunctiva reflects on itself, covering the undersurface of the eyelids and then onto the eyeball. This is similar to visceral and parietal layers found elsewhere in the body. The fat in the lower orbit is behind the septum but in front of the retractor system. Hence it may be termed precapsulopalpebral fat. All orbital fat is linked by septa so that traction placed on anterior extraconal fat produces a disturbance in the deep extraconal and intraconal fat. Note the coalescence of the inferior orbital septum with the capsulopalpebral fascia is well below the inferior tarsal plate. This zone of coalescence is a favored access route to the important potential space. We call this the postorbicularis precapsulopalpebral fascial space, which is important in deftly executing both transconjunctival and transcutaneous blepharoplasties.

The lower lid retractors are intimately linked to the inferior extraocular muscles, the inferior rectus muscles, and the inferior oblique muscles. Capsulopalpebral fascial extensions connect these muscles to the inferior edge of the lower lid tarsal plate, which is analogous to the levator aponeurosis of the upper lid. This capsulopalpebral fascia is a voluntary retractor of the lower lid, allowing the lid to be pulled away when the globe is depressed, and is an important structure that is divided during any transconjunctival approach to the orbit. Both the upper and lower lid retractors have a reorientation of their direction of pull within the orbit as they course anteriorly. The levator palpebrae superioris changes its vector from the anterior/posterior direction to the cephalad/caudad direction by way of a pulley system allowing the upper lid to raise, much like a garage door. This fascial condensation or ligamentous band is Whitnall's ligament (Fig. 54-3) and should be visualized during all upper lid blepharoplasties. Its fibers connect to the trochlea medially and laterally. They extend to join the lacrimal gland stroma, which divides the gland into palpebral and orbital lobes. It finally inserts on the key surgical structure known as Whitnall's tubercle, which is a bony excrescence within the orbital rim and below the zygomaticofrontal junction. This is also the place where the lateral canthal tendon inserts; it is placed 6 mm below the lacrimal fossa and 2 mm within the orbit (Fig. 54-4). It is important to accurately realign the anatomic structures in this area to prevent lateral upper lid retraction or lag on attempted closure as well as a loss of upper lid sweep.

The origin of most extraocular muscles is at a fibrous thickening of periosteum known as the annulus of Zinn, which is located at the apex of the orbit. The superior oblique and levator muscles also arise at the apex but originate outside the annulus. The orbital apex is delineated by the greater sphenoid wing, which separates the middle

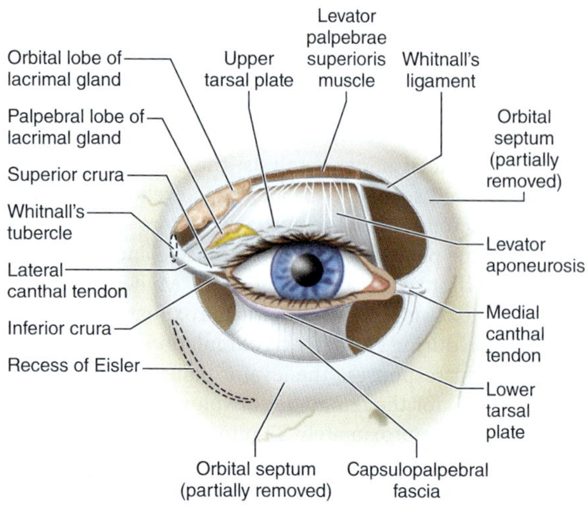

Figure 54-3 The upper and lower eyelids are suspended in space, tethered medially and laterally by the canthal tendons; and these in turn are linked to Whitnall's and Lockwood's ligaments. The orbital and palpebral lobes of the lacrimal gland are divided by Whitnall's ligament. The orbital septum inserts at the orbital rim, except inferolaterally where it inserts beyond the rim forming the Eisler recess.

cranial fossa from the orbit and is the juncture at which a number of nerves pass between the intracranial compartment and the orbit. These include the optic, oculomotor, trochlear, and abducens nerves. The function of the extraocular muscles include abduction, addiction, intorsion, and extortion, and they derive their blood supply from the ophthalmic artery, with each muscle receiving two anterior ciliary arteries except for the lateral rectus that receives only one. The anterior ciliary artery penetrates the sclera to contribute to nourishing the anterior segment of the globe and thus disinsertion of more than two rectus muscles can result in anterior segment necrosis. The inferior oblique muscle is responsible for elevation, abduction, and extortion or rotation of the globe clockwise and is the most frequently damaged muscle during a blepharoplasty, especially during a transconjunctival approach, as it divides the medial and central fat pads. The superior oblique muscle arises superomedial to the annulus and functions to depress, abduct, and intorse the globe and also divides the medial and central fat pads in the upper compartment. To a lesser extent, it is also vulnerable to injury during an upper lid blepharoplasty.

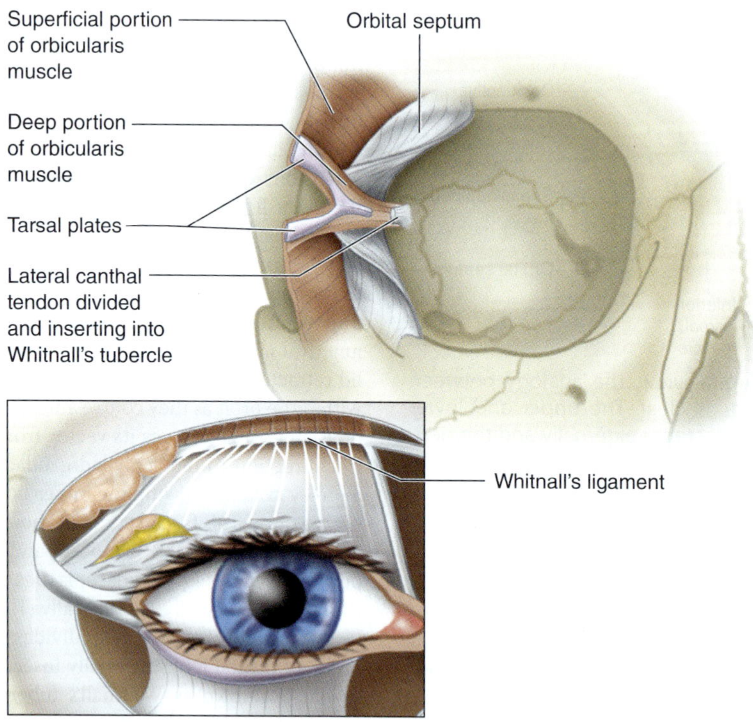

Figure 54-4 The anatomy of the lateral canthal region shows the integration of muscular, tendinous, and other components of the lateral retinaculum. The pretarsal orbicularis muscle follows the deep portion of the lateral retinaculum. The pretarsal orbicularis muscle follows the deep portion of the lateral canthal tendon behind the septum inserting on Whitnall's tubercle. The preseptal orbicularis muscle moves superficially with the superficial aspects of the lateral canthal tendon, just anterior to the orbital septum. Note the orbital septum dividing into anterior and posterior leaflets in continuity with the periosteum and periorbita. Whitnall's ligament, seen through the septum (insert), sends a small component superiorly and a main component to split the lacrimal gland and insert on Whitnall's tubercle.

Orbital fat is generally the focus of much of the cosmetic surgery in the periocular region. On the upper lid, the fat to be addressed is anterior to the levator aponeurosis and is termed preaponeurotic. Analogously, in the lower eyelid the fat is in the precapsulopalpebral fascial plane. Due to linkage of fat within the orbit by way of septa that transgress the extraocular muscle cone, there is a small but definitive risk of orbital hemorrhage and even blindness when addressing anterior orbital fat in surgical procedures.

EVALUATION OF THE PATIENT

Every patient should have a detailed history not only focusing on the chief complaint but also ascertaining preexisting ocular complaints. These should include a query regarding such conditions as dry eyes, contact lens wear, thyroid or Graves' disease, previous refractive surgery, recurrent acute or chronic blepharitis, or any other relevant ocular complaints. Physical examination should start with gross inspection at a comfortable distance with particular note taken of any gross abnormalities or asymmetries. The upper lid should divide the width of the upper iris in half and the lower lid should lie above or at the corneoscleral junction. Visual acuity, papillary reactivity, intrinsic lid tone, lower eyelid support, baseline tear production, and lid position should also be assessed during the presurgical consultation.

Eyelid position and, more importantly, malposition is one topic that must be further elucidated prior to moving on to describe specific procedures. Malpositions of the eyelid, specifically the lower lid, include ectropion, or turning out of the lid margin, entropion, turning in of the lid margin, and retraction or scleral show. Classically, ectropion and entropion have been classified as cicatricial, senile/involutional, mechanical, paralytic, and congenital, but oftentimes it is more helpful to identify the pathophysiology in order to correctly address the problem. Involutional or senile lid malpositions are most common and are secondary to progressive laxity of the medial and lateral canthal tendons over time (Fig. 54-5).

Repositioning of the lateral canthal tendon specifically is addressed with a lateral cathopexy, which is a tightening or resuspension of the canthal tendon, or a canthoplasty, a division or disinsertion coupled with a resuspension procedure. Another technique aimed at repositioning and tightening the lateral canthal tendon is the tarsal strip.

UPPER LID BLEPHAROPLASTY

Blepharoplasty has become one of the more common aesthetic surgical procedures. Preoperative evaluation, as previously discussed, should focus on a complete eye examination as well as explore the patient's desires and his or her perception of what needs to be corrected. It is important to point out preexisting asymmetries as well as conditions such as dry eyes or herpes zoster or simplex infections. The physical examination should include a Schirmer test, tear film break-up time, visual acuity with and without correction, and eyelid retraction or laxity. In the patient undergoing upper lid blepharoplasty, it is extremely important to assess eyebrow position and the presence or absence of ptosis. It is also important to note the presence of blepharochalasis or dermatochalasis. The former is defined as redundant upper lid tissue secondary to an underlying pathophysiology such as chronic edema, which may be found in renal failure or congestive heart failure. Dermatochalasis is the redundant upper eyelid tissue commonly seen secondary to the aging process with or without ptotic eyebrow changes.

The eyebrow hairline and sub-brow fat pad should also be evaluated in relationship to the upper orbital rim. It is important to note that a surgeon who attempts to correct significant brow ptosis with an upper lid blepharoplasty alone will meet with an unsatisfactory result. Typically, this procedure by itself will result in a blending of thinner eyelid skin with the thicker eyebrow skin giving the patient the appearance of having his/her eyelids directly sutured to his/her eyebrows. Hence, in this situation, one should refer this patient to a surgeon more facile in performing complex periorbital procedures.

The amount of horizontal lid laxity is also an important factor that should be appreciated preoperatively. Absence of lid lag, or lagophthalmos, should be noted because asymptomatic lagophthalmos can easily be converted to the symptomatic variety with very small amounts of skin excision.

An important concept in appreciating upper eyelid functional and cosmetic surgery is illustrated by contrasting nuances in the anatomy and pathophysiology between racial and age groups (Fig. 54-6). For example, the upper eyelid crease lies 6 to 8 mm from the lid margin in a young Caucasian patient. The lid fold is created by extensions of

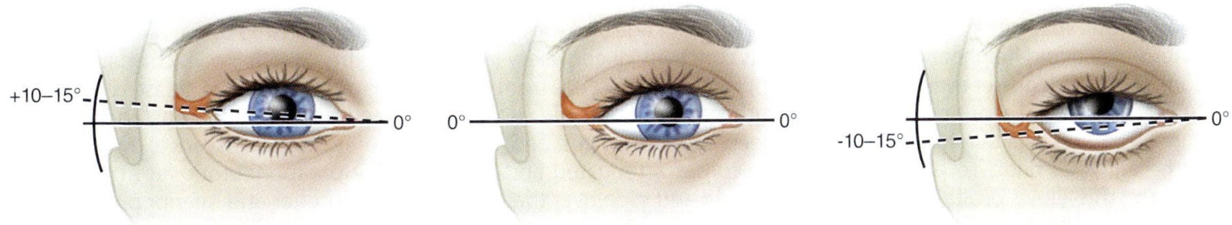

A B C

Figure 54-5 A–C. The lateral canthus is normally inclined cephalad by 10 to 15 degrees compared with the medial canthus. Attenuation with aging produces a descent of the lateral canthus so that the lateral canthus rotates (clockwise on the left and counterclockwise on the right) around the medial canthus. The end result is a lateral canthus that is coplanar or declined compared with the medial canthus. As the lateral canthus sags inferiorly, the intercommissure distance shortens (distance between medial and lateral canthus) and the lower lid and inferior lateral septum become lax. This produces scleral show, ectropion or entropion, orbital fat prominence especially laterally, and tear film distribution and drainage problems.

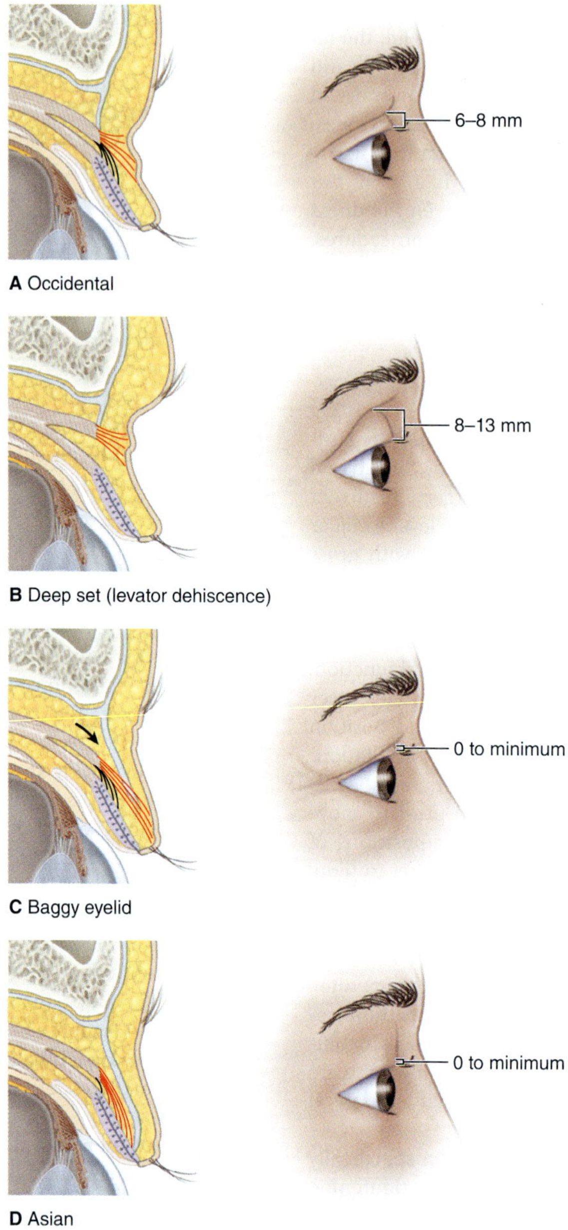

Figure 54-6 The anatomic variations in the upper eyelid displayed by different ethnic groups and the changes associated with senescence within each group allow for a convergence of anatomy. Many of these ethnic differences are erased by again and/or attenuation of structures, allowing for what the author likes to call a unified upper lid concept. **A.** The normal youthful occidental upper eyelid has levator extensions inserting onto the skin surface to define a lid fold that averages 6 to 8 mm above the lid margin. Note the orbital septum coalescing with the levator aponeurosis creating the fat-containing preaponeurotic space. The position of the levator-skin linkage and the anteroposterior relationship of the preaponeurotic fat determine lid fold height and degree of sulcus concavity or convexity (as shown on the right half of each anatomic depiction). **B.** In the deep-set eyelid or in the case of levator dehiscence from the tarsal plate, the upper lid crease is displaced superiorly. The orbital septum and preaponeurotic fat linked to the levator are displaced superiorly and posteriorly. These anatomic changes create a high lid crease, a deep superior sulcus, and, in the case of levator dehiscence, eyelid ptosis. **C.** In the aging or baggy eyelid, the septum becomes attenuated and stretches. The preaponeurotic fat attachments loosen, and this allows orbital fat to prolapse forward and slide over the levator into an anterior and inferior position. The net result is an inferior displacement of the levator skin attachments and a low and anterior position of the preaponeurotic fat pad. Clinically, this results in a low lid crease that is only a few millimeters from the lid margin and may not be visible owing to the overhanging lid. **D.** The youthful Asian eyelid anatomically resembles the baggy or senescent upper lid with a low levator skin zone of adhesion and inferior and anteriorly located preaponeurotic fat. The characteristic, but variable, low eyelid crease and convex upper eyelid and sulcus are classic.

the levator muscle onto the lid skin. This lid fold is significantly elevated in the deep-set eye or an eyelid in which a levator dehiscence has occurred. In both instances, preaponeurotic fat is retracted or located more cephalad. In the senescent or "baggy" Caucasian upper eyelid, septal laxity and tissue relaxation allow preaponeurotic fat to prolapse anteriorly, lowering the eyelid fold and moving it closer to the lid margin. This age-related pathophysiology is analogous to the normal anatomy in the youthful Asian upper eyelid. Here, the eyelid fold is low and variable closer to the lid margin, with fullness created above it owing to prolapsed preaponeurotic fat extending to the insertion of the levator aponeurotic elements on the overriding lid skin.

The procedure of an upper eyelid blepharoplasty essentially involves the removal of redundant or excessive skin of the upper eyelids along with a small portion of the orbicularis muscle and preaponeurotic fat. It is, therefore, important that the surgeon and patient choose the appropriate technique based on the pathophysiology and the patient's desires after assessing the "relative" dermatochalasis, or skin redundancy, as contributed from the eyelid versus the eyebrow.

The first important anatomic landmark is the upper eyelid crease. In Caucasians, the crease is 6 to 10 mm above the eyelid margin and is typically slightly higher in females. In the Asian eyelid, by contrast, the lid crease may be considerably lower although some patients may request a more Caucasian eyelid, which means raising the endogenous upper eyelid fold. Once this margin has been marked preoperatively, the next step is to perform a pinch test to determine the extent of upper eyelid skin excision. The design of the upper and lower limbs of the incision should be curvilinear, with the medial aspect being convex superiorly and the lateral aspect being convex inferiorly. Every attempt should be made to assure that the lateral aspect of the lower skin incision is placed within a skin crease, which is upwardly inclined to meet the upper aspect of the incision and then extended laterally. The lateral extent of the incision is dictated by the degree of lateral eyebrow ptosis or hooding, if present (Fig. 54-7). Local anesthetic with epinephrine is infiltrated and adequate time for hemostasis is allowed to elapse. Upper and lower lid eyelid incisions are made in a medial-to-lateral direction through the skin and orbicularis muscle. The skin muscle flap is elevated, this time in a lateral-to-medial direction with digital retraction laterally. The orbital septum is then tented upward with a forceps, unroofed from lateral to medial, using a sharp scissors or needle-tip cautery at the level of the upper extent of the eyelid incision. Preaponeurotic fat (medial and central fat pads) can be accessed by opening the orbital septum as cephalad as possible where the levator aponeurosis lies most posteriorly with interposed preaponeurotic fat. This can be dissected out using a fine hemostat and light digital pressure on the globe to tease the fat free of adhesions and allow for spontaneous prolapse. The fat can then be resected using a fine tip cautery. By using light inferior traction on the upper lid, one should be able to visualize the levator aponeurosis and Whitnall's ligament. It is easy to obtain complete access to the anterior one-third of the orbit above the levator muscle using these simple techniques (Fig. 54-8A–E).

More advanced procedures such as modifying the levator aponeurosis can be carried out at this time depending on level of expertise. It may be freed from the tarsal plate and advanced in a formal levator advancement procedure for ptosis or plicated for milder degrees of ptosis. Closure, for which there have been numerous techniques described, is then performed. For the sake of simplicity, only our preferred closure method is described here. Using a 5-0 nonabsorbable monofilament suture the incision is closed in a running fashion. Laterally, the incision can be closed with interrupted 6-0 monofilament sutures to assure adequate skin eversion along the canthal line, and to avoid unsightly depressed scarring particularly for female patients.

Suture removal is performed at 5 to 10 days as deemed appropriate by the surgeon.

LOWER LID BLEPHAROPLASTY

The lower lid blepharoplasty has traditionally been viewed as the more technically challenging blepharoplasty to perform. The perception of difficulty likely lies more in the numerous decision-making processes the surgeon and patient are forced to undergo to achieve a satisfactory lower lid result. During the initial consultation, a thorough history, including the features that the patient feels are the most problematic, should be obtained and the patient should be evaluated for the presence and degree of horizontal lid laxity and the position of the lateral and medial canthal angles. The presence of scleral show, entropion, ectropion, or other underlying pathologic processes should also be thoroughly evaluated prior to surgery. Once the patient has been evaluated, the surgeon has many more choices as to how to approach the lower lid blepharoplasty and less margin for error. There are numerous surgical approaches to address excess skin, such as performing a simple skin trim, laser resurfacing, or performing a skin peel. Similarly, the surgical approaches to excess fat can be addressed with simple resection, redistribution, or both. Other decisions to be made include whether to perform a transcutaneous or transconjunctival approach, whether to perform a canthal procedure such as a tarsal tuck or tarsal strip procedure, or whether to reposition the entire lateral canthus (common canthoplasty).

The transcutaneous lower lid blepharoplasty is a powerful technique for addressing lower lid cosmetic abnormalities. It allows for a number of adjuvant procedures to be performed easily and more accurately than with the transconjuctival approach. The transcutaneous approach can be considered more technically challenging, taking more time with a more extensive dissection, which would lead to greater secondary fibrosis leading to scleral show and/or ectropion. This approach, however, is better for addressing fat alone, while approaching the skin and/or muscle separately, with the lower lid tightened thereafter by way of a direct approach to the lateral lower lid tarsus or inferior crus of the lateral canthal tendon. The transcutaneous route also allows access to the midface and can allow for some elevation of the medial cheek at the nasolabial junction.

The lower eyelid may be delineated for blepharoplasty by drawing an incision line extending from the lateral canthus posteriorly in a natural skinfold. This is usually

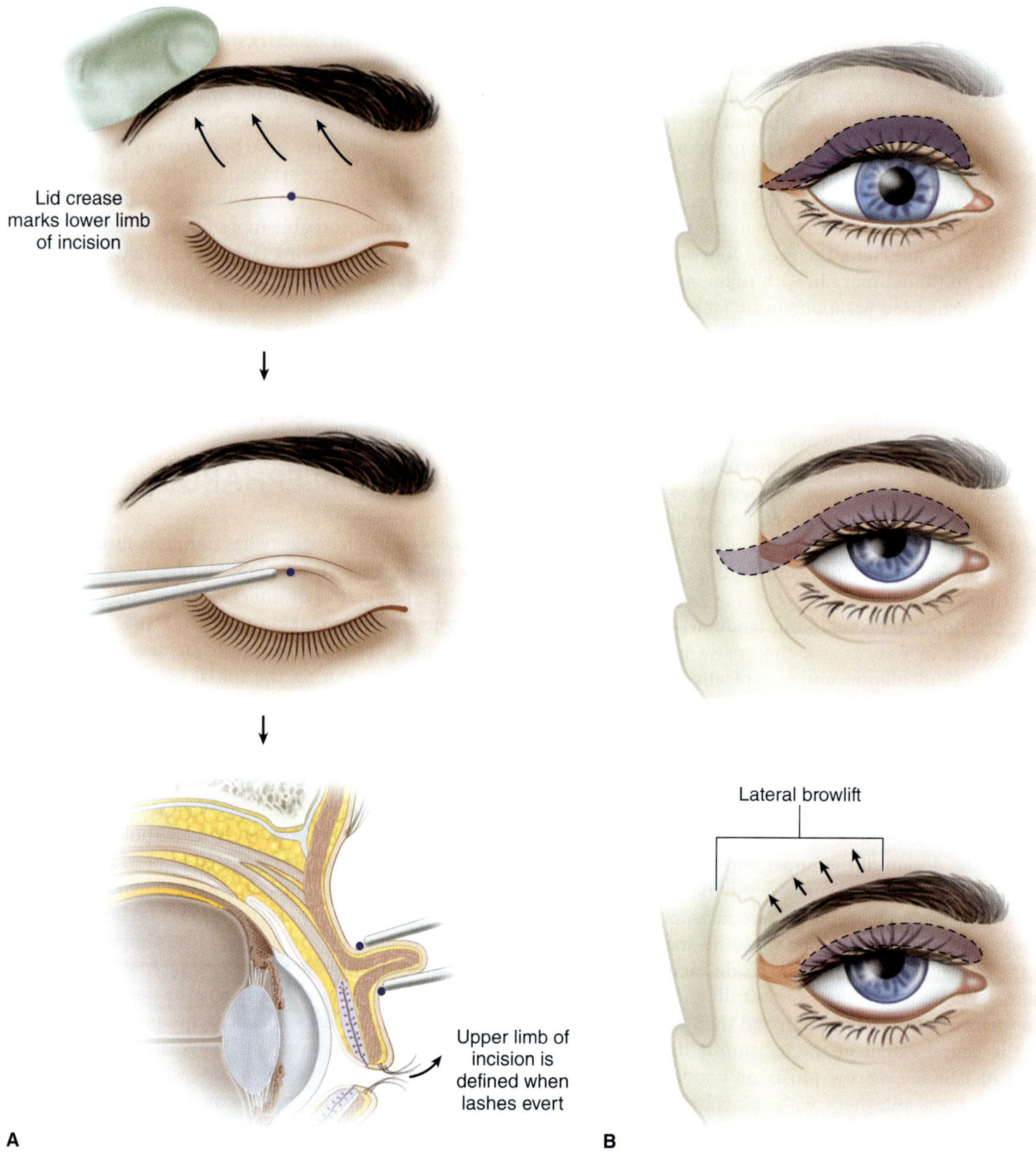

Figure 54-7 The key points in planning and executing the upper lid blepharoplasty are as follows: **A.** Determination of the endogenous lid crease or height at which to create a new lid crease (if different from the existing crease). The latter would require supratarsal fixation. The level of this crease will serve as the lower limb of the blepharoplasty incision and the height of supratarsal fixation, should that be necessary. The width or extent of skin excision is determined by pinching the lid skin between forceps using slight lash line eversion as the end point. This superior point will determine the location for the superior limb of the skin incision (left). **B.** Determination of the extent of lateral eyebrow ptosis and, hence, the amount of lateral upper eyelid hooding. The greater the hooding the more lateral the extent of the incision (top, dark to lighter shades of color). In general, incisions that extend beyond the orbital rim are not well tolerated (middle). The unequal lengths of the upper and lower limbs are effectively Burow's triangles to eliminate dog-ears and must be exaggerated as one widens the lateral skin excision. Also a brow that lacks stability may be pulled down by tension induced by a wide lateral excision. Here a balance must be made between the extent of lateral hooding and the drive to maintain incision lines within the confines of the orbital rim. Once the lateral extent of the incision becomes excessive a lateral brow suspension should be entertained.

subtly declined inferiorly to appear more natural and to avoid encroaching on the upper lid. As in the upper lid blepharoplasty, it is better to minimize the lateral extent of the incision line, and we choose to make a limited incision that is extended if necessary for skin and muscle redraping and/or suspension. The incision line will extend medial to the lateral canthus in the natural fold below the lower eyelid. It is preferable to leave a cuff of pretarsal orbicularis below the lash margin, which is theoretically responsible for eyelash orientation (Riolan's muscle).

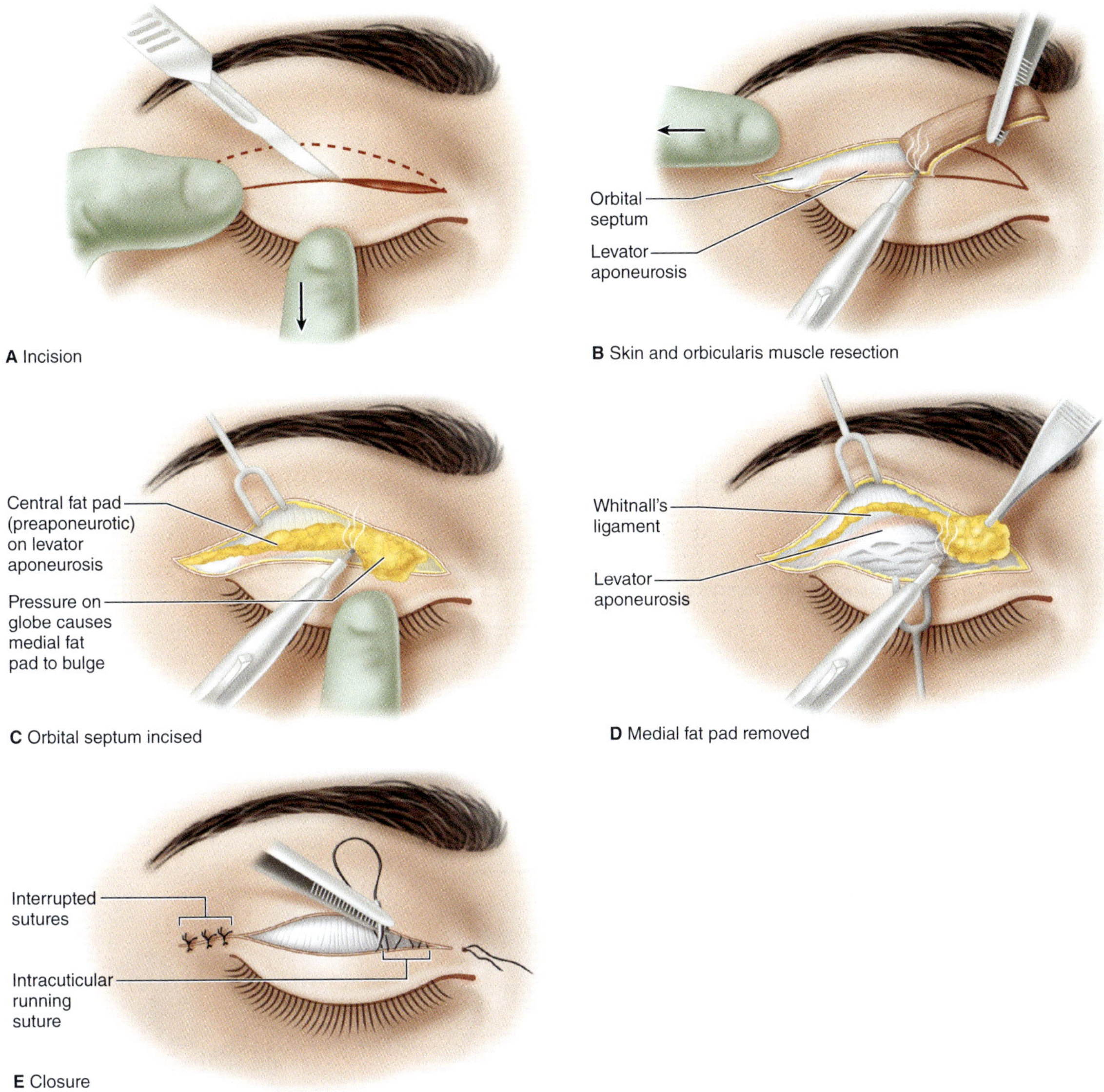

Figure 54-8 In practice the upper lid blepharoplasty can be efficiently performed using a few technical manipulations consistent with the anatomy. Digital traction and light pressure by the surgeon and/or assistant allow smooth quick skin incisions. **A.** Slightly more pressure must be exerted on the scalpel laterally as the skin thickens around and lateral to the orbital rim. **B.** The skin may be elevated with the orbicularis muscle in one maneuver using an instrument on the skin-muscle section to be resected and pulling this superonasally while providing digital traction laterally. A needle-tipped insulated cautery can be the most advantageous in this and other succeeding steps, especially in avoiding any delaying hemostasis problems. The orbital septum is the widely opened, exposing the preaponeurotic space. **C.** The underlying levator aponeurosis is protected by opening the septum as cephalad as possible, because the levator and septum diverge as one moves superiorly. **D.** The medial fat pad may require some digital pressure to expose and grasp; however, care should be taken not to overly resect fat when using digital pressure techniques. Excessive traction and manipulation of fat could cause a deep orbital hemorrhage and should, therefore, be avoided. **E.** Closure may then be performed with 6-0 nylon interrupted sutures laterally and 5-0 nylon intracuticular sutures medially.

Local anesthetic of choice (lidocaine with epinephrine) is infiltrated, and adequate time for hemostasis is allowed to elapse. An incision is made in the lateral extent of the delineated incision through the skin and orbicularis muscle. A curved sharp Steven's or tenotomy scissors is inserted in the postorbicularis/preseptal plane. This is the potential space just anterior to the orbital septum. As one enters this space from lateral to medial, the scissors are opened gently and a true space is developed extending from the preseptal to the pretarsal suborbicularis regions. The scissors are withdrawn and a fine small sharp scissors (iris scissors) reinserted with one limb of the scissors in the incision and the other overlying the skin of the lower lid. The marginal aspect of the incision is then made just below the last-line margin of the lid with the scissors beveled inferiorly (lower limb inferior) (Fig. 54-9). The incision should extend up to a point lateral to the medial punctum. The lower lid is then placed in cephalic traction

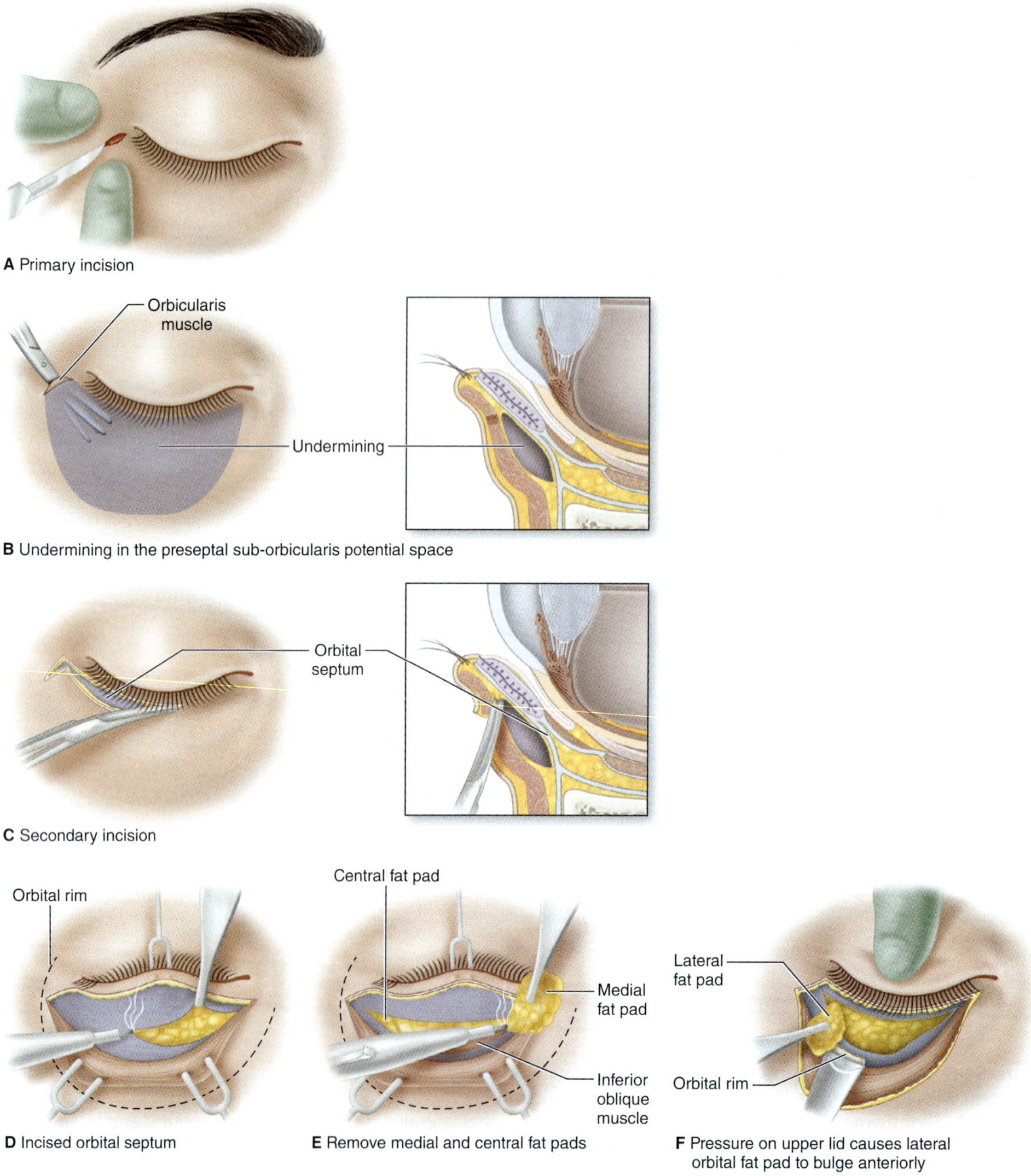

Figure 54-9 As with the upper lid, the successful completion of the lower lid blepharoplasty requires a few technical steps that will simplify and speed its execution. The anatomy of the lower eyelid can be advantageous to the surgeon in properly performing these steps. **A.** The primary incision should be in a desired fold or potential fold at and lateral to the lateral canthus. The incision should be limited but able to admit a small curved scissors. The scissors should be passed through the incision into the suborbicularis preseptal space. **B.** This plane is developed from lateral to medial while gently pushing and separating the scissors. Once this plane is developed, the myocutaneous flap can be mobilized with ease. The scissors are withdrawn and only one limb is inserted into the preseptal postorbicularis plane, with the other over the skin surface. The scissors may be beveled toward the eyeball (less skin, more muscle). **C.** The second incision is completed lateral to medial with the assistance of inferior digital traction, ending just lateral to the lower lid punctum. The flap should be mobilized to the orbital rim without violating the septum. This is best achieved with a combination of digital cheek traction inferiorly and instrument elevation of the myocutaneous flap. **D.** The septum may be opened either widely or with stab incisions. **E.** In either case the inferior oblique muscle should be visualized and protected. We usually identify the oblique muscle before resection or repositioning fat. The muscle is most anterior medially, adjacent to the medial fat pad, and this is the best place to identify it using an instrument to spread or probe while concomitantly applying light digital pressure. **F.** Remember that over-resection of fat, especially in the lateral compartment, can lead to less than acceptable cosmetic results. Skin resection should be conservative and involve lateral and cephalic vectors.

with an eyelid hook, and with countertraction on the skin muscle flap, the myocutaneous flap is elevated to the level of the orbital rim inferiorly. If a corneal shield or contact lens has not been used, the lower eyelid hook should be placed on the conjunctival side of the lower eyelid so as to avoid corneal or globe injury. Once the myocutaneous flap is elevated to the orbital rim, the orbital septum will be easily visualized and may be incised to address orbital fat when appropriate.

The orbital septum can be incised to visualize all three fat pads along with the inferior oblique muscle. The fat can then be conservatively resected with a needle cautery. Over-resection can lead to concavity or a "sickly appearance," to the lower lid and inferior orbital region. Fat redistribution techniques may be used alone or in combination with fat resection depending on which compartment is thought to be prominent or deficient. In general, when approaching fat resection alone, only fat that spontaneously herniates with light digital pressure to the globe should be removed and the amputation point should not extend within the orbital rim. Special care should be taken to directly observe the lateral fat compartment because this is the most frequently missed or inappropriately addressed (Fig. 54-9A–F).

Once fat has been addressed and the surgeon has suspended the lower lid and/or midface if appropriate, the skin muscle flap is redraped and adjusted. Every attempt should be made to elevate the skin muscle flap cephalad and laterally so as to create a vector force that runs superiorly from the nasojugal groove through the lateral canthal area. This orientation is important in eliminating the line of force that links the lower eyelid directly to the malar tissue in one plane. This technique, however, may be slightly less advantageous in eliminating lower eyelid skin rhytides. The flap may be backcut at the point of insertion to the lateral canthal region, and skin may be trimmed from lateral to medial as a tapered wedge so that very little, if any, skin is resected from the level of the papillary axis to the medial canthus. The area of the skin muscle flap that lies lateral to the lateral canthus can be appropriately resected without tension, with the possibility of extending the incision line temporarily depending on the amount of redundancy, or dog-ear, created. A separate closure of the muscular layer may be performed when a larger amount of myocutaneous resection is employed.

A single absorbable suture through the orbicularis muscle that engenders cephalic lateral suspension forces can be useful not only in eliminating or reducing tension on the skin closure but also in further supporting the lower lid against distraction forces. This is especially useful when one performs a formal lower lid tightening procedure such as a canthopexy. Orbicularis repair may be achieved with a small (5-0) absorbable suture, such as polyglycolic acid. Before skin closure one may consider resecting a 2 to 3 mm, cuff of orbicularis muscle from the undersurface of the myocutaneous flap extending from the lateral canthal region medially. This maneuver can be fraught with hemostasis issues, but it is useful in eliminating or avoiding an orbicularis bulge inferior to the lid margin, which many patients will indicate as a preoperative concern.

Finally, the skin is closed using a running 6-0 silk suture from medial to the lateral canthus and interrupted 6-0 nylon sutures are used lateral to that. Only the nylon sutures are tied down, which enables the silk to be easily removed early in the postoperative period, in approximately 3 to 5 days (Fig. 54-10)

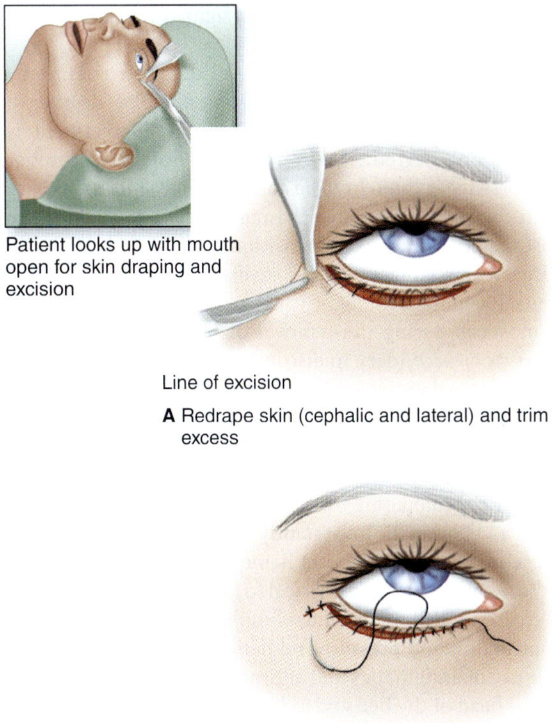

Figure 54-10 Lower lid blepharoplasty closure. **A.** This will render the most tension under the canthus and the smallest distraction force on the mid lower lid. It is helpful to have the patient look up and open his or her mouth to add conservation to the skin excision step (insert). Before closure, it is sometimes helpful to resect a few millimeters of orbicularis muscle at the superior aspect of the flap. This does not affect function and avoids the annoying post-blepharoplasty bulge or roll. **B.** Complete closure after hemostasis is controlled with running 6-0 silk medially and interrupted nylon laterally.

Various techniques to assist the surgeon in avoiding overexcision of skin have been described, and these may be useful but should not be entirely depended on. The amount of skin resected and the degree of cephalic lateral suspension should be judged based on the patient's history, physical examination, and appearance. That is, most of the decision-making is made preoperatively. In patients who have minimal tolerance for over-resection based on these parameters, one might want to evoke distraction tests, such as forcibly opening the patient's mouth and/or having the patient look up, prior to finally trimming the skin muscle flap (Fig. 54-10).

COMPLICATIONS AFTER BLEPHAROPLASTY

The continuous rise in demand for blepharoplasty in the United States has predictably coincided with an increased number of early as well as late complications resulting from the procedure. It is imperative, therefore, that the surgeon be familiar not only with the undesirable cosmetic outcomes but also with sight-threatening complications and their management.

Retrobulbar hemorrhage is one of the most commonly feared complications of blepharoplasty. The degree of visual loss can be profound if appropriate treatment is delayed or deferred. The overall incidence of retrobulbar hemorrhage is thought to be approximately 1 in 2000 cases with the risk of permanent visual loss at 1 in 10,000. The vast majority of cases occur within the first 24 hours after surgery (96%), but can occur several days after the procedure. Bleeding is thought to be secondary to inadequate hemostasis during the removal of the superficial orbital fat pads or secondary to disruption of deep orbital vessels from manipulation of superficial fat pads because these are linked to deep orbital fat. Bleeding can also be a result of trauma to the vasculature during injection of local anesthetic. Patient-related factors include hypertension and certain coagulopathies, as well as the use of medications such as vitamin E. Importantly, there are several steps a surgeon can take to prevent hemorrhage, namely by doing a thorough history and physical to identify individuals at an increased risk for bleeding complications, intraoperative control of blood pressure and hemostasis, and postoperative use of antiemetics and antitussives as well as elevation of the head of the bed and judicious use of ice packs.

It is important to recognize the signs of retrobulbar hemorrhage as early as possible to avoid permanent visual impairment or compromise. On the operating room table, these include sudden papillary changes, proptosis, visual loss, and/or loss of ocular motility. Patients who are discharged after routine blepharoplasty should be instructed to contact their surgeon immediately in the event of severe eye pain or loss of vision. For these reasons, the eyes of blepharoplasty patients should not be patched and their vision should be checked after surgery and before discharge.

Should retrobulbar hemorrhage occur during the procedure, the status of the globe, including intraocular pressure, as well as the optic nerve should be properly assessed, preferably by an ophthalmologist. However, all surgeons who perform blepharoplasty should be familiar with Schiøtz tonometry and basic techniques for assessing the globe. Mild hemorrhage can be controlled by head elevation and close observation. For more severe hemorrhage a stepwise approach must be undertaken to decompress the globe. These include lysis of one or both crura of the lateral canthal ligament. This procedure allows the globe to move forward and protects the globe and optic nerve from ischemic and/or compressive damage. In addition, the intraocular pressure can be reduced by means of topical medications such as timolol 0.5%, dorzolamide 2%, and brimonidine 5% or systemic hyperosmolar agents such as mannitol. Finally, in cases of severe hemorrhage uncontrolled by the previously described measures, one may choose to decompress the inferior orbital wall and/or explore the retro-orbital space surgically to control the hemorrhage. The sequence for treatment in the event of orbital hemorrhage should usually be canthotomy with concomitant medical treatment: systemic corticosteroids, hyperosmolar agents, and carbonic anhydrase inhibitors along with topical β-adrenergic blockers. All surgeons who perform blepharoplasty should be familiar with these treatment modalities.

Inadvertent globe perforation during anesthesia is a rare but potentially devastating complication. This is best avoided by protecting the globe with a corneal shield before injecting the anesthetic agent and by directing the needle away from the globe. Should this complication occur; however, it is important to recognize it early and intervene quickly. Ophthalmic consultation should immediately be obtained, and the procedure should be aborted. Indicative signs of globe perforation include a sudden change in vision or change in the position of or circular symmetry of the pupil.

Extraocular muscles may also be damaged during local anesthetic injection, resulting in temporary or permanent strabismus. This complication occurs more commonly with blind retrobulbar or peribulbar injections. More commonly, however, is the damage that occurs to extraocular muscles during surgical dissection. The inferior oblique muscle is at the highest risk for injury, which typically occurs from failure to adequately identify the muscle during a lower lid blepharoplasty. This muscle is the only extraocular muscle that originates anteriorly in the orbit. Its insertions are on the maxillary bone approximately one-third of the way from the junction of the medial and inferior walls. It then courses posteriorly and laterally to insert on the globe near the corresponding region on the macula. Superior oblique palsy has also been reported from damage to the trochlea during an upper lid blepharoplasty. This is best avoided by careful nasal dissection, avoidance of excessive cautery in the region of the trochlea, and proper identification of the superior medial palpebral artery inferonasal to the medial fat pad.

One of the more common complications following blepharoplasty is trauma to the corneal epithelium. Although the majority of "abrasions" heal spontaneously within 24 hours or less, this is a cause of significant discomfort to the patient and a potential source of infection in some. This complication commonly occurs from abrasive movements of instruments and sutures as well as traumatic insertion and removal of protective corneal lenses. The best way to avoid this complication is to pay close attention to the various instruments used during the procedure, fill the corneal protective shield with lubricant prior to insertion, as well as irrigate the lens surface with a balanced salt solution before and after placement. Should an abrasion occur, however, antibiotic ointment can be prescribed and the patient should be observed daily until healing occurs. It is imperative to avoid using topical anesthetic solutions to alleviate the patient's pain because this will significantly delay healing and put the patient at a higher risk for the development of a neurotrophic corneal ulcer.

Wound dehiscence may occur immediately after the surgery or subacutely within days to weeks postoperatively. Besides inadequate closure or disruption of sutures, one of the most common causes of wound dehiscence is the formation of a hematoma. This may occur slowly as vessels recover from the effects of epinephrine used with the local anesthetic, or it may be secondary to a lysis of the coagulum. In general, small quantities of "oozing" can be observed carefully in the recovery room, and the patient can be reassured about the temporary nature of the bleeding. If one encounters more brisk bleeding, however, the situation is best reassessed in the operating room. Lower lid fat excision may be associated with "flash" hemorrhage from vessels deep in the orbit. This may present as a retrobulbar hemorrhage or a continuous serosanguinous discharge through the lower lid incision. Again, this scenario is best assessed in the operating room.

Eyelid malposition, as briefly discussed earlier in this chapter, is another possible consequence following blepharoplasty. The final positioning of the lower eyelid relies heavily on the adequate understanding of lower lid anatomy. Malposition results when abnormal downward forces are applied to the lower eyelid such as with excessive skin resection, scarring, hematoma, edema, or imbrication of the orbital septum. Patients with dematochalasis have variable degrees of eyelid laxity and can have malpositions appear more apparent after the removal of skin and fatty tissue. This is why it is imperative that the surgeon carefully examine the relative position of the eyelid margin and tarsal consistency prior to surgery with tests like the snap-back test or eyelid distraction test. Conjunctival chemosis with prolapse may occur secondary to significant tightening of the lower eyelid with resultant edema, or it may occur when repositioning severely and chronically malpositioned eyelids such as with ectropion repairs.

Upper eyelid malpositions tend to be less common than those of the lower lids and typically occur secondary to excessive skin excision or damage to the levator complex. Preoperatively, any lagophthalmos must be carefully noted as it has a tendency to worsen after surgery. In deciding on the amount of skin to remove, care must be taken not to confuse excessive upper eyelid skin with brow ptosis, especially in men. After the brow is held in its desirable anatomic location, smooth forceps can be used to determine the amount of upper skin to be removed. An inadequate preoperative assessment of eyelid movement and anatomy may result in lagophthalmos and corneal dryness or decompensation after surgery. Ptosis is a rare complication after blepharoplasty that may result from damage to the levator aponeurosis muscle during dissection or excessive stretching of an already rarified muscle during surgery. Finally, it may result from lack of recognition of preoperative ptosis in a patient with significant dermatochalasis. Regardless of the etiology, it is important to resist the urge to quickly intervene after a case of eyelid malposition as many will disappear or improve significantly over time.

The loss of lashes after blepharoplasty is a more common complication in patients undergoing a combined procedure with a ptosis correction as the anterior tarsal surface is exposed. Excessive inferior dissection 2 to 3 mm from the lid margin of the upper lid can lead to damage of the hair follicles with subsequent atrophy and loss of lashes in the postoperative period.

Postoperative complaints of dry eye typically occur in patients with preoperative tear insufficiency. By widening the palpebral fissure and increasing exposure to the environment, blepharoplasty can result in decompensation in the predisposed patient. Dryness may also be the sequela of cicatricial changes in the skin or conjunctiva. Finally, the lacrimal gland may be damaged during an upper eyelid blepharoplasty, where it can be mistaken for upper lid fat. This is best avoided by avoiding aggressive dissection laterally where the lacrimal gland is located. Often the symptoms of dryness can be addressed by the use of artificial tears and lubricants, but should symptoms persist, a referral to an ophthalmologist is warranted to evaluate the status of the corneal tear film.

Infection is an extremely rare complication after blepharoplasty owing to the extensive vascularity of the eyelids and orbit. Nevertheless, once the orbital septum has been violated, pathogens can easily gain access to the deep orbital structures. A common source of infection is thought to be the nasolacrimal outflow system in patients with postlacrimal sac stenosis in whom bacteria can multiply and reflux toward the conjunctiva. Signs of orbital cellulitis include pain, redness, decreased vision, restricted ocular motility, and proptosis. Systemic antibiotics are warranted as well as close monitoring in a hospital setting.

Postoperative scarring is a relatively rare complication and is generally well managed with massage and topical corticosteroid application. More severe scars can be managed with intralesional corticosteroids or excision and radiation. As with eyelid malposition, the surgeon should resist the urge at an early intervention, as many scars will improve with time.

Excessive removal of upper eyelid fat, especially in the midportion, can result in a "hollow" appearance while excessive resection of fat from the lower lid can lead to a tear trough deformity. The most prudent way to treat this complication is to avoid it with careful and limited fat excision intraoperatively.

Blepharoplasty is a seemingly straightforward procedure, but even the most experienced and skilled surgeons can be faced with complications. Many of the complications are avoidable through a comprehensive preoperative evaluation, adequate preoperative patient education, a thorough knowledge of eyelid anatomy and meticulous surgical technique. Despite all efforts, every surgeon will eventually encounter postoperative complications and must be prepared to handle them or risk-causing serious functional and/or cosmetic morbidity to the patient.

SUGGESTED READINGS

1. Aiache A. The suborbicularis oculi fat pad: an anatomic and clinical study. *Plast Reconstr Surg.* 2001;107:1602–1604; discussion 1605–1606.
2. Alster TS, Lupton JR. An overview of cutaneous laser resurfacing. *Clin Plast Surg.* 2001;28:37–52.
3. Aldave AJ, Maus M, Rubin PA. Advances in the management of lower eyelid retraction. *Facial Plast Surg.* 1999;15:213–224.
4. Allen MV, Cohen KL, Grimson BS. Orbital cellulitis secondary to dacryocystitis following blepharoplasty. *Ann Ophthalmol.* 1985;17:498–499.
5. Bartisch S, Swartz KA, Spinelli HM. Lateral canthoplasty using the Mitek anchor system. *Aesthetic Plast Surg.* 2012; 36(1):3–7.
6. Barretto RL, Mathog RH. Orbital measurement in black and white populations. *Laryngoscope.* 1999;109(7 pt 1):1051–1054.
7. Bas CT, Perez-Guisado J. A new approach: resection and suture of orbicularis oculi muscle to define the upper eyelid fold and correct asymmetries. *Aesthetic Plast Surg.* 2013; 37(1):46–50.
8. Berke A, Mueller S. The kinetics of lid motion and its effects on the tear film. *Adv Exp Med Biol.* 1998;438:417–424.
9. Berman M. Rejuvenation of the upper eyelid complex with autologous fat transplantation. *Dermatol Surg.* 2000;26: 1113–1116.
10. Bernardi C, Dura S, Amata PL. Treatment of orbicularis oculi muscle hypertrophy in lower lid blepharoplasty. *Aesthetic Plast Surg.* 1998;22:349–351.
11. Borodic G, Townsend D. *Atlas of Eyelid Surgery.* Philadelphia, PA: WB Saunders; 1994.

12. Bosniak S. *Principles and Practice of Ophthalmic Plastic and Reconstructive Surgery*. Vols. 1 and 2. Philadelphia, PA: WB Saunders; 1996.
13. Brown SM, Coats DK, Collins ML, Underdahl JP. Second cluster of strabismus cases after periocular anesthesia without hyaluronidase. *J Cataract Refract Surg*. 2001;27:1872–1875.
14. Caldato R, Lauande-Pimentel R, Sabrosa NA, et al. Role of reinsertion of the lower eyelid retractor on involutional entropion. *Br J Ophthalmol*. 2000;84:606–608.
15. Carruthers J. Brow lifting and blepharoplasty. *Dermatol Clin*. 2001;19:531–533.
16. Carter SR, Seiff SR, Grant PE, Vigneron DB. The Asian lower eyelid: a comparative anatomic study using high-resolution magnetic resonance imaging. *Ophthalmic Plast Reconstr Surg*. 1998;14:227–234.
17. Castro E, Foster JA. Upper lid blepharoplasty. *Facial Plast Surg*. 1999;15:173–181.
18. Cheng J, Xu FZ. Anatomic microstructure of the upper eyelid in the Oriental double eyelid. *Plast Reconstr Surg*. 2001;107:1665–1668.
19. Chia CT, Swartz KA, Spinelli HM. Transcutaneous lower lid blepharoplasty. In: Lin SJ, Mustoe TA. eds. *Aesthetic Head and Neck: An Operative Atlas*. New York, NY: McGraw-Hill; 2012.
20. Codner MA. Reduction of lower palpebral bulge by placating attenuated orbital septa: a technical modification in cosmetic blepharoplasty. *Plast Reconstr Surg*. 2000;105:2559–2560.
21. Craig JP, Singh I, Tomlinson A, Morgan PB, Efron N. The role of tear physiology in ocular surface temperature. *Eye*. 2000;14(pt 4):635–641.
22. Dagum AB, Antonyshyn O, Hearn T. Medial canthopexy: an experimental and biomechanical study. *Ann Plast Surg*. 1995;35:262–265.
23. Della Rocca R, Bedrossian E, Arthurs B. *Ophthalmic Plastic Surgery: Decision Making and Techniques*. New York, NY: McGraw-Hill; 2002.
24. Della Rocca R, Nesi F, Lisman R. *Ophthalmic Plastic and Reconstructive Surgery*. Vol. 1. St. Louis, MO: CV Mosby; 1997.
25. DeMere M, Wood T, Austin W. Eye complications with blepharoplasty or other eyelid surgery. A national survey. *Plast Reconstr Surg*. 1974;53:634–637.
26. Dutton J. *Atlas of Clinical and Surgical Orbital Anatomy*. Philadelphia, PA: WB Saunders; 1994.
27. Elahi E, Spinelli HM. Eyelid and orbit reconstruction. Chapter 65. In: Guyuron B, Eriksson E, Persing J, Chung K, Disa J, Gosain A, Kinney BM, Rubin JP, eds. *Plastic Surgery*. London: Elsevier Limited; 2009.
28. Ettl A, Koornneef L, Daxer A, Kramer J. High resolution magnetic resonance imaging of the orbital connective tissue system. *Ophthal Plast Reconstr Surg*. 1998;14:323–327.
29. Ettl A, Kramer J, Daxer A, Koornneef L. High resolution magnetic resonance imaging of the normal extraocular musculature. *Eye*. 1997;11(pt 6):793–797.
30. Ettl A, Priglinger S, Kramer J, Koornneef L. Functional anatomy of the levator palpebrae superioris muscle and its connective tissue system. *Br J Ophthalmol*. 1996;80:702–707.
31. Friedland JA, Jacobsen WM, Terkonda S. Safety and efficacy of combined upper blepharoplasties and open coronal browlift: a consecutive series of 600 patients. *Aesthetic Plast Surg*. 1996;20:453–462.
32. Fu S, Fan J, Chen W, Yang Z, Yin Z. Aesthetic correction of severe sicatricial upper-eyelid ectropion with a Retrograde Postauricular Island Flap. *Aesthetic Plast Surg*. 2013;37(1):95–101.
33. Hamra S. *Composite Rhytidectomy*. St. Louis, MO: Quality Medical Publishing; 1993.
34. Haramoto U, Kubo T, Tamatani M, Hosokawa MK. Anatomic study of the insertions of the levator aponeurosis and Muller's muscle in oriental eyelids. *Ann Plastic Surg*. 2001;47:528–533.
35. Hwang K, Joong Kim D, Chung RS. Pretarsal fat compartment in the lower eyelid. *Clin Anat*. 2001;14:179–183.
36. Hwang K, Kim DJ, Chung RS, Lee SI, Hiraga Y. An anatomical study of the junction of the orbital septum and the levator aponeurosis in Orientals. *Br J Plast Surg*. 1998;51:594–598.
37. Gallo SA, Wesley RE, Klippenstein KA, Biesman BS. Cosmetic eyelid surgery. *Ophthalmol Clin North Am*. 2000;13:749–764.
38. Glatt HJ. Follow-up methods and the apparent success of entropion surgery. *Ophthal Plast Reconstr Surg*. 1999;15:396–400.
39. Gorla MS, Gorla RS. Nonlinear theory of tear film rupture. *J Biomech Eng*. 2000;122:498–503.
40. Guyuron B, Knize DM. Corrugator supercilii resection through blepharoplasty incision. *Plast Reconstr Surg*. 2001;107:606–607.
41. Januszkiewicz JS, Nahai F, Zarem HA. Transconjunctival upper blepharoplasty. *Plast Reconstr Surg*. 1999;103:1015–1019.
42. Jeong S, Lemke BN, Dortzbach RK, Park YG, Kang HK. The Asian upper eyelid: an anatomical study with comparison to the Caucasian eyelid. *Arch Ophthalmol*. 1999;117:907–912.
43. Kim P, Berdoukas P, Francis IC, Coroneo MT, Kappagoda MB. Kinetic observational exophthalmometry: a simple clinical method of assessing the relative axial positions of the eyes. *Ophthalmic Surg Lasers*. 2001;32:257–259.
44. Kim JW, Kikkawa DO, Lemke BN. Donor site complications of hard palate mucosal grafting. *Ophthalmic Plast Reconstr Surg*. 1997;13:36–39.
45. Kim JW, Lee JO. Asian blepharoplasty with a short-pulsed contract Nd-YAG laser: limited-incision resectable laser double fold with internal medial and lateral functional epicanthoplasty. *Aesthetic Plast Surg*. 1998;22:433–438.
46. Lee Y, Kwon S, Hwang K. Correction of sunken and/or multiply folded upper eyelid by fascia-fat graft. *Plast Reconstr Surg*. 2001;107:15–19.
47. Lee Y, Lee E, Park WJ. Anchor epicanthoplasty combined with out-fold type double eyelidplasty for Asians: do we have to make an additional scar to correct the Asian epicanthal fold? *Plast Reconstr Surg*. 2000;105:1872–1880.
48. Lelli G, Lisman R. Blepharoplasty complications. *Plast Reconstr Surg*. 2010;125:1007–1010.
49. Lemke BN, Cook BE Jr, Lucarelli MJ. Canthus sparing ectropion repair. *Ophthalmic Plast Reconstr Surg*. 2001;17:161–168.
50. Leone C, Grove A, Lloyd W, Wojno T. *Atlas of Orbital Surgery*. Philadelphia, PA: WB Saunders; 1992.
51. Lisman R, Campbell J. Tarsal suspension canthoplasty. *Aesthetic Surg J*. 1999;19:412–424.
52. Lisman RD, Campbell JP. Complications of blepharoplasty. *Facial Plast Surg Clin North Am*. 2000;8:303–327.
53. Lisman RD, Spinelli HM. Soft tissue trauma and orbital fractures. Section VI, #2. In: Boyd BF, ed. *World Atlas Series of Ophthalmic Surgery, Highlights of Ophthalmology*. Panama: El Dorado; 1995:237–253.
54. Lisman RD, Spinelli HM. Injectible collagen. In: Byron Smith BC, ed. *Ophthalmic Plastic and Reconstructive Surgery*. St Louis, MO: CV Mosby; 1987:357–361.
55. Lisman RD, Spinelli HM. Orbital adnexal injuries. In: Foster CA, Sherman JE, eds. *Surgery of Facial Bone Fractures*. New York, NY: Churchill Livingstone; 1987:93–122.
56. Malbouisson JM, Baccega A, Cruz AA. The geometrical basis of the eyelid contour. *Ophthalmic Plast Reconstr Surg*. 2000;16:427–431.
57. Matsuo K. Stretching of the Mueller muscle results in involuntary contraction of the levator muscle. *Ophthalmic Plast Reconstr Surg*. 2002;18:79–83.
58. Mommaerts MY, DeRiu G. Prevention of lid retraction after lower lid blepharoplasties: an overview. *J Craniomaxillofacial Surg*. 2000;28:189–200.
59. Mulliken JB, Godwin SL, Prachanktam N, Altobelli DE. The concept of the sagittal orbital-globe relationship in craniofacial surgery. *Plast Reconstr Surg*. 1996;97:700–706.
60. Nesi F, Lisman R, Levine M. *Smith's Ophthalmic Plastic and Reconstructive Surgery*. St. Louis, MO: CV Mosby; 1998.
61. Nguyen XC. Guidelines to avoid lid retraction following lower transcutaneous blepharoplasty. *Int J Cosmetic Surg Aesthetic Dermatol*. 2000;2:231–233.
62. Olver JM, Barnes JA. Effective small-incision surgery for involutional lower eyelid entropion. *Ophthalmology*. 2000;107:1982–1988.

63. Olver JM, Sathia PJ, Wright M. Lower eyelid medial canthal tendon laxity grading: an interobserver study of normal subjects. *Ophthalmology*. 2001;102:2321–2325.
64. Papas E. Tear break-up time: clinical procedures and their effects. *Ophthalmic Physiol Opt*. 1999;19:274–275.
65. Patel BC, Patipa M, Anderson RL, McLeish W. Management of postblepharoplasty lower eyelid retraction with hard palate grafts and lateral tarsal strip. *Plast Reconstr Surg*. 1997;99:1251–1260.
66. Patipa M. The evaluation and management of lower eyelid retraction following cosmetic surgery. *Plast Reconstr Surg*. 2000;106:438–453; discussion 454–459.
67. Pessa JE, Zadoo VP, Adrian EK, et al. Anatomy of a "black eye": a newly described fascial system of the lower eyelid. In: Fagien S, ed. *Putterman A: Cosmetic Oculoplastic Surgery*. 2nd ed. Philadelphia, PA: WB Saunders; 1993.
68. Portnof JE, Spinelli HM. Penetrating orbital trauma: case report. *Oral Surg*. 2009;2(2):99–102.
69. Rhee SC, Woo KS, Kwon B. Biometric study of eyelid shape and dimensions of different races with references to beauty. *Aesthetic Plast Surg*. 2012;36(5):1236–1245.
70. Reiffel AJ, Cohen B, Spinelli HM. Browpexy through the upper lid (BUL): a new technique of stabilizing and/or lifting the brow using a standard blepharoplasty incision. *Aesthet Surg J*. 2011;31(2):163–169.
71. Rougraff PM, Tse DT, Johnson TE, Feuer W. Involutional entropion repair with fornix sutures and lateral tarsal strip procedure. *Ophthalmic Plast Reconstr Surg*. 2001;17:281–287.
72. Schoenwald RD, Vidvauns S, Wurster DE, Barfknecht CF. The role of tear proteins in tear film stability in the dry eye patient and in the rabbit. *Adv Exp Med Biol*. 1998;438:391–400.
73. Schwartz GS, Spinelli HM. The correction of upper eyelid retraction using deep temporal fascia spacer grafts. *Plast Reconstr Surg*. 2008;122(3):765–774.
74. Shinohara H, Taniguchi Y, Kominami R, Yasutaka S, Kawamata S. The lacrimal fascia redefined. *Clin Anat*. 2001;14:401–405.
75. Spinelli HM. Pre-expansion of mucosa-lined flap for lower eyelid reconstruction. *Plast Reconstr Surg*. 2005;116(5):83–84.
76. Spinelli HM. Aesthetic surgery of the lower eyelid. *J Cutan Laser Therapy*. 2000;2:106–107.
77. Spinelli HM. *Atlas of Aesthetic Eyelid and Periocular Surgery*. Philadelphia, PA: Saunders-An imprint of Elsevier, Inc; 2004.
78. Spinelli HM, Ali-Salaam P. Reconstruction of the orbit. *Surg Oncol Clin N Am*. 1997;6:45–69.
79. Spinelli HM, Carraway JH, Grant MP, Lisman RD. Panel discussion on "Correction of lower lid laxity." *Aesthet Surg J*. 2005;25(2):159–168.
80. Spinelli HM, Falcone S, Lee G. Orbital venous approach to the cavernous sinus-an analysis of the facial and orbital venous system. *ACTA, Volume of the V International Congress of the International Society of Craniomaxillofacial Surgery*. Monduzzi Editore: Santiago De Compostela, Bologna; 1993, 1994.
81. Spinelli HM, Farris RL. The tear film. In: Byron Smith BC, ed. *Opthalmic Plastic and Reconstructive Surgery*. St. Louis, MO: CV Mosby; 1987:535–545.
82. Spinelli HM, Jelks GW. Periocular reconstruction-a systematic approach. *Plast Reconstr Surg*. 1993;91(6):1017–1024.
83. Spinelli HM, Jelks GW. Periocular reconstruction-a systematic approach. In: Miller SH, ed. *Yearbook of Plastic, Reconstructive and Aesthetic Surgery*. St Louis, MO: Mosby-Yearbook, Inc; 1994:88–90.
84. Spinelli HM, Riou JP. Lower lid anatomy and aesthetic surgery. *Am Acad Ophthalmol* Focal Points Clinical Modules for Ophthalmologists. San Francisco, CA. 1995;13(7):1–10.
85. Spinelli HM, Sherman JE, Smith B, Lisman RD. Human bites of the eyelid. *Plast Reconstr Surg*. 1986;75(5):610–614.
86. Spinelli HM, Newman MI. Reconstruction of eyelids, correction of ptosis, and canthoplasty. Chapter 39. In: Thorne CH, ed. *Grabb and Smith's Plastic Surgery*. 6th ed. Philadelphia, PA: Lippincott Williams & Wilkins; 2006: 397–416.
87. Suzman MS, Spinelli HM. Soft-tissue deformities in orbital trauma. Evaluation and repair of medial and lateral canthal injury. *J Oper Tech Plast Reconstr Surg*. 2003;8(4):249–258.
88. Swartz KA, Spinelli HM. Ptosis. In: Lin SJ, Mustoe TA, eds. *Aesthetic Head and Neck: An Operative Atlas*. New York, NY: McGraw-Hill; 2012.
89. Swartz KA, Newman MI, Spinelli HM. Canthal fixation. In: *Aesthetic Head and Neck: An Operative Atlas*. New York, NY: McGraw-Hill; 2012.
90. Swartz KA, Silich R, Spinelli HM. Transconjunctival lower lid blepharoplasty. In: *Aesthetic Head and Neck: An Operative Atlas*. New York, NY: McGraw-Hill; 2012.
91. Thale A, Paulsen F, Rochels R, Tillmann B. Functional anatomy of the human efferent tear ducts: A new theory of tear outflow mechanism. *Graefes Arch Clin Exp Ophthalmol*. 1998;236: 674–678.
92. Tiffany JM, Pandit JC, Bron AJ. Soluble mucin and the physical properties of tears. *Adv Exp Med Biol*. 1998;438:229–234.
93. Tsubota K. Tear dynamics and dry eye. *Prog Retin Eye Res*. 1998; 17:565–596.
94. Ullmann Y, Levi Y, Ben-Izhak O, Har-Shai Y, Peled IJ. The surgical anatomy of the fat in the upper eyelid medial compartment. *Plast Reconstr Surg*. 1997;99:658–661.
95. Van Den Bosch WA, Leenders I, Mulder P. Topographic anatomy of the eyelids and the effects of sex and age. *Br J Ophthalmol*. 1999;83:347–352.
96. Weber PJ, Wulc AE, Foster J. Transconjunctival upper blepharoplasty. *Plast Reconstr Surg*. 1999;104:2333–2334.
97. Wesley RE, Pollard ZF, McCord CD Jr. Superior oblique paresis after blepharoplasty. *Plast Reconstr Surg*. 1980;66:283–286.
98. Wilhelmi BJ, Mowlavi A, Neumeister MW. Upper blepharoplasty with bony anatomical landmarks to avoid injury to trochlea and superior oblique muscle tendon with fat resection. *Plast Reconstr Surg*. 2001;108:2137–2140; discussion 2141–2142.
99. Wolfort FG, Vaughan TE, Wolfort SF, Nevarre DR. Retrobulbar hematoma and blepharoplasty. *Plast Reconstr Surg*. 1999;104:2154–2162.
100. Yamamoto H, Morikawa K, Uchinuma E, Yamashina S. An anatomical study of the medial canthus using a three dimensional model. *Aesthetic Plast Surg*. 2001;25:189–193.
101. Yip CC, Choo CT. The correction of oriental lower lid involutional entropion using the combined procedure. *Ann Acad Med Singapore*. 2000;29:463–466.

CHAPTER 55

Facial Rejuvenation

Jenny C. Hu & Jenny Kim

INTRODUCTION

Aging in the face is a multifactorial process involving one's genetic make-up as well as exogenous factors, and leads to various changes in the skin including vascular and pigmentary alterations, rhytide formation, volume loss, and bony structural changes of the face. To better understand how to globally rejuvenate the skin, it is helpful to understand the various changes in the skin that contribute to the appearance of aging. With the advancement in aesthetic therapeutics available to physicians, these changes can be targeted with various procedures including the use of botulinum toxin, injectable fillers, and light and laser therapies.

SKIN AND AGING

INTRINSIC AND EXTRINSIC AGING

With aging, skin undergoes physiologic and morphologic changes that can be categorized as intrinsic aging due to endogenous factors and extrinsic aging due to exogenous factors. Intrinsic aging is influenced mainly by genetics, cellular metabolism, and hormone environment. Histopathologically, intrinsic aging exhibits decreased amounts of normal collagen and elastic fibers, atrophy of the extracellular matrix, diminution of the dermal thickness with decreased number of fibroblasts, thinning of the subcutaneous fat, slow replacement of lipids, reduced function of skin appendages (e.g., sebaceous glands, sweat glands, apocrine glands), and epidermal atrophy.[1–4] Extrinsic aging mostly involves sun-exposed skin and is primarily caused by ultraviolet radiation, ionizing radiation, toxins, chemicals, and pollutants. Among these, cumulative ultraviolet light exposure and tobacco use appear to be more influential in aging skin.[5,6] The morphologic changes demonstrated in extrinsic aging include impaired proliferation and differentiation of keratinocytes, increased levels of dysfunctional glycosaminoglycans and proteoglycans, increased collagen degradation with sparse distribution of collagen fibers, accumulation of abnormal elastic tissue in the dermis, reduced number of anchoring fibrils, and thickening of the epidermis in the early stages.[1–4] The thickened epidermis is thought to be due to a chronic wound-like state in which there is a continual attempt to repair the skin.[3,4] These changes of both intrinsic and extrinsic aging ultimately lead to the decrease in skin elasticity, overall volume loss caused by both dermal and subcutaneous atrophy, and fine wrinkle formation seen with aging in the skin.

RHYTIDES

The presence of rhytides, whether dynamic or static, contributes to the appearance of aging in facial skin. Rhytides are formed as a result of both cumulative ultraviolet light exposure and repetitive muscle contractions. With exposure to ultraviolet light over time, there is an accumulation of abnormal elastic tissue in the dermis,[1,3] which leads to reduced elasticity and subsequent impaired retightening of the skin—seen clinically as rhytides. In early photoaging, these rhytides are apparent only with dynamic movement of the face, often on the forehead, the lateral canthi (crow's feet), near the oral commissures, and over the zygomatic arch and malar eminences. In more advanced photoaging, with the added influence of repetitive muscle contractions, these rhytides are visible when the face is at rest and are known as static rhytides.

VOLUME LOSS

Clinically when evaluating changes in an aged face, there is some loss of volume evident in older patients, particularly in the regions of the temples and midface. There have been a number of studies examining the loss of facial volume and fat as related to aging using various imaging techniques. A study using computed tomography scans of cadaveric heads specifically examining the midfacial fat compartments demonstrated volume loss of the deep medial cheek fat, in addition to migration of the midfacial fat compartments inferiorly and shifting of the volume within the compartments inferiorly with aging.[7] Another study using photographic three-dimensional surface imaging techniques to evaluate periorbital aging found atrophy and regression of the soft tissues in the nasojugal groove of the infraorbital area and the medial canthal region.[8]

BONY CHANGES

More recently, knowledge regarding how the bony structure of the face changes with age has added further insight into the overall pathology of an aging face and implications for facial rejuvenation. Various studies have evaluated these bony changes using computed tomography imaging.[9–11] With age, the maxillary angle (as measured by the angle between the orbital floor and anterior maxillary wall or the angle between the superior and inferior maxilla) decreases, leading to regression of the anterior maxillary wall and an appearance of deflation of the mid face.[9–11] Furthermore, the glabellar angle (the angle measured between the maximal prominence of the glabella to the nasofrontal suture) also decreases with age, adding to the appearance of a regressed orbital and mid face region.[10,11] Changes in the mandible include decreases in the mandibular length and height as well as an increase in the mandibular angle (angle between the inferior border of the mandibular body and posterior border of the ramus), resulting in the appearance of a protruding mandible as compared to the mid face.[10] Another study evaluated bone mineral density changes of the facial skeleton with aging and found a significant reduction in the bone mineral density of the maxilla and mandible in middle-aged individuals as compared to younger individuals.[12] These changes, altogether, may contribute to the appearance of an aged face and a regressed midface.

PIGMENTARY ALTERATIONS

Pigmentary changes in the skin, another sign of aging, can result from chronic sun exposure. Skin that is chronically sun exposed demonstrates an approximate twofold increase in the density of melanocytes as well as increased dopa positivity of individual melanocytes when compared to sun-protected skin.[13] In addition, when compared to younger sun-exposed skin, the pigmentation that results from sun-exposed aging skin is more unevenly distributed.[14]

VASCULAR ALTERATIONS

Ultraviolet light exposure also contributes to vascular alterations seen in aging skin. These changes differ depending on whether the skin is chronically or acutely irradiated with ultraviolet light. In chronically sun-exposed skin as well as in sun-protected aging skin, vessels in the upper dermis become obliterated over time.[15] In comparison, skin that undergoes more acute irradiation with ultraviolet light exhibits vasodilation of the dermal blood vessels, vascular hyperpermeability, and angiogenesis.[15–17] These changes that are observed clinically as increased erythema further adds to the aged appearance of facial skin.

TREATMENTS

BOTULINUM TOXIN

Botulinum toxin, derived from the gram-positive bacteria *Clostridium botulinum*, is a neurotoxin that causes neuromuscular paralysis. Among its medical uses include treatment for strabismus, blepharospasm, hemifacial spasm, hyperhidrosis, and more recently chronic migraines. Its use cosmetically has become very popular, as it is effective in temporarily treating dynamic rhytides. There are seven serotypes of botulinum toxin, which include types A, B, C (C1, C2), D, E, F, and G. Of these, type A has been shown to have the longest duration of neuromuscular paralysis (4 months), followed by types B and E.[18] Botulinum toxin type A (BTX-A) preparations have been the most commonly used clinically, given its prior availability, safety profile, efficacy, and immunologic aspects.[19] BTX-A acts as a neuromuscular paralytic agent by cleaving SNAP-25 (synaptosomal-associated protein of 25 kDa), a protein that mediates the fusion of presynaptic vesicles with the plasma membrane of neurons at the neuromuscular junction that results in the release of the acetylcholine neurotransmitter.[20] Therefore, BTX-A inhibits the release of acetylcholine causing a chemical denervation.

Currently, there are three United States Food and Drug Administration (FDA)-approved BTX-A agents for the temporary improvement of moderate-to-severe glabellar lines: OnabotulinumtoxinA (Botox Cosmetic, Allergan, Inc.), AbobotulinumtoxinA (Dysport, Medicis Aesthetics, Inc.), and IncobotulinumtoxinA (Xeomin, Merz Aesthetics, Inc.) (Table 55-1). IncobotulinumtoxinA differs from the others in that it is a BTX-A without complexing proteins and thus does not have temperature restrictions for storage; both OnabotulinumtoxinA and AbobotulinumtoxinA must be stored at temperatures between 2°C and 8°C.[21] In order to assess how these three BTX-A products can be used interchangeably, many studies have attempted to determine the conversion ratio of OnabotulinumtoxinA to AbobotulinumtoxinA and IncobotulinumtoxinA that would provide an equivalent comparison of their efficacy, and have used OnabotulinumtoxinA as the basis of comparison since it has had the longest history of clinical use. The conversion ratio for OnabotulinumtoxinA:AbobotulinumtoxinA ranges widely from 1:1 to 1:6.[22–25] However, the more common conversion ratio that many practitioners use at this time is between 1:3 and 1:4, though many practitioners are beginning to vary the conversion ratio based on their anecdotal experience with the product. Of note, these ratios are based mostly on studies evaluating their comparative efficacies in treating cervical dystonia, blepharospasm, and hemifacial spasm.[24,25] The conversion ratio for OnabotulinumtoxinA:IncobotulinumtoxinA is approximately 1:1. Diffusion characteristics between

TABLE 55-1
Food and Drug Administration-Approved Botulinum Toxin Type A Agents

FDA-Approved BTX-A Agents	Brand Name	Company	Potency Ratio (Compared to OnabotulinumtoxinA)	Average Months of Duration
OnabotulinumtoxinA	Botox Cosmetic	Allergan, Inc.	N/A	3–4
AbobotulinumtoxinA	Dysport	Medicis Aesthetics, Inc.	1:3 or 1:4	3–4
IncobotulinumtoxinA	Xeomin	Merz Aesthetics, Inc.	1:1	3–4

FDA, Food and Drug Administration; BTX-A, Botulinum toxin type A.

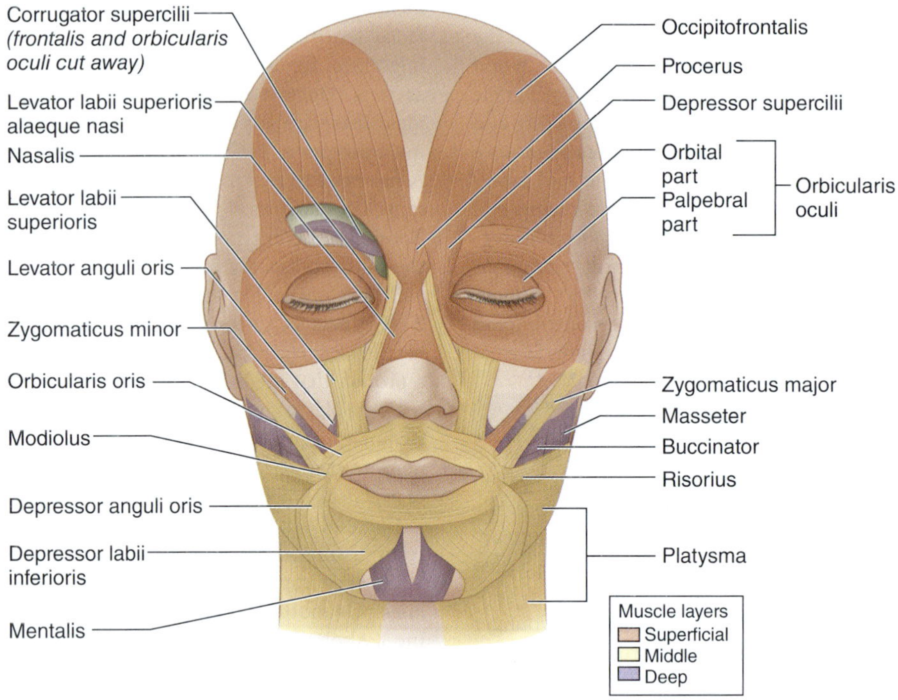

Figure 55-1 Main muscles of facial expression that contribute to facial rhytides that can be treated with botulinum toxin type A.

OnabotulinumtoxinA, AbobotulinumtoxinA, and IncobotulinumtoxinA appear to be similar.[25,26]

Being able to use BTX-A appropriately and effectively requires an understanding of the muscle anatomy of the face that contributes to rhytide formation. Furthermore, the use of BTX-A of the lower face has become more popularized in recent years. Rejuvenation of the lower face had traditionally focused on correcting folds and creases with injectable fillers, but with the new paradigm of combination cosmetic therapy many practitioners are increasingly using BTX-A on the lower face in conjunction with injectable fillers.

FOREHEAD RHYTIDES

The transverse forehead rhytides are caused by the action of the frontalis muscle (Fig. 55-1). The frontalis muscle originates superiorly in the galeal aponeurotic layer and extends inferiorly toward the procerus, corrugator, and orbicularis oculi muscles, interdigitating with these muscles. Contraction of the frontalis retracts the scalp and elevates the brows, thereby producing transverse rhytides across the forehead.

To treat the forehead lines, BTX-A is injected in the regions where rhytides are present. Different practitioners have different methods of placing BTX-A injections. Because BTX-A diffuses, injections can be placed along a single horizontal line across the mid forehead or staggered across the forehead with two or more horizontal lines (Fig. 55-2). The authors prefer to stagger the injections across the forehead with multiple horizontal lines and using smaller units per injection. For older patients who already have some degree of ptosis of the eyelids, caution should be taken with injecting lower on the forehead or treating with higher units of BTX-A, as too much weakening of the

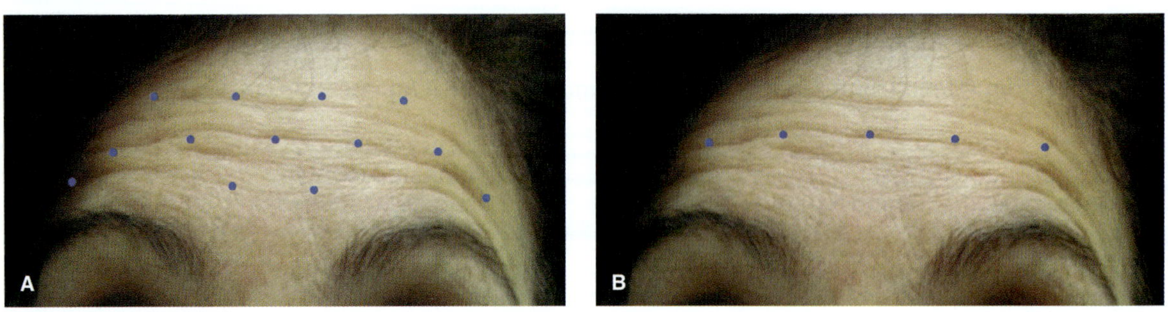

Figure 55-2 Injection points for treatment of forehead lines, with injections staggered across the forehead with smaller amount of units per injection site (authors' preference) **(A)** versus in a horizontal line across the midforehead with larger amount of units per injection site **(B)**.

frontalis muscle may lead to further ptosis of the eyelids and a dissatisfied patient. Furthermore, in patients who do not have a pretarsal crease (the crease of the upper eyelid that forms a "double eyelid"), such as that frequently observed in Asian individuals, injecting lower on the forehead may cause an unpleasant sensation of heaviness of the brow and upper eyelids.

GLABELLAR RHYTIDES

The muscles that contribute to dynamic rhytides seen in the glabella are the depressor muscles of this region: procerus, corrugator supercilii, depressor supercilii, and medial orbital portion of the orbicularis oculi muscles (Fig. 55-1). The procerus is located 1 to 4 mm beneath the skin surface and lies vertically between the frontalis muscles of the forehead and the lower portion of the nasal root. As the procerus contracts, it brings the eyebrows inferiorly and causes the horizontal glabellar rhytides. The corrugator supercilii lies deep to the frontalis muscle, originating in the superior portion of the nasal dorsum and inserting just above the medial eyebrows. The depressor supercilii lies superficially to the corrugator muscle and just lateral to the procerus, also originating on the superior nasal dorsum and inserting at the medial eyebrow. The medial fibers of the orbicularis oculi originate from the medial orbital rim and its fibers interdigitate with the frontalis, procerus, and corrugator muscles. The corrugator supercilii, depressor supercilii, and medial orbital portion of the orbicularis oculi muscles displace the medial eyebrows inferomedially and produce the vertical glabellar rhytides.

Treatment of the glabellar lines is achieved with either 3 or 5 injection sites (Fig. 55-3), though the authors prefer five injection sites to minimize the risk of the "Spock" look, in which the lateral brows become raised upward inadvertently. One injection is placed in the mid glabella in the area of the procerus muscle, each of two injections are placed just superior to the medial brow to affect the corrugator supercilii, depressor supercilii, and medial fibers of the orbicularis oculi, and each of the last two injections are placed about 0.5 to 1 cm above the mid brow. If these last two injections above the mid brow are placed too close to the brow itself, then the diffusion of the BTX-A can consequently cause some eyelid ptosis. For women who would like to maintain the same curvature of their brow arch, the last two injections can be placed just lateral to the mid brow rather than just above the mid brow where the arch of the brow is typically the highest.

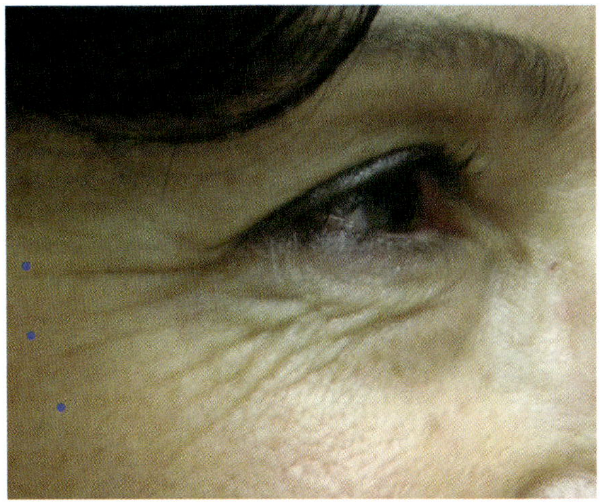

Figure 55-4 Injection points for treatment of crow's feet.

CROW'S FEET

Crow's feet are the lines that radiate laterally and inferolaterally from the lateral canthi and are accentuated with smiling. These lines are caused by the contraction of the lateral fibers of the orbicularis oculi (Fig. 55-1). Because the orbicularis oculi muscle is diffusely innervated, multiple injections are placed along the lateral orbital rim to treat the crow's feet more effectively (Fig. 55-4). It is important to place the injections along the lateral orbital rim and not too medially, as the goal is to target only the lateral fibers of the orbicularis oculi. Injecting too medially will cause an inability to close the eyelids completely. In addition, caution must be taken to not inadvertently weaken the zygomaticus major muscle, which will lead to a partial upper lip ptosis. The zygomaticus major lies adjacent and inferior to the orbicularis oculi muscle, partially contributing to the more inferior and medial crow's feet (Fig. 55-1).

BUNNY LINES

The bunny lines are the lines that form across the dorsal and lateral aspects of the nasal root. The main muscle that causes these lines is the transverse nasalis, although the levator labii superioris alaeque nasi also contributes (Fig. 55-1). To treat these lines, one injection should be placed on each side of the superior portion of the transverse nasalis (Fig. 55-5). Placing the injections too inferiorly at

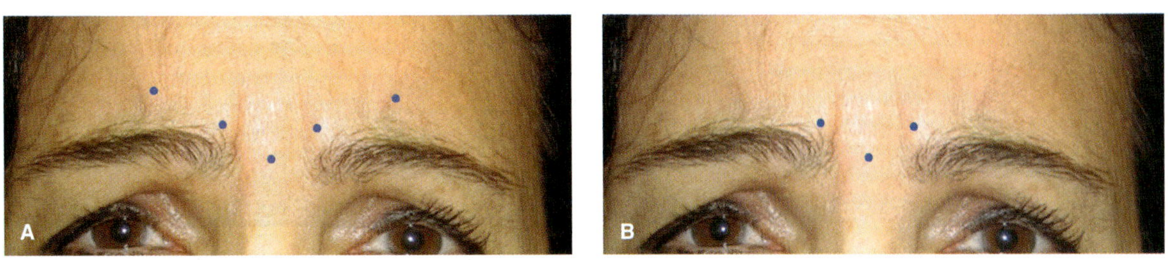

Figure 55-3 Injection points for treatment of glabellar lines, with five injection points (authors' preference) (**A**) versus three injection points (**B**).

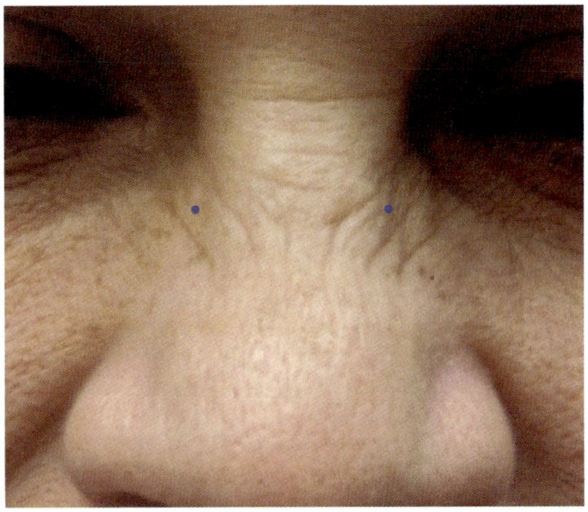

Figure 55-5 Injection points for treatment of bunny lines.

the nasofacial groove can cause paresis of the levator labii superioris alaeque nasi and levator anguli oris muscles, resulting in an ipsilateral lip ptosis and subsequently an asymmetric smile (Fig. 55-1).

PERIORAL RHYTIDES

Static rhytides can form periorally with aging and repetitive contraction of the orbicularis oris muscle (Fig. 55-1). BTX-A can be injected in the upper and lower cutaneous lips in the area of the orbicularis oris muscle to improve static rhytides in these areas, especially when used in combination with injectable filler into the creases (Fig. 55-6). It is important, however, to not overtreat the perioral area with BTX-A as the goal is to reduce the rhytides but maintain the sphincteric function of this muscle.

MENTAL CREASE

A prominent mental crease can be partially caused by strong contraction of the mentalis muscle, which elevates the central lower lip. The mentalis muscle has two bellies,

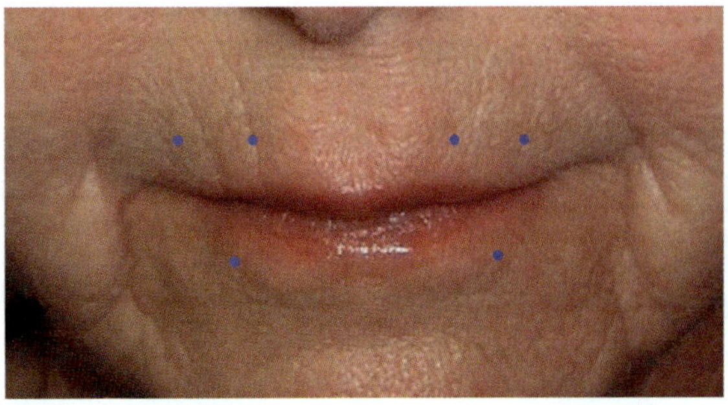

Figure 55-6 Injection points for treatment of perioral rhytides.

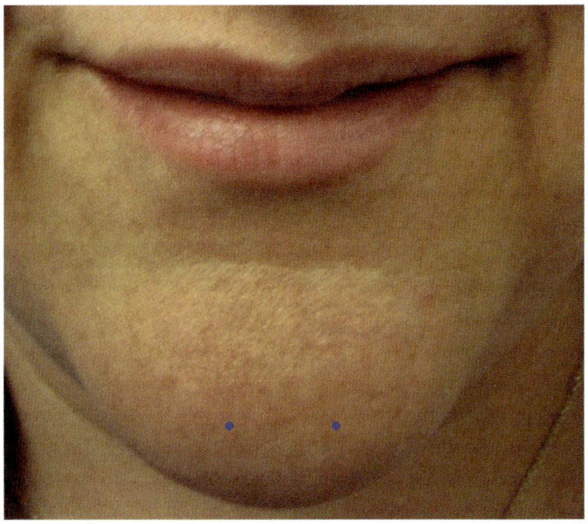

Figure 55-7 Injection points for treatment of mental crease.

each of which originate from either side of the mandible and insert into the deep dermis of the chin pad (Fig. 55-1). The crease can be softened by placing an injection of BTX-A into each belly of the mentalis muscle (Fig. 55-7). Using injectable filler into the mental crease can further soften its appearance.

DEPRESSOR ANGULI ORIS

The depressor anguli oris originates in the oblique line of the mandible and inserts into the area at the corner of the mouth (Fig. 55-1). It is responsible for the inferior and lateral movement of the angle of the mouth and, therefore, can contribute to the downturned appearance of the corners of the mouth. Injection of BTX-A into the posterior aspect of the depressor anguli oris muscle just above the mandible can further improve downturned corners of the mouth when used in combination with injectable filler just beneath the lateral sides of the lower lip (Fig. 55-8).

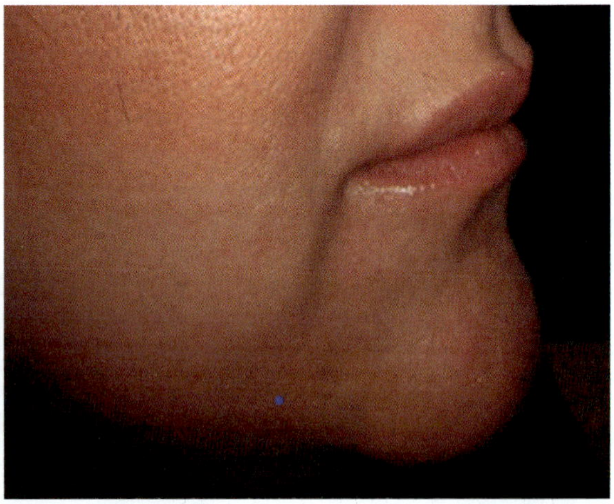

Figure 55-8 Injection points for treatment of depressor anguli oris.

TABLE 55-2
Injectable Fillers

Injectable Filler Material	Brand Name	Company	FDA Indication	Depth of Injection	Average Months of Duration
Nonpermanent					
Hyaluronic acid	Hylaform, Hylaform Plus	Genzyme Corporation	Moderate-to-severe facial rhytides and folds such as nasolabial folds	Dermis or dermal-subcutaneous junction	3–5
	Juvéderm Ultra, Juvéderm Ultra XC,	Allergan, Inc.	Moderate-to-severe facial rhytides and folds such as nasolabial folds	Dermis or dermal-subcutaneous junction	6–12
	Juvéderm Ultra Plus, Juvéderm Ultra Plus XC	Allergan, Inc.	Moderate-to-severe facial rhytides and folds such as nasolabial folds	Dermis or dermal-subcutaneous junction	6–12
	Restylane, Restylane-L	Medicis Aesthetics, Inc.	Moderate-to-severe facial rhytides and folds such as nasolabial folds, lip enhancement	Dermis or dermal-subcutaneous junction	6–9
	Perlane, Perlane-L	Medicis Aesthetics, Inc.	Moderate-to-severe facial rhytides and folds such as nasolabial folds	Dermis or dermal-subcutaneous junction	6–10
	Belotero Balance	Merz Aesthetics, Inc.	Moderate-to-severe facial rhytides and folds such as nasolabial folds	Dermis or dermal-subcutaneous junction	6–9
	Prevelle Silk	Mentor Corporation	Moderate-to-severe facial rhytides and folds such as nasolabial folds	Dermis or dermal-subcutaneous junction	3–5
	Hydrelle	Anika Therapeutics, Inc.	Moderate-to-severe facial rhytides and folds such as nasolabial folds	Dermis or dermal-subcutaneous junction	6–12
Semipermanent					
Calcium hydroxylapatite	Radiesse	Merz Aesthetics, Inc.	Moderate-to-severe facial wrinkles and folds such as nasolabial folds, HIV-associated lipoatrophy	Subcutaneous plane or the epi-periosteal plane	12–15
Poly-L-lactic acid	Sculptra	Dermik Laboratories	Shallow-to-deep smile lines such as the nasolabial folds, other facial wrinkles, HIV-associated lipoatrophy	Dermal-subcutaneous junction or upper hypodermis	12–24
Permanent					
Polymethyl methacrylate	Artefill	Suneva Medical, Inc.	Nasolabial folds	Dermal-subcutaneous junction	Permanent

INJECTABLE FILLERS

The advent of injectable fillers has revolutionized how facial rejuvenation can be achieved non-surgically. In this new era of facial rejuvenation, fillers are often combined with BTX-A as well as cosmetic laser treatments to achieve a more global rejuvenation of the face. Since the introduction of bovine collagen fillers in the early 1980s, there has been a rapid growth in the development and use of new injectable fillers. The current United States FDA-approved injectable fillers are discussed later and can be categorized as nonpermanent, semi-permanent, and permanent fillers (Table 55-2).

NONPERMANENT FILLERS

HYALURONIC ACID

Hyaluronic acid (HA) is a glycosaminoglycan found in the extracellular matrix of connective tissue as well as in synovial fluid, vitreous of the eye, cartilage, fascia, and umbilical cord. It is composed of repeating disaccharide units of D-glucuronic acid and N-acetylglucosamine and is identical in both molecular and chemical form in all tissues and mammals.[27–29] Because of this species' nonspecific nature of HA, there is low risk of a hypersensitivity reaction when using HA fillers.[30] Residing in dermal ground substance, HA fills the extracellular spaces between collagen fibers while providing structure and volume. HA is extremely water-soluble, with 1 g of HA being able to bind 6 L of water.[31] Due to its potent hydrophilic quality, it attracts and maintains moisture while creating a volumizing effect. With aging, there is a reduction in the amount of HA in the skin, which has been shown to directly correlate with moisture loss, dermal volume loss, and the formation of rhytides.[32]

HA fillers have a dual mechanism of action: they first integrate into the dermal tissue and then, through their hydrophilic properties, bind water to sustain the augmentation. Furthermore, HA fillers have been shown to stimulate the production of type I collagen in the skin.[33] The two broad categories of HA fillers include: (1) animal-derived from rooster combs and (2) non–animal-derived synthetic hyaluronic acid (NASHA) derived from *Streptococcus equi* bacterium. Rare allergic reactions to HA fillers can occur if the patient is sensitive to the residual trace amounts of avian proteins in the animal-derived HA fillers or bacterial proteins in NASHA HA fillers. FDA-approved HA fillers derived from rooster combs include Hylaform (Hylaform, Hylaform Plus; Genzyme Corporation). The FDA-approved NASHA fillers include Juvéderm (Juvéderm Ultra, Juvéderm Ultra Plus, Juvéderm Ultra XC, Juvéderm Ultra Plus XC; Allergan, Inc.), Restylane (Restylane, Restylane-L; Medicis Aesthetics, Inc.), Perlane (Perlane, Perlane-L; Medicis Aesthetics, Inc.), Belotero Balance (Merz Aesthetics, Inc.), Prevelle Silk (Mentor Corporation), and Hydrelle (Anika Therapeutics, Inc.). These injectable fillers are indicated for the correction of moderate-to-severe facial rhytides and folds such as nasolabial folds; Restylane is also indicated for lip enhancement. HA fillers are very versatile and have been used widely off-label in the lips, tear troughs, glabellar creases, Marionette lines, oral commissures, chin, prejowl sulcus, cheeks, temples, lateral brow, as well as for correction of acne scars, nasal augmentation and contouring, and correction of human immunodeficiency virus (HIV)-associated lipoatrophy.[34–42] The authors caution against the use of HA fillers in the glabellar region due to the reported serious adverse effect of retinal artery occlusion. HA fillers should be injected into the dermis or dermal-subcutaneous junction. Injections placed too superficially in the dermis can cause visible nodules with a bluish discoloration due to the Tyndall effect, caused by scattering of light.[43] Injections placed too deeply in the subcutaneous plane result in reduced efficacy of the HA filler. Juvéderm Ultra Plus, Juvéderm Ultra Plus XC, and Perlane are useful in areas of deeper folds and for more volumetric correction. The approximate duration of the HA fillers varies based on the particular product.

SEMIPERMANENT FILLERS

CALCIUM HYDROXYAPATITE

Calcium hydroxyapatite (CaHA) or Radiesse (Merz Aesthetics, Inc.) is a synthetic semipermanent injectable filler composed of 30% CaHA microspheres suspended in a 70% aqueous carboxymethylcellulose gel carrier. CaHA is a normal constituent of human bone and teeth and has been used in bone reconstruction as well as dental implants or coating materials. Due to its calcium density, it can sometimes be detected on routine radiographic studies.[44] As an injectable filler, it is indicated for the correction of moderate-to-severe facial wrinkles and folds such as nasolabial folds and facial wasting due to HIV-associated lipoatrophy. It has been used off-label for aging of the hand, acne scars, temporal hollowing, correction of marionette lines and prejowl sulcus, augmentation of the malar, submalar, and zygomatic areas, and nasal augmentation and contouring.[41,45–48] The use of CaHA off-label in the lips and periocular area is avoided due to the reported formation of nodules in these areas; the authors highly suggest avoiding its use in the lips.[49–51] CaHA should be injected into the subcutaneous plane or the epi-periosteal plane, and overcorrection is not recommended.[34,52]

Similar to the HA fillers, the filling effects of CaHA are twofold. The CaHA filler causes immediate filling effects when injected, but it also stimulates neocollagenesis around the microspheres as the gel is phagocytized.[53] It is broken down slowly, accounting for the prolonged filling effects of CaHA of approximately 12 to 15 months as compared to HA fillers.

POLY-L-LACTIC ACID

Poly-L-Lactic Acid (PLA) or Sculptra (Dermik Laboratories) is a synthetic biodegradable polymer that is composed of microparticles of PLA suspended in a sodium carboxymethylcellulose gel. It requires reconstitution with sterile water before it is injected. PLA is FDA-approved for the correction of shallow to deep smile lines such as the nasolabial folds, other facial wrinkles, and HIV-associated lipoatrophy. Off-label, it has been used to correct volume loss in the face, chest, and hands as well as for acne scars, but should be avoided in the lips and periocular areas due to possible nodule formation.[37,52,54–61] PLA should be injected into the plane of the dermal-subcutaneous junction or upper hypodermis in order to stimulate fibroblastic production of collagen as well as to avoid nodule formation with more superficial injections.[52,54] There is a high incidence of subcutaneous nodule formation associated with PLA that can occur as result of insufficient reconstitution, injection techniques, amount of volume injected, muscle movement causing concentration of the PLA injected, or an allergic or inflammatory response.[60–63]

The filling effect of PLA is mainly through its gradual stimulation of collagen production, although there is some immediate volumizing effect from fluid that becomes absorbed over several days.[64,65] As the PLA microparticles are degraded over weeks to months, a foreign body reaction occurs associated with a fibrous-tissue response that deposits collagen around it.[64,65] It is thought that this fibrous tissue response accounts for the sustained correction of 12 to 24 months seen with PLA.[65]

PERMANENT FILLERS

POLYMETHYL METHACRYLATE. Polymethyl methacrylate (PMMA) or Artefill (Suneva Medical, Inc.) is composed of 20% PMMA mircrospheres suspended in 80% bovine collagen with the addition of lidocaine and buffers. Due to the bovine collagen component, an Artefill skin test is required prior to its use in a patient and should not be used in patients with known allergy to bovine collagen or lidocaine as well as in patients with a history of severe allergies, as indicated by having multiple severe allergies or an anaphylactic episode. It is FDA-indicated for the correction of nasolabial folds, but has been used off-label in the glabellar creases, corners of the mouth, and perioral rhytides.[52,66–68] Its use should be avoided in the lips. PMMA injections should occur in the plane of the dermal-subcutaneous junction.

After PMMA is injected into the skin, the bovine collagen constituent is rapidly degraded within 1 to 3 months while the PMMA microspheres remain permanently as the microspheres are too large to be phagocytized. New collagen is also deposited around the PMMA microspheres through fibroplasia, further adding to its augmentation properties.[69,70]

TECHNIQUES

There are a variety of injection techniques when using fillers, and different practitioners will have a preference for different techniques. The most common injection techniques include linear threading (either retrograde or anterograde), serial puncture, fanning, cross-hatching, or a combination of any of these (Fig. 55-9). These techniques can be implemented in virtually any area of soft-tissue augmentation, including the nasolabial folds, marionette lines, and tear trough deformity. Prior to injection, it is advised that the practitioner pull back on the plunger to ensure that there is no flashback of blood indicating that the tip of the needle is not within a vessel. Injection directly into a vessel, particularly an artery, may cause vascular occlusion and consequent necrosis to the anatomic area which the vessel supplies.

When using the linear threading technique, many practitioners prefer threading in a retrograde fashion as there is less risk of unintentionally pushing the tip of the needle directly into a vessel and injecting directly into it as what may occur when injecting in an anterograde fashion. However, some practitioners believe that the vessels are pushed out of the way by the filler material when injecting in an anterograde fashion, if the filler is expelled from the

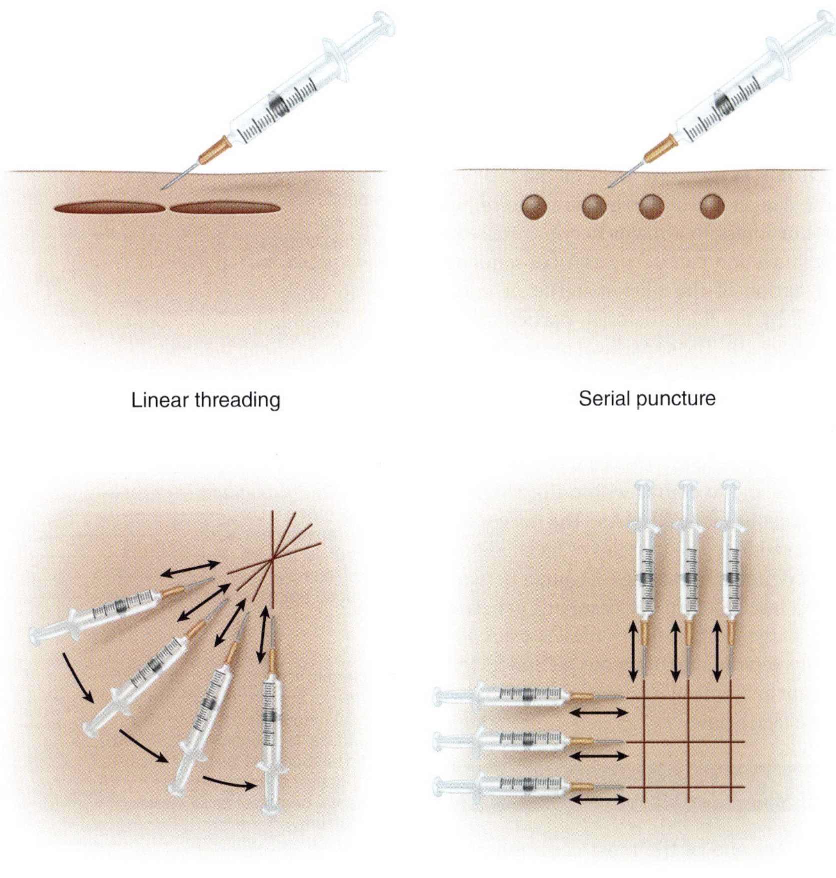

Figure 55-9 Different injection techniques for injectable fillers.

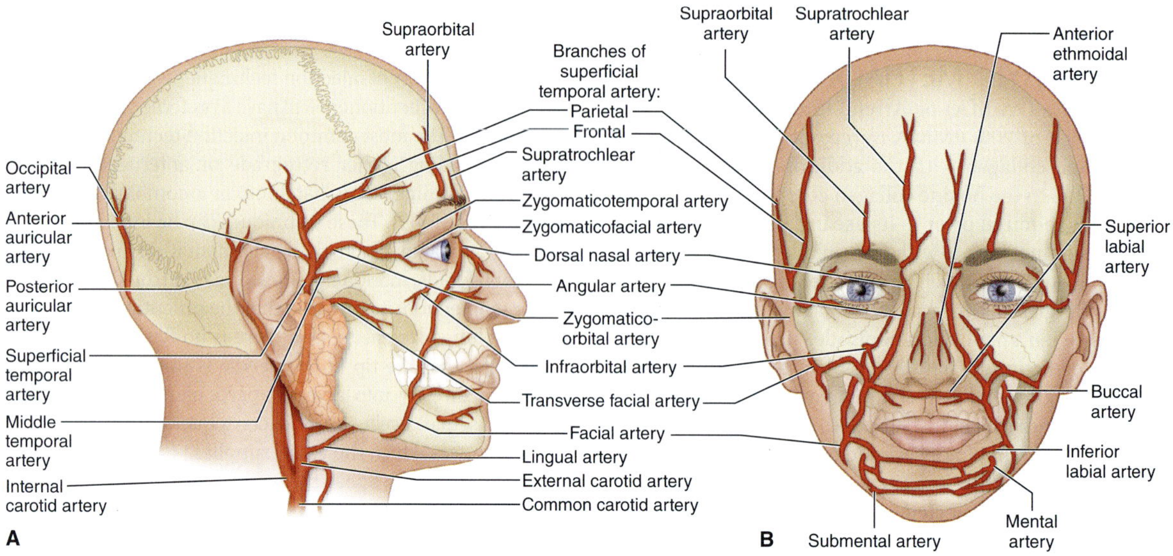

Figure 55-10 Arterial supply of the face, front view **(A)** and profile **(B)**.

needle before the needle is pushed forward. With serial puncture, there may be increased risk of bleeding and bruising at the injection site, particularly if the patient is on any medications or supplements that cause anticoagulation. Both fanning and cross-hatching are particularly useful for filling larger and deeper defects and for facial shaping.

OVERVIEW OF FACIAL ANATOMY

When using injectable fillers, it is essential to understand the underlying anatomy in different areas of the face and be familiar with the danger and watershed areas to reduce the risk of necrosis or injury to a major nerve. Cutaneous necrosis from filler injection can occur as a consequence of intra-arterial injection of the filler material or extra-arterial compression by the filler material, particularly in watershed areas (Fig. 55-10). The superficial muscular aponeurotic system (SMAS), which is the superficial fascia of the head and neck region beneath the subcutaneous fat, is an important structure that provides protection of key structures (Fig. 55-11). In general, the axial blood vessels that supply the face ascend to course within the SMAS or between the subcutaneous fat and SMAS. The nerves that provide motor innervation to the muscles of facial expression – the facial nerve and its branches – course between the SMAS and deep fascia before the branches penetrate the facial muscles. Large facial sensory nerves track in a superficial plane between the subcutaneous fat and SMAS. Particularly important anatomical landmarks are discussed in each region of the face below.

NASOLABIAL FOLDS

The nasolabial folds are one of the most common areas where injectable fillers are used. The linear threading technique is very useful in this area, threading serially along the nasolabial fold. At the superior edge of the

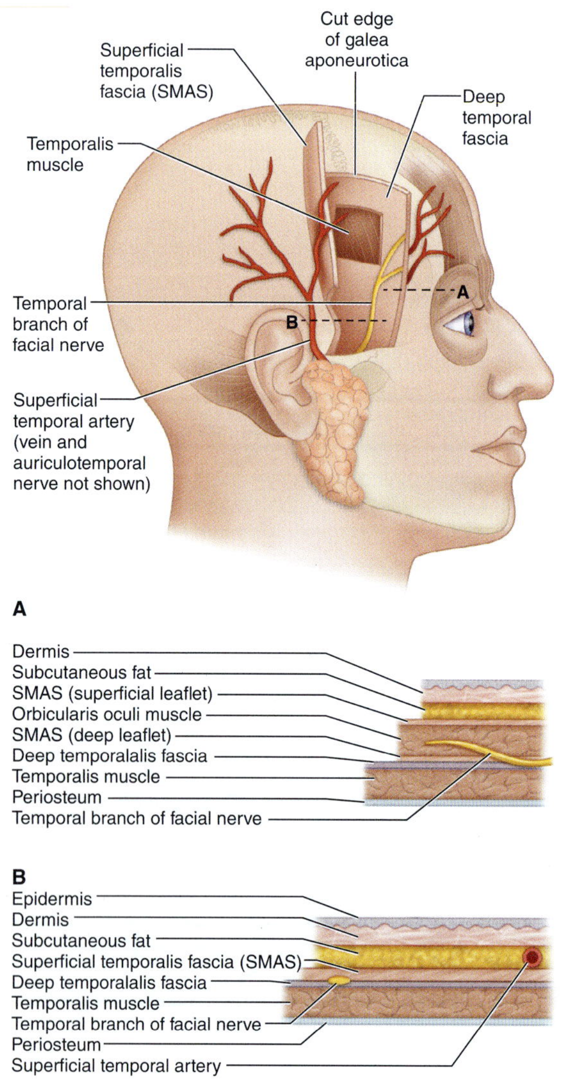

Figure 55-11 Cross-section anatomy of the superficial musculoaponeurotic system (SMAS) and its general relation to facial arteries and motor nerves.

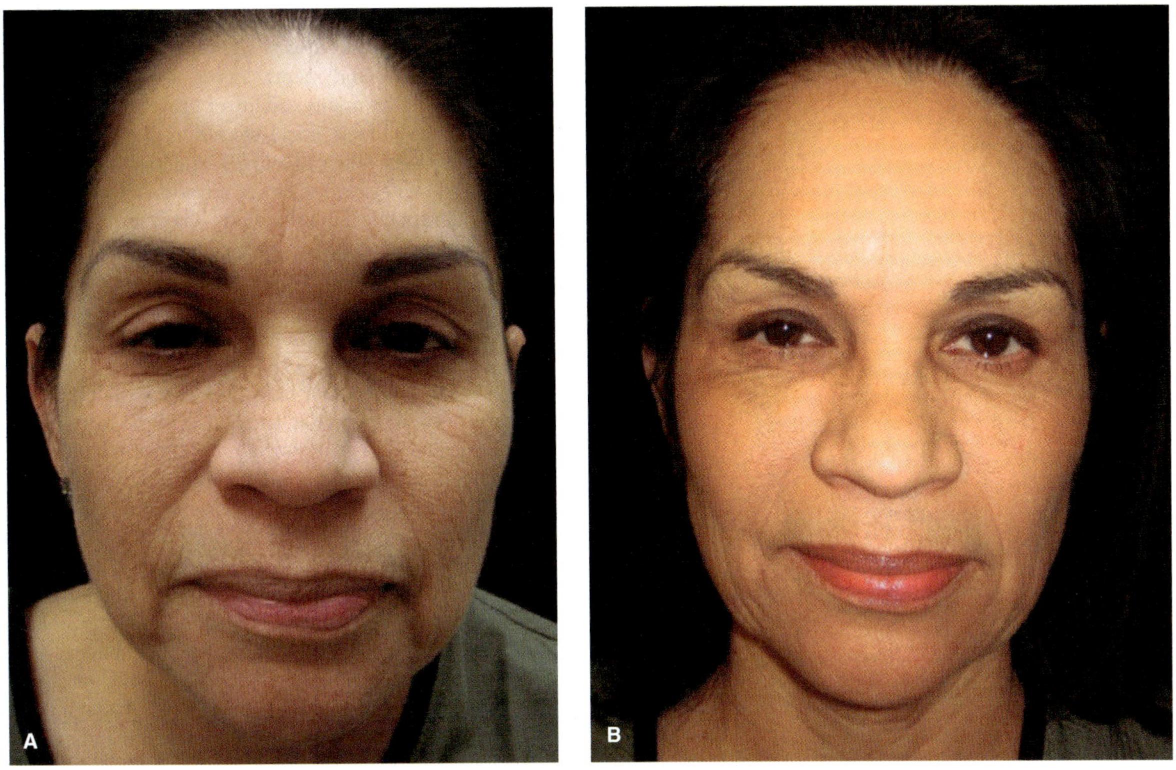

Figure 55-12 A patient before **(A)** and after hyaluronic acid filler injections in the nasolabial folds, marionette lines, tear trough deformity, mid face, and jowls as well as BTX-A into the bunny lines **(B)**.

nasolabial fold, the fanning technique may be employed for any relatively increased loss of volume between the nasolabial fold and the alar-facial groove. For overall deeper nasolabial folds, the fanning technique can be used along the entire length of the fold itself. When filling the nasolabial fold, filler should be placed into the fold itself and also medial to the fold if needed. It is important not to inject filler in the area lateral to the nasolabial fold as this will increase the volume of the medial cheek and, therefore, cause accentuation of the fold itself (Fig. 55-12).

The important anatomic consideration in the area of the nasolabial fold is the course of the facial artery (Fig. 55-10). As this artery runs obliquely from the mandible toward the nasal ala, it passes beneath the zygomaticus muscles as it crosses the nasolabial fold. It then runs along the alar crease and lateral nasal sidewall, where it terminates as the angular artery and continues toward the medial orbital rim. Since injectable fillers, when used appropriately in this area, are not injected deep to the subcutaneous fat, injection directly into the angular artery is uncommon. However, if a large volume of injectable filler is used particularly near the superior portion of the nasolabial fold, then a mass effect of the filler material can cause external compression of the angular artery and risk necrosis of the nasal ala.[71]

MARIONETTE LINES

Marionette lines are the creases that run vertically downward from the oral commissures and outline the chin. Fanning and cross-hatching techniques are often used here particularly if the folds are deeper as well as to form a buttress for the corners of the lower lip. The majority of the filler should be injected medial to the marionette lines to avoid accentuating the lines themselves, similar to the nasolabial folds, although a small amount of filler can be laid across the Marionette lines to help create a buttress of support (Fig. 55-12).

TEAR TROUGH DEFORMITY

The tear trough, also known as the nasojugal groove, is a depression that extends inferolaterally from the medial canthus to the region of the midpupillary line and naturally occurs even in individuals of young age. When it becomes more prominent with aging, it is known as the tear trough deformity. Although multiple factors likely contribute to the deformity, the predominating factor is the loss of subcutaneous fat in the infraorbital area. Other age-related factors that contribute to accentuation of the deformity include herniation of orbital fat above the deformity, inferior shifting of the malar fat pad below the deformity (also known as midface descent), and skin laxity.

Injectable fillers can be used to soften the tear trough deformity as well as help lessen the shadowing – or "dark circles" – of the infraorbital area that is often made more noticeable by the deformity and the general loss of subcutaneous fat (Fig. 55-12). Unless there is significant herniation of the orbital fat above the tear trough deformity, cosmetic correction of the deformity can be performed with a nonsurgical approach in the current era of facial rejuvenation.

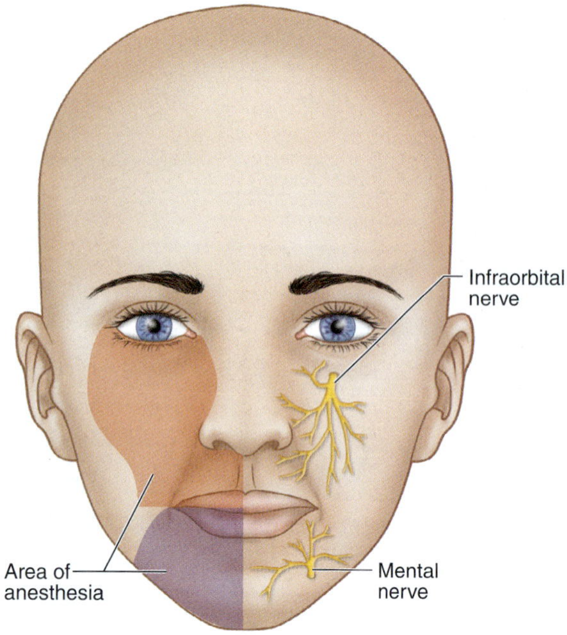

Figure 55-13 Areas of anesthesia of infraorbital and mental nerve blocks.

Given the thinness of the periorbital skin, filler should be injected deep to the orbicularis muscle in the plane of the periosteum to reduce the risk of nodularity and lumpiness if the filler is injected too superficially. To inject in the plane of the periosteum, the tip of the needle should be just touching the bone. The authors suggest the use of a cannula to prevent bruising. Linear threading is useful in this area; serial puncture may also be utilized but may increase the risk of bruising given the multiple punctures in an area of thin skin. It is important to avoid injecting in the area of the infraorbital foramen, where the infraorbital artery, vein, and nerve exit. It is located approximately 1 cm inferior to the infraorbital rim along the midpupillary line.

LIPS

For volumization of the lips with injectable filler, consideration should be taken regarding performing nerve blocks prior to the cosmetic procedure as filler injections into the lips is typically associated with significant pain. An infraorbital nerve block and mental nerve block are used for augmentation of the upper and lower lips, respectively. An infraorbital nerve block blocks sensation to the upper lip, medial cheek, nasal sidewall and ala, and lower eyelid (Fig. 55-13). It can be performed either intraorally (the authors' preferred approach) or extraorally via the infraorbital foramen. Using the intraoral approach, local anesthesia is injected into the mucobuccal fold in the area of the canine and first premolar of the upper teeth with the needle directed toward the midpupillary line and positioned parallel to the maxilla (Fig. 55-14A). About 0.5 to 1 cc of local anesthesia can be injected. Using the extraoral approach, local anesthesia is injected in the region of the infraorbital foramen located approximately 1 cm inferior to the infraorbital rim along the midpupillary line (Fig. 55-14B). As the needle is in close proximity to the infraorbital artery using this approach, it may be advised to use local anesthesia without any vasoconstrictive agents. The mental nerve block affects sensation to the chin and the lower lip (Fig. 55-13) and is performed using an intraoral approach. Local anesthesia is injected into the mucobuccal fold between first and second premolars of the lower teeth with a total of 0.5 to 1 cc of local anesthesia. Massaging the anesthesia into the tissue following infraorbital and mental nerve blocks can assist with ensuring adequate anesthesia.

There is a multitude of methods for augmentation of the lips and every practitioner has or will develop their preferred methods. It is best to use smaller particle fillers for lip augmentation, such as Restylane/Restylane-L (FDA-approved for lip augmentation) or Juvéderm Ultra/Juvéderm Ultra XC (off-label use), as patients can sometimes feel the larger particle fillers, which may be uncomfortable. To define and evert the lips, filler is injected along the vermillion border but within the red portion of the lip with linear threading. Oftentimes, filler does not need to be injected into the most lateral portion of the vermillion border close to the oral commissures, as a more natural appearance is achieved when the filler is tapered off laterally. It is helpful in giving the lips a more defined appearance if the needle is beveled up toward the red surface of the lip, being careful to not inject too superficially to cause the Tyndall effect. Filler can also be injected into the white roll, along the plane of the potential space between

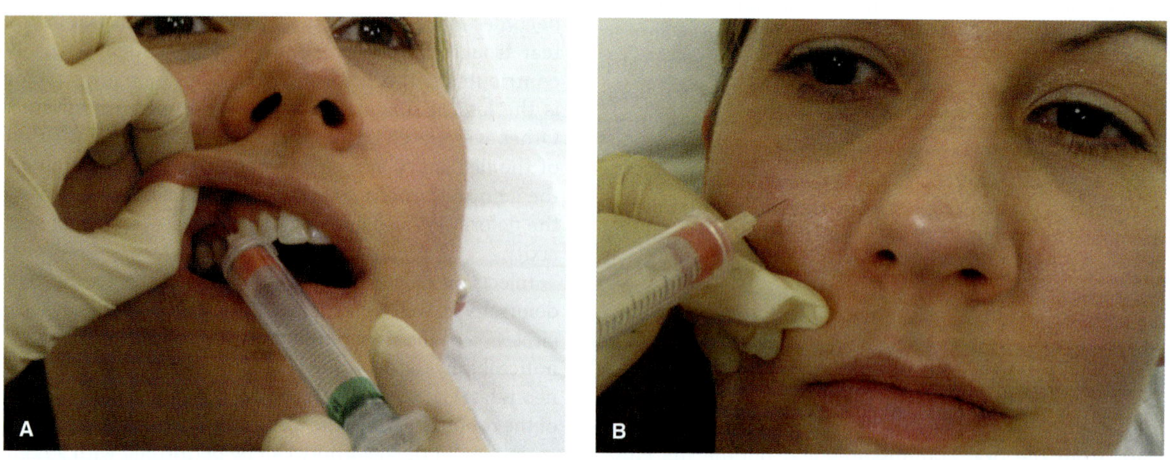

Figure 55-14 Infraorbital nerve block for lip rejuvenation using the intraoral approach **(A)** and extraoral approach **(B)**.

the mucosal lip and orbicularis oris muscle, if this area appears blunted with age. For lip augmentation, it is useful to begin with the vermillion border and the white roll if needed, as sometimes filling of these areas is enough to give the lip an eversion that a patient may be satisfied with. Additional definition of the cupid's bow may be created by injecting a very conservative amount of filler along the mucosal edge, being careful not to overfill this area as often only a minimal amount of filler is needed. Filler can then be injected into the remainder of the mucosal lips for further augmentation through a combination of various techniques including linear threading, serial puncture, and small depot injections in which a small bolus of filler is injected. The volume of filler injected can, again, be tapered off as injection approaches the oral commissures to give a more natural appearance to lip augmentation. To give a pouty appearance, small depot injections can be injected into both areas just lateral to the midline lip in the upper and lower lips. When there is volume loss in the philtral columns, filler can be injected into the philtral columns as linear threading throughout the entire length of the philtral column or as triangles at the inferior portion of the philtral column depending on where the volume is needed.

To avoid the potential complication of necrosis of the lips, it is advised to pull back on the plunger of the syringe to ensure the needle is not within a vessel before injecting. Furthermore, it is best to inject the filler into the anterior half of the lips to avoid injecting into the superior or inferior labial arteries of the upper and lower lips, respectively. These arteries are located in the posterior one-third of the lips and run approximately parallel to the vermillion border (Fig. 55-10). In addition, CaHA and permanent fillers should be avoided in the lips due to nodule formation that has been reported.

TEMPLES

With aging, volume loss can also be seen in the temporal areas causing a wasted and gaunt appearance. Common methods utilized for correcting hollowing of the temples include the depot technique, in which a single bolus of injectable filler is deposited and then massaged throughout the temples, or through the fanning technique both injected in the plane of the periosteum just above the temporal bone.

Filler should be injected in the plane of the periosteum to avoid potential complications involving the superficial temporal artery or the temporal branch of the facial nerve (Fig. 55-11). The tissue layers in the temporal region from superficial to deep include skin, subcutaneous fat, superficial temporalis fascia (SMAS), deep temporalis fascia, and temporalis muscle, which lie atop the periosteum and temporal bone. In the temple region, the superficial temporal artery courses within the subcutaneous fat above the superficial temporalis fascia. The temporal branch of the facial nerve (which supplies motor innervation to the frontalis, corrugator supercilii, orbicularis oculi, and temporoparietalis muscles) runs within the superficial temporalis fascia in the temple region superior to the zygomatic arch. The devastating complication of blindness, resulting from central retinal artery embolization, can occur when using injectable fillers in the temples and, therefore, the practitioner must be careful when volumizing this area. This complication has also been reported when using injectable fillers in the glabellar area, nose, periorbital area, and nasolabial fold. Central retinal artery embolization occurs via retrograde arterial displacement of injectable products with embolization to the ophthalmic artery, causing blindness.

GLABELLAR CREASES

Injectable filler can be used in conjunction with BTX-A in the glabellar region for deep vertical rhytides. However, it is the most frequently reported site of necrosis irrespective of the type of injectable filler used and, therefore, it is advised that the injector be very familiar with the anatomy of the glabella. The danger lies in the path of the supratrochlear artery and its smaller branches that supply the glabella and the forehead (Fig. 55-10). The supratrochlear artery exits the orbit at the superior and medial corner, coursing superiorly just medial to the brow where glabellar creases may be located.[72] Its smaller branches course more superficially and medial to the brow as well. Because of the limited collateral circulation, the glabella is a particular danger area for vascular compromise and impending necrosis along the distribution of the supratrochlear artery.

To reduce the risk of necrosis, the needle tip should be placed superficially and pointed medially to avoid injecting into the supratrochlear artery or its branches. Also, it is critical to pull back on the plunger to ensure that there is no flashback of blood, confirming that the needle tip is not located within a vessel. Furthermore, it is best to not overcorrect and to inject only small aliquots of filler as larger amounts of filler may cause external compression of the arteries and compromise vascular flow.[73]

BROW

The combination of BTX-A and injectable filler can be used to achieve a lateral brow lift. First, BTX-A is injected just beneath the end of the lateral brow to weaken the depressors of the brow, which include the orbicularis oculi and depressor supercilii muscles. Then to further enhance the brow lift and brow fullness, filler is injected in the area of the lateral brow fat pad just beneath the lateral brow along the superior orbital rim using either linear threading or serial puncture techniques (Fig. 55-15). However, it is crucial to start the injection lateral to the palpable supraorbital notch and not inject into the area of the notch, where the supraorbital artery, vein, and nerve pass through.

MID FACE

Injectable fillers can be used to restore volume loss that often occurs in the mid face with aging. Use of larger particle fillers, such as the HA fillers Perlane/Perlane-L and Juvéderm Ultra Plus/Juvéderm Ultra Plus XC or CaHA, can provide more volumization as compared to using smaller particle fillers. Volume loss in this area can be

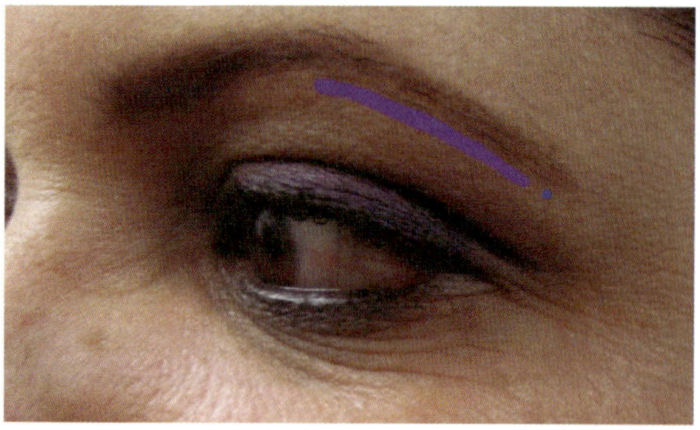

Figure 55-15 Injection sites for creating a brow lift using combination of BTX-A (*blue dot*) and injectable filler (*purple line*).

visible as subtle grooves along the mid upper cheek as well as reduced prominence and fullness of the malar cheeks. The fanning and cross-hatching techniques are useful here for correction of larger and deeper volume deficits and for facial shaping particularly of the malar cheeks (Fig. 55-12).

JOWLS

Jowls in the mandibular area are mainly due to skin laxity and sagging. Injectable fillers can lessen the appearance of mild jowls, but will be ineffective in camouflaging more significant jowls in which a lower facelift may be recommended. For mild jowls, filler can be injected into the defect itself as depot injections or can be strewn across the defect with the linear threading technique (Fig. 55-12).

When using injectable fillers along the jawline, it is important to avoid injury to the marginal mandibular branch of the facial nerve. The marginal mandibular branch crosses over the mandible at an area along the jawline just lateral to the oral commissures up to 2 cm posterior to the oral commissures. The nerve branch is susceptible to injury in this area as it is covered only by fascia, a thin platysma muscle, and skin.

ACNE SCARS

The appearance of acne scars, particularly the deeper scars, can be minimized with the use of smaller particle fillers, such as Restylane/Restylane-L and Juvéderm Ultra/Juvéderm Ultra XC. To treat acne scars, the filler should be injected into the dermal layer of the skin being cautious of not to inject so superficially as to cause nodule formation (Fig. 55-16).

LIGHT AND LASER THERAPIES

Various devices have been developed to treat different signs of aging, including vascular lesions (e.g., erythema, telangiectasias, cherry angiomas), pigmented lesions (e.g., lentigines), and rhytides (Table 55-3). These devices work by emitting specific wavelengths of lights that are targeted by particular chromophores within the skin, including blood vessels, pigment, or water, respectively. The introduction

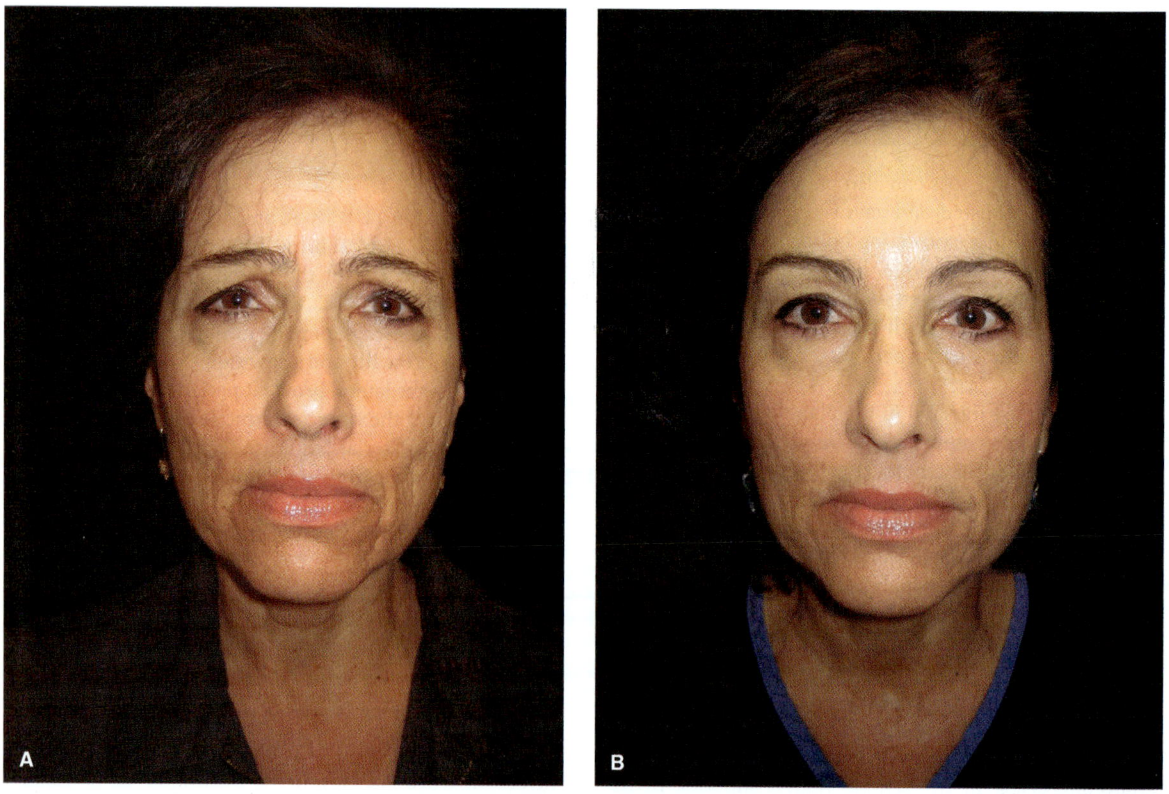

Figure 55-16 A patient before **(A)** and after hyaluronic filler injections into acne scars of the mid and lower cheeks and chin as well as botulinum toxin to the glabella, forehead, and crow's feet **(B)**.

TABLE 55-3
Vascular and Pigment Light and Laser Devices

Device	Indications
Intense pulsed light (500–1200 nm)	Superficial vascular lesions, lentigines, poikiloderma
Pulsed dye laser (585–595 nm)	Superficial vascular lesions
KTP laser (532 nm)	Superficial telangiectasias
Nd:YAG laser (1064 nm)	Deeper vascular lesions
Q-switched lasers Frequency-doubled Nd:YAG (532 nm) Ruby (694 nm) Alexandrite (755 nm) Nd:YAG (1064 nm)	Lentigines, tattoos

KTP, Potassium-Titanyl-Phosphate; Nd:YAG, Neodymium: Yttrium-Aluminum-Garnet.

of light and laser therapies has further reformed how facial rejuvenation can be achieved with noninvasive, nonsurgical methods.

VASCULAR AND PIGMENT LIGHT AND LASER DEVICES

INTENSE-PULSED LIGHT. Intense-pulsed light (IPL) is a high-intensity noncoherent light source, as opposed to lasers that are highly coherent light sources, which emits a range of light wavelengths and is commonly used to treat vascular and pigmented lesions. This device includes filters that exclude certain wavelengths so that specific wavelengths of light can be applied. These various filters are used to allow the practitioner to treat vascular lesions, pigmented lesions, or both. The ability of the IPL to treat both vascular and pigmented lesions simultaneously is due to its capacity to emit various wavelengths at the same time that are preferentially absorbed by chromophores both within the blood vessels and pigmented area. Because of this ability as well as the minimal downtime, the IPL is a commonly used device for photorejuvenation of the skin. When using the IPL for pigmented lesions, the practitioner should be aware that it also targets the pigment in the hair and thus is also used for hair removal. Therefore, it should be carefully used around areas of the eyebrows as well as the beard and mustache areas of men when used for photorejuvenation.

PULSED DYE LASER. The pulsed dye laser (PDL) has become the treatment of choice for vascular conditions, including facial telangiectasias, port-wine stains, and some superficial infantile hemangiomas, as well as for cutaneous erythema such as that seen in rosacea and poikiloderma of Civatte. The wavelengths of PDL, 585 nm and 595 nm, are near the peak of absorption of oxyhemoglobin and thus are selective for vascular injury while leaving the surrounding tissue intact. Posttreatment side effects, including textural abnormality and scarring, are rare. Post-inflammatory hyperpigmentation may occur if purpuric settings are used in darker skinned patients, but this usually resolves. In addition, PDL has been also shown to soften scars and improve rhytides by inducing collagen remodeling as supported by the histologic findings of thickened collagen in the superficial dermis as well as increases in type III procollagen, type I collagen mRNA, and chondroitin sulfate.[74–79] The mechanism for improving rhytides is not fully understood, but it is thought that certain mediators are released into the surrounding tissue when the blood vessels are targeted by the PDL.

POTASSIUM-TITANYL-PHOSPHATE LASER. The potassium-titanyl-phosphate (KTP) laser is a vascular laser having a wavelength of 532 nm. Its use in dermatologic conditions is limited, but it can be effective in treating fine facial telangiectasias when these lesions are traced out with the laser. Results are seen immediately, but recurrences may occur.

NEODYMIUM:YTTRIUM-ALUMINUM-GARNET LASER. Treatment of deep cutaneous vascular lesions can be challenging. The long-pulsed neodymium:yttrium-aluminum-garnet (Nd:YAG) laser, with its wavelength of 1064 nm, can be used to treat deeper vascular lesions that may not be as effectively treated with other vascular lasers. It can also be used in combination with other vascular lasers, such as the PDL laser, to treat the deeper component of a mixed vascular lesion. It has been shown effective in treating facial veins and venous lakes, as well as other vascular tumors and malformations.[80–82]

Q-SWITCHED LASERS. Q-switched lasers include the Q-switched frequency-doubled Nd:YAG (532 nm), Q-switched ruby (694 nm), Q-switched alexandrite (755 nm), and Q-switched Nd:YAG (1064 nm) and are used primarily for the treatment of pigmented lesions, lentigines and tattoos. These short-pulsed, pigment-specific lasers allow for the highly selective targeting of subcellular pigment, whether endogenous or exogenous, with minimal injury to surrounding tissues, thereby reducing the risk of complications such as scarring. The Q-switched lasers are the most effective in treating pigmented lesions, as their very short pulse durations more effectively target the melanosome. Epidermal pigment is targeted by the Q-switched frequency-doubled Nd:YAG with its 532 nm wavelength; both epidermal and dermal pigment are targeted by the Q-switched ruby and Q-switched alexandrite with their 694 nm and 755 nm wavelengths, respectively, and deeper dermal pigment is targeted by the Q-switched Nd:YAG with its 1064 nm wavelength.

NONABLATIVE RESURFACING

PHOTODYNAMIC THERAPY. Photodynamic therapy (PDT) is a nonablative treatment for actinic keratoses as well as for photoaging that requires a photosensitizer, light with an appropriate wavelength, and oxygen that are present simultaneously.[83] When used for photorejuvenation, it has been shown to reduce erythema, dyspigmentation, and fine wrinkles associated with photoaging.[84]

The photosensitizing agents that are FDA-approved for use in PDT for the treatment of actinic keratoses, but also used for off-label cosmetic applications, are 5-aminolevulinic acid (5-ALA) and the methyl ester of ALA (mALA). These agents are applied to the area of skin being treated for an appropriate incubation time before a light source is applied to the skin. ALA, after being applied to the skin, is converted to protoporphyrin IX, which is absorbed into actinically damaged skin cells and pilosebaceous units.[84,85] Upon exposure to an appropriate visible light source (400– 800 nm), the formation of reactive oxygen species occurs that leads to the destruction of the cells that have accumulated protoporphyrin IX.[83,85] Blue light (417 nm) had been conventionally chosen as the light source for PDT as its wavelength corresponds to the largest absorption band of protoporphyrin IX known as the Soret band (maximum at 412 nm).[84] However in more recent years, other light and laser sources have been used efficaciously in conjunction with PDT that overlap with the other absorption peaks of protoporphyrin IX of 504, 538, 576, and 635 nm.[84,85] These sources include red light (632 nm), IPL (400–1200 nm), and PDL (585 and 595 nm).[84,85] Although blue light is the most potent wavelength for activation of the PDT effect, the longer and deeper penetrating visible light wavelengths of the IPL and PDL more effectively reach and thermally target chromophores of the blood vessels, pigment, and to a lesser degree collagen and, therefore, are thought to be more effective when used in PDT for the treatment of photoaging.[86,87]

NONABLATIVE FRACTIONATED LASER RESURFACING. Ablative laser resurfacing yields excellent outcomes in photorejuvenation of the skin, but is associated with longer downtime for the patient and a higher risk of postprocedure complications. Nonablative laser therapies offer reduced downtime, but have limited clinical efficacy in skin rejuvenation. Nonablative fractionated laser resurfacing was subsequently developed to present a more efficacious treatment for facial rejuvenation with consistent results as compared to the nonablative laser therapies, while associated with minimal downtime and reduced complications as compared to the ablative laser resurfacing treatments.

The nonablative fractionated laser is an erbium-doped fiber laser with a wavelength of 1550 nm that targets water as its chromophore. It produces microthermal treatment zones (MTZ) of controlled width, depth, and density in the dermis, which are microscopic columns of thermally denatured tissue with water as the primary energy-absorbing molecule. The untreated tissue surrounding the MTZ facilitates the rapid repair of the treatment zones.[88] It has also been suggested that these MTZ allow for the passage of microscopic epidermal necrotic debris (MENDs), which may also contain melanin pigment, to be eliminated through the stratum corneum and, therefore, render nonablative fractionated laser resurfacing potentially useful in treating cutaneous disorders involving pigment deeper in the epidermis.[89,90] Furthermore, elastin fibers have been demonstrated to be eliminated through the MENDs.[91] As photoaging comprises a combination of epidermal pigmentation and solar elastosis, the 1550 nm fractionated laser may exert its effects by eliminating these products from the skin. This laser has been shown to effectively treat photodamage and rhytides with minimal patient downtime and side effects.[92] More recently, it has also demonstrated improvements in treating atrophic scars.[93]

ABLATIVE RESURFACING

Ablative laser resurfacing is highly effective for rejuvenating photodamaged skin, but is associated with higher risks of undesirable side effects including infection, dyspigmentation, and scarring. These lasers target intracellular water and include the carbon dioxide (CO_2) laser and the erbium:yttrium-aluminum-garnet (Er:YAG) laser. The CO_2 laser was the first ablative laser created and the Er:YAG laser was later introduced to offer an ablative laser that would require less downtime for recovery as well as less risk of untoward side effects as compared to the CO_2 laser.

The CO_2 laser emits a wavelength of 10,600 nm and has a maximum penetration depth of approximately 250 μm, corresponding to ablation of the epidermis and superficial portion of the papillary dermis. It has been demonstrated to yield improvements in wrinkle severity and overall skin tone of 50% or greater[2,75,94]; but these improvements are more pronounced for fine wrinkles – particularly those in the periorbital and perioral areas—and less marked for the deeper rhytides.[95] However, this laser is associated with significant downtime for patient recovery until reepithelialization occurs, typically taking at least 1 month. Furthermore, it has been shown to be effective in treating mild-to-moderate acne scars, showing improvements of up to 81%.[96] It has not shown to be as effective in treating severe acne scars.[97]

The Er:YAG laser emits a wavelength of 2940 nm, which is close to the absorption peak of water. As a result, it has a higher affinity for water as compared to the CO_2 laser but has a reduced depth of penetration. The depth of penetration for the Er:YAG laser is 1 to 3 μm of tissue per J/cm^2, whereas the depth of penetration for the CO_2 laser is 20 to 30 μm per J/cm^2.[98] These features make the Er:YAG laser a popular ablative laser as it is capable of more accurate ablation with minimal thermal damage of the surrounding tissues. Because there is less coagulation of the surrounding tissue, it is associated with more bleeding post procedure. However as compared to the CO_2 laser, the Er:YAG laser demonstrates less tissue contraction and is thus slightly less efficacious than the CO_2 laser though still fairly comparable.

Fractional delivery systems have also been developed for these ablative lasers in an effort to achieve similar clinical results as the conventional ablative resurfacing lasers but with quicker patient recovery and reduced scarring risk. These lasers cause microscopic columns of complete epidermal ablation with varying amounts of dermal ablation. Similar to the fractionated nonablative lasers, the untreated tissue surrounding the MTZ allows for more rapid recovery of the treatment zones.[88] Significant improvements in rhytides, pigmentation, skin texture, and skin laxity have been achieved after a series of one to three treatments with the fractional CO_2 laser or Er:YAG laser.[99–101]

REFERENCES

1. Zouboulis CC, Makrantonaki E. Clinical aspects and molecular diagnostics of skin aging. *Clin Dermatol.* 2011;29(1):3–14.
2. Rabe JH, Mamelak AJ, McElgunn PJ, Morison WL, Sauder DN. Photoaging: mechanisms and repair. *J Am Acad Dermatol.* 2006;55(1):1–19.
3. Makrantonaki E, Zouboulis CC. Molecular mechanisms of skin aging: state of the art. *Ann N Y Acad Sci.* 2007;1119:40–50.
4. Gilchrest BA. A review of skin ageing and its medical therapy. *Br J Dermatol.* 1996;135(6):867–875.
5. Green AC, Hughes MC, McBride P, Fourtanier A. Factors associated with premature skin aging (photoaging) before the age of 55: a population-based study. *Dermatology.* 2011;222(1):74–80.
6. Martires KJ, Fu P, Polster AM, Cooper KD, Baron ED. Factors that affect skin aging: a cohort-based survey on twins. *Arch Dermatol.* 2009;145(12):1375–1379.
7. Gierloff M, Stöhring C, Buder T, Gassling V, Açil Y, Wiltfang J. Aging changes of the midfacial fat compartments: a computed tomographic study. *Plast Reconstr Surg.* 2012;129(1):263–273.
8. Camp MC, Wong WW, Filip Z, Carter CS, Gupta SC. A quantitative analysis of periorbital aging with three-dimensional surface imaging. *J Plast Reconstr Aesthet Surg.* 2011;64(2):148–154.
9. Mendelson BC, Hartley W, Scott M, McNab A, Granzow JW. Age-related changes of the orbit and midcheek and the implications for facial rejuvenation. *Aesthetic Plast Surg.* 2007;31(5):419–423.
10. Shaw RB Jr, Katzel EB, Koltz PF, et al. Aging of the facial skeleton: aesthetic implications and rejuvenation strategies. *Plast Reconstr Surg.* 2011;127(1):374–383.
11. Shaw RB Jr, Kahn DM. Aging of the midface bony elements: a three-dimensional computed tomographic study. *Plast Reconstr Surg.* 2007;119(2):675–681; discussion 682–683.
12. Shaw RB Jr, Katzel EB, Koltz PF, Kahn DM, Puzas EJ, Langstein HN. Facial bone density: effects of aging and impact on facial rejuvenation. *Aesthet Surg J.* 2012;32(8):937–942.
13. Gilchrest BA, Blog FB, Szabo G. Effects of aging and chronic sun exposure on melanocytes in human skin. *J Invest Dermatol.* 1979;73(2):141–143.
14. Longo C, Casari A, Beretti F, Cesinaro AM, Pellacani G. Skin aging: in vivo microscopic assessment of epidermal and dermal changes by means of confocal microscopy. *J Am Acad Dermatol.* 2013;68(3):e73–e82.
15. Chung JH, Eun HC. Angiogenesis in skin aging and photoaging. *J Dermatol.* 2007;34(9):593–600.
16. Bielenberg DR, Bucana CD, Sanchez R, Donawho CK, Kripke ML, Fidler IJ. Molecular regulation of UVB-induced cutaneous angiogenesis. *J Invest Dermatol.* 1998;111(5):864–872.
17. Yano K, Kadoya K, Kajiya K, Hong YK, Detmar M. Ultraviolet B irradiation of human skin induces an angiogenic switch that is mediated by upregulation of vascular endothelial growth factor and by downregulation of thrombospondin-1. *Br J Dermatol.* 2005;152(1):115–121.
18. Shukla HD, Sharma SK. Clostridium botulinum: a bug with beauty and weapon. *Crit Rev Microbiol.* 2005;31(1):11–18.
19. Dressler D, Hallett M. Immunological aspects of Botox, Dysport and Myobloc/NeuroBloc. *Eur J Neurol.* 2006;13(suppl 1):11–15.
20. Schiavo G, Santucci A, Dasgupta BR, et al. Botulinum neurotoxins serotypes A and E cleave SNAP-25 at distinct COOH-terminal peptide bonds. *FEBS Lett.* 1993;335(1):99–103.
21. Grein S, Mander GJ, Taylor HV. Xeomin is stable without refrigeration: complexing proteins are not required for stability of botulinum toxin type A preparations. *Toxicon.* 2008;51:13.
22. Dressler D, Mander G, Fink K. Measuring the potency labelling of onabotulinumtoxinA (Botox((R))) and incobotulinumtoxinA (Xeomin ((R))) in an LD50 assay. *J Neural Transm.* 2012;119(1):13–15.
23. Wohlfarth K, Schwandt I, Wegner F, et al. Biological activity of two botulinum toxin type A complexes (Dysport and Botox) in volunteers: a double-blind, randomized, dose-ranging study. *J Neurol.* 2008;255(12):1932–1939.
24. Sampaio C, Costa J, Ferreira JJ. Clinical comparability of marketed formulations of botulinum toxin. *Mov Disord.* 2004;19(suppl 8):S129–S136.
25. Rosales RL, Bigalke H, Dressler D, Pharmacology of botulinum toxin: differences between type A preparations. *Eur J Neurol.* 2006;13(suppl 1):2–10.
26. Carli L, Montecucco C, Rossetto O. Assay of diffusion of different botulinum neurotoxin type a formulations injected in the mouse leg. *Muscle Nerve.* 2009;40(3):374–380.
27. Fraser JR, Laurent TC, Laurent UB. Hyaluronan: its nature, distribution, functions and turnover. *J Intern Med.* 1997;242(1):27–33.
28. Laurent TC, Laurent UB, Fraser JR. The structure and function of hyaluronan: an overview. *Immunol Cell Biol.* 1996;74(2):A1–A7.
29. Price RD, Berry MG, Navsaria HA, Hyaluronic acid: the scientific and clinical evidence. *J Plast Reconstr Aesthet Surg.* 2007;60(10):1110–1119.
30. Hamilton RG, Strobos J, Adkinson NF Jr. Immunogenicity studies of cosmetically administered nonanimal-stabilized hyaluronic acid particles. *Dermatol Surg.* 2007;33(suppl 2):S176–S185.
31. Sutherland IW. Novel and established applications of microbial polysaccharides. *Trends Biotechnol.* 1998;16(1):41–46.
32. Ghersetich I, Lotti T, Campanile G, Grappone C, Dini G. Hyaluronic acid in cutaneous intrinsic aging. *Int J Dermatol.* 1994;33(2):119–122.
33. Wang F, Garza LA, Kang S, et al. In vivo stimulation of de novo collagen production caused by cross-linked hyaluronic acid dermal filler injections in photodamaged human skin. *Arch Dermatol.* 2007;143(2):155–163.
34. Redbord KP, Busso M, Hanke CW. Soft-tissue augmentation with hyaluronic acid and calcium hydroxyl apatite fillers. *Dermatol Ther.* 2011;24(1):71–81.
35. Skeie L, Bugge H, Negaard A, Bergersen BM. Large particle hyaluronic acid for the treatment of facial lipoatrophy in HIV-positive patients: 3-year follow-up study. *HIV Med.* 2010;11(3):170–177.
36. Gooderham M, Solish N. Use of hyaluronic acid for soft tissue augmentation of HIV-associated facial lipodystrophy. *Dermatol Surg.* 2005;31(1):104–108.
37. Kuhne U, Imhof M. Treatment of the ageing hand with dermal fillers. *J Cutan Aesthet Surg.* 2012;5(3):163–169.
38. Epstein RE, Spencer JM. Correction of atrophic scars with artefill: an open-label pilot study. *J Drugs Dermatol.* 2010;9(9):1062–1064.
39. Beer KR. Nasal reconstruction using 20 mg/ml cross-linked hyaluronic acid. *J Drugs Dermatol.* 2006;5(5):465–466.
40. Bray D, Hopkins C, Roberts DN. Injection rhinoplasty: non-surgical nasal augmentation and correction of post-rhinoplasty contour asymmetries with hyaluronic acid: how we do it. *Clin Otolaryngol.* 2010;35(3):227–230.
41. Humphrey CD, Arkins JP, Dayan SH. Soft tissue fillers in the nose. *Aesthet Surg J.* 2009;29(6):477–484.
42. Tanaka Y, Matsuo K, Yuzuriha S. Westernization of the asian nose by augmentation of the retropositioned anterior nasal spine with an injectable filler. *Eplasty.* 2011;11:e7.
43. Cohen JL. Understanding, avoiding, and managing dermal filler complications. *Dermatol Surg.* 2008;34(suppl 1):S92–S99.
44. Valiyaparambil J, Rengasamy K, Mallya SM. An unusual soft tissue radiopacity–radiographic appearance of a dermal filler. *Br Dent J.* 2009;207(5):211–212.
45. Busso M, Applebaum D. Hand augmentation with Radiesse (Calcium hydroxylapatite). *Dermatol Ther.* 2007;20(6):385–387.
46. Goldberg DJ, Amin S, Hussain M. Acne scar correction using calcium hydroxylapatite in a carrier-based gel. *J Cosmet Laser Ther.* 2006;8(3):134–136.
47. Siclovan HR, Jomah JA. Injectable calcium hydroxylapatite for correction of nasal bridge deformities. *Aesthetic Plast Surg.* 2009;33(4):544–548.

48. Becker H. Nasal augmentation with calcium hydroxylapatite in a carrier-based gel. *Plast Reconstr Surg.* 2008;121(6):2142–2147.
49. Sadick NS, Katz BE, Roy D. A multicenter, 47-month study of safety and efficacy of calcium hydroxylapatite for soft tissue augmentation of nasolabial folds and other areas of the face. *Dermatol Surg.* 2007;33(suppl 2):S122–S126; discussion S126–S127.
50. Requena L, Requena C, Christensen L, Zimmermann US, Kutzner H, Cerroni L. Adverse reactions to injectable soft tissue fillers. *J Am Acad Dermatol.* 2011;64(1):1–34; quiz 35–36.
51. Duffy DM. Complications of fillers: overview. *Dermatol Surg.* 2005;31(11 Pt 2):1626–1633.
52. Jones DH. Semipermanent and permanent injectable fillers. *Dermatol Clin.* 2009;27(4):433–444, vi.
53. Coleman KM, Voigts R, DeVore DP, Termin P, Coleman WP 3rd. Neocollagenesis after injection of calcium hydroxylapatite composition in a canine model. *Dermatol Surg.* 2008; 34(suppl 1):S53–S55.
54. Goldman MP. Cosmetic use of poly-L-lactic acid: my technique for success and minimizing complications. *Dermatol Surg.* 2011;37(5):688–693.
55. Rendon MI, Cardona LM, Pinzon-Plazas M. Treatment of the aged hand with injectable poly-l-lactic acid. *J Cosmet Laser Ther.* 2010;12(6):284–287.
56. Mazzuco R Hexsel D. Poly-L-lactic acid for neck and chest rejuvenation. *Dermatol Surg.* 2009;35(8):1228–1237.
57. Peterson JD, Goldman MP. Rejuvenation of the aging chest: a review and our experience. *Dermatol Surg.* 2011;37(5): 555–571.
58. Butterwick K, Lowe NJ. Injectable poly-L-lactic acid for cosmetic enhancement: learning from the European experience. *J Am Acad Dermatol.* 2009;61(2):281–293.
59. Sadick NS, Palmisano L. Case study involving use of injectable poly-L-lactic acid (PLLA) for acne scars. *J Dermatolog Treat.* 2009;20(5):302–307.
60. Apikian M, Roberts S, Goodman GJ. Adverse reactions to polylactic acid injections in the periorbital area. *J Cosmet Dermatol.* 2007;6(2):95–101.
61. Stewart DB, Morganroth GS, Mooney MA, Cohen J, Levin PS, Gladstone HB. Management of visible granulomas following periorbital injection of poly-L-lactic Acid. *Ophthal Plast Reconstr Surg.* 2007;23(4):298–301.
62. Hamilton DG, Gauthier N, Robertson BF. Late-onset, recurrent facial nodules associated with injection of poly-L-lactic acid. *Dermatol Surg.* 2008;34(1):123–126; discussion 126.
63. Palm MD, Woodhall KE, Butterwick KJ, Goldman MP. Cosmetic use of poly-l-lactic acid: a retrospective study of 130 patients. *Dermatol Surg.* 2010;36(2):161–170.
64. Gogolewski S, Jovanovic M, Perren SM, Dillon JG, Hughes MK. Tissue response and in vivo degradation of selected polyhydroxyacids: polylactides (PLA), poly(3-hydroxybutyrate) (PHB), and poly(3-hydroxybutyrate-co-3-hydroxyvalerate) (PHB/VA). *J Biomed Mater Res.* 1993; 27(9):1135–1148.
65. Bentkover SH. The biology of facial fillers. *Facial Plast Surg.* 2009;25(2):73–85.
66. Lemperle G, Knapp TR, Sadick NS, Lemperle SM. ArteFill permanent injectable for soft tissue augmentation: i. Mechanism of action and injection techniques. *Aesthetic Plast Surg.* 2010;34(3):264–272.
67. Hilinski JM, Cohen SR. Soft tissue augmentation with ArteFill. *Facial Plast Surg.* 2009;25(2):114–119.
68. Cohen SR, Berner CF, Busso M, et al. ArteFill: a long-lasting injectable wrinkle filler material–summary of the U.S. Food and Drug Administration trials and a progress report on 4- to 5-year outcomes. *Plast Reconstr Surg.* 2006;118(3 suppl):64S–76S.
69. Lemperle G, Ott H, Charrier U, Hecker J, Lemperle M. PMMA microspheres for intradermal implantation: part I. Animal research. *Ann Plast Surg.* 1991;26(1):57–63.
70. Lemperle G, Morhenn V, Charrier U. Human histology and persistence of various injectable filler substances for soft tissue augmentation. *Aesthetic Plast Surg.* 2003;27(5):354–366; discussion 367.
71. Grunebaum LD, Bogdan Allemann I, Dayan S, Mandy S, Baumann L. The risk of alar necrosis associated with dermal filler injection. *Dermatol Surg.* 2009;35(suppl 2): 1635–1640.
72. Shumrick KA, Smith TL. The anatomic basis for the design of forehead flaps in nasal reconstruction. *Arch Otolaryngol Head Neck Surg.* 1992;118(4):373–379.
73. Glaich AS, Cohen JL, Goldberg LH. Injection necrosis of the glabella: protocol for prevention and treatment after use of dermal fillers. *Dermatol Surg.* 2006;32(2):276–281.
74. Alster TS, Williams CM. Treatment of keloid sternotomy scars with 585 nm flashlamp-pumped pulsed-dye laser. *Lancet.* 1995;345(8959):1198–1200.
75. Alster TS, McMeekin TO. Improvement of facial acne scars by the 585 nm flashlamp-pumped pulsed dye laser. *J Am Acad Dermatol.* 1996;35(1):79–81.
76. Nouri K, Elsaie ML, Vejjabhinanta V, et al. Comparison of the effects of short- and long-pulse durations when using a 585-nm pulsed dye laser in the treatment of new surgical scars. *Lasers Med Sci.* 2010;25(1):121–126.
77. Hsu TS, Zelickson B, Dover JS, et al. Multicenter study of the safety and efficacy of a 585 nm pulsed-dye laser for the nonablative treatment of facial rhytides. *Dermatol Surg.* 2005;31(1):1–9.
78. Moody BR, McCarthy JE, Hruza GJ. Collagen remodeling after 585-nm pulsed dye laser irradiation: an ultrasonographic analysis. *Dermatol Surg.* 2003;29(10):997–999; discussion 999–1000.
79. Zelickson BD, Kilmer SL, Bernstein E, et al. Pulsed dye laser therapy for sun damaged skin. *Lasers Surg Med.* 1999;25(3):229–236.
80. Eremia S, Li CY. Treatment of face veins with a cryogen spray variable pulse width 1064 nm Nd:YAG Laser: a prospective study of 17 patients. *Dermatol Surg.* 2002;28(3):244–247.
81. Bekhor PS. Long-pulsed Nd:YAG laser treatment of venous lakes: report of a series of 34 cases. *Dermatol Surg.* 2006;32(9):1151–1154.
82. Groot D, Rao J, Johnston P, Nakatsui T. Algorithm for using a long-pulsed Nd:YAG laser in the treatment of deep cutaneous vascular lesions. *Dermatol Surg.* 2003;29(1):35–42.
83. Henderson BW, Dougherty TJ. How does photodynamic therapy work? *Photochem Photobiol.* 1992;55(1):145–157.
84. Goldberg DJ. Photodynamic therapy in skin rejuvenation. *Clin Dermatol.* 2008;26(6):608–613.
85. Uebelhoer NS, Dover JS. Photodynamic therapy for cosmetic applications. *Dermatol Ther.* 2005;18(3):242–252.
86. Anderson RR, Parish JA. In: Fitzpatrick RE, Goldman MP, eds. *Cosmetic Laser Surgery*. St. Louis, MO: Mosby; 2000.
87. Goldberg D, Tan M, Dale Sarradet M, Gordon M. Nonablative dermal remodeling with a 585-nm, 350-microsec, flashlamp pulsed dye laser: clinical and ultrastructural analysis. *Dermatol Surg.* 2003;29(2):161–163; discussion 163–164.
88. Manstein D, Herron GS, Sink RK, Tanner H, Anderson RR. Fractional photothermolysis: a new concept for cutaneous remodeling using microscopic patterns of thermal injury. *Lasers Surg Med.* 2004;34(5):426–438.
89. Tierney EP, Hanke CW. Review of the literature: treatment of dyspigmentation with fractionated resurfacing. *Dermatol Surg.* 2010;36(10):1499–1508.
90. Sherling M, Friedman PM, Adrian R, et al. Consensus recommendations on the use of an erbium-doped 1,550-nm fractionated laser and its applications in dermatologic laser surgery. *Dermatol Surg.* 2010;36(4):461–419.
91. Hantash BM, Bedi VP, Sudireddy V, Struck SK, Herron GS, Chan KF. Laser-induced transepidermal elimination of dermal content by fractional photothermolysis. *J Biomed Opt.* 2006;11(4):041115.
92. Wanner M, Tanzi EL, Alster TS, Fractional photothermolysis: treatment of facial and nonfacial cutaneous photodamage with a 1,550-nm erbium-doped fiber laser. *Dermatol Surg.* 2007;33(1):23–28.
93. Alster TS, Tanzi EL, Lazarus M. The use of fractional laser photothermolysis for the treatment of atrophic scars. *Dermatol Surg.* 2007;33(3):295–399.

94. Fitzpatrick RE, Goldman MP, Satur NM, Tope WD. Pulsed carbon dioxide laser resurfacing of photo-aged facial skin. *Arch Dermatol.* 1996;132(4):395–402.
95. Grover R, Grobbelaar AO, Morgan BD, Gault DT. A quantitative method for the assessment of facial rejuvenation: a prospective study investigating the carbon dioxide laser. *Br J Plast Surg.* 1998;51(1):8–13.
96. Alster TS, West TB. Resurfacing of atrophic facial acne scars with a high-energy, pulsed carbon dioxide laser. *Dermatol Surg.* 1996;22(2):151–154; discussion 154–155.
97. Apfelberg DB. A critical appraisal of high-energy pulsed carbon dioxide laser facial resurfacing for acne scars. *Ann Plast Surg.* 1997;38(2):95–100.
98. Miller LD. The erbium laser gains a role in cosmetic surgery. *Biophoton Int* 1997;38–43.
99. Tierney EP, Hanke CW. Fractionated carbon dioxide laser treatment of photoaging: prospective study in 45 patients and review of the literature. *Dermatol Surg.* 2011;37(9):1279–1290.
100. Tierney EP, Hanke CW, Petersen J. Ablative fractionated CO_2 laser treatment of photoaging: a clinical and histologic study. *Dermatol Surg.* 2012;38(11):1777–1789.
101. Trelles MA, Mordon S, Velez M, Urdiales F, Levy JL. Results of fractional ablative facial skin resurfacing with the erbium:yttrium-aluminium-garnet laser 1 week and 2 months after one single treatment in 30 patients. *Lasers Med Sci.* 2009;24(2):186–194.

CHAPTER 56

Hand Rejuvenation

Nils Krueger & Neil S. Sadick

INTRODUCTION

The hand is the most visible unclothed body part, besides the face and neck, and is, therefore, of major aesthetic importance. Because of its form and function, the hand has become a symbol of beauty and is widely accepted as an indicator of character.[1] However, it is also a visual marker of age that is difficult to conceal. Like every part of the body, the hands are subject to the intrinsic aging process.[2] In addition, they are constantly exposed to extrinsic environmental factors such as UV radiation; climatic influences; and the stress of intense, continuous use. These factors together can accelerate the aging process, resulting in premature aging of the hands. Together with the face, the hands are often the part of the body where aging is most visible.

Hand aging has to be understood as a three-dimensional (3D) process that involves bones, vessels, and skin. With aging, the wrinkling pattern of the skin increases and gives hands a wrinkly, often leather-like appearance. Dermal changes, muscle atrophy and loss of subcutaneous fat together result in pronounced dorsal veins that present as a bluish color through the skin. Age spots emerge on the back of the hand, due to the lifetime accumulation of UV radiation, and give the hands a mottled and uneven appearance. Dermal atrophy and volume loss result in a more visible skeleton, commonly mistaken as significant joint thickening of the proximal interphalangeal joints.[3]

Considering the different factors of hand aging, a multidimensional approach that addresses all issues is necessary for successful treatment. This 3D rejuvenation approach must include the treatment of skin laxity and prominent veins, augmentation of volume loss, and removal of discolorations. A combination approach utilizing multiple modalities is often beneficial and yields optimal treatment results.

TREATMENT OF HAND VEINS

Large veins with diameters from 1 to 6 mm on the dorsal aspect of the hands often become more prominent with aging and are a common source of patient dissatisfaction. This phenomenon is only partially due to intrinsic changes in the veins themselves. With age, they may become enlarged and tortuous, but of equal importance is volume loss within the surrounding tissue. Volume loss is a result of muscle atrophy, bone demineralization, and loss of adipose tissue.[3] Consequently, vessels protrude to an increasing extent on the backs of the hands, and their bluish color is visible through the skin, giving the hands a fragile and unsightly appearance.

Dorsal hand veins represent the equivalent of varicose veins of the lower extremities.[3] Thus, the same treatment options are available as for leg veins, including sclerotherapy with or without foam, endovenous laser therapy for hands (EVLH), and ambulatory phlebectomy. However, the treatment of hand veins for cosmetic reasons remains controversial as the vessels are necessary to provide intravenous access should medical emergencies occur.[4] Furthermore, complications can result in motor deficits with a significant influence on a patient's life.

The choice of the right sclerosant depends primarily on the vein diameter. Thin-walled veins with a diameter <2 mm are best treated with 0.5% polidocanol solution, 0.25% to 0.5% polidocanol foam, or 0.25% sodium tetradecyl sulfate (STS) solution or foam. By contrast, thick-walled veins with a diameter of 2 to 5 mm should be treated with 1% polidocanol foam or 0.5% to 1% STS foam. An important association exists between high concentrations of sclerosant and the development of extensive, uncomfortable thromboses extending beyond the desired treatment area. Contraindications to sclerotherapy (Table 56-1) should be strictly observed and patients should be adequately informed about the risks of the procedure (Table 56-2) prior to treatment. The hand receiving treatment should be positioned below the table to facilitate vein distention and clenched to a fist to stretch the skin and stabilize the veins. An elevated position of the hand is recommended after the cannulation to facilitate slow injection. The vein should always be filled to the dorsum of the wrist, while the vessel is manually occluded at the wrist to minimize thrombosis (Fig. 56-1). After withdrawing the needle, the treated areas should be gently massaged in a cephalad or proximal direction before release of the occlusion. Cotton swabs or foam pads should be applied over the treatment site and an elastic bandage should be placed over these to wrap the treated hand. Patients must be instructed to carefully monitor changes in sensation, temperature, and color and to be attentive to

TABLE 56-1
Contraindications for Hand Sclerotherapy

Abnormal venous distribution on the hands
Foreseeable need for future intravenous access at treatment sites
Carpal tunnel syndrome
Radical mastectomy
Presence of dialysis shunts
Chronic hand pain, weakness, edema, severe arthritis, or functional abnormalities

TABLE 56-2
Risks of Hand Sclerotherapy

Always	Loss of intravenous access sites
Often	Intravascular thrombi Dysesthesia, paresthesia, pain
Rare	Postoperative (permanent) vascular matting Motor deficits
Never	Postoperative pigmentation

decreased motion of the fingers and to loosen the bandage if necessary.

The minimally invasive EVLH utilizes laser technology to archive nonthrombotic vein occlusion through placement of a small laser fiber within the vessel. The laser generates heat and induces the formation of steam bubbles at the tip of the laser fiber. These bubbles cause thermal damage to endothelial cells of the inner vein wall, resulting in occlusion of the lumen with a clot. A variety of wavelengths are available for this approach, as several chromophores are targeted. These include 810, 940, and 980 nm for hemoglobin, and 1319, 1320, and 1470 nm for both water and collagen. The diminishment of the vein is proportional to the delivered linear endovenous energy density (LEED), which depends on the output of the laser and the pullback speed of the catheter. A range of 60 to 80 J/cm was found to be safe and to produce a successful ablation.[5] The advantages of EVLH are its efficacy with a single treatment, reduced bruising, and high patient satisfaction. Disadvantages include the difficulty of treating multiple veins at once, the risk of skin injury (burn), high cost, the need for local anesthesia, the potential for long recovery times and the need for veins to be relatively straight. The EVLH treatment protocol includes outlining of the vessel in a lowered position, placement of a topical anesthetic such as benzocaine, lidocaine or tetracaine, microincision (24G 0.75 in needle) and insertion of an angiocatheter as well as tumescent anesthesia using 12.5 cc 1% lidocaine mixed in 250 cc lactated Ringer's solution. The laser fiber should be advanced to the lateral aspect of the treatment area and slowly but steadily withdrawn at a defined speed depending on the output of the laser. The treatment should cease as the distal tip of the sheath approaches the puncture site. This will keep the tip of the laser fiber within the vein and prevent thermal injury to the subcutaneous tissues or skin.[6] EVLH is a relatively simple office procedure that is effective in reducing large, dark, tortuous dorsal hand veins. The procedure ensures high patient and physician satisfaction and has low complication rates without long-term adverse sequelae.[7]

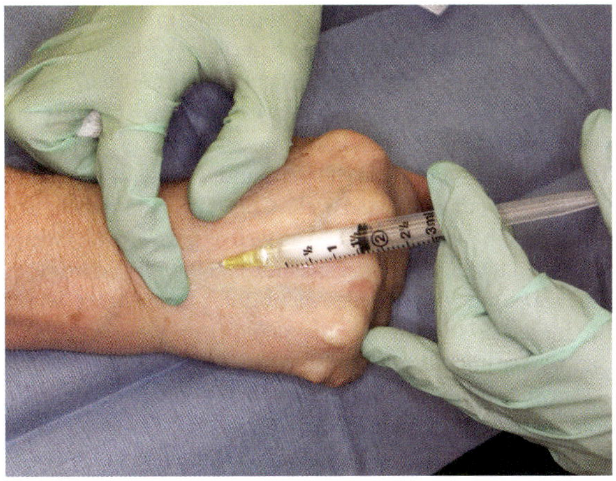

Figure 56-1 Filling of the vein with sclerosant, while the vessel is manually occluded with the index finger.

VOLUME AUGMENTATION

Several suitable filler materials are available for the augmentation of lost volume in the hands, including poly-L-lactic acid (PLLA), calcium hydroxyapatite (CaHA), autologous fat (AF), and hyaluronic acid (HA). The injection of the material can be completed with either a single bolus approach or with multiple microbolus injections. With both approaches, the filler material can be mixed with 1% lidocaine prior to injection to reduce injection pain. An intensive massage of at least 5 minutes is necessary to spread the material evenly throughout the tissue. For the injection itself, it is advisable to use blunt cannulas instead of sharp needles to minimize bleeding, reduce pain, and lower the risk of nerve injuries. After placement of a lidocaine bleb, an 18G needle is used to create an entry point in the skin, where the 27G cannula is inserted after the needle is removed (Fig. 56-2).

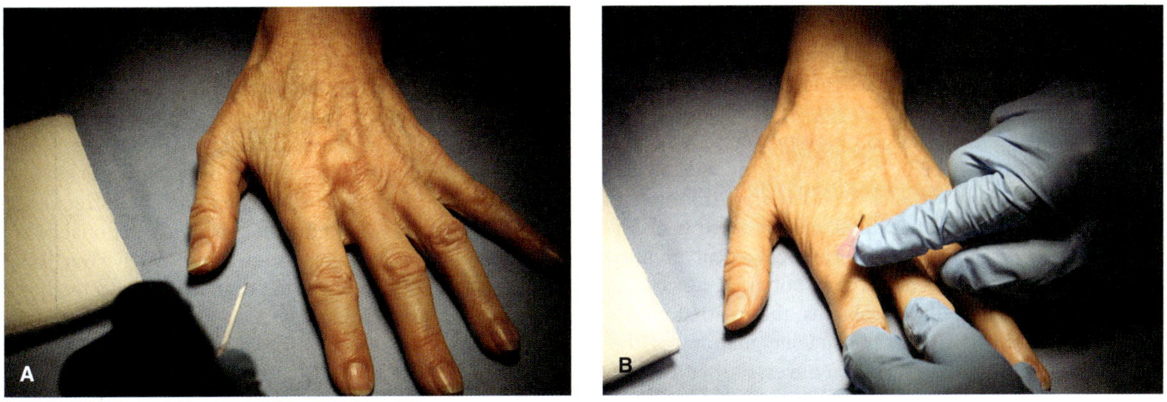

Figure 56-2 **A.** Lidocaine bleb. **B.** Creation of an entry point in the skin with 18G needle.

When using PLLA for hand augmentation, 2 to 3 treatment sessions 4 weeks apart are necessary for an optimal treatment result that lasts upward of 24 months.[8,9] Each vial of PLLA should be diluted in 7 to 10 mL bacteriostatic water mixed with 2 mL lidocaine 24 hours prior to use. The average usage is one vial per hand. A large central bleb is injected and massaged well. Common side effects are bruising and swelling (30.8%) as well as pain (15.4%) while itching (3.8%) and arterial spasm (3.8%) are less common. The appearance of papules or nodules is very rare when the material is vigorously massaged from wrist to tips of digits after injection.[8]

Another semipermanent filler that is particularly suitable for hand augmentation is CaHA.[10,11] The filler consists of CaHA microspheres with a diameter of 25 to 45 μm dispersed in a carboxymethyl cellulose carrier gel. While the carrier gel gradually absorbs and degrades within weeks, the calcium microspheres stay in the dermis for several months to years and induce a local fibroblastic response resulting in fibrous encapsulation.[12] Before injecting CaHA into the hands, the 1.3 mL vial has to be reconstituted with 0.5 mL of lidocaine 2%. Therefore, the syringe is attached via a Luer-Lok to Luer-Lok connector to a 3 mL Luer-Lok syringe containing the lidocaine.[11] After admixing back and forth 10 times, the completely smooth airless CaHA–lidocaine mixture can be injected using a needle or cannula.[13] After the injection, the area must be firmly massaged with the patient's hand in a fist, to disperse the filler. Adverse events including ecchymosis, erythema, and occasional edema are rare and resolve within 2 weeks, when CaHA is injected and massaged properly. Improvement in treated sites can be seen for up to 12 months after treatment.[14]

A natural filler that can be used for volume augmentation of the hands is AF. It has the benefit of not eliciting any antigenicity. However, its placement requires a two-stage procedure and this material has unpredictable longevity.[15] AF may be injected using a 1 mm cannula or a 20G needle through the web spaces of each digit and creasing over the ulnar and radial heads at the wrist. It is important to stay in the superficial plane over the joints.

Another popular choice for the treatment of volume loss in the hands is HA fillers. HA is a naturally occurring glycosaminoglycan with an elastic and viscous matrix. HA fillers have an overall low immunogenic profile and reactions are extremely rare.[16] The differences between the various HA fillers include the amount of molecular cross-linking, gel consistency properties and HA concentration. In general, HA fillers with a higher level of cross-linking or a greater particle size have a higher lifting power and longevity and are, therefore, particularly suitable for hand augmentation.[17]

Most problems that can occur when augmenting lost volume of the hands are independent of the filler material used. These problems include discomfort from injection, nodules secondary to thin skin, increased bruising secondary to dorsal veins, long-term mechanical mobility issues, persistent hand edema, and potential functional aberrations. To avoid these problems, the treating physician must be well versed in the specific anatomy of the hand including the complex system of vessels, nerves, and tendons, and must be appropriately cautious when performing these procedures.

TREATMENT OF DISCOLORATIONS

Discolorations on the dorsal surfaces of the hands are another main complaint of aesthetic hand patients, besides prominent veins and volume loss. Next to the face, the hands are the area of the body with the highest exposure to sun. While the daily use of sun protection for the face is widely accepted, the hands are still not always covered consistently, resulting in an increased risk for solar lentigo and discolorations in general.

Unlike the fluctuant absorption curves of blood or water, the melanin absorption curve decreases gradually from 400 to 1200 nm[18] allowing a wide range of lasers and light sources to be effective for the treatment of discolorations. Devices with wavelengths between 600 nm and 1300 nm seem to be ideal for the targeting of melanin, as the absorption of hemoglobin and water is low in this range. Accordingly, Q-switched Nd:YAG (532/1064 nm), ruby (694 nm) and alexandrite (755 nm) lasers along with intense pulsed light (IPL) (500–1200 nm) are the most commonly used light sources for the treatment of hand pigmentation. However, recent studies show that fractional erbium diode fiber laser of 1550 nm[19] as well as ablative, fractional CO_2 laser of 10,600 nm[20] can also be effective and safe for the removal of discoloration on the hands.

In preparation for a laser procedure for pigmented lesions, the use of isotretinoin should be avoided for 6 months, as prolonged healing and scarring has been reported when isotretinoin was used concomitant with laser treatment.[21,22] Patients should further be advised to avoid sun exposure for at least 1 week before and after the laser treatment. The careful use of broad-spectrum sunscreen or covering gloves is recommended for up to 4 weeks after treatment. For best results, 3 to 5 treatments are indicated. In some cases, complete clearance is not possible.

THREE-DIMENSIONAL APPROACH TO HAND REJUVENATION

Because of the multidimensional aging process of the hands that involves bones, vessels, and the skin, a 3D approach to hand rejuvenation is advised for optimal results and high patient satisfaction. This approach must be based on the three types of aging, which appear on the hands. Type I, which includes solar lentigines, prominent vascular lesions and vessels, skin roughness and rhytides, can be targeted with a combination of Q-switched lasers or fractional lasers, IPL, endovenous laser treatment for the hands (EVLH), and sclerotherapy with polidocanol or STS. Type II aging is characterized by redundant skin and skin laxity and can best be targeted with radiofrequency and broadband IPL as well as nonablative fractional lasers (1550 nm) and second-generation microablative fractional lasers (1927 nm). Finally, aging type III includes the bony appearance and prominent veins of the hands due to volume loss. Suitable fillers for the augmentation of the hands are HA, CaHA, PLLA or AF. The individual anatomic conditions as well as the patient's concerns should be considered when choosing the right filler material.

The thin epidermis of the skin of the hands requires cautious and conservative ablative resurfacing. Resurfacing of the dorsal aspect of the hands can been performed with fractional CO_2 lasers with a penetration depth of 50 to 100 µm. Typically a single pass of 150 to 200 mJ/pulse can be used. Otherwise an erbium:YAG laser with a more superficial ablation depth of 5 to 20 µm has been proven to be efficacious for hand resurfacing.

IPL utilizes polychromatic light between 515 and 1200 nm for achieving photorejuvenation and dermal heating resulting in collagen stimulation. Although no studies have been conducted to show this on nonfacial skin, this effect can lead to improvement in skin texture, rhytides, and pore size.

Radiofrequency devices designed specifically for skin tightening have been recently used for the treatment of facial as well as total body skin laxity. The electrical current emitted by the devices generates a diathermic effect which results in immediate collagen denaturation leading to remodeling as well as long-term collagen stimulation by fibroblasts. The authors advise practitioners to begin with low settings and gradually increase depending on patient tolerance. Several treatments are often necessary for optimal patient satisfaction.

CONCLUSION

The hands are the most visible, unclothed body part, besides the face and neck, and, therefore, of major aesthetic importance. As they are difficult to conceal, they are also a visual marker of age and, therefore, a main concern of many patients in aesthetic dermatology. Over the last few decades, several procedures have been found to be effective and safe for the treatment of aging hands. Nevertheless, the treatment remains a challenge due to the specific anatomy of this region. The understanding and matching of patient concerns with treatment plans must be the highest priority for the treating physician to yield optimal patient satisfaction. A 3D approach utilizing multiple modalities to target the different types of hand aging is often beneficial and therefore highly recommended.

REFERENCES

1. Jakubietz RG, Jakubietz MG, Kloss D, Gruenert JG. Defining the basic aesthetics of the hand. *Aesthetic Plast Surg.* 2005;29(6):546–551.
2. Jenkins G. Molecular mechanisms of skin ageing. *Mech Ageing Dev.* 2002;123(7):801–810.
3. Duffy DM, Garcia C, Clark RE. The role of sclerotherapy in abnormal varicose hand veins. *Plast Reconstr Surg.* 1999;104(5):1474–1479; discussion 1480–1481.
4. Park U-J, Do Y-S, Park K-B, et al. Treatment of arteriovenous malformations involving the hand. *Ann Vasc Surg.* 2012;26(5):643–648.
5. Johnson CM, McLafferty RB. Endovenous laser ablation of varicose veins: review of current technologies and clinical outcome. *Vascular.* 2007;15(5):250–254.
6. Ash JL, Moore CJ. Laser treatment of varicose veins: order out of chaos. *Semin Vasc Surg.* 2010;23(2):101–106.
7. Shamma AR, Guy RJ. Laser ablation of unwanted hand veins. *Plast Reconstr Surg.* 2007;120(7):2017–2024.
8. Sadick NS, Anderson D, Werschler WP. Addressing volume loss in hand rejuvenation: a report of clinical experience. *J Cosmet Laser Ther.* 2008;10(4):237–241.
9. Lowe NJ, Maxwell CA, Lowe P, Shah A, Patnaik R. Injectable poly-l-lactic acid: 3 years of aesthetic experience. *Dermatol Surg.* 2009;35(Suppl 1):344–349.
10. Bank DE. A novel approach to treatment of the aging hand with Radiesse. *J Drugs Dermatol.* 2009;8(12):1122–1126.
11. Edelson KL. Hand recontouring with calcium hydroxylapatite (Radiesse). *J Cosmet Dermatol.* 2009;8(1):44–51.
12. Flaharty P. Radiance. *Facial Plast Surg.* 2004;20(2):165–169.
13. Busso M, Voigts R. An investigation of changes in physical properties of injectable calcium hydroxylapatite in a carrier gel when mixed with lidocaine and with lidocaine/epinephrine. *Dermatol Surg.* 2008;34(Suppl 1):S16–S23; discussion S24.
14. Sadick NS. A 52-week study of safety and efficacy of calcium hydroxylapatite for rejuvenation of the aging hand. *J Drugs Dermatol.* 2011;10(1):47–51.
15. Sommer B, Sattler G. Current concepts of fat graft survival: histology of aspirated adipose tissue and review of the literature. *Dermatol Surg.* 2000;26(12):1159–1166.
16. Kim J-E, Sykes JM. Hyaluronic acid fillers: history and overview. *Facial Plast Surg.* 2011;27(6):523–528.
17. Beasley KL, Weiss MA, Weiss RA. Hyaluronic acid fillers: a comprehensive review. *Facial Plast Surg.* 2009;25(2):86–94.
18. König K. Multiphoton microscopy in life sciences. *J Microsc.* 2000;200(Pt 2):83–104.
19. Sadick NS, Smoller B. A study examining the safety and efficacy of a fractional laser in the treatment of photodamage on the hands. *J Cosmet Laser Ther.* 2009;11(1):29–33.
20. Stebbins WG, Hanke CW. Ablative fractional CO2 resurfacing for photoaging of the hands: pilot study of 10 patients. *Dermatol Ther.* 2011;24(1):62–70.
21. Bernestein LJ, Geronemus RG. Keloid formation with the 585-nm pulsed dye laser during isotretinoin treatment. *Arch Dermatol.* 1997;133(1):111–112.
22. Zachariae H. Delayed wound healing and keloid formation following argon laser treatment or dermabrasion during isotretinoin treatment. *Br J Dermatol.* 1988;118(5):703–706.

CHAPTER 57

Laser Treatment of Asian Skin

Samantha Yee Nam Shek & Henry Hin Lee Chan

INTRODUCTION

Ethnic skin is often classified by the Fitzpatrick Skin Type classification with a scale that ranges from type I (ivory white skin) to type VI (dark brown skin) Table 57-1. Asian skin color is often characterized as types III to V. This reflects the person's complexion and tolerance to sunlight, which is determined by the melanin content and melanosome dispersion. It is well established that there are no racial differences in the number of melanocytes.[1] Melanosomes in keratinocytes of light skin as in Caucasians are distributed as membrane-bound clusters, whereas the melanosomes in keratinocytes of dark skin as in African individuals tend to be distributed individually.[2] A study analyzed the melanosomes extracted from the epidermis in subjects of different skin types from various ethnicities. Epidermal melanin content is significantly greater in chronically photoexposed skin than it is in corresponding photoprotected skin (up to twofold). Analysis of melanosome size revealed a significant and progressive variation in size with ethnicity: African skin having the largest melanosomes followed in turn by Indian, Mexican, Chinese, and European.[3] Skin pigmentation is strongly influenced by both the amount and composition of the melanin in the epidermis. Variation in melanosome size may also play a significant role.

TABLE 57-1
Fitzpatrick Skin Type Classification

Type	Scores	Description
I	0–7	White; very fair; freckles; typical albino skin Always burns, never tans
II	8–16	White; fair Usually burns, tans with difficulty
III	17–24	Beige; very common Sometimes mild burn, gradually tans to a light brown
IV	25–30	Beige with a brown tint; typical Mediterranean Caucasian skin Rarely burns, tans with ease to a moderate brown
V	>30	Dark brown Very rarely burns, tans very easily
VI		Black Never burns, tans very easily, deeply pigmented

The function of melanin in the skin is to absorb and scatter rays of ultraviolet (UV) light. The larger, individually dispersed melanosomes have a higher melanin content and are able to absorb more UV light energy than the aggregated, smaller melanosomes with less melanin content found in fair-skinned white subjects.[4] This means that the degree of protection corresponds to the degree of pigmentation. This sun protection offers significant prevention of photoaging, which is the cosmetic advantage of skin types IV to VI. The downside is that skin of color has a tendency to develop hyperpigmentation or hypopigmentation. Indeed, pigment disorders are one of the most frequent concerns in skin types IV to VI.[5] Although melanin protects skin from UV radiation, all skin types with prolonged sun exposure develop clinical abnormalities, consisting of textural changes and hyperpigmentation.[6]

Each culture has different standards of what it considers to be beautiful. Therefore, a clear understanding and awareness of the patient's perception of beauty is essential. In Asian culture, flawless fair skin free of scars and pigment is thought to be ideal as opposed to a tanned healthy complexion amongst Americans. These differences would influence the choice of procedures offered to patients. For example, Asian patients may be unhappy with the outcome of phototherapy if tanning results. The patient's skin color is an important factor to consider when determining which procedures would be most appropriate or assessing the risk involved with treatments. Anything that has a potential to cause skin irritation or erythema can lead to pigment alterations in ethnic skin.

Knowing where the patient is situated on the Fitzpatrick skin type classification scale helps the physician to assess which procedures are most suitable for that skin type. For example, those with Fitzpatrick skin types I to II would have more difficulty undergoing intense pulsed light (IPL) for laser hair removal because the melanin cells at the hair shafts may not absorb sufficient light energy to be destroyed. Those with darker skin types have a higher chance of developing hyperpigmentation from procedures such as laser, IPL, or chemical peel. Thus, the types of lasers and the parameters used must be different in Asian skin from those used on fair skin. In this chapter, we aim to focus on laser treatments for pigmentary conditions and nonablative skin rejuvenation in Asian skin.

CLINICAL EXAMINATION AND PATIENT HISTORY

The correct clinical diagnosis is the first and vital step before initiating any treatment. The patient's concerns and expectations should be addressed. As mentioned previously, the patient's cultural background should be taken into consideration. A detailed patient history is important, followed by careful physical examination. The use of oral retinoids within the previous 6 months can increase the risk of scarring from light source treatment. Anyone with infection, recent sun exposure to the treatment site, photosensitivity, a tendency to develop keloids or scarring, immunocompromise, pregnancy, and a personal or family history of melanoma should not undergo treatment with lasers or light sources. Asking whether the patient has a tendency to tan or burn helps to gain an understanding of the patient's skin photoype. A previous history of hyper- or hypopigmentation after minor injuries such as an insect bite or acne may also help the physician to assess the patient's skin phototype. A Wood's light can help the physician to determine the epidermal or dermal components of a pigmented lesion and reveal the presence of subclinical melasma. Photographs should be taken to monitor the condition and assess pre- and posttreatment results.

It is vital for patients to have realistic expectations of what any procedure will and will not do for them. The length of recovery, duration of treatment, possible side effects, and expected outcome should be discussed. The factors to consider when determining which procedure is best for the individual patient include recovery time, risk of side effects, realistic expectations of improvement, and cost.

Patient compliance should be emphasized. The use of daily sun protection throughout the course of treatment (preferably adopting it as a daily habit posttreatment) and avoiding the sun for at least 2 weeks prior to laser treatment should be enforced. This is recommended to reduce the risk of posttreatment dyschromia. Any photosensitizing agents such as tetracycline and oral contraceptives must not be taken. Avoidance of the sun is encouraged for at least 4 weeks postoperatively. Bleaching agents can be administered to prevent the development of postinflammatory hyperpigmentation (PIH).

PIGMENT LASERS

FRECKLES AND SOLAR LENTIGINES

Freckles and solar lentigines are the more frequently encountered pigmentary complaints. Freckles present as multiple small round smooth-surfaced brown patches on sun-exposed areas of the face, neck, and forearms. They tend to darken with sun exposure in summer and fade in winter. Freckles tend to run in families and are uniform in their distribution, size, and color whereas lentigines are nonuniformly distributed and tend to vary in size and color.

In a review article looking at the management of freckles and lentigines using four different pigment lasers on Asian skin, there was significant improvement with the use of 595 nm LPDL, 532 nm LP KTP lasers, and 532 nm QS Nd:YAG.[7] Although most patients in these groups showed improvement, the 532 nm QS Nd:YAG was associated with a 10% risk of PIH. The 755 nm LP alexandrite laser has been shown to be effective in Type II skin,[8] but failed to achieve significant results in Asian skin with a risk of PIH of 20%. In contrast, there did not appear to be any risk of PIH in patients treated with 595 nm LPDL and 532 nm LP KTP lasers. This observation is due to the short bursts (nanoseconds) of wavelength-specific energy by QS lasers, which cause destruction of melanin by means of photothermal and photomechanical effects. The photomechanical effect also causes undesirable damage to the surrounding oxyhemoglobin, leading to inflammation of superficial vessels. The epidermal inflammatory response results in the release and oxidation of arachidonic acid to prostaglandins and leukotrienes. These mediators alter the activity of melanocytes and immune cells by stimulating epidermal melanocytes thereby increasing the synthesis of melanin and pigment transfer to surrounding keratinocytes.[9]

Another study by Wang et al.[10] came to the same conclusion, with QS alexandrite laser being associated with greater risk of PIH than IPL for the treatment of freckles and lentigines in Chinese skin. It is now recognized that long pulse lasers and IPL carry a relatively lower risk of PIH when used on ethnic skin (Figs. 57-1 and 57-2). Although IPL can be effective in the removal of lentigines in Asians, the number of treatment sessions (4–6) required means it is less cost-effective compared to laser treatment. The advantage of IPL is that there is minimal downtime. While QS lasers have a higher risk of PIH, they have the advantage of significant clearance after only 1 to 2 sessions (Fig. 57-2). As a result, Chan[11] suggested an approach in the treatment of freckles and lentigines. After discussing the advantages and disadvantages of the various treatment options, the choice ultimately depends on cost-effectiveness, possible complications, and patient expectations. Patients are informed that with the more aggressive QS lasers, the number of treatment sessions is minimal (1–2 sessions) but carries a downtime of 1 week and a PIH risk of 5% to 10%. Alternatively, patients can choose a less aggressive approach using a long-pulsed laser requiring 3 to 4 treatment sessions at 4 to 6 weekly intervals. There is less downtime and the risk of PIH is about 1%.

The following is a step-by-step approach of a typical procedure carried out in our practice after physician consultation and signing an informed consent.

1. Photographic documentation (Canfield System®)
2. Application of topical anesthetic (lidocaine 2.5% and prilocaine 2.5%, EMLA®) under cling-film occlusion to treatment sites for 1 hour
3. Removal of topical anesthetic
4. Protect patient's eyes with a laser eye shield or intraocular laser eye shield
5. Physician and physician assistants should wear wavelength appropriate laser safety glasses or goggles
6. Calibrate the device to the desired parameters
7. Treatment

In our practice, a long-pulsed 532 nm KTP is often used. A typical setting would be 6.5 to 8.0 J/cm^2 without cooling or 12 to 14 J/cm^2 with the cooling sapphire window, 2 mm spot size, and 2 ms pulse duration (8–9 J/cm^2 if a 3 mm spot size is used). The end point would be defined as the lowest fluence that can achieve an ash-gray appearance without purpura (Fig. 57-3).

For the 532 nm QS Nd:YAG laser, the ideal end point would be immediate whitening with the lowest fluence without bleeding. The parameters of 0.6 J/cm^2, 2 mm

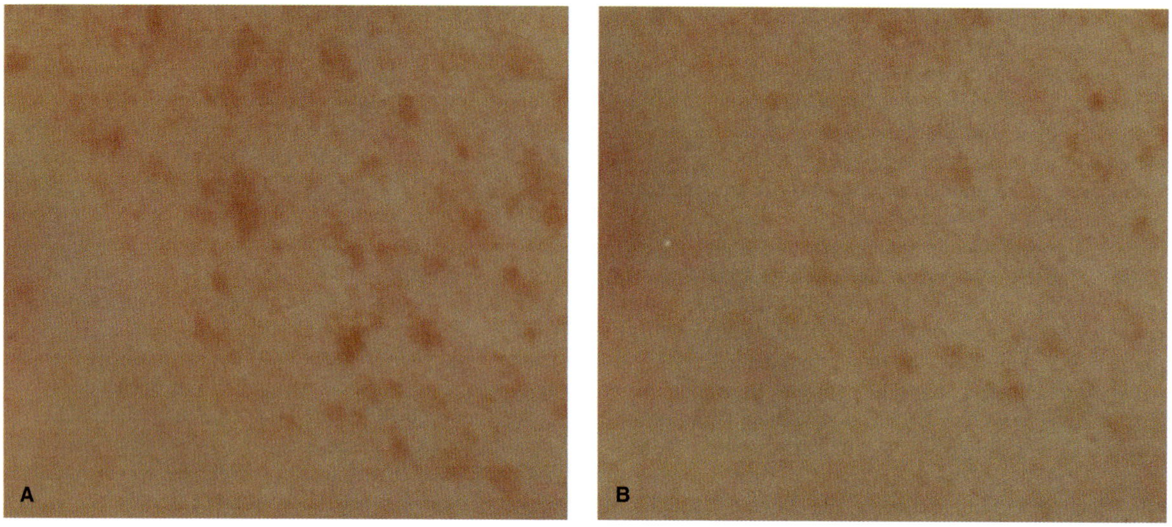

Figure 57-1 A. Baseline lentigines. B. After one treatment with QS alexandrite laser.

spot size, 10 Hz are frequently used. Wet wrap with mometasone ointment 1:4 for 15 minutes after treatment is applied followed by clobetasone butyrate twice daily for up to 3 days. IPL can also be used with a handpiece of 400 to 700 nm or 70 to 1200 nm, used at 40 ms, 0.4 Hz, 18 to 20 J/cm^2. There will be crusting over the irradiated lesions 1 to 2 days after treatment which will resolve within a week. Patients should be advised to avoid direct sunlight. The use of UV protection should always be emphasized as part of their regular skin care regimen. For large handpiece devices, the contrast between lesional and nonlesional skin should be assessed and a small spot size should be used if the contrast is significant. If there is low contrast between the lesional and nonlesional skin, then the operator should use a low fluence with minimal impact. If the above threshold fluence is used, this will lead to excessive injury to the surrounding area.

NEVUS OF OTA

Nevus of Ota was originally described by Ota and Tanino in 1939 and is a hamartoma of dermal melanocytes. Clinically, it appears as blue-black or slate gray macules within the distribution of the opththalmic and maxillary branches of the trigeminal nerve. The nevus can be unilateral or bilateral and may involve ocular and oral mucosa. It affects between 0.014% and 0.034% of the Asian population.[12] Goldberg and Nychay[13] and Geronemus[14] were among the first to report the use of lasers to treat nevus of Ota. QS ruby 694 nm, QS alexandrite 755 nm, and QS 1064 Nd:YAG lasers have all been reported to be effective (Fig. 57-4). Watanabe and Takahashi[15] looked at 114 nevus of Ota patients treated with the QS ruby laser and confirmed excellent improvement after three or more treatment sessions Kono et al.[16] reviewed 101 patients at 12 months post QS ruby treatment and found that 56% of the patients had over 75% clearance with 36% achieving complete clearance Complications observed were hypopigmentation and hyperpigmentation in 17% and 6% of patients, respectively.

Chan et al.[17] compared the use of QS alexandrite and QS 1064 Nd:YAG lasers and found that the QS alexandrite laser was better tolerated. However, the latter was shown to be superior in efficacy after three or more treatment sessions. A recent retrospective review compared the

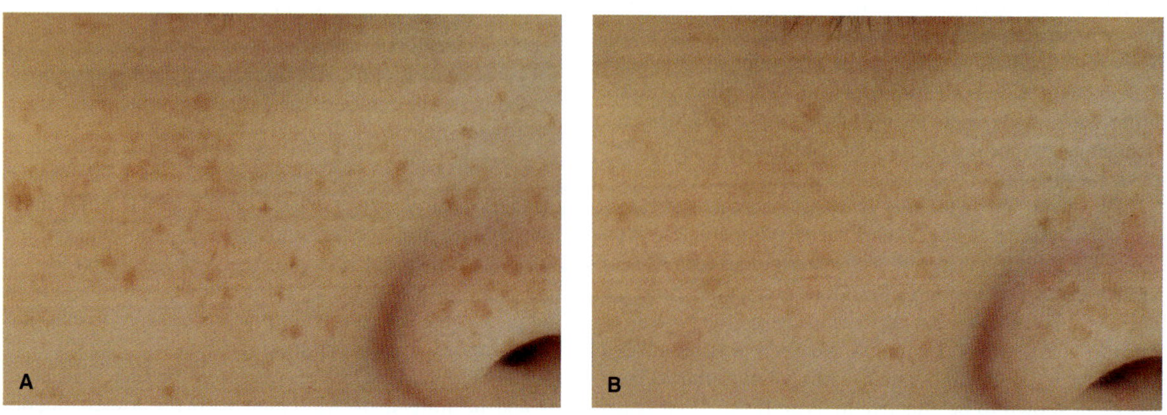

Figure 57-2 A. Baseline ephelides. B. After three treatments with IPL.

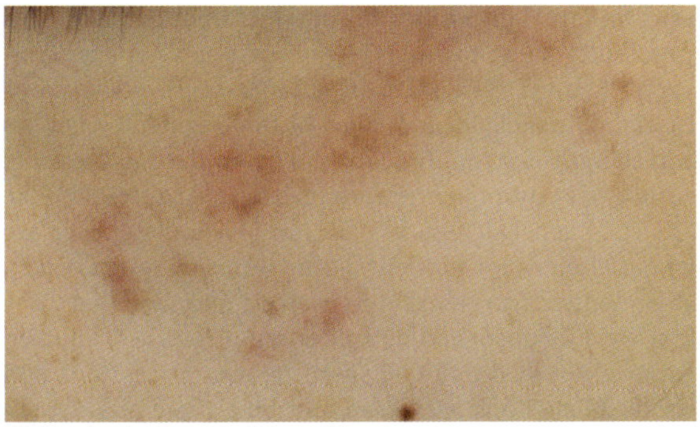

Figure 57-3 Immediately after treatment with 532 nm LP KTP laser for freckles.

effectiveness of QS ruby laser with QS Nd:YAG laser in 94 patients. The group that received treatment with QS ruby laser had statistically significant improvement (p-value of 0.044) in their clearance response compared to the group that received QS Nd:YAG laser treatment.[18]

Another study looked into laser treatment of nevus of Ota in different age groups. The number of treatment sessions required for complete clearance and the degree of complications in children and adults were compared.[19] The treatment of nevus of Ota in children can achieve an excellent result in fewer sessions and at a lower complication rate than laser treatment. However, risk of recurrence is a concern. The risk of such recurrence is estimated to be 0.6% to 1.2%.[20] Therefore, the pros and cons of treating pediatric patients should be addressed during consultation. In our practice, QS ruby laser is most commonly used for treating nevus of Ota. The laser parameters are 694 nm wavelength, 30 ns pulse duration, 4 mm spot size, 5 to 7 J/cm^2 at 3 to 4 month intervals.

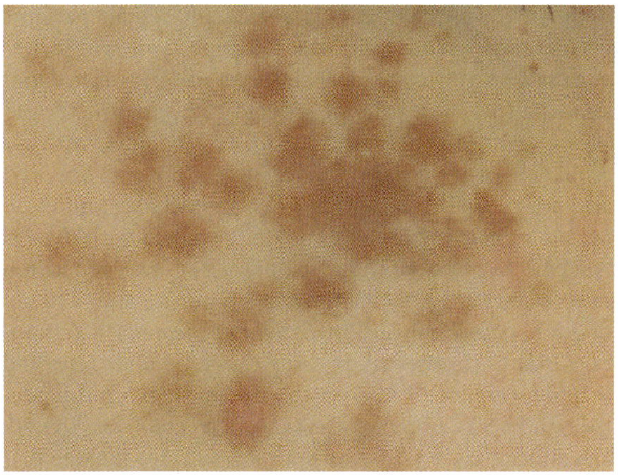

Figure 57-5 Hori's macules.

ACQUIRED BILATERAL NEVUS OF OTA-LIKE MACULES (ABNOM)/ HORI'S MACULES

Acquired bilateral nevus of Ota-like macules (ABNOM), or Hori's macules, is a common dermal hyperpigmentation in Asians that is characterized by bluish macules in the bilateral malar regions (Fig. 57-5). It was first described by Hori in 1984.[21] Unlike nevus of Ota, ABNOM is an acquired condition that often develops after 20 years of age, involves both sides of the face and does not involve the mucosa. QS ruby laser, QS Nd:YAG laser, and QS alexandrite laser have all been shown to be effective for the treatment of Hori's macules. However, transient pigmentary changes are not uncommon after laser treatment.

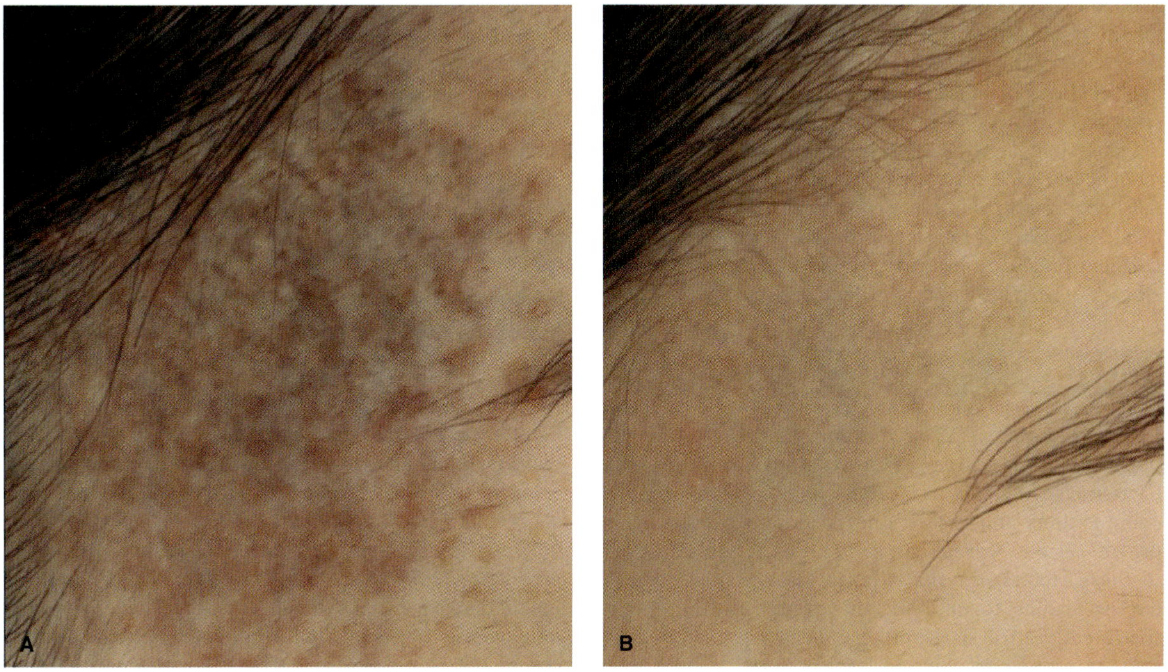

Figure 57-4 **A.** Baseline nevus of Ota. **B.** After fifth treatment with laser.

In 1999, Kunachak et al.[22] treated 140 female patients with Hori's macules with the QS ruby laser with a fluence of 7 to 10 J/cm^2, repetition rate of 1 Hz, and a spot size of 2 to 4 mm, with an average of 2.3 treatment sessions. Over 90% achieved complete clearance with no recurrence after a mean follow-up of 2.5 years. The PIH rate was 7%. The following year, Kunachak studied 68 female subjects with Hori's macules treated with the QS Nd:YAG laser (8–10 J/cm^2, spot size 2–4 mm, repetition rate of 10 Hz). 100% clearance was reported after a mean of 2.8 sessions but 50% of patients experienced temporary PIH.[23] Another study using the same laser reported a 70% incidence of PIH posttreatment.[24] In a retrospective study, 32 Chinese patients were treated with the QS alexandrite laser (755 nm, spot size 3 mm, fluence 8 J/cm^2), and 80% had over 50% clearance, with 28% having complete clearance. 12.5% developed PIH.[25] Two studies looked into combination treatments to improve the efficacy of QS lasers. One study compared the use of CO_2 laser followed by QS ruby laser on one side of the face versus using QS ruby laser alone.[26] Another study published by Ee et al.[27] compared QS 532 Nd:YAG laser followed by QS 1064 nm Nd:YAG laser versus QS 1064 nm Nd:YAG laser alone. Both studies showed that the degree of pigmentary clearance was significantly higher in the combination arm. The mechanism behind the success of combination treatment is the following: By synergistically eliminating epidermal pigmentation, more dermal penetration is achieved, and dermal pigmentation can be more effectively eradicated. As Hori's macules tend to be more resistant to therapy compared to nevus of Ota, our approach is to treat more frequently with repeated laser sessions every 4 weeks. The idea is to treat the area before epithelial repigmentation occurs. Side effects such as postlaser hyperpigmentation and hypopigmentation can be minimized but not eliminated by sun avoidance and the prophylactic use of topical bleaching cream before and after laser treatment. The use of low fluence QS 1064 nm Nd:YAG laser has been advocated for the treatment of Hori's macules as a procedure with decreased down time. Although such an approach can lighten Hori's macules, the large numbers of treatment sessions (>10) make it an impractical option.[28]

Picosecond lasers have recently been used for the treatment of tattoos. If successful, these lasers may have potential impact upon the treatment of dermal pigmentation including nevus of Ota or Hori's macules in the future. Further studies are necessary to examine the safety and efficacy of such devices in skin of color.[29]

TATTOOS

Laser technology has revolutionized the removal of tattoos without scarring. However, not all tattoos can be removed. Tattoos are often composed of multiple compositions and colors, and treatment requires the use of various wavelength modalities.[30,31] In addition to these factors, the ink is located at variable dermal depths leading to unpredictable responses after laser treatment. Tattoo darkening has been reported due to reduction of ferric oxide to ferrous oxide.[32] Test spots can be performed prior to treatment to avoid this complication. It is important for patients to understand this possibility so as to manage their expectations accordingly. The QS 694 nm ruby laser is highly efficacious in removing black and blue tattoo pigments, but its wavelength is strongly absorbed by epidermal melanin, resulting in dyspigmentation in ethnic skin tones.[33] The QS 1064 nm Nd:YAG or 755 nm alexandrite laser are better choices for black and blue tattoo pigments given their longer wavelength, as well as the fact that they are less well absorbed by epidermal melanin.[33,34] Tattoo removal often requires 6 to 10 treatment sessions and up to 20 sessions for green and blue pigments. Green tattoo pigment is particularly difficult to remove, but QS ruby and QS alexandrite can at times be successful. A method called R20 has been described, whereby the tattoo is treated repeatedly with a QS laser for 20 minutes for up to 4 treatment sessions. Studies have indicated its efficacy as compared to a single treatment. However, in our hands, such an approach is associated with increased treatment time as well as a higher risk of pigmentary and texture changes (Fig. 57-6).[35]

A picosecond laser was first reported to be effective for tattoo clearance in a porcine model in 2010.[36] Brauer et al.[35] looked at a series of 10 patients with 12 blue and/or green tattoos that were multicolored or resistant to previous treatment. All treatments were performed with a 755 nm alexandrite laser with variable pulse duration of 750 to 900 picoseconds, repetition rate 5 Hz, spot sizes 3.0 to 3.6 mm, and fluence 2.0 to 2.83 J/cm^2. After a single treatment, 11 of the 12 treated tattoos achieved greater than 75% clearance at 1 months' follow-up, with over two-thirds of those approaching 100% clearance. Postinflammatory pigmentary change was observed in a minority of patients. A prospective study by Saedi et al.[37] reported more than 75% clearance in 12 patients, of whom 9 obtained over 75% clearance after 2 to 4 treatments. The average number of treatment sessions required to obtain this level of clearance was 4.25. Pigmentary changes were also reported in this study. Further studies are necessary to confirm the safety and efficacy of tattoo removal in darker skin types. At our center, the approach to tattoo removal is as follows: The picosecond 755 nm laser is used with a 3 to 4.5 mm spot size, using immediate whitening as an end point. Mometasone ointment is then applied to the lesion under a wet wrap dressing twice a day for 2 to 3 days to reduce excessive swelling and blister formation.

MELASMA

Melasma is an acquired disorder of hyperpigmentation that can cause significant psychosocial stress and is difficult to treat. It is characterized by symmetrical facial hyperpigmented macules. The incidence in Asia has been reported to be 0.25% to 4%[38] with a female predominance, suggesting a hormone-related etiology. It is further demonstrated by an increased incidence of presentation at pregnancy, hence the term "the mask of pregnancy". Hormonal therapy and diseases affecting the female hormones have been associated with the onset of melasma. It is more common in skin types IV to VI and in patients with extensive UV exposure. The role of UV exposure is further

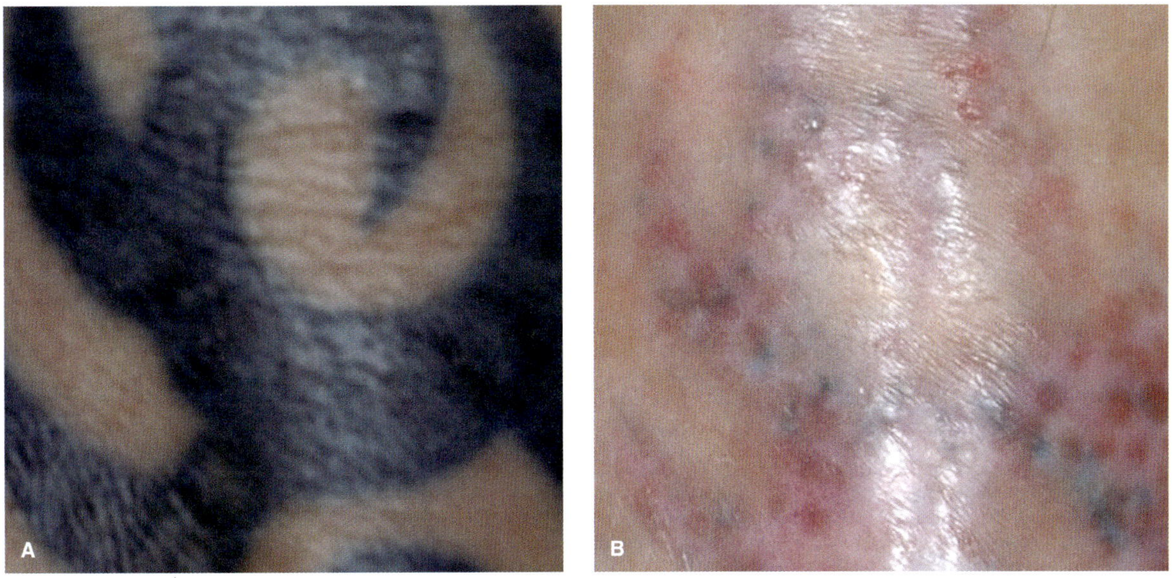

Figure 57-6 **A.** Baseline tattoo. **B.** After 12th treatment with QS ruby laser.

supported by the location of melasma being in sun-exposed facial areas. Many patients have a family history, indicating a genetic predisposition. It may be composed of epidermal, dermal, or mixed components. A Wood's light can be used to determine the level of pigment change with respect to normal skin.

Sun protection must be emphasized with any therapy directed toward melasma. A broad-spectrum sunscreen should be worn during the day and physical protection should be used when outdoors. Topical therapy is the gold standard for treatment. Combination topical therapy such as hydroquinone 4%/6%, azelaic acid 20%, and monometamesone ointment 0.1% is used most frequently at our center. Another popular combination is hydroquinone 5%, tretinoin 0.1%, and demxamethasone 0.1% or hydrocortisone 1%. Topical regimens should be applied once daily. Should irritation occur, patient should decrease application to every other day and slowly step up to once daily. Hydroquinone decreases pigment production and increases the breakdown of melanosomes by inhibiting the activity of tyrosinase, DNA and RNA synthesis in melanotic cells; it thereby degrades melanosomes and destroys melanocytes.[39,40] There have been concerns over the carcinogenicity of hydroquinone when administered in large oral doses in rodents; however, there are no known associations of cancer development in humans related to the use of topical hydroquinone. Azelaic acid is a reversible inhibitor of tyrosinase and may have cytotoxic and antiproliferative effects on melanocytes.[41,42] Tretinoin, a retinoid, inhibits tyrosinase transcription and interrupts melanin synthesis.[43] While tretinoin may be effective, it takes at least 24 weeks to see clinical improvement.[44] It is also more irritating than other agents, and may therefore cause PIH. Observable clinical improvement generally requires 2 to 4 months of topical treatment.

Since most Asian patients with melasma have both epidermal and dermal pigmentation, topical therapy alone is often insufficient to clear melasma. We recommend that patients undergo microdermabrasion, vitamin C iontophoresis, and chemical peels as adjunctive therapies.

Laser and IPL are considered to be secondary treatment options for melasma because of their risk of producing postlaser dyschromia that can clinically make the problem worse. The experience with IPL for the treatment of laser has been mixed. Initial studies using IPL (570 and 590–615 nm filters, 4 treatments at 4 week intervals) showed 39.8% improvement compared to 11.6% improvement in the control group.[45] Two patients had PIH. Microcrust formation tends to develop 2 to 3 days after treatment. Long-pulsed pigment lasers can be used to treat mixed type melasma. The clinical end point is an ash-gray appearance. The QS 1064 nm Nd:YAG laser (8 mm spot size, 2.3 J/cm^2) can also be used and mild erythema is the end point. Patients often require one to two treatments per month, since depigmentation can occur when patients are treated too frequently. Ablative laser is another option, as it removes abnormal melanocytes at the epidermal basal layer. Combining CO_2 laser and QS alexandrite laser produced greater improvement but was associated with more adverse effects.[46] Fractional skin resurfacing with the use of a 1540 nm laser to create microscopic injury can be used effectively for the treatment of epidermal melasma.[47] However, there is a 10% chance of developing a generalized increase in pigmentation.

More recently nonablative fractional resurfacing has been advocated for the treatment of melasma. While it can lead to transient improvement, the relapse rate 3 months after the last treatment session is high.[48] Regardless of which laser/IPL device is used, the main challenge is that approximately 10% of patients experience an increase in pigmentation, which can make them very unhappy. Test spots should be performed before full face treatment is offered. The use of topical bleaching agents during IPL and laser therapies along with UV protection often improves the clinical outcome.

REFERENCES

1. Szabo G. Pigment cell biology. In: Gordon M, ed. *Mitochondria and Other Cytoplasmic Inclusions.* New York, NY: Academic Press; 1959.
2. Rosdahl IK, Szabo G, Thymidine labeling of epidermal melanocytes in UV-irradiated skin. *Acta Derm Venereol.* 1976;56(2):159–161.
3. Alaluf S, Atkins D, Barrett K, Blount M, Carter N, Heath A. Ethnic variation in melanin content and composition in photoexposed and photoprotected human skin. *Pigment Cell Res.* 2002;15(2):112–118.
4. Kaidbey KH, Agin PP, Sayre RM, Kligman A. Photoprotection by melanin - a comparison of black and Caucasian skin. *J Am Dermatol.* 1979;1:249–260.
5. Grimes PE. Skin and hair cosmetic issues in women of color. *Dermatol Clin.* 2000;18(4):659–665.
6. Kotrajaras R, Kligman AM. The effect of topical tretinoin on photodamaged facial skin: the Thai experience. *Br J Dermatol.* 1993;129:302–309.
7. Ho SG, Chan NP, Yeung CK, Shek SY, Kono T, Chan HH. A retrospective analysis of the management of freckles and lentigines using four different pigment lasers on Asian skin. *J Cosmet Laser Ther.* 2012:14(2):74–80.
8. Trafeli JP, Kwan JM, Meehan KJ, et al. Use of a long-pulse alexandrite laser in the treatment of superficial pigmented lesions. *Dermatol Surg.* 2007;33:1477–1482.
9. Masu S, Seiji M. Pigmentary incontinence in fixed drug eruptions. Histologic and electron microscopic findings. *J Am Acad Dermatol.* 1983;8:525–532.
10. Wang CC, Sue YM, Yang CH, Chen CK. A comparison of Q-switched alexandrite laser and intense pulsed light for the treatment of freckles and lentigines in Asian persons: a randomized, physician-blinded, split face comparative trial. *J Am Acad Dermatol.* 2006;54(5):804–810.
11. Chan H. The use of lasers and intense pulsed light sources for the treatment of acquired pigmentary lesions in Asians. *J Cosmet Laser Ther.* 2003;5(3–4):198–200.
12. Chan HH, Kono T. Nevus of Ota: clinical aspects and management. *SKINmed.* 2003;2(2):89–98.
13. Goldberg DJ, Nychay SG. Q-switched ruby laser treatment of nevus of Ota. *J Dermatol Surg Oncol.* 1992;18:817–821.
14. Geronemus RG. Q-switched ruby laser therapy of nevus of Ota. *Arch Dermatol.* 1992;128:1618–1622.
15. Watanabe S, Takahashi H. Treatment of nevus of Ota with the Q-switched ruby laser. *N Engl J Med.* 1994;331(26):1745–1750.
16. Kono T, Nozaki M, Chan HH, Mikashima Y. A retrospective study looking at the long-term complications of Q-switched ruby laser in the treatment of nevus of Ota. *Lasers Surg Med.* 2003;32(2):148–151.
17. Chan HH, Ying SY, Ho WS, Kono T, King WW. An in vivo trial comparing the clinical efficacy and complications of Q-switched 755nm alexandrite and Q-switched 1064 nm Nd:YAG lasers in the treatment of nevus of Ota. *Dermatol Surg.* 2000;26(10):919–922.
18. Chang CJ, Kou CS. Comparing the effectiveness of Q-switched Ruby laser treatment with that of Q-switched Nd:YAG laser for oculodermal melanosis (Nevus of Ota). *J Plast Reconstr Aesthet Surg.* 2011;64(3):339–345.
19. Kono T, Chan HH, Ercocen AR, et al. Use of Q-switched ruby laser in the treatment of nevus of Ota in different age groups. *Lasers Surg Med.* 2003;32(5):391–395.
20. Chan HH, Leung RS, Ying SY, Lai CF, Chua J, Kono T. Recurrence of nevus of Ota after successful treatment with Q-switched lasers. *Arch Dermatol.* 2000;136:1175–1176.
21. Hori Y, Kawashima M, Oohara K, Kukita A. Acquired, bilateral nevus of Ota-like macules. *J Am Acad Dermatol.* 1984;10(6):961–964.
22. Kunachak S, Leelaudomlipi P, Sirikulchayanota V. Q-Switched ruby laser therapy of acquired bilateral nevus of Ota-like macules. *Dermatol Surg.* 1999;25(12):938–941.
23. Kunachak S, Leelaudomlipi P. Q-switched Nd:YAG laser treatment for acquired bilateral nevus of ota-like maculae: a long-term follow-up. *Lasers Surg Med.* 2000;26(4):376–379.
24. Polnikorn N, Tanrattanakorn S, Goldberg DJ. Treatment of Hori's necus with the Q-switched Nd:YAG laser. *Dermatol Surg.* 2000;26(5):477–480.
25. Lam AY, Wong DS, Lam LK, Ho WS, Chan HH. A retrospective study on the efficacy and complications of Q-switched alexandrite laser in the treatment of acquired bilateral nevus of Ota-like macules. *Dermatol Surg.* 2001;27(11):937–941; 41–42.
26. Manuskiatti Q, Sivayathorn A, Leelaudomlipi P, Fitzpatrick RE. Treatment of acquired bilateral nevus of Ota-like macules (Hori's nevus) using a combination of scanned carbon dioxide laser followed by Q-switched ruby laser. *J Am Acad Dermatol.* 2003;48(4):584–591.
27. Ee HL, GOh CL, Khoo LS, Chan ES, Ang P. Treatment of acquired bilateral nevus of Ota-like macules (Hori's nevus) with a combination of the 532 nm Q-switched Nd:YAG laser followed by the 1064 nm Q-switched Nd:YAG laser is more effective: prospective stud. *Dermatol Surg.* 2006;32(1):34–40.
28. Cho S, Park SJ, Kim MJ, Bu TS. Treatment of acquired bilateral nevus of Ota-like macules (Hori's nevus) using 1064-nm Q-switched Nd: YAG laser with low fluence. *Int J Dermatol.* 2009;48(12):1308–1312.
29. Saedi N, Metelitsa A, Petrell K, Arndt KA, Dover JS. Treatment of tattoos with a picoseconds alexandrite laser: a prospective trial. *Arch Dermatol.* 2012;148(12):1306–1303.
30. Kilmer SL. Laser treatment of tattoos. *Dermatol Clin.* 1997;15(3):409–417.
31. Alster TS. Q-switched alexandrite (755-nm) laser treatment of professional and amateur tattoos. *J Am Dermatol.* 1995;33:69–73.
32. Anderson RR, Geronemus R, Kilmer SL, Farinelli W, Fitzpatrick RE. Cosmetic tattoo ink darkening. A complication of Q-switched and pulsed-laser treatment. *Arch Dermatol.* 1993;129(8):1010–1014.
33. Grevelink JM, Duke D, van Leeuwen RL, Gonzales E, DeCoste SD, Anderson RR. Laser treatment of tattoos in darkly pigmented patients: efficacy and side effects. *J Am Acad Dermatol.* 1996;34(4):653–656.
34. Jones A, Roddey P, Orengo I, Rosen T. The Q-switched ND:YAG laser effectively treats tattoos in darkly pigmented skin. *Dermatol Surg.* 1996;22(12):999–1001.
35. Brauer JA, Reddy KK, Anolik R, et al. Successful and rapid treatment of blue and green tattoo pigment with a novel picoseconds laser. *Arch Dermatol.* 2012;148(7):820–823.
36. Izikson L, Farinelli W, Sakamoto F, Tannous Z, Anderson RR. Safety and effectiveness of black tattoo clearance in a pig model after a single treatment with a novel 758 nm 500 picosecond laser: a pilot study. *Lasers Surg Med.* 2010;42(7): 640–646.
37. Saedi N, Metelista A, Petrell K, Arndt KA, Dover JS. Treatment of tattoos with a picosecond alexandrite laser: a prospective trial. *Arch Dermatol.* 2012;148:1360–1363.
38. Goh CL, Diova CN. A retrospective study on the clinical presentation and treatment outcome of melasma in a tertiary dermatological referral centre in Singapore. *Sing Med J.* 1999;40:455–458.
39. Palumbo A, D'Lschia M, Misuraca G, Prota G. Mechanism of inhibition of melanogenesis by hydroquinone. *Biochim Biophys Acta.* 1991;1073:85–90.
40. Jimbow K, Obata H, Pathak MA, Fitzpatrick TB. Mechanism of depigmentation by hydroquinone. *J Invest Dermatol.* 1974;62:436–449.
41. Nazzaro-PorroM.Azelaicacid.*JAmAcadDermatol.*1987;17(6): 1033–1041.
42. Fitton A, Goa KL. Azelaic acid. A review of its pharmacological properties and therapeutic efficacy in acne and hyperpigmentary skin disorders. *Drugs.* 1991;41(5):780–798.
43. Romero C, Aberdam E, Larnier C, Ortonne JP. Retinoic acid as modulator of UVB-induced melanocyte differentiation. Involvement of the melanogenic enzymes expression. *J Cell Sci.* 1994;107(Pt 4):1095–1103.
44. Griffiths CE, Finkel LJ, Ditre CM, Hamilton TA, Ellis CN, Voorhees JJ. Topical tretinoin (retinoic acid) improves melasma. A vehicle-controlled, clinical trial. *Br J Dermatol.* 1993;129(4): 415–421.

45. Wang CC, Hui CY, Sue YM, Wong WR, Hong HS. Intense pulsed light for the treatment of refractory melasma in Asian Persons. *Dermatol Surg.* 2004,30:1196–1200.
46. Angsuwarangee S, Polnikorn N. Combined ultrapulse CO2 laser and Q-switched alexandrite laser compared with Q-switched alexandrite laser alone for refractory melasma:spli-face design. *Dermatol Surg.* 2003;29:59–64.
47. Rokhsar C, Fitzpatrick RE. The treatment of melasma with photothermolysis: a pilot study. *Dermatol Surg.* 2005;31: 1645–1650.
48. Kossida T, Rigopoulos D, Katsambas A, Anderson RR. Optimal tattoo removal in a single laser session based on the method of repeated exposures. *J Am Acad Dermatol.* 2012;66(2):271–277.

CHAPTER 58

African Skin

Valerie D. Callender, Cherie M. Young, & Susan C. Taylor

INTRODUCTION

Patients of African descent, like those of Asian and European descent, are interested in corrective aesthetic procedures to improve the appearance of their skin and hair. Facial aesthetic problems of concern for this population include dyspigmentation, benign facial growths, rhytides, laxity, and aging. Alopecia and facial hypertrichosis are additional aesthetic problems for which these patients seek treatment.

Many widely performed aesthetic procedures are appropriate for individuals of African ancestry. However, given the increased propensity for many of these patients to experience adverse events such as pigmentary alterations or keloidal scarring after aesthetic procedures, knowledge of proper techniques, selection of appropriate tools, agents and/or devices is critically important to achieve successful outcomes in this population.

Microdermabrasion and chemical peels may be used safely and effectively for the treatment of dyschromias, scarring, acne, and textural changes in skin of color (SOC) patients. In general, superficial and medium depth chemical peels are appropriate for individuals with darker skin tones, but deep chemical peels should be avoided. Among superficial and mid-depth peels, careful selection of appropriate peeling agents and concentrations as well as slow titration upward, when appropriate, are important to avoid postinflammatory hyperpigmentation (PIH) or hypopigmentation.

A variety of modalities exist for the removal of facial dermatosis papulosa nigra (DPN), common benign growths of aesthetic concern that commonly occur in African American women. Whereas light electrodesiccation, curettage, scissor excision, and laser may safely remove the lesions, cryotherapy should be avoided in darker skin, as it may produce hypopigmentation or depigmentation of the skin.

The selection of appropriate lasers for the SOC patient is critically important to avoid adverse events. For example, selection of the long-pulsed 1064 nm Nd:YAG for hair removal or the 1550 nm erbium-fractionated lasers for acne scarring can lead to success in individuals of color with appropriate treatment settings. In contrast, hair removal with the alexandrite laser or with intense pulsed light will likely lead to pigmentation problems, given the stronger selectivity for pigment of these devices.

Neurotoxins and fillers can be used to ameliorate the signs of aging in darker-skinned patients. Minimizing cutaneous trauma during injection by keeping the number of entry points to a minimum and delivering dermal injections is important to avoid pigmentary changes.

For hair transplantation, an understanding of the curved structure of the African hair follicle, the propensity for keloidal scar formation and the selection of appropriate tools for graft preparation is important for transplantation success in this population.

Being armed with the proper knowledge, skills and tools for the execution of aesthetic procedures in individuals of African descent will lead to success.

MICRODERMABRASION

Microdermabrasion is a treatment that was first introduced to the United States in 1996 and is primarily used for skin resurfacing.[1] Its noninvasive approach makes it a safe procedure to use in all Fitzpatrick skin types, with essentially no down time and limited risk for the patient.[2] Indications for the use of microdermabrasion include superficial acne scarring, hyperpigmentation, photodamage, facial rejuvenation, enlarged pores, and textural changes.[1,2] In combination with other procedures and treatments, the role of microdermabrasion has expanded over the years. Additional indications include treatment for vitiligo as well as keratosis pilaris, with promising results when combined with other treatment modalities.[3–5]

The majority of microdermabrasion systems use aluminum oxide crystals, whereas other systems use sodium chloride and sodium bicarbonate crystals that are less abrasive. Crystal-free systems are also available. These systems use a diamond wand for treatment. The actual procedure for microdermabrasion consists of superficial abrasion of the skin with a diamond chip or fine crystals. The depth of ablation is dependent on several factors, including the amount of force used to spray the crystals onto the skin, the flow rate of the crystals, crystal size, and the angle used to apply the crystals to the skin.[6]

There are three levels of microdermabrasion used for treatment and they include[6]:

Level one: Superficial abrasion of the epidermis for gentle exfoliation of the skin

Level two: Extends to the papillary dermis for treatment of fine wrinkles, striae, and superficial scars

Level three: Extends to the upper reticular dermis and treats striae

Levels two and three must be used with caution in all skin types, but especially in darker skin types.

CHEMICAL PEELS

Chemical peeling is the process of applying chemical agents to the skin to exfoliate the epidermis or dermis

TABLE 58-1
Types of Chemical Peels

Superficial Peels	Medium-Depth Peels
Glycolic acid	Trichloroacetic acid 35–40%
Polyhydroxy acid	Jessner's solution + TCA 35%
Salicylic acid	Glycolic acid 70% + TCA 35%
Trichloroacetic acid (TCA)	
Tretinoin	
Jessner's solution	

leading to re-epithelialization. This cosmetic procedure is used commonly in SOC patients and has many indications, including dyschromias, acne vulgaris, and scarring. There are several types of chemical agents used for chemical peeling and special consideration must be taken when choosing the correct agent for patients of African descent.

The types of chemical peels that are available fall into three major categories: superficial, medium-depth, and deep chemical peels. For patients with Fitzpatrick skin types IV to VI, superficial and medium-depth peels are mainly used for cosmetic treatment and have been found to be safe in this patient population. Superficial peeling agents penetrate the stratum corneum and extend down to the papillary dermis and are listed in Table 58-1. Glycolic acid is a very popular chemical agent and is considered an alpha-hydroxy acid.[7] It is used to treat several conditions found in SOC patients including acne, melasma, and hyperpigmentation. Glycolic acid peels improve these conditions by thinning the stratum corneum and interrupting intercellular bonding.[8] They also allow for improved penetration of topical agents into the skin and increase collagen synthesis within the dermis.[9] The glycolic acid concentrations that are used most frequently range from 30% to 70%, with increased concentrations of glycolic acid resulting in deeper peels, and a concomitant risk for adverse side effects. Fifty percent to 70% glycolic acid solutions are used for pigmentary disorders, whereas 30% to 50% concentrations are used for the treatment of acne.[7] Salicylic acid is an older peeling agent, a beta-hydroxy acid that is found in willow tree bark.[7] Salicylic acid can be an effective adjunctive agent in 3% to 5% concentrations and improves the penetration of other peeling agents. It is also an effective comedolytic agent and is used for the treatment of acne in a 20% to 30% concentration. Salicylic acid peels are also beneficial for the treatment of melasma and PIH in SOC patients.[10]

Trichloroacetic acid (TCA) is a crystalline inorganic compound that is used alone or in combination with glycolic acid or salicylic acid. It is an effective peeling agent for the treatment of acne scarring in SOC patients. Initial treatment with TCA peels should be done using lower concentrations in order to prevent complications. Twenty-five percent TCA peels have been used in combination with 70% glycolic acid gel.[8] The use of glycolic acid gel assists in decreasing the harshness of the TCA.

TECHNIQUE

Prior to treatment with chemical peeling agents, a thorough history and skin examination should be performed. It is important to counsel the patient to avoid certain procedures 1 week before treatment and to discontinue certain products 2 to 3 days prior to the procedure. Patients should not have electrolysis, waxing, or laser hair removal done for 1 week prior to treatment, and patients should avoid the use of topical retinoids, alpha-hydroxy acids, beta-hydroxy acids, and benzoyl peroxide containing products 2 to 3 days prior to the procedure. If patients have a history of herpes simplex, prophylactic treatment with antiviral therapy should be initiated.

The skin should be thoroughly cleansed with a gentle cleanser and degreased with acetone. The eyes should be protected with moistened pads or eye shields. Aquaphor™ or petrolatum is applied to sensitive areas of the skin prior to treatment, including the perinasal area, lateral canthi, lateral commissures, and lips. Typically the peels are applied to the skin with a sponge applicator and remain on the skin anywhere from 2 to 5 minutes depending on the type of peeling agent being used. Twenty percent to 30% salicylic acid peels used to treat acne remain on the skin for approximately 2 to 5 minutes, depending on the nature of the treatment. Tingling occurs before a white frost appears, which signals the end of the peel. The white frost of the salicylic acid represents a crystalline precipitation rather than the protein agglutination associated with a deep peel frost in glycolic acid and TCA peels, which signals a concerning endpoint. Glycolic acid and TCA peels are usually left on the skin for 2 to 4 minutes before being rinsed off with cool water. Following a chemical peel, patients are instructed to wash with gentle cleansers and to apply bland emollients twice a day. Daily sun protection with SPF 30 is also advised. The procedure can be repeated 4 to 6 weeks later. Jessner's solution is a superficial peeling agent that consists of resorcinol 14 g, which is a phenolic skin lightening agent, salicylic acid 14 g and lactic acid 14 g in ethanol 95%. This solution penetrates the papillary dermis and is well tolerated in SOC patients. When used in combination with TCA 35%, it is very effective as a treatment for acne scarring in patients with darker skin types.

COMPLICATIONS

The proper use of chemical peeling agents in SOC patients is very important and helps in decreasing the risk of complications. Superficial peeling agents usually present a low risk of complications; however if not used properly, scarring, hyperpigmentation, or hypopigmentation can occur (Fig. 58-1). Erythema, milia formation, and infection are also complications that can be observed, especially with more aggressive treatments.

It is recommended that a test area be performed prior to a full session to help prevent complications. Starting with lower, more conservative concentrations also help to prevent adverse events. Deeper peels, such as the Baker phenol peel, are not recommended in SOC patients because they can result in complications such as scarring, hyperpigmentation, and hypopigmentation.

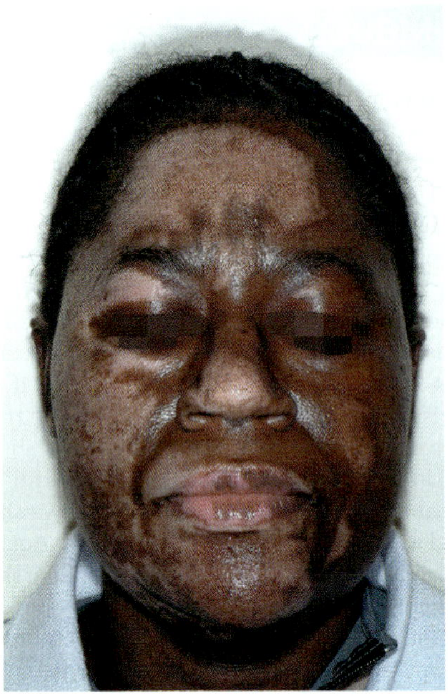

Figure 58-1 African American patient with postinflammatory hypopigmentation from chemical peeling. (Reproduced with permission from Kelly AP, Taylor S, eds. *Dermatology for Skin of Color*. Copyright © McGraw-Hill Education LLC.; 2009:517).

REMOVAL OF DERMATOSIS PAPULOSA NIGRA

DPN is a benign tumor that is considered to be a variant of seborrheic keratosis. These epithelial growths are very common in blacks and Asians (particularly women) and occur in 35% to 77% of the black population.[11] DPNs present clinically as multiple smooth brown-black papules or pedunculated lesions on the face, neck, and trunk (Fig. 58-2).

Because of the benign nature of these growths, treatment of DPNs is recommended only if symptomatic (they become inflamed from trauma) or are a cosmetic concern. The removal can be performed by electrodesiccation, curettage,[12] cryotherapy, scissor excision (with or without local anesthesia), or laser surgery.[13–15] Hypopigmentation or depigmentation can occur from cryotherapy in patients with darker skin types, so the preferred method is by electrodesiccation with a low-energy setting and without curettage, allowing the skin lesions to gradually fall off in 1 to 2 weeks. A topical anesthetic cream can be applied to the area 1 hour before treatment to enhance patient comfort; local anesthesia can be used for larger DPNs.[16] In addition, application of a topical corticosteroid to the treated areas immediately after the procedure to reduce the erythema and potential risk of PIH is recommended, as temporary hyperpigmentation and more long-lasting hyperpigmentation are realistic potential concerns. Taylor et al.[17] demonstrated that postprocedural treatment with Aquaphor™ twice daily was safe and effective in healing associated with DPN removal in African American subjects.

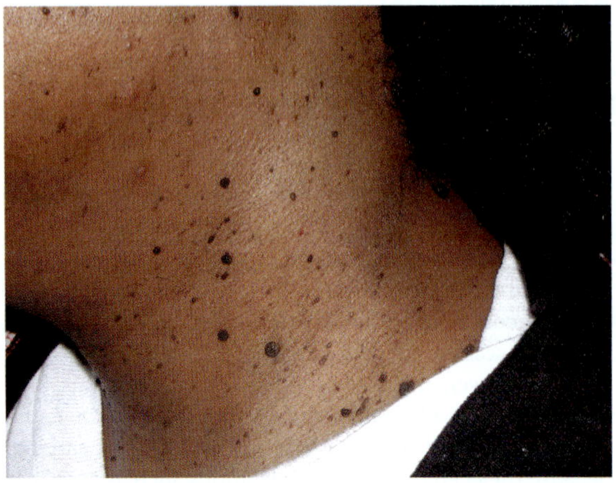

Figure 58-2 Dermatosis papulosa nigra.

LASER THERAPY

There are many different laser modalities available for the treatment of dermatologic conditions, yet approaching treatment in SOC patients can be challenging. It is essential to consider the Fitzpatrick skin type of the patient and the condition being treated when choosing an appropriate laser for treatment. The goal is to strive for optimal results while minimizing posttreatment side effects. Several indications for laser treatment in SOC patients include hair removal, dyschromias, psoriasis, vitiligo, and hypertrophic/keloidal scars.[18]

DYSCHROMIAS

The use of laser therapy for the treatment of hyperpigmentary disorders in SOC patients presents challenges relating to worsening of the hyperpigmentation. The treatment of melasma with lasers has shown limited beneficial results, and they are therefore not commonly used for treatment. Early studies using the 510 nm pigmented lesion dye laser and the Q-switched ruby laser did not show much improvement.[19–22] The ablative lasers carry the risk of PIH, which can persist for months, if not longer. A study using the Erbium:YAG laser treating melasma in 10 patients, including those with darker skin types (Fitzpatrick skin types II to V) resulted in PIH.[23] Fractional photothermolysis has shown improvement in the treatment of melasma without major side effects in a majority of patients with lighter skin phototypes.[24] This nonablative form of treatment causes areas of thermal damage called microthermal treatment zones (MTZs).[25,26] This procedure works well because it penetrates the skin deeply causing extraction of dermal pigment without affecting the surrounding tissue. Rapid re-epithelialization occurs within 1 day following treatment.[27,28] In darker skin types, there is a major risk of hyperpigmentation. Often, no improvement is seen at all. When there is improvement, recurrence of the melasma, as with other treatments, is common. Although PIH has not shown great improvement with laser therapy, medication-induced hyperpigmentation has improved with treatment of Q-switched lasers, especially the long wavelength 1064 nm Q-switched Nd:YAG in darker skin types.[29]

HAIR REMOVAL

Laser hair removal is a very common procedure performed in SOC patients. Since the inception of lasers in 1996, there has been an increase in the number of lasers being used for hair removal. Laser technology has improved to the degree that it has been found to be a very safe procedure in darker skin types.[18,30] The long-pulsed Nd:YAG laser (1064 nm) is the laser of choice for hair removal in SOC patients. Its increased wavelength allows for decreased melanin absorption. Longer pulse durations produce slower heating and decrease the potential for adverse pigmentary side effects. The most important feature of the Nd:YAG laser is its cooling device, which decreases thermal damage.[30] Selective cooling has been achieved by using cryogen spray or cold sapphire contact handpieces.[31] These devices selectively cool the epidermis to lower temperatures without affecting the target chromophore temperature before the laser pulse is delivered.[31]

Studies in SOC patients have shown that the long-pulsed Nd:YAG laser is very effective in hair reduction and it is considered to be a safe procedure.[32] If complications arise, the most common ones observed are hyperpigmentation, hypopigmentation, blistering, and scarring (Fig. 58-3).

PSORIASIS AND VITILIGO

The 308 nm excimer laser is an effective method used for the treatment of psoriasis and vitiligo in SOC patients. This laser type is very similar to narrowband UVB therapy. Side effects with the excimer laser are minimal due to its targeted nature and the use of a lower dosage than that used in narrowband UVB therapy. The patients exhibiting the best results after vitiligo treatment with the excimer laser include those with small- to medium-sized lesions in UV-sensitive areas, such as the face, neck, and chest.[33] Lesions that have been present for a shorter duration, 3 years or less, have better results.[33] The recommended treatment for vitiligo with the excimer laser is three times weekly for the first 3 weeks and then twice per week. Minimal response to treatment is usually seen after 10 treatments, with the average treatment course being 16 to 25 treatments. As with most conditions, treatment with combination therapy shows enhanced improvement for the treatment of vitiligo. Studies have shown that the combination of calcineurin inhibitors with the excimer laser has improved vitiligo treatment efficacy.[34] The most common side effects with this laser are erythema, blistering, hyperpigmentation, and reactivation of herpes labialis. If a patient experiences moderate to severe erythema following treatment, a mid- to high-potency topical corticosteroid should be applied for several days and the subsequent treatment dose should be reduced by 50 to 100 mJ/cm^2.

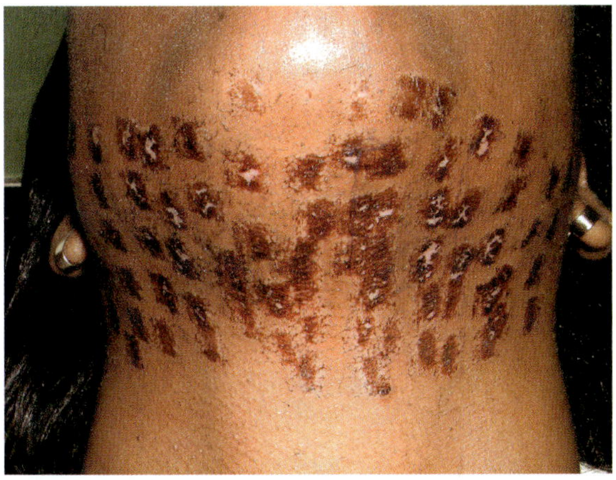

Figure 58-3 Laser hair removal complication, consisting of patterned hyperpigmentation.

KELOIDAL/HYPERTROPHIC SCARS

Improvement with keloidal and hypertrophic scars has been observed with laser treatment postoperatively. Pulsed dye laser treatment has shown improvement in treating these scars by reducing erythema.[35,36] The laser of choice for treating SOC patients with keloidal or hypertrophic scars is the 595 nm long-pulsed dye laser. Low fluences, appropriate cooling, and careful inspection of clinical endpoints are essential for safe and effective treatment. The ablative fractional CO_2 laser has also proven to be efficacious in the treatment of keloids following surgical removal. When compared to radiotherapy, the use of the CO_2 laser has produced improvement without recurrence and without the risk of carcinogenesis.[37] As with most treatments, the earlier the laser treatment begins following surgical removal of a keloid, the better the outcome. For more improvement, it is recommended that concomitant therapy be performed with intralesional injections of corticosteroids and/or 5-fluorouracil (5-FU) following laser treatment.[38]

SYRINGOMAS

Of note, lasers have been used to treat other conditions in darker skin. Syringomas are benign hereditary adnexal neoplasms found predominantly on the face, neck, chest, and axilla, which can be challenging to treat (Fig. 58-4). A study was performed using combination therapy with a TCA peel and CO_2 laser resurfacing for the treatment of eruptive syringomas in an African American patient.[39] This patient was pretreated with TCA, which decreased the bulk of the lesions and enabled a decrease in the number of laser passes required to flatten the remainder of the lesions.[39] Although the syringomas did not completely resolve with this combination treatment, the patient did exhibit improved results without major side effects.[39]

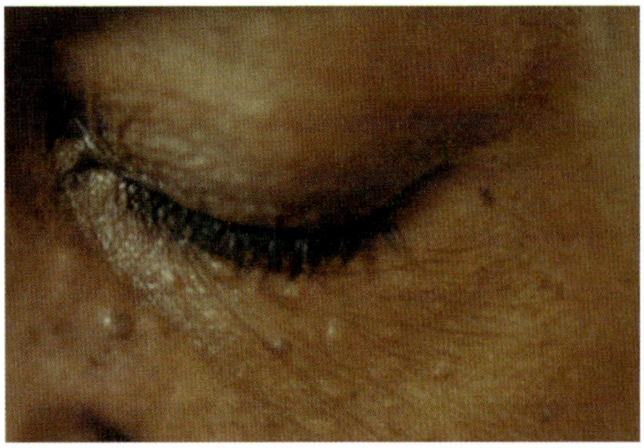

Figure 58-4 Syringomas in an African American woman.

SKIN TIGHTENING

Nonablative skin tightening devices have been found to be safe and effective in the treatment of SOC patients. There are two main types of these devices: radiofrequency energy and infrared light. Radiofrequency devices are classified as unipolar, bipolar, or multipolar depending on the number of electrodes used.[40] The mechanism of action of these devices is heating the dermis, which in turn causes collagen denaturation, collagen contraction, and long-term collagen remodeling, leading to skin tightening.[41] This is done while protecting the epidermis with a cooling tip. Radiofrequency waves are not absorbed by melanin, and therefore this procedure is safe to use in African skin. The best results are seen when several treatments are performed at 1 to 3 month intervals. A clinical trial was performed evaluating the safety and efficacy of infrared skin tightening in the treatment of skin laxity in patients with Fitzpatrick skin types IV and V.[42] Twenty-one patients received 3 monthly treatments and a final assessment was performed 6 months following the last treatment. Physician final assessments revealed improvement in skin laxity in 86% of the patients.[42] Side effects were minimal with the main one being superficial blistering occurring in 7 out of 63 treatments performed. No subsequent scarring was observed.[42]

ACNE SCARRING

Treatment of acne scarring in patients with darker skin types with the use of lasers is a challenging balance between achieving efficacy while minimizing adverse effects. It has been known that ablative lasers, although effective in the treatment of acne scars, can lead to severe complications in SOC patients. Fractional lasers have been found to be effective in the treatment of acne scars in darker skin types with less severe side effects.[43] A study was performed treating acne scars in patients with skin types IV to VI using a 1550 nm erbium fractionated laser. Patients were divided into two groups, with one group being treated with 10 mJ and the other group being treated with 40 mJ.[43] Five monthly sessions were performed. Interestingly, the results revealed significant improvement in acne scarring, with no significant difference between the treatment groups despite the different depths of laser penetration.[43] The side effects observed were significant PIH and pain with the procedure.[43] Pain is common in all skin types with this treatment.[43]

NEUROTOXINS AND FILLERS

Dark-skinned patients manifest the signs of skin aging differently than patients with lighter skin. This difference is due to the inherent protective effects of melanin in darker skin, which has an average sun protective factor (SPF) of 13.4.[44] Because of this difference, patients of African descent exhibit more intrinsic facial aging, and less extrinsic (or photo-damaged skin) facial aging. The latter can be delayed by 10 to 20 years as compared to Caucasians. Mid-facial aging predominates in patients of color and signs include descent of the malar fat pads, tear trough deformity, infraorbital hollowing, and deepening of the nasolabial folds (Fig. 58-5).[45]

Common cosmetic procedures, such as neurotoxins for dynamic rhytides and fillers for static rhytides and volumization can be used safely in darker-skinned patients to treat the signs of aging, as these treatments do not in any way target pigmentation, unlike lasers and chemical peels (Fig. 58-6). According to the American Society for Aesthetic Plastic Surgery Statistic Report, SOC patients comprised 30% of all surgical and nonsurgical cosmetic procedures in the United States in 2012 (Fig. 58-7).[46] African Americans composed 8% of these procedures, and notably, there was a 6% rise in these procedures as compared to 2011. With the proper knowledge of how to

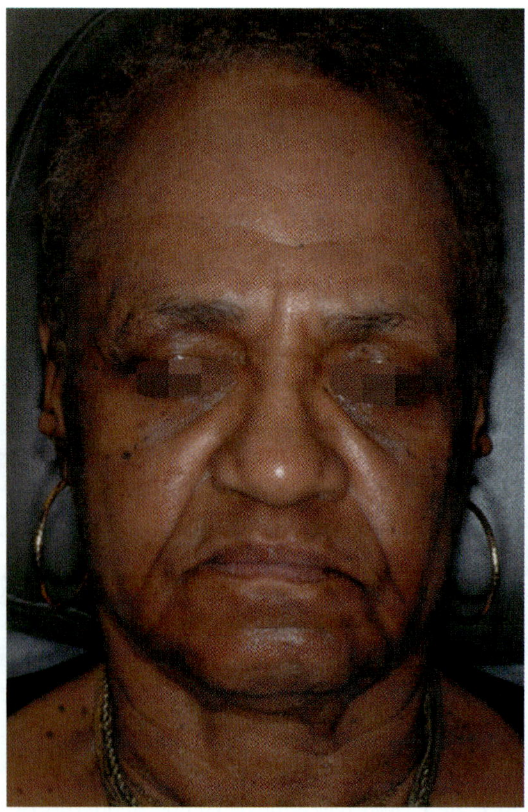

Figure 58-5 Facial skin aging in skin of color.

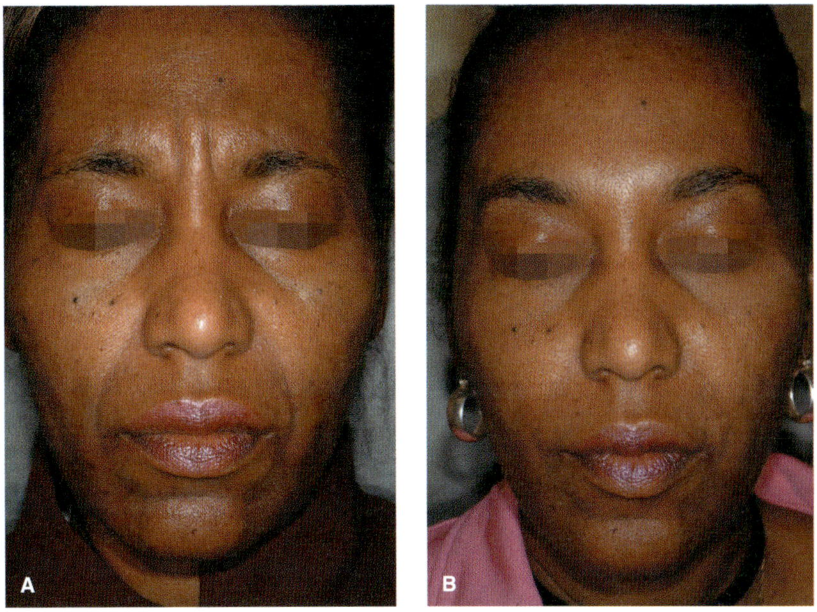

Figure 58-6 Before **(A)** and after **(B)** HA filler treatment for nasolabial folds and BTX-A injections for glabellar brow furrows. (Reproduced with permission from Kelly AP, Taylor S, eds. *Dermatology for Skin of Color*. Copyright © McGraw-Hill Education LLC.; 2009: Figure 69–10 A&B, p. 524.)

treat and manage complications of aging African skin, the physician can provide the benefits of cosmetic procedures while minimizing their risks.[47]

Safety data, although limited, is available for neurotoxins in patients with darker skin (Fitzpatrick skin types IV to VI).[48–50] Recently, a meta-analysis (pooled data from six clinical trials) was performed to examine the safety and effectiveness of botulinum toxin type A injections for the reduction of glabellar lines in patients with SOC.[51] The results demonstrated a similar onset of effect and adverse event rates in white patients and SOC patients; however, the response rate at 30 days after treatment was greater in the SOC patients.[51]

An important consideration for patients with darker skin is the potential for the development of pigmentary

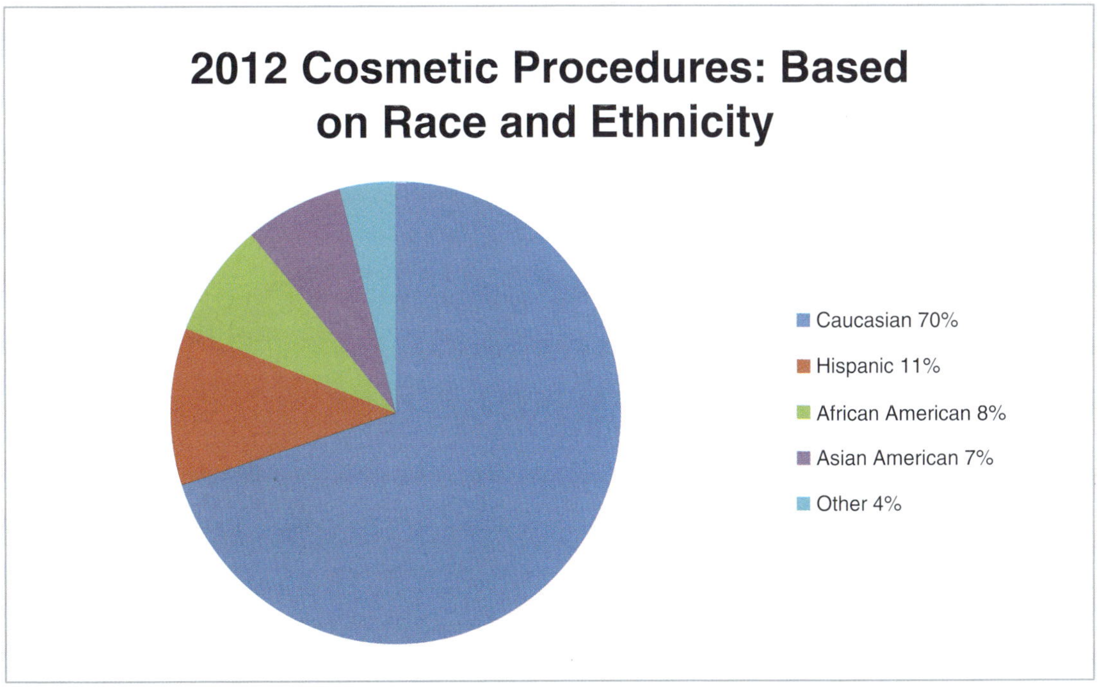

Total ethnic population = 30%

Figure 58-7 2012 ASPS Statistic Report on Cosmetic Procedures in the United States (pie chart). (*Source:* American Society of Aesthetic Plastic Surgery; www.plasticsurgery.org/documents;news-resources/statistics/2011).

TABLE 58-2
Clinical Studies Evaluating Safety of Dermal Fillers in Skin of Color

Author	Agent	Pigmentary Changes	HTS/Keloid
Grimes[52]	HA (Juvederm)	7.5%	None
Grimes[52]	HA (Hylaform)	2.5%	None
Taylor[53]	HA (Restylane)	9%	None
Taylor[53]	HA (Perlane)	6%	None
Marmur[54]	CaHa (Radiesse)	None	None

HTS, hypertrophic scarring; HA, hyaluronic acid; CaHa, calcium hydroxyapatite.

changes, hypertrophic scarring, and keloids from cosmetic and surgical procedures. Several studies have been conducted to elucidate the occurrence of those adverse events from dermal filler injections in SOC (Table 58-2) that significantly differ from those of lighter skin phototypes. Pigmentary changes were noted in 2.5% to 9% of SOC patients who received hyaluronic acid fillers and there were no pigmentary changes in those patients receiving calcium hydroxylapatite (CaHa).[52–54] In the latter study, the authors concluded that the lack of dyspigmentation noted in the SOC patients was due to the deeper injection technique with CaHa, which allows for less trauma at the dermal–epidermal junction as compared to a more superficial injection.[54] In all studies, there were no reports of hypertrophic scars or keloids.

INJECTION TECHNIQUE

There are various injection techniques that are used to inject dermal fillers. These include linear threading, serial puncture, fanning, and cross hatching. In order to minimize adverse events in darker skin types, proper injection techniques must be used to lessen skin trauma. These include minimizing the number of entry points, delivering product deep to the dermal–epidermal junction, avoiding the fanning technique and using a slow rate of injection.[53–56]

HAIR TRANSPLANTATION

Hair transplantation in African skin patients varies in surgical technique, indications, and complications as compared to Caucasians. The most common indication for hair transplant surgery in all races is androgenetic alopecia; however, in black females, traction alopecia and central centrifugal cicatricial alopecia (CCCA) are the most common reason for hair replacement.[57–60] Both conditions produce a permanent form of hair loss that can be corrected by a surgical procedure, such as hair transplantation, after alterations in hair grooming and medical therapy have been completed. There are two chapters in this text that have been devoted to hair transplantation, so this section will focus only on the racial differences that exist between Caucasians/Asians and blacks (Table 58-3).

TABLE 58-3
Hair Transplantation Differences in Persons of Color

	Blacks	Caucasians	Asians
Hair shape	Curly	Straight, wavy	Straight
Hair follicle	Curved	Straight	Straight
Hair density	0.6 FU/mm^2	1 FU/mm^2	1 FU/mm^2
Hair groupings	Three	Two	Two
Indications	AGA, TA, CCCA	AGA	AGA
Recipient sites	>1.2 mm	<1.2 mm	<1.2 mm
Keloid risk	High	Low	Moderate

FU, follicular units; AGA, androgenetic alopecia; TA, traction alopecia; CCCA, central centrifugal cicatricial alopecia.
Source: Reproduced with permission from Kelly AP, Taylor S, eds. *Dermatology for Skin of Color*. Copyright © McGraw-Hill Education LLC.; 2009: Table 69–2, p. 519.

Ethnic differences in hair characteristics play a major role in the surgical technique of hair transplantation.[57–60] Africans have a curved hair follicle (Fig. 58-8), and a coiled, spiraled, or helical hair structure, which makes donor harvesting and graft preparation more challenging due to the increased risk of follicular transection that may occur.[57–60] In addition, there are racial differences in hair densities that exist, which may play a role in the number

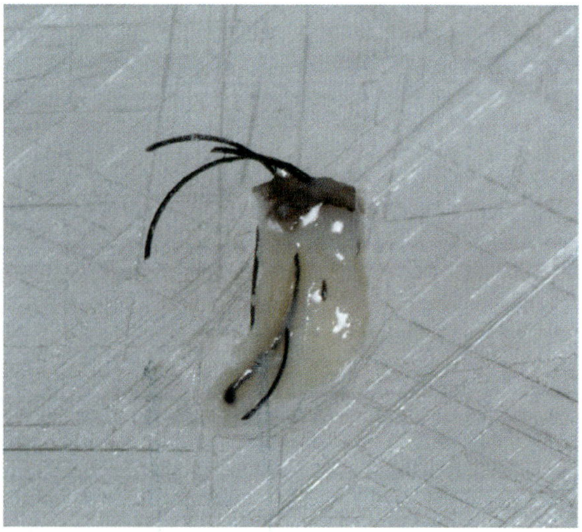

Figure 58-8 Hair follicles and hair shafts from an African American patient demonstrating the curly nature of African hair. (Reproduced with permission from Kelly AP, Taylor S, eds. *Dermatology for Skin of Color*. Copyright © McGraw-Hill Education LLC.; 2009: Figure 69–5, p. 520).

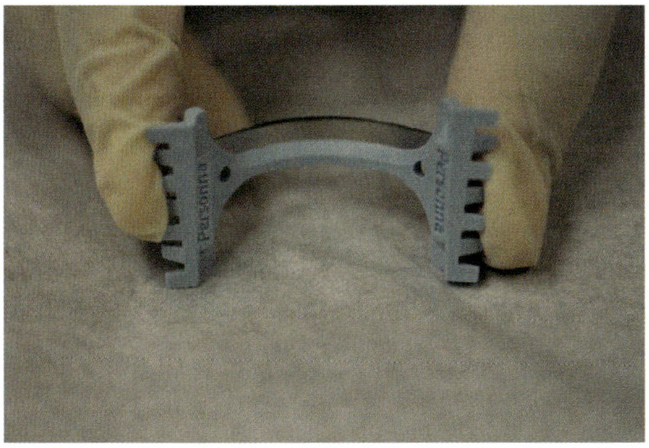

Figure 58-9 Flexible blade used for preparing curly hair grafts.

of donor grafts needed to provide adequate coverage of the recipient site.[61] Patients of African descent have lower hair densities (0.6 FU/mm^2) as compared to Caucasians and Asians (1 FU/mm^2).[62]

A flexible blade (Dermablade, Personna Medical, Verona, VA) can be used during graft preparation of curly hair when meticulous accuracy is needed while dissecting individual follicular units during hair transplant surgery (Fig. 58-9).[63] This blade can easily bend to match the natural curvature of the hair follicle and hair shaft, thereby minimizing the rate of transection, improving graft survival, and graft preparation time.

COMPLICATIONS

Keloids and hypertrophic scarring from hair transplant surgery are uncommon. In fact, patients of African descent typically have excellent results from this procedure. However, keloid formation from hair transplantation has been reported in the literature and therefore, a detailed history of keloids must be performed to avoid this complication.[64] If the patient has a history of scarring, a test procedure and observation for at least 3 months is recommended.[65] If a hypertrophic scar or keloid develops postoperatively at the donor graft site, it should be treated immediately without delay. Triamcinolone 20 to 40 mg/mL can be injected intralesionally every 2 to 4 weeks until flat.[58,59]

TREATMENT OF POSTINFLAMMATORY HYPERPIGMENTATION

PIH can develop from any form of skin trauma, whether induced by inflammation of the skin or from a procedure, particularly in individuals with darker skin types. Thus PIH is a common sequela of microdermabrasion, chemical peels, removal of DPNs, and dermal filler injections. Mid to high-potency topical corticosteroids can be used immediately postoperatively for 1 to 3 days to the affected areas to minimize erythema. The anti-inflammatory effect of cortisones may prevent the development of PIH. Table 58-4 lists some of the common therapies used for treating hyperpigmentation in SOC.[66,67]

TABLE 58-4
Treatment Options for Postinflammatory Hyperpigmentation

Sun protection and strict sun avoidance
Observation and time
Skin lightening agents Hydroquinone Azaleic acid Topical retinoids Kojic acid Arbutin Soy Vitamin C Niacinamide (Vitamin B3) N-acetyl glucosamine Licorice
Lignin peroxidase
Microdermabrasion
Chemical peels
Lasers

CONCLUSION

The desire to have an even skin tone, a full head of hair, fewer wrinkles, and absence of aging skin or moles is universal; however, corrective aesthetic procedures pose a risk of adverse events in patients with darker skin. Proper technique and awareness of racial differences between patients are key to successful outcomes for the aesthetic SOC patient.

REFERENCES

1. Rajan P, Grimes PE. Skin barrier changes induced by aluminum oxide and sodium chloride microdermabrasion. *Dermatol Surg.* 2002;28:390–393.
2. Shim EK, Barnette D, Hughes K, Greenway HT. Microdermabrasion: a clinical and histopathologic study. *Dermatol Surg.* 2001;27:524–530.
3. Patel NS, Paghdal KV, Cohen GF. Advanced treatment modalities for vitiligo. *Dermatol Surg.* 2012;38:381–391.
4. Garg T, Chander R, Jain A. Combination of microdermabrasion and 5-fluorouracil to induce repigmentation in vitiligo: an observational study. *Dermatol Surg.* 2011;37:1763–1766.
5. Lee SJ, Chung WS, Kim J, Cho SB. Combination of 595-nm pulsed dye laser, long-pulsed 755-nm alexandrite laser and microdermabrasion treatment for keratosis pilaris. *J Dermatol.* 2012;39:479–480.
6. Lim JT. Microdermabrasion. In: Grimes PE, ed. *Aesthetic and Cosmetic Surgery for Darker Skin Types.* Philadelphia, PA: Lippincott Williams & Wilkens; 2008:147–153.
7. Roberts WE. Chemical peeling in ethnic/dark skin. *Dermatol Ther.* 2004;17:196–205.
8. Van Scott EJ, Yu RJ. Hyperkeratinization, corneocyte cohesion, and alpha hydroxyl acids. *J Am Acad Dermatol.* 1984;11:867–879.
9. Tung RC, Bergfeld WF, Vidimos AT, Remzi BK. Hydroxy acid-based cosmetic procedures: guidelines for patient management. *Am J Clin Dermatol.* 2000;1:1–88.
10. Grimes PE. The safety and efficacy of salicylic acid chemical peels in darker racial-ethnic groups. *Dermatol Surg.* 1999;25:18–22.

11. Grimes PE, Arora S, Minus HR, Kenney JA Jr. Dermatosis papulosa nigra. *Cutis*. 1983;32(4):385–386.
12. Kauh YC, McDonald JW, Rapaporty JA, Ruschak PJ, Luscombe HA. A surgical approach for dermatosis papulosa nigra. *Int J Deramtol*. 1983;22:590–592.
13. Schweiger ES, Kwasniak L, Aires DJ. Treatment of dermatosis papulosa nigra with q 1064 nm Nd:YAG laser: report of two cases. *J Cosmet Laser Ther*. 2008;10:120–122.
14. Kundu RV, Joshi SS, Suh KY, et al. Comparison of electrodessication and potassium-titanyl-phosphate laser for treatment of dermatosis papulosa nigra. *Dermatol Surg*. 2009;35: 1079–1083.
15. Katz TM, Goldberg LH, Friedman PM. Dermatosis papulosa nigra treatment with fractional photothermolysis. *Dermatol Surg*. 2009;35:1840–1843.
16. Carter EL, Coppola CA, Barsanti FA. A randomized, doulble-blind comparison of two topical anesthetic formulations prior to electrodessication of dermotesis papulos nigra. *Dermatol Surg*. 2006;32:1–6.
17. Taylor SC, Averyhart AN, Heath CR. Postprocedural wound-healing efficacy following removal of dermatosis papulosa nigra lesions in an African American population: a comparison of a skin protectant ointment and a topical antibiotic. *J Am Acad Dermatol*. 2011;64(3 Suppl):S30–S35.
18. Callender VD, Narukar VA, Davis EC. Cosmetic Treatment. In: Taylor SC, Badreshia-Bansals S, Callender VD, Gathers RC, Rodriguez DA, eds. *Treatments for Skin of Color*. New York, NY: Elsevier Saunders; 2011:309–347.Table 17.9; p. 333.
19. Fitzpatrick RE, Goldman MP, Ruiz-Esparza J. Laser treatment of benign pigmented epidermal lesions using a 300 nsecond pulse and 510 nm wavelength. *J Dermatol Surg Oncol*. 1993;19:341–347.
20. Grekin RC, Shelton RM, Geisse JK, Frieden I. 510-nm pigmented lesion dye laser: its Characteristics and clinical uses. *J Dermatol Surg Oncol*. 1993;19:380–387.
21. Goldberg DJ. Benign pigmented lesions of the skin: treatment with the Q-switched ruby laser. *J Dermatol Surg Oncol*. 1993;19:376–379.
22. Taylor CR, Anderson RR. Ineffective treatment of refractory melasma and postinflammatory hyperpigmentation by Q-switched ruby laser. *J Dermatol Surg Oncol*. 1994;20:592–597.
23. Manaloto RM, Alster T. Erbium:YAG laser resurfacing for refractory melasma. *Dermatol Surg*. 1999;25:121–123.
24. Katz TM, Glaich AS, Goldberg LH, Firoz BF, Dai T, Friedman PM. Treatment of melasma using fractional thermolysis: a report of eight causes with long-term follow-up. *Dermatol Surg*. 2010;36:1273–1280.
25. Fisher GH, Geronemus RG. Short-term side effects of fractional photothermolysis. *Dermatol Surg*. 2005;31:1245–1249; discussion1249.
26. Manstein D, Herron GS, Sink RK, Tanner H, Anderson RR. Fractional photothermolysis: a new concept for cutaneous remodeling using microscopic patterns of thermal injury. *Lasers Surg Med*. 2004;34:426–438.
27. Narurkar VA. Non-ablative fractional resurfacing for total body rejuvenation. *J Drugs Dermatol*. 2008;7:352–355.
28. Rokhsar C, Fitzpatrick RE. The treatment of melasma with fractional photothermolysis: a pilot study. *Derm Surg*. 2005;31: 1645–1650.
29. Ke MS, Soriano T. Laser therapies for disorders of hyperpigmentation. In: Grimes PE, ed. *Aesthetics and Cosmetic Surgery for Darker Skin Types*. Philadelphia, PA: Lippincott Williams and Wilkins; 2008:117–124.
30. Tanzi EL, Alster TS. Long-pulsed 1064-nm Nd:YAG laser-assisted hair removal in all skin types. *Derm Surg*. 2004;30: 13–17.
31. Nelson JS, Majaron B, Kelly KM. Active skin cooling in conjunction with laser dermatologic surgery. *Semin Cutan Med Surg*. 2000;19:253–266.
32. Nanda S, Bansal S. Long pulsed Nd:YAG laser with inbuilt cool sapphire tip for long term hair reduction on type IV and V skin: a prospective analysis of 200 patients. *Indian J Dermatol Venereol Leprol*. 2010;76:677–681.
33. Alhowaish AK, Dietrich N, Onder M, Fritz K. Effectiveness of a 308-nm excimer laser in treatment of vitiligo: a review. *Lasers Med Sci*. 2013;28(3):1035–1041.
34. Hossani-Madani AR, Halder RM. Topical treatment and combination approaches for vitiligo: new insights, new developments. *G Ital Dermatol Venereol*. 2010;145:57–78.
35. Alster TS, Handrick C. Laser treatment of hypertrophic scars, keloids, and striae. *Semin Cutan Med Surg*. 2000;19: 287–292.
36. Bouzari N, Davis SC, Nouri K. Laser treatment of keloids and hypertrophic scars. *Int J Dermatol*. 2007;46:80–88.
37. Scrimali L, Lomeo G, Tamburino S, Catalani A, Perrotta R. Laser CO_2 versus radiotherapy in treatment of keloid scars. *J Cosmet Laser Ther*. 2012;14:94–97.
38. Manuskiatti W, Fitzpatrick RE. Treatment response of keloidal and hypertrophic sternotomy scars: comparison among intralesional corticosteroid, 5-FU (5-fluorouracil) and 585 flashlamp-pumped pulsed dye laser treatments. *Arch Dermatol*. 2002;138:1149–1155.
39. Frazier CC, Camacho AP, Cockerell CJ. The treatment of eruptive syringomas in an African American patient with a combination of trichloroacetic acid and CO_2 laser destruction. *Dermatol Surg*. 2001;27:489–492.
40. Krueger N, Sadick NS. New generation radiofrequency technology. *Cutis*. 2013;91:39–46.
41. Woolery-Lloyd H, Kammer JN. Skin tightening. *Curr Probl Dermatol*. 2011;42:147–152.
42. Chua S, Ang P, Khoo L, Goh CL. Nonablative infrared skin tightening in type IV and V Asian skin: a prospective clinical study. *Dermatol Surg*. 2007;33:146–151.
43. Mahmoud BH, Srivastava D, Janiga JJ, Yang JJ, Lim HW, Ozog DM. Safety and efficacy of erbium-doped yttrium aluminum garnet fractionated laser for treatment of acne scars in type IV to VI skin. *Dermatol Surg*. 2010;36:602–609.
44. Kaidbey KH, Agin PP, Sayre RM, Kligman AM. Photoprotection by melanin–a comparison of black and Caucasian skin. *J Am Acad Dermatol*. 1979;1:249–260.
45. Harris MO. The aging face in patients of color: minimally invasive surgical facial rejuvenation–a targeted approach. *Dermatol Ther*. 2004;17:206–211.
46. 2012 ASAPS Statistics. Complete charts. American Society for Aesthetic Plastic Surgery [online]. Available from http://www.plasticsurgery.org/Media/Statistics.html. Accessed July 24, 2014.
47. Callender VD, Davis EC. Aesthetic dermatology for aging ethnic skin. *Dermatol Surg*. 2011;37(7):901–917.
48. Grimes PE, Shabazz D. A four-month randomized, double-blind evaluation of the efficacy of botulinum toxin type A for the treatment of glabellar lines in women with skin types V and VI. *Dermatol Surg*. 2009;35:429–436.
49. Kane MA, Brandt F, Rohrich RJ, et al; Reloxin Investigational Group. Evaluation of variable-dose treatment with a new U.S. Botulinum Toxin Type A (Dysport) for correction of moderate to severe glabellar lines: results from a phase III, randomized, double-blind, placebo-controlled study. *Plast Reconstr Surg*. 2009;124:1619–1629.
50. Brandt F, Swanson N, Baumann L, Huber B. Randomized, placebo-controlled study of a new botulinum toxin type A for treatment of glabellar lines: efficacy and safety. *Dermatol Surg*. 2009;35:1893–1901.
51. Taylor SC, Callender VD, Albright CD, Coleman J, Axford-Gatley RA, Lin X. AbobotulinumtoxinA for reduction of glabellar lines in patients with skin of color: post hoc analysis of pooled clinical trial data. *Dermatol Surg*. 2012;38:1804–1811.
52. Grimes PE, Thomas JA, Murphy DK. Safety and effectiveness of hyaluronic acid fillers in skin of color. *J Cosmet Dermatol*. 2009;8:162–168.
53. Taylor SC, Burgess CM, Callender VD. Safety of nonanimal stabilized hyaluronic acid dermal fillers in patients with skin of color: a randomized, evaluator-blinded comparative trial. *Dermatol Surg*. 2009;35:1653–1660.
54. Marmur ES, Taylor SC, Grimes PE, Boyd CM, Porter JP, Yoo JY. Six-month safety results of calcium hydroylapatite for treatment of nasolabial folds in Fitzpatrick skin types IV to VI. *Dermatol Surg*. 2009;35:1641–1645.

55. Odunze M, Cohn A, Few JW. Restylne and people of color. *Plast Reconstr Surg*. 2007;120:2011–2016.
56. Glogau R, Kane M. Effect of injection techniques on the rate of local adverse events in patients implanted with nonanimal hyaluronic acid gel dermal fillers. *Dermatol Surg*. 2008;34:S105–S109.
57. Callender VD, McMichael AJ, Cohen GF. Medical and surgical therapies for alopecias in black women. *Dermatol Ther*. 2004;17:164–176.
58. Callender VD. Hair transplantation for pigmented skin. In: Halder RM, ed. *Dermatology and Dermatological Therapy of Pigmented Skins*. Boca Raton, FL: Taylor & Francis; 2006:245–257.
59. Callender VD, Young CM. Alopecias and hair restoration in women. In: Grimes PE, Soriano T, Hexsel DM, Kim J, eds. *Aesthetics and Cosmetic Surgery for Darker Skin Types*. Philadelphia, PA: Lippincott Williams & Wilkins; 2008:287–295.
60. Callender VD, Davis EC. Hair transplantation. In: Alexis AF, Barbosa VH, eds. *Skin of Color*. New York, NY: Springer; 2013:P351–P370.
61. Sperling LC. Hair density in African Americans. *Arch Dermatol*. 1990;135:656–658.
62. Bernstein RM, Rassman WR. The aesthetics of follicular transplantation. *Dermatol Surg*. 1997;23:785–799.
63. Callender VD, Davis EC. Hair transplantation technique: a flexible blade for preparing curly hair grafts. *Dermatol Surg*. 2011;37(7):1032–1034.
64. Brown MC, Johnson T, Swanson NA. Extensive keloids following hair transplantation. *J Dermatol Surg Oncol*. 1990;16:867–869.
65. Meyer M. Hair restoration in patients of African descent. In: Unger W, Shapiro R, eds. *Hair Transplantation*, 4th ed. New York, NY: Marcel Decker; 2004:595–602.
66. Davis EC, Callender VD. Postinflammatory hyperpigmentation: a review of the epidemiology, clinical features and treatment options in skin of color. *J Clin Aesthet Dermatol*. 2010;3(7):20–31.
67. Callender VD, St Surin-Lord S, Davis EC, Maclin M. Postinflammatory hyperpigmentation: etiologic and therapeutic considerations. *Am J Clin Dermatol*. 2011;12(2):87–99.

INDEX

Note: Page numbers followed by *f* and *t* indicate figures and tables respectively.

B

Index

D

E

M

N

O

P

T

U

V

W

X

Z